MOSBY'S COMPREHENSIVE REVIEW OF NURSING

MOSBY'S COMPREHENSIVE REVIEW OF NURSING

TENTH EDITION

Illustrated

The C. V. Mosby Company

ST. LOUIS • TORONTO • LONDON   1981

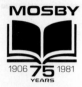

MOSBY

1906 **75** 1981
YEARS

A TRADITION OF PUBLISHING EXCELLENCE

TENTH EDITION

Copyright © 1981 by The C. V. Mosby Company

Previous editions copyrighted 1949, 1951, 1955, 1958, 1961, 1965, 1969, 1973, 1977

Printed in the United States of America

The C. V. Mosby Company
11830 Westline Industrial Drive, St. Louis, Missouri 63141

Library of Congress Cataloging in Publication Data

Mosby (C. V.) Company.
  Mosby's Comprehensive review of nursing.

  Bibliography: p.
  Includes index.
  1. Nursing—Examinations, questions, etc. 2. Nursing
—Outlines, syllabi, etc. I. Title. II. Title: Compre-
hensive review of nursing. [DNLM: 1. Nursing—Examina-
tion questions. 2. Nursing—Outlines. WY 100 M894c]
RT55.M6 1981   610.73'076   80-26510
ISBN 0-8016-3530-6

AC/D/D 9 8 7 6 5 4 3 2   03/B/308

EDITORIAL PANEL

EDITOR

Dolores F. Saxton, R.N., B.S. in Ed., M.A., Ed.D.

Dean of Instruction, Health Sciences/Physical Education, Nassau Community College, Garden City, New York

ASSOCIATE EDITORS

Patricia M. Nugent, R.N., A.A.S., B.S., M.S.

Instructor, Department of Nursing, Nassau Community College, Garden City, New York

Phyllis K. Pelikan, R.N., A.A.S., B.S., M.A.

Professor and Chairman, Department of Nursing, Nassau Community College, Garden City, New York

CONTRIBUTING AUTHORS

JoAnn Festa, R.N., A.A.S., B.S., M.S.

Instructor, Department of Nursing, Nassau Community College, Garden City, New York

MaryAnn Hellmer, R.N., A.A.S., B.S., M.S.

Instructor, Department of Nursing, Nassau Community College, Garden City, New York

Mildred L. Montag, R.N., B.A., B.S., M.A., Ed.D., LL.D.

Professor Emeritus, Teachers College, Columbia University, New York, New York

Peter Pilchman, B.A., Ph.D.

Associate Professor, Department of Biology, Kingsborough Community College, City University of New York, Brooklyn, New York

Mary Sirotnik, Reg. N., B.Sc.N.

Year II Coordinator, Mack Centre of Nursing Education, Niagara College of Applied Arts and Technology, St. Catharines, Ontario, Canada

Donna L. Wong, R.N., M.N., P.N.P.

Nursing Counselor and Consultant in Private Practice, Tulsa, Oklahoma

REVISION AUTHORS

Norma Alkon, R.N., M.S.

Board Certified N.Y.S.N.A. Psychotherapist; Faculty, Canterbury Group/Family Institute, Great Neck, New York

Irene Pagel, R.N., B.S., M.A., M.Ed., Ed.D.

Professor, School of Nursing, Adelphi University, Garden City, New York

CONTRIBUTORS OF ADDITIONAL TEST QUESTIONS

Helen M. Arnold, R.N., B.S., M.S., Ph.D.

Associate Professor, School of Nursing, Adelphi University, Garden City, New York

Natalie Asouline, R.N., B.S., M.A.

Associate Professor, Department of Nursing, Nassau Community College, Garden City, New York

Norita Halvorsen, R.N., A.A.S., B.S., M.A.

Associate Professor, Department of Nursing, Nassau Community College, Garden City, New York

PREFACE

The previous material in *Mosby's Comprehensive Review of Nursing* has undergone major revision for this, the tenth, edition. The progression of subject matter in each area reflects the consistent approach that has been used throughout the book. Selected information incorporates the latest knowledge, newest trends, and current practices in the profession of nursing.

The material that previously appeared in the supportive areas has been updated and placed within the most applicable clinical area. This permits the individual to study an entire area as a complete, self-contained unit.

The medical-surgical chapter has been completely revised and now contains the material previously included under fundamentals of nursing and rehabilitation nursing. Pharmacology, the sciences, and nutrition have been integrated throughout all the clinical areas, and the legal aspects material has been added to the section on history and trends in nursing. A chapter providing directions on how to study and use the review to prepare for the current and proposed state boards is included.

The move to incorporate all the material into the traditional clinical groupings was decided on after consultation with many of our readers. It is believed that, even in preparing for the comprehensive examination, the average student will study all the distinct parts before attempting to put them together. With this thought in mind we have expanded the number of questions following each clinical area and have included a rationale for why the answer is correct.

The comprehensive tests at the back of the book provide the reader with the opportunity to apply material from the specific clinical areas to any nursing situation. With both Canada and the United States changing to comprehensive examinations, these tests will help the student prepare for this experience. The movement from specific learning to general application is educationally sound, and the reader should follow this approach in studying.

All the questions used in this book have been submitted by outstanding educators and practitioners of nursing. Initially the editorial panel reviewed all questions, selecting the most pertinent for inclusion in a mass field-testing project. Graduating students from baccalaureate, associate degree, and diploma nursing programs in various locations in the United States and Canada provided a diverse testing group. The results were statistically analyzed. This analysis was used to select questions for inclusion in the book and to provide the reader with a general idea of each question's level of difficulty. Letters indicating the difficulty of the questions appear next to the answers. The letter *a* signifies that more than 75% of the students answering the question answered it correctly; *b* signifies that between 50% and 75% of the students answering the question answered it correctly; and *c* signifies that between 25% and 50% of the students answering the question were correct. Perforated answer sheets, for the convenience of the student, appear after the index at the back of the book.

We would like to take this opportunity to express our sincere appreciation to our many colleagues for their contributions and support: to Jerry G. Simotas for his help with the computer; to Janet Tischler, Winifred Hennessy, Vicki Staehle, Sally Festa, and Jean Keppler for their careful typing of the manuscript; to Kelly and Heather Nugent for their clerical help; and last, but not least, to our families, who survived without our assistance for a prolonged period of time.

Dolores F. Saxton
Patricia M. Nugent
Phyllis K. Pelikan

CONTENTS

1 **Introduction for students preparing for the licensing examination,** 1

Examples, 2
Preparing for the examination, 2
Taking the examination, 2
How to use this book in studying, 2
General clues for answering multiple choice
   questions, 3

2 **Medical-surgical nursing,** 4

Conceptual introduction, 4
  The health-illness continuum, 4
  Health resources, 5
  The nurse's role, 7
Preoperative and postoperative care, 18
  Review of microbiology, 18
  Review of physical principles related to preoperative
    and postoperative care, 23
  Review of pharmacology related to preoperative and
    postoperative care, 25
  Related procedures, 28
  General nursing care, 29
Controlling infection, 31
  Nursing responsibilities to prevent
    cross-contamination, 31
  Drugs that control infection, 32
Antineoplastic drugs, 38
  General information, 38
  Implications for nurses, 38
  Drugs used, 38
Maintenance of fluid, electrolyte, and acid-base
  balance, 40
  Fluid and electrolyte balance, 40

Acid-base balance, 43
Chemical principles related to fluid and
  electrolytes, 46
Circulatory system, 48
  Review of anatomy and physiology of the circulatory
    system, 48
  Review of physical principles related to the circulatory
    system, 55
  Review of chemical principles related to the circulatory
    system, 58
  Review of microbiologic principles related to the
    circulatory system, 62
  Pharmacology related to circulatory system
    disorders, 64
  Related procedures, 71
  Major diseases, 73
Respiratory system, 86
  Review of anatomy and physiology of the respiratory
    system, 86
  Review of physical principles related to the respiratory
    system, 89
  Review of chemical principles related to the respiratory
    system, 91
  Review of microorganisms related to the respiratory
    system, 91
  Pharmacology related to respiratory system
    disorders, 91
  Related procedures, 93
  Major diseases, 96
Gastrointestinal system, 105
  Review of anatomy and physiology of the
    gastrointestinal system, 105
  Review of physical principles related to the
    gastrointestinal system, 111

Review of chemical principles related to the
gastrointestinal system, 112
Review of microorganisms related to the
gastrointestinal system, 117
Pharmacology related to gastrointestinal system
disorders, 118
Related procedures, 121
Major diseases, 124
Genitourinary system, 140
Review of anatomy and physiology of the
genitourinary system, 140
Review of physical principles related to the
genitourinary system, 148
Review of chemical principles related to the
genitourinary system, 149
Review of microorganisms related to the
genitourinary system, 149
Pharmacology related to urinary system
disorders, 150
Related procedures, 150
Major diseases, 150
Pharmacology related to reproductive system
disorders, 156
Related procedures, 158
Major diseases, 158
Endocrine system, 166
Review of anatomy and physiology of the
endocrine system, 166
Pharmacology related to endocrine system
disorders, 173
Major diseases, 175
Neuromusculoskeletal systems, 183
Review of anatomy and physiology of the
neuromusculoskeletal systems, 183
Review of physical principles related to the
neuromusculoskeletal systems, 206
Review of chemical principles related to the
neuromusculoskeletal systems, 214
Review of microorganisms related to the
neuromusculoskeletal systems, 215
Pharmacology related to neuromusculoskeletal
system disorders, 215
Related procedures, 219
Major diseases, 223
Integumentary system, 248
Review of anatomy and physiology of the
integumentary system, 248
Review of physical principles related to the
integumentary system, 249

Review of chemical principles related to the
integumentary system, 249
Pharmacology related to integumentary system
disorders, 250
Related procedures, 251
Major diseases, 252
Medical-surgical nursing review questions, 258

3 Psychiatric nursing, 322

Background information from the behavioral
sciences, 322
Basic concepts from anthropology, 322
Basic concepts from sociology, 323
Basic concepts from psychology, 326
Nursing in psychiatry, 332
Basic principles of psychiatric nursing, 332
The therapeutic nursing relationship, 332
Deviate patterns of behavior, 334
Classification of mental disorders, 336
Pathology, symptoms, therapies, and nursing
approaches for the major diagnostic entities
in psychiatry, 337
Additional pharmacology, 352
Psychiatric nursing review questions, 354

4 Maternity nursing, 370

Puberty, 370
Maternity cycle, 371
The newborn, 377
Deviations from the normal maternity cycle in the
mother, 383
Deviations from the normal maternity cycle in the
newborn, 388
Infertility and sterility, 391
Family planning, 393
Abortion, 394
Grief responses in pregnancy, 394
Menopause, 394
Agencies providing parent-child health services, 395
Maternity nursing review questions, 395

5 Pediatric nursing, 414

Basic concepts, 414
The family, 414
Human growth and development, 414
Play, 416

The infant, 416
    Growth and development, 416
    Play during infancy (solitary play), 418
    Health promotion during infancy, 418
    Acute and chronic health problems, 422
The toddler, 438
    Growth and development, 438
    Play (parallel play), 439
    Health promotion during childhood, 440
    Acute and chronic health problems, 440
The preschool-age child, 450
    Growth and development, 450
    Play (cooperative play), 450
    Acute and chronic health problems, 451
The school-age child, 454
    Growth and development, 454
    Play, 455
    Acute and chronic health problems, 455
The adolescent, 460
    Growth and development, 460
    Health promotion, 461
Pediatric nursing review questions, 461

6 Historical and legal aspects of nursing in the United States and Canada, 480

    Nursing in the United States, 480
    Nursing in Canada, 491
    Nursing practice and the law—United States and Canada, 506

Comprehensive test 1, 510

Comprehensive test 2, 522

Comprehensive test 3, 534

Comprehensive test 4, 547

Answers and rationales, 559

    Review questions, 559
        Medical-surgical nursing, 559
        Psychiatric nursing, 588
        Maternity nursing, 594
        Pediatric nursing, 602
    Comprehensive test 1, 611
    Comprehensive test 2, 615
    Comprehensive test 3, 619
    Comprehensive test 4, 623

Bibliography, 628

MOSBY'S COMPREHENSIVE REVIEW OF NURSING

1 INTRODUCTION FOR STUDENTS PREPARING FOR THE LICENSING EXAMINATION

The professional nurse licensing examination has traditionally consisted of five tests, one in each of the major clinical fields: medical, surgical, obstetric, pediatric, and psychiatric nursing. However, both Canada and the United States have recognized that these fragmented examinations presented some difficulty in evaluating whether the candidates have the minimum overall cognitive ability to practice nursing. To overcome these problems, comprehensive examinations based on normally encountered nursing situations that cross clinical disciplines have been developed by both countries. As of 1980 in Canada and 1982 in the United States, comprehensive examinations will replace the five examinations based on clinical areas.

The candidates will find that both forms of the examination emphasize the nursing care of patients with representative common national health problems. The questions are designed to evaluate a candidate's skill in recognizing and using pertinent principles from the physical, biologic, and social sciences, as well as her understanding of specific nursing skills and abilities involved in meeting the needs of a patient safely and effectively. To answer the questions appropriately, a candidate needs to understand and correlate certain aspects of anatomy and physiology, behavioral sciences, basic nursing, the effects of medications administered, the patient's attitude toward illness, and other pertinent factors such as legal responsibility. Most questions are based on nursing situations similar to those with which candidates have had experience. Some, however, require candidates to apply basic principles and techniques to clinical situations with which they have had little, if any, experience.

Both forms of the test are objective and multiple choice, offering the candidate four possible answers to each question. One of the answers is most correct and most complete. The three other answers are rarely totally wrong but usually are not as complete as the correct answer. These three answers are called distractors and are designed to entice the student away from the correct answer.

The comprehensive form of the examination has been developed to test the cognitive abilities of the candidate as classified by B. S. Bloom, et al.* The classifications include knowledge (recall), comprehension (understand and use material with limits), application (use and apply abstractions), analysis (break down material into parts), synthesis (put parts into a whole), and evaluation (make quantitative and qualitative judgments). It is expected that most of the questions will be from the comprehension and application classifications. This means that candidates should expect questions which require an understanding of the information given to be able to choose the correct answer. Other questions require the recall and application of principles and theories that are only alluded to by the question.

---

*Taxonomy of educational objectives: the classification of educational goals. Handbook 1: cognitive domain, New York, 1956, David McKay Co., Inc.

EXAMPLES
Question requiring understanding in decision making

1 Mr. Jones has congestive heart failure and is receiving 0.25 mg digoxin daily. You take his pulse and find it is irregular and 100 beats per minute. You would
1. Administer the medication as ordered
2. Notify the physician immediately
3. Give the medication in divided doses
4. Withhold the medication

The correct answer is *1*, based on the knowledge that the pulse is usually both rapid and irregular in patients with congestive heart failure. In this question you are required to demonstrate your understanding of both congestive heart failure and the action of digoxin and to use this understanding in making your decision.

Question requiring recall and application of principles

2 Jamey, age 4, has been hospitalized for fever of undetermined origin (FUO). He screams and becomes uncontrollable as his mother leaves after visiting hours. The best approach is to
1. Ignore this outburst
2. Sit quietly at his bedside
3. Hold and pat him even though he struggles
4. Give him a favorite toy to hold

The correct answer is *2*, since, based on your knowledge of separation anxiety, you recognize that the child needs nonthreatening companionship. In this question you are required to demonstrate your understanding of the principles of growth and development and apply these principles to reject answers *1* and *4*, since they ignore the basic problem of a feeling of abandonment, as well as answer *3*, since restraining and holding him would only serve to make the child more upset.

PREPARING FOR THE EXAMINATION

A few individuals can improve their scores significantly by a highly concentrated period of study immediately before taking an examination. The majority, however, profit more by spreading their review over a much longer period of time, and the best time to begin studying for state boards is the first class attended in the school. Many candidates profit from devoting the evening immediately preceding the examination to a pleasant diversion that is completed in time to permit a good night's rest.

TAKING THE EXAMINATION

The most crucial requisite for doing well in this examination is to bring to it a sound understanding of the subject and a high level of reading comprehension. Determination to do well and a degree of confidence will further enhance the well-prepared individual's chances of earning high scores.

At least three other requirements must be met if an individual's performance is to accurately reflect professional competence. First, the candidate must follow explicitly all the directions given by the examiner and those printed at the beginning of each test, as well as any that refer to a specified group of questions. Second, the candidate must read each question carefully before deciding how to answer it. Third, the candidate must record the answers in the space and manner specified. Some candidates find it helpful to glance over a test before starting to answer the questions. It enables them to answer the questions in the order most efficient and comfortable for them. Others find it more efficient to go through the test answering all questions they are sure of first, then going back to the more difficult questions.

The score candidates earn on each test is the number of questions answered correctly minus a deduction for each incorrect answer given. Therefore candidates reduce their scores if they give more than one reply to any question. Although there is a possibility of lowering the score by answering any question about which they are uncertain, it is generally advantageous to answer such questions, since a general knowledge and understanding of nursing increases the likelihood of giving the expected (best) answer more often than would be expected by chance alone. Accordingly, candidates increase their chances of earning the highest score by omitting only those questions about which they have absolutely no information and making certain that they give one reply to each question answered.

The comprehensive examination, as well as the traditional five-part examination, is given over a 2-day period, but instead of five distinct scores there is only one overall score on the comprehensive form.

HOW TO USE THIS BOOK IN STUDYING

A. Start in one area. Study the material covered by the section. Refer to other textbooks to find additional details if you are unsure of a specific fact.
B. Take the test questions following the area. As you answer each question, write a few words about why

you think that answer was correct; in other words, simply justify why you selected the answer you did. Do you make wild guesses.

C. Mark your paper.

D. Review the questions you answered incorrectly or did not answer. Look up the material covered by these questions and review the rationale for the selection of the correct answer.

E. Next to the correct answer you will find a letter—*a*, *b*, or *c*—in parentheses. These letters indicate the difficulty of the question and can serve as a guide in your studying. The letter *a* signifies that more than 75% of the graduating students in the testing group answered this question correctly; *b* signifies that between 50% and 75% of the students answering the question answered it correctly; and *c* signifies that between 25% and 50% of the students answering the question answered it correctly.

F. A few days later you should review the area again and retake the test questions following it. If you miss the same questions again, you should recognize that you need further study of the material.

G. In the back of the book you will find four comprehensive tests. After you have completed all the area tests, begin taking the comprehensive tests, since they will assist you in applying knowledge and principles from the specific clinical area to any nursing situation.

H. The clinical area tested by the question has been identified in the margin next to the question. This has been done to assist you in finding the material in which you need additional review work.

GENERAL CLUES FOR ANSWERING MULTIPLE CHOICE QUESTIONS

A. Read the question carefully before looking at the answers.
   1. Attempt to determine what the question is really asking; look for key words.
   2. Read each answer thoroughly and see if it completely covers the material asked by the question.

   3. Narrow the choices by immediately eliminating those answers which you know are incorrect.

B. Because few things in life are absolute without exceptions, avoid selecting answers that include words such as *always*, *never*, *all*, *every*, and *none*, since they are rarely correct.

C. Attempt to select the answer that is most complete and includes the other answers within it. An example follows:

   1 A child's intelligence is influenced by
   1. Heredity and environment
   2. Environment and experience
   3. A variety of factors
   4. Education and economic factors

   The most correct answer is *3* because it includes all the other answers.

D. Make certain that the answer you select is reasonable and obtainable under ordinary circumstances and that the action can be carried out in the given situation.

E. Avoid selecting answers that state hospital rules or regulations as a reason or rationale for action.

F. Look for answers that focus on the patient or are directed toward feelings.

G. If the question asks for an immediate action or response, all the answers may be correct, so base your selection on identified priorities for action.

H. Do not select answers that contain exceptions to the general rule, controversial material, or degrading responses.

I. Reread the question if the answers do not seem to make sense, since you may have missed the word *not* or *except* in the statement.

J. Do not worry if you select the same numbered answer repeatedly, since there is usually no pattern to the answers.

K. Make certain you mark the correct space on the answer sheet for the question you are answering.

L. Mark the space completely with a dark line but do not extend your answer over the lines.

2 MEDICAL-SURGICAL NURSING

Medical-surgical nursing is concerned with those aspects of nursing care which are related to the physical and emotional needs of patients with specific types of health problems. The concepts, principles, and skills included here will assist the practitioner in all aspects of nursing care.

Medical-surgical content has been developed by using a systems approach with examples of major diseases. The areas covered include a general conceptual introduction, preoperative and postoperative care, and cardiovascular, respiratory, gastrointestinal, genitourinary, endocrine, neurologic, musculoskeletal, and integumentary systems. The format for each section follows a similar pattern, beginning with a review of anatomy and physiology, related pharmacology, and related procedures, and moving into the major diseases. Etiology and pathophysiology, subjective and objective symptomatology, treatment, and nursing care are included for each disease presented.

Conceptual introduction

THE HEALTH-ILLNESS CONTINUUM
Introduction
A. Health is a generally accepted right; well-being is the norm toward which most governments and all health personnel direct their efforts
B. One of the primary functions of the nursing and medical professions is to help individuals, families, and groups reach the highest level of wellness of which they are capable

Definition
A. The World Health Organization states, "Health is a state of complete physical, mental and social well-being and not just the absence of disease or infirmity"
B. This definition implies there is
   1. Interaction between self and environment
   2. Preservation of structure and function
   3. Maintenance of adaptive potential
C. Significance of definition
   1. Accepted right of all rather than privilege

2. Reciprocal relationships between individual health and community health
3. Increasing public expectation of government support for health services and the extent of care provided
4. Need for nursing and medical practice to move toward maintenance and promotion of health and rehabilitation of the ill rather than merely focusing on provision of episodic care

Basic concepts
A. Health is a continually changing phenomenon
   1. Moves on a continuum between optimal wellness (where potential is maximized and used with purpose) and death
   2. Change may be gradual or abrupt
   3. Level of health attainable depends on adaptive energy, genetic, and environmental factors
      a. Fluctuates throughout life cycle
      b. Varies among individuals
   4. Individual may or may not be aware of change
   5. A person's position on the continuum is determined by
      a. Ability to adapt

b. Level of adaptation

c. Culture's view of health

d. Ability to carry out social, family, and job responsibilities

B. A variety of stresses affect physical, emotional, and social health

1. May be internal or external

2. Can be beneficial or detrimental to life

a. Tension is essential to life

b. Stress of life and living cause wear and tear

(1) Produces a nonspecific response that Hans Selye identifies as the general adaptation syndrome (GAS)

(2) Three stages—alarm, resistance, and exhaustion

3. They elicit some response from or change in the individual

4. Sources of stress vary widely for different individuals or within the same individual at different times

5. Tolerance for stress is individual

6. Stress may be

a. Physical—e.g., thermal, acoustic

b. Chemical—e.g., gas, hormone, nutrient

c. Microbiologic—e.g., virus, bacteria

d. Physiologic—e.g., neoplasms, hypofunctions, hyperfunctions

e. Developmental—e.g., genetic, aging

f. Psychologic—e.g., values, self-image

C. Rehabilitation assists people to attain their maximum level of wellness on the continuum

1. Rehabilitation is particularly concerned with establishing function that is lost while at the same time expanding, maintaining, and supporting the limited remaining function

2. Immediate or potential rehabilitation needs are exhibited in all health problems

3. The patient is the primary rehabilitator—professional health team members only assist the patient and family with the process of self-rehabilitation

4. Rehabilitation is not an isolated process; it involves the patient, the family, the health team, the community, and society

5. The rehabilitation process is concerned with all levels of prevention—primary, secondary, and tertiary

6. Health problems that cause disabilities are socially significant because of the number of people affected, the economic cost and loss, the distress of personal suffering, and the conditions in society that increase their incidence

D. The ability to maintain and return to a relative level of health is influenced by the availability of health resources

HEALTH RESOURCES

A. Government agencies

1. Definition—associations functioning at the international, national, state, and local levels, providing a variety of services to meet the health, education, and welfare needs of the people; these programs are funded by the government, and services are rendered by professionals

2. Examples of government agencies

a. International—World Health Organization

b. National

(1) United States—Department of Health and Human Resources; United States Public Health Service

(2) Canada—Department of National Health and Welfare

c. State or provincial

(1) United States—state health departments

(2) Canada—provincial departments of health

d. Local—county or city department of health, fire department, police department

B. Voluntary agencies

1. Definition—organizations consisting of lay and professional persons dedicated to the prevention and solution of health problems by providing educational, research, and service programs; these agencies are dependent on voluntary donations for funds, are often concerned with specific health problems, and are national organizations that function through state and/or provincial and local chapters

2. Examples of voluntary agencies

a. International—Rockefeller Foundation; international branches of professional organizations

b. National—The American Heart Association, The American Cancer Society, National Multiple Sclerosis Society

c. State and/or provincial—chapters of national organizations

d. Local—branches of national voluntary organizations, community hospitals, volunteers

(a league of women supporting a community hospital, a Girl Scout troop visiting a nursing home, a church group visiting an orphanage)

C. Crises intervention groups
1. Services of crises intervention groups
a. Provide assistance for people in crises—clients' previous methods of adaptation are inadequate to meet present needs
b. The focus of some groups is specific; e.g., poison control, drug addiction centers, suicide prevention; others are general; e.g., walk-in mental health clinics, hospital emergency rooms
c. Depending on the community's needs and facilities, these services can be offered by the government; e.g., state hospitals, Department of Health; or voluntary organizations; e.g., community hospitals, community drug councils
d. Some crises intervention groups provide service over the phone; e.g., poison control, suicide prevention centers; others provide services for the physically present; e.g., hospital emergency rooms, walk-in mental health clinics
2. Crises intervention group success factors
a. The client or family is seeking help
b. The client is provided an immediate opportunity to explore feelings
c. The client is assisted in investigating alternative approaches to solving the problem
d. Information is provided about other health resources where the client may receive additional assistance

D. Self-help groups
1. Services of self-help groups
a. Groups organized by patients or their families to provide services that are not adequately supplied by previous organizations
b. Meets needs of patients and families with chronic problems requiring intervention over an extended period of time
c. The focus of some groups is specific; e.g., Gamblers Anonymous; others deal with a range of problems; e.g., Association for Children with Learning Disabilities
d. Some organizations are nonprofit; e.g., Alcoholics Anonymous; others are profitmaking; e.g., Weight Watchers International, Inc.
e. Provides services to people who frequently are

not accepted by society (the individual who is a drug addict, an alcoholic, a child abuser, mentally ill, obese, or brain injured)
2. Self-help group success factors
a. All members are accepted as equals
b. All members have experienced similar problems
c. They deal with behavior and changes in behavior rather than the underlying causes of the behavior
d. A ready supply of human resources is available
(1) Personal resources
(2) Assistance from peers
(3) Finally, extension of self to others
e. Each member has identified the problem and wants help in meeting needs—self-motivation
f. The group has a ritual and language specific to the group and specific to the problems
g. Leadership of the group remains with the membership
h. Group interaction
(1) Identification with peers—a sense of belonging
(2) Group expectations—discipline required of members
(3) Small steps are encouraged and, when attained, reinforced by the group
i. As a member achieves success within the group, the individual will frequently start to receive reinforcement from outside the group

E. Acute care facilities—the general hospital provides care for the short-term ill patient undergoing treatment for a health problem
1. Intensive care—provides services and equipment to meet the needs of the acutely ill patient undergoing intensive treatment for a health problem; e.g., intensive care unit, coronary care unit, burn unit, psychiatric unit
2. Intermediate care—provides services for the moderately ill patient who is overcoming a health crisis but still has special needs that cannot be adequately met in a general unit; e.g., intermediate care unit, progressive coronary care unit, isolation units
3. Self-care—provides services for the patient and family who need little assistance with health care but have a greater need for teaching, motivation, and control over own care

F. Extended care facilities—the extended care facility

provides services to persons who require either short- or long-term convalescence; these patients need a wide range of services beyond acute care (nursing care, physical therapy, social and psychologic services); extended care facilities can be self-contained or function as an extension of a hospital that utilizes its facilities when needed; the expense of extended care services is usually less than hospital care because of larger nursing units, less building support systems, increased paramedical personnel, and smaller range of services

G. Long-term services—facilities provide services over an extended period of time and most deal with chronic or long-term health problems

  1. Nursing home—where a person goes to live, either for an extended period of time or for permanent residency; the resident is generally well but elderly and can function fairly independently; however, for physical or psychosocial reasons, requires the medical and nursing services and environmental facilities offered by the nursing home

  2. Adult facility—a residence where an individual goes to live; meals and recreational programs may often be supplied; however, medical and nursing supervision are generally not provided on a full-time basis

  3. Rehabilitation center—an institution that provides multiple services and facilities which assist a patient and family to make an adjustment to living; the patient can obtain an optimal level of health by developing personal abilities to their fullest potential and utilizing the following resources

    a. Medical and nursing—total health assessment and planning, physical therapy, occupational therapy, and speech therapy

    b. Psychosocial—personal counseling, social service, and psychiatric service

    c. Vocational—work evaluation, vocational counseling, vocational training, trial employment in sheltered workshops, terminal employment in sheltered workshops, and placement

  4. Continued patient care—includes those facilities and services that are available for people with health needs who are living at home

    a. Outpatient or ambulatory care—diagnosis, treatment, and follow-up care are provided by patient care facilities for people on an outpatient basis; e.g., emergency room, outpatient clinics, mobile health units

    b. Home care—provides comprehensive care for people who do not need to be hospitalized and yet require more care than an outpatient facility can provide; e.g., public health nurses, homemaker services, medical home care programs

    c. Community resources—special services provided by organizations to meet specific client needs; e.g., Meals on Wheels, FISH

    d. Day-care facilities—provide supervised activities and other services to individuals on a daily basis; individual comes to the center for the day and returns home in the evening

H. Health services personnel

  1. Roles and functions

    a. Variety of health professionals can result in overlapping and/or fragmentation of patient care; e.g., nurse, physician, therapist, nutritionist, social worker, physician's assistant, paramedic

    b. Requirements for quality care

      (1) Clarification of role and function

      (2) Development of standards for licensure

      (3) Better utilization of personnel

      (4) Enforcement of present health practice acts

  2. Team approach often used—provides optimal, unified care to the patient who is the focus of the team

    a. Professional health team includes registered professional nurse and physician as colleagues

    b. Other members—social worker, nutritionist, therapists, chaplains, etc., utilized as necessary

    c. The registered nurse leads the nursing team

THE NURSE'S ROLE
Introduction

A. General responsibilities

  1. Recognize the right of persons to receive necessary help

  2. Know and understand self as a person, including personal attitudes, values, and exhibited behavioral responses

  3. Understand the pathophysiologic and psychosocial processes involving the patient's and family's health problem

  4. Encourage and preserve the patient's individual-

ity, self-identity, and inalienable right to be the center of the health team

5. Utilize the problem-solving approach to meet patient needs in achieving full potential
6. Function as collaborator with team members

B. Methods of delivery of nursing care
1. Functional—specific tasks (e.g., medicine administration, treatments, vital signs) are assigned to individual nurses
2. Team nursing—patient assigned to specific group of nurses responsible for that patient's total care
3. Primary nursing—a specific nurse is responsible for a specific patient's total care

Problem-solving approach

A. Introduction
1. The basis of personalized patient care is planned rather than intuitive intervention
2. The most efficient way to accomplish this in a future of exploding knowledge and rapid social change is by the use of the problem-solving process
   a. A theoretical framework used by the nurse
   b. Assists in solving or alleviating both simple and complex nursing problems
3. A changing, expanding, more responsible role demands knowledgeably planned, purposeful, and accountable action by nurses
4. Better prepared health professionals and more efficient use of health facilities can meet increasing demands for health care
5. A decision-making process that systematically selects and uses relevant information is a requisite for individualized patient care
6. The composite of cognitive, affective, and activity components that is nursing can best be integrated by the problem-solving process
7. The process consists of assessing, planning, implementing, and evaluating a problem

B. Steps in process
1. Assessment
   a. Collection of personal, social, medical, and general data
      (1) Sources—primary (patient, family, and chart) and secondary (colleagues, Kardex, literature)
      (2) Methods
         (a) Interviewing formally (nursing health history) or informally during various nurse-patient interactions

         (b) Observation
         (c) Review of records
   b. Classification of data—screening, organizing, and grouping significant and related information
   c. Definition of problem—making a nursing diagnosis that is the scientific identification of patient needs
      (1) Use of judgment
         (a) Inductive reasoning—specific data to generalizations
         (b) Deductive reasoning—generalizations to specific data
      (2) Identification of stresses in environments (external and internal)
      (3) Awareness of patient and patient's reactions to stress
2. Intervention
   a. Making a hypothesis or formulating a nursing care plan—a blueprint for action
      (1) Individualized prescription for care
      (2) Synonymous with nursing orders
   b. Implementation of plan or chosen solution
      (1) Actual administration of planned care
      (2) Adjusted as necessary to immediate needs
   c. Awareness that nursing functions are both independent and interdependent
3. Evaluation and revision include nursing prognosis as to effectiveness of and response to care

C. Advantages
1. Makes allowance for individual responses to problems
2. Determines priority of care, permitting organization of individual needs in order of importance
3. Permits independent, creative, and flexible nursing intervention
4. Facilitates team cooperation by promoting
   a. Communication between team members
   b. Contribution of team members
   c. Coordination of care
   d. Continuity of approach
5. Provides for patient input

D. Extension to medical records
1. Problem oriented medical record (POMR) consists of standardized data base, problem list, assessment and plan for each problem, and progress notes
   a. Updated by appropriate team members on single progress note
   b. Each problem described according to specific

format, which includes *s*ubjective data, *o*bjective findings, *a*ssessment, and a *p*lan for diagnosis, therapy, or teaching (SOAP)
2. Problem oriented records have become the basis for peer review
3. Justifies nursing function
4. Focuses on patient rather than task
5. Improves patient care

Maintenance of effective communication

A. Introduction
1. The need to communicate is universal
2. People communicate to satisfy needs
3. Recognition of what is communicated is basic for the establishment of a therapeutic nurse-patient relationship
4. Clear, accurate communication among members of the health team, including the patient, is vital to support the patient's welfare
B. Nursing responsibilities in promotion of productive communication
1. Be aware that effective communication requires skill in both sending and receiving messages
   a. Verbal—words, tone of voice, etc.
   b. Written
   c. Nonverbal—facial expression, eye contact, posture, tension, etc.
2. Recognize the high stress—anxiety potential of most health settings created in part by
   a. The health problem itself
   b. Treatments and procedures
   c. Exclusive behavior of personnel
   d. Foreign environment
   e. Change in life-style, body image, and self-concept
3. Recognize the individual intrinsic worth of each person
   a. Listen, consider wishes when possible, explain when necessary
   b. Avoid stereotyping, snap judgments, unjustified comparisons
   c. Be nonjudgmental and nonpunitive in response and behavior
4. Be aware that each individual must be treated as a whole person
5. Recognize that all behavior has meaning and usually results from coping with stress or anxiety
   a. Be aware of importance of value systems

b. Be aware of significance of cultural differences
c. Be sensitive to personal meaning of experiences to patients
d. Recognize that giving information may not alter patient's behavior
e. Recognize the defense mechanisms the individual is using
f. Recognize own anxiety and cope with it
g. Search for patterns of adaptation on which to base action
h. Recognize that adequate behavior patterns may become inadequate under stress
   (1) Health problems may produce a change in family or community constellations
   (2) Health problems may lead to change in self-perception and role identity
i. Be aware that behavioral changes are possible only when the individual has a replacement behavior to maintain equilibrium
6. Help the patient to accept the health problem and its consequences
7. Identify the individual's needs and determine their priority for care
8. Maintain an accepting, open environment
   a. Permissive rather than authoritarian
   b. Identify and face problems honestly
   c. Value the expression of feelings
   d. Be nonjudgmental
9. Where possible, encourage patient participation in decision making
10. Recognize the patient as a person
    a. Use names rather than labels such as room numbers or diagnoses
    b. Maintain patient's dignity
    c. Be courteous toward patient, family, and visitors
    d. Protect privacy by use of curtains, avoidance of probing
    e. Permit personal possessions where practical; e.g., own nightclothes, pictures, toys
    f. Explain at patient's level of understanding and tolerance
    g. Encourage expression of feelings
    h. Approach the patient as a person with difficulties, not as a "difficult" person
11. Support a social environment that focuses on patient needs
    a. Use problem-solving techniques in assessment, intervention, and recording

    b. Be flexible in carrying out routines and policies

    c. Be discreet in use of power

    d. Recognize that use of medical jargon can isolate the patient

C. Patient factors influencing communication

  1. Hierarchy of needs

    a. Need to survive—physiologic needs for air, food, water, etc.

    b. Need for safety and comfort—physical and psychologic security

    c. Interpersonal needs—social needs for love, acceptance, status, and recognition

    d. Intrapersonal needs—self-esteem, self-actualization

  2. Developmental level

    a. Infant—the infant must adapt to a totally new environment; the stress from this culture shock is compounded for the infant with a congenital defect

    b. Child—maturation involves physical, functional, and emotional growth; it is an ever-changing process that produces stress; disabilities will provide additional factors that may quantitatively or qualitatively affect maturation

    c. Adolescent—the adolescent is experiencing a physical, psychologic, and social growth spurt; the individual is asking: "Who am I?" on the way to developing a self-image; limitations provide additional stress during identity formation

    d. Adult—in society the adult is expected to be independent and productive, to provide for self and family; if one cannot assume this role totally or partially, it can cause additional stress

    e. Aged—our society tends to venerate youth and deplore old age; all elderly persons are experiencing multiple stresses (loss of loved ones, change in usual life style, loss of physical vigor, and, for many, the thought of approaching death) at a time when their ability to adapt is compromised by the anatomic, physiologic, and psychologic alterations that occur during the aging process

  3. Type of condition affecting patient

    a. Acute illness—caused by a health problem that produces signs and symptoms abruptly, runs a short course, and from which there is usually a full recovery; an acute illness may leave an individual with a loss of a body part or function and may develop into a long-term illness

    b. Chronic illness—caused by a health problem that produces signs and symptoms over a period of time, runs a long course, and from which there is only partial recovery

      (1) Exacerbation—a period of time when a chronic illness becomes more active and there is a recurrence of pronounced signs and symptoms of the disease

      (2) Remission—a period of time when a chronic illness is controlled and signs and symptoms are reduced or not obvious

      (3) Degenerative—a continuous deterioration or increased impairment of a person's physical state

    c. Terminal illness—an illness that has no cure; death is inevitable in the near future

    d. Primary health problem—an original condition developing independently of another health problem

    e. Secondary health problem—a condition or disorder that develops as a direct result of another health problem

  4. Personal resources

    a. Level of self-esteem—an attitude that reflects the individual's perception of self-worth; it is a personal subjective judgment of one's self

    b. Experiential background—knowledge derived from one's own actions, observations, or perceptions; maturation, culture, and environment influence the individual's experiential foundation

    c. Intelligence

      (1) Genetic intellectual potential

      (2) Amount of formal and informal education

      (3) Level of intellectual development; e.g., child versus adult

      (4) Ability to reason, conceptualize, and translate words into actions

    d. Level of motivation—an internal desire or incentive to accomplish something

    e. Values—factors that are important to the individual

    f. Religion—a deep personal belief in a higher force than humanity

  5. Extent of actual or perceived change in body image

a. Obvious reminder of disability to self and others
   (1) Loss of a body part
   (2) Need for a prosthesis; e.g., breast, leg, eye
   (3) Need for hardware; e.g., pacemaker, braces, hearing aid, wheelchair
   (4) Extent of disability or limitation
   (5) Need for medication
b. Value placed on loss by self or society
   (1) "No longer whole," "a cripple"
   (2) Type of loss—perceptions of body part or function as being good, pleasing, repulsive, clean, dirty, etc.
      (a) Symbols of sexuality—breast, uterus, prostate, heart
      (b) May lack social acceptability—colostomy, mental illness, incontinence, cancer, tuberculosis
      (c) Impairment of senses and/or ability to communicate—laryngectomy, stroke, deafness, blindness
      (d) Altered body image resulting from anatomic changes—amputation of limb or breast, colostomy
6. Patient's and family's stage of adaptation
   a. Self-protection—disbelief, denial, avoidance, and/or intellectualization; with developing awareness of implications of illness the individual defends the self further—anger, depression, and/or joking
   b. With developing realization of implications of illness the individual reorganizes self-feelings and restructures relationships with family and society
   c. As the losses are resolved, the individual begins to accept the consequences of the illness and acknowledges feelings about the self and further changes that must be made
7. Patient's previous history
   a. Health history
      (1) Physiologic—what physical adaptations were manifested in the past
      (2) Psychologic—what psychologic methods of adaptation were exhibited in the past
   b. Sociocultural history
      (1) Religion—particular denomination, specific belief; e.g., agnostic, atheist, "energy force"
      (2) Ethnic group
      (3) Occupation
      (4) Economic status
      (5) Family members and their personal resources
      (6) Race
      (7) Educational background
      (8) Environment—urban versus rural, private home versus apartment
      (9) Social status

Establishment of a teaching-learning environment

A. Definitions
   1. Teaching is communication especially structured and sequenced to produce learning
   2. Learning is the activity by which knowledge, attitudes, and skills are acquired, resulting in a change in behavior; goals of learning
      a. Understanding or acquiring knowledge—cognitive learning; e.g., What is diabetes and how does it affect me?
      b. Feeling or developing attitudes—affective learning; e.g., What does this health problem mean to me?
      c. Doing or developing psychomotor skills—conative learning; e.g., How do I give myself an injection?
B. Principles of the teaching-learning process and related nursing approaches
   1. Learning occurs best when there is a felt need or readiness to learn
      a. Identify the patient's emotional or motivational readiness—is the person ready to put forth the effort necessary to learn
      b. Identify the patient's experiential readiness—does the person have the necessary background of experience, skills, attitudes, and ability to learn what is needed
      c. Determine the patient's level of adaptation—it is usually difficult to teach during the beginning stages of adaptation because the patient is expressing denial, anger, and/or depression; once the initial defensive compensatory reactions have passed, the individual is more receptive to teaching
      d. Assess the patient's level of human needs; the patient whose physical and safety needs are not met will not be concerned with interpersonal and intrapersonal needs

e. Specific signs of the patient's readiness to learn
   (1) The patient is adapting to the initial crisis
   (2) The patient has a developing awareness of the health problem and its implications
   (3) The patient is asking direct questions
   (4) The patient is presenting clues that indicate indirect seeking of information
   (5) The patient's physical condition or behavior invites the nurse to intervene through teaching
f. Once a need is recognized, readiness is determined, and the time and place are appropriate, develop a plan and teach

2. The method of presentation of material influences the patient's ability to learn
   a. A tentative teaching plan should be developed and communicated to all members of the health team
   b. Information presented should be organized, accurate, and concise; e.g., simple to the complex, general to the specific
   c. Appropriate teaching methods should be instituted
      (1) Concepts are best taught with lectures, audiovisual materials, and discussion
      (2) Attitudes are taught by exploring feelings, role models, discussions, and atmosphere of acceptance
      (3) Skills are taught by illustrations, models, demonstration, return demonstration, and practice
   d. Teaching tools should be used when indicated; e.g., models, filmstrips, illustrations
   e. The patient and family should be encouraged to ask questions, which should be answered directly
   f. Opportunities should be provided for evaluation

3. Learning is made easier when material to be learned is related to what the learner already knows
   a. Find out what the patient knows about the problem
   b. Begin the teaching program at the patient's level of understanding
   c. Avoid the use of technical terminology; use simple terms or ones with which the patient feels comfortable

4. Learning is purposeful; short- and long-term goals are important because they identify the behavior to be attained
   a. With the patient, set short- and long-term goals
   b. Goal should meet the following criteria
      (1) Specific—state exactly what is to be accomplished
      (2) Measurable—set a minimum acceptable level of performance
      (3) Realistic—the goal must be potentially achievable

5. Learning is an active process and takes place within the learner
   a. Utilize a teaching approach that includes the learner; e.g., programed instruction books, discussion, questions and answers, return demonstration
   b. Provide opportunities for the patient to practice motor skills
   c. Encourage self-directed activities

6. Every individual has capabilities and strengths (physical strengths, emotional maturity, a supportive family) that can be utilized to help the patient learn
   a. Identify the patient's personal resources
   b. Build on the identified strengths
   c. Utilize these personal resources when and where appropriate

7. Energy and endurance levels will affect the patient's ability to learn and perform
   a. During instructions, balance teaching with sufficient rest periods
   b. Provide teaching at opportune times; e.g., earlier in the day rather than at night, after periods of rest
   c. Present instruction in a manner the patient can comprehend and at a pace that can be maintained
   d. Be flexible and adjust plan according to patient's rest and activity needs

8. Learning does not always progress on a straight line forward and upward; the patient may experience plateaus and remissions with a resulting change in adaptation and needs
   a. Accept patient's feelings regarding lack of progress
   b. Point out progress that has been made
   c. Be patient and do not cause additional stress for the patient

    d. Try alternative approaches for achieving goals

    e. Identify short-term objectives for meeting goals

    f. Alter long-term goals as necessary

  9. Learning from previous experience can be transferred to new situations

    a. When teaching something new, relate the commonalities or similarities of previously learned experiences

    b. Base the plan of instructions on the foundation of the patient's knowledge

    c. Once the known is reinforced, then the unknown can be explored and the differences taught

C. Motivation

  1. Definition—motivation is the process of stimulating a person to assimilate certain concepts or behavior

  2. Principles of motivation and related nursing approaches

    a. People are complex products of self, family, and culture; the nurse must care for the patient as a unified being

      (1) Respect the patient as a person

      (2) Accept the patient's feelings without minimizing them

      (3) Assist the patient and family in accepting that the person's individuality and wholeness continue despite the changed physical or emotional state

      (4) Involve the person in deciding what to do and how to do it

      (5) The person must take precedence over the purpose of the lesson

    b. Learning is fostered when the plan of instruction is designed to operate within the individual's personal attitude and value system

      (1) Provide an atmosphere that allows for acceptance of differing value systems

      (2) Let the patient explore personal values, attitudes, and feelings concerning the health problem and its implications

      (3) Explore with the family the possibilities of carrying out instruction and how to individualize it so it is acceptable and practical for the patient and family

    c. A motivated learner assimilates what is learned more rapidly than one who is not motivated

      (1) The patient needs an opportunity to explore and discover personal learning needs and feelings concerning them

      (2) Awareness of a need to know can cause mild anxiety, which in itself is motivating

      (3) Motivation that is too intense may reduce the effectiveness of learning

      (4) Determine patient's readiness for learning

    d. Intrinsic motivation (stimulated from within the learner) is preferable to extrinsic motivation (stimulated from outside the learner)

      (1) Identify those factors which are essential for the individual to have a feeling of meaningful achievement; e.g., being able to care for own health needs, respect and appreciation from others, acquiring new knowledge, receiving a reward

      (2) Satisfaction with learning progress promotes additional learning; therefore design nursing care which will assist the patient in attaining that feeling of meaningful achievement

      (3) Encourage the patient to participate as a member of the health team and to be self-directed

    e. Information is learned more readily when it is relevant and meaningful to the learner

      (1) Help the patient interpret why the information is important and how the information gained will be useful

      (2) Relate the information by building the teaching plan on the patient's foundation of knowledge, experience, attitudes, and feelings

    f. Learning motivated by success or rewards is preferable to learning by failure or punishment

      (1) Help patient to set realistic goals within the motivation zone (goals set too high may be too challenging, whereas goals set too low may lead to no action)

      (2) Focus on a patient's strengths and abilities rather than on failures and disabilities

      (3) Select learning tasks in which the patient is likely to succeed

      (4) Assist the patient to master or feel successful at one stage of instruction before moving on to the next

      (5) Errors must be accepted as part of the learning process

      (6) Tolerance for failure is best taught

through providing a backlog of success that compensates for experienced failure

g. Planned reinforcement is essential for learning; operant conditioning is based on the theory that satisfaction motivates learning and that those events which occur together are associated
(1) For each patient identify and utilize those factors which are stimulants or incentives for action; e.g., praise, smile, rewards, rest, specific privileges, being able to care for self
(2) Provide visible reinforcements; e.g., progress charts, graphs
(3) Repetition is a form of reinforcement; therefore repeated activities tend to become habitual
(a) Provide opportunities for the patient to practice old and new skills
(b) Review information previously taught before introducing new information
(4) Involve the patient in groups with people with the same health problems but at various stages of convalescence
(a) To be successful it is helpful for the patient to associate with successful people
(b) Individuals can often learn more by teaching than in any other way

h. Evaluation of performance aids in learning
(1) Purpose of evaluation
(a) Involves measuring behavior and interpreting the results with regard to what degree the set goals are being attained
(b) Reinforces correct behavior
(c) Assists the learner to realize how to change incorrect behavior
(d) Helps the teacher to determine the adequacy of the teaching
(2) Together the teacher and learner should observe and evaluate the learner's response in light of the desired behavior
(3) Explain the "whys" of a good or poor evaluation
(4) Value judgments, especially "poor" or "inadequate," must relate to the performance rather than the individual

Administration of medications

A. Introduction
1. The scientific age has introduced an increasing number of pharmaceuticals appropriate for relief of stress and symptoms, support of defense systems, and adjuncts to other supplemental and curvative therapies
2. Increasingly, as part of the nursing care, the nurse assumes the dependent function of administering these medications, either singly or in combinations
3. In the interest of patient welfare and safety, it is imperative that the independent and collaborative responsibilities inherent in this function be understood and practiced

B. Basic concepts
1. Legally, the administration of medications is a dependent function requiring a physician's written order and knowledge of cause and effect
2. Legally, morally, and ethically, independent judgment is required before prescribed medications are administered
3. Certain chemical agents alter, inactivate, or potentiate other medications when mixed either prior to or after administration
4. Medications may be given for local or systemic effects
5. Pharmacologic actions of drugs tend to stimulate or depress physiologic activity
6. Medications may be given in a variety of ways, depending on factors such as the effect desired, rapidity of action desired, or the effect of the chemical on the tissues

C. Common terms
1. Chemotherapy—use of drugs to destroy invading organisms or abnormal tissue in the host
2. Drug—chemical agent that interacts with living systems and is employd to prevent, diagnose, or treat disease
3. Drug legislation—laws that provide the standards for drug manufacture and distribution and protect the public against fraudulent claims about drug action; e.g., Federal Controlled Substances Act, regulations of the Federal Bureau of Narcotics and Dangerous Drugs, and regulations by specific states
4. Drug standards—criteria for drug composition established by chemical or bioassay and pub-

lished in official publications; e.g., United States Pharmacopeia, National Formulary, Pharmacopoeia Internationalis

5. Pharmacodynamics—the biochemical and physiologic effects of drugs and their mechanisms of action on living tissue
6. Pharmacology—the analysis of properties of chemicals that have a biologic action
7. Pharmacotherapeutics—the planned use and evaluation of the effect of drugs employed to prevent and treat disease
8. Toxicology—the analysis of poisons and poisonings caused by drugs

D. Terms that describe drug effects
1. Adverse effect—an action differing from the planned effect
2. Side effect—an often predictable outcome that is unrelated to the primary action of the drug
3. Toxic effect—a pathologic extension of the primary action of the drug
4. Cumulation—elevation of circulating levels of a drug consequent to slowing of metabolic pathways or excretory mechanisms
5. Drug dependence—driving need for continued use of a behavior or mood altering drug that leads to abuse
   a. Psychic dependence—craving requiring periodic or continued use of a drug for pleasure or relief of discomfort
   b. Physical dependence—appearance of characteristic symptoms when drug use is suspended or terminated (withdrawal or abstinence symptoms)
6. Hypersusceptibility—a response to a drug action which is higher than that occurring when the same dosage is given to 90% of the population
7. Idiosyncrasy—genetically conditioned enzymatic or receptor responsiveness that interferes with metabolic degradation of a drug
8. Paradoxic response—an action of a drug producing a response that contrasts sharply with the usual therapeutic effect obtained with the same dosage of the drug
9. Receptor—cellular site where union between a drug and a cellular constituent produces a reversible action
10. Tolerance—lowering of effect obtained from an established dosage of a drug that necessitates raising the dosage to maintain the effect
11. Tachyphylaxis—rapidly developing tolerance to a drug
12. Drug allergy—response occurring when drugs are from protein sources or combine with body protein and induce an allergen-antibody reaction which releases vasoactive intermediates that cause fluid transudation into tissues
    a. Anaphylaxis—life threatening episode of bronchial constriction and edema which obstruct the airway and cause generalized vasodilation that depletes circulating blood volume; occurs when a drug allergen is administered to an individual having antibodies produced by prior use of the drug
    b. Urticaria—generalized pruritic skin eruptions or giant hives; occurs when a drug is administered to an individual having antibodies produced by prior use of the drug
    c. Angioedema—fluid accumulation in periorbital, oral, and respiratory tissues with lengthening of the expiratory phase and wheezing as bronchial constriction gradually progresses; occurs when a drug is administered to an individual having antibodies produced by prior use of the drug
    d. Serum sickness—gradually emerging intermittent episodes of dyspnea, hypotension, generalized edema, joint pain, rash, swollen lumph glands; occurs 7 or more days after initial administration of a drug causing gradual low-level (titer) production of antibodies that interact with circulating drug to produce symptoms as long as the drug remains in the body
    e. Arthus reaction—a localized area of tissue necrosis caused by disruption of blood supply; occurs when spasticity, occlusion, and degeneration of blood vessels are precipitated by injection of a drug into a site having large quantities of bivalent antibodies
    f. Delayed-reaction allergies—rash and fever occurring during drug therapy

E. Drug actions
1. Local—drug acts at the site of application
2. Systemic—drug is distributed to selected internal receptor sites after being absorbed from tissues

following administration; these routes include oral, sublingual, buccal, rectal, parenteral (intradermal, subcutaneous, intramuscular, intravenous, intraspinal, intracardiac)

F. Mechanisms
   1. Replacement—administration of insulin required for cellular utilization of glucose
   2. Interruption—antimetabolic drugs trick the cell into utilizing an inactive component in building protein
   3. Potentiation—sulfonylurea group of oral hypoglycemic agents stimulate pancreatic beta cells to produce insulin

G. Factors influencing dosage-response relationships
   1. Age, weight, sex, size, physiologic status, genetic and environmental factors affect responses and dosage required for therapeutic effect
   2. The ratio between the median toxic dose and the median effective dose (TD50/ED50) of a drug provides the therapeutic index (T.I.), which is used as a guide to the safe dosage range; a low T.I. provides a narrow margin of safety, and the patient's status is monitored closely for evidence of drug-related adverse effects; e.g., antineoplastic drugs
   3. Concentration of active drug at receptors and duration of drug action are affected by
      a. Characteristics of the drug and the rate of absorption, distribution, biotransformation, and excretion
      b. Drug affinity for particular tissues, immaturity of enzymes required for metabolism of the drug, or depressed function of tissues naturally metabolizing or excreting the drug
   4. Membrane barriers, placental or blood-brain barrier, may block or selectively pass drug from circulating fluids to protected areas
   5. Plasma protein binding of drugs maintains tissue levels by liberating drug when stores are lowered and by slowing renal clearance until the drug is freed from binding sites

H. Drug interactions
   1. Drugs and foods may interact to adversely affect the therapeutic plan; e.g., ingestion of foods or vitamin preparations containing vitamin K may inhibit the hypothrombinemic effect of oral anticoagulants
   2. Drug antagonism—opposing effects of 2 drugs at receptor sites in body tissues
      a. Chemical antagonism—combining or binding of 2 drugs causing inactivation of the chemicals
      b. Pharmacologic antagonism—competition of 2 drugs for a receptor that may allow the weaker drug to block access by the more potent drug
      c. Physiologic antagonism—opposing action on physiologic systems that allows cancellation of action by either drug
   3. Drug action summation—combined or concurrent action of drugs that increases therapeutic effects or incidence of adverse effects
      a. Synergism—interaction of drugs at common receptor sites that alters metabolism or excretion and enhances the effect of drugs
      b. Addition—action of 2 drugs at different receptors which produces an effect twice that possible when either drug is used alone
      c. Potentiation—an intensified action occurring when 2 drugs are administered concurrently that is greater than when either drug is used alone

I. General information
   1. Drug nomenclature
      a. Official name (generic, nonproprietary)—designated title under which a drug is listed in official publications
      b. Chemical name—descriptive name identifying chemical composition and placement of atoms
      c. Trade name (brand, proprietary)—manufacturer's registered and legally owned name for a drug
   2. Sources of drugs
      a. Active constituents of plants—alkaloids, glycosides, gums, resins, tannins, waxes, volatile or fixed oils
      b. Animal sources of biologic products—enzymes, sera, vaccines, antitoxins, toxoids, hormones
      c. Mineral sources—iron, iodine, Epsom salt
   3. Drug dosage forms
      a. Prepared by manufacturers in units for convenience of administration
      b. Forms used include capsules, extended-release capsules, tablets (enteric-coated, extended-release), troche, pills, suppositories, powders, ampules, vials, delayed-release (repository) suspensions, prefilled cartridges, liniment, lotion, cream, ointments, pastes
      c. Chemical preparations—solutions (waters,

true solutions, syrups), aqueous suspensions (mixtures, emulsions, magmas, gels), spirits, elixirs, tinctures, fluidextracts, extracts

J. Nursing responsibilities

1. Ascertain the presence and correctness of a physician's order

2. Know the common symbols and equivalents in the apothecary and metric systems

3. Know the common abbreviations denoting frequency and route of administration

4. Know the usual dosage of a drug, the usual route of administration, and the expected, unusual, untoward, or toxic effects of a drug

5. Use independent judgment before administering a medication by assessing

   a. The patient's need relative to factors such as prn medications and expected effects of the medication; e.g., diuresis or sleep

   b. Untoward or toxic manifestations of prior doses; e.g., pruritus following an antibiotic, bradycardia below 60, or visionary disturbances with digoxin

   c. Compatibility of medications administered at the same time; e.g.,

      (1) The presence of clouding or a precipitate when mixing injectables; e.g., phenobarbital (Luminal Sodium) and meperidine (Demerol)

      (2) Inhibition of medication; e.g., antacids or milk given with tetracycline interferes with absorption, resulting in decreased serum levels of the antibiotic

      (3) Potentiation of another medication; e.g., A.S.A. given when a patient is on anticoagulants intensifies the anticoagulant effect

   d. Effects on living tissues; e.g.,

      (1) Iron can discolor tissue and must be given through a straw in liquid form or by the Z-track method intramuscularly

      (2) Abscess formation can occur when the same area is used too frequently for intramuscular administration; thus rotation of site is necessary

      (3) Pain, irritation, or inflammation can occur during intravenous administration and may necessitate adjustments such as greater dilution or slower flow rate

6. Assist the patient to accept ordered medications by independent actions such as

   a. Crushing tablets that cannot be swallowed

   b. Disguising unpalatable tastes with fruit juices

   c. Reinforcing the need for medication

7. Ensure that the right medication is given to the right patient at the right time in the right dose and by the right route

   a. Verify orders

   b. Read labels

   c. Calculate the dosage accurately when prescribed dose is not available

   d. Pour or draw up correct amounts

   e. Identify the patient correctly by checking the arm band

   f. Prepare the patient psychologically by providing explanations as indicated

   g. Prepare the patient physically by

      (1) Positioning appropriately for oral and parenteral medications

      (2) Disinfecting the skin when it is to be punctured

   h. Use clean or sterile technique as indicated by route of administration

   i. Use the route specified as appropriate for the ordered medication and dosage

8. For assistance with calculation of solutions and dosages refer to a programed text (see Bibliography)

9. Use the appropriate technique for administration

   a. Preparations such as tablets, capsules, pills, powders, or liquids may be swallowed; in addition

      (1) Tablets; e.g., nitroglycerine may be held sublingually

      (2) Powders may be inhaled with Medihaler; e.g., cromolyn sodium

      (3) Liquids may be nebulized and inhaled or they may be swabbed, sprayed, or instilled

   b. Parenteral preparations such as ampules or vials containing dosage in solution or powder to which sterile water or saline must be added may be given in several ways

      (1) Subcutaneously or hypodermically in small volume (0.5 to 2 ml)

         (a) Pinch the tissue on the outer surface of the upper arm or the anterior aspect of the thigh or the abdomen

         (b) Insert a 25- to 26-gauge needle ⅝ to

1 inch in length at a 45- to 60-degree angle and inject the medication
   - (c) Massage to increase absorption (contraindicated when giving heparin)
- (2) Intramuscularly in slightly larger volume (up to 5 ml)
  - (a) Spread the tissue taut or pinch if necessary
  - (b) Use the upper outer quadrant of the buttock or ventral gluteal muscle, the lateral aspect of the thigh, or the deltoid area of the arm
  - (c) When using the gluteal muscle, promote relaxation of the muscle whenever possible by placing the patient in a prone position with toes pointing inward or on the side with the leg flexed
  - (d) Insert a 19- to 22-gauge needle 1 to 2 inches in length at a 90-degree angle quickly and smoothly
  - (e) Depth of insertion depends on factors such as the weight of the patient and the size of the muscle used
  - (f) Aspirate when the needle is in place and tissue is released (unless giving a substance such as iron-dextran [Imferon], for which it is contraindicated)
    - (1) If no blood returns, continue injection
    - (2) If blood is aspirated withdraw and prepare a fresh dose
  - (g) Apply pressure or massage area after injection as required (unless contraindicated; e.g., **Z**-track technique)
- (3) Intradermally with very small volume for local effect
  - (a) Use syringe with appropriate calibrations; e.g., tuberculin
  - (b) Inject at a 15-degree angle using a 26-gauge needle, ⅜ to ½ inch in length with the bevel up
- (4) Piggyback administration using intravenous tubing in place
  - (a) Dilute medication according to directions—usually with 50 to 150 ml of fluid
  - (b) Remove air from tubing of piggyback
  - (c) Cleanse diaphragm on intravenous tubing already in place with alcohol
  - (d) Insert needle in rubber diaphragm on tubing leading from the infusion that is keeping the vein open
  - (e) Stop flow of or lower solution below level of piggyback
  - (f) Adjust rate of flow on piggyback medication to complete absorption in time designated—usually about 30 minutes
  - (g) Remove the piggyback and readjust flow rate
10. Clearly and accurately record and report the administration of medications and the patient's response

---

Preoperative and postoperative care

REVIEW OF MICROBIOLOGY
Bacteria

A. Definition—bacteria are unicellular microbes without chlorophyll
B. Some examples of medically important bacteria
   1. Eubacteriales ("true bacteria")—typically unicellular microbes having a rigid cell wall; the morphologic types are
      a. Rod-shaped bacilli—variations of the rod shape may be curved or clubbed (some of the gram-positive rods form endospores)
      b. Spherical cocci
      c. Eubacteriales are divided into 5 families based on shape, Gram stain, and endospore formation
         (1) Gram-positive cocci include
            (a) Diplococci—occurring predominantly in pairs; e.g., *Diplococcus pneumoniae*
            (b) Streptococci—occurring predominantly in chains; e.g., *Streptococcus pyogenes*
            (c) Staphylococci—occurring predominantly in grapelike bunches; e.g., *Staphylococcus aureus*

(2) Gram-negative cocci include *Neisseria gonorrhoeae* and *Neisseria meningitidis*

(3) Gram-negative rods include enterobacteria such as *Escherichia*, *Salmonella*, and *Shigella* species

(4) Gram-positive rods that do not produce endospores include *Corynebacterium diphtheriae*

(5) Gram-positive rods producing endospores include *Bacillus anthracis*, *Clostridium botulinum*, and *Clostridium tetani*

2. Actinomycetales (actinomycetes)—moldlike microbes with elongated cells, frequently filamentous; e.g., *Mycobacterium tuberculosis* and *Mycobacterium leprae*

3. Spirochaetales (spirochetes)—flexuous, spiral organisms; e.g., *Treponema pallidum*

4. Mycoplasmatales (mycoplasmas)—delicate, nonmotile microbes displaying a variety of sizes and shapes
   a. Commonly referred to as pleuropneumonialike organisms (PPLO)
   b. Mycoplasmas are the smallest organisms known that are capable of growth and reproduction outside living cells

C. Bacterial cell
   1. Size—from 0.5 to 15 mm
   2. Cell wall—gram-positive species are rich in muramic acid and low in lipids; the opposite is true of the gram-negative species
   3. Capsule—a thickened protective material (generally a polysaccharide) that is secreted by the cell, thereby protecting it from being phagocytized and increasing its virulence; e.g., *Diplococcus pneumoniae*
   4. Spores—the inactive resistant structures into which bacterial protoplasm can transform under adverse conditions (under favorable conditions a spore germinates into an active and growing vegetative cell)
      a. The endospores are resistant to heat and desiccation
      b. Spore formers *Clostridium tetani* and *Clostridium botulinum* are difficult to destroy; therefore their destruction is used to set the standards of sterilization for the hospital and food industries
   5. Flagella—organelles of locomotion possessed by all motile bacteria; some species have 1 flagellum

(monotrichous), whereas others have flagella over their entire surface (peritrichous)

6. Reproduction—bacteria reproduce by binary fission, an asexual process dividing the cell into new daughter cells; bacteria are also able to conjugate and exchange genetic material

D. Growth needs
   1. Nutrition
      a. Autotrophic organisms—may do well on simple diet of carbon dioxide, inorganic salts, and water
      b. Heterotrophic organisms—demand organic nutrients
         (1) Saprophytes—derive nourishment from dead or decaying organic matter
         (2) Parasites—derive nourishment from living tissue; obligate parasites cannot be cultured except in living tissue
   2. Culturing
      a. Culture—growth of large numbers of microbes on suitable food media; e.g., broth, agar, milk
      b. Culture media—food substances in or on which cultures are grown
      c. Colony—cluster of millions of microbes, presumably all descendants from single bacterium, visible to naked eye
      d. Ways in which cultures are studied
         (1) Smears made and organisms studied microscopically either with or without staining
         (2) Cultural characteristics observed
            (a) Media most favorable to growth
            (b) Appearance of colonies—the color, shape, and texture, whether large or small, smooth or rough, opaque or translucent
            (c) Molecular oxygen requirement (anaerobic, aerobic, or facultative)

E. Biochemical reactions
   1. Fermentation—anaerobic oxidation reactions by which some organisms use carbohydrates to generate energy-rich adenosine triphosphate (ATP) molecules; various kinds of fermentation reactions are useful for identifying different groups of microorganisms
      a. Nonfermenters
      b. Fermenters that produce only acid
      c. Fermenters that produce acid and gas; e.g.,

Escherichia coli, a normal inhabitant of intestinal tract

    d. Lactose fermenters; e.g., *Escherichia coli* and other nonpathogens in intestinal tract

    e. Nonlactose fermenters; e.g., *Shigella* and *Salmonella* pathogens in intestinal tract

  2. Urea-splitting reaction—identifies organisms as

    a. Urease-positive organisms (contain enzyme urease, which catalyzes conversion of urea to ammonia); e.g., *Proteus bacilli* (gram-negative, normal inhabitants of intestinal tract)

    b. Urease-negative organisms—do not contain urease so cannot convert urea to ammonia; e.g., *Salmonella* and *Shigella,* pathogens in intestinal tract

F. Hydrogen ion concentration (pH)—majority of bacteria grow and culture best at a pH of about 7.5; most fungi (molds and yeasts) culture best at a pH of about 5

G. Oxygen utilization

  1. Obligate aerobes—organisms that cannot grow without free (molecular) oxygen

  2. Obligate anaerobes—organisms that cannot grow in the presence of free (molecular) oxygen

  3. Facultative—organisms that can grow with or without free oxygen

H. Temperature

  1. Psychrophiles—organisms growing best at low temperatures (10° to 20° C [50° to 68° F])

  2. Mesophiles—organisms growing best at "middle temperatures" (20° to 45° C [68° to 113° F]); this range includes human pathogens that have an optimum temperature of 37° C [98.6° F]

  3. Thermophiles—organisms growing best at high temperatures (45° to 65° C [113° to 149° F])

I. Staining—artificial coloration to facilitate visualization and identification of tissues and microorganisms.

  1. Gram stain—gram-positive organisms retain the crystal violet color when treated with ethyl alcohol; gram-negative organisms are decolorized with ethyl alcohol

  2. Acid-fast stain—after being stained with carbolfuchsin, acid-fast organisms resist decolorization with dilute acid alcohol and do not take counterstain (usually methylene blue); non-acid-fast organisms decolorize and take counterstain

J. Pathogenicity—some 2000 species of bacteria, most of which are harmless; those causing disease (pathogens) are usually heterotrophic mesophiles

Viruses

A. Definition—obligate intracellular parasite of unknown relationship to other forms of life

B. Characteristics—virions (virus particles)—range in size from 1 to 350 nanometers (nm); 1 nm equals 1 billionth of a meter or $^1/_{1000}$ of a millimeter; some cuboidal and others rod shaped; unlike rickettsiae and chlamydiae, composed of either ribonucleic acid (RNA) or deoxyribonucleic acid (DNA), not both

C. Classification

  1. Animal viruses—some contain RNA and others DNA; divided into 14 categories on the basis of particle size, symmetry, and nucleic acid content

  2. Plant viruses—contain RNA

  3. Bacterial viruses—most contain DNA; those which destroy bacterial cells called bacteriophages

D. Culturing—being obligate parasites, viruses demand living tissues such as embryonated hen's eggs, tissue cultures, and animal inoculation

E. Pathogenicity—viruses cause cancer in animals and Burkitt's lymphoma, mumps, rubeola, rubella, smallpox, chickenpox, herpes simplex, encephalitis, yellow fever, and many other infections in humans

Fungi

A. Definition—higher protists; include morels, truffles, cup fungi, mildews, mushrooms, puffballs, smuts, rusts, molds, and yeasts (molds and yeasts are of medical concern)

B. Molds—fuzzy growths of interlacing filaments called hyphae

  1. Hyphae—filaments of a mold; in some species hyphae divided by partial septa and appear to be multicellular, whereas in others they are nonseptate

  2. Mycelium—a tuft of interwoven hyphae

  3. Spores—means by which molds reproduce; a single spore in the proper environment gives rise to new mycelium; spores produced sexually and asexually

C. Yeasts—organisms that usually are single celled and usually reproduce by budding

  1. Yeast cell—round or ovoid and much larger and more complex than bacterial cell

  2. Reproduction—usually by the asexual process of budding, but many species also reproduce sexually by means of ascospores

  3. True yeasts—reproduce sexually as well as asexually (by budding); many species, such as *Sac-*

charomyces cerevisiae (baker's yeast), convert glucose into alcohol and carbon dioxide (alcoholic fermentation); *Candida albicans,* another type of yeast, causes ''thrush'' in humans (this yeast is part of the normal flora but may become an opportunistic pathogen in persons with low resistance)
4. Pathogenicity—certain species of molds cause infection, particularly those belonging to the class Fungi Imperfecti (Deuteromycetes), which account for diseases such as athlete's foot, ringworm of the scalp and axillary regions, and systemic mycosis

Microbial control

A. Definitions
  1. Disinfection—the removal of or destruction of pathogenic microbes
  2. Sterilization—the removal or destruction of all microbes
B. Physical methods
  1. Heat sterilization
    a. Moist heat
      (1) Steam under pressure (autoclave)—usually operated at 121° C (250° F) (15 lb pressure per square inch); time needed for procedure depends on material(s) being sterilized
      (2) Boiling water—object(s) to be sterilized immersed in water and boiled for 15 minutes; because some spores resist boiling, procedure not suitable for surgical instruments
    b. Dry heat (hot-air oven)
      (1) Operating temperature—160° to 170° C (310° to 338° F) (usually for 2 hours)
      (2) Items sterilized—petrolatum gauze dressings and other items that might be damaged by steam or water
    c. Pasteurization—the disinfection of milk and other substances by use of moderate heat; pathogenic organisms killed and microbial development considerably delayed (thus retarding spoilage)
      (1) Holding method—heating to 63° C (145° F) for 30 minutes, followed by rapid cooling
      (2) Flash method—heating to 71.7° C (161° F) for not less than 15 seconds, followed by rapid cooling

2. Radiation—all types of radiation injurious to microbes
  a. Gamma rays—used to sterilize food and drugs
  b. Ultraviolet light—used to inhibit microbial population of air in operating rooms, nurseries, laboratories, school rooms, and food establishments (the disadvantage of ultraviolet light is that it has little penetration power)
3. Filtration—removal of microbes from liquids by means of porous materials (diatomaceous earth, asbestos, porcelain) used to sterilize drugs, culture media, and certain other heat-sensitive substances
4. Refrigeration—low temperature inhibits microbial multiplication; used for food preservation
5. Hypertonicity—by their osmotic effects hypertonic solutions inhibit microbial multiplication; e.g., brine and syrups
6. Desiccation (drying)—removal of water; bacterial spores and certain vegetable cells resistant to such treatment; commonly used in food preservation
C. Chemical agents (for body surfaces and inanimate objects)
  1. Definitions—many terms used to describe action of chemical agents on microorganisms; in actual practice such terms often have little meaning because of variables
    a. Antiseptic—inhibits microbial growth
    b. Disinfectant—destroys pathogenic microbes
    c. Germicide—destroys pathogenic microbes
    d. Bactericide—destroys bacteria
    e. Fungicide—destroys fungi
    f. Virucide—destroys viruses
  2. Conditions (variables) affecting action of chemical agents
    a. Types and number of microbes—microbes respond differently to different agents; spores are resistant to most agents
    b. Concentration—typically the greater the concentration of chemical, the greater the effect
    c. Time—a certain time needed for maximum effect
    d. Temperature—a rise usually hastens action
    e. Organic matter—presence inhibits action
  3. Evaluation—various tests used to evaluate antiseptics and disinfectants; all have limitations
    a. Phenol coefficient—bactericidal activity of a chemical agent in relation to the bactericidal action of phenol

b. Culture inhibition—filter paper disks impregnated or saturated with chemical agent placed on agar plates previously inoculated with test organism; clear zone observed around disk (following incubation) if agent is inhibitory to organism (this is the same procedure used in determining the sensitivity of a culture to chemotherapeutic agents)

4. Commonly used chemical agents
   a. Ethyl alcohol (70%)
   b. Isopropyl alcohol (80%)
   c. Benzalkonium (Zephiran) (1:1000)
   d. Hydrogen peroxide (3%)
   e. Silver nitrate (1%)
   f. Iodine and iodine-releasing compounds
   g. Chlorine and chlorine-releasing compounds
   h. Substituted phenols
   i. Cresols
   j. Ethylene oxide

D. Chemotherapy—the systemic use of chemical agents (anti-infectives) in the treatment of infection
   1. Anti-infectives
      a. Antibiotics
      b. Sulfonamides
      c. Anthelmintics
      d. Antiprotozoals
      e. Tuberculostatics
   2. Antibiotic sensitivity—determined by 2 general techniques
      a. Paper disks—multilobed disk impregnated with different antibiotics placed on surface of inoculated plate; zones of inhibition (following incubation) surround lobes containing antibiotics to which microbe is sensitive
      b. Tube dilution—antibiotic in question diluted out in growth broth and tubes then inoculated with the organisms in question; minimal inhibitory concentration (MIC) determined (following incubation) by noting minimal concentration preventing growth

Infection

A. Definition—invasion of the body by pathogenic microorganisms (pathogens) and the reaction of the tissues to their presence and to the toxins generated by them

B. Types
   1. Local, focal, or systemic
      a. Local infection—one in which etiologic agent is limited to one locality of the body, such as a boil; often a local infection may have systemic repercussions such as fever and malaise
      b. Focal infection—a local infection such as an abscess from which the organisms themselves spread to other parts of body; e.g., a tooth abscess that continues to seed organisms into blood
      c. Systemic infection—one in which the infectious agent is spread throughout the body; e.g., typhoid fever
   2. Acute or chronic
      a. Acute infection—one that develops rapidly, usually resulting in a high fever and severe sickness
      b. Chronic infection—one that develops slowly, with mild but longer lasting symptoms; sometimes an acute infection may become chronic and vice versa
   3. Primary or secondary
      a. Primary infection—the initial infection unrelated to other health problems
      b. Secondary infection—an infection occasioned when invaders (or opportunists) take advantage of the weakened defenses resulting from the primary infection; e.g., staphylococcal pneumonia as a sequela of measles
   4. Bacteremia—the presence of nonmultiplying bacteria in the blood
   5. Septicemia—bacterial cells actively multiplying in the blood
   6. Toxemia—the presence of microbial toxins in the blood
   7. Viremia—the presence of viruses in the blood

C. Proof of etiology (Koch's postulates)—4 requirements must be fulfilled to establish a given microbe as the etiologic agent of a given disease
   1. Particular microbe must be found in every case of the particular disease
   2. Particular microbe must be isolated and grown in pure culture
   3. Particular microbe must cause particular disease when inoculated into susceptible animal
   4. Particular microbe must be recovered from inoculated animal and its identity established

D. Source and transmission of pathogens
   1. Source—ultimate source (or reservoir) of almost all pathogens are humans or animals; human sources include

a. Persons exhibiting symptoms of disease
b. Carriers—persons who harbor a pathogen in the absence of a discernible clinical disease
   (1) Types of carriers
       (a) Healthy carriers—those who never had the disease in question
       (b) Incubatory carriers—those in the incubation period of a disease
       (c) Chronic carriers—those who have recovered from a disease but continue to harbor pathogen
   (2) Diseases commonly spread by carriers
       (a) Typhoid fever
       (b) Diphtheria
       (c) Meningitis
       (d) Pneumonia
       (e) Dysentery
2. Transmission
   a. Direct
      (1) Body contact
      (2) Droplets (droplet infection)
   b. Indirect
      (1) Food
      (2) Water
      (3) Air
      (4) Soil
      (5) Fomites
      (6) Vectors (insects)
          (a) Mechanical transfer—insects' feet
          (b) Biologic transfer—microbe undergoes part of its life cycle in insect's body
3. Portals of entry and exit
   a. Portal of entry—where microbe enters body
      (1) Nose
      (2) Mouth
      (3) Urogenital tract
      (4) Skin: wounds, abrasions, and insect bites
   b. Portal of exit—where microbe leaves body
      (1) Nose
      (2) Mouth
      (3) Feces
      (4) Urine
      (5) Vaginal discharges
      (6) Pus and exudates
      (7) Vomitus
      (8) Blood
E. Development
   1. Definitions

a. Pathogenicity—the ability of a microbe to cause disease
b. Virulence—the degree of pathogenicity
2. Determinants of pathogenicity
   a. Chemical products
      (1) Exotoxins—heat-labile proteins readily released from bacterial cell; most deadly of all biologic poisons; e.g., botulism, tetanus, and diphtheria
      (2) Endotoxins—heat-stable lipopolysaccharide-protein complexes released from gram-negative bacteria; less deadly than exotoxins; e.g., typhoid fever and dysentery
      (3) Other toxic products
          (a) Hemolysins—destroy red cells
          (b) Leukocidins—destroy white cells
          (c) Coagulase—clots blood plasma
          (d) Hyaluronidase—dissolves intercellular cement
          (e) Kinases—dissolve clots or inhibit their formation
          (f) Collagenase—disintegrates collagen
   b. Cellular destruction—some microbes damage tissues and cause disease by direct mechanical injury to the cells, particularly intracellular parasites; e.g., viruses and rickettsiae
   c. Capsules—increase virulence apparently by making microbes possessing them less vulnerable to destruction by phagocytosis

REVIEW OF PHYSICAL PRINCIPLES RELATED TO PREOPERATIVE AND POSTOPERATIVE CARE
Electricity

Static electricity
A. Substances can be charged by friction whereby a negatively charged object picks up positive charges, which it discharges via a spark when touching an object that is a good conductor
B. Applications
   1. Removing blankets and sheets from a bed will build up electric charges through the hands that should be discharged by touching a grounded object before touching others
   2. Wool, silk, nylon, and dacron may set off sparks caused by static electric charges and should not be used around combustible gases or monitoring equipment

3. Electric equipment and operating room tables should be grounded to allow static charges to drain off, thus preventing sparks

Current electricity

A. Direct current (DC)—the flow of electric charge is in only one direction; e.g., the electric system of an automobile
B. Alternating current (AC)—electric charge in the circuit moves first in one direction and then in the opposite direction with the voltages and currents alternating back and forth; e.g., the outlets in homes and hospitals
C. Concept of electric energy and work
  1. The potential energy of the electric field is called electric potential and is measured in volts (V)
  2. The rate of flow of electric current is measured in amperes (amp); 1 amp is a current flow of 1 coulomb/second; a coulomb is 6.25 billion electrons
  3. Ohm's law—electric potential (volts), rate of flow of electric charge (amperes), and resistance are related; the rate of flow of electricity between 2 points is directly proportional to the impressed voltage and inversely proportional to the resistance between the 2 points; thus the rate of flow of electricity can be increased by either increasing the voltage or decreasing the resistance
    a. Dry fingers or hands touching an ungrounded or faulty electric source can result in a definite shock; the source touched with wet fingers or while standing in water can result in enough electric energy to be fatal
    b. As little as 0.05 amp can be fatal, and 0.1 amp is practically always fatal, since the electric currents upset the natural electric rhythms of the heart and can result in fibrillation and also stop the breathing center from working
    c. The shock obtained via alternating current is not caused by electrons pouring from the socket into the body but by the powerful vibrations of electrons and ions already inside the body, which are energized via the electric field that is flowing from the outlet

Power

A. Power represents the quantity of energy used per unit of time and is expressed in watts (W)
B. The kilowatt (kW) is 1000 W; power companies compute the number of kilowatt hours of power used for billing purposes; a kilowatt hour is the quantity of electric power consumed in 1 hour at a rate of 1 kW per hour

Application

A. Electronic cardiac pacemakers—battery-operated devices supplement or replace defective electric stimulation in the human heart and thus help to maintain the individual's heartbeat at a selected rate
B. Electrosurgery—an extremely high-frequency device called an oscillator is utilized to generate high temperatures in a small area to coagulate or desiccate tissue, thus preventing bleeding during surgery; electric cutting (using the oscillator) vibrates the tissues apart and simultaneously cauterizes the small blood vessels, thus preventing bleeding
C. Electronic thermometers—in this device, temperature change in a crystal alters the resistance of the crystal to electric flow; an individual's temperature changes the resistance of the crystal, allowing a certain amount of current to flow through and the amount read on a scale calibrated for temperature readings; these thermometers give readings more accurate than mercury thermometers in about 5 to 7 seconds
D. Electrocardiograms measure and record the electric activity of the heart as this activity is carried to the surface of the body by the ions of the body fluids; this information provides an electric picture of the heart's activity

Heat

A. Temperature measures the intensity of heat
  1. The 3 common measures of temperature are
    a. Celsius or centigrade
    b. Fahrenheit
    c. Absolute or Kelvin
  2. Conversions
    If
      T_f = temperature in Fahrenheit degrees,
      T_c = temperature in Celsius degrees, and
      T_k = temperature in absolute (Kelvin) degrees,
    then
      $T_f = (9/5\ T_c) + 32$
      $T_c = (T_f - 32) \times 5/9$
      $T_k = T_c + 273°$
B. The unit which expresses the quantity of thermal energy or the amount of heat that could be produced in a body is the calorie

C. The British Thermal Unit (BTU) is defined as the quantity of heat required to change the temperature of 1 lb of water 1° F
D. Specific heat is the quantity of heat required to raise the temperature of a substance 1° C
E. Water has a high specific heat, which means that a relatively large quantity of energy must be added to water to bring about small temperature changes; e.g., a hot water bottle stays hot for a long time because water possesses a great deal of thermal energy
F. Heat is used to kill all living organisms on medical instruments and other materials; dry heat at a temperature of 170° C (338° F) for 30 minutes is considered sufficient for sterilization; dry heat sterilization has an advantage over steam sterilization in that no damage is done to the fine cutting edges of surgical instruments or to ground glass surfaces

Change of state

A. Evaporation—molecules of a liquid become molecules of gas; since the most energetic molecules leave the surface of a liquid during evaporation, the average kinetic energy and temperature of the remaining liquid molecules are lower; thus evaporation causes cooling
  1. Rubbing alcohol applied to the skin will rapidly evaporate, cooling the body
  2. Sweating is an important physiologic process because evaporation helps to control body temperature
B. Boiling—the evaporation occurring beneath the surface of a liquid; the gas bubbles so formed are buoyed to the liquid's surface and escape into the atmosphere; this evaporation can be speeded up by (1) adding heat to the liquid molecules so that they possess enough energy to burst out from the surface of the liquid, and (2) reducing the atmospheric pressure above the liquid
  1. Autoclave—by increasing the pressure inside the autoclave (which is like a giant pressure cooker), higher water temperatures can be reached and bacteria and their spores can be readily destroyed by the steam generated; thus the autoclave sterilizes materials placed in it for specified lengths of time
  2. Distillation (all chemical and drug solutions are made in distilled water)—purifying water by boiling and collecting the vapor; impurities are left behind during water evaporation

REVIEW OF PHARMACOLOGY RELATED TO PREOPERATIVE AND POSTOPERATIVE CARE
Drugs that produce anesthesia

A. Inhalation anesthetics
  1. General implications for nurses
    a. Ascertain an accurate history of allergies and other medical problems that could alter a patient's response to the drugs used during surgery
    b. Be aware of the stages of anesthesia
      (1) Stage I—euphoria, gradual loss of consciousness
      (2) Stage II—hyperexcitement (thrashing of extremities), hyperactivity of reflexes (eyelids, swallowing), dilation of pupils
      (3) Stage III—depression of corneal reflex and pupillary response to light, voluntary control absent, muscle tone decreased
      (4) Stage IV—medullary paralysis, death
    c. In the operating room be aware of flammable agents and use grounded equipment
    d. Observe patient for side effects
      (1) Excitement and restlessness
      (2) Nausea and vomiting
      (3) Respiratory distress
  2. Actions—in general, balanced anesthesia includes use of several drugs and provides control of pain, consciousness, and muscle relaxation
  3. Examples
    a. Cyclopropane, trimethylene
    b. Enflurane (Ethrane)
    c. Ether, diethyl ether
    d. Ethyl chloride
    e. Ethylene
    f. Fluroxene (Fluoromar)
    g. Halothane (Fluothane)
    h. Methoxyflurane (Penthrane)
    i. Nitrous oxide, nitrogen monoxide
    j. Trichloroethylene (Trilene)
    k. Vinyl ether (Vinethene)
B. Intravenous barbiturates as anesthetics
  1. General implications for nurses
    a. Obtain a detailed health history to reduce the possibility of untoward effects
    b. Carefully monitor vital signs postoperatively

    c. Observe patient for adverse effects
      (1) Respiratory depression
      (2) Hypotension and tachycardia
      (3) Laryngospasm
  2. Action—high lipoid affinity provides prompt effect on cerebral tissue and rapid induction with ultrashort action
  3. Examples
    a. Methohexital sodium (Brevital Sodium)
    b. Thiamylal sodium (Surital Sodium)
    c. Thiopental sodium (Pentothal Sodium)
C. Intravenous and intramuscular nonbarbiturates as anesthetics
  1. General implications for nurses
    a. Decrease stimulation, since psychic disturbances may occur when patient emerges from anesthesia
    b. Observe patient for adverse effects
      (1) Respiratory failure
      (2) Increased blood pressure
      (3) Rigidity
  2. Action—induce a cataleptic state (patient appears to be awake but dissociated from the environment); abort pain response; amnesia for the procedure
  3. Example—ketamine hydrochloride (Ketaject)
D. Local anesthetics
  1. General implications for nurses
    a. Observe patient for side effects
      (1) Allergic reactions
      (2) Cardiac arrest
      (3) Convulsions
      (4) Hypotension
    b. Be aware of sites of administration
      (1) Surface (topical)
      (2) Infiltration (local)—solution injected in limited area where nerve fibers have no sheath and weak solution blocks nerve endings
      (3) Field block—solution injected close to nerves around area to be anesthetized
      (4) Nerve block—solution injected at perineural site distant from desired anesthesia site; stronger solutions are required to allow filtration through the nerve sheath
      (5) Peridural (epidrual, extradural, caudal)—solution is injected at a site blocking the paravertebral and peridural sections of spinal nerves controlling sensory stimuli at the manipulation site

      (6) Spinal (intrathecal, subarachnoid)—solution is injected into the spinal subarachnoid space to anesthetize nerve roots emerging from the spinal cord; hypobaric solutions (drug diluted with distilled water) gravitate caudad, and hyperbaric solutions (drug diluted with dextrose) gravitate cephalad
  2. Action—there is a decrease in the permeability of the nerve membrane to the influx of sodium ions required for depolarization of the neuron
  3. Examples
    a. Local anesthetics used topically
      (1) Benoxinate hydrochloride (Drosacaine)
      (2) Benzocaine
      (3) Butacaine sulfate (Butyn Sulfate)
      (4) Butyl aminobenzoate (Butesin Picrate)
      (5) Cocaine
      (6) Cyclomethycaine (Surfacaine)
      (7) Dibucaine (Nupercaine); also used for spinal anesthesia
      (8) Dimethisoquin hydrochloride (Quotane Hydrochloride)
      (9) Diperodon Hydrochloride (Diothane Hydrochloride)
      (10) Dyclonine hydrochloride (Dyclone)
      (11) Hexylcaine hydrochloride (Cyclaine Hydrochloride); also used for nerve block
      (12) Lidocaine hydrochloride (Xylocaine); also used for nerve block
      (13) Phenacaine hydrochloride (Holocaine Hydrochloride)
      (14) Piperocaine hydrochloride (Metycaine Hydrochloride)
      (15) Pramoxine hydrochloride (Tronothane Hydrochloride)
      (16) Proparacaine hydrochloride (Ophthetic, Ophthaine)
      (17) Tetracaine hydrochloride (Tetracel, Anacel, Pontocaine Hydrochloride); also used for nerve block
    b. Local anesthetics used primarily for nerve block
      (1) Bupivacaine hydrochloride (Marcaine Hydrochloride)
      (2) Chloroprocaine hydrochloride (Nesacaine, Nesacaine-CE)
      (3) Mepivacaine hydrochloride (Carbocaine Hydrochloride)

(4) Prilocaine hydrochloride (Citanest Hydrochloride)

(5) Procaine hydrochloride (Novocain)

(6) Propoxycaine hydrochloride (Blockain
Hydrochloride)

Drugs that produce sedation and sleep

1. General implications for nurses
   a. Check with pharmacist for drug compatibility if
      patient is receiving other medications
   b. Observe patient for adverse effects specific to each
      medication
2. Barbiturate sedatives
   a. Action—drug depresses the central nervous sys-
      tem, starting with the diencephalon
   b. Examples
      (1) Hexobarbital (Sombucaps, Sombulex)
      (2) Pentobarbital sodium (Nembutal)
      (3) Secobarbital (Seconal)
      (4) Amobarbital (Amytal)
      (5) Aprobarbital (Alurate)
      (6) Butabarbital sodium (Bubartal Sodium, Bu-
          tisol Sodium)
      (7) Probarbital calcium (Ipral)
      (8) Talbutal (Lotusate)
      (9) Barbital (Neuronidia)
      (10) Phenobarbital (Luminal)
   c. Adverse effects
      (1) Drowsiness
      (2) Photosensitivity
      (3) Hypotension
3. Trichloroacetic acid
   a. Action—produces a natural sleep by depressing
      the central nervous system
   b. Examples
      (1) Chloral betaine (Beta-Chlor)
      (2) Chloral hydrate (Felsules, Lorinal, Noctec,
          Somnos)
      (3) Petrichloral (Periclor)
   c. Adverse effects
      (1) Gastric irritation
      (2) Diarrhea
4. Phenothiazine derivatives
   a. Action—relaxation of skeletal muscles; act on
      central and autonomic nervous systems
   b. Examples
      (1) Methotrimeprazine hydrochloride
          (Levoprome)
      (2) Promazine hydrochloride (Sparine)

(3) Propiomazine hydrochloride (Largon)
   c. Adverse effects
      (1) Hypotension
      (2) Dry mouth
      (3) Pseudoparkinsonian symptoms
      (4) Agranulocytosis
5. Other sedatives and hypnotics
   a. Action—generally, depression of the central
      nervous system and skeletal muscle relaxation are
      the principal actions of these drugs
   b. Specific drugs and their adverse effects
      (1) Ethchlorvynol (Placidyl)—morning drowsi-
          ness, blurring vision, transient hypotension
      (2) Ethinamate (Valmid)—morning drowsiness
      (3) Flurazepam hydrochloride (Dalmane)—dizzi-
          ness, tachycardia, gastrointestinal distur-
          bances
      (4) Methaqualone (Quaalude, Sopor)—morning
          drowsiness, gastrointestinal disturbances
      (5) Methyprylon (Noludar)—morning drowsi-
          ness, gastrointestinal disturbances
      (6) Sodium bromide used primarily for daytime
          sedation—gastric irritation, generalized rash,
          tremulousness of hands, lips, and tongue, im-
          paired mental processes, auditory and visual
          hallucinations, or coma with long-term use of
          excess levels of drug
      (7) Glutethimide (Doriden)
          (a) Adverse effects—morning drowsiness,
              transient hypotension, and, infrequently,
              pharyngeal and laryngeal reflex depres-
              sion
          (b) Drug interactions—acts synergistically
              with oral anticoagulants to decrease their
              effectiveness

Drugs that control pain

A. Nonnarcotic agents
   1. General implications for nurses
      a. Observe for side effects of each drug
      b. Explain the importance of maintaining a thera-
         peutic dosage when discharged
      c. Observe for toxicity characterized by central
         nervous system stimulation, excitement, delir-
         ium
   2. Salicylates
      a. Action
         (1) Action unclear but involves many mecha-
             nisms

(2) Antipyretic activity—lowers hypothalamic "thermostat" and dissipates heat by vasodilation and diaphoresis

(3) Anti-inflammatory

b. Examples

(1) Acetylsalicylic acid (A.S.A., aspirin, Asteric, Ecotrin)

(2) Carbaspirin calcium (Calurin)

(3) Choline salicylate (Arthropan)

(4) Salicylamide (Amid-Sal, Liquiprin, Rasberin, Salamide, Salicim, Salrin)

(5) Sodium salicylate

c. Adverse effects

(1) Gastric irritation

(2) Visual disturbances

(3) Decreased clotting time

(4) Tinnitus

3. Nonsalicylates

a. Action—similar to salicylates; used for patients with salicylate allergy, gastric ulcers, or those receiving anticoagulants

b. Examples

(1) Acetaminophen (Apamide, Febrolin, Fendon, Lyteca, Nebs, Tempra, Tylenol); also has muscle relaxant properties

(2) Acetophenetidin (used as component of preparations to allow lower dosage because higher dosage causes agranulocytosis, anemia, hepatotoxicity, and methemoglobinemia)

(3) Dipyrone (Dimethone, Narone, Nartate, Novaldin, Pydirone, Pyrilgin)

(4) Mefenamic acid (Ponstel); also has anti-inflammatory properties

c. Adverse effects

(1) Vertigo

(2) Skin rash

(3) Depression of leukocyte and erythrocyte production

4. Propoxyphene hydrochloride (Darvon)

a. Action—functions as an analgesic without anti-inflammatory effects

b. Adverse effects

(1) Constipation

(2) Skin rash

(3) Psychic dependence

5. Carbamazepine (Tegretol)

a. Actions

(1) Controls trigeminal neuralgia by decreasing synaptic transmission in the nerve nucleus

(2) Has sedative, anticholinergic, and muscle relaxant properties

b. Adverse effects

(1) Dry mouth

(2) Weakness

(3) Lethargy

B. Narcotic analgesics

1. General implications for nurses

a. Request physician to rewrite orders for narcotics q 24 h

b. Observe for respiratory depression prior to and following administration of narcotics

c. Utilize nursing judgment in evaluating patient needs for narcotic analgesics

d. Evaluate effectiveness of medication

2. Actions

a. Raise the pain threshold and interfere with pain perception centers

b. Have antitussive and sedative actions

3. Examples

a. Codeine sulfate

b. Hydromorphone hydrochloride (Dilaudid)

c. Levorphanol tartrate (Levo-Dromoran)

d. Meperidine hydrochloride (Demerol)

e. Morphine sulfate

f. Oxycodone (used in Percodan)

g. Oxymorphone hydrochloride (Numorphan)

h. Pantopium (Pantopon)

i. Pentazocine hydrochloride (Talwin)

4. Adverse effects

a. Decreased gastric motility

b. Euphoria

c. Urine retention

d. Respiratory depression

e. Hypotension

RELATED PROCEDURES
Intravenous (IV) therapy

A. Purpose

1. Replace fluid and electrolyte loss

2. Provide route for other medications

3. Maintain nutrition when patient is unable to tolerate feedings (see hyperalimentation procedure under gastrointestinal disorders)

B. Nursing responsibilities

1. Explain procedure to patient
2. Assist patient with care, since mobility will be limited
3. Check solution for clarity and correct type
4. Assist qualified person to start IV
5. Regulate flow rate

$$\frac{\text{Total number of milliliters to be infused} \times \text{Drop factor}}{\text{Number of hours} \times 60 \text{ minutes}} =$$

Per minute drop rate

6. Monitor intake and output
7. Observe for signs of complications
   a. Infiltration—pain, swelling, coldness, and decreased flow of IV
   b. Phlebitis—pain, redness, and heat at site
   c. Air embolisms are rare, since the tubing does not contain sufficient air to cause an embolism
   d. Circulatory overload—dyspnea, cough, frothy sputum, rales evident on auscultation
8. Change tubing and site at intervals specified by agency or if infiltration or phlebitis occurs
C. Physical principle involved—gravity

Blood transfusion

A. Purpose
   1. Restore blood volume after hemorrhage
   2. Maintain hemoglobin levels in severe anemias
   3. Replace specific blood components
B. Nursing responsibilities
   1. Check that blood or blood components have been typed and cross matched, indicating that the blood of the donor and recipient are compatible
   2. Blood should not be administered straight from the refrigerator
   3. A baseline of the patient's temperature, blood pressure, pulse, and respirations should be determined prior to administration
   4. An IV with normal saline and a blood administration set containing a filter are used to start the infusion; solutions containing glucose may cause the blood to clot in the tubing and should not be used
   5. Before starting the infusion, it is advisable for 2 nurses to verify the blood type, Rh factor, patient and blood numbers, as well as the expiration date

6. The container should be inverted gently to suspend the red cells within the plasma
7. Observe for signs of hemolytic reaction, which generally occur early in the transfusion (within the first 10 to 15 minutes)
   a. Shivering
   b. Headache
   c. Lower back pain
   d. Increased pulse and respiratory rate
   e. Hemoglobinuria
   f. Oliguria
   g. Hypotension
8. Observe for signs of febrile reaction, which usually occur within 30 minutes
   a. Shaking
   b. Headache
   c. Elevated temperature
   d. Back pain
   e. Confusion
   f. Hematemesis
9. Observe for allergic reaction
   a. Hives
   b. Wheezing
   c. Pruritus
   d. Joint pain
10. If any reaction occurs
    a. Stop infusion immediately
    b. Notify physician
    c. Maintain patency of IV with normal saline
    d. Send blood to the laboratory
    e. Montior vital signs frequently
    f. Send a urine specimen to the laboratory if a hemolytic reaction is suspected
C. Physical principle involved—gravity

GENERAL NURSING CARE
Preoperative care

A. Prior to day of surgery
   1. Allow patient time to ask questions about procedures and surgery
   2. Explain all procedures to the patient and give reasons and objectives for them
   3. Determine patient's level of understanding of operative procedure to ascertain whether signature on permit represents informed consent
   4. Allow and encourage patient to ventilate feelings about diagnosis and surgery
   5. Tell patient what to expect in the operating

room, recovery, and/or intensive care units if indicated

6. Inform patient if the plan is to be returned to other than the present room
7. Provide spiritual counselor if desired by patient or family
8. Consider needs of the family when discussing surgery
9. Teach patient the activities that will be instituted after surgery; e.g., deep breathing, coughing, turning
10. Teach patient physical exercises that will be used to promote circulation after surgery; e.g., isometric leg exercises, ambulation routines
11. Inform patient to expect some discomfort after surgery and teach the importance of requesting medication for pain
12. Make certain that history, physical examination results, recent laboratory tests, and chest x-ray report are entered on the chart
13. Inform all members of the medical team, especially the anesthesiologist, of the patient's allergies and other health problems and prominently mark the chart
14. Carry out ordered preoperative preparation; e.g., shave, Betadine, pHisoHex washes, enemas, douches
15. Remove nail polish from fingers and toes
16. Administer prescribed sleeping medication
17. Inform patient not to take anything by mouth after midnight, remove fluid, and place obvious signs at bedside

B. Day of surgery
1. In the morning, check patient's vital signs and assess overall physical status; record and report any deviations to physician
2. Have patient void
3. See that any drainage tubes (catheter or Levin tube) which were ordered are inserted
4. Make certain that name identification band is on patient's wrist
5. Have patient remove dentures and other prosthetic devices and store valuables
6. Administer prescribed preoperative medication
7. Put side rails up after administering medications
8. Transfer patient to stretcher when operating room calls, and fasten stretcher strap in place before transporting
9. Consider the needs of the family on the day of surgery

Postoperative care

A. Be aware of surgical stresses
1. Depression of the central nervous system from general or regional anesthesia
2. An interruption in the integrity of the skin
3. Depressed respiratory functioning
4. Alterations in circulation and fluid and electrolyte balance
5. Depression of gastrointestinal and urinary functioning
6. Emotional trauma
7. Change in body image

B. Minimize postoperative complications
1. Maintain patent airway by keeping artificial airway in place until gag reflex returns, suctioning trachea as needed, keeping head extended and turned to the side, and observing rate and character of respirations
2. Assess patient's physical status—note and record level of consciousness, vital signs, color and temperature of skin, condition of surgical site, presence and functioning of intravenous and drainage tubes, and return of sensorimotor functioning; report significant changes
3. Protect patient from injury by keeping under close observation, keeping side rails in place, positioning patient to prevent excessive pressure on body parts or on tubing, controlling restlessness and preventing patient from pulling on tubes or dressing, and making certain all equipment is in safe working condition and that it is properly used
4. Turn patient frequently and encourage deep breathing and coughing to prevent the development of atelectasis or hypostatic pneumonia
5. Perform or encourage range of motion and isometric exercises and early ambulation to prevent phlebitis, paralytic ileus, and circulatory stasis
6. Maintain patency of tubing (catheter, gastric tubes, T-tube, chest tubes, etc.) to promote drainage and maintain decompression to reduce pressure on suture line
7. Monitor patient's overall physical status, vital signs, dressing, and drainage to observe for early signs of hemorrhage and to prevent excessive blood loss and shock
8. Use surgically aseptic technique when changing dressings or as necessary when irrigating tubing to prevent infection

9. Monitor intake and output to prevent dehydration, fluid and electrolyte imbalance, and urinary suppression or retention
10. Observe for abdominal distention to prevent discomfort and intestinal obstruction
11. Give medication for pain as ordered to prevent discomfort and restlessness
12. Regulate IV therapy to prevent circulatory overload
13. Support or encourage patient to support and splint incisional site when coughing, moving, or turning to prevent tension on suture line
14. Position patient as required by type of surgery to prevent misalignment and prevent the accumulation of fluid or the blocking of drainage tubes
C. Immediate care in the recovery room
1. Monitor vital signs
2. Reorient patient to time, place, and situation
3. Call patient by name
4. Answer questions as honestly and as simply as possible and avoid complicated, involved explanations
5. Medicate for pain and restlessness
6. Expect and accept repetitious questions and give patient necessary reassurance
7. Maintain patency of all tubing and attach to appropriate drainage as ordered
8. Maintain patency of airway; observe for return of gag reflex
D. Consider postoperative nutritional needs
1. Initial IV therapy for water and electrolytes, but oral intake needed as soon as possible for adequate nutrition
2. Hyperalimentation—parenteral nutrition of high-nutrient density; solutions of amino acids, glucose, electrolytes, minerals, vitamins; usually inserted into larger veins (inferior or superior vena cava) to avoid thrombosis in peripheral veins; used in cases of major tissue trauma, injury, or extensive surgery
3. Gradually increase oral intake as permitted
  a. Liquid diets
    (1) Clear liquid—clear broth, bouillon, juices, plain gelatin, fruit-flavored water ices, ginger ale, coffee, tea
    (2) Full liquid—may add milk and items made with milk, such as cream soups, milk drinks, sherbet, ice cream, puddings, custard

  b. Soft diet—may add all soft cooked foods, such as refined cereals, pasta, rice, white bread and crackers, eggs, cheese, meat, potatoes, cooked whole vegetables, cooked fruits, few soft ripe plain fruits without membranes or skins, simple desserts
  c. Light diet—same as soft with few additional whole cooked foods, light raw foods such as fruit; mainly avoid heavily seasoned or fried foods
  d. Full (or general) diet—full, well-balanced diet of all foods as desired and tolerated, including a wide variety for interest and flavor
4. Provide for special nutritional needs
  a. Protein—increased protein need caused by protein losses and catabolic period of recovery and tissue healing; a period of negative nitrogen balance initially
  b. Calories—adequate amount to supply energy and spare protein for tissue building
  c. Water—adequate fluid therapy to prevent dehydration caused by large fluid losses
  d. Minerals—replacement of deficiencies and ensurance of continued adequacy essential to maintain electrolyte balance; zinc needed for wound healing in deficient individuals
  e. Vitamins—vitamin C especially needed for tissue synthesis and wound healing; B complex essential in energy production and tissue building

Controlling infection
NURSING RESPONSIBILITIES TO PREVENT CROSS-CONTAMINATION
A. Recognize that microorganisms can be transferred directly by fomites and insects and indirectly by airborne particles
B. Use medical aseptic techniques
1. Handwashing before and after patient care, after handling excreta, etc.
2. Bacteriostatic chemicals—antiseptics and disinfectants
  a. To inhibit or destroy pathogens
  b. In concurrent and terminal disinfections of contaminated articles
3. Barriers such as gowns, gloves, and masks to

protect personnel when caring for persons with infections

4. Correct disposal of contaminated materials; e.g., linens, tissues, dressings, secretions, and excretions

C. Use surgical aseptic techniques
   1. Sterilize by autoclaving, boiling, etc. to destroy all microorganisms
   2. Barriers such as gowns, gloves, and masks to protect the patient against microbiologic hazards in the environment
   3. Sterile equipment and technique when caring for wounds, irrigating sterile cavities, giving injections, inserting instruments or devices into body cavities or areas that are normally sterile

DRUGS THAT CONTROL INFECTION
Definition of terms

A. Antibiotic—a metabolic product of an organism used to destroy another organism
B. Bactericidal effect—capable of destroying bacteria at low concentrations; e.g., disrupt building of cell membrane or wall and allow leak of cytoplasm
C. Bacteriostatic effect—slows reproduction of bacteria; natural physiologic mechanisms are required for phagocytic abolition of the bacteria
D. Superinfection—emergence of microorganism growth; e.g., yeast and fungi, when natural protective flora is destroyed by anti-infective drug
E. Bacterial resistance—a natural characteristic of an organism or one acquired by mutation preventing destruction by a drug to which it was previously susceptible

General implications for nurses administering anti-infective drugs

A. Knowledge of why patient is receiving specific anti-infective medication
   1. Check culture and sensitivity reports
   2. Observe for inflammatory response, including elevated temperature and WBC count
B. Be aware that certain foods and other medications may affect the action of the anti-infective
C. Prevent superinfection by providing yogurt or Bacid capsules
D. Administer antibiotics at equal intervals during the day
E. Increase fluid intake
F. Observe for common adverse effects such as skin

rashes and GI disturbances, as well as the specific effects listed under each classification

Penicillin preparations

A. Actions
   1. Disrupt bacterial cell wall synthesis when new cells are forming by interfering with the synthesis and cross-linkage of mucopeptides in the final stage of cell wall synthesis
   2. Broad spectrum of pathogen susceptibility except to *Staphylococcus aureus*
B. Examples
   1. Amoxicillin (Amoxil, Larocin)
   2. Ampicillin (Omnipen, Penbritin, Polycillin, Principen)
   3. Carbenicillin disodium (Geopen, Pyopen)
   4. Methicillin sodium (Staphcillin)
   5. Nafcillin sodium (Unipen)
   6. Oxacillin sodium (Bactocill, Prostaphlin)
   7. Penicillin G potassium (Dramicillin, Pedacillin, Pentids, Pfizerpen)
   8. Penicillin G procaine (Crysticillin A.S., Diurnal-Penicillin, Duracillin A.S., Pentids-P, Wycillin)
   9. Penicillin V (Pen-Vee, V-Cillin)
C. Adverse effects
   1. Allergic reactions
      a. Range from skin rash to anaphylactic shock
      b. Penicillinase (Neutrapen) is used to inactivate circulating penicillin by its enzymatic action
   2. Superinfection; e.g., *Candida* or *Pseudomonas* species in vagina or respiratory and intestinal tracts

Cephalosporins

A. Actions
   1. Disrupt synthesis of bacterial cell wall by inactivating transpeptidase required for cross-linkage of peptidoglycan chains
   2. Minor structural difference from penicillin allows therapy for penicillin-sensitized patients
   3. Broad spectrum limited by sensitivity to action of cephalosporinase of some gram-negative rods *(Enterobacter, Pseudomonas)*
B. Examples
   1. Cefazolin sodium (Ancef, Kefzol)
   2. Cephacetrile (Celospor)
   3. Cephalexin monohydrate (Keflex)
   4. Cephaloglycin (Kafocin)
   5. Cephaloridine (Loridine)

6. Cephalothin sodium (Keflin)
7. Cephradine (Velosef, Anspor)
C. Adverse effects
  1. Allergic reactions (minor rashes, urticaria, fever, eosinophilia)
  2. Superinfections
  3. Diarrhea
  4. Nephrotoxicity with large doses
D. Special considerations—metabolites cause a false positive reaction for glycosuria in tests with Clinitest and Fehling's and Benedict's solutions

Erythromycins and similar drugs

A. Actions
  1. Compete for receptor sites on the ribosome unit to inhibit mRNA synthesis of protein required for reproduction
  2. Excretion route is in the bile through the intestine (90%), which allows use with compromised renal function
B. Examples
  1. Clindamycin hydrochloride (Cleocin Hydrochloride)
  2. Erythromycin (E-Mycin, Erythrocin, Ilotycin)
  3. Erythromycin ethylsuccinate (Erythrocin Ethylsuccinate, Pediamycin)
  4. Lincomycin hydrochloride monohydrate (Lincocin)
C. Adverse effects
  1. Nausea and vomiting
  2. Diarrhea
  3. Abdominal pain
  4. Black tongue

Tetracyclines

A. Actions
  1. Block tRNA attachment to ribosomes to inhibit protein synthesis
  2. Provide broad-spectrum effect
B. Examples
  1. Chlortetracycline hydrochloride (Aureomycin)
  2. Demeclocycline (Declomycin)
  3. Doxycycline hyclate (Vibramycin Hyclate)
  4. Oxytetracycline (Terramycin)
  5. Tetracycline (Achromycin, Panmycin, Sumycin, Tratracyn)
C. Adverse effects
  1. Gastroenteritis—caused by superinfection
  2. Hepatotoxicity—lethargy, anorexia, jaundice, fatty necrosis

3. Phototoxicity
4. Nephrotoxicity
5. Hyperuricemia
6. Enamel hypoplasia, dental caries, and bone defects in children under 8 years of age and in fetus after the fourth month of gestation
D. Other considerations
  1. Drugs delay blood coagulation and potentiate effect of oral anticoagulants
  2. Oral drug forms insoluble mixture with iron and the calcium, magnesium, and aluminum salts of foods and drugs; e.g., absorption of drug is erratic when milk and antacids taken concurrently
  3. Oral sodium bicarbonate decreases dissolution of capsules that require acid media in stomach
  4. Parenteral drugs contain ascorbic acid, causing false positive test with Benedict's solution and Clinitest and false negative test with Clinistix and Tes-Tape

Aminoglycosides

A. Actions
  1. Disrupt protein synthesis by providing substitute for essential nucleotide required by mRNA
  2. Have broad-spectrum effect but are used only in the treatment of serious infections
B. Examples
  1. Gentamicin sulfate (Garamycin)
  2. Kanamycin sulfate (Kantrex)
  3. Neomycin sulfate (Mycifradin Sulfate, Neobiotic)
  4. Streptomycin sulfate (Strycin)
  5. Amikacin sulfate (Amiken)
  6. Tobramycin sulfate (Nebcin)
C. Adverse effects
  1. Ototoxicity (tinnitus, vertigo, hearing loss)
  2. Rapid emergence of resistant bacteria
  3. Nausea and vomiting
  4. Nephrotoxicity
  5. Blood dyscrasias

Polymycin group

A. Actions
  1. Detergent effect on bacterial cell membrane increases permeability, which disrupts intracellular osmotic gradient
  2. Oral forms of both drug groups are used to suppress bacterial growth in the intestine (decrease ammonia production or "sterilize bowel")

B. Examples
  1. Colistimethate sodium (Coly-Mycin M)
  2. Colistin sulfate (Coly-Mycin S)
  3. Polymyxin B sulfate (Aerosporin)
C. Adverse effects
  1. Circumoral or lingual paresthesias
  2. Nephrotoxicity
D. Other considerations
  1. Potentiation of neuromuscular blocking agents, general anesthetics, or parenterally administered magnesium
  2. Suppression of intestinal bacteria that synthesize vitamin K by oral forms decreases available vitamin K and potentiates action of oral anticoagulants

Chloramphenicol

A. Actions
  1. Substitutes for essential amino acid phenylalanine, which prevents mRNA activity
  2. Used in severe drug-resistant infections
B. Examples
  1. Amphicol
  2. Chloromycetin
  3. Mychel
  4. Novochlor
C. Adverse effects
  1. Aplastic anemia
  2. Leukopenia
  3. Thrombocytopenia
  4. Headache
  5. Confusion
  6. Peripheral neuropathy
  7. Optic neuritis
  8. GI disturbances
  9. Gray baby syndrome (abdominal distention, pallid cyanosis, vasomotor collapse, ashen gray color, death)
  10. Interference with metabolism of phenytoin, oral antidiabetic agents, and dicumarol, leading to cumulative effects of these drugs

Antiviral—amantadine hydrochloride

A. Actions
  1. Primary use is prophylaxis when exposure to viral infection, e.g., A_2 influenza virus, has occurred
  2. Drug acts by preventing entrance of virus into host cells

B. Adverse effects
  1. Insomnia
  2. Dizziness
  3. Tremor
  4. Psychosis
  5. Orthostatic hypotension
  6. Constipation
  7. Urinary retention

Sulfonamides

A. Actions
  1. Act by substitution of a false metabolite for para-aminobenzoic acid required for bacterial synthesis of folic acid
  2. Plasma protein binding maintains tissue levels by liberating drug when tissue levels are low
  3. Tenacious plasma protein-binding may hold drug until it reaches renal sites, producing high levels in tubular urine
  4. Many forms require alkalinization of urine and high fluid intake to maintain urine volume and decrease incidence of nephron crystals
  5. Recycling of drug in nephron delays excretion and maintains blood levels of drug
     a. Tubule cells excrete drug into tubular urine after removal from plasma protein-binding sites
     b. Tubule cells also reabsorb drug from tubule urine, and it returns to tissue and liver sites to be metabolized
     c. Alkalinization of urine slows recycling and increases excretion rate
B. Examples
  1. Phthalylsulfathiazole (Cremothalidine, Rothalid, Sulfathalidine)
  2. Succinylsulfathiazole (Rolsul, Sulfasuxidine)
  3. Sulfasalazine (Azulfidine)
  4. Sulfadiazine
  5. Sulfamethizole (Thiosulfil)
  6. Sulfamethoxazole (Gantanol)
  7. Sulfaphenazole (Sulfabid)
  8. Sulfisomidine (Elkosin)
  9. Sulfisoxazole (Gantrisin, SK-Soxazole, Sodizole, Sosol, Soxomide, Sulfisocon, Unisulf)
C. Adverse effects
  1. Anorexia
  2. Nausea and vomiting caused by gastric irritation and action at vomiting centers in medulla
  3. Malaise

4. Blood dyscrasias (leukopenia, thrombocytopenia, erythrocytopenia)
5. Fever
6. Headache
7. Stomatitis
8. Conjunctivitis
9. Hepatotoxicity

Kidney-specific drugs

A. Nalidixic acid (NegGram)
  1. Action—urinary bactericidal that provides high concentration in nephron
  2. Adverse effects
    a. Nausea and vomiting
    b. Rash, urticaria
    c. Dizziness
    d. Diplopia
    e. Headache
  3. Causes false positive results with Clinitest
B. Nitrofurantoin (Cyantin, Furadantin, Furalan, Macrodantin, Trantoin)
  1. Actions
    a. Acts as a diffusible acid when tubular urine is acidic
    b. Provides a high concentration of drug in nephrons for antibacterial action
  2. Adverse effects
    a. Nausea and vomiting
    b. Skin rashes
    c. Hemolytic anemia
C. Methenamines
  1. Action—exert antibacterial activity by liberating ammonia and formaldehyde by hydrolysis in acid urine
  2. Examples
    a. Methenamine (Uritone)
    b. Methenamine hippurate (Hiprex)
    c. Methenamine mandelate (Mandelamine)
  3. Adverse effects
    a. Nausea and vomiting
    b. Pruritus
    c. Rash
D. Sulfa drugs specific for urinary tract infections
  1. Action and adverse effects same as other sulfa drugs
  2. Examples
    a. Sulfisoxazole (Gantrisin)
    b. Sulfamethoxazole (Gantanol)

Sulfones that control *Mycobacterium leprae* (Hansen's disease)

A. Actions
  1. Deprives bacteria of the nucleotide required for folic acid synthesis and growth
  2. Slow elimination and wide tissue distribution of the drug permit daily administration; mucosal lesions improve in 3 to 6 months; nerve tenderness decreases in 6 to 9 months; however, skin lesions require 1 to 3 years for bacilli clearance
B. Examples
  1. Acedapsone (repository form with few adverse effects)
  2. Acetosulfone sodium (Promacetin)
  3. Clofazimine (Lamprene)—a red compound that colors the skin, conjunctiva, urine, sputum, and sweat red-brown
  4. Dapsone (Avlosulfon)
  5. Sulfoxone sodium (Diasone Sodium)
  6. Thiazolsulfone (Promizole)
C. Adverse effects
  1. Hemolytic anemia at start of therapy
  2. Gastrointestinal disturbances
  3. Serum sickness–like symptoms and exacerbation of lesions

Drugs that control *Mycobacterium tuberculosis*

A. General considerations
  1. Primary triad of drugs for therapy includes isoniazid, streptomycin sulfate, aminosalicylic acid or ethambutol
  2. Bacterial resistance to single drugs develops rapidly, and combination decreases resistance and adverse effects
B. Isoniazid (INH, Hyzyd, Niconyl, Nydrazid)
  1. Actions
    a. Interferes with synthesis of the lipoprotein cell wall of *Mycobacterium*
    b. Competes for enzyme required for synthesis of pyridoxine, resulting in a vitamin B_6 deficiency causing neurologic symptoms (hyperreflexia, paresthesia of extremities, vertigo) unless this vitamin is supplied during therapy
    c. Used for prophylaxis of 1 year's duration for individuals who change from a negative to a positive reaction to the tuberculin test and to individuals living with a newly diagnosed tubercular patient

2. Adverse effects
   a. Hepatotoxicity
   b. Bone marrow depression
   c. Skin rash
   d. Exacerbation of rheumatoid arthritis
3. May cause false positive reactions with Clinitest

C. Para-aminosalicylic acid preparations
   1. Action—interfere with bacterial synthesis of folic acid by providing a substitute nucleotide
   2. Examples
      a. Calcium aminosalicylate (Teebacin Calcium)
      b. Para-aminosalicylic acid (P.A.S.)
      c. Potassium aminosalicylate (Teebacin, Paskalium)
      d. Sodium aminosalicylate (Parasal Sodium, Pasdium)
   3. Adverse effects
      a. Gastric irritation
      b. Abdominal pain
      c. Nausea, vomiting, and diarrhea
      d. Blood dyscrasias

D. Streptomycin sulfate (see amino glycosides)

E. Drugs used as substitutes for streptomycin sulfate
   1. Examples
      a. Capreomycin sulfate (Capastat Sulfate)
      b. Cycloserine (Seromycin)
      c. Rifampin (Rifadin, Rimactane)
      d. Viomycin sulfate (Viocin)
   2. Other considerations
      a. Dosage spacing (2 to 3 times per week) after initial intensive therapy decreases incidence of neurotoxicity to these drugs
      b. Drug interactions with rifampin—absorption delayed by aminosalicylates (drugs administered on a schedule allowing 8 to 12 hours between them); inhibits activity of oral anticoagulants; phenobarbital interferes with rifampin activity when used concomitantly

F. Second line drugs used in therapy
   1. Actions
      a. Inhibit cell metabolism
      b. Prevent multiplication of cells
   2. Examples
      a. Ethambutol hydrochloride (Myambutol)
      b. Ethionamide (Trecator S.C.)
      c. Pyrazinamide (PZA)

Antifungals

A. Griseofulvin, micronized (Fulvicin-U/F, Grifulvin V, Grisactin)
   1. Action—acts as an analog of purine and is incorporated into new epithelial cells during synthesis of nucleic acids
   2. Adverse effects
      a. Peripheral neuritis
      b. Vertigo
      c. Fever
      d. Arthralgia
      e. Nausea
      f. Diarrhea
      g. Headache

B. Nystatin (Mycostatin, Nilstat)
   1. Action—binds tenaciously to cell wall sterols and causes a detergent effect that increases permeability of membrane and causes cell to rupture
   2. Adverse effects
      a. Nausea
      b. Vomiting

C. Amphotericin B (Fungizone)
   1. Action—detergent-like effect on cell wall that increases permeability of membrane and causes cell to rupture
   2. Adverse effects
      a. Paresthesia and muscle weakness (caused by drug effect on normal cells containing sterols)
      b. Chills
      c. Hyperpyrexia
      d. Nephrotoxicity
      e. Nausea and vomiting
      f. Flushed skin
      g. Generalized pain
      h. Convulsions

Antiparasitics

A. Metronidazol (Flagyl)
   1. Actions
      a. Acts as a trichomonacidal and amebacidal agent
      b. Used in the treatment of trichomoniasis, intestinal amebiasis, and amebic liver abscess
   2. Adverse effects
      a. Nausea and vomiting
      b. Diarrhea
      c. Abdominal cramps
      d. Metallic taste

e. If taken with alcohol, nausea, vomiting, head-ache, and hypotension

B. Emetine hydrochloride
  1. Actions
    a. Causes degeneration of the nucleus and re-ticulation of the ameba cytoplasm
    b. Used in the treatment of acute amebic dy-sentery, amebic hepatitis, and abscess
  2. Adverse effects
    a. Nausea and vomiting
    b. Dizziness
    c. Tachycardia
    d. Muscular weakness
    e. Dyspnea
    f. Precordial pain
    g. Local myositis at injection site

C. Antimalarial drugs
  1. Definition of terms
    a. Causal prophylaxis—drugs used to intercede at primary tissue sites to eradicate *Plasmodium* before it begins reproduction cycles
    b. Radical cure—drugs used to destroy tissue parasites
    c. Suppressive prophylaxis and suppressive cure—drugs used to interrupt the blood cycle phase
    d. Clinical cure—drugs provide relief of symptoms in an acute exacerbation of malaria
  2. Primaquine phosphate
    a. Actions
      (1) Primary drug for radical cure of *Plasmodium vivax* and also has a gametocytocide action in 3 days
      (2) Control requires 14 days; therapy is continued for 8 weeks
    b. Adverse effects
      (1) Leukopenia
      (2) Agranulocytosis
      (3) Intravascular hemolysis
      (4) Visual disturbances
      (5) Nausea and vomiting
  3. Chloroquine phosphate (Aralen Phosphate, Roquine) and hydroxychloroquine sulfate (Plaquenil Sulfate)
    a. Actions
      (1) Inhibit oxygen uptake and interfere with nucleic acid synthesis in plasmodia
      (2) Modify gametocytes of *P. vivax* to prevent completion of reproduction cycle

      (3) Used with primaquine phosphate for suppressive prophylaxis of *P. vivax* for individuals traveling to endemic areas
    b. Adverse effects
      (1) Blood dyscrasias
      (2) Dizziness
      (3) Convulsions
      (4) Visual disturbances
      (5) Ototoxicity
      (6) GI distress
  4. Amodiaquine hydrochloride (Camoquin Hydrochloride, Flavoquin)
    a. Actions
      (1) Used with chloroquine hydrochloride for clinical cure of *P. vivax* or *P. falciparum*
      (2) Rapid-acting schizonticide providing negative peripheral blood samples in 48 to 72 hours; afebrile in 24 to 48 hours; continuation of therapy provides suppressive cure of *P. falciparum*
    b. Adverse effects
      (1) Blood dyscrasias
      (2) Headache
      (3) Fatigue
      (4) Psychosis
      (5) Visual disturbances
      (6) Ototoxicity
      (7) Nausea and vomiting
  5. Chloroguanide hydrochloride (Paludrine) and pyrimethamine (Daraprim)
    a. Actions
      (1) Used for suppressive prophylaxis
      (2) Act as folic acid antagonists and prevent nucleic acid synthesis by plasmodia; sterilizing effect that inhibits gametocyte development in mosquito breeder of *P. falciparum* and *P. vivax*
      (3) Slow acting; therapy continued 4 weeks after last exposure
    b. Adverse effects
      (1) Blood dyscrasias
      (2) Headache
      (3) Convulsions
      (4) Visual disturbances
      (5) Ototoxicity
      (6) GI disturbances
  6. Quinine sulfate
    a. Actions

(1) Acts as schizonticidal and gametocidal agent

(2) Used for radical cure and for suppression

b. Adverse effects

(1) Blood dyscrasias (hemolytic anemia, thrombocytopenia, agranulocytosis)

(2) Severe headache

(3) Convulsions

(4) Hypothermia

(5) Hypotension

(6) Visual disturbances

(7) GI distress

(8) Renal damage

Antineoplastic drugs

GENERAL INFORMATION

A. Drugs act primarily by action on malignant cells during reproduction of proteins

B. One drug or a combination of drugs may be used to increase specificity of action and decrease drug tolerance

C. Administration routes delivering drug to involved organs

1. Isolation or regional perfusion that requires extracorporeal perfusion

2. Intra-arterial infusion at organ site that allows uptake of drug before it enters the venous route

3. Intracavity instillation

D. Antineoplastic drugs have a low therapeutic index (T.I.), and evidence of cytotoxic effects occurs in normal tissues

E. General adverse effects—anorexia, nausea, vomiting, lassitude, hyperuricemia (caused by rapid breakdown of tumor tissue), epithelial tissue lesions (stomatitis, abdominal cramps, diarrhea), bone marrow depression (bleeding, infections), alopecia

IMPLICATIONS FOR NURSES

A. Protect patient from communicable diseases and use strict asepsis

B. Observe patient for adverse effects of each antineoplastic drug

C. Provide emotional support

D. Allow patient to ventilate feelings

E. Help set realistic goals

DRUGS USED

Hormones in chemotherapy

A. Actions

1. Change hormonal balance and slow growth rate of certain tumors

2. Especially useful in treatment of neoplasms involving the reproductive organs

B. Examples

1. Estrogen (Premarin, Diethylstilbestrol, Feminone, Lynoral)

2. Androgen (Drolban, Halotestin, Teslac, Oreton)

3. Progesterone (Delalutin, Depo Provera, Megace)

C. Adverse effects

1. Emergence of characteristics of the opposite sex

2. Edema

3. Changes in libido

4. Irritability

5. Uterine bleeding

Antimetabolites

A. Action—interfere with production of purine precursors (guanine, adenine) required for DNA or RNA synthesis; pyrimidine precursors (cytosine, thymine) required for DNA synthesis or the precursors (cytosine, uracil) required for RNA synthesis; or the folic acid conversion required for DNA or RNA protein construction

B. Analogs used to interfere in cell reproduction

1. Purine antagonist (adenine analog)

a. Azathioprine (Imuran) action as sulfhydryl enzyme inhibitor makes it useful as immunosuppressive drug

b. Mercaptopurine (Purinethol)

2. Purine antagonist (guanine analog)—Thioguanine

3. Pyrimidine antagonist (thymine analog)

a. Fluorouracil (also uracil analog)

b. Floxuridine (also uracil analog)

c. Hydroxyurea (Hydrea)

4. Pyrimidine antagonist (cytosine analog)—cytarabine (Cytosar)

5. Folic acid antagonist—methotrexate

C. Adverse effects

1. Liver dysfunction

2. Intractable vomiting

3. Leukopenia

4. Alopecia

Alkylating agents

A. Action—cause chromatin disruptive effects similar to those of x rays by transferring their side chains to molecules in the cell and reacting selectively with phosphate groups of DNA
B. Examples
   1. Busulfan (Myleran)
   2. Carmustine
   3. Chlorambucil (Leukeran)
   4. Cyclophosphamide (Cytoxan, Endoxan)
   5. Mechlorethamine hydrochloride (Caryolysine, Mustargen)
   6. Melphalan (Alkeran)
   7. Pipobroman (Vercyte)
   8. Thio-tepa (Thio-TEPA)
   9. Uracil mustard
C. Adverse effects
   1. Persistent vomiting
   2. Ataxia
   3. Convulsions

Plant alkaloids

A. Action—disorganize the mitotic spindle to decrease cell reproduction
B. Examples
   1. Vinblastine sulfate (Velban)
   2. Vincristine sulfate (Oncovin)
C. Adverse effects
   1. Constipation
   2. Peripheral neuropathy
   3. Ataxia
   4. Muscle weakness
   5. Paresthesia

Antineoplastic antibiotics

A. Action—act by binding to DNA to slow RNA production and interfere with cell building (these drugs are highly toxic and are not useful as anti-infectives)
B. Examples
   1. Dactinomycin (Cosmegen)
   2. Daunomycin
   3. Mithramycin (Mithracin)
   4. Mitomycin (Mutamycin)
   5. Bleomycin sulfate (Blenoxane)
   6. Doxorubicin hydrochloride (Adriamycin)
C. Adverse effects
   1. Irritation of vein on administration
   2. Leukopenia
   3. Alopecia
   4. Nausea and vomiting

Radioactive antibiotics

A. Action—these drugs destroy neoplasms by irradiation
B. Examples
   1. Gold (^{198}Au) used for pleural effusions and ascites secondary to cancer
   2. Sodium iodide (^{131}I) avidly taken up by thyroid cells
   3. Sodium phosphate (^{32}P) reduces the erythrocyte count; e.g., in polycythemia vera
C. Adverse effects
   1. Radiation sickness
   2. Low-grade fever
   3. Skin rash

Cancer immunotherapy

A. Actions
   1. Nonspecific immunotherapy involves the introduction of noncancerous antigens into the body to stimulate the production of lymphocytes and antibodies
   2. Passive immunotherapy involves the transfer of antibodies from an individual who has been cured of cancer to someone with that same cancer
   3. Active specific immunotherapy involves injection of tumor cells intradermally to stimulate the patient's immune system
B. Examples of nonspecific immunotherapy
   1. BCG (bacillus of Calmette-Guérin)
   2. *Corynebacterium parvulum*
C. Adverse effects
   1. Fever
   2. Chills
   3. Malaise
   4. Enlarged lymph nodes
   5. Local abscess formation

Common combinations of chemotherapeutic agents

A. MOPP
   1. Mechlorethamine (nitrogen mustard)
   2. Vincristine (Oncovin)
   3. Procarbazine (Matulane)
   4. Prednisone

B. COP
   1. Cyclophosphamide (Cytoxan)
   2. Vincristine (Oncovin)
   3. Prednisone
C. MAC
   1. Methotrexate
   2. Dactinomycin (Actinomycin D)
   3. Cyclophosphamide (Cytoxan)
D. POMP
   1. 6-Mercaptopurine (Purinethol)
   2. Vincristine (Oncovin)
   3. Methotrexate
   4. Prednisone
E. COMFU-P
   1. Cyclophosphamide (Cytoxan)
   2. Vincristine (Oncovin)
   3. Methotrexate
   4. 5-Fluorouracil (5-FU)
   5. Prednisone
F. CODFU
   1. Cyclophosphamide (Cytoxan)
   2. Vincristine (Oncovin)
   3. Dactinomycin (Actinomycin D)
   4. 5-Fluorouracil (5-FU)

Maintenance of fluid, electrolyte, and acid-base balance

FLUID AND ELECTROLYTE BALANCE
Basic concepts

A. Total volume of fluid and total amount of electrolytes in body normally remain relatively constant
B. Volume of blood plasma, interstitial fluid, and intracellular fluid and the concentration of electrolytes in each remain relatively constant
C. Fluid balance and electrolyte balance are interdependent
D. Intake must equal output
E. Fluid and electrolyte balance maintained primarily by mechanisms that adjust output to intake; secondarily by mechanisms that adjust intake to output
F. Fluid balance is also maintained by a physical mechanism that controls movement of water between fluid compartments (osmosis)
G. Average adult male (150 lb) contains about 40 L of water, comprising 60% body weight; 25 L intracellular and 15 to 17 L extracellular

H. Extracellular fluid divided among
   1. Interstitial fluid—10 to 12 L
   2. Plasma—3 L
   3. Small fluid compartments 1 L; e.g., cerebrospinal fluid, aqueous humor, serous and synovial fluid, lymphatic channels
   4. Gastrointestinal tract—1 L at any given time for all gastrointestinal organs
I. All body fluids are related and mix well with each other: plasma becomes interstitial fluid as it filters across capillary wall; interstitial fluid can return to capillary by osmosis or enter lymphatic channel becoming lymph; interstitial fluid and intracellular fluid are in osmotic equilibrium across the cell membranes, regulated by Na^+ concentration of interstitial fluid and K^+ concentration of intracellular fluid
   1. Mechanism of fluid flow between plasma and interstitial fluid involves several forces
      a. Blood hydrostatic pressure
      b. Blood osmotic pressure
      c. Interstitial fluid hydrostatic pressure
      d. Interstitial fluid osmotic pressure
   2. Blood hydrostatic pressure, interstitial fluid osmotic pressure, and interstitial fluid hydrostatic pressure (normally a negative value) tend to move fluid out of the blood in the capillaries and into the interstitial fluid
   3. Blood osmotic pressure moves fluid back into the capillary blood from the interstitial fluid
   4. Starling's law of the capillaries states that equal amounts of water move back and forth between blood and interstitial fluid only when blood hydrostatic pressure plus interstitial fluid osmotic pressure plus interstital fluid hydrostatic pressure equals blood osmotic pressure; under these conditions fluid balance exists between blood and interstitial fluid
      a. Blood gains liquid from interstitial fluid whenever blood hydrostatic pressure plus interstitial fluid osmotic pressure and interstitial fluid hydrostatic pressure are less than blood osmotic pressure
      b. Blood loses liquid to interstitial fluid whenever blood osmotic pressure is less than blood hydrostatic pressure plus interstitial fluid osmotic pressure and interstitial fluid hydrostatic pressure
J. Chemically, extracellular fluid and intracellular fluid are strikingly different: sodium is the main cation of extracellular fluid; potassium is the main cation of

Table 2-1. Average concentrations of major ions in extracellular and intracellular fluids (usually expressed in milliosmols per liter [mOsm/L of H_2O])

Ion	Intracellular fluid	Extracellular fluid	
		Plasma	Interstitial
Na^+	10	144.0	137.0
K^+	141	5.0	4.7
Cl^-	4	107.0	112.7
HCO_3^-	10	27.0	28.3
Ca^{+2}	0	2.5	2.4
Mg^{+2}	31	1.5	1.4
SO_4^{-2}	1	0.5	0.5
Phosphates ($H_2PO_4^-$; $H_2PO_4^{-2}$)	11	2.0	2.0
Proteins	4	1.2	0.2

intracellular fluid; chloride is the main anion of extracellular fluid; phosphate is the main anion of intracellular fluid; protein concentration is much higher in intracellular fluid than in interstitial fluid (see Table 2-1)

K. Chemically, plasma and interstitial fluid are almost identical except that plasma contains slightly more electrolytes, considerably more proteins, somewhat more sodium, and fewer chloride ions that interstitial fluid (see Table 2-1)

Major ions (electrolytes)

A. Cations (+)
  1. Sodium (Na^+)
    a. Most abundant cation in extracellular fluid
    b. Sodium pump in most body cells pumps sodium out of intracellular fluid
    c. Regulates cell size by osmotically drawing water from cells to balance flow of water into cells due to osmotically active intracellular proteins
    d. Action potential of nervous and muscle fibers requires sodium; sodium is basic to body's communication system
    e. Helps to regulate acid-base balance by exchanging hydrogen ions for sodium ions in kidney tubules; excess hydrogen ions (acid) are excreted
  2. Potassium (K^+)
    a. Most abundant cation of intracellular fluid
    b. Potassium pump brings potassium into cells of body
    c. Resting polarization and repolarization of nervous and muscle fibers depend on potassium
      (1) If potassium concentration of extracellular fluid rises above normal (hyperkalemia), the force of the contracting heart weakens; with extremely high concentrations the heart will not contract
      (2) If potassium concentration of extracellular fluid drops below normal (hypokalemia), resting polarization in nerve and muscle fibers increases, resulting in weakness and eventual paralysis
  3. Calcium (Ca^{++})
    a. Forms salts with phosphates, carbonate, and fluoride in bones and teeth to make them hard
    b. Required for correct functioning of nerves and muscles
      (1) If calcium concentrations rise above normal levels (hypercalcemia), nervous system becomes depressed and sluggish
      (2) If calcium concentrations fall below normal levels (hypocalcemia), nervous system becomes extremely excitable, resulting in cramps and tetany
    c. Calcium is required for blood clotting, acting as a cofactor in formation of prothrombin activator and thrombin
  4. Magnesium (Mg^{++})
    a. Cofactor for many enzymes involved in energy metabolism
    b. Normal constituent of bone
B. Anion (−)
  1. Chloride (Cl^-)

a. Most abundant anion in extracellular fluid
b. In great part balances sodium
c. Major component of gastric secretions
2. Bicarbonate (HCO_3^-)
   a. Part of bicarbonate buffer system
   b. Reacts with a strong acid to form carbonic acid and a basic salt, thus limiting the drop in pH
3. Phosphate (HPO_4^- and $HPO_4^=$)
   a. Part of phosphate buffer system
   b. Function in cellular energy metabolism: phosphate + ADP → ATP (the energy currency of the cell)
   c. Combines with Ca^{++} in bone, providing hardness
   d. Involved in structure of genetic material, DNA and RNA

Major avenues by which water enters and leaves body

A. Water enters body through digestive tract both in liquids (drinking) and in foods (preformed water)
B. Water is formed in the body by metabolism of foods (oxidative water)
C. Water leaves body via kidneys (as urine), intestines (with feces), and lungs and skin (insensible water losses)

Mechanisms that maintain total fluid volume

A. Osmoreceptor system
   1. Regulates water output volume to balance fluid intake volume
   2. Most important mechanism for regulation of water output, since other fluid losses through skin, lungs, and gastrointestinal system have no feedback mechanism relative to water loss
   3. Cells in hypothalamus synthesize ADH, which is then stored in posterior pituitary prior to release into circulation
   4. Osmoreceptors respond to dehydration by increasing frequency of nerve impulses to posterior pituitary, resulting in an increase in the amounts of ADH released; this increases water reabsorption in the kidney tubules and decreases urinary output
   5. Osmoreceptors respond to overhydration by decreasing nerve impulses to posterior pituitary, which decreases the release of ADH, resulting in an increase in urinary output

B. Interaction of circulatory system
   1. Regulation of blood volume (extracellular fluid volume)
   2. Increased fluid intake increases blood volume
   3. Increased blood volume results in an increase in cardiac output, blood pressure, and therefore glomerular filtration
   4. Increased glomerular filtration results in an increase in urinary output and a decrease in blood volume
C. Regulation of fluid intake—thirst mechanism
   1. Dehydration of cells in thirst center of hypothalamus gives rise to thirst sensation
   2. Thirst sensations also induced by dryness of oral mucosa
   3. Fluid intake stretches stomach and moistens the mouth and throat; these sensations cancel thirst sensation prior to actual hydration of body fluids
D. Various factors such as hyperventilation, hypoventilation, vomiting, diarrhea, and circulatory failure may alter the volume of fluid lost

Mechanisms that maintain electrolyte concentrations

A. Aldosterone feedback mechanism
   1. Adrenal cortex secretes steroid hormone aldosterone when extracellular fluid sodium concentrations decrease or potassium concentrations increase
   2. Aldosterone stimulates kidney tubules to reabsorb sodium; potassium reabsorption decreases as sodium reabsorption increases; sodium is salvaged while potassium is excreted
   3. This mechanism helps preserve normal sodium and potassium concentrations in extracellular fluid
   4. Secondary effects of aldosterone
      a. Chloride conserved with sodium
      b. Water conserved, since it is reabsorbed by osmosis as tubules reabsorb salt
B. Parathyroid regulation of calcium
   1. Parathyroid glands secrete parathormone when extracellular fluid calcium concentrations decrease
   2. Parathormone stimulates release of calcium from bone, calcium reabsorption in small intestine (also requires vitamin D), and calcium reabsorption in kidney tubules
   3. Increased extracellular fluid calcium concentra-

tions result in decreased secretion of parathormone and gradual loss of excess calcium

ACID-BASE BALANCE
Basic concepts

A. Healthy survival depends on the body maintaining a state of acid-base balance; more specifically, healthy survival depends on the maintenance of a relatively constant, slightly alkaline pH of blood and other fluids

B. When the body is in a state of acid-base balance, it maintains a stable hydrogen ion concentration in body fluids; specifically, blood pH remains relatively constant between 7.35 and 7.45

C. The body has 3 devices or mechanisms for maintaining acid-base balance; named in order of the speed with which they act, they are the buffer mechanism, the respiratory mechanism, and the renal or urinary mechanisms

D. A state of uncompensated acidosis exists if blood pH decreases below 7.35

E. A state of uncompensated alkalosis exists if blood pH increases above 7.45

F. The pH of body fluids shifts from the ideal of 7.35 to 7.45 for several reasons
   1. Glucose, utilized by almost all body cells, is oxidized with O_2, producing energy, H_2O, and CO_2; CO_2 combines with H_2O to produce carbonic acid
   2. Metabolism of sulfur amino acids results in formation of sulfuric acid
   3. Metabolism of phospholipids and phosphoproteins results in formation of phosphoric acid
   4. Muscle metabolism under anaerobic conditions produces lactic acid
   5. Rapid weight loss results in extra fat metabolism, producing ketone bodies that include alpha keto acids
   6. The acid produced by the normal mechanisms just mentioned requires neutralization to avoid acidosis, coma, and death

Buffer mechanisms for maintaining acid-base balance

A. The buffer mechanism consists of chemicals called buffers, which are present in the blood and other body fluids and which combine with relatively strong acids or bases to convert them to weaker acids or bases; hence, buffers function to prevent marked changes in blood pH when either acids or bases enter the blood

B. A buffer is often referred to as a buffer pair because it consists of not 1 but 2 substances; the chief buffer pair in the blood consists of the weak acid, carbonic acid (H_2CO_3), and its basic salts, collectively called base bicarbonate (B · HCO_3); sodium bicarbonate ($NaHCO_3$) is by far the most abundant base bicarbonate present in blood plasma

C. When the body is in a state of acid-base balance, blood contains 27 mEq base bicarbonate per liter and 1.35 mEq carbonic acid per liter; usually this is written as a ratio, referred to as the base bicarbonate/carbonic acid ratio:

$$\frac{27 \text{ mEq B} \cdot \text{HCO}_3}{1.35 \text{ mEq H}_2\text{CO}_3} = \frac{20}{1}$$

D. Whenever the base bicarbonate/carbonic acid ratio of blood equals 20/1, blood pH equals 7.4

E. Base bicarbonate buffers nonvolatile acids that are stronger than carbonic acid; it reacts with them to convert them to carbonic acid and a basic salt

F. Some facts about the changes in capillary blood produced by the buffering of blood by base bicarbonate
   1. Buffering does not prevent blood pH from decreasing, but it does prevent it from decreasing as markedly as it would without buffering
   2. Buffering removes some sodium bicarbonate from blood and adds some carbonic acid to it; this necessarily decreases the base bicarbonate/carbonic acid ratio, which in turn necessarily decreases the pH of blood as it flows through capillaries (from its arterial level of about 7.4 to its venous level of about 7.38)
   3. Anything that decreases blood's base bicarbonate/carbonic acid ratio necessarily decreases blood pH and thus tends to produce acidosis; the corollary is also true: anything that increases the base bicarbonate/carbonic acid ratio necessarily increases blood pH and thus tends to produce alkalosis

G. Other buffer systems in body fluids
   1. Protein buffer
      a. Most plentiful; three fourths of all chemical buffering power lies in proteins of the body fluids
      b. Provides support to other buffering systems such as bicarbonate buffer and phosphate buffer

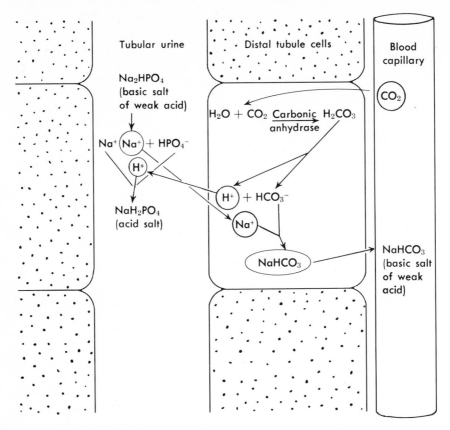

Fig. 1. Acidification of urine and conservation of base by distal renal tubule excretion of H ions into the urine and reabsorption of Na ions into the blood in exchange for the H ions excreted from it. (From Anthony, C. P., and Kolthoff, N. J.: Textbook of anatomy and physiology, ed. 9, St. Louis, 1975, The C. V. Mosby Co.)

2. Phosphate buffer system
   a. One sixth as concentrated as bicarbonate buffer in extracellular fluid
   b. More important in intracellular fluids, where its concentration is considerably higher
   c. Helps to buffer pH of urine in kidney tubules
3. Hemoglobin buffer system—buffers intracellular fluid of the erythrocyte
H. Bicarbonate buffer is the most important buffer in human body fluids because its components, base bicarbonate and carbonic acid, are actively and constantly regulated by the action of the respiratory and urinary systems

Respiratory mechanism for controlling acid-base balance

A. Respiratory system controls acid-base balance by controlling rate of CO_2 exhalation from lungs; during normal body metabolism CO_2 is produced, which reacts with water to form carbonic acid, resulting in a decrease in pH (as acidity increases, pH decreases); when the respiratory system blows CO_2 out of the body, carbonic acid breaks down into CO_2 and water, resulting in an increase in pH (as acidity decreases, pH increases)
B. Respiratory acidosis
   1. Conditions impairing the ability of the respiratory

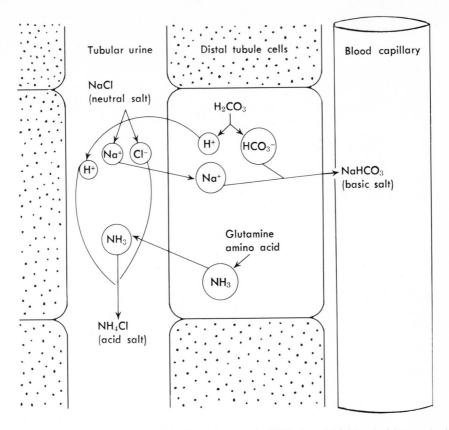

Fig. 2. Acidification of urine by tubule excretion of ammonia (NH$_3$). An acid (glutamine) leaves the blood, enters a tubule cell, and is deaminized to form ammonia that is excreted into urine, where it combines with hydrogen to form NH$_4$ ion. In exchange for NH$_4$ ion, the tubule cell reabsorbs Na ion. (From Anthony, C. P., and Kolthoff, N. J.: Textbook of anatomy and physiology, ed. 9, St. Louis, 1975, The C. V. Mosby Co.)

system to blow off CO$_2$ will result in a buildup of CO$_2$ in the body; excess CO$_2$ combines with water to form carbonic acid and hydrogen ions, resulting in a decrease in pH

2. Signs of respiratory acidosis include dyspnea, irritability, tachycardia, and cyanosis
3. Common causes include emphysema, pneumonia, asthmatic attack, atelectasis, pneumothorax, drug overdose

C. Respiratory alkalosis
   1. Less frequently, hyperventilation blows off too much CO$_2$ from the body, causing an excessive breakdown of carbonic acid, resulting in an increase of pH

2. Signs of respiratory alkalosis include deep or deep and rapid breathing, light-headedness, tetany, convulsions, and unconsciousness
3. Common causes include hysteria, prolonged crying, and mechanical ventilation

Renal mechanism for maintaining acid-base balance

A. The renal mechanism is the most effective device the body has for maintaining acid-base balance; unless it operates adequately, acid-base balance cannot be maintained
B. The renal mechanism for maintaining acid-base bal-

ance makes the urine more acidic and the blood more alkaline; this neutralizes the constant production of acid products from cells; the mechanism consists of 2 functions performed by the distal renal tubule cells, both of which remove hydrogen ions from blood to urine and in exchange reabsorb sodium ions from tubular urine to blood

1. Distal tubule cells secrete hydrogen ions and reabsorb sodium ions (Fig. 1)
2. Distal tubule cells form ammonia, which combines with hydrogen ions they have secreted to form ammonium (NH_4) ions, which are excreted in the urine in exchange for sodium ions, which are reabsorbed into the blood (Fig. 2)

C. The distal tubule functions produce the following results
1. They increase blood's sodium bicarbonate content and decrease its carbonic acid content, thereby increasing the base bicarbonate/carbonic acid ratio and blood pH
2. They acidify urine (decrease urine pH)

D. Metabolic acidosis
1. Excess acid, other than carbonic acid, which is a respiratory acid, accumulates in the body beyond the body's ability to neutralize it
2. Signs of metabolic acidosis include weakness, malaise, headache, disorientation, deep rapid breathing, fruity odor to breath, coma
3. Common causes include diabetes mellitus, salicylate poisoning, severe diarrhea, vomiting of intestinal contents, infection

E. Metabolic alkalosis
1. Excess base bicarbonate in the body
2. Signs of metabolic alkalosis include muscle hypertoxicity, tetany, confusion, shallow slow respirations, convulsions, coma
3. Common causes include vomiting of stomach contents or prolonged gastric suction, excessive ingestion of alkaline drugs, potent diuretics

F. Compensation
1. In respiratory acidosis the urinary system excretes increased hydrogen ions to compensate for the respiratory system's inability to blow off CO_2
2. In respiratory alkalosis the urinary system may decrease excretion of hydrogen ions to compensate and maintain the body's pH in the normal range
3. In metabolic acidosis the respiratory system compensates by hyperventilation in an attempt to blow off CO_2 and raise the pH

4. In metabolic alkalosis the respiratory system compensates by decreasing the rate and depth of breathing in an attempt to retain CO_2 and decrease the pH

CHEMICAL PRINCIPLES RELATED TO FLUID AND ELECTROLYTES
Ionization
Ion
A. When an atom loses or gains an electron (electrons), it is no longer a neutral atom but a charged particle—an ion
B. The charge on this particle depends on whether electrons are lost ($+$) or gained ($-$) and the number of electrons lost or gained
C. An electron is a negative particle; the loss of 1 electron makes ion positive (less negative) by 1; with loss of 2 electrons, ion is 2^+, etc.
D. The gain of 1 electron makes ion negative by 1; with 2 electrons gained, the ion is 2^-, etc.

Ionization and water
A. When certain compounds are placed in water, the polar water molecules dissociate the molecules of the compound into ions—a process called ionization
B. A substance that will ionize when placed in water is called an electrolyte
C. A substance that will ionize in water (an electrolyte) will allow the passage of an electric current through its solution
D. Acids, bases, and salts ionize in water and conduct an electric current

Factors affecting strength of electrolytes
A. Amount of electrolyte present in solution
B. How well the electrolyte dissociates in solution—degree of ionization
1. Weak electrolytes are substances that dissociate into ions to only a slight degree
2. Strong electrolytes are substances that dissociate into ions to a larger degree

Bases, acids, and salts
Bases
A. Definition—a base is a substance that usually adds an OH^- (hydroxyl) ion to any solution in which it is placed; e.g.,

$$NaOH \xrightarrow{\text{in water}} Na^+ + OH^-$$

B. Properties of a base
1. Bitter taste
2. Slippery feeling
3. Electrolyte in water
4. Reacts with indicators, giving a base color
   a. Methyl orange—yellow
   b. Litmus—blue
   c. Phenolphthalein—red
5. Reacts with acids to form water and a salt (neutralization)
6. Reacts with certain metals to release hydrogen gas
7. Combines with organic acids (fatty acids) to form soaps
8. In high concentration destroys organic material; corrosive
C. Names and formulas of common bases
1. Calcium hydroxide ($Ca[OH]_2$)—water solution, called lime water
2. Sodium hydroxide (NaOH)—caustic soda
3. Potassium hydroxide (KOH)—soap making
4. Ammonium hydroxide (NH_4OH)—household cleaner
5. Magnesium hydroxide ($Mg[OH]_2$)—water solution marketed under trade name Milk of Magnesia—antacid, mild laxative
6. Aluminum hydroxide ($Al[OH]_3$)—component of antacid pills

Acids
A. Definition—an acid is ordinarily thought of as a substance that liberates an H^+ (hydrogen ion) to a solution in which it is placed; e.g.,

$$\text{in water} \downarrow$$
$$H_2CO_3 \rightarrow H^+ + HCO_3^-$$

B. Properties of an acid
1. Sour taste
2. Reacts with indicators, giving an acid color
   a. Methyl orange—red
   b. Litmus—red
   c. Phenolphthalein—colorless
3. Combines with certain metals, releasing hydrogen gas
4. Reacts with bases to form water and a salt (neutralization)
5. Reacts with carbonates to give carbon dioxide gas
6. Acts as an electrolyte in water
7. In high concentration destroys organic materials—corrosive

C. Names and formulas of common acids
1. Hydrochloric acid (HCl)—secreted by the parietal cells of the stomach; transforms pepsinogen into pepsin, which is a protein-digesting enzyme of gastric juice
2. Nitric acid (HNO_3)—used in test for proteins
3. Sulfuric acid (H_2SO_4)—in storage batteries
4. Carbonic acid (H_2CO_3)
   a. One form in which CO_2 is transported in the blood
   b. Part of the bicarbonate buffer system, which is the most important buffer system regulating the pH of body fluids
5. Boric acid (H_3BO_3)—mild antiseptic
6. Acetic acid ($C_2H_3O_2H$)—vinegar
7. Lactic acid ($CH_3CHOHCOOH$)—builds up in muscle tissue during exercise; most lactic acid is then transported to the liver via the circulatory system where it is completely oxidized into CO_2, water, and energy (as ATP)

General considerations concerning acids and bases
A. Weak acids produce few hydrogen ions in solution, whereas strong acids produce many
B. Weak bases produce few hydroxyl ions in solution, whereas strong bases produce many
C. Strong acids and bases can cause serious damage to human tissue
D. Acids and bases can be used to neutralize each other—therefore, in the event of acid or base burn, flood with water and add the opposite chemical in weak, diluted form

Salts
A. Definition—the compound (besides water) formed when an acid is neutralized by a base is a salt; e.g.,

$$HCl + KOH \rightarrow H_2O + KCl$$
$$\textbf{Acid} \quad \textbf{Base} \quad \textbf{Water} \quad \textbf{Salt}$$

B. Properties of a salt
1. Crystalline in nature
2. Ionic even in the dry crystal
3. Electrolyte in solution
4. "Salty" taste
C. Names and formulas of common salts
1. Sodium chloride (NaCl)—salt of intercellular and extracellular spaces
2. Calcium phosphate ($CaPO_4$)—bone and tooth formation
3. Potassium chloride (KCl)—salt of intracellular spaces

4. Calcium carbonate ($CaCO_3$)—limestone
5. Barium sulfate ($BaSO_4$)—when taken internally, outlines internal structures for x-ray studies
6. Silver nitrate ($AgNO_3$)—antiseptic
7. Iron (II) sulfate ($FeSO_4$)—treatment of anemia
8. Sodium bicarbonate ($NaHCO_3$)—antacid
9. Calcium sulfate ($CaSO_4$)—hydrated form is plaster of paris (casts for broken bones)
10. Magnesium sulfate ($MgSO_4$)—Epsom salt

Hydrogen ion concentration (pH)

A. The *p* in pH comes from the French word *puissance*, meaning power
B. The *H* in pH stands for *hydrogen*
C. Thus pH denotes the power or strength of hydrogen (ions) in a solution
D. A neutral solution has the same amount of acid-reacting ions, H^+ (actually H_3O^+), as basic-reacting ions, OH^-
E. An acid-reacting solution has more H^+ than OH^-
F. A basic-reacting solution has more OH^- than H^+
G. pH is used to represent these conditions
   1. A neutral solution has a pH of 7.00
   2. An acid solution would have a pH in the range from 0 to 6.99; the lower the pH, the more acid the solution
   3. A basic solution would have a pH in the range from 7.01 to 14.00; the higher the pH, the more basic the solution
   4. The pH of the extracellular (vascular and interstitial) fluid is in the narrow range of 7.35 to 7.45; fluctuations in pH of 0.4 unit above or below this range can result in body distress; a prolonged blood pH of 7 or less or 7.8 or more can result in death
   5. Certain body fluids have a pH different from 7.4; gastric juice has a pH of 1 or 2 caused by the presence of hydrochloric acid; bile is basic; urine may be acidic or basic

Circulatory system

REVIEW OF ANATOMY AND PHYSIOLOGY OF THE CIRCULATORY SYSTEM
Functions

A. Primary function—provides communication between widely separated body parts through transportation of hormones, nutrients, wastes, respiratory gases, vitamins, minerals, enzymes, water, leukocytes, antibodies, and buffers
B. Secondary functions—contributes directly or indirectly to all the body's metabolic functions: tissue perfusion with O_2 and nutrients, water balance, immunity, enzymatic reactions, and pH and temperature regulation

Structures

Blood

A. Blood components
   1. Serum—plasma with fewer or no coagulating proteins
   2. Plasma
      a. Water—3 L in average adult; constitutes 90% of plasma
      b. Ions—see fluid and electrolytes and Table 2-2

Table 2-2. Plasma constituents

Constituent	Normal concentration range
Water	Approximately 90% by volume
Ions	
Sodium (Na^+)	135 to 145 mEq/L
Potassium (K^+)	4.0 to 5.5 mEq/L
Calcium (Ca^{++})	4.5 to 5.0 mEq/L
Magnesium (Mg^{++})	1.5 to 2.5 mEq/L
Chloride (Cl^-)	100 to 106 mEq/L
Bicarbonate (HCO_3^-)	23 to 28 mEq/L
Phosphate ($HPO_4^=$; $H_2PO_4^-$)	1.5 to 2.5 mEq/L
Plasma proteins	
Albumin	3.5 to 5.5 g/100 ml
Globulins (alpha, beta, and gamma)	1.5 to 3.6 g/100 ml
Glucose	70 to 110 mg/100 ml
Nitrogenous substances	
Blood urea nitrogen (BUN)	5 to 25 mg/100 ml
Uric acid	2 to 8 mg/100 ml
Creatinine	0.7 to 1.5 mg/100 ml
Amino acids	0.1 to 3.0 mg/100 ml
Bilirubin	0.0 to 1.5 mg/100 ml
Lipids	
Cholesterol	150 to 300 mg/100 ml
Fatty acids	200 to 400 mg/100 ml
Triglycerides	15 to 25 mg/100 ml
Other constituents	
Respiratory gases (O_2 and CO_2)	Variable concentrations
Hormones	
Vitamins	
Enzymes	

c. Proteins—all act as buffers; fractionated and separated from each other by electrophoretic and ultracentrifugation techniques
  (1) Albumin
    (a) Largest component of plasma proteins
    (b) Principally responsible for plasma colloid osmotic pressure (COP)
    (c) Reversibly combines with and transports certain lipids, bilirubin, thyroxin, and certain drugs, such as barbiturates
  (2) Alpha and beta globulins
    (a) Help establish COP
    (b) Transport certain vitamins, iron, copper, and cortisol
    (c) Hemostasis (prothrombin and fibrinogen are in this blood fraction)
  (3) Gamma globulins—antibodies
d. Glucose—prime oxidative metabolite of body cells
3. Formed elements
  a. Erythrocytes
    (1) Shape—pliable biconcave disc that maximizes surface area proportional to volume for ease of diffusion of respiratory gases
    (2) Number—males: 4.5 to $6.2 \times 10^6/mm^3$; females: 4.0 to $5.5 \times 10^6/mm^3$
    (3) Formation
      (a) Location—red marrow of vertebrae, sternum, ribs, iliac crests, clavicles, scapulae, and skull
      (b) Maturation process—mature erythrocytes are mainly sacs of hemoglobin without a nucleus, mitochondria, ribosomes, endoplasmic reticula, or Golgi bodies; process requires folic acid and vitamin B_{12}; vitamin B_{12} plus intrinsic factor from the parietal cells of the stomach form hemopoietic factor, which stimulates erythrocyte formation (see pernicious anemia)
      (c) Under conditions of low O_2 tension, liver and kidneys secrete proteins into blood that combine to form erythropoietin, which stimulates erythrocyte production
    (4) Principal component is hemoglobin
      (a) Conjugated protein—globulin plus 4 molecules of heme
      (b) Formed within the erythrocyte utilizing copper, cobalt, iron, nickel, and vitamin B_6
      (c) Functions to bind O_2 through iron in heme and CO_2 through globulin portion; can carry both simultaneously
    (5) Erythrocytes live for about 125 days; old or deteriorated erythrocytes removed by reticuloendothelial cells of the liver, spleen, and bone marrow; 3.5×10^6 die and are replaced daily; heme converted to bilirubin, which is excreted from liver as a part of bile
  b. Leukocytes
    (1) Types
      (a) Granulocytes (polymorphonuclear)—originate in red marrow and consist of neutrophils (50% to 70% of total), eosinophils (1% to 4% of the total), and basophils (0% to 1% of the total)
      (b) Agranulocytes (mononuclear)—originate in red marrow and lymphatic tissue and consist of monocytes (3% to 8% of the total), which become macrophages in tissue spaces, and lymphocytes (25% to 40% of the total)
    (2) Functions
      (a) Phagocytosis of bacteria by neutrophils and macrophages; phagocytosis of antibody-antigen complexes by eosinophils
      (b) Antibody synthesis—B lymphocytes produce antibodies; they also become plasma cells, which produce most circulatory antibodies
      (c) Destruction of transplanted tissues and cancer cells by T lymphocytes, which form in lymphoid tissue and mature in thymus gland
    (3) Leukocytes live for a few hours or days; some T lymphocytes live for many years and provide long-term immunity
  c. Thrombocytes—anucleate cellular fragments associated with hemostasis
    (1) Origin—fragmentation of megakaryocytes in bone marrow
    (2) Number—150,000 to $500,000/mm^3$
    (3) Function in blood coagulation

      (a) Adhere to each other and to damaged areas of circulatory system to limit or prevent blood loss

      (b) Release chemicals that constrict damaged blood vessels

B. Physical properties of blood
  1. Volume
    a. Male: 5 to 6 L; female: 4.5 to 5.5 L
    b. Hematocrit: percent blood volume occupied by red cells (normal range: 36% to 45%)
  2. Specific gravity (sp gr)—normal range: 1.05 to 1.06
  3. Viscosity—about 5.5 times as viscous as pure water
C. Blood groups
  1. Names—indicate type antigens on or in red cell membrane; e.g., type A blood means that red cells have A antigens; type O means that red cells have no antigens
  2. Every person's blood belongs to one of the 4 blood groups—type A, type B, type AB, or type O—and is either Rh positive or Rh negative
  3. Plasma—normally contains no antibodies against antigens present on its own red cells but does contain antibodies against other A or B antigens not present on its red cells; e.g., type A plasma does not contain antibodies against A antigen but does contain antibodies against B antigen
  4. Blood does not normally contain anti-Rh antibodies; Rh-positive blood never contains them; Rh-negative blood will contain anti-Rh antibodies if the individual has been transfused with Rh-positive blood or has carried an Rh-positive fetus
  5. The potential danger in transfusing blood is that the donor's blood may be agglutinated (clumped) by the recipient's antibodies
D. Hemostasis—arrest of bleeding
  1. Vasoconstriction—reflex spasm in cut or ruptured vessel's smooth muscles
  2. Aggregation of platelets—adhere to damaged blood vessel walls forming plugs
  3. Blood coagulation (clotting)—blood becomes gel as soluble fibrinogen is converted to insoluble fibrin; process brought about by at least a dozen different chemical clotting factors operating in sequence after mechanism is triggered
    a. Extrinsic clotting mechanism—trigger for mechanism is blood contacting damaged tissue

    b. Intrinsic clotting mechanism—trigger for mechanism is release of chemicals (platelet factors) from platelets aggregated at either the site of a wound or at a rough spot on blood vessel wall
  4. Some facts about the blood proteins essential for clotting
    a. Liver cells synthesize prothrombin, fibrinogen, and other clotting factors; adequate amounts of vitamin K must be present in blood for the liver to make normal amounts of prothrombin, Stuart factor, factor VIII, and Christmas factor
    b. Normal blood prothrombin content—10 to 15 mg/100 ml of plasma
    c. Normal blood fibrinogen content—350 mg/100 ml of plasma
    d. Both prothrombin and fibrinogen are soluble proteins normally present in blood in adequate amounts for clotting to occur at the normal rapid rate
    e. Fibrin is an insoluble protein formed from the soluble protein fibrinogen, in the presence of the enzyme thrombin; fibrin appears as a tangled mass of threads having a jellylike texture; blood cells become enmeshed in these threads, and red cells give the clot its red color
  5. Clinical applications
    a. Hemophilia—hereditary sex-linked disease characterized by defect in clotting ability of blood caused by lack of a blood protein essential for clotting (factor VIII)
    b. Thrombosis—partial or complete occlusion of a blood vessel, caused by presence of a stationary clot (thrombus)
    c. Embolism—partial or complete occlusion of a blood vessel by a moving clot (embolus)
    d. Atherosclerosis—plaques of lipoid material deposited in endothelium act as rough spots, causing platelet disintegration and thrombus formation

Heart
A. Location—in pericardial cavity within the mediastinum with apex on diaphragm and pointing to left (apical beat may be counted by placing stethoscope in fifth intercostal space on line with left midclavicular point); two thirds of bulk of heart lies to left of midline of body, one third to right
B. Covering—pericardium

1. Structure
   a. Fibrous pericardium—loose-fitting, inextensible sac around heart
   b. Serous pericardium—consists of 2 layers
      (1) Parietal layer—lines inner surface of fibrous pericardium
      (2) Visceral layer (epicardium)—adheres to outer surface of the heart; pericardial space, lying between parietal and visceral layers, contains a few drops of lubricating pericardial fluid
2. Function—protects heart against friction and erosion by providing well-lubricated, smooth sac in which the heart beats

C. Structure of heart
   1. Heart wall
      a. Myocardium—composed of cardiac muscle cells
      b. Endocardium—delicate endothelial lining of myocardium
      c. Cardiac skeleton—continuous dense connective tissue regions at the heart's base and in the interventricular septum serving as points of origin and insertion for cardiac muscle fibers and as supports for the heart's valves
   2. Cavities
      a. Upper 2 called atria
      b. Lower 2 called ventricles
   3. Valves and openings
      a. Openings between atria and ventricles known as atrioventricular orifices
         (1) Guarded by cuspid valves
            (a) Tricuspid on right
            (b) Mitral (bicuspid) on left
         (2) Valves consist of 3 parts
            (a) Flaps or cusps
            (b) Chordae tendineae
            (c) Papillary muscles
      b. Opening from right ventricle into pulmonary artery guarded by pulmonary semilunar valves
      c. Opening from left ventricle into the aorta guarded by aortic semilunar valves
   4. Blood supply to myocardium (heart muscle)
      a. By way of only 2 small vessels: the right and left coronary arteries, the first branches of the aorta
      b. Both coronary arteries send branches to both sides of the heart
      c. Right coronary branches supply right side of heart mainly but also carry some blood to left ventricle
      d. Left coronary branches supply left side of heart mainly but also carry some blood to right ventricle
      e. Most abundant blood supply goes to the myocardium of the left ventricle
      f. Greatest flow of blood into myocardium occurs when heart relaxes due to decreased arterial compression
      g. Relatively few anastomoses (branches from one artery to another artery) exist between the larger branches of the coronary arteries (poor collateral circulation); hence, if one of these vessels becomes occluded, little or no blood can reach the myocardial cells supplied by that vessel; deprived of an adequate blood supply, cells soon die (myocardial infarction)
   5. Nerve supply to heart
      a. Sympathetic fibers (in cardiac nerves) and parasympathetic fibers (in vagus nerves) form cardiac plexuses
      b. Fibers from cardiac plexuses terminate mainly in sinoatrial node
      c. Sympathetic impulses tend to accelerate and strengthen heartbeat
      d. Parasympathetic (vagal) impulses slow the heartbeat
   6. Conduction system of heart
      a. Sinoatrial node (SA node)—a cluster of cells located in the right atrial wall near the opening of the superior vena cava
      b. Atrioventricular node (AV node)—a small mass of special conducting cells located in the base of the right atrium at the top of the interventricular septum
      c. AV bundle of His—special conducting fibers that originate in the AV node and extend by 2 branches down the 2 sides of the interventricular septum (right and left bundle branches)
      d. Purkinje fibers—special conducting fibers that extend from the AV bundles throughout the wall of the ventricles
      e. Normally a nerve impulse begins its course through the heart in the heart's own pacemaker, the SA node; it quickly spreads through both atria, via special conducting fibers, to the AV node; after a short delay at this node, the impulse is conducted by 2 branches

of the AV bundle of His down both sides of the interventricular septum; from there, the impulse travels over Purkinje fibers to the lateral walls of the ventricles

f. Impulse conduction through heart generates electric currents that spread through surrounding tissues to the skin, from which visible records of conduction can be made with the electrocardiograph or oscillograph; conduction from the SA node through the atria causes atrial contraction and gives rise to the so-called P wave of the electrocardiogram; conduction from the AV node down the bundle of His and out the Purkinje fibers causes ventricular contraction and gives rise to the QRS wave; ventricular repolarization is associated with the T wave

g. Refractory period—particularly long (¼ second) to ensure against extra beats arising as electrical energy flows around the surface of heart; only SA node depolarizations, occurring after refractory period, produce next beat

D. Physiology of heart
1. Function—to pump varying amounts of blood through vessels as needs of cells change
2. Cardiac cycle
   a. Consists of systole (contraction) and diastole (relaxation) of atria and of ventricles; atria contract, and as they relax ventricles contract
   b. Time required—about ⁴/₅ second from one cardiac cycle; so 70 to 80 cycles or heartbeats per minute
3. Auscultatory events (heart sounds)—first sound (I), "lub," occurs at beginning of ventricular systole due to closing of the atrioventricular valves (tricuspid and mitral); second sound (II), "dub," occurs at end of ventricular systole due to closing of semilunar valves

Blood vessels
A. Kinds
1. Arteries—vessels that carry blood away from heart (all arteries except pulmonary artery carry oxygenated blood); arteries branch into smaller and smaller vessels called arterioles, which branch into microscopic vessels, the capillaries
2. Veins—vessels that carry blood toward heart (all veins except the pulmonary veins carry deoxygenated blood); veins branch into venules, which collect blood from capillaries; veins in cranial cavity formed by dura mater called sinuses

3. Capillaries—microscopic vessels that carry blood from arterioles to venules; capillaries unite to form small veins or venules, which, in turn, unite to form veins; exchange of substances between blood and interstitial fluid occurs in capillaries

B. Structure of blood vessels
1. Arteries
   a. Lining (tunica intima) of endothelium
   b. Middle coat (tunica media) of smooth muscle, elastic, and fibrous tissues; this coat permits constriction and dilation
   c. Outer coat (tunica adventitia or externa) of fibrous tissue; its firmness makes arteries stand open instead of collapsing when cut
2. Veins
   a. Same 3 coats, but thinner and fewer elastic fibers
   b. Veins collapse when cut
   c. Semilunar valves present in most veins over 2 mm in diameter
3. Capillaries
   a. Only lining coat present (intima)
   b. Wall only 1 cell thick

C. Fetal circulation—structures essential for fetal circulation but normally cease to exist after birth
1. Umbilical arteries—2 extensions of hypogastric arteries (internal iliacs) carry fetal blood to placenta
2. Placenta—attached to uterine wall
3. Umbilical vein—extends from placenta back to fetus' body; returns oxygenated blood from placental to fetal circulation; 2 umbilical arteries and 1 umbilical vein constitute umbilical cord
4. Ductus venosus—small vessel that connects umbilical vein with inferior vena cava in fetus
5. Foramen ovale—opening in fetal heart septum between right and left atria
6. Ductus arteriosus—small vessel connecting pulmonary artery with descending thoracic aorta
7. Only 2 fetal blood vessels carry oxygenated blood—umbilical vein and ductus venosus; as soon as blood enters inferior vena cava from ductus venosus it becomes mixed with venous blood

Physiology of circulation
A. Definitions
1. Circulation—blood flow through circuit of vessels
2. Systemic circulation—blood flow from left ven-

tricle into aorta, other arteries, arterioles, capillaries, venules, and veins to right atrium of heart

3. Pulmonary circulation—blood flow from right ventricle to pulmonary artery to lung arterioles, capillaries, and venules, to pulmonary veins, to left atrium

4. Hepatic portal circulation—blood flow from capillaries, venules, veins of stomach, intestines, spleen, pancreas, and gallbladder into portal vein, liver sinusoids, to hepatic veins, to inferior vena cava

5. Cardiac output (CO)—volume of blood pumped per minute by either left or right ventricle; average for male at rest: 5 L/minute; cardiac output is the stroke volume (systolic discharge) times heart rate; CO increases if heart rate increases or if stroke volume increases, as by sympathetic stimulation

B. Regulation of cardiac output

1. Starling's law of the heart—within physiologic limits the heart, when stretched by an increased returning volume of blood, contracts more strongly and pumps out the extra returned blood; heart pumps in proportion to peripheral demand

2. Autoregulation—volume of blood returning to heart and subsequently pumped by the heart is determined by the tissues; precapillary sphincters, which precede every capillary bed of body, relax and permit more blood flow when O_2 tension falls; they constrict and restrict flow when O_2 tension rises

3. Venous return—sum of all volumes of blood flowing through all capillary beds of body; initiates Starling's law of the heart

4. Nervous and hormonal influences on heart—physiologic limit on heart's ability to increase output as venous return increases; maximum at about 15 L/minute; sympathetic stimulation and epinephrine raise upper limit of cardiac output to 25 to 30 L/minute in normal individuals and to 35 L/minute in athletes; parasympathetic stimulation decreases heart rate and stroke volume

5. Neural influence on veins—venous constriction due to sympathetic stimulation milks blood toward heart, increasing venous return and cardiac output

C. Principles of circulation

1. Blood circulates because a blood pressure gradient exists in the vessels; like all fluids, blood moves from regions where its pressure is greater

to regions where pressure is less; because blood pressure is highest in the left ventricle and aorta, successively lower in arteries, arterioles, capillaries, venules, veins, and lowest in the central veins (venae cavae and right atrium), blood flows through the circulatory system in this order

2. Normal range of systolic blood pressure is 100 to 139 mm Hg; consistent readings in 140s and 150s are borderline high; readings 160 and above are high; difference between systolic and diastolic pressures is the pulse pressure, normally between 30 and 40 mm Hg

3. Blood pressure normally remains relatively constant over a wide range of activities due to

a. Neural regulation—maintains blood pressure on a minute-by-minute basis; increase in arterial pressure stimulates baroreceptors in aorta and carotid sinus, which leads to increased parasympathetic impulses to heart via vagus nerve, which slow the heart rate; a decrease in arterial pressure inhibits baroreceptors in aorta and carotid sinus and thereby leads to decreased parasympathetic impulses and increased sympathetic impulses to heart, which in turn cause a faster heart rate

b. Intrinsic circulatory regulation—maintains blood pressure on hour-to-hour basis; increased blood pressure raises hydrostatic pressure of plasma, leading to increased filtration of plasma from circulatory system to interstitial spaces; results in reduced venous return, decreased cardiac output, and decreased blood pressure

c. Kidney regulation—provides long-term day-to-day regulation of blood pressure; increased blood pressure drives more blood through kidneys, which in turn make and excrete more urine; as a result venous return, cardiac output, and blood pressure all decrease

4. Blood flow through the capillary bed—plasma filters through capillary wall at arterial end of capillary bed and becomes interstitial fluid; fluid flows over cells in capillary bed, and diffusion of nutrients and wastes occurs between fluid and cells; about half the interstitial fluid filters back into venous end of capillary bed, becoming plasma again; remaining half of interstitial fluid enters lymphatic channels along with leaked plasma proteins and returns to venous system

5. Regulation of blood flow in circulatory system—rate of flow in liters per minute directly proportional to blood pressure gradient and diameter of blood vessels; as pressure gradient and vessel diameter increase, flow rate increases; rate of flow is inversely proportional to blood vessel length and blood viscosity; as vessel length and blood viscosity increase, flow rate decreases; peripheral resistance refers to combined effects of blood vessel radius and length and blood viscosity

6. Under nonpathologic conditions blood pressure remains relatively constant; since vessel length and blood viscosity are constant, rate of flow depends almost entirely on blood vessel radius (constriction and dilation)
   a. Sympathetic discharge constricts muscular arteries and arterioles leading to viscera, kidneys, and skin and dilates those leading to skeletal muscle
   b. Postural reflexes (baroreceptor system)—arterioles are constricted when one suddenly stands after sitting or lying down; this raises blood pressure and ensures adequate perfusion of brain cells with oxygen and nutrients
   c. Sympathetic discharge constricts blood reservoirs, such as the veins, and propels blood toward the heart

D. Pulse
   1. Definition—alternate expansion and elastic recoil of blood vessel
   2. Cause—variations in pressure within vessel caused by intermittent injections of blood from heart into aorta with each ventricular contraction; pulse can be felt because of elasticity of arterial walls
   3. Pulse can be felt wherever artery lies near surface and over firm background such as bone; some of those most easily palpated are
      a. Radial artery—at wrist
      b. Temporal artery—in front of ear, or above and to outer side of eye
      c. Common carotid artery—along anterior edge of sternocleidomastoid muscle, at level of lower margin of thyroid cartilage
      d. Facial artery—at lower margin of lower jaw bone, on line with corners of mouth, in groove in mandible about one third of way forward from angle of bone
      e. Brachial artery—at bend of elbow, along inner margin of biceps muscle
      f. Posterior tibial artery—behind medial malleolus (inner "ankle bone")
      g. Dorsalis pedis—on anterior surface of foot, just below the bend of the ankle
   4. Venous pulse—in large veins only; produced by changes in venous pressure brought about by alternate contraction and relaxation of atria rather than of ventricles, as in arterial pulse

Lymphatic system
Lymphatic vessels
A. Structure—lymph capillaries similar to blood capillaries in structure; larger lymphatics similar to veins but are thinner walled, have more valves, and have lymph nodes in certain places along their course
B. Names—largest lymphatic known as thoracic duct; drains lymph from entire body except upper right quadrant into left subclavian vein (where it joins the internal jugular); right lymphatic ducts drain lymph from upper right quadrant into right subclavian vein
C. Functions
   1. Lymphatics return fluid and proteins to blood from interstitial fluid; about 60% of fluid filtered out of blood capillaries returns to circulation via lymphatics rather than by osmosis into venous ends of capillaries; about 50% of total blood proteins leak out of capillaries per day; the only way these large molecules can return to blood is via lymphatics
   2. Adequate lymph return is essential for maintaining homeostasis of blood proteins and therefore of blood volume
   3. Interference with the return of proteins to the blood results in edema caused by the loss of protein and changes in colloid osmotic pressure

Lymph nodes
A. Structure—lymphatic tissue, separated into compartments by fibrous partitions; afferent lymphatic vessels enter each node; 1 (usually) efferent vessel drains lymph out of node
B. Location—usually in clusters; some of more important groups, from nursing viewpoint, follow
   1. Submental and submaxillary groups in floor of mouth; lymph from nose, lips, and teeth drains through these nodes
   2. Superficial cervical nodes in neck, along sterno-

cleidomastoid muscle; lymph from head and neck drains through these nodes

3. Superficial cubital nodes at bend of elbow; lymph from hand and forearm drains through these nodes

4. Axillary nodes in axilla; lymph from arm and upper part of chest wall, including breast, drains through these nodes (frequently removed during mastectomy for carcinoma)

5. Inguinal nodes in groin; lymph from legs and external genitals drains through these nodes

C. Functions

1. Help defend body against injurious substances (notably, bacteria and tumor cells) by filtering them out of lymph and thereby preventing their entrance into bloodstream; leukocytes in lymph nodes destroy many of these substances by phagocytosis and antibody action

2. Lymphatic tissue of lymph nodes carries on process of hemopoiesis; specifically, it forms T and B lymphocytes

Lymph

A. Lymph—fluid in lymphatics

B. Source of lymph is interstitial fluid that has entered the lymphatic capillaries

1. Interstitial fluid is the fluid in the microscopic tissue spaces

2. Interstitial fluid is formed by plasma filtering out of the blood capillaries into the tissue spaces

Spleen

A. Location—left hypochondrium, above and behind cardiac portion of stomach

B. Structure—lymphatic tissue, similar to lymph nodes; size varies, contains numerous spaces filled with venous blood

C. Functions

1. Defense—phagocytosis of particles such as microbes, red cell fragments, and platelets by reticuloendothelial cells of spleen (reticuloendothelial system—phagocytic cells, located mainly in liver, spleen, bone marrow, and lymph nodes; also, macrophages of connective tissue and microglia in brain and cord); antibody formation by plasma cells of spleen

2. Hemopoiesis—lymphatic tissue of spleen, like that of the lymph nodes, forms lymphocytes and possibly monocytes

3. Spleen serves as blood reservoir; sympathetic

stimulation causes constriction of its capsule, squeezing out an estimated 200 ml of blood into general circulation within 1 minute

REVIEW OF PHYSICAL PRINCIPLES RELATED TO THE CIRCULATORY SYSTEM
Principles of mechanics

Newton's laws of motion

A. First law: A body remains at rest or in uniform motion in a straight line unless forces act on the body making it change its state of rest or uniform motion; in other words, bodies continue to do whatever they are doing unless some force acts on them

EXAMPLE: The heart produces the force that propels the blood through the vessels; without such a force the blood would not flow

B. Second law: If a body is accelerated, the greater the force applied to the body, the greater the acceleration; the greater the mass of the body, the more force needed to produce a desired acceleration

EXAMPLE: In polycythemia, the greater cell mass of each unit volume of blood requires greater force of cardiac contraction to produce a desired rate of blood flow

C. Third law: For every action there is an equal and opposite reaction

EXAMPLE: As blood flows through an artery, it exerts an action force on the walls of the artery; the walls of the artery exert a reaction force on the blood, which helps to provide the pressure to keep the blood flowing

Law of gravitation

Any 2 objects in the universe are attracted to each other with a force equal to the product of the masses of the 2 objects divided by the square of the distance between them; i.e., the greater the mass of the bodies, the greater the gravitational force; the closer they are together, the greater the gravitational force

EXAMPLE: When a person is standing, blood tends to pool in the lower extremities, resulting in bulging of veins in lower parts of the body and requiring greater pumping force from the heart to overcome such pooling; orthostatic hypotension and recovery by the baroreceptor reflex are a direct result of gravitational forces; the evolutionary development of valves in the venous system (particularly in the legs) is due to gravitational forces

Momentum

A. Basic concept—an object's momentum is dependent on its mass and the velocity at which it is moving

EXAMPLE: A 250-lb person in a heavy motorized wheelchair moving down a corridor at 3 miles per hour has greater momentum than a 100-lb person in a light wheelchair rolling along at 5 miles per hour

B. Changes in momentum—an object's momentum can be changed by applying a force to an object for a certain length of time; the greater the force applied and/or the longer the time that the force is applied, the greater is the change in momentum of the object

EXAMPLE: During exercise, the contracting heart imparts great momentum to the blood because the force of contraction of the myocardium is great, and the duration of contraction of the myocardium is relatively long

Energy

A. Basic concept—a property that enables a body to perform work

EXAMPLE: The heart possesses energy because it is capable of doing the work of circulating the blood

B. Work—the product of the force exerted and the distance through which the force moves

EXAMPLE: The heart exerts a force that moves the blood a certain distance

C. Laws concerning energy

1. First law of thermodynamics (law of conservation of energy)—energy cannot be created or destroyed but may be transformed from one form into another

EXAMPLE: The potential energy of the ATP molecule is transformed into the kinetic energy of cardiac muscle contraction during the cardiac cycle

2. Second law of thermodynamics—all systems in the universe have a natural tendency to become disorderly or randomized; the energy of the system continually becomes more spread out and dilute

a. Molecules tend to move from areas where they are in high concentration to areas where they are in low concentration; this is usually stated as the law of diffusion

EXAMPLES

(1) The diffusion of oxygen and carbon dioxide between the air sacs and capillaries of the lungs

(2) The diffusion of water through the membrane systems of cells (osmosis)

b. Heat always flows from a hot body into a colder one

EXAMPLES

(1) Some of the chemical energy stored in muscles is transformed into heat when muscles contract; this heat flows from the hot body (the muscles) into cooler bodies (the surrounding tissues, including blood) and helps to maintain the human body temperature of 37° C (98.6° F)

(2) When the human body is too hot, vasodilation occurs in the skin and heat radiates from the body into the cooler surrounding air

Efficiency

Efficiency—never total, since friction that occurs when two surfaces rub together produces resistance and heat; the greater the efficiency, the less heat produced; friction causes mechanical devices to eventually be worn away

EXAMPLE: If friction did not operate, the human heart would only have to beat once in a lifetime, since the initial force would propel the blood indefinitely through the blood vessels; friction continuously slows blood flow, and consequently the adult heart beats an average of 72 times each minute

Principles of physical properties of matter

Solids

Concept of elasticity—because of external or internal stresses, solids may change their shape or size

EXAMPLE: Heart and blood vessels constantly change shape as blood pressure and degree of neural stimulation undergo change

Liquids

A. Hydrostatic pressure—pressure (force per unit area) caused by the weight of the fluid on matter submerged in the fluid

EXAMPLE: The weight of blood in a capillary exerts a hydrostatic force that helps to filter the blood through the capillary wall, forming interstitial fluid

B. Pascal's principle—when pressure is applied to a fluid in a closed, nonflexible container, that pressure is transmitted undiminished throughout all parts of the fluid and the pressure acts in all directions

EXAMPLES: In the circulatory system the pressure

exerted as a result of the contracting ventricles is transmitted throughout the blood vessels of the circulatory system; this pressure is responsible for blood flow

1. Pressure—fluid always flows from regions of higher pressure to those of lower pressure; the pressure in the human circulatory system is highest in the ventricles during systole, decreases throughout the length of the circulatory system, and is lowest in the atria; the normal pressure of blood in the circulatory system varies with age and disease
2. Lumen of the tube—the flow of fluid through a tube is directly proportional to the radius of the tube; e.g., the degree of constriction of the arterioles for the most part determines the quantity of blood entering the capillary beds and returning to the heart
3. Length of the tube—the longer the tube, the less fluid flow there is through the tube in a unit of time; when blood circulation to the skin is greatly increased, the heart must increase its output to maintain normal circulation, since many more miles of tubing (capillaries) have been added to the system
4. Viscosity—the molecular components of a fluid exert forces of attraction on each other; as the fluid flows along, an internal friction, caused by the molecular attractions of the fluid's components, tends to impede fluid flow; this internal resistance to fluid flow is viscosity
   a. Anemia—because of a reduced number of red blood cells, the viscosity of the blood is decreased; therefore blood returns to the heart more rapidly, increasing cardiac output, which may overwork the heart during periods of increased exercise
   b. Polycythemia—an increased number of red blood cells in the blood increases its viscosity; blood flows more sluggishly and the blood pressure will increase to compensate
C. Capillarity—when a small-diameter tube is dipped into water or other fluid, the water will rise in the tube because of adhesion of the water molecules to the components of the glass; surface tension then causes the film of water to contract and pull itself up the tube; the water continues to rise until the weight of the water balances the adhesive force; this rise of the fluid level in a tube is called capillarity or capillary action

EXAMPLE: Capillarity draws blood into a capillary tube when a technician takes a small blood sample for various analyses

Gases

Gases are carried in circulatory system by combining with other molecules

Principles of acoustics

Basic concept—sound is a mechanical vibration that cannot occur in a vacuum; it is propagated best through solids and through liquids better than gases; sound travels in waves from a vibrating source such as human vocal cords, a loudspeaker, or a dropped object

EXAMPLES

1. A very faint heartbeat might be heard by placing the ear on the chest; even strong heartbeats cannot be heard distinctly with just the ears
2. The sound vibrations (waves) pass readily through the tissue of the human body to the surface of the skin where a stethoscope can pick them up
3. Ultrasonic fetal heart monitors can detect the fetal heart beat in as early as the twelfth week of gestation
4. Echocardiography—a sound wave–constructed picture of the heart helps in the identification of cardiac diseases

Principles of electricity

Electric force

A. The atoms composing all matter represent an almost perfect balance of protons and electrons; the attraction of a positive proton for a negative electron (opposite charges attracting) is the electric force that also results in like charges repelling
B. Electric forces hold atoms and molecules together and thus hold solid matter together; electric forces also provide the source for all chemical energy; the molecular rearrangements associated with cellular metabolism derive their energy from electric forces between enzymes, substrates, and cofactors

Conductors and insulators

A. Conductors are good transferrers of electric fields and the energy they contain; copper and aluminum are good conductors and are commonly used for all electric wiring, including the electrodes for cardiac monitoring
B. Insulators—rubber and most nonmetals are good insulators, as is the connective tissue separating the atria and ventricles of the heart and electrically insu-

lating these regions; consequently the only way electrical energy can flow from the AV node to the ventricles is through the heart's specialized conducting system (bundles of His) in the interventricular septum

C. Water as a conductor—distilled water is a poor conductor, although tap water contains enough charged particles (ions) to make it a fairly good electric conductor; the ions (electrolytes) of body fluids make them excellent conductors of electrical energy

Application of electricity

A. Electronic devices used in health care
  1. Electronic cardiac pacemakers—battery-operated devices supplement or replace defective electric stimulation in the human heart and thus help to maintain the individual's heartbeat at a selected rate
  2. Defibrillator—electronic device that delivers electrical energy through electrodes strategically placed on an individual whose heart is in atrial or ventricular fibrillation; the use of such a device is based on the premise that the sustaining mechanism of the fibrillation process is different from the initiating mechanism; thus, if the initiating mechanism is no longer present and the sustaining mechanism is terminated by the defibrillating electric current, sinus rhythm will ensue

B. Applications to the human body—the contraction of all types of muscle is preceded by depolarization of the muscle fibers; ions carry the electric charges
  EXAMPLE: Electrocardiograms measure and record the electric activity of the heart as this activity is carried to the surface of the body by the ions of the body fluids; this information provides an electric picture of the heart's activity

Principles of light (electromagnetic waves)

Basic concept—high-frequency electromagnetic waves emitted as a result of the excitation of the innermost orbital electrons of atoms; to excite the innermost orbital electron, considerable energy must be expended
EXAMPLE: Angiography—observation of motion picture x-ray images

REVIEW OF CHEMICAL PRINCIPLES RELATED TO THE CIRCULATORY SYSTEM
Water
General information

A. A chemical combination of oxygen and hydrogen
B. Most abundant compound

C. Essential to life
D. Sixty percent of the average adult human body weight is water; this percentage may be as high as 80% in infants and as low as 40% to 50% in the elderly

Physical properties

A. Colorless, tasteless, odorless liquid
B. Exists chiefly as ice at low temperatures, liquid at moderate temperatures, and gas at elevated temperatures
  1. Water changes from liquid to solid at the freezing point (0° C [32° F])
  2. Water changes from liquid to gas at the boiling point (100° C [212° F])
  3. These transition points in the physical states of water are the basis of the Celsius and Fahrenheit temperature scales
  4. Conversion from one temperature scale to the other is accomplished by using the formula

$$C° = \frac{5}{9}(F° - 32)$$

Chemical properties

A. Water molecule is a polar molecule and because of this molecular shape, water is an excellent solvent for ionic or slightly ionic substances
B. Water is a very stable compound; dissociates very slightly to H^+ and OH^- ions under normal conditions
C. Electrolysis can dissociate water into its components, hydrogen and oxygen
D. Many chemical reactions need water as a solvent before reaction will occur
E. Process of splitting a substance with the addition of water is called hydrolysis, which is the basis for the digestion of food
F. Crystals formed with water in their molecule are called hydrates

Importance

A. Necessary for life; universal solvent
B. Essential for many chemical reactions
C. Needed for digestion (hydrolysis) of food
D. Forms large percentage of plant and animal tissue
E. Necessary for circulation of blood; plasma is a water solution
F. Necessary for elimination; urine, sweat, feces contain water
G. Lubricating fluid at joints (synovial fluid) contains water
H. Water has a great capacity for absorbing heat or giv-

ing off absorbed heat; useful in ice packs, hydrotherapy, and hot compresses

Water as a standard

A. Thermometer scales—the freezing and boiling points of water are used to standardize Celsius and Fahrenheit scales
B. Specific gravity—compares the density of a volume of water to the density of the same volume of another substance
C. Weight—1 g is the weight of 1 ml of water at 4° C
D. Calorie—the heat needed to raise 1 g of water 1° C
E. pH—water acts as neutrality point on acid-base scale

Body regulation of water content

A. The osmoreceptors of the hypothalamus influence the neurohypophysis in its release of ADH (antidiuretic hormone or vasopressin); working through the kidney tubules, this hormone regulates water reabsorption from urine
B. The thirst center of the hypothalamus detects body dehydration and produces the sensation of thirst

Proteins

A. Polymers of alpha amino acids connected by peptide bonds
B. Characteristics of proteins
  1. Protein molecules are very large
  2. Proteins form colloid particles in solution
  3. Synthesis of proteins is in ribosomes of cell, according to specific genetic patterns under direction of the nucleic acids DNA and RNA
  4. Structure patterns of proteins are extremely specific; proteins differ from species to species, individual to individual, organ to organ; present problems for transplant operations
  5. Proteins are the tissue builders of the body
C. Classification of proteins
  1. Simple proteins—give amino acids on hydrolysis
    a. Albumins—water soluble, coagulated by heat; e.g., lactalbumin (milk), serum albumin (blood), egg white; albumin is most important in the development of the plasma colloid osmotic pressure, which helps control (through osmosis) the flow of water between the plasma and interstitial fluid; during a condition such as starvation, a fall in the albumin level of the blood results in a fall in the plasma colloid osmotic pressure; this results in edema caused by less fluid being drawn by osmosis into the capillaries from the interstitial spaces
    b. Globulins—insoluble in water, soluble in di-

lute salt solutions, coagulated by heat; e.g., lactoglobulin (milk), serum globulin (blood), gamma serum globulin (form antibodies of blood)

Enzymes

A. Organic catalysts that enter into reactions and are reformed at end of reaction
B. Needed in minute amounts
C. Protein in nature and inactivated by all factors that denature proteins; e.g., high temperature, changes in pH
D. Substrate is the substance acted on by an enzyme; e.g., CO_2 and H_2O are the substrate for the enzyme carbonic anhydrase, found in the erythrocyte, which catalyzes the conversion of CO_2 and H_2O into carbonic acid
E. Enzymes usually have ending "ase" added on to name of substrate or to action of enzyme; e.g., sucrase—enzyme hydrolyzing sucrose; lactic acid dehydrogenase—enzyme removing hydrogen from lactic acid
F. Enzymes, being proteins, are usually quite specific in action
  1. One enzyme will usually catalyze only 1 reaction—substrate specificity
  2. Enzyme activity will be high at temperature specific for the enzyme and low at other temperatures—temperature specificity
  3. Enzyme activity will be high at the pH specific for the enzyme and low at the other pH values—pH specificity
G. Certain inorganic ions act to speed up or slow down enzyme activity—enzyme activators and enzyme inhibitors
H. Enzymes acting within cells are called intracellular enzymes; e.g., the enzymes bringing about the breakdown of glucose and other sugars, the synthesis of carbohydrates, proteins, and nucleic acids all function within cells and are intracellular enzymes
I. Enzymes acting outside cells are called extracellular enzymes; e.g., the digestive enzymes found in the mouth, stomach, and small intestine all function outside of cells and are extracellular enzymes
J. Some enzymes exist in 2 parts
  1. Apoenzyme—protein part of enzyme
  2. Coenzyme—nonprotein part of enzyme
  3. Holoenzyme—the apoenzyme and the coenzyme together

Solutions

Basic concepts

A. Substances that dissolve in other substances form solutions
B. A solution can be classified as a homogeneous mixture
C. Solids, liquids, and gases can be dissolved in other solids, liquids, and gases
   1. Substance dissolved is called the solute
   2. Substance in which the solute is dissolved is called the solvent
   3. Common solution is one where a solid, liquid, or gas is dissolved in a liquid; e.g., blood is mainly a liquid (water) containing dissolved ions, sugars, amino acids, and respiratory gases

Factors affecting solubility

A. Chemical and physical nature of the solvent
B. Chemical and physical nature of the solute
C. Amount of solvent versus amount of solute
D. Temperature—warming aids some solutes (solids) to dissolve; cooling aids others (gases) to dissolve
E. Presence or absence of mixing; mixing usually speeds solution reaction
F. Pressure—especially when one of the components is a gas

Types of solutions

A. Dilute—a small amount of solute in a relatively large amount of solvent
B. Concentrated—a large amount of solute in a relatively small amount of solvent
C. Unsaturated—a solution holding less solute than is possible for it to dissolve at a certain temperature and pressure
D. Saturated—a solution holding all the solute that it can dissolve at a certain temperature and pressure
E. Supersaturated solution—unique case of a solution holding more solute than it normally should for a particular temperature and pressure
   1. Very unstable condition
   2. Excess solute easily precipitates from solution
F. Percent solution—grams of solute per gram of solution
G. Molar solution (M)—the number of gram-molecular weights of solute per liter of solution
H. Normal solution (N)—the number of gram-equivalent weights of solute per liter of solution
I. Molal solution—a gram-molecular weight of solute in 1000 g of solvent

Osmosis

A. Process of selective diffusion
B. More concentrated solution is separated from a less concentrated solution by a membrane that is permeable only to the solvent—a semipermeable membrane
C. Solvent moves more rapidly from the dilute solution into the concentrated solution than in the reverse direction
D. Pressure forcing the solvent across the membrane is called osmotic pressure
E. Isotonic solutions—when the osmotic pressures of 2 liquids are equal, the flow of solvent is equalized and the 2 solutions are said to be isotonic to each other
   1. Physiologic saline—0.89% NaCl in distilled water—is isotonic to blood and body tissues
   2. Five percent dextrose in water is isotonic to blood and body tissues
   3. When isotonic solutions are administered intravenously, the blood cells remain intact
F. Hypertonic solutions—when one solution has less osmotic pressure (is more concentrated) than another, it draws fluid from the other and is said to be hypertonic to it
G. Hypotonic solutions—when one solution has more osmotic pressure (is more dilute) than another, it forces fluid into the other and is said to be hypotonic to it
H. Both hypertonic and hypotonic types of solution are destructive to body cells and should not be used in intravenous injections
I. Osmosis constantly occurs as part of the normal physiology of human beings
   1. Capillary membrane—the colloid osmotic pressure of the plasma draws fluid from the tissue spaces back into the capillaries; edema results when disease states upset the normal colloid osmotic pressure (starvation, kidney disease)
   2. Plasma membranes—water freely flows from interstitial fluid into intracellular fluid and vice versa, depending on the relative concentration of water in these 2 fluid compartments

Size of the particle of solute determines type of solution

A. Atomic, ionic, and most molecular-sized particles are extremely small—submicroscopic
   1. Particles are freely dispersed by solvent

2. Particles are kept in solution by movement and attraction of solvent molecules
3. Substances of this class are called *crystalloids*
4. Crystalloids form true solutions
   a. Clear in appearance—particles cannot be seen
   b. Solute stays in solution as long as the solvent is not removed by evaporation or other means
   c. Solute accompanies solvent as it passes through filters and most membranes; e.g., the ions Na^+, K^+, Cl^-, HCO_3^- dissolved in plasma are in true solution
B. Large particles of matter do not form solutions in the real sense of the term
   1. Solute particles easily settle out of solvent
   2. Solute particles can be seen by naked eye or with microscope when suspended in solvent
   3. Solute can be removed by ordinary filtration
   4. Substances of this class are called coarse suspensions; e.g., the erythrocytes are suspended in plasma and can be seen microscopically and removed by fine filters or centrifugation
C. The colloid particle
   1. Intermediate in size between the crystalloid and the coarse suspensoid
   2. Particle size much larger than that of crystalloid although smaller than particle of coarse suspensoid; diameter of colloid around 0.0000001 to 0.00001 mm
   3. Solutions of colloids
      a. Solute particles dispersed by solvent
      b. Solution—clear, cloudy, or opalescent
      c. Show bright path of reflected light when a beam of light is passed through solution—the Tyndall effect
      d. More stable than coarse suspensoids, less stable than true solutions
      e. With time, the colloid particles will settle out
      f. Affect osmotic pressure less than crystalloids
      g. Most of the proteins in plasma are dispersed as colloidal particles
      h. Blood is classified as a colloid and a suspension
   4. Colloid particles will pass through ordinary filters but will be held back by most membranes
   5. Colloid particles carry electric charges on their surfaces—not to be confused with ionic charges
   6. Importance of colloid suspensions

a. Proteins, fats, and many carbohydrates form molecules in the colloid range in size
b. These form colloid solutions in the cells and body fluids
c. Protoplasm of cell itself is a colloid

Buffers

A. A poorly ionized acid or base, plus a salt formed from that acid or base, acts as a buffer in solution; e.g., a typical buffer of the blood is carbonic acid (H_2CO_3) plus its salt, sodium bicarbonate ($NaHCO_3$)
B. A buffer allows the addition of acid ions (H_3O^+) and basic ions (OH^-) without a change occurring in the pH of the solution to which the addition is made
C. The body regulates its pH through buffer systems; e.g., during normal metabolism, the body builds up CO_2, which forms carbonic acid with water; the subsequent ionization of carbonic acid would tend to lower the body fluid pH; but through increased rate and depth of breathing, the excess CO_2 is expelled from the body; thus the circulatory and respiratory systems interacting with buffer systems help to regulate the body's pH
D. Blood buffers
   1. Proteins, amino acids, bicarbonates, phosphates all act to prevent changes in the pH of the blood
   2. Blood buffers are necessary to prevent changes in the pH of the blood that are incompatible with life

Radioactive elements

A. Certain elements (such as radium) have atoms whose nuclei are naturally unstable and are constantly breaking down at a set rate
B. In the breakdown process these elements emit high-energy particles and rays that can penetrate other materials—radioactive rays
   1. Alpha particle—fast-moving helium nucleus
      a. Weight—4 atomic weight units (awu)
      b. Charge—2^+
      c. Penetration—slight
   2. Beta particle—fast-moving electrons
      a. Weight—practically 0 awu
      b. Charge—1^-
      c. Penetration—moderate
   3. Gamma ray—penetrating ray, similar to light ray
      a. Weight—none
      b. Charge—none
      c. Penetration—high

C. Uses of radioactivity
   1. Leukemia, polycythemia, and bone cancer treatments with radioactive phosphorus (^{32}P); radiophosphorus has also been useful in localizing breast tumors because of the uptake of the ^{32}P into the rapidly growing, cancerous tissue
   2. Studies on red cells (erythrocytes) and hemoglobin formation with radioactive iron (^{59}Fe) and radioactive chromium (^{51}Cr)

REVIEW OF MICROBIOLOGIC PRINCIPLES RELATED TO THE CIRCULATORY SYSTEM
Major pathogens

A. *Streptococcus pyogenes*—a gram-positive streptococcus; the most virulent strain (Group A beta hemolytic streptococci) causes scarlet fever, septic sore throat, tonsillitis, cellulitis, puerperal fever, erysipelas, rheumatic fever, and glomerulonephritis
B. *Streptococcus viridans*—gram-positive streptococcus; distinguishable from *S. pyogenes* by its alpha hemolysis (rather than beta) of red blood cells; the most common cause of subacute bacterial endocarditis

Resistance

A. Nonspecific—resistance directed against all invading microbes; varies considerably from one species to another and even among individuals of same species
   1. Body surface barriers
      a. Intact skin and mucosa
      b. Cilia and secretion of mucus
   2. Antimicrobial secretions
      a. Oil of skin—contains fatty acids effective against many bacteria and fungi
      b. Tears—contain lysozyme, a bactericidal (gram-positive) enzyme
      c. Gastric juice—contains highly bactericidal hydrochloric acid
      d. Vaginal secretions—low pH acts to inhibit microbial growth
   3. Internal antimicrobial agents
      a. Interferon—an antiviral substance produced within the cells in response to a viral attack; it inhibits viral growth and multiplication
      b. Properdin—a protein agent in blood that destroys certain gram-negative bacteria and viruses
      c. Lysozyme—ubiquitous; destroys mainly gram-positive bacteria

   4. Phagocytosis—part of the role of the reticuloendothelial system
      a. Phagocytes—cells that ingest and destroy microbes
         (1) Microphages—the polymorphonuclear leukocytes of the blood, of which the neutrophils are the most active; in the inflammatory response they pass through the intact capillary wall (diapedesis) into the intercellular area
         (2) Macrophages
            (a) Fixed (or sessile) macrophages—phagocytes lining the capillary endothelium and sinuses of liver (Kupffer's cells), spleen, bone marow, lymph nodes, and other organs where they remove microbes from the blood
            (b) Wandering macrophages (histiocytes)—blood monocytes that enter the tissues (via diapedesis) and devour intercellular debris, including debilitated microphages
B. Specific resistance—resistance directed against a specific pathogen (foreign protein) or its toxin
   1. Antigen—any substance, including allergens, that stimulates the production of antibodies when introduced into the body; typically, antigens are foreign proteins, the most potent being microbial cells and their products
      a. Plasma cells—the antibody-producing cells that arise from B lymphocytes in the presence of antigens; a specific antigen provokes the production of a specific antibody (homologous antibody), which is considered to be ineffective against any other antigen
      b. Memory cells—a large population of antibodies that develops on first encounter with an antigen; they become somewhat dormant until stimulated by subsequent encounters with the antigen; this phenomenon explains the dramatic rise in antibody titer following a booster shot of a vaccine (anamnestic reaction)
   2. Antibody—an immune substance produced by plasma cells; antibodies are gamma globulin molecules and are commonly referred to as immunoglobulin (Ig)
      a. Chemical structure—the antibody molecule is made up of 4 polypeptide chains in 2 pairs
      b. Classification—there are 5 major classes of antibodies

(1) Immunoglobulin G (IgG) antibodies—most important class making up more than 80% of the total immunoglobulins; only immunoglobulin that passes the placental barrier, providing natural passive immunity to the newborn

(2) Immunoglobulin A (IgA) antibodies—present in blood, mucus, and human milk secretions; play an important role against respiratory pathogens

(3) Immunoglobulin M (IgM) antibodies—the first antibodies to be detected after an injection of antigen; bactericidal for gram-negative bacteria under specific conditions

(4) Immunoglobulin D (IgD) antibodies—present in small numbers in normal individuals; specific immunologic role presently under investigation

(5) Immunoglobulin E (IgE) antibodies—responsible for hypersensitivity and allergies; these antibodies exist tightly bound to the surface of mast cells (large basophilic connective tissue cells)

   (a) Upon introduction of their homologous antigens (allergens), they cause the mast cells to release histamine and other pharmacologic agents

   (b) The release of histamine and other pharmacologic agents causes the symptoms of hypersensitive reactions

   (c) This process explains the relief of symptoms by the administration of antihistamines

3. Antigen-antibody reactions
   a. Agglutination—the clumping together of cells and specific antigens by homologous antibodies called agglutinins
   b. Cytolysis—the disruption or dissolution of cells (lysis) by homologous antibodies called cytolysins or lysins
   c. Opsonification—the rendering of bacteria and other cells susceptible to phagocytosis by homologous antibodies called opsonins
   d. Neutralization (viral)—the rendering of viruses noninfective by homologous antibodies called neutralizing antibodies
   e. Neutralization (toxin)—the chemical neutralization of a toxin by homologous antibodies called antitoxins
   f. Precipitation—the formation of an insoluble complex (precipitate) in the reaction between a soluble antigen and its homologous antibodies called precipitins
4. Complement-fixation—a group of blood serum proteins needed in certain antigen-antibody reactions; both the complement and the antibody must be present for a reaction to occur

Immunity

A. Species immunity—certain species are naturally immune to specific microorganisms; e.g., humans are immune to distemper, dogs are immune to measles

B. Active immunity—antibodies formed in the body
   1. Natural active immunity—antibodies formed by the individual during the course of the disease; in some instances the antibodies provide lifelong immunity; e.g., measles, chickenpox, yellow fever, smallpox
   2. Artificial active immunity—the use of a vaccine or toxoid to stimulate the formation of homologous antibodies; revaccination (booster shots) are often needed to sustain antibody titer (anamnestic effect)
      a. Killed vaccines—antigenic preparations containing microbes grown in the laboratory separated from growth medium and killed by heat or a chemical agent; usually injected subcutaneously; less often given by intramuscular or oral routes; e.g., pertussis vaccine, typhoid vaccine
      b. Live vaccines—antigenic preparations containing microbes weakened (attenuated) by drying, continued and prolonged passage through culture media or animals (to induce mutations), or by other means; tyically such vaccines are more antigenic than killed preparations; e.g., oral (Sabin) poliomyelitis vaccine, measles vaccine
      c. Toxoids—antigenic preparations composed of inactivated bacterial toxins (generally an exotoxin treated with formaldehyde); e.g., tetanus, diphtheria toxoids

C. Passive immunity—antibodies acquired from an outside source
   1. Natural passive immunity—the passage of preformed antibodies from mother through the placenta or colostrum to the baby; therefore during the first few weeks of life the newborn is immune

to certain diseases to which the mother has active immunity

2. Artificial passive immunity—the injection of antisera derived from immunized animals or humans; antisera (antiserums) provide immediate and often complete protection in susceptible exposed persons and also are of value in treatment; e.g., diphtheria antitoxin, tetanus antitoxin (individuals may be hypersensitive to certain sera such as horse serum, and pretesting for hypersensitivity must be carried out before administration)

PHARMACOLOGY RELATED TO CIRCULATORY SYSTEM DISORDERS

A. Cardiac glycosides
  1. General implications for nurses
    a. Check apical pulse for 1 minute before administration; if pulse is below 60 or above 120 beats per minute, the dose should be withheld and the physician notified
    b. Observe for signs of digitalis toxicity, which include nausea and vomiting, visual disturbances, bigeminal rhythm, and muscle weakness
    c. Increase potassium in diet because digitalis toxicity is more common if the patient is hypokalemic
    d. Patient teaching regarding the above factors
    e. Observe patient for adverse effects
      (1) Most frequent—nausea, vomiting, headache, drowsiness, insomnia, vertigo, confusion are all attributable to drug action at central nervous system sites; oral forms also cause nausea and vomiting by irritation of gastric mucosa
      (2) Bradycardia attributable to drug-induced slowing of the sinoatrial (SA) node firing; arrhythmias are first evidence of toxicity in one third of patients; premature nodal or ventricular impulses are varying degrees of heart block caused by drug action that slows transmission of impulses through the atrioventricular (AV) node
      (3) Xanthopsia (yellow vision) caused by drug effect on visual cones
      (4) Gynecomastia (mammary enlargement) in males resulting from estrogen-like steroid portion of digitalis glycosides

2. Action
  a. Positive inotropic action (increased force of contraction) is achieved by increasing permeability of muscle membranes to the calcium and sodium ions required for contraction of muscle fibrils
  b. Negative chronotropic effect (decreased rate of contraction) is achieved by an action mediated by the vagus nerve that slows firing of the SA node and impulse transmission through the AV node
3. Examples of drugs
  a. Digitalis
  b. Digitoxin (Crystodigin, Digitaline)
  c. Digoxin (Lanoxin)
  d. Gitalin (Gitaligin)
  e. Lanatoside C (Cedilanid)
  f. Ouabain
4. Digitalization
  a. Provides an initial loading dose for acute effect on the heart
  b. After desired effect is achieved, the dosage is lowered to maintenance level, replacing drug metabolized and excreted each day

B. Antiarrhythmic drugs
  1. General implications for nurses
    a. Observe for variations in cardiac rhythm
    b. If medication given intravenously, maintain patient on monitor
    c. Observe for specific adverse effects of each drug
    d. Patient teaching regarding drug action, specific side effects, and the need for continued medical supervision
  2. Quinidine preparations
    a. Actions
      (1) Control atrial arrhythmias by prolonging the effective refractory period and slowing depolarization
      (2) Quinidine has a mild depressant effect on the hepatic enzyme system, which synthesizes coagulation factors; therefore concomitant use with oral anticoagulants may cause excess hypoprothrombinemia with bleeding
      (3) Quinidine has anticholinergic properties, and excess cholinergic blocking (excess dryness of mouth, constipation) may result with concomitant use of belladonna

alkaloids or other drugs with anticholinergic properties (phenothiazines, antihistamines, tricyclic antidepressants, procainamide hydrochloride)
b. Examples
(1) Quinidine gluconate (Quinaglute)
(2) Quinidine hydrochloride
(3) Quinidine polygalacturonate (Cardiaquin)
(4) Quinidine sulfate (Quinidex, Quinora)
c. Adverse effects
(1) Heart block caused by drug depression of AV node and ventricular conduction tissue
(2) Accelerated AV conduction or ventricular tachycardia occurring with initial dose is caused by vagolytic action (may be lessened by digitalis administration)
(3) Vasodilation with syncope and hypotension caused by depressant effect on all muscle tissue may occur with high dosage or IV use
(4) Gastric irritation with nausea, vomiting, and diarrhea may occur with oral use
3. Lidocaine hydrochloride
a. Action—controls ventricular irritability by shortening the refractory period and suppresses ectopic foci
b. Adverse effects
(1) Drowsiness
(2) Nervousness
(3) Blurred vision
(4) Nausea
(5) Tremor
(6) Hypotension
(7) Generalized paresthesias
(8) Convulsions
(9) Respiratory arrest
4. Procainamide hydrochloride (Pronestyl)
a. Actions
(1) Controls ventricular and atrial arrhythmias by prolonging the refractory period of the heart and slowing the conduction of cardiac impulses
(2) Has some anticholinergic effects
b. Adverse effects
(1) Hypotension
(2) Bradycardia
(3) Decreased motility of gastrointestinal tract (paralytic ileus)

5. Phenytoin (Dilantin)
a. Action—controls atrial or ventricular arrhythmias by reducing automaticity without decreasing conduction
b. Adverse effects
(1) Lack of coordination
(2) Dizziness
(3) Nausea
(4) Vomiting
(5) Nystagmus
(6) Megaloblastic anemia
(7) High alkalinity requires infusion in large veins at maximum rate of 50 mg per minute
6. Disopyramide phosphate (Norpace)
a. Actions
(1) Exerts antiarrhythmic effect by decreasing the rate of diastolic depolarization
(2) Primarily used to treat ventricular arrhythmias
b. Adverse effects
(1) Contraindicated in the presence of cardiogenic shock or heart block
(2) Urinary retention
(3) Constipation
(4) Dry mouth
(5) Hypotension
(6) Diarrhea
(7) Nausea
7. Propranolol hydrochloride (Inderal)
a. Actions
(1) Used effectively in the treatment of supraventricular arrhythmias and is currently used for therapy of angina pectoris and hypertension
(2) Has a negative inotropic effect by depressing cardiac response to sympathetic nervous system stimuli via blocking action at beta receptors
(a) Some vasodilation of coronary arteries occurs
(b) Reduces inotropic and chronotropic effect of exercise, and patient may be light-headed, weak, and fatigued after exercise
b. Adverse effects
(1) Bradycardia
(2) Cardiac arrest
(3) AV block

    (4) Nausea, vomiting, and diarrhea

    (5) Visual disturbances and hallucinations

C. Drugs that increase the heart rate

  1. General implications for nurses

    a. Monitor vital signs frequently

    b. Awareness of drug effect on preexisting conditions

    c. Observe for adverse effects, such as tachycardia and those specific to each drug

  2. Atropine sulfate

    a. Actions

      (1) Suppresses parasympathetic nervous system control at SA and AV nodes

      (2) Administer IV by bolus to increase the heart rate in severe bradycardia

    b. Adverse effects

      (1) Decreased bladder emptying

      (2) Decreased glandular secretions

      (3) Depression of gastrointestinal motility

  3. Isoproterenol hydrochloride (Isuprel Hydrochloride)

    a. Actions

      (1) Stimulates beta-adrenergic receptors of sympathetic nervous system, thereby also improving tissue perfusion

      (2) Used in cardiogenic shock and Adams-Stokes and carotid sinus syndromes

    b. Adverse effects

      (1) Hypotension

      (2) Tachycardia and palpitation

      (3) Flushing of skin

      (4) Headache

      (5) Anxiety and restlessness

  4. Epinephrine hydrochloride

    a. Actions

      (1) Acts via sympathetic nervous system to stimulate the rate and force of cardiac contraction; used in cardiogenic shock and heart block

      (2) Reduces blood flow to abdominal viscera

      (3) Bronchodilation

    b. Examples

      (1) Adrenaline Hydrochloride

      (2) Vaponefrin

    c. Adverse effects

      (1) Palpitation, cardiac arrhythmias

      (2) Throbbing headache

      (3) Urinary retention

D. Drugs that dilate the coronary arteries—nitrates

  1. General implications for nurses

    a. Instruct patient to take sublingual medication only when sitting or lying down because of postural hypotension

    b. Instruct patient to store medication correctly

    c. Observe for adverse effects

      (1) Facial blushing

      (2) Hypotension, which may be sudden if drug is taken with alcohol

      (3) Vertigo, fainting

      (4) Headache

  2. Actions

    a. Decrease resistance of smooth muscle of large-capacity vessels (veins, venules) and high-resistance vessels, which decrease cardiac work and myocardial oxygen requirements

    b. Decrease the incidence of anginal attacks and improve work tolerance

    c. Decrease central venous pressure, left ventricle end-diastolic pressure, and pulmonary wedge pressure and lower blood pressure, causing a reflex increase in heart rate

    d. Increase blood flow through coronary arteries and collateral channels with increased blood flow to ischemic areas of the heart

  3. Examples

    a. Nitrates for sublingual use

      (1) Erythrityl tetranitrate (Cardilate)

      (2) Isosorbide dinitrate (Isordil, Sorbitrate)

      (3) Nitroglycerin

        (a) Effect in 1 to 2 minutes; repeat dose in 5 minutes if pain persists

        (b) When taken 3 minutes before activity known to cause anginal pain, pain-free exercise tolerance increases

        (c) Tablets deteriorate rapidly in heat, light, moisture (potency loss by sublimation)

        (d) Sublingual use causes slight stinging, burning, tingling under the tongue, and absence of these signs can indicate deterioration of the drug

    b. Nitrates for oral use

      (1) Erythrityl tetranitrate (Cardilate)

      (2) Mannitol hexanitrate (Nitranitol)

      (3) Pentaerythritol tetranitrate (Peritrate)

      (4) Trolnitrate phosphate (Metamine)

(5) Isosorbide dinitrate (Sorbitrate, Iso-Bid, Isordil)

   c. Nitrates for topical use

      (1) Nitro-Bid ointment

      (2) Nitrol ointment

      (3) Nitrong ointment

E. Drugs that dilate the peripheral blood vessels

  1. General implications for nurses

    a. Observe for common side effects, such as postural hypotension, weakness, and dizziness, as well as those specific to drugs

    b. Monitor blood pressure in standing and prone positions

    c. Teach patient and family side effects and necessity of continued medical supervision

  2. Rauwolfia alkaloids

    a. Actions

      (1) Inhibit the stimulation of vascular smooth muscles

      (2) Cross the blood-brain barrier and act on medullary vasomotor centers and on central nervous tissue to cause sedative effect

    b. Examples

      (1) Reserpine (Rau-Sed, Reserpoid, Sandril, Serpasil)

      (2) Syrosingopine (Singoserp)

      (3) Deserpidine (Harmonyl)

      (4) Rauwolfia serpentina (Raudixin, Rautina, Wolfina)

      (5) Rescinnamine (Moderil)

    c. Adverse effects

      (1) Bizarre dreams, drowsiness

      (2) Nasal congestion

      (3) Bradycardia, lethargy

  3. Guanethidine sulfate (Ismelin)

    a. Action—depresses activity of sympathetic nervous system

    b. Adverse effects

      (1) Persistent diarrhea

      (2) Hypotension

      (3) Bradycardia

      (4) Dizziness and weakness

      (5) Inhibits ejaculation

  4. Methyldopa (Aldomet)

    a. Action—depletes norepinephrine at peripheral and central sites

    b. Adverse effects

      (1) Bradycardia

      (2) Dizziness, drowsiness

      (3) Orthostatic hypotension

      (4) Diarrhea

  5. Hydralazine hydrochloride

    a. Actions

      (1) Relaxes small muscles of arteries, causing vasodilation and a lowering of blood pressure

      (2) Increases cardiac output

    b. Examples

      (1) Apresoline Hydrochloride

      (2) Dralzine

    c. Adverse effects

      (1) Postural hypotension

      (2) Tachycardia

      (3) Numbness and tingling of extremities

      (4) Localized edema

      (5) Gastrointestinal disturbances

  6. Sodium nitroprusside (Nipride)

    a. Actions

      (1) Causes peripheral dilation to lower blood pressure in a hypertensive crisis

      (2) Must be administered by continuous IV infusion and must be protected from heat, light, and moisture

    b. Adverse effects

      (1) Sweating, muscular twitching, and apprehension associated with rapid reduction of blood pressure

      (2) Skin rash

      (3) Psychosis, if toxic levels are reached

  7. Diazoxide (Hyperstat IV)

    a. Action—dilates peripheral arterioles, producing an immediate fall in blood pressure

    b. Adverse effects

      (1) Hyperglycemia

      (2) Marked sodium and water retention

      (3) Transient tachycardia

      (4) Gastrointestinal disturbances

  8. Clonidine hydrochloride (Catapres)

    a. Actions

      (1) Decreases cardiac output

      (2) Reduces peripheral resistance

    b. Adverse effects

      (1) Orthostatic hypotension

      (2) Dry mouth

      (3) Sedation

      (4) Rapid rise in blood pressure if therapy is discontinued abruptly

9. Prazosin hydrochloride (Minipress)
   a. Actions
      (1) Smooth muscle relaxant
      (2) Relaxation of peripheral arterioles results in decreased peripheral resistance
   b. Adverse effects
      (1) Dizziness, drowsiness
      (2) Weakness
      (3) Palpitation and syncope
      (4) Vertigo
10. Cyclandelate (Cyclospasmol)
    a. Action—smooth muscle relaxant causing decreased peripheral resistance
    b. Adverse effects
       (1) Flushing
       (2) Tachycardia
       (3) Nausea
11. Isoxsuprine hydrochloride (Vasodilan)
    a. Actions
       (1) Vasodilator due to smooth muscle relaxation
       (2) Uterine relaxant
    b. Adverse effects
       (1) Palpitation, tachycardia
       (2) Dizziness, weakness
F. Drugs that decrease circulating blood volume (diuretics)
   1. General implications for nurses
      a. Assess intake and output
      b. Weigh patient daily under standard conditions
      c. Observe for signs of electrolyte imbalance and weakness, as well as specific adverse effects of drugs
      d. Administer in morning
      e. Encourage foods high in potassium if indicated
   2. Thiazides
      a. Actions
         (1) Wide use includes therapy of hypertension to decrease circulating blood volume, counteract sodium-retaining effects of antihypertensives, and improve blood flow from capillaries
         (2) Interfere with sodium ion transport at ascending limb of Henle's loop and inhibit carbonic anhydrase activity at distal tubule sites
      b. Examples
         (1) Chlorothiazide (Diuril)
         (2) Chlorthalidone (Hygroton)
         (3) Hydrochlorothiazide (Esidrix, HydroDiuril, Oretic)
         (4) Methyclothiazide (Enduron)
      c. Adverse effects
         (1) Hypokalemia caused by rapid exchange of potassium ions for sodium ions at collecting tubules
         (2) Initial diuresis may cause weakness, fatigue, dizziness
         (3) Drug-induced hyperglycemia may convert prediabetic to diabetic state
         (4) Headache, dizziness, vertigo, paresthesia
         (5) Gastrointestinal irritation
         (6) Long-term therapy may induce symptoms of gout secondary to increased uric acid reabsorption and asymptomatic hyperuricemia
   3. Potassium-sparing drugs
      a. Action—interfere with aldosterone-induced reabsorption of sodium ions at distal nephron sites to increase sodium chloride excretion and decrease potassium ion loss (potassium sparing)
      b. Examples
         (1) Spironolactone (Aldactone)
         (2) Triamterene (Dyrenium)
      c. Adverse effects
         (1) Hyponatremia, tissue dehydration
         (2) Mild headache
         (3) Mild acidosis resulting from decreased excretion of ammonium
         (4) Long-term use causes low serum sodium ion concentrations that stimulate aldosterone secretion
   4. Mercurials
      a. Actions
         (1) Mercurial diuretics block sulfhydryl-containing enzymes that control tubule transport systems for sodium ions in the nephron by release of mercurial ions in tubule cells
         (2) Act chiefly at proximal and distal tubule sites for active transport; also affect passive transport of chloride and water
      b. Examples
         (1) Mercaptomerin sodium (Thiomerin)
         (2) Mersalyl with theophylline (Salyrgan-Theophylline)

c. Adverse effects
   (1) Hypokalemic alkalosis caused by potassium and hydrogen ion exchange for sodium ions at collecting tubules, which increases output of K^+ and H^+ with prolonged therapy
   (2) Destruction of tubule cells with excess use
   (3) Hypersensitivity reactions (pruritus, skin rash, gastrointestinal disturbances, stomatitis, vertigo, headache)

5. Other potent diuretics
  a. Actions
    (1) Interfere with active transport of sodium ions in ascending limb of Henle's loop
    (2) Action at proximal tubule sites inhibits sodium chloride and water reabsorption
  b. Examples
    (1) Ethacrynic acid (Edecrin)
    (2) Furosemide (Lasix)
    (3) Metolazone (Zaroxolyn)
  c. Adverse effects
    (1) Hypokalemia and alkalosis (drugs exchange sodium ions at collecting tubules, causing K^+ and H^+ loss)
    (2) Hyperuricemia with long-term oral use
    (3) Elevated blood urea nitrogen
    (4) Ototoxicity (rare)

G. Drugs that constrict peripheral blood vessels
1. General implications for nurses
  a. Careful monitoring of blood pressure at frequent intervals
  b. Infiltration may cause local vasoconstriction and tissue necrosis
  c. Titrate IV with blood pressure to prevent hypertension
  d. Observe for hypertensive headache and abdominal distress, as well as adverse effects listed under specific drugs
2. Alpha-adrenergic stimulators
  a. Actions
    (1) Alpha receptors cause constriction that elevates the blood pressure
    (2) Increase arterial constriction, which increases the work load of the left ventricle and may reflexively slow cardiac rate, causing reduced cardiac output and less effective blood flow
    (3) Venous alpha receptors cause constriction that improves blood flow toward the heart

b. Examples
    (1) Hydroxyamphetamine hydrobromide (Paredrine)
    (2) Methoxamine hydrochloride (Vasoxyl)
    (3) Phenylephrine hydrochloride (Neo-Synephrine Hydrochloride)
    (4) Levarterenol bitartrate (Levophed Bitartrate); also has a positive inotropic and chronotropic effect on the heart
    (5) Mephentermine sulfate (Wyamine Sulfate); also stimulates cardiac beta receptors
    (6) Metaraminol bitartrate (Aramine); also stimulates cardiac beta receptors
c. Adverse effects
    (1) Constriction of resistance vessels without action on capacitance vessels may increase venous pooling and reduce venous return to the heart
    (2) Adrenergic stimulation inhibits intestinal motility, and gaseous distention or constipation may occur with prolonged administration

3. Vasopressin (Pitressin)
  a. Action—musculotropic effect that constricts small vessels when infused by a route delivering the drug to bleeding sites
  b. Adverse effects
    (1) Tremors
    (2) Diaphoresis
    (3) Pounding in head
    (4) Urticaria
    (5) Abdominal cramps

H. Plasma volume expanders
1. General implications for nurses
  a. Must be administered slowly to prevent circulatory overload
  b. Observe for signs of pulmonary edema caused by circulatory overload, as well as specific adverse effects
  c. Monitor intake and output
2. Osmotic agents
  a. Action—cause movement of fluid from interstitial spaces into bloodstream
  b. Examples
    (1) Dextran 40 (Rheomacrodex)
    (2) Dextran 70 (Macrodex)
    (3) Dextran (Expandex)
  c. Adverse effects

(1) Anaphylactic reaction
(2) Pulmonary edema
3. Albumin preparations
  a. Actions
    (1) Expand blood volume
    (2) May provide clotting factors (except plasma protein fraction)
    (3) Decrease the hematocrit
  b. Examples
    (1) Normal human serum albumin
    (2) Normal human serum albumin (salt-poor)
    (3) Plasma protein fraction
  c. Adverse effects
    (1) Rash
    (2) Nausea and vomiting
    (3) Increased salivation
    (4) Hepatitis
I. Drugs that prevent intravascular clot formation (anticoagulants)
  1. General nursing implications
    a. Observe for signs of bleeding, such as hemoptysis and hematuria, and other adverse effects specific to the drug
    b. Check appropriate laboratory tests
    c. Have antidote available—vitamin K for warfarin sodium (Coumadin) and protamine sulfate for heparin
    d. Patient teaching
      (1) Signs of bleeding
      (2) Use of electric razor
      (3) Carrying a medical alert card
      (4) Effects of diet and other medications on therapy
  2. Oral anticoagulants
    a. Actions
      (1) Interfere with synthesis of prothrombin by liver
      (2) Cause an increased prothrombin time
      (3) Effects are counteracted by vitamin K
    b. Examples
      (1) Dicumarol
      (2) Warfarin sodium (Coumadin, Panwarfin)
  3. Heparin sodium
    a. Action—must be administered parenterally and inhibits conversion of prothrombin to thrombin
    b. Examples
      (1) Depo-Heparin Sodium
      (2) Lipo-Hepin

      (3) Meparin
      (4) Panheprin
    c. Adverse effects
      (1) Chills, fever, pruritus
      (2) Asthmalike reactions
      (3) Local irritation and hematoma from IM or SC injections
J. Drugs that affect red blood cell building
  1. General implications for nurses
    a. Use Z-track procedure for IM administration
    b. Patient teaching about side effects of hematinics; adverse effects of vitamin replacement are rare
    c. Mouth care to prevent staining of teeth
  2. Vitamin replacements
    a. Action—provide components for protein framework of cells by supplying cofactors for DNA synthesis of nucleotides
    b. Examples
      (1) Vitamin B_{12} replacement
        (a) Cyanocobalamin
        (b) Hydroxocobalamin
        (c) Vitamin B_{12} with intrinsic factor concentrate
        (d) Liver injection
      (2) Tetrahydrofolic acid
        (a) Folate sodium (Folvite Sodium)
        (b) Folic acid (Folvite)
        (c) Leucovorin calcium
  3. Hematinics
    a. Action—provide a component of hemoglobin for erythroblasts
    b. Examples
      (1) Oral iron sources
        (a) Ferrocholinate (Chel-Iron, Ferrolip)
        (b) Ferrous fumarate (Ircon, Toleron)
        (c) Ferrous gluconate
        (d) Ferrous lactate (Ferro Drops)
        (e) Ferrous sulfate
      (2) Parenteral iron sources
        (a) Iron-dextran injection (Imferon)
        (b) Iron sorbitex (Jectofer)
    c. Adverse effects
      (1) Injectable preparation causes tissue staining
      (2) Fever
      (3) Urticaria
      (4) Nausea and vomiting
      (5) Black stools

RELATED PROCEDURES
Cardiac monitoring

A. Definition
1. Electric observation of the conductivity patterns of the heart by the use of skin electrodes and a monitoring device; the heart's electric activity is conducted to the surface of the skin by the salty fluids bathing the cells and tissues
2. Utilized in heart disease, during surgery and intrusive procedures, or when danger of arrhythmias (cardiac irregularities in rhythm) is apparent
3. P, Q, R, S, and T segments are parts of the normal electrocardiogram (ECG); P wave represents atrial depolarization, QRS waves (QRS complex) ventricular depolarization, and T wave ventricular depolarization

B. Nursing responsibilities
1. Explain procedure to patient and attempt to allay anxiety
2. Prepare skin on chest for electrode attachment
   a. Cleanse area with alcohol swab to remove dirt and oils
   b. Shave area if hairs are present to improve skin-electrode contact
3. Place electrodes on skin and attach to monitor cable as indicated
   a. Right arm (on chest)
   b. Left arm (on chest)
   c. Center (or ground)
4. Turn on monitor scope and set machine's sensitivity when clear picture is obtained
5. Observe monitor for changes in rate and rhythm
6. Set alarm and readout attachment (if available) so that an electric printout will be made if there is a change in cardiac activity
7. If arrhythmia occurs, act appropriately
   a. Emergency arrhythmias require immediate intervention
   b. If arrhythmia is nonemergency, document occurrence with rhythm strip and notify physician
8. Life-threatening arrhythmias require immediate intervention
   a. Ventricular fibrillation—repetitive rapid stimulation from ectopic ventricular foci to which the ventricles are unable to respond; ventricular contraction is replaced by uncoordinated twitching; circulation ceases, and death ensues
      (1) Defibrillate immediately
      (2) Inject lidocaine
      (3) Institute cardiopulmonary resuscitation
      (4) Document arrhythmia and notify physician
   b. Ventricular tachycardia—a series of three or more bizarre premature ventricular beats that occur in a regular rhythm; this electric activity results in decreased cardiac output and may rapidly convert to ventricular fibrillation
      (1) Use lidocaine intravenously to convert rhythm
      (2) Be prepared to administer defibrillation and cardiopulmonary resuscitation
      (3) Document arrhythmia and notify physician
   c. Premature ventricular contractions of greater than 5 per minute—a PVC is a beat that originates in the ventricles and occurs before the next expected sinus beat; it can be life threatening when it occurs close to the T wave, since cardiac repolarization is interfered with and ventricular fibrillation may ensue
      (1) Administer lidocaine intravenously
      (2) Document arrhythmia and notify physician
      (3) Long-term institution of oral antiarrhythmics may be indicated
   d. Complete heart block—occurs when there is no electric communication between the atria and ventricles and each beats independently; this activity will not provide long-term adequate circulation, and syncope, congestive failure, or cardic arrest may ensue
      (1) Document arrhythmia and notify physician
      (2) Use of intravenous isoproterenol is generally indicated
      (3) Prepare for pacemaker insertion (see procedure)
   e. Asystole—occurs when there is no cardiac activity demonstrated on ECG tracing as a flat line; this terminates in death unless intervention is begun immediately
      (1) Institute cardiopulmonary resuscitation
      (2) Document arrhythmia and notify physician
      (3) Cardiac stimulants may be given via IV or intracardiac route
      (4) Pacemaker insertion may be indicated (see procedure)

Cardiac pacemaker insertion

A. Definition—artificial pacemakers replace natural electric stimulation of the heart and are indicated in the treatment of
1. Complete heart block—impulses generated from the SA node of the heart do not reach the ventricles; the atria and ventricles beat independently of each other
2. Second-degree AV (atrioventricular) block—there is intermittent failure of impulse to reach the ventricles
3. Adams-Stokes syndrome—a sudden drop in ventricular rate that causes syncope and temporary loss of consciousness
B. Pacemakers—involve the insertion of an electrode catheter into the right ventricle, which transmits the impulses generated by the pacing unit
1. Demand pacemakers are most frequently used; the pacemaker will stimulate the ventricles to contract only if the patient's ventricular rate falls below the rate set on the pacemaker
2. Fixed-rate pacemakers will stimulate the heart a specific amount of times per minute regardless of the patient's rhythm
3. Pacemakers may be temporary and worn externally or permanent and surgically placed under the skin
C. Nursing responsibilities
1. Explain procedure to patient
2. Observe cardiac monitor before, during, and after procedure to verify pacemaker capture, and observe for arrhythmias
3. Have emergency medications (lidocaine, atropine sulfate, and isoproterenol) available, as well as defibrillator
4. Teach patient how to take pulse, to keep a diary of pulse, and to notify physician immediately if rate falls below the rate set on pacemaker
5. Teach patient to remain under physician's supervision, since batteries must be replaced approximately every 2 years; pacemaker function may be checked by special telephone devices
6. Encourage patient to wear bracelet or carry medical alert card

Angiography

A. Definition—angiography is an x-ray examination using contrast dye to visualize the patency of an artery

B. Nursing responsibilities
1. Patient should be informed of the risks involved in this procedure (allergic reaction, embolus, cardiac arrhythmia)
2. Administer mild sedative as ordered prior to procedure
3. Observe patient for complications
4. Postprocedure care involves checking the injection site for bleeding and inflammation, assessing circulatory status of extremities, and enforcing bed rest

Bone marrow aspiration

A. Definition—puncture to collect tissue from bone marrow
1. Sites used include sternum, vertebral body, iliac crest, or the tibia in infants
2. Performed to study the cells involved in blood production
B. Nursing responsibilities
1. Obtain informed consent
2. Attempt to allay anxiety of patient
3. Assist physician in maintaining a sterile field and positioning patient
4. Send specimen to laboratory in proper container with appropriate label

Swan-Ganz catheter procedure

A. Definition—catheter used to measure pulmonary capillary wedge pressure, pulmonary artery pressure, and right atrial pressure
1. The double-lumen catheter with a balloon tip is inserted into the brachial vein and advanced through the superior vena cava, into the right atrium and ventricle, and into the pulmonary artery; the catheter is guided further until, when the balloon is inflated, it is wedged in the distal arterial branch
2. This catheter functions to yield information on the patient's circulatory status, left ventricular pumping action, and vascular tone
B. Nursing responsibilities
1. Obtain informed consent for procedure
2. Assist physician in inserting catheter using surgical aseptic technique
3. Observe insertion site for inflammation
4. Observe line for patency and air bubbles
5. Take readings with transducer at the level of the patient's sternal notch

6. Change dressing as ordered using surgical asepsis
7. Notify physician if waveform changes of pressure readings are altered
8. Normal readings
   a. Pulmonary capillary wedge pressure: 5 to 13 mm Hg
   b. Pulmonary artery pressure
      (1) Systolic: 16 to 30 mm Hg
      (2) Diastolic: 0 to 7 mm Hg
   c. Right atrial pressure: 5 mm Hg

Central venous pressure (CVP) monitoring

A. Definition
   1. CVP measures the right atrial pressure, which is normally 2 to 8 mm Hg
   2. A catheter is passed from the subclavian vein into the superior vena cava or right atrium
B. Nursing responsibilities
   1. Obtain informed consent
   2. Assist physician with insertion of catheter using surgical aseptic technique
   3. Obtain chest x-ray film after insertion to ascertain position of catheter
   4. Take readings as ordered
      a. Place patient in supine position
      b. Place stopcock of manometer at midaxillary line (which is approximately the level of the right atrium) and fill with fluid from line
      c. Allow fluid to enter catheter by placing stopcock in ''off'' position toward IV bottle
      d. If patient is on a respirator, remove it during readings
   5. Record and report changes in CVP readings; often CVP readings are used to regulate the rate of administration of IVs (high readings are present in congestive heart failure and low readings in hypovolemia)

MAJOR DISEASES
Hypertension

A. Etiology and pathophysiology
   1. Hypertension increases the risk of coronary artery disease, heart failure, myocardial infarction, cerebral vascular accidents (CVAs), and renal failure
   2. Essential hypertension
      a. Anxiety and other stresses are believed to play a role in releasing a pressor from kidneys, which causes chronic vasoconstriction, thereby raising blood pressure
      b. Individuals with essential hypertension have difficulty handling hostile feelings, are less assertive, and have more obsessive-compulsive traits than nonhypertensive individuals
      c. Onset is generally between 25 and 55 years of age
   3. Renal hypertension
      a. Narrowing of the lumen of a renal artery as a result of atherosclerosis causes release of renin
      b. Renin sets off series of reactions, which cause sodium retention and subsequent rise in blood pressure
      c. Onset is generally after 50 years of age
   4. Malignant hypertension results from sustained hypertension of any form, which causes necrosis of the arterioles and proliferative changes of the renal arteries leading to renal failure, CVA, and heart failure, if untreated
   5. Hypertension may also be caused by endocrine disorders (pheochromocytoma) and increased intracranial pressure
B. Signs and symptoms
   1. Subjective
      a. Headache (occipital area)
      b. Light-headedness
      c. Tinnitus
      d. Easy fatigue
      e. Visual disturbances
   2. Objective
      a. Blood pressure greater than 140/90 mm Hg in person younger than 50 years of age; World Health Organization defines hypertension as greater than 160/95 mm Hg
      b. Retinal changes
      c. Possible hematuria
      d. Epistaxis
      e. Cardiac hypertrophy
C. Treatment
   1. Antihypertensive drugs to decrease peripheral resistance
   2. Diuretics to decrease amount of water and sodium retained by the body
   3. Sedatives to control tension
   4. Weight reduction
   5. Smoking discouraged
   6. Physical as well as psychologic rest (psychotherapy is often helpful for patients with essential hypertension)

7. Sodium-restricted diet (1 to 3 g daily)
8. A sympathectomy (cutting of sympathetic nerve fibers) may be done to cause dilation of arteries

D. Nursing care
1. Encourage early detection by participation in community screening programs
2. Monitor vital signs with patient in both upright and recumbent positions (orthostatic hypotension is a common adverse effect of antihypertensive drugs)
3. Check weight daily
4. Educate patient regarding drugs, follow-up care, diet and activity restrictions (caution: salt substitutes often contain potassium and should not be suggested without physician approval)
5. Reassure and support in expressing emotions
6. If epistaxis occurs, place an ice pack on the back of the neck, which may alleviate it; packing is sometimes required
7. Nursing care related to specific medications should also be included

Arterioatherosclerosis

A. Etiology and pathophysiology
1. Atherosclerosis is the deposition of fatty plaques along the inner wall of the artery; most often affects the peripheral arteries, aorta, coronary arteries, and arteries supplying the brain
2. Arteriosclerosis is considered a loss of elasticity of the arteries, or ''hardening of the arteries''

B. Signs and symptoms (depends on arteries affected)
1. Subjective
a. Intermittent claudication
b. Pain, depending on degree circulation is impaired
c. Forgetfulness
2. Objective
a. Decreased skin temperature
b. Pallor
c. Diminished pulsations
d. May lead to ulcerations and gangrene
e. Elevated serum cholesterol and lipids
f. Objective memory loss on testing

C. Treatment
1. Drugs that cause vasodilation
2. Weight loss
3. Dietary restrictions of fat and cholesterol

D. Nursing care

1. Evaluate all pulses, color, and temperature of involved area
2. Discourage positions that hamper circulation; e.g., cross-legged
3. Teach patient the hazards of smoking (nicotine causes vasoconstriction)
4. Dietary teaching for family as well as patient
5. Teach importance of warm clothing
6. No vigorous massages of involved area

Angina pectoris

A. Etiology and pathophysiology
1. Atherosclerosis is a common cause of narrowed coronary arteries (coronary artery disease)
2. Patients with aortic stenosis or extremely low pressure may also have impaired coronary artery blood flow
3. Increased metabolic demands caused by strenuous exercise, emotional stress, hyperthyroidism, or severe anemia may also precipitate angina pectoris
4. When oxygen supplied by the blood cannot meet the metabolic demands of the muscle, hypoxia occurs
5. Pain is thought to occur as a result of anaerobic metabolic end products

B. Signs and symptoms
1. Subjective
a. Chest pain associated with activity; generally subsides after a few minutes of rest
b. Pain is usually substernal and is described as ''crushing'' or ''pressure''
c. Pain may radiate to the left shoulder and arm, jaw, epigastric area, or right shoulder
d. Palpitation
e. Faintness
f. Dyspnea
2. Objective
a. Diaphoresis
b. Blood pressure may be elevated
c. Signs of underlying disease may be evident (cardiac enlargement, valvular disease, arrhythmias)
d. ECG often indicates a previous infarction

C. Treatment
1. Restricted activity
2. Drugs, such as nitroglycerin, and slower acting vasodilators
3. Weight loss
4. Oxygen therapy during attack

5. Coronary artery bypass surgery if medical regimen not successful
6. Cholesterol and fat restrictions in diet

D. Nursing care
1. Provide physical and mental rest
2. Relieve pain by administration of vasodilators
3. Assess activity tolerance
4. Discourage smoking
5. Educate patient regarding diet, medication, and activity
6. Provide necessary emotional support due to required alterations in life-style

Myocardial infarction

A. Etiology and pathophysiology
1. An acute necrosis of an area of heart muscle caused by the interruption of the oxygen supply to the area resulting in altered functioning and reduced cardiac output
2. Possible causes include atherosclerosis, thrombus formation, or decreased blood flow

B. Signs and symptoms
1. Subjective
   a. Sudden, severe, crushing, or viselike pain in the substernal region; may radiate to the arms, neck, and back
   b. Nausea and vomiting
   c. Severe anxiety and dyspnea
   d. Patient's health history, including smoking and drinking habits, obesity, high-cholesterol diet, physical and emotional stresses, chest pain, hypertension
2. Objective
   a. Signs of shock: cold clammy skin, profuse diaphoresis, decreased blood pressure, rapid thready pulse
   b. Slight elevation of temperature
   c. Blood serum enzyme and isoenzyme levels
      (1) Creatinine phosphokinase (CPK)—elevated on days 1 to 3
      (2) Serum glutamic oxaloacetic transaminase (SGOT)—elevated day 2 to 4
      (3) Lactic dehydrogenase (LDH)—elevated on day 1, reaching a peak on days 3 to 4, and then gradually subsiding
   d. Complete blood studies, particularly white blood cells and sedimentation rate, to determine presence of inflammatory process
   e. Coagulation studies—prothrombin time (PT) and partial thromboplastin time (PTT)

C. Treatment
1. Admit patient to coronary care unit
2. Morphine sulfate IV or SC to relieve pain and reduce apprehension
3. Bed rest with cardiac precautions to reduce demand for oxygen
4. Oxygen as necessary
5. Cardiac monitoring for continued surveillance of the heart's electric activity
6. Frequent monitoring of vital signs, including temperature, pulse (apical and radial), respirations, blood pressure, intake and output
7. One or more of the following medications to prevent or reduce complications: antiarrhythmic agents, digitalis, diuretics, anticoagulants, potassium salts, vasopressors or vasodilators, sedatives, and stool softeners
8. IV fluids at slow rate to keep vein open for administration of medications
9. Clear liquid diet is prescribed initially to decrease oxygen consumption, and then advanced to low sodium
10. A Swan-Ganz catheter is used to monitor pressure in pulmonary artery, which reflects function of left ventricle
11. Intra-aortic balloon pump that inflates during diastole and deflates during systole may be used to decrease cardiac work load

D. Nursing care
1. Observe cardiac monitor and immediately document and report changes in rate, conductivity, and rhythm
2. Observe for ventricular fibrillation and asystole and take appropriate life-saving actions if they occur; e.g., cardiopulmonary resuscitation, electric defibrillation
3. Observe for other variations, such as PVCs close to a T wave, ventricular tachycardia, and atrial fibrillation; if they occur, administer prescribed medications, document the rhythm, and notify the physician
4. Observe patient's vital signs every 15 minutes until stable
5. Closely observe patient's intake and output
6. Observe for pulmonary congestion and dependent edema
7. Observe for pain and restlessness and administer medication as ordered
8. Observe for cyanosis and dyspnea and administer oxygen as necessary

9. Recognize that the patient is subject to sensory overload
   a. Orient to unit and machinery
   b. Allow patient time to express feelings and fears
10. Provide gradual increase in activity
11. Apply antiembolism stockings

Inflammatory diseases of the heart (pericarditis, myocarditis, subacute bacterial endocarditis)

A. Etiology and pathophysiology
   1. Pericarditis is an acute or chronic inflammation of the pericardium caused by bacterial or viral invasion, trauma, heart disease, or an autoimmune process
      a. The inflammatory process can result in loss of pericardial elasticity or an accumulation of fluid within the sac
      b. Heart failure or cardiac tamponade (the compression of the heart due to a collection of fluid within the pericardial sac) may result
   2. Myocarditis is an inflammation of the myocardium due to pericarditis, systemic infection, or allergic response
      a. The contractility of the heart is impaired due to the inflammatory process
      b. Myocardial ischemia and necrosis are critical complications
   3. Subacute bacterial endocarditis is an inflammation of the inner lining of the heart and valves generally caused by *Streptococcus viridans* or other nonhemolytic streptococci spreading through blood to heart from infected teeth, gums, and tonsils; structural damage to the valves may occur in a matter of days, and pump failure will ensue
B. Signs and symptoms
   1. Subjective
      a. Precordial or substernal pain
      b. Shortness of breath
      c. Chills
      d. Fatigue and malaise
   2. Objective
      a. Arrhythmias
      b. Increased cardiac enzymes
      c. Fever
      d. Positive blood cultures
      e. Friction rubs evident on auscultation

C. Treatment
   1. Administer oxygen
   2. Bed rest
   3. Antibiotics to relieve underlying infection
   4. Corticosteroids
   5. Antiarrhythmics
   6. Pericardectomy (surgical removal of scar tissue and the pericardium), if indicated
D. Nursing care
   1. Carefully observe patient for signs of shock, heart failure, and arrhythmias
   2. Maintain a tranquil environment and help patient achieve maximum rest
   3. If patient has surgical intervention, care of chest tubes and routine postoperative chest surgery care (see cardiac surgery)
   4. Explain posthospitalization therapy to patient to improve compliance (life-long doses of penicillin prophylactically)

Congestive heart failure (CHF)

A. Etiology and pathophysiology
   1. Heart failure refers to inability of the heart to meet the demands of the body
   2. Pump failure may be caused by cardiac abnormalities or conditions that place increased demands on the heart
      a. Myocardial infarctions
      b. Valvular defects
      c. Hypertension
      d. Anemia
      e. Hyperthyroidism
      f. Obesity
      g. Circulatory overload
   3. When one side of a heart "fails," there is essentially a buildup of pressure in the vascular system feeding into that side of the heart: signs of right-sided failure will be evident in the systemic circulation; signs of left-sided failure will first be evident in the pulmonary system
B. Signs and symptoms
   1. Right-sided failure
      a. Dependent, pitting edema; ankle edema is frequently the first sign of CHF; often subsides at night when legs are elevated
      b. Ascites from increased pressure within the portal system
      c. Respiratory distress if ascites is severe
      d. Fatigue

2. Left-sided heart failure
   a. Dyspnea from fluid within the lungs
   b. Orthopnea
   c. Frothy, blood-tinged sputum
   d. Fatigue
   e. Apprehension, restlessness
C. Treatment
   1. Morphine sulfate is often given to decrease anxiety and dyspnea
   2. Oxygen is generally administered by mask or cannula; however, if acute left-sided failure exists, the patient may require endotracheal intubation and placement on a ventilator
   3. Digitalis is generally prescribed to increase the efficiency of the heart's pumping action
   4. Diuretics such as furosemide (Lasix) are often ordered to remove excess fluid, thereby decreasing cardiac work load
   5. Potassium supplements are usually prescribed to prevent digitalis toxicity and hypokalemia
   6. Rotating tourniquets (dry phlebotomy) may be used to decrease venous return; generally tourniquets are applied to 3 of the extremities, and every 15 minutes a tourniquet is removed and rotated in a clockwise direction; when patient is stable, tourniquets are removed one at a time in 15-minute intervals
   7. A paracentesis may be performed if ascites exists and is causing respiratory distress
   8. Sodium-restricted diet
D. Nursing care
   1. Maintain patient in high Fowler's position
   2. Elevate extremities
   3. Frequently monitor vital signs
   4. Change position frequently
   5. Monitor intake and output and daily weight
   6. Observe for electrolyte imbalances (hyponatremia, hypokalemia)
   7. Provide patient and family teaching and emotional support
   8. Nursing implications for digitalis therapy and diuretics should also be considered

Cardiac surgery

A. May be used to correct
   1. Mitral stenosis or regurgitation
   2. Aortic stenosis or insufficiency
   3. Coronary occlusion
   4. Ventricular aneurysm

B. Preoperative procedures
   1. Vital signs and weight
   2. Coughing and deep breathing exercises are taught and practiced
   3. Inhalation therapy to improve pulmonary function
   4. Coagulation studies in addition to routine laboratory tests
   5. Chest x-ray examination
   6. ECG to assess electric pattern of heart
   7. Echocardiography, which uses sound, is especially helpful in evaluating valvular defects
   8. Cardiac catheterization involves insertion of a radiopaque catheter into the heart; blood samples and pressure readings may be obtained
C. Types of procedures—open or closed heart surgery (when extracorporeal circulation or the heart-lung machine is used, it is called open heart surgery; hypothermia may be used in either open or closed heart surgery to decrease the metabolic demands of the body)
   1. Mitral commissurotomy or valvotomy involves splitting the joined portions of the mitral valve that are present in mitral stenosis
   2. Mitral valve replacement is done for mitral insufficiency, which occurs when the mitral valve does not close properly to block reflux of blood from the ventricle into the atrium during systole (regurgitation)
   3. Coronary bypass surgery is done when severe arteriosclerotic disease causes severe angina pectoris; a segment of vessel (often the saphenous vein) is anastomosed, bypassing the diseased portion of a coronary artery
   4. Aneurysmectomy is done to correct a ventricular aneurysm that occurs in approximately 10% to 30% of patients with myocardial infarctions when a weakened ventricular wall balloons out, causing decreased cardiac efficiency
D. Postoperative nursing care
   1. Monitor cardiac functioning
   2. Evaluate vital signs, including peripheral pulses and neurologic signs
   3. Utilize rectal probe to monitor temperature
   4. Maintain airway; patient will have an endotracheal tube in place postoperatively and require mechanical ventilation; suction as necessary
   5. Monitor intake and output
   6. Assess state of hydration by frequent checks on

CVP readings, electrolytes, specific gravity, and observation of patient

7. Care for chest tubes
    a. Milk tubing to maintain patency
    b. Avoid kinked tubing
    c. Drainage should not be more than 200 ml/hour
8. Maintain Foley catheter in place; in addition to output, monitor specific gravity
9. Assess pain (nature, site, duration, and type) and provide relief
10. Encourage coughing and deep breathing; change position frequently
11. Evaluate arterial blood gases
12. Administer parenteral therapy, including electrolytes and blood
13. Plan with patient and family for meeting both short- and long-term goals
14. Provide relief of anxiety and fear by staying with patient and explaining procedures; encourage verbalization of feelings; provide emotional support

E. Complications
1. Hemorrhage that can lead to hypovolemia
    a. Decreased BP, increased pulse rate
    b. Restlessness, apprehension
    c. Lowered CVP readings
    d. Pallor
2. Cardiac tamponade caused by collection of fluid or blood within pericardium
    a. Decreased arterial pressure
    b. Elevated CVP
    c. Rapid, thready pulse
    d. Diminished output
3. Congestive heart failure
    a. Dyspnea
    b. Elevated CVP
    c. Tachycardia
    d. Edema
4. Myocardial infarction
5. Renal failure
6. Embolism
7. Psychosis resulting from an inability to cope with anxiety associated with cardiac surgery

Thrombophlebitis and emboli

A. Etiology and pathophysiology
1. Thrombophlebitis is the inflammation of a vein and is associated with clot formation (thrombus)
2. An embolus is a clot or solid particle carried by the bloodstream that may interfere with circulation to vital organs
3. Risk factors thought to contribute to this disorder include immobilization, venous stasis, trauma to vessels, and pregnancy
4. Surgical procedures involving the pelvic area increase the risk of phlebitis because of the vascularity of the area and subsequent vascular impairment

B. Signs and symptoms
1. Subjective
    a. Pain on dorsiflexion of affected extremity (Homans' sign)
    b. Sometimes no signs are present until embolus is released and lodges in a vessel supplying a vital organ
2. Objective
    a. Swollen limb with hard veins that are sensitive to pressure
    b. Redness and warmth of area along the vein
    c. If emboli are released, pulse may be lost in area and severe pain may persist

C. Treatment
1. Bed rest with elastic stockings to promote venous return
2. Warm moist heat to promote vasodilation; however, some feel this may dislodge clot, and ice packs are ordered
3. Elevation of extremity to reduce edema
4. Anticoagulants to prevent recurrence of deep vein involvement
5. Vasodilators to prevent vascular spasm
6. Amputation of an extremity when vascular supply is severely impaired; may also be indicated for a neoplasm or following trauma
    a. Below-the-knee amputation provides patient with a more natural gait, since knee movement is maintained
    b. Above-the-knee amputation limits patient's movement, since prosthesis contains knee joint
    c. A guillotine amputation, in which the wound is left open and skin traction is applied, is performed when the area is infected, gangrenous, extensively traumatized, or the patient is a poor surgical risk
    d. A flap-type amputation is less prone to infection, since the skin covers the area and healing

occurs within 2 weeks; may be above or below the knee

D. Nursing care
1. Associated with medical management
   a. Observe patient frequently for signs of vascular impairment, such as pallor, cyanosis, coolness, diminished pulses
   b. Assist patient in understanding the rationale for prolonged bed rest and minimal activity
   c. Apply antiembolitic stockings and remove for 15 minutes every 8 hours
   d. Observe and record vital signs, including peripheral pulses
   e. Instruct the patient to avoid tight and constricting clothing, cigarette smoking, or maintaining one position for long periods
   f. Observe for signs of embolism, such as sudden pain, cyanosis, hemoptysis, and shock
2. Associated with amputation
   a. Observe patient for bleeding
   b. Keep tourniquet at bedside
   c. Allow patient to express emotional reactions to procedure
   d. Elevate stump for 24 to 48 hours
   e. Keep patient's extremities close to the body to prevent abduction deformity
   f. Encourage patient to move stump
   g. Place the patient with a lower extremity amputation in a prone position twice daily to stretch the flexor muscles
   h. Start range of motion exercises to the stump after about 10 days
   i. Encourage the patient not to sit in any position for prolonged periods, since this inactivity can cause hip flexion contractures
   j. Provide and teach good care of the stump
      (1) Stump shrinkage (a change in size and shape of stump) is caused by reduction of subcutaneous fat by pressure of constrictive bandage and socket of prosthesis as well as disuse atrophy occurring in the involved muscles; maximum shrinkage usually takes a minimum of 1 to 1½ years and sometimes longer
      (2) Keep the stump clean: wash with mild soap but do not soak; use clean bandages and socks
      (3) Physical preparation for a prosthesis
         (a) Apply compression bandage to prevent edema and promote stump shrinkage
         (b) Massage the stump to soften the scar, decrease tenderness, and improve vascularity
         (c) Teach and encourage the patient to do stump conditioning exercises to harden the stump (push stump against pillow and then progress to harder surfaces)
   k. With the physical therapist, assist the patient with a lower extremity amputation to learn crutch walking
   l. For patients fitted with a prosthesis immediately after surgery, ambulation instruction is begun on the first postoperative day
   m. Explain and discuss phantom limb phenomenon with the patient
      (1) Phantom limb—a physiologic reaction of the nerves in the stump causing an unpleasant feeling that the limb is still there; this response may or may not be precipitated by a psychologic overlay
      (2) Phantom limb pain—when the unpleasant feelings become painful or disagreeable
      (3) Characteristics of phantom limb—sensations may be constant or intermittent, and of varying severity
      (4) Approaches that may help relieve phantom limb—have the patient look at the stump or close eyes and put the stump through range of motion as if the full limb were still there; if the patient continues to have severe pain of long duration, the medical therapy may include
         (a) Injecting the nerve endings in the stump with alcohol to give temporary relief
         (b) Surgical revision of the stump
   n. Consider special needs related to upper extremity amputation
      (1) Mastery of an upper extremity prosthesis is more complex than that of a lower extremity prosthesis
      (2) The patient must do bilateral shoulder exercises to prepare for fitting the prosthesis
      (3) The artificial arm cannot be used above the head or behind the back because of the harnessing

(4) There is no artificial hand that can dupli-
cate all the fine movements of the fingers
and thumb of the normal hand, although
the development of electronic limbs does
not negate this possibility for the future

(5) There is a loss of sensory feedback;
therefore the patient must use visual control at all times (a blind person could not
adequately use a functional prosthesis)

Varicose veins

A. Etiology and pathophysiology
1. The veins in the lower trunk and extremities become dilated, congested, and tortuous due to
weakness of valves or loss of elasticity of vessel
walls
2. A positive Trendelenburg test is diagnostic of
varicose veins: the patient lies down with legs
elevated until veins empty completely; the patient
then stands, and observation of filling of veins is
made; a normal vein fills from below, whereas a
varicose vein fills from above
B. Treatment
1. Surgical intervention involves ligation of the vein
above the varicosity and removal of the involved
vein; the great saphenous vein may be ligated
near the femoral junction
2. Postoperative early ambulation is essential to
prevent formation of thrombi
C. Nursing care
1. Elevate foot of bed for first 24 hours
2. Observe vital signs and incisions for indications
of hemorrhage
3. Assist patient with ambulation
4. Administer analgesics as ordered

Peripheral vascular disorders

A. Etiology and pathophysiology
1. Buerger's disease (thromboangiitis obliterans)
a. Peripheral circulation is impaired by inflammatory occlusions of the peripheral arteries
b. Thromboses of both arteries and veins may
occur
c. Incidence is highest in young adult males who
smoke
2. Raynaud's disease
a. Spasms of digital arteries thought to be caused
by abnormal response of sympathetic nervous
system to cold or emotional stress

b. Primarily occurs in young females
c. Rarely leads to gangrene
3. Atherosclerosis is a contributing factor
B. Signs and symptoms
1. Subjective
a. Paresthesia
b. Aching pain
2. Objective
a. Pallor or cyanosis
b. Gangrenous ulcers (more common in Buerger's disease)
c. Diminished pulses in Buerger's disease
C. Treatment
1. Vasodilators may be given
2. Sympathectomy to sever the sympathetic ganglia supplying the area; there is local vasodilation
and improved circulation
a. Lumbar sympathectomy deprives the leg and
foot of innervation
b. Cervicothoracic sympathectomy relieves vaso-
spasm in the arms and hands
3. Femoropopliteal bypass grafting
a. Saphenous vein grafting from femoral artery
to the area below the obstruction
b. Polyester fiber grafts in aortic iliac obstructions
D. Nursing care
1. Associated with medical management
a. Instruct patient not to smoke or wear constrictive garments
b. Extremities should be kept warm; instruct patient to wear gloves when exposed to cold
c. Protect from injury since there is decreased
wound healing ability; lubricants may be applied to keep skin supple
d. Assess color, temperature, pulses, and sensation of involved extremities
2. Associated with sympathectomy
a. Monitor vital signs frequently, since shock
can occur
b. Change position gradually, since dizziness
might be a problem
c. Apply elastic bandages if ordered
3. Associated with femoropopliteal bypass grafting
a. Assess circulation of involved extremity by
checking pulses, color, temperature, and
neurologic function
b. Observe blood pressure frequently, since hy-

potension increases the possibility of thrombus formation
c. Observe for signs of hemorrhage, including
pain, change in skin color, and alteration of
vital signs
d. Ambulate patient as ordered; sitting should be
avoided in femoropopliteal bypass surgery

Aneurysms

A. Etiology and pathophysiology
1. An aneurysm is a distention at the site of a weakness in the arterial wall
a. Saccular aneurysm—a pouchlike projection
at one side of the artery
b. Fusiform aneurysm—the entire circumference
of the artery wall is dilated
c. Mycotic aneurysm—tiny weaknesses in the
arterial wall that result from infection
d. Dissecting aneurysm—a tear in the inner
lining of an arteriosclerotic aorta wall cause
blood to form a hematoma between layers of
the artery, and actually compress the lumen of
the artery
2. Causes
a. Congenital weakness
b. Atherosclerosis (most common cause of both
thoracic and abdominal aortic aneurysm)
c. Syphilis
d. Trauma
B. Signs and symptoms
1. Thoracic aortic aneurysm
a. Subjective
(1) May be asymptomatic
(2) Pain resulting from pressure against the
nerves or vertebrae
(3) Dyspnea
(4) Dysphagia
b. Objective
(1) Hoarseness, aphonia from impingement
of laryngeal nerve
(2) Cough
(3) Unequal pulses and arterial pressure in
upper extremities
(4) Trachea may be displaced from midline
due to adhesions between trachea and
aneurysm
2. Abdominal aortic aneurysm
a. Subjective
(1) May be asymptomatic
(2) Lower back pain

b. Objective
(1) Hypertension
(2) Pulsating abdominal mass
3. Dissecting aortic aneurysm
a. Subjective
(1) Restlessness and anxiety
(2) Severe pain
b. Objective
(1) Diminished pulses
(2) Signs of shock
C. Treatment
1. Resection of aneurysm and use of Teflon or Dacron graft
2. Surgical procedures involving the aorta would
necessitate use of heart-lung device (cardiopulmonary bypass)
3. Medical treatment is aimed at decreasing cardiac
output and blood pressure through use of drugs
D. Postoperative nursing care
1. Vital signs and pulses of all extremities, including posterior tibial and dorsalis pedis
2. Monitor central venous pressure frequently
3. Accurate intake and output, since renal failure
may occur after surgery
4. Administer narcotics as ordered to alleviate pain
5. Apply abdominal binders to provide support
while coughing, deep breathing, and ambulating
6. Prevent flexion of hip and knees to eliminate
pressure on arterial wall
7. Apply elastic stockings and encourage dorsiflexion of foot to help decrease the risk of thrombophlebitis
8. Maintain patency of nasogastric tube if present

Shock

A. Etiology and pathophysiology
1. Hypovolemic shock occurs when there is a loss
of fluid resulting in inadequate tissue perfusion;
caused by
a. Excessive bleeding
b. Excessive diarrhea or vomiting
c. Fluid loss from fistulas or burns
2. Cardiogenic shock occurs when pump failure
causes inadequate tissue perfusion; caused by
a. Congestive heart failure
b. Myocardial infarction
c. Cardiac tamponade
3. Neurogenic shock is caused by rapid vasodilation

and subsequent pooling of blood within the peripheral vessels; caused by
   a. Spinal anesthesia
   b. Emotional tension
   c. Drugs that inhibit the sympathetic nervous system
 4. Anaphylactic shock is caused by an allergic reaction that causes a release of histamine and subsequent vasodilation
 5. Septic shock is similar to anaphylaxis and is the body's reaction to bacterial toxins (generally gram-negative infections), which results in the leakage of plasma into tissues
B. Signs and symptoms
 1. Subjective
   a. Apprehension
   b. Restlessness
   c. Paresis of extremities
 2. Objective
   a. Weak, rapid, thready pulse
   b. Diaphoresis
   c. Cold, clammy skin
   d. Decreased blood pressure
   e. Decreased urine output
   f. Pallor
   g. Progressive loss of consciousness
   h. Lowered CVP readings
C. Treatment
 1. Aimed at correcting the underlying cause
 2. Fluid and blood replacement
 3. Oxygen therapy
 4. Vasoconstricting drugs to increase blood pressure
 5. Cardiac monitoring
 6. Cardiotonics, such as digitalis preparations, for cardiogenic shock
 7. Antihistamines for anaphylactic shock
 8. Antibiotics for septic shock based on blood cultures
 9. Trendelenburg position to ensure circulation to vital organs
 10. Intra-aortic balloon pump may be used to aid the failing heart
D. Nursing care
 1. Keep patient warm
 2. Check vital signs and CVP frequently
 3. Monitor urine output and specific gravity
 4. Allay anxiety
 5. Carefully observe response to therapy

Anemia
A. Iron deficiency anemia
 1. Etiology and pathophysiology
   a. Poor dietary habits leading to inadequate intake of iron
   b. Iron is essential for the formation of hemoglobin and erythrocytes needed to carry oxygen to cells
 2. Signs and symptoms
   a. Subjective
     (1) Fatigue
     (2) Headache
     (3) Paresthesia
   b. Objective
     (1) Ankle edema
     (2) Dry, pale mucous membranes
     (3) Pearly white sclera
     (4) Decreased hemoglobin and RBC
     (5) Increased iron binding capacity
 3. Treatment
   a. Improve diet; include ascorbic acid, which stimulates iron uptake
   b. Iron supplements
 4. Nursing care
   a. Diet teaching
   b. Teach patient about side effects of medications
B. Pernicious anemia
 1. Etiology and pathophysiology
   a. The lack of intrinsic factor in the stomach prevents the absorption of vitamin B_{12} in the lower portion of the ileum
   b. There is a subsequent reduced number of erythrocytes formed, leading to anemia
 2. Signs and symptoms
   a. Subjective
     (1) Weakness
     (2) Sore mouth
     (3) Paresthesia
     (4) Dyspnea
   b. Objective
     (1) Pallor
     (2) Beefy red tongue
     (3) Positive Romberg test (loss of balance when eyes close)
     (4) Gastric analysis—no intrinsic factor
     (5) Schilling test—urine test for B_{12} absorption
 3. Treatment—lifetime cyanocobalamin (B_{12}) injections

4. Nursing care
   a. Explain disease process and need for continued treatment
   b. Teach family member how to give IM injections or make referral to visiting nurse
C. Aplastic anemia (hypoplastic anemia)
   1. Etiology and pathophysiology
      a. Bone marrow is depressed or destroyed by a chemical or drug
      b. Leukopenia, thrombocytopenia, and decreased erythrocytes
   2. Signs and symptoms
      a. Subjective
         (1) Headache
         (2) Weakness
         (3) Anorexia
         (4) Dyspnea
      b. Objective
         (1) Fever
         (2) Bleeding from mucous membranes
         (3) Decreased leukocytes, erythrocytes, and platelets
   3. Treatment
      a. Identify and eliminate causative agent
      b. Blood transfusions
      c. Maintenance of fluid and electrolyte balance
   4. Nursing care
      a. Support patient and family in understanding illness
      b. Prevent infection by reverse isolation

Blood dyscrasias

A. Thrombocytopenic purpura
   1. Etiology and pathophysiology—a bleeding disorder of unknown origin (possibly autoimmune) in which there is a reduction of platelets
   2. Signs and symptoms
      a. Subjective
         (1) History of epistaxis
         (2) History of gum bleeding
      b. Objective
         (1) Low platelet count
         (2) Ecchymotic areas
         (3) Hemorrhagic petechiae
   3. Treatment
      a. Corticosteroids
      b. Immunosuppressive agents
      c. Splenectomy
      d. Platelet transfusions

4. Nursing care
   a. Prevent injury and bruises
   b. Encourage patient to adhere to medical regimen
   c. Teach the side effects of medications, particularly proness to infection
   d. Provide postoperative care related to splenectomy
B. Polycythemia vera
   1. Etiology and pathophysiology—a disorder of unknown origin that results in an increased number of erythrocytes, leukocytes, and platelets
   2. Signs and symptoms
      a. Subjective
         (1) Headache
         (2) Weakness
         (3) Itching
      b. Objective
         (1) Increased hemoglobin
         (2) Purple-red complexion
         (3) Dyspnea
         (4) Bleeding from mucous membranes
   3. Treatment
      a. Phlebotomy several times yearly
      b. Diet low in iron
      c. Radioactive phosphorus; busulfan (Myleran)
   4. Nursing care
      a. Discuss diet with patient and family
      b. Supportive care and prevention of hemorrhage
      c. Assist with phlebotomy
C. Agranulocytosis
   1. Etiology and pathophysiology
      a. A disease that results in a decreased number of leukocytes
      b. Thought to result from physical agents, such as heavy metals, and cytotoxic drugs
   2. Signs and symptoms
      a. Subjective
         (1) Fatigue
         (2) Malaise
      b. Objective
         (1) High fever
         (2) Necrotic ulcers of mucosa
         (3) Rapid weak pulse
   3. Treatment
      a. Removal of causative agent
      b. Transfusions
      c. Antibiotics
   4. Nursing care

a. Prevent infection and observe for signs of infection
b. Careful oral hygiene
c. Bed rest
d. High-vitamin diet
D. Disseminated intravascular coagulation (DIC)
1. Etiology and pathophysiology
  a. The body's response to injury or disease in which microthrombi obstruct the blood supply of organs
  b. The disorder is further complicated by hemorrhage at various sites throughout the body
2. Signs and symptoms
  a. Subjective
    (1) Restlessness
    (2) Anxiety
  b. Objective
    (1) Laboratory tests indicate low fibrinogen and prolonged prothrombin and partial thromboplastin times
    (2) Hemorrhage, both subcutaneous and internal
3. Treatment
  a. Goal is to relieve underlying cause of DIC
  b. Heparin to prevent the formation of thrombi
  c. Transfusion of blood products
4. Nursing care
  a. Observe for bleeding
  b. Minimize skin punctures
  c. Prevent injury
  d. Provide emotional support

Leukemia

A. Etiology and pathophysiology
1. Incidence is highest in children ages 3 to 4; declines until age 35, at which point there is a steady increase
2. Etiology is unknown, although exposure to certain toxic substances such as radiation seems to increase the incidence
3. There is, in general, an uncontrolled proliferation of white blood cells
4. Classified according to the type of white cell affected
  a. Acute lymphocytic leukemia
    (1) Primarily occurs in children
    (2) Most favorable prognosis with chemotherapy
    (3) Results from abnormal leukocytes in blood-forming tissue
  b. Acute myelogenous leukemia
    (1) Occurs throughout life cycle
    (2) Prognosis is poor with or without chemotherapy
    (3) Results from inability of leukocytes to mature; those which do are abnormal
  c. Chronic myelogenous leukemia
    (1) Occurs after the second decade
    (2) Prognosis is poor
    (3) Results from abnormal production of granulocytic cells
  d. Chronic lymphocytic leukemia
    (1) Occurs after age 35
    (2) Life expectancy is approximately 4 to 5 years
    (3) Results from increased production of leukocytes and lymphocytes and proliferation of cells within bone marrow, spleen, and liver
B. Signs and symptoms
1. Subjective
  a. Malaise
  b. Bone pain
2. Objective
  a. Anemia
  b. Thrombocytopenia
  c. Elevated WBC
  d. Decreased platelets
  e. Petechiae
  f. Gingival bleeding
C. Treatment
1. Chemotherapy
2. Transfusions of whole blood or blood fractions
3. Analgesics
4. Bone marrow transplant
D. Nursing care
1. Discuss the importance of follow-up care with patient and/or family
2. Emotional support for patient and family
3. Specific nursing responsibilities related to particular chemotherapeutic therapy, transfusion, or diagnostic tests

Infectious mononucleosis

A. Etiology and pathophysiology
1. Acute infectious disease of the lymphatic system due to Epstein-Barr (EB) herpes virus
2. Transmitted by respiratory droplets
3. Incubation period is uncertain; probably 28 to 42 days

4. Incidence highest between ages 15 and 35
5. Complications include hepatitis, ruptured spleen, pericarditis, and meningoencephalitis

B. Signs and symptoms
  1. Subjective
    a. Sore throat
    b. Malaise
    c. Stiff neck
    d. Nausea
  2. Objective
    a. Elevated temperature
    b. Enlarged, tender lymph nodes (generally, posterior cervical nodes are involved first)
    c. Splenomegaly in approximately 50% of patients
    d. Elevated lymphocyte and monocyte counts
    e. Positive heterophile antibody agglutination test

C. Treatment
  1. Generally directed toward symptoms (recovery is approximately 3 weeks)
  2. A.S.A.; steroids, if severely ill
  3. If spleen ruptures, splenectomy and blood transfusions necessary

D. Nursing care
  1. Provide rest
  2. Administer A.S.A. as indicated
  3. Assessment for signs of complications; spleen should not be palpated once diagnosis is made
  4. Increased fluid intake

Hodgkin's disease

A. Etiology and pathophysiology
  1. Cause is unknown
  2. Higher incidence in females and young adults
  3. Proliferation of malignant cells (Reed-Sternberg cells) within lymph nodes
  4. All tissues may eventually be involved, but chiefly lymph nodes, spleen, liver, tonsils, and bone marrow
  5. Classification by staging and presence or absence of systemic symptoms

B. Signs and symptoms
  1. Subjective
    a. Dyspnea and dysphagia resulting from pressure from enlarged nodes
    b. Pruritus
    c. Anorexia
  2. Objective

    a. Enlarged lymph nodes (generally cervical nodes are involved first)
    b. Diagnosis confirmed by histologic examination of lymph node
    c. Progressive anemia
    d. Elevated temperature
    e. Enlarged spleen and liver may occur
    f. Pressure from enlarged lymph nodes may cause symptoms of edema and obstructive jaundice
    g. Thrombocytopenia if spleen and bone marrow are involved

C. Treatment
  1. Radiotherapy
    a. Vital organs must be shielded
    b. Potential side effects
      (1) Nausea
      (2) Skin rashes
      (3) Dry mouth
      (4) Dysphagia
  2. Surgical intervention
    a. Excision of node for biopsy
    b. Excision of masses to relieve pressure on other organs
    c. Laparotomy or laparoscopy for staging
  3. Chemotherapy
    a. Nitrogen mustard
    b. Thiophosphoramide (Thiotepa)
    c. Chlorambucil
    d. Vincristine
    e. Doxorubicin (Adriamycin)
    f. Prednisone

D. Nursing care
  1. Provide emotional support for patient and family
  2. Protect from infection
  3. Monitor temperature
  4. Observe for signs of anemia; provide adequate rest
  5. Examine sclera and skin for signs of jaundice
  6. Provide diet as tolerated; observe for anorexia and nausea

Lymphosarcoma

A. Etiology and pathophysiology
  1. Malignant tumors of lymph nodes and lymphatic tissue
  2. Gastrointestinal tract, tonsils, spleen, and liver frequently involved
  3. Cause unknown; incidence is increased in patients who have immunologic disorders

B. Signs and symptoms
   1. Subjective
      a. Malaise
      b. Lethargy
   2. Objective
      a. Painless lymphadenopathy
      b. Fever
      c. Diaphoresis
      d. Weight loss
      e. Decreased resistance to disease
C. Treatment similar to that for Hodgkin's disease
D. Nursing care similar to that for Hodgkin's disease

Respiratory system

REVIEW OF ANATOMY AND PHYSIOLOGY OF THE RESPIRATORY SYSTEM
Functions
A. To make possible exchange of gases between blood and air
B. To make possible cellular respiration

Organs
Nose
A. Structure
   1. Portions
      a. Internal—in skull, above roof of mouth
      b. External—protruding from face
   2. Cavities
      a. Divisions—right and left
      b. Meati—superior, middle, and lower; named for turbinates located above each meatus
      c. Openings
         (1) To exterior—the anterior nares
         (2) To nasopharynx—the posterior nares
      d. Conchae (turbinates)
         (1) Superior and middle processes of ethmoid bone; inferior conchae, separate bones
         (2) Conchae partition each nasal cavity into 3 passageways or meati
      e. Floor—formed by palatine bones and maxillae; these also act as roof of mouth
   3. Lining—ciliated mucosa
   4. Sinuses draining into nose (paranasal sinuses)
      a. Frontal
      b. Maxillary (antrum of Highmore)

c. Sphenoidal
d. Ethmoidal
B. Functions
   1. Serves as passageway for incoming and outgoing air, filtering, warming, moistening, and chemically examining it
   2. Organ of smell (olfactory receptors located in nasal mucosa)
   3. Aids in phonation

Pharynx
A. Structure—composed of muscle with mucous lining
   1. Divisions
      a. Nasopharynx—behind nose
      b. Oropharynx—behind mouth
      c. Laryngopharynx—behind larynx
   2. Openings
      a. In nasopharynx—4 openings: 2 auditory (eustachian) tubes and 2 posterior nares
      b. In oropharynx—1 opening: fauces, archway into mouth
      c. In laryngopharynx—2 openings: into esophagus and into larynx
   3. Organs in pharynx
      a. In nasopharynx—nasopharyngeal tonsils (adenoids)
      b. In oropharynx—palatine and lingual tonsils
B. Functions
   1. Serves as passageway and entrance to both respiratory and digestive tracts
   2. Aids in phonation
   3. Tonsils function to destroy incoming bacteria and to detoxify certain foreign proteins

Larynx
A. Location—at upper end of trachea, just below pharynx
B. Structure
   1. Cartilages—9 pieces arranged in boxlike formation, thyroid largest of cartilages, "Adam's apple"; epiglottis, "lid" cartilage; cricoid, "signet ring" cartilage
   2. Vocal cords
      a. False cords—folds of mucous lining
      b. True cords—fibroelastic bands stretched across hollow interior of larynx; the paired vocal cords (folds) and the posterior arytenoid cartilages make up the glottis; the slit between the vocal cords, through which air enters and leaves the lower respiratory passages, is the rima glottidis
   3. Lining—ciliated mucosa

C. Functions
1. Voice production—during expiration, air passing through larynx causes vocal cords to vibrate; vibration of short, tense cords produces high pitch; long, relaxed cords, low pitch
2. Serves as part of passageway for air; entrance to lower respiratory tract

Trachea

A. Structure
1. Walls—smooth muscle; contain C-shaped rings of cartilage at intervals; these keep tube open at all times but do not constrict the esophagus, which is directly behind the trachea
2. Lining—ciliated mucosa
3. Extent—from larynx to bronchi; about 4½ inches long
B. Function—furnishes open passageway for air going to and from lungs

Lungs

A. Structure
1. Size—large enough to fill pleural divisions of thoracic cavity
2. Shape—cone shaped, with base downward
3. Location—in pleural divisions of thorax; extend from slightly above clavicle to diaphragm; base of each lung rests on diaphragm
4. Divisions
   a. Lobes—3 in right lung, 2 in left
   b. Root—consists of primary bronchus, pulmonary artery and veins bound together by connective tissue
   c. Hilum—vertical slit on medial surface of lung, through which root structures enter lung
   d. Apex—pointed upper part of lung
   e. Base—broad, inferior surface of lung
5. Bronchial tree—consists of the following
   a. Bronchi—right and left bronchi formed by branching of trachea; right bronchus slightly larger and more vertical than left; each primary bronchus branches, on entering lung, into 10 segmental bronchi in each lung; bronchi and segmental bronchi all contain C-shaped cartilage rings
   b. Bronchioles—small branches off secondary bronchi; distinguished by lack of C-shaped cartilage and a duct diameter of about 1 mm
   c. Terminal bronchioles—last bronchioles possessing a ciliated mucosa
   d. Respiratory bronchioles—composed of cuboidal nonciliated cells

   e. Alveolar ducts—microscopic branches off bronchioles composed of a thin squamous epithelium
   f. Alveoli—microscopic sacs composed of single layer of extremely thin squamous epithelial cells; each alveolar duct terminates in cluster of alveoli, often likened to bunch of grapes; each alveolus enveloped by network of lung capillaries
6. Covering of lung—visceral layer of pleura
B. Function—place where air and blood can come in close enough contact for rapid diffusion of gases to occur
1. Bronchi, bronchioles, alveolar ducts—lower part of airway through which air moves into and out of alveoli
2. Alveoli—microscopic sacs in which gases are exchanged very rapidly between air and blood; membranous walls of the millions of alveoli provide surface area large enough and thin enough to make possible rapid gas exchange
3. Alveolar surfaces coated with group of substances called surfactant; effect is to lower alveolar surface tension to facilitate breathing, since sacs have less tendency to collapse with their walls adhering to each other

Physiology of respiration

A. Mechanism of inspiration
1. Respiratory muscles contract
2. Thorax increases in size
3. Intrathoracic pressure decreases
4. Lungs increase in size
5. Intrapulmonic pressure decreases
6. Air rushes from positive pressure in atmosphere to negative pressure in alveoli
7. Inspiration is completed
B. Mechanism of expiration
1. Respiratory muscles relax
2. Thorax decreases in size
3. Intrathoracic pressure increases
4. Lungs decrease in size
5. Intrapulmonic pressure increases
6. Air expelled from higher pressure in the lung to lower pressure in the atmosphere
7. Expiration is completed
C. Neural control
1. Alveolar stretch receptors respond to inspiration (lung inflation) by sending inhibitory impulses to

inspiratory neurons in brainstem; this is the Hering-Breuer inflation reflex, and it prevents lung overdistention

2. During expiration (lung deflation) the stretch receptors no longer inhibit inspiratory neurons, and inspiration may begin again; this is the Hering-Breuer deflation reflex

D. Chemical control
   1. Blood pH—decrease in pH stimulates respiration by direct stimulation of neurons of respiratory center and indirectly by stimulation of carotid and aortic chemoreceptors
   2. Blood P_{CO_2}—increase in arterial P_{CO_2} results in decrease in pH and mimics effects in number 1 above
   3. Stimulation of respiratory center neurons or chemoreceptors results in hyperventilation; hypoventilation occurs when the arterial pH rises or the arterial P_{CO_2} falls

E. Amount of air exchanged in breathing
   1. Directly related to gas pressure gradient between atmosphere and alveoli and inversely related to resistance opposing air flow; the greater the difference between atmospheric pressure and alveolar pressure, the greater the amount of air exchanged in breathing; the greater the resistance opposing air flow to or from the lungs, the less air exchanged

   2. Measured by apparatus called spirometer
   3. Tidal air—average amount expired after normal inspiration; approximately 500 ml
   4. Expiratory reserve volume (ERV)—largest additional volume of air that can be forcibly expired after a normal inspiration and expiration; normal ERV 1000 to 1200 ml
   5. Inspiratory reserve volume (IRV)—largest additional volume of air that can be forcibly inspired after a normal inspiration; normal IRV 3000 to 3300 ml
   6. Residual air—that which cannot be forcibly expired from lungs; about 1200 ml
   7. Minimal air—that which can never be removed from alveoli if they have been inflated even once, even though lungs are subjected to atmospheric pressure that squeezes part of residual air out
   8. Vital capacity—approximate capacity of lungs as measured by amount of air that can be forcibly expired after forcible inspiration; varies with size of thoracic cavity, which is determined by various factors; e.g., size of rib cage, posture, vol-

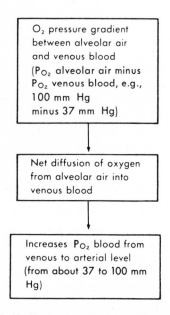

Fig. 3. Mechanism of oxygen diffusion.

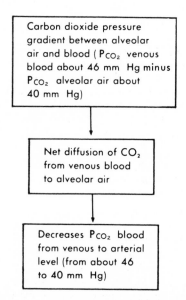

Fig. 4. Mechanism of carbon dioxide diffusion.

ume of blood and interstitial fluid in lungs, size of heart

9. Maximal expiratory flow rate—an individual should be able to exhale 70% of his vital capacity in the first second and empty more than 90% in 3 seconds; asthma and emphysema prevent such normal, forced expiratory rates; measurable with a spirometer

F. Diffusion of gases between air and blood occurs across alveolar-capillary membranes; i.e., in lungs between air in alveoli and venous blood in lung capillaries

1. Direction of diffusion
   a. Oxygen—net diffusion toward lower oxygen pressure gradient; i.e., from alveolar air to blood
   b. Carbon dioxide—net diffusion toward lower carbon dioxide pressure gradient; i.e., from blood to alveolar air
2. Mechanism of oxygen diffusion (Fig. 3)
3. Mechanism of carbon dioxide diffusion (Fig. 4)

G. How blood transports oxygen

1. As solute—about 0.5 ml of oxygen is dissolved in 100 ml of blood; produces the blood P_{O_2} (pressure of oxygen in the blood)
2. As oxyhemoglobin—each gram of hemoglobin can combine with 1.34 ml of oxygen; hence, with normal hemoglobin content (e.g., 15 g per 100 ml of blood) and 100% oxygen saturation, about 20 ml (15×1.34) of oxygen is transported as oxyhemoglobin
3. Various factors influence rate at which oxygen assciates with hemoglobin to form oxyhemoglobin, including
   a. Increasing pressure of oxygen in the blood
   b. Decreasing pressure of carbon dioxide in the blood
4. Various factors influence rate at which oxygen dissociates from hemoglobin, including
   a. Decreasing pressure of oxygen in the blood
   b. Increasing pressure of carbon dioxide in the blood
   c. Increased blood temperature

H. How blood transports carbon dioxide

1. As solute—small amount dissolves in plasma
2. As bicarbonate ion—more than half of CO_2 in blood is present in the plasma as bicarbonate ion, formed by ionization of carbonic acid
3. As carbhemoglobin—less than one third of CO_2 is transported in combination with hemoglobin

I. Diffusion of gases between arterial blood and tissues occurs in tissue capillaries

1. Oxygen—net diffusion of dissolved O_2 out of blood into tissues because of lower P_{O_2} there (perhaps 30 mm Hg compared with arterial P_{O_2} of 100 mm Hg); diffusion of dissolved oxygen out of blood lowers blood P_{O_2} from arterial to venous level (from 100 to 40 mm Hg); decreasing P_{O_2} as blood moves through tissue capillaries causes oxygen to dissociate from hemoglobin, thereby releasing more oxygen for diffusion out of blood to tissue cells
2. Carbon dioxide—net diffusion of CO_2 into blood because of lower P_{CO_2} there (40 mm Hg compared with probably over 50 mm Hg in tissues); diffusion of CO_2 into tissue capillaries increases blood P_{CO_2} from arterial to venous level (from 40 to 46 mm Hg); increasing P_{CO_2} like decreasing P_{O_2}, tends to accelerate oxygen dissociation from hemoglobin

REVIEW OF PHYSICAL PRINCIPLES RELATED TO THE RESPIRATORY SYSTEM
Principles of mechanics
Law of gravitation
EXAMPLES

1. Postural drainage—positioning of individual so that the throat is below level of lungs to help drain fluid from the lungs
2. Rocking beds—abdominal viscera alternately push against and then away from the diaphragm, thus aiding in respiration
3. Position of head postoperatively—head is placed on one side; thus, the force of gravity pulls the tongue down, breathing remains unobstructed and allows for drainage in case of vomiting
4. Use of chest tubes to restore negative pressure to intrapleural space

Momentum
EXAMPLES

1. During a cough or a sneeze, the abdominal and intercostal muscles apply a large force on the air in the lungs; the sudden opening of the vocal cords and epiglottis results in the explosive propulsion of air from the lungs; in this case momentum of the air stream is great, not because of the mass of the particles (since the molecules of gasses in air are light), but because of their high velocity
2. When a person speaks, the vocal cords vibrate and in turn produce vibrations in the air molecules sur-

rounding them; the momentum in these vibrating molecules is transferred from air molecule to air molecule all the way to the ear of the listener, where the vibrations are converted into nerve impulses that the brain interprets as sound

Energy

EXAMPLES
1. Epithelial cells of the human respiratory tract possess energy because their cilia beat back and forth and thus do the work of pushing mucus and foreign matter up toward the throat
2. Every living cell in the body possesses energy because it does work to maintain certain water and electrolyte concentrations within itself
3. The cilia exert a force that moves them through a certain distance in the fluid surrounding them
4. The cell membranes exert a force that moves ions a certain distance through the membrane
5. Second law of thermodynamics

Principles of physical properties of matter

Solids

Concept of elasticity
EXAMPLE: The elastic recoil of the lungs during quiet respiration provides the entire force necessary to effect expiration

Liquids

Surface tension—the molecules of a liquid exert forces of attraction on one another; at the surface of the liquid the molecules are attracted by other molecules at the bottom and sides, but not at the top since air is there; this results in a force of contraction at the liquid surface called surface tension
EXAMPLE: The alveoli and respiratory passages of the human lungs have a mixture of surface tension-reducing substances collectively called surfactant that reduce surface tension and the pull that the water molecules would ordinarily have on each other if these surface active agents were absent; breathing is therefore much easier because of this agent

Gases

The molecules composing gases are so far apart that they do not exert any cohesive forces on each other; consequently, the gas will expand to fill any container and will exert pressure on the container because of elastic rebound of the gas molecules with the walls of the container
A. Boyle's law—at constant temperature, the pressure exerted by a gas is inversely proportional to its

volume; as the volume of a gas is decreased, its pressure increases, and as the volume is increased, the pressure decreases
1. Respiration—the contraction and downward movements of the dome-shaped diaphragm increase the volume of the thoracic cavity containing the lungs; since the volume of air in the lungs is increased, the pressure exerted by the air is decreased; air now flows from the area of higher pressure outside the body to the area of lower pressure inside the lungs; conversely, during expiration, the upward movement of the diaphragm and the elastic recoil of the lungs themselves decrease the volume of air in the thoracic cavity and lungs as air flows out
2. Pneumothorax—an opening connecting the outside air with the intrapleural space results in air flowing into the intrapleural space; this eliminates the pressure gradient between the thoracic cavity and the atmosphere, and the lungs cannot inflate
3. Intermittent positive pressure breathing (IPPB) apparatus—a special valve is operated by the individual's own respirations; on inspiration, one part of the valve opens and oxygen or a mixture of gases is forcefully pushed under greater than atmospheric pressure (positive pressure) into the lungs through a special mouthpiece or face mask
B. Dalton's law—the pressure exerted (in millimeters of of mercury [mm Hg]) by a gas in a mixture of gases is proportional to its percentage in the mixture; e.g., partial pressure of O_2 in alveoli is 104 mm Hg; partial pressure of O_2 in pulmonary artery and alveolar capillaries is 40 mm Hg; therefore O_2 diffuses from alveoli air sacs into capillaries
C. Henry's law—the quantity of gas dissolving in a liquid is proportional to the partial pressure of the gas at a given temperature; i.e., a person overcome by smoke inhalation or who has some obstruction to normal breathing can benefit from inhalation of either pure O_2 or a mixture of gases having a higher partial pressure of O_2 than is found in air
D. Bernoulli's principle

Principles of light

A. X rays use high-frequency electromagnetic waves
EXAMPLE: The chest x-ray examination permits observation of a variety of lung disorders, such as pneumonia, tumors, and tuberculosis
B. Total internal reflection—at a certain critical angle,

light between two media is not refracted (bent) through the two media, but is reflected back into the first medium

EXAMPLE: Fiberoptics allows illumination and visualization of trachea and bronchi (bronchoscopy); the image picked up by the lens internally reflects along fiberoptic tubing (even if bent) until it reaches the eye of the observer

REVIEW OF CHEMICAL PRINCIPLES RELATED TO THE RESPIRATORY SYSTEM

(Same as cardiovascular)

REVIEW OF MICROORGANISMS RELATED TO THE RESPIRATORY SYSTEM

A. Bacterial pathogens
  1. *Bordetella pertussis*—small, gram-negative coccobacillus; causes pertussis or whooping cough
  2. *Diplococcus pneumoniae*—gram-positive, encapsulated diplococcus; on the basis of the antigenic nature of the capsule there are about 100 types, the most important being Types I, II, and III; causes pneumococcal pneumonia (most commonly lobar) and often responsible for sinusitis, otitis media, and meningitis
  3. *Haemophilus influenzae*—small gram-negative, highly pleomorphic bacillus; causes acute meningitis and upper respiratory tract infections
  4. *Klebsiella pneumoniae* (Friedländer's bacillus)—gram-negative, encapsulated, non-spore-forming bacillus; causes pneumonia and urinary tract infections
  5. *Mycobacterium tuberculosis* (tubercle bacillus)—acid-fast actinomycete (thin, waxy rods, often bent, nonmotile, non-spore forming); causes tuberculosis
B. Rickettsial pathogen
  1. *Coxiella burnetii*—the only species of rickettsiae not associated with a vector; causes Q fever, an infection clinically similar to primary atypical pneumonia
C. Viral pathogens
  1. DNA viruses
    a. Adenoviruses—spherical and 70 to 80 nm in diameter; cause acute respiratory disease, adenoidal-pharyngeal conjunctivitis, and other respiratory infections
  2. RNA viruses
    a. Coronaviruses—enveloped pleomorphic viruses; frequently associated with a mild upper respiratory infection
    b. Picornaviruses—spherical and 20 to 30 nm in diameter; cause poliomyelitis, Coxsackie disease, common cold, and various diseases of animals
    c. Reoviruses—double-stranded RNA virus involved in mild respiratory infections of humans
D. Fungal pathogen
  1. *Histoplasma capsulatum*—dimorphic fungus producing characteristic spores (chlamydospores) in infected tissue; causes histoplasmosis (a primary lung infection)

PHARMACOLOGY RELATED TO RESPIRATORY SYSTEM DISORDERS

A. Bronchodilators
  1. General implications for nurses
    a. Administer via correct route (oral, rectal, parenteral, inhalation)
    b. Monitor vital signs for changes
    c. Observe for signs of adequate oxygenation such as warmth and color
    d. Teach patient action and side effects of therapy
    e. Observe for side effects
      (1) Dizziness, nervousness
      (2) Gastric irritation
      (3) Palpitations
  2. Theophylline derivatives
    a. Actions
      (1) Act directly on bronchial smooth muscle to decrease spasm and relax smooth muscle of the vasculature
      (2) Direct stimulatory effect on myocardium increases cardiac output, which improves blood flow to kidneys
      (3) Direct action on renal tubules provides diuretic effect by increasing excretion of sodium and chloride ions
    b. Examples
      (1) Aminophylline
      (2) Dyphylline (Dilor, Neothylline)
      (3) Oxtriphylline (Choledyl)
      (4) Theophylline (Aqualin, Elixophyllin)
  3. Sympathetic amines
    a. Actions
      (1) Act at beta-adrenergic receptors in bron-

chus to relax smooth muscle and increase respiratory volume

(2) Inhalants have a local action causing vasoconstriction that reduces congestion or edema

(3) With large doses the myocardium is stimulated, which results in an increased cardiac output

b. Examples

(1) Epinephrine hydrochloride (Adrenalin, Epifrin)

(2) Epinephrine, aqueous (Sus-Phrine)

(3) Ethylnorepinephrine hydrochloride (Bronkephrine)

(4) Ephedrine sulfate

(5) Pseudoephedrine hydrochloride (Sudafed)

(6) Metaproterenol sulfate (Alupent, Metaprel)

(7) Terbutaline sulfate (Brethine)

(8) Aminophylline

(9) Isoproterenol hydrochloride (Isuprel)

B. Mucolytic agents and expectorants

1. General implications for nurses

a. Observe for respiratory distress

b. Have mechanical suction apparatus available in the event the patient is unable to cough up secretions

c. Wash the patient's face after administration, since stickiness is common

d. Administer drugs diluted as ordered; do not directly follow expectorants with other fluid intake

e. Observe patient for adverse effects

(1) Nausea

(2) Skin eruptions

(3) Jitteriness

f. Increase fluid intake to loosen secretions

g. Encourage coughing and deep breathing

2. Mucolytic agents

a. Action—raise osmolality of bronchial glandular secretions, causing fluid to dilute the secretions

b. Examples

(1) Calcium iodide

(2) Glyceryl guaiacolate (Robitussin)

(3) Iodinated glycerol (Organidin)

(4) Potassium iodide (SSKI, Pima Syrup)

3. Expectorants

a. Action—increase production of thinner, less viscid secretions that protect bronchial tissues

b. Examples

(1) Acetylcysteine (Mucomyst)

(2) Glyceryl guaiacolate (Guaifenesin, Robitussin)

(3) Terpin hydrate elixer

C. Antitussives

1. General implications for nurses

a. Explain side effects to patient

b. Advise patient not to take liquids for 15 minutes after administration

c. Provide adequate fluids and put in semi- or high Fowler's position to support respiratory processes

d. Observe patient for adverse effects

(1) Hypersensitivity

(2) Nausea

(3) Drowsiness

2. Narcotic antitussives

a. Actions

(1) Act on medullary control center to suppress cough

(2) Are usually used when cough is not productive

b. Examples

(1) Dextromethorphan hydrobromide (Dormethan, Romilar)

(2) Hydrocodone bitartrate (Codone, Dicodid)

(3) Levopropoxyphene napsylate (Novrad)

(4) Noscapine (Nectadon)

3. Nonnarcotic antitussives

a. Action—act to inhibit cough reflex at afferent endings of vagus nerve and at medullary transmission sites

b. Examples

(1) Benzonatate (Tessalon)

(2) Dextromethorphan hydrobromide (Romilar HBr, Sucrets)

4. Antihistaminic cough suppressants

a. Action—act at tissue level to prevent histamine-induced edema causing irritation of cough-sensitive nerve endings in tracheobronchial structures

b. Examples

(1) Chlophedianol hydrochloride (Ulo)

(2) Diphenhydramine hydrochloride (Benadryl)

D. Drugs that antagonize the effects of narcotics

1. General implications for nurses
   a. Carefully monitor vital signs, especially respirations
   b. Prepare for emergency resuscitative measures
   c. Be alert to withdrawal symptoms
   d. Observe patient for adverse effects
      (1) Respiratory depression when drug used alone
      (2) Lethargy, dizziness
      (3) Nausea and vomiting
      (4) Miosis (constriction of pupils)
2. Actions
   a. Compete with narcotics for receptors at respiratory center
   b. Lower threshold for carbon dioxide stimulation of respiration (increases respiratory rate and tidal volume, which decreases blood CO_2 level)
3. Examples
   a. Levallorphan tartrate (Lorfan)
   b. Nalorphine hydrochloride (Nalline)
   c. Naloxone hydrochloride (Narcan)
E. Drugs that have an antihistaminic effect
   1. General implications for nurses
      a. Caution the patient regarding operating machinery and driving while taking this medication
      b. Advise patient to report side effects to the physician
      c. If given IM, inject deep into tissue to prevent irritation to tissue
      d. Observe patient for adverse effects
         (1) Inability to concentrate
         (2) Insomnia
         (3) Ataxia
         (4) Tremors
         (5) Headache
         (6) Nausea, anorexia
         (7) Diarrhea
   2. Actions
      a. Interfere with histaminic action by competing for extravascular receptors at arteriole sites
      b. Block histamine-induced irritation of nerve endings, causing itching or burning, dilation of arterioles, and constriction of venules, which causes transudation of fluid into tissues
      c. Prevent progression but have no effect on existing problems
      d. Also have antiemetic, anticholinergic, and central nervous system depressant effect

3. Examples
   a. Brompheniramine maleate (Dimetane)
   b. Chlorpheniramine maleate (Chlor-Trimeton, Histaspan, Teldrin)
   c. Cyproheptadine hydrochloride (Periactin Hydrochloride)
   d. Methdilazine hydrochloride (Tacaryl)
   e. Chlorothen citrate (Tagathen)
   f. Methapyrilene hydrochloride (Histadyl)
   g. Pyrilamine maleate
   h. Tripelennamine citrate (Pyribenzamine Citrate)
   i. Carbinoxamine maleate (Clistin)
   j. Diphenhydramine hydrochloride (Benadryl)
   k. Doxylamine succinate (Decapryn)
   l. Hydroxyzine hydrochloride (Atarax)
   m. Hydroxyzine pamoate (Vistaril)

RELATED PROCEDURES
Administration of oxygen

A. Definition
   1. Administration of supplemental oxygen when patient's respiratory system is compromised and tissue hypoxia is threatened
   2. May be administered via catheter, cannula, mask, or tent
B. Nursing responsibilities
   1. Explain procedure to patient and family
   2. Attach ''no smoking'' signs to door of room and instruct patients and visitors to adhere to this ruling, since oxygen supports combustion
   3. Assess patient's color (nail beds, general appearance) and vital signs prior to and during therapy
   4. Ascertain if patient has chronic lung disease before administering high concentrations of oxygen
   5. Attach appropriate apparatus to oxygen source and fill humidification cannister with water to prevent drying of mucous membranes

Bronchoscopy

A. Definition
   1. Visualization of the tracheobronchial tree via a scope advanced through the mouth into the bronchi
   2. Procedure may be performed to remove foreign body, to remove secretions, or to obtain specimens of tissue or mucus for further study
B. Nursing responsibilities
   1. Obtain an informed consent

2. Maintain patient NPO prior to procedure and remove dentures and jewelry
3. Administer ordered preprocedure medications to produce sedation and decrease anxiety
4. Postprocedure responsibilities
   a. Monitor vital signs until stable
   b. Do not allow patient to drink until gag reflex returns
   c. Inform patient to expect some hemoptysis after procedure
   d. Observe patient for signs of hemorrhage and/or respiratory distress

Suctioning of airways

A. Definition
   1. Mechanical aspiration of mucous secretions from the bronchotracheal tree by application of negative pressure
   2. Utilized to maintain patent airway, obtain sputum specimen, or stimulate coughing
   3. May be nasotracheal, oral-pharyngeal, or directly through trachea or endotracheal tube
B. Nursing responsibilities
   1. Maintain surgical asepsis
   2. Assess proper functioning of equipment
   3. Lubricate suction catheter with sterile water
   4. Insert catheter
      a. If tracheal suction is being utilized, catheter is inserted approximately 4 inches
      b. If nasotracheal suction is being utilized, catheter is inserted until cough reflex is induced
   5. Apply no suction while the catheter is being inserted
   6. Rotate and withdraw catheter while suction is applied; suction should not exceed 10 to 15 seconds
   7. Clear catheter with sterile solution and encourage patient to breathe deeply
   8. If deeper suction is required, ask patient to turn head to the side to permit entry of the suction catheter into the opposite bronchus

Tracheostomy care

A. Definition—the removal of dried secretions from the cannula to maintain a patent airway, prevent infection, and prevent irritation
B. Nursing responsibilities
   1. Trach care should be done at least every 8 hours
   2. Suction to remove secretions from the lumen of the tube (see procedure for suctioning of airways)

3. If an inner cannula is present
   a. Remove and place in container of hydrogen peroxide and rinse with normal saline, using surgical aseptic technique
   b. Remove dried secretions within cannula, using sterile pipe cleaners or brush
   c. Drain excess saline before reinserting tube, which is then locked in place
4. Clean the area around the stoma with peroxide and saline, using aseptic technique; apply antiseptic ointment if ordered
5. Change trach string or tape, being careful not to dislodge cannula
6. Place a trach dressing or fenestrated 4 × 4-inch (unfilled) dressing below the stoma to absorb expelled secretions
7. Humidify inhaled air mechanically or by the use of a moistened 4 × 4-inch bandage over the trach, since air is bypassing normal humidification process in the nasopharynx

Mechanical ventilation

A. Definition—the use of a mechanical device to instill a mixture of air and oxygen into the lungs using positive pressure
B. Types of ventilators
   1. Volume control—delivers a preset tidal volume at various pressures
   2. Pressure control—delivers preset pressure at various volumes
C. Types of ventilation
   1. Controlled—the patient receives a specified volume at a specific pressure with no triggering of the machine by the patient; the nurse may have to administer drugs such as curare or morphine to decrease the patient's own respiratory response
   2. Assisted—the patient triggers the machine so that the rate may vary; however, if the patient has periods of apnea, the machine will take over initiation of respirations
D. Nursing responsibilities
   1. Keep respirator at settings as ordered and notify respiratory therapy department and physician if distress occurs
   2. Maintain a sealed system between respirator and patient so that volume to be delivered is kept constant and air is not lost around tubing; this is accomplished by inflating the cuff of the endotracheal tube or tracheostomy tube to minimum occlusive volume

3. Suction the patient frequently, since humidified oxygen helps to liquefy secretions that must be removed
4. Observe patient for signs of respiratory insufficiency, such as tachypnea, cyanosis, and changes in sensorium
5. Ascertain blood gases as ordered to determine effectiveness of ventilation
6. Establish a means of communication, since patient will be unable to speak while on a ventilator

Pulmonary function tests

A. Definition
   1. A series of tests used to detect problems in the performance capabilities of the pulmonary system
   2. A spirometer is used to measure amounts of gas exchanged between the patient and the atmosphere; nose clips are used to allow only mouth breathing and prevent air leakage
   3. Measurement studies include
      a. Tidal volume—amount of air inhaled or exhaled during one respiration
      b. Vital capacity—volume of air that can be forcefully exhaled after a maximum inspiration
      c. Total lung capacity—volume of air in the lungs following a maximum inspiration
B. Nursing responsibilities
   1. Explain procedure to patient to allay anxiety and promote compliance at time of test
   2. Notify respiratory therapist of all medications that patient is receiving which affect respiratory function

Thoracentesis

A. Definition
   1. A surgically aseptic procedure in which the chest wall is punctured with a trocar to remove fluid or air; this is done for diagnostic purposes or to alleviate respiratory embarrassment
   2. No more than 1000 ml of fluid should be removed at a time; fluid withdrawn should be sent to the laboratory for culture and sensitivity tests
   3. Complications include pneumothorax from trauma to the lung and pulmonary edema as a result of sudden fluid shifts
B. Nursing responsibilities
   1. Obtain informed consent
   2. Explain procedure to the patient

3. Ensure that chest x-ray examination is done prior to and after procedure
4. Assist and support patient in the sitting position
5. Set up sterile field for physician
6. Assess pulse and respirations prior to, during, and after procedure
7. Inform patient not to cough during procedure to prevent trauma to the lungs
8. After procedure, label and send specimens for laboratory tests
9. Note and record the amount, color, and clarity of the fluid withdrawn
10. Place patient on opposite side for approximately 1 hour to prevent leakage of fluid through thoracentesis site
11. Observe patient for coughing, bloody sputum, and rapid pulse rate and report their occurrence immediately

Chest tubes

A. Definition
   1. Use of tubes and suction to return negative pressure to the intrapleural space
   2. To drain air from the intrapleural space, the chest tube is placed between the second or third intercostal space; to drain blood or fluid, the catheter would be placed at a lower site, usually the eighth or ninth intercostal space
   3. One-bottle underwater system—allows air or fluid to drain from the pleural cavity by gravity via a glass rod, which extends approximately 2 cm below the surface of the water within the collection bottle
   4. Two-bottle drainage system—involves 1 bottle that acts as a collection chamber and provides the water seal while a second bottle can be connected to a suction apparatus; the bubbling of water within the second bottle indicates that the desired suction is maintained
   5. Three-bottle system—includes 1 bottle that serves to collect drainage, 1 that acts as the water-seal chamber, and 1 that controls suction
   6. Pleurevac—a commercially prepared plastic unit designed for closed chest suction; it combines the features of the other systems and may or may not be attached to suction
B. Nursing responsibilities
   1. Ensure that tubing is not kinked; tape all connections to prevent separation

2. Milk tubing in direction of drainage system to maintain patency
3. Maintain level of drainage system below level of chest
4. Turn frequently, making sure patient does not lie on chest tubes
5. Report drainage on dressing immediately, since this is not a normal occurrence
6. Observe for fluctuation of fluid in glass tube; the level will rise on inhalation and fall on exhalation; if there are no fluctuations, either the lung has expanded fully or the chest tube is clogged
7. Palpate area around chest tube drainage for subcutaneous emphysema or crepitus, which indicate that air is leaking into the subcutaneous tissue
8. Situate the drainage bottles or pleurevac to avoid breakage
9. Place 2 clamps at the bedside for use if the underwater seal bottle is broken; clamp the chest tube immediately to prevent air from entering the intrapleural space, which would cause pneumothorax to recur or extend
10. Encourage coughing and deep breathing every 2 hours, splinting the area as needed
11. When the physician removes the chest tube, instruct the patient to exhale or strain (Valsalva maneuver) as the tube is withdrawn; apply a gauze dressing immediately and firmly secure with tape to make an airtight dressing
12. Encourage movement of the arm on the affected side

MAJOR DISEASES
Pulmonary embolism and infarction

A. Etiology and pathophysiology
1. Postoperative patients, as well as those confined to bed, are prone to venous stasis, which causes peripheral thrombus formation
2. When an embolus lodges in the pulmonary artery causing hemorrhage and necrosis of lung tissue, it is called a pulmonary infarction
B. Signs and symptoms
1. Subjective
a. Severe dyspnea that occurs suddenly
b. Anxiety
c. Restlessness
d. Sharp upper abdominal or thoracic pain
2. Objective

a. Violent coughing with hemoptysis
b. On auscultation, dullness over area of infarction
c. Increased temperature
C. Treatment
1. Anticoagulant therapy
2. Maintenance of blood pressure
3. Angiogram may be performed, and, if condition is severe, an embolectomy may be indicated
D. Nursing care
1. Place in high Fowler's position to aid respiration
2. Monitor vital signs
3. Administer medications and oxygen as ordered

Pulmonary edema

A. Etiology and pathophysiology
1. An acute emergency condition characterized by a rapid accumulation of fluid in the alveolar spaces resulting from increased pressure within the pulmonary system
2. Possible causes include valvular disease, left ventricular failure, circulatory overload, or congestive heart disease
B. Signs and symptoms
1. Subjective
a. History of premonitory symptoms such as shortness of breath, paroxysmal nocturnal dyspnea, wheezing, and orthopnea
b. Acute anxiety, apprehension, restlessness
2. Objective
a. Rapid thready pulse
b. Pink frothy sputum
c. Elevated central venous pressure (CVP)
d. Decreased circulation time
e. Cyanosis
f. Wheezing
g. Stertorous respirations
C. Treatment
1. Medications aimed at decreasing cardiac work load and improving cardiac output, such as morphine sulfate, digitalis, diuretics, bronchodilators
2. Oxygen in high concentration or by IPPB as necessary
3. Phlebotomy to remove approximately 500 ml of blood or the application of rotating tourniquets to reduce the volume of circulating blood
4. Cardiac monitoring
D. Nursing care
1. Support patient in a high or semi-Fowler's position

2. Observe and record vital signs and monitor cardiac activity and intake and output
3. Provide reassuring environment to allay anxiety
4. Suction as needed to maintain patent airway
5. Apply rotating tourniquets when ordered
   a. Tourniquets are generally applied to extremities without completely obliterating the pulse
   b. One touniquet is moved in a clockwise direction every 15 minutes
   c. When patient is no longer in distress, tourniquets are removed 1 at a time at 15-minute intervals to prevent sudden cardiac overload; legs are rotated off last

Pleural effusion

A. Etiology and pathophysiology
   1. Pleural effusion refers to the collection of fluid in the pleural space
   2. This generally occurs secondary to diseases such as cancer of the lung, tuberculosis, and congestive heart failure
B. Signs and symptoms
   1. Subjective
      a. Pleuritic pain that is sharp and increases on inspiration
      b. Dyspnea
      c. Malaise
   2. Objective
      a. Tachycardia
      b. Elevated temperature
      c. Cough (may be productive or nonproductive, depending on cause)
      d. Decreased breath sounds
      e. Chest x-ray examination shows obliteration of the angle between the ribs and diaphragm; it may also reveal a mediastinal shift away from the fluid
C. Treatment
   1. Thoracentesis is generally performed (see procedure)
   2. Treatment of underlying cause
D. Nursing care
   1. Monitor vital signs, particularly temperature and respirations
   2. Auscultate lung fields
   3. Encourage coughing and deep breathing
   4. Increase fluid intake
   5. Place patient in high Fowler's position for maximum air exchange

Pleurisy

A. Etiology and pathophysiology
   1. An inflammation of the visceral and parietal membranes, which rub together during respiration and cause pain
   2. Caused by chest trauma, tuberculosis, pneumonia, or chest surgery
B. Signs and symptoms
   1. Subjective
      a. Knifelike pain on inspiration
      b. Apprehension
      c. Dyspnea
   2. Objective
      a. Decreased excursion of involved chest wall
      b. Pleural friction rub is discernible on auscultation of chest wall
C. Treatment
   1. Treat underlying condition
   2. Analgesics for pain
   3. Applications of heat or cold to thoracic area
D. Nursing care
   1. Instruct patient to lie on affected side to splint chest wall and lessen pain on inspiration
   2. Administer medications as ordered
   3. Allay anxiety
   4. Observe for signs of shock or pulmonary emboli

Empyema

A. Etiology and pathophysiology
   1. A collection of pus within the thoracic cavity
   2. May occur following staphylococcal pneumonia, tuberculosis, chest trauma, or surgery
B. Signs and symptoms
   1. Subjective
      a. Unilateral chest pain
      b. Malaise
      c. Anorexia
      d. Dyspnea
   2. Objective
      a. Chest x-ray examination shows pleural exudate
      b. Elevated temperature
      c. Cough
      d. Unequal chest expansion
C. Treatment
   1. A thoracentesis is performed to obtain a specimen of exudate to culture
   2. Chest tubes are inserted to drain thoracic cavity
   3. Antibiotics may be instilled through the chest tube or may be given systemically

4. If condition is long-standing, the area of inflammation is surgically removed; this is known as decortication
D. Nursing care
   1. Monitor chest tube (see procedure)
   2. Provide emotional support
   3. Administer antibiotics as ordered
   4. Monitor vital signs, particularly temperature and character of respirations

Pneumonia

A. Etiology and pathophysiology
   1. Inflammatory disease usually caused by an infectious agent (bacterial, viral, or fungal) but may also be caused by inhalation of chemicals and aspiration of gastric contents
   2. Pneumonia is commonly spread by respiratory droplets
   3. Pneumococcal pneumonia is most common type of bacterial pneumonia and occurs in winter and spring; other bacterial pneumonias include *Klebsiella pneumoniae*, *Haemophilus influenzae*, species of *Pseudomonas*, *Proteus*, and *Streptococcus*, and *Staphylococcus aureus*
   4. Aspiration pneumonia occurs when gastric contents and the normal flora of the upper respiratory tract are aspirated into the lung
B. Signs and symptoms
   1. Subjective
      a. Lassitude
      b. Chest pain that increases on inspiration
      c. Dyspnea
   2. Objective
      a. Elevated temperature
      b. Increased WBC
      c. Cough
      d. Chest x-ray examination shows pulmonary infiltration
      e. Sputum production
         (1) Pneumococcal pneumonia—purulent, rusty sputum
         (2) Staphylococcal pneumonia—yellow, blood-streaked sputum
         (3) Klebsiella pneumonia—red gelatinous sputum
         (4) Mycoplasma pneumonia—nonproductive that advances to mucoid
C. Treatment
   1. If bacterial pneumonia, culture and sensitivity

tests will be done of blood and sputum to determine appropriate antibiotic therapy
   2. Oxygen therapy usually via nasal cannula
   3. Inhalation therapy such as IPPB or the use of incentive spirometer
D. Nursing care
   1. Encourage coughing and deep breathing, splinting the chest as necessary
   2. Observe amount and characteristics of sputum
   3. Collect sputum specimen for culture and sensitivity tests in sterile container; notify physician if organism is resistant to the antibiotic being given
   4. Increase fluid intake
   5. Monitor vital signs
   6. Observe for signs of respiratory distress, such as labored respirations, cool clammy skin, and cyanosis

Atelectasis

A. Etiology and pathophysiology
   1. Atelectasis occurs when respirations are shallow and ineffective, as in postoperative patients
   2. Bronchioles are obstructed by secretions, and alveoli distal to the bronchioles collapse; many small bronchioles or a stem of the bronchus may be involved
   3. Causes include compression due to large pleural effusion, empyema, or pneumothorax, obstruction of a bronchus by a tumor, and deficiency of surfactant in an infant
B. Signs and symptoms
   1. Subjective
      a. Restlessness
      b. Anxiety
   2. Objective
      a. Rapid shallow respirations
      b. Diminished breath sounds in lower lobes
      c. Productive cough
      d. Temperature elevation
C. Treatment
   1. Oxygen therapy
   2. IPPB
   3. Prophylactic antibiotics
D. Nursing care
   1. Encourage coughing and deep breathing
   2. Monitor respirations closely
   3. Auscultate breath sounds for signs of decreased ventilation
   4. Place in high Fowler's position; turn every 2 hours

Sarcoidosis

A. Etiology and pathophysiology
1. Characterized by epithelioid cell tubercles, most commonly in the lung
2. Cause is unknown, although 80% have high titers of Epstein-Barr virus
3. Incidence is highest in blacks and young adults
B. Signs and symptoms
1. Subjective
a. Fatigue
b. Malaise
c. Dyspnea
2. Objective
a. Night sweats
b. Fever
c. Weight loss
d. Cough
e. Nodules of face
f. Polyarthritis
g. Mild anemia
h. Elevated serum calcium
i. Kveim test—sarcoid node antigen is injected intradermally and causes local nodular lesion in approximately 1 month
j. Biopsy of skin, lymph node, or liver
k. X-ray findings include bilateral hilar and paratracheal adenopathy
C. Treatment
1. No specific treatment
2. Corticosteroids to control symptoms
D. Nursing care
1. Monitor temperature and other vital signs
2. Increase fluid intake
3. Provide frequent periods of rest
4. Provide small nutritious meals, taking into consideration patient's preferences

Pulmonary tuberculosis

A. Etiology and pathophysiology
1. Infection of lungs caused by *Mycobacterium tuberculosis,* an acid-fast bacterium
2. Causes tubercles, fibrosis, and calcification within the lungs
3. The tubercle bacillus may be communicated to others by means of droplet formation (inhalation), ingestion, or inoculation
4. Predisposing factors include debilitating diseases such as alcoholism, cardiovascular disease, diabetes mellitus, and cirrhosis, as well as poor nutrition and crowded living conditions
5. Chronic, progressive, and reinfection phase is most frequently encountered in adults and involves progression or reactivation of primary lesions after months or years of latency
6. Swallowing infected sputum may lead to laryngeal, oropharyngeal, and intestinal tuberculosis
B. Signs and symptoms
1. Subjective
a. Malaise
b. Pleuritic pain
c. Easy fatigue
2. Objective
a. Fever
b. Night sweats
c. Cough that progressively becomes worse
d. Hemoptysis
e. Weight loss
f. Chest x-ray examination to determine presence of calcified lesions
g. Analysis of sputum and gastric contents for presence of acid-fast bacilli
h. Tuberculin testing
(1) Examples
(a) Tine
(b) Heaf
(c) Mantoux, which frequently involves the use of purified protein derivative (PPD)
(2) Determines antibody response to tubercle bacillus
(3) Indicates prior exposure to bacillus, which may or may not indicate active disease state (a sudden change from negative to positive requires follow-up testing)
(4) In each test, either old tuberculin (OT) or PPD is injected intradermally; redness and edema present 48 to 72 hours later indicate a positive finding
C. Treatment
1. Determine and prescribe a program of combined antituberculin drugs such as INH, PAS, streptomycin, PZA
2. Encourage bed rest until symptoms abate or therapeutic regimen is established
3. Determine whether surgical resection of the involved lobe is necessary if symptoms such as hemorrhage develop or chemotherapy is unsatisfactory

4. Provide prophylactic therapy to immediate contacts (all cases and follow-up of contacts must be reported to public health agency)
5. Place the patient on high-carbohydrate, high-protein, high-vitamin diet with supplemental vitamin B_6

D. Nursing care
   1. Teach patient to provide for scheduled rest periods
   2. Teach patient which foods to include in diet and the use of nutritious between-meal supplements
   3. Teach patient the importance of maintaining the drug program that has been established without variation
   4. Teach patient the proper techniques to prevent spread of infection
      a. Frequent hand washing
      b. Cover mouth when coughing
      c. The proper use and disposal of tissues
      d. The proper cleansing of eating utensils and disposal of food wastes
      e. The use of isolation when sputum is positive for the organism
   5. Encourage patient to participate in developing a schedule of activities and therapy and following the schedule once established
   6. Instruct patient to be alert to the early symptoms of hemorrhage such as hemoptysis and to contact the physician immediately if any occur
   7. Instruct patient to be alert to the early symptoms of adverse drug reactions (e.g., neuritis, ringing in the ears, ataxia, dermatitis) and to contact the physician immediately if any occur
   8. Encourage patient to follow prescribed program for productive coughing and deep breathing
   9. Instruct patient to avoid any medications such as cough syrups without physician's approval
   10. Explain the need for and instruct the patient to continue follow-up care and supervision
   11. Encourage patient to express feelings about disease and the many ramifications (stigma, isolation, fear) it creates
   12. Expect and accept patient's expression of hostility and depression
   13. Encourage patient to limit activities until physician gives approval for gradual increase
   14. Help patient plan a realistic schedule for taking the large number of necessary medications

Chronic obstructive pulmonary disease (COPD)

A. Etiology and pathophysiology
   1. COPD refers to a group of diseases that result in an obstruction of airflow; etiology includes air pollution, smoking, chronic respiratory infections, exposure to molds and fungi, and allergic reactions
   2. Diseases classified under this category
      a. Asthma—obstruction of the bronchioles characterized by attacks that occur suddenly and last from 30 to 60 minutes; an asthmatic attack that is difficult to control is referred to as status asthmaticus
      b. Bronchitis—inflammation of the bronchial walls with hypertrophy of the mucous goblet cells; characterized by a chronic cough
      c. Emphysema—characterized by distended, inelastic, or destroyed alveoli and a bronchiolar obstruction and collapse; these alterations greatly impair the diffusion of gases through the alveolocapillary membrane
   3. Patients with COPD become accustomed to an elevated CO_2 and do not respond to high CO_2 levels as the normal respiratory stimulant; these patients respond to a drop in oxygen concentration in the blood

B. Signs and symptoms
   1. Subjective
      a. Fatigue and weakness
      b. Headache, impaired sensorium
      c. Dyspnea
   2. Objective
      a. Orthopnea, expiratory wheezing, stertorous breathing sounds, cough
      b. Barrel chest, cyanosis, and clubbing of fingers
      c. Distention of neck veins
      d. Edema of extremities
      e. Increased P_{CO_2} and decreased P_{O_2} of arterial blood gases
      f. Polycythemia

C. Treatment
   1. Antibiotics and cortisone to prevent and reduce inflammation
   2. Bronchodilators to reduce muscular spasm
   3. Mucolytics and expectorants to liquefy secretions and to facilitate their removal
   4. Oxygen at 2 to 3 L even if hypoxia is severe

5. Respiratory therapy program to include IPPB, postural drainage, exercise, and blow bottles
6. High-protein, soft diet

D. Nursing care
1. Advise the elimination of smoking and other external irritants, such as dust, as much as possible
2. Teach or supervise patient's respiratory exercises, such as pursed lip or diaphragmatic breathing
3. Teach patient proper use of nebulizer and other special equipment
4. Carefully monitor patient for symptoms of carbon dioxide intoxication if oxygen is being administered
5. Teach patient to adjust activities to avoid overexertion
6. Teach patient to avoid people with respiratory infections
7. Teach patient to maintain resistance by getting proper rest, eating proper food, dressing properly for existing weather conditions
8. Teach patient to be alert to early symptoms of infection, hypoxia, hypercapnea, or adverse response to medications
9. Encourage patient to continue with close medical supervision
10. Encourage patient to express feelings about disease and therapy
11. Accept patient's feelings about life-long restrictions in activity
12. Encourage patient to take an active role in planning therapy
13. Encourage patient to take medications as ordered
14. Support patient's efforts to give up smoking by poviding diversional activities such as eating hard candies
15. Encourage family to support patient's efforts to give up smoking

Silicosis (black lung)

A. Etiology and pathophysiology
1. Fibrotic disease of lungs caused by inhalation of inorganic dusts over long periods
2. Common in people whose professions expose them to free silica, such as miners and sandblasters
3. Tuberculosis is a frequent complication

B. Signs and symptoms
1. Subjective
   a. Exertional dyspnea
   b. Anxiety
2. Objective
   a. Frequent respiratory infections
   b. Sputum may be blood streaked
   c. Cough
   d. Chest x-ray examination reveals nodular lesions and enlarged hilar nodes
   e. Biopsy to establish diagnosis

C. Treatment
1. Relieve cough with antitussives
2. Prescribe medications for complications such as tuberculosis
3. Eliminate toxic substances from environment

D. Nursing care
1. Assess patient's ability to meet oxygen needs
2. Encourage coughing and deep breathing
3. Involve patient and family in programs aimed at improved occupational health and safety

Pneumothorax

A. Etiology and pathophysiology
1. A pneumothorax is a collapse of a lung as a result of the disruption in the negative pressure that normally exists within the intrapleural space due to the presence of air in the pleural cavity
2. Collapse of a lung will reduce the surface area for gaseous exchange and lead to hypoxia and retention of carbon dioxide (hypercarbia)
3. Types
   a. Spontaneous pneumothorax—thought to occur when a weakened area of the lung (bleb) ruptures; air then moves from the lung to the intrapleural space causing collapse; highest incidence is in men 20 to 40 years of age
   b. Open pneumothorax—an opening (such as a stab wound) through the chest wall into the intrapleural space
   c. Hemothorax—collection of blood within the pleural cavity
   d. Hydrothorax—an accumulation of fluid in the pleural cavity
   e. Tension pneumothorax—buildup of pressure as air accumulates within the pleural space; as pressure increases, a mediastinal shift is likely to occur

4. Mediastinal shift may occur toward the uninvolved side as a result of increased pressure within the pleural space; this involves the trachea, esophagus, heart, and great vessels
B. Signs and symptoms (depend on extent of collapse)
   1. Subjective
      a. Chest pain, usually described as sharp and increasing on exertion
      b. Dyspnea
   2. Objective
      a. Rapid, shallow respirations (nonsymmetrical)
      b. Breath sounds on affected side will be diminished or absent
      c. Chest x-ray examination will reveal extent of pneumothorax
      d. Tachycardia
      e. Hypotension
C. Treatment
   1. Bed rest is initially prescribed
   2. Analgesics
   3. Negative pressure is returned to the intrapleural space by the insertion of chest tubes attached to underwater drainage
D. Nursing care
   1. Assess respiratory status
      a. Vital signs
      b. Color
      c. Chest motion during respirations
      d. Auscultate lung fields
   2. Maintain patency of chest tubes (see procedure)

Chest injuries

A. Etiology and pathophysiology
   1. Chest injuries are penetrating or crushing wounds of the chest wall generally caused by acts of violence (stabbing, gunshot wounds) or motor vehicle accidents
   2. Flail chest—occurs when ribs are fractured in more than one area; the chest wall on the involved side becomes unstable; the portion of lung below the injury moves in the opposite direction to the remainder of the lung, which results in hypoxia
B. Signs and symptoms
   1. Subjective
      a. Dyspnea
      b. Anxiety
   2. Objective
      a. Presence of a wound with a sucking sound on inspiration

b. Presence of cyanosis and symptoms of mild to profound shock, depending on size of wound
c. Mediastinal shift may occur toward the unaffected side caused by the pressure exerted by a pneumothorax or hemothorax, causing a change in the site of the apical pulse and paradoxic respirations
d. Absence of breath sounds on affected side
C. Treatment
   1. Apply a pressure dressing over wound
   2. Aspiration of the pleural cavity to promote lung expansion
   3. Establish a water-sealed suction drainage
   4. Reduce the oxygen demand by ordering bed rest and limitation of activity
   5. Oxygen as necessary
   6. Restore blood volume and treat shock
   7. Antibiotics and mild analgesics
   8. Respiratory therapy to promote lung expansion
   9. Volume-controlled respirator is utilized in cases of severe chest trauma
D. Nursing care
   1. Maintain chest tubes if present (see procedure)
   2. Observe patient's respiratory status
   3. Encourage patient to move and cough
   4. Teach patient to self-splint with hands and arms
   5. Explain purpose and functioning of chest tubes and water-sealed drainage
   6. Administer oxygen and analgesics as ordered and as necessary
   7. Encourage patient to follow directions of respiratory therapists; e.g., blow bottles, IPPB

Bronchogenic carcinoma

A. Etiology and pathophysiology
   1. Carcinoma of the lungs may be primary or metastatic
   2. Etiology is unknown, but is much more common in smokers than nonsmokers
   3. Incidence is highest in men over the age of 40
   4. Symptoms may occur after metastasis to other organs such as the ribs, liver, adrenal glands, mediastinal organs, kidney, and brain
B. Signs and symptoms
   1. Subjective
      a. Dyspnea
      b. Chills
      c. Fatigue
      d. Chest pain

2. Objective
   a. Persistent cough
   b. Hemoptysis
   c. Unilateral wheeze detected by auscultation
   d. Weight loss
   e. Clubbing of fingers
   f. Pleural effusion
   g. "Coin" lesions detected by x-ray examination of chest
   h. Cytologic test of sputum positive
C. Treatment
   1. Surgical
      a. Lobectomy—removal of 1 lobe of the lung when the lesion is limited to 1 area
      b. Wedge section—removal of a small confined lesion; may also be done for biopsy
      c. Pneumonectomy—removal of an entire lung
      d. Exploratory thoracotomy—opening of the thoracic cavity to confirm diagnosis
      e. Thoracoplasty—removal of ribs to reduce the size of the pleural cavity; may be done to prevent complications after resection of lung
   2. Radiation therapy may be used as an adjunct therapy or to alleviate symptoms of pain, dyspnea, and hemoptysis
   3. Chemotherapy
D. Nursing care
   1. Maintain open communication between self, patient, and family; refer to community agencies and mental health practitioner as necessary
   2. Monitor temperature and vital signs
   3. Encourage coughing and deep breathing
   4. Change position frequently; semi- or high Fowler's positions promote greater lung expansion
   5. Specific care based on therapy being used
      a. Care of patient with chest tubes (see procedure)
      b. Radiation therapy
         (1) Adjust diet to patient's preference; provide small frequent feedings
         (2) Avoid washing off port marks used for radiation therapy
         (3) Do not apply powders and ointments that might contain metals
         (4) Apply a nonadherent dressing to areas of skin breakdown
      c. Chemotherapy (refer to specific drugs)

Cancer of the larynx

A. Etiology and pathophysiology
   1. Most tumors of the larynx (vocal cords, epiglottis, laryngeal cartilages, and ventricle) are squamous cell carcinoma
   2. Cigarette smoking and heavy alcohol consumption appear to be related to increased incidence
   3. More common in men 50 to 65 years of age
B. Signs and symptoms
   1. Subjective
      a. Sore throat
      b. Dyspnea
      c. Dysphagia
      d. Weakness
   2. Objective
      a. Increasing hoarseness
      b. Weight loss
      c. Enlarged cervical lymph nodes
      d. Foul breath
C. Treatment
   1. Radiation therapy
   2. Chemotherapy (i.e., methotrexate, bleomycin, and fluorouracil)
   3. Surgical intervention
      a. Thyrotomy—removal of tumor from the larynx via an incision through the thyroid cartilage
      b. Total laryngectomy—removal of total larynx with construction of a permanent tracheostomy
      c. Radical neck dissection (used when tumor has metastasized into surrounding tissue and lymph nodes)—removal of larynx, surrounding tissue and muscle, lymph nodes, and glands with a permanent tracheostomy
D. Nursing care of a patient with a total laryngectomy
   1. Provide patient with time to discuss diagnosis and the ramifications of surgery
   2. Assist and encourage patient to express feelings
   3. Answer patient's questions as thoroughly and honestly as possible
   4. Arrange for individuals with laryngectomies to visit patient and discuss rehabilitative process
   5. Instruct patient as to method of communication that will be used postoperatively; e.g., slate board and chalk, pencil and paper, sign language
   6. Observe for obstruction of airway by mucous plugs, edema, or blood; e.g., air hunger, dyspnea, cyanosis, gurgling

7. Observe for signs of hemorrhage; e.g., increased pulse rate, drop in blood pressure, cold clammy skin, appearance of blood on dressing
8. Stay with patient but provide a bell or other system for patient to signal for help
9. Provide, at patient's bedside, suction apparatus and catheters (additional laryngectomy tube and a surgical instrument set with additional hemostats should be immediately available in case tube becomes dislodged or blocked)
10. Suction tracheostomy tube that is left in place for approximately 3 days (see procedure)
11. Provide humidity to compensate for loss of normal humidification of air in the nasopharynx; later the tracheostomy may be covered with a moistened unfilled gauze pad
12. Prevent cross infection and contamination of the wound by providing special oral hygiene, cleanliness at tracheal site, avoidance of people with respiratory infections, use of clean equipment
13. In patients receiving radiation or chemotherapy, observe for signs of adverse reactions
14. Expect and accept a period of mourning but prevent withdrawal from reality by
    a. Involving patient in laryngectomy care
    b. Keeping channels of communication open
    c. Supporting patient's strengths
    d. Encouraging return to activities of daily living
    e. Allowing patient time to write responses or use sign language
15. Encourage patient to become involved in speech therapy and realistically support efforts and gains
16. Teach patient the skills necessary to handle altered body functioning
    a. Method of tracheobronchial suctioning to maintain patency of airway emphasizing pressure, depth, frequency, and safety
    b. Method of changing, cleaning, and securing laryngectomy tube
    c. Care of skin around opening
    d. Importance of providing humidified air for inspiration to prevent drying of secretions (can be achieved by use of moist dressing)
17. Teach patient to avoid activities that may permit water or irritating substances to enter the trachea, since the usual defensive mechanisms (glottis and cilia) are absent; patient should avoid showers, swimming, dust, hair spray, and other volatile substances
18. Teach patient to avoid wearing clothes with tight collars or constricting necklines
19. Teach patient that certain other activities will be interrupted; e.g., sipping through a straw, whistling, blowing the nose

Adult respiratory distress syndrome (ARDS)

A. Etiology and pathophysiology
   1. ARDS is respiratory failure that occurs in patients with previously healthy lungs as a complication of conditions such as trauma, aspiration, prolonged mechanical ventilation, severe infection, or open heart surgery
   2. The pathophysiology of ARDS involves
      a. Pulmonary capillary damage with loss of fluid and interstitial edema
      b. Impaired alveolar gas exchange and tissue hypoxia due to pulmonary edema
      c. An alteration in surfactant production and alveoli collapse
      d. Atelectasis resulting in labored and inefficient respiration
B. Signs and symptoms
   1. Subjective
      a. Restlessness
      b. Anxiety
      c. Dyspnea
   2. Objective
      a. Increased P_{CO_2} and decreased P_{O_2} arterial blood gases
      b. Tachypnea
      c. Cyanosis
C. Treatment
   1. Relieve underlying cause
   2. Mechanical ventilation
   3. Positive end expiratory pressure (PEEP)—this setting on a mechanical ventilator maintains positive pressure within the lungs on expiration, which increases the residual capacity, reducing hypoxia
   4. Monitoring arterial blood gases
   5. Corticosteroids may be used
D. Nursing care
   1. Allow frequent rest periods between therapeutic interventions
   2. Provide tranquil supportive environment because

sedation is contraindicated due to its depressant effect on respirations

3. Observe behavioral changes and vital signs, since confusion and hypertension may indicate cerebral hypoxia
4. Auscultate breath sounds to observe for signs of pneumothorax when patient is on PEEP (lung tissue that is frail may not withstand increased intrathoracic pressure, and pneumothorax occurs)
5. Monitor arterial blood gases, as ordered; use a heparinized syringe to obtain specimen
6. Maintain patent airway
7. Care of patient on mechanical ventilation (see procedure)

Carbon monoxide poisoning

A. Etiology and pathophysiology
   1. Caused by inadequately vented combustion devices
   2. Carbon monoxide combines with hemoglobin more readily than with oxygen, causing tissue anoxia
B. Signs and symptoms
   1. Subjective
      a. Headache
      b. Faintness
      c. Vertigo
      d. Tinnitus
   2. Objective
      a. Color may be normal, cyanotic, or flushed, but is usually cherry pink
      b. Paralysis
      c. Loss of consciousness
      d. ECG changes
C. Treatment
   1. Administer artificial respiration
   2. 100% oxygen until carboxyhemoglobin is reduced and respirations are normal
   3. Administer 50% glucose or mannitol
   4. Administer synthetic red cells (Fluosol), which deliver oxygen to cells in the presence of carbon monoxide
D. Nursing care
   1. Remove individual from immediate area
   2. Evaluate for cardiopulmonary function
   3. Institute cardiopulmonary resuscitation, if necessary, and maintain until additional help arrives
   4. Administer oxygen, if available
   5. Maintain respirations with assistance, if necessary

6. Maintain body temperature
7. Observe vital signs with special concern for respirations
8. Maintain oxygen flow at prescribed levels

Gastrointestinal system

REVIEW OF ANATOMY AND PHYSIOLOGY OF THE GASTROINTESTINAL SYSTEM
Functions

A. Digestion of food, essential preparation for absorption and metabolism
B. Absorption of digested food
C. Elimination of wastes of digestion

Organs
Mouth (buccal cavity)

A. Lips
B. Cheeks
C. Hard palate—formed by 2 palatine bones and palatine processes of maxillae
D. Soft palate—formed of muscle in shape of arch that forms partition between mouth and nasopharynx; fauces, archway, or opening, from mouth into oropharynx; uvula, conical process; possess numerous mucus-secreting glands
E. Gums (gingivae)
F. Teeth
   1. Deciduous or "baby teeth"—10 in each jaw or 20 in set
   2. Permanent—16 per jaw or 32 in set
   3. Eruption
      a. Deciduous—first 1 erupts usually at 6 months of age; rest follow at intervals of 1 or more months; however, great individual variation in time of eruption of teeth; deciduous teeth shed between 6 and 13 years of age
      b. Permanent—usually between 6 years and about 17 years; third molars (wisdom teeth) last to erupt
G. Tongue
   1. Papillae—many rough elevations on tongue's surface
   2. Taste buds—specialized receptors of cranial nerves VII and IX; located in papillae
   3. Frenum (or frenulum)—fold of mucous membrane that helps anchor tongue to mouth floor

H. Tonsils—lymphatic tissue connected to surface epithelium by a channel (crypt); produces lymphocytes; defense against infection

I. Salivary glands—produce saliva, a mixture of water, mucin, salts, enzyme (salivary amylase)
1. Parotid—below and in front of ear
2. Submandibular—posterior part of floor of mouth
3. Sublingual—anterior part of floor of mouth, under tongue

Pharynx

See Respiratory system discussion

Esophagus

A. Location and extent
1. Posterior to trachea; anterior to vertebral column
2. Extends from pharynx through opening in diaphragm (hiatus) to stomach

B. Structure—collapsible muscular tube; about 10 inches (25 cm) long and 0.05 inch (0.13 cm) wide

C. Secretions and functions—secretes mucus; facilitates movement of food

Stomach

A. Size, shape, position
1. Size—varies in different persons and according to degree of distention
2. Shape—elongated pouch, with greater curve forming lower left border
3. Position—in epigastric and left hypochondriac portions of abdominal cavity

B. Divisions
1. Fundus—portion above esophageal opening
2. Body—central portion
3. Pylorus—constricted lower portion

C. Curves
1. Lesser—upper right border
2. Greater—lower left border

D. Sphincters
1. Cardiac—guarding opening of esophagus into stomach
2. Pyloric—guarding opening of pylorus into duodenum

E. Glands of stomach—secrete gastric juice composed of mucus, hydrochloric acid, and enzymes
1. Simple columnar epithelial cells form surface of gastric mucosa; goblet cells secrete mucus
2. Millions of microscopic gastric glands embedded in gastric mucosa composed of different types of cells; mainly chief cells (zymogen cells) that secrete gastric juice enzymes, and parietal cells that secrete hydrochloric acid and intrinsic factor

F. Functions—food storage and liquefaction (chyme)

Small intestine

A. Size—approximately 1 inch (2.5 cm) in diameter, 20 feet (6.1 m) in length when relaxed

B. Divisions
1. Duodenum—joins pylorus of stomach; about 10 inches (25 cm) in length; C shaped
2. Jejunum—middle section about 8 feet (2.4 m) in length
3. Ileum—lower section about 12 feet (3.6 m) in length; no clear boundary between jejunum and ileum

C. Functions—digestion and absorption

D. Process—mixing movements; peristalsis; secretion of water, ions, and mucus; receives secretions from liver, gallbladder, and pancreas

Large intestine

A. Size—approximately 2½ (6.3 cm) inches in diameter, but only 5 or 6 feet (1.5 m) in length when relaxed

B. Divisions
1. Cecum—the first 2 or 3 inches (5 to 7.6 cm) of large intestine
2. Colon
a. Ascending—extends vertically along right border of abdomen up to level of liver
b. Transverse colon—extends horizontally across abdomen, below liver and stomach and above small intestine
c. Descending colon—extends vertically down left side of abdomen to level of iliac crest
d. Sigmoid colon—S-shaped part of large intestine curving downward below iliac crest to join rectum; lower part of sigmoid curve that joins rectum bends toward left
3. Rectum—last 7 or 8 inches (17.7 or 20.3 cm) of intestines
4. Anus—terminal opening of alimentary tract

C. Functions—water and sodium ion absorption; temporary storage of fecal matter; defecation

D. Process—weak mixing movements, mass movements, and peristalsis

Vermiform appendix

A. Size, shape, location—about size and shape of large angleworm; blind-end tube off cecum just beyond ileocecal valve; 3 to 4 inches (7.6 to 10 cm) long; ¼ inch (0.6 cm) in diameter

B. Structure—same coats as compose intestinal wall

C. Function—part of immune system; submucosa unique in the large size of its lymphatic modules

Liver
A. Location and size—occupies most of right hypochondrium and part of epigastrium; largest gland in body
B. Lobes—divided into thousands of lobules by blood vessels and fibrous partitions
   1. Right lobe—subdivided into 2 smaller lobes (caudate and quadrate) and right lobe proper
   2. Left lobe—single lobe
C. Ducts
   1. Hepatic duct—from liver
   2. Cystic duct—from gallbladder
   3. Common bile duct—formed by union of hepatic and cystic ducts in Y formation; drains bile into duodenum at hepatopancreatic papilla surrounded by sphincter of Oddi
D. Functions—liver is one of most vital organs because of its role in metabolism of proteins, carbohydrates, and fats
   1. Carbohydrate metabolism by liver cells
      a. Glycogenesis—conversion of glucose to glycogen for storage
      b. Glycogenolysis—conversion of glycogen to glucose and release of glucose into blood; epinephrine and glucagon accelerate glycogenolysis
      c. Gluconeogenesis—formation of glucose from proteins or fats; glucocorticoids (hydrocortisone, corticosterone) have accelerating effect on gluconeogenesis
   2. Fat metabolism by liver cells
      a. Ketogenesis—first step in fat catabolism occurs mainly in liver cells; consists of series of reactions by which fatty acids are converted to ketone bodies (acetoacetic acid, acetone, beta-hydroxybutyric acid)
      b. Fat storage
      c. Synthesis of triglycerides, phospholipids, cholesterol, and the B complex factor choline
   3. Protein metabolism by liver cells
      a. Anabolism—synthesis of various proteins, notably blood proteins; e.g., prothrombin, fibrinogen, albumins, alpha and beta globulins, and clotting factors V, VII, IX, and X
      b. Deamination—first step in protein catabolism; chemical reaction by which amino group is split off from amino acid to form ammonia and a keto acid
      c. Urea formation—liver cells convert most of the ammonia formed by deamination to urea

4. Secretes bile, substance important for emulsifying fats prior to digestion and as vehicle for excretion of cholesterol and bile pigments
5. Detoxifies various substances; e.g., drugs, hormones
6. Vitamin metabolism—stores vitamins A, D, K, and B_{12}; synthesizes B_3 from tryptophan

Gallbladder
A. Size, shape, location—approximately size and shape of small pear; lies on undersurface of liver
B. Structure—sac made of smooth muscle, lined with mucosa arranged in rugae (expandable longitudinal folds)
C. Functions—concentrates and stores bile

Pancreas
A. Size, shape, location—larger in men than in women, but considerable individual variation; fish shaped, with body, head, and tail, extending from duodenal curve to spleen
B. Structure—both duct and ductless gland
   1. Pancreatic cells—pour secretion, pancreatic juice, into duct that runs length of gland and empties into duodenum at hepatopancreatic papilla
   2. Islands of Langerhans (or islet cells)—clusters of cells not connected with pancreatic ducts; 2 main types of cells compose islets, namely, alpha and beta cells; constitute endocrine glands
C. Functions
   1. Pancreatic cells connected with pancreatic ducts secrete pancreatic juice, enzymes of which help digest all three kinds of foods
   2. Islet cells constitute endocrine gland
      a. Alpha cells secrete hormone glucagon, which accelerates liver glycogenolysis; hence, tends to increase blood sugar
      b. Beta cells secrete insulin, one of most important metabolic hormones, which exerts profound influence over the metabolism of carbohydrates, proteins, and fats (Fig. 5)
         (1) Insulin accelerates active transport of glucose (along with potassium and phosphate ions) through cell membranes; therefore it tends to decrease blood glucose (hypoglycemic effect) and to increase glucose utilization by cells either for catabolism or for anabolism
         (2) Insulin stimulates liver cell glucokinase;

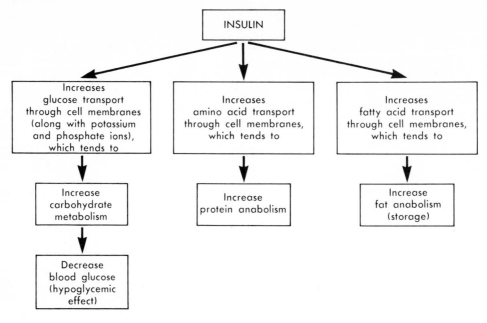

Fig. 5. Major insulin effects.

therefore it promotes liver glycogenesis, another effect that tends to lower blood glucose

(3) Insulin inhibits liver cell phosphatase and therefore inhibits liver glycogenolysis

(4) Insulin accelerates rate of amino acid transfer into cells, so promotes protein anabolism within them

(5) Insulin accelerates rate of fatty acid transfer into cells, promotes fat anabolism (also called fat desposition or lipogenesis), and inhibits fat catabolism

Digestion

A. Definition—all changes that food undergoes in alimentary canal

B. Purpose—conversion of foods into chemical and physical forms that can be absorbed and metabolized

C. Kinds
 1. Mechanical digestion—all movements of alimentary tract that
    a. Change physical state of foods from comparatively large solid pieces into minute dissolved particles

    b. Propel food forward along alimentary tract, finally eliminating digestive wastes from body
       (1) Deglutition—swallowing
       (2) Peristalsis—wormlike movements that squeeze food downward in tract
       (3) Mass peristalsis—entire contents moved into sigmoid colon and rectum; usually occurs after meal
       (4) Defecation—emptying of rectum, so-called bowel movement
    c. Churn intestinal contents so all become well mixed with digestive juices and all parts of contents come in contact with surface of intestinal mucosa to facilitate absorption
 2. Chemical digestion—series of hydrolytic processes dependent on specific enzymes; hydrolysis, decomposition of complex compound into 2 or more simple compounds by means of chemical reaction with water

D. Control of digestive gland secretion
 1. Secretion of saliva—neural control of this reflex results from parasympathetic impulses to glands, initiated by taste, smell, and sight of food (cephalic phase of digestion)

Table 2-3. Absorption of protein, carbohydrate, and fat

Substance	Structures into which absorbed	Circulation
Protein—amino acids	Into blood in intestinal capillaries	Portal vein, liver, hepatic vein, inferior vena cava to heart, etc.
Carbohydrate—monosaccharides (glucose and fructose)	Same as amino acids	Same as amino acids
Fat—glycerol and fatty acids; fatty acids are insoluble and must first combine with bile salts to form water-soluble substance	Chiefly into lymph in intestinal lacteals; some into blood	During absorption while in epithelial cells of intestinal mucosa, glycerol and fatty acids recombine to form microscopic particles of fats (chylomicrons); lymphatics carry them by way of thoracic duct to left subclavian vein, superior vena cava, heart, etc.

2. Gastric juice
   a. Neural control similar to that of salivary glands
   b. Hormonal control—partially digested proteins cause gastric mucosa to release hormone (gastrin) into blood; gastrin stimulates gastric mucosa to secrete juice with high pepsin and hydrochloric acid content
3. Pancreatic juice
   a. Hormonal control—hydrochloric acid in chyme entering duodenum from stomach causes intestinal mucosa to release hormone (secretin) into blood; secretin stimulates pancreatic cells to secrete juice high in sodium bicarbonate content to neutralize hydrochloric acid but low in enzymes; products of protein digestion (e.g., proteoses, peptones, and amino acids) cause intestinal mucosa to release another hormone, pancreozymin, which stimulates pancreatic cells to secrete enzymes
   b. Neural control—reflex secretion of pancreatic juice results from parasympathetic impulses via vagus nerve
4. Bile
   a. Although bile is secreted continuously, secretin increases amount of bile secreted
   b. Presence of fats in intestine causes intestinal mucosa to release hormone, cholecystokinin, into blood; cholecystokinin stimulates smooth muscle of gallbladder to contract, ejecting bile into duodenum

5. Intestinal juice—control obscure but believed to be both reflex and hormonal; food in small intestine causes mucosa to release hormone (enterocrinin) into blood; enterocrinin stimulates intestinal glands to secrete

Absorption

A. Definition—passage of substances through intestinal mucosa into blood or lymph
B. Accomplished mainly through active transport by intestinal cells; makes it possible for both water and solutes to move through intestinal mucosa in direction opposite that expected in osmosis and diffusion
C. Absorption occurs in duodenum and jejunum of small intestine, with exception of alcohol, certain drugs, and some water, which are absorbed from stomach; largest amount of water absorbed from small intestine
D. Absorption of protein, carbohydrate, and fat (Table 2-3)

Metabolism

A. Definition—sum of all the chemical reactions in the body
B. Catabolism
   1. Consists of complex series of chemical reactions that take place inside cells and yield energy, carbon dioxide, and water; about half of energy released from food molecules by catabolism is put back in storage in unstable, high-energy bonds of ATP molecules, and the rest is transformed to

heat; energy in high-energy bonds of ATP can be released as rapidly as needed for doing cellular work

2. Two processes involved; glycolysis and Krebs' citric acid cycle

3. Purpose—to continually provide cells with utilizable energy

C. Anabolism

1. Synthesis of various compounds from simpler compounds

2. Cellular work that uses some of energy made available by catabolism

D. Metabolism of carbohydrates

1. Consists of the following processes

a. Glucose transport through cell membranes and phosphorylation

(1) Insulin promotes this transport through cell membranes

(2) Glucose phosphorylation—conversion of glucose to glucose-6-phosphate, catalyzed by enzyme glucokinase; insulin increases activity of glucokinase and promotes glucose phosphorylation, which is essential prior to both glycogenesis and glucose catabolism

b. Glycogenesis—conversion of glucose to glycogen for storage; occurs mainly in liver and muscle cells

c. Glycogenolysis

(1) In muscle cells glycogen is changed back to glucose-6-phosphate, which is then catabolized in the muscle cells

(2) In liver cells glycogen is changed back to glucose; enzyme, glucose phosphatase, is present in liver cells and catalyzes final step of glycogenolysis, the changing of glucose-6-phosphate to glucose; glucagon and epinephrine accelerate liver glycogenolysis

d. Glucose catabolism

(1) Glycolysis—series of anaerobic reactions that break 1 glucose molecule down into 2 pyruvic acid molecules with conversion of about 5% of energy stored in glucose to heat and ATP molecules

(2) Krebs' citric acid cycle—series of aerobic chemical reactions by which 2 pyruvic acid molecules (from 1 glucose molecule) are broken down to 6 carbon dioxide and

6 water molecules with release of some energy as heat and some stored again in ATP; citric acid cycle releases about 95%, and glycolysis only about 5% of energy stored in glucose; citric acid cycle occurs in the mitochondria of cells

e. Gluconeogenesis—sequence of chemical reactions carried on in liver cells; process converts protein or fat compounds into glucose

f. Principles of normal carbohydrate metabolism

(1) Principle of preferred energy fuel—cells first catabolize glucose, sparing fats and proteins; when their glucose supply becomes inadequate, they next catabolize fats, sparing proteins; and finally, when fats are used up, they catabolize their own cell proteins

(2) Principle of glycogenesis—glucose in excess of about 120 to 140 mg per 100 ml blood brought to liver by portal veins enters liver cells where it undergoes glycogenesis and is stored as glycogen

(3) Principle of glycogenolysis—when blood glucose decreases below midpoint of normal, liver glycogenolysis accelerates and tends to raise blood glucose concentration back toward midpoint of normal

(4) Principle of gluconeogenesis—when blood glucose decreases below normal or when amount of glucose entering cells is inadequate, liver gluconeogenesis accelerates and tends to raise blood glucose concentration

(5) Principle of glucose storage as fat—when blood insulin content is adequate, glucose in excess of amount used for catabolism and glycogenesis is converted to fat and stored in fat depots

E. Control of metabolism—primarily by hormones

1. Pancreatic hormones

a. Insulin—exerts predominant control over carbohydrate metabolism but also affects protein and fat metabolism; in general, insulin accelerates carbohydrate metabolism by cells, thereby decreasing blood glucose

b. Glucagon secreted by alpha cells of islands of Langerhans—accelerates liver glycogenolysis only

2. Anterior pituitary hormones

a. Growth hormone tends to
   (1) Accelerate protein anabolism; hence promotes growth of skeleton and soft tissues
   (2) Accelerate fat mobilization from adipose cells, which tends to bring about a shift from use of glucose to use of fats for catabolism
   (3) Accelerate liver gluconeogenesis from fats, which tends to increase blood glucose
   (4) Stimulate glucagon secretion, which in turn stimulates liver glycogenolysis and glucose release into blood
b. ACTH (adrenocorticotropic hormone)—stimulates adrenal cortex secretion, especially of glucocorticoids

3. Adrenal cortex hormones—glucocorticoids, mainly cortisol and corticosterone, tend to
   a. Accelerate fat mobilization and catabolism, thereby promoting shift to fat catabolism from glucose catabolism whenever latter is inadequate for energy needs
   b. Accelerate tissue protein mobilization (catabolism)
   c. Accelerate liver gluconeogenesis; presumably secondary effect; results from protein mobilization and tends to increase blood sugar

4. Adrenal medulla hormones—the catecholamines, epinephrine and norepinephrine, tend to accelerate both liver and muscle glycogenolysis with release of glucose from liver into circulation; therefore tend to increase blood sugar

5. Male sex gland hormone—testosterone, secreted by interstitial cells of testes, tends to accelerate protein anabolism

F. Metabolic rate—calories of heat energy produced and expended per hour or per day
   1. Basal metabolic rate (BMR)—calories of heat produced when individual is awake but resting in a comfortably warm environment 12 to 18 hours after last meal
      a. Factors determining basal metabolic rates
         (1) Size—BMR is directly related to square meters of surface area of body; the larger the surface area, the higher the BMR
         (2) Sex—5% to 7% higher in male than in female of same size and age
         (3) Age—BMR inversely related to age; as age increases, BMR decreases
         (4) Amount of thyroid hormones secreted; thyroid hormones accelerate BMR
         (5) Body temperature—BMR directly related to body temperature; 1° C increase in body temperature above normal is accompanied by about 13% increase in BMR
         (6) Miscellaneous factors such as sleep (decreases BMR), pregnancy, and emotions (increase BMR)
      b. Measurement
         (1) Determined by measuring the amount of oxygen inspired in a given time
         (2) Reported as normal or as a definite percentage above or below normal
   2. Total metabolic rate—calories of heat energy expended per day; equal to basal metabolic rate plus number of calories of energy used for muscular work, eating and digesting food, and adjusting to cool temperatures
   3. Some principles about the metabolic rate and its relation to body weight
      a. For body weight to remain constant except for variations in water content, energy balance must be maintained; body weight remains constant when energy input equals energy output
      b. Whenever energy input (food intake) is greater than the energy output (total metabolic rate) body weight increases
      c. Whenever energy input (food intake) is less than the energy output (total metabolic rate), body weight decreases

REVIEW OF PHYSICAL PRINCIPLES RELATED TO THE GASTROINTESTINAL SYSTEM
Principles of mechanics
Law of motion
EXAMPLE: The greater the force of contraction of the intestinal wall and the more frequent the contractions, the more rapid the propulsion of food and fecal matter through digestive tract; under irritating conditions, rapid powerful peristalsis leads to abdominal cramps and diarrhea
Gravity
EXAMPLE: Colostomy irrigations and enemas
Energy
A. Potential and kinetic energy
   EXAMPLE: The potential energy in glucose (food) molecules is captured in the bonds of the high-

energy molecule ATP; such potential energy is released as kinetic energy when ATP powers the contraction of muscle and the beating of cilia and flagella

B. First law of thermodynamics

EXAMPLE: The energy stored in an ATP molecule exactly equals the energy of work (of muscles, cilia, etc.) and heat energy liberated during the process

C. Second law of thermodynamics

EXAMPLE: The diffusion of nutrients and enzymes in the various digestive juices results in their collisions and chemical interactions because it is the natural tendency of molecules and systems to become more randomized

Principles of physical properties of matter

Solids

EXAMPLE: The elastic properties of the connective and muscular tissues of the stomach permit distention during a meal and the consequent storage and slow digestion and absorption of food over the next several hours

Liquids

A. Pascal's principle

EXAMPLE: The voluntary contraction of muscles of the abdominal wall, such as the external and internal oblique, applies pressure on the fluids of the abdominal cavity, which is transmitted undiminished throughout the abdominopelvic cavity and aids in defecation; chronic constipation with chronic straining during defecation may predispose to hemorrhoids

B. Surface tension

EXAMPLE: Bile salts partly combine with fats and with water; this dual combination lowers the surface tension of the water molecules surrounding large fat droplets, which disperse into thousands of smaller droplets whose greater total surface area promotes more rapid hydrolysis (digestion) by pancreatic lipase

Gases

Boyle's law

EXAMPLES

1. During gastric analysis, the volume of gas in the tube is increased as the barrel of the syringe attached to the tube is pulled out; the result is a flow of gastric contents from the stomach due to the decreased pressure exerted by the gas in the tube as compared with gas pressure in the stomach

2. The same applies during paracentesis
3. During gastric gavage the process is reversed

Heat

A. Body temperature maintained by heat produced as by-product of biochemical reactions; basal metabolism rate is a measure of heat production under specified conditions

B. The normal metabolism in each of the cells of the human body produce heat; in addition, heat is a by-product of muscular contraction

Light

A. Refraction

EXAMPLE: Total internal reflection in fiberoptics permits viewing of interior walls of stomach and intestines for diagnostic purposes such as endoscopic procedures, gastroscopy, sigmoidoscopy, and proctoscopy

B. X rays

EXAMPLES

1. GI series and barium enemas allow visualization of the soft tissues of the upper and lower gastrointestinal tract; the barium salts coat the inner walls of the alimentary tube and absorb the x rays striking them; as a result, the organ surfaces are outlined

2. Fluoroscopy can be considered the observation of "live" x-ray images; after the x rays pass through the individual, they strike a fluorescent screen that absorbs the x rays and emits visible light; with x-ray–opaque chemicals the intestinal and biliary tracts can be observed

REVIEW OF CHEMICAL PRINCIPLES RELATED TO THE GASTROINTESTINAL SYSTEM

Oxidation and reduction

A. Uniting oxygen with a substance results in oxidation
B. Uniting hydrogen with a substance results in reduction

Oxidation-reduction reactions in the body

A. Important in body chemistry as a source of energy through cellular oxidation of foods in cytoplasm and mitochondria; oxidation of nutrients like glucose results in the formation of high-energy ATP molecules and heat—both useful to the body

B. Oxygen is the usual oxidizing agent in cells

C. Some forms of life (anaerobes) can use substances other than oxygen for cellular oxidation; e.g., *Clostridium perfringens* found in gangrenous tissue

Diffusion and osmosis

EXAMPLES

1. Diffusion of nutrients and enzymes results in the collisions necessary to promote chemical (metabolic) reactions
2. Absorption of water by osmosis occurs through the mucosa of the GI tract

Active transport

The movement of molecules against a concentration gradient due to energy (ATP) expenditure

EXAMPLE: The absorption of most simple sugars and amino acids in the small intestine involves active transport processes

Buffers

Pairs of chemical substances that resist changes in pH

EXAMPLE: The sodium bicarbonate part of the bicarbonate buffer system secreted from the pancreas into the duodenum acts as a buffer to prevent acidification of intestinal juices due to the presence of HCl from gastric juice

Types of compounds

Organic acids

$$O$$
$$\|$$

All organic acids contain the $C-OH$ (carboxyl) group

EXAMPLES

1. Lactic acid—end product of anaerobic muscle metabolism; converted to pyruvic acid and oxidized completely to CO_2 and H_2O aerobically
2. Citric acid—one of the intermediates in Krebs' citric acid cycle; cycle occurs in mitochondria as a major oxidation—reduction pathway for the generation of ATP (potential chemical energy)
3. Salicylic acid—synthesis of aspirin

Amino acids

A. Amino acids possess 2 functional groups: an amine group and an acid or carboxyl group
B. Amino acids are amphoteric—act as both acids or bases; therefore proteins act as buffers in body fluids
C. Reactions of amino acids
   1. Amino acids are able to act as an acid and as a base (amphoteric character)
   2. Condense via peptide bond to form proteins
D. Essential amino acids cannot be synthesized well enough in the body to maintain health and growth and must be supplied in the food

Carbohydrates

A. Aldehyde or ketone derivatives of single oxidation of polyhydric alcohols, or compounds yielding aldehyde or ketone derivatives on hydrolysis
B. Include simple sugars, starches, celluloses, gums, and resins
C. Widespread in plant and animal tissue
D. Contain carbon, hydrogen, and oxygen with the hydrogen and oxygen present in approximately the ratio of 2 to 1
E. Synthesis—plants synthesize carbohydrates from carbon dioxide and water with the aid of the green pigment chlorophyll (which acts as an enzyme) and solar energy
F. Classification
   1. By functional group
      a. Carbohydrates having the aldehyde group are called aldoses; e.g., glucose
      b. Carbohydrates having the ketone group are called ketoses; e.g., fructose
   2. By complexity of the molecule
      a. Carbohydrate having a single ketose or aldose molecule is called a monosaccharide—a simple sugar; e.g., glucose, fructose
      b. Carbohydrate formed by combining 2 aldose molecules or an aldose and a ketose molecule is called a disaccharide; e.g., sucrose, lactose, maltose
      c. Carbohydrate having more than 2 simple sugars joined in a molecule is called a polysaccharide; e.g., starch, glycogen
G. Tests for glucose in urine
   1. Benedict's test and Clinitest tablets use copper ions in basic medium—show presence of sugar in urine by change in color
   2. Positive reaction gives colors from green (very little sugar) to brick red (more than 2 g of sugar per 100 ml of urine)
   3. Iron ions and silver ions can be used instead of copper to give a test for sugar
   4. Most monosaccharides and disaccharides except sucrose are reducing sugars; therefore sucrose put into urine will not produce a reaction
H. Important carbohydrates
   1. Glycerose and dihydroxyacetone—triose intermediates in cellular metabolism of carbohydrates
   2. Ribose and deoxyribose—pentose constituents in nucleic acids

3. Glucose (dextrose)—hexose monosaccharide; a sugar found abundantly in body fluids, fruits, and vegetables; the pancreatic hormones insulin and glucagon regulate the blood glucose concentration in the normal range of 70 to 105 mg/100 ml of blood; glucose is the basic food molecule that is broken down first in glycolysis (in the cytoplasm of cells) and then in the Krebs' cycle (in mitochondria); the breakdown of each molecule of glucose results in the release of 38 molecules of ATP, which can be used in almost all cellular energy requiring functions
4. Fructose (levulose)—ketose monosaccharide; found in fruits and honey, sweetest sugar known; important intermediate in cellular metabolism of carbohydrates
5. Galactose—hexose monosaccharide; present in brain and nervous tissue
6. Lactose (milk sugar)—disaccharide of glucose and galactose molecules; bacterial fermentation of lactose to lactic acid causes milk to sour
7. Sucrose (cane sugar)—disaccharide of glucose and fructose molecules; nonreducing sugar, common table sugar used in sweetening and baking
8. Maltose—disaccharide of 2 glucose molecules; found in grains and malt
9. Starch—mixed polysaccharide of glucose molecules found in plants
   a. Amylose—straight-chained glucose polymer
   b. Amylopectin—branched-chain glucose polymer
   c. Chief food carbohydrate in human nutrition
   d. Starch polymers react with iodine to form a blue complex; used as a test for starch
      (1) Test becomes colorless as starch is hydrolyzed
      (2) Starch (blue) → amylodextrin (purple) → erythrodextrin (red) → achroodextrin (colorless) → maltose (colorless) → glucose (colorless)
10. Glycogen—polysaccharide polymer of glucose molecules found in human and animal tissue; storage compound in body; hydrolyzes to glucose, maintaining blood glucose levels
11. Cellulose—polysaccharide polymer of glucose found in plants; not digestible by humans; important in manufacture of cotton cloth, paper, and cellulose acetate synthetics
12. Inulin—polysaccharide polymer of fructose, used in kidney function test (inulin clearance test)
13. Agar-agar—polysaccharide polymer of galactose used as a solid medium for bacteriologic studies

Lipids

A. Organic substances essentially insoluble in water but soluble in organic solvents (ether, chloroform, acetone, etc.)
B. Fatty acids—important constituents of all lipids (except sterols)
   1. Usually straight-chained carboxylic acids
   2. Naturally occurring fatty acids contain even numbers of carbon atoms
   3. Saturated fatty acids—have no double bonds (points of unsaturation) between their carbon atoms
   4. Unsaturated fatty acids—have 1 or more points of unsaturation between their carbon atoms
   5. Essential fatty acids—cannot be synthesized by body; must be taken in by diet
C. Classification of lipids
   1. Simple lipids—esters of fatty acids and alcohols
      a. Fats—the alcohol of fats is the trihydric alcohol glycerol
         (1) Solid fats—fats that are solid at room temperature contain long-chained, saturated fatty acids
         (2) Liquid fats (oils)—fats that are liquid at room temperature contain short-chained, unsaturated fatty acids
      b. Waxes—esters of long-chained fatty acids and an alcohol other than glycerol; lanolin, a mixed wax from wool, is used in creams and salves
      c. Reactions of simple lipids
         (1) Hydrolysis—splitting into fatty acid(s) and alcohol by breaking ester bond is effected by acid, base, or enzymatic action
         (2) Saponification—basic hydrolysis; soap is formed from organic salts of fatty acid and metal ion of base
         (3) Addition—fats containing unsaturated fatty acids will form addition products at points of unsaturation
            (a) Addition of oxygen will cause fat to become rancid; antioxidants slow this reaction in packaged foods

(b) Unsaturated oils used in paints add oxygen and oils become hard and glossy

(c) Hydrogenation—liquid fats can form solid fats by adding in hydrogen at double bonds

2. Compound lipids—fats containing chemical substances other than fatty acids and alcohols
   a. Phospholipids—contain alcohol, fatty acids, phosphoric acid, and a nitrogenous base (or inositol)
      (1) Lecithins—contain the alcohol glycerol, fatty acids, phosphoric acid, and the nitrogenous base choline; are found in brain and nervous tissue; in blood, lecithin serves to render fats soluble in plasma (a lipotropic agent)
      (2) Cephalins—similar in structure to lecithin except base is ethanolamine; important in brain and nerve tissue; help blood-clotting mechanism
      (3) Sphingomyelins—made from amino alcohol (sphingosinol), a fatty acid, phosphoric acid, and choline; important in brain and nerve tissue
   b. Cardiolipids—made from unsaturated fatty acids, glycerol, and phosphoric acid; found in heart tissue
   c. Glycolipids (cerebrosides) structure contains the monosaccharide galactose, amino alcohol (sphingosinol), and a fatty acid; found in brain tissue and the myelin sheaths of nerves
3. Steroids—complex monohydroxy alcohols found in plant and animal tissues—basic structure, the phenanthrine structure plus a cyclopentane ring; characteristic side chains determine specific steroids
   a. Cholesterol—a sterol found in human and animal tissue, chiefly in brain and nerve tissue; an important, normal component of membranes; found in blood within a normal range of 150 to 300 mg/100 ml; high blood cholesterol seems associated with coronary thrombosis
   b. Ergosterol—a plant sterol that can be converted to vitamin D by ultraviolet light
   c. Bile acids—sterols that aid in digestion and absorption of fats
   d. Steroid hormones—sex and adrenal gland hormones (glucocorticoids, mineralocorticoids)
   e. Vitamin D—steroid helping to control calcium metabolism by regulating calcium uptake from the gastrointestinal tract

Proteins

A. Classification of proteins
   1. Simple proteins—give amino acids on hydrolysis
      a. Albumins—water soluble, coagulated by heat; e.g., lactalbumin (milk), serum albumin (blood), egg white; albumin is most important in the development of the plasma colloid osmotic pressure, which helps control (through osmosis) the flow of water between the plasma and interstitial fluid; during a condition such as starvation, a fall in the albumin level of the blood results in a fall in the plasma colloid osmotic pressure; this results in edema caused by less fluid being drawn by osmosis into the capillaries from the interstitial spaces
      b. Globulins—insoluble in water, soluble in dilute salt solutions, coagulated by heat; e.g., lactoglobulin (milk), serum globulin (blood), gamma serum globulin—forms antibodies of blood
      c. Glutelins—soluble in dilute bases or acids, insoluble in neutral solutions; coagulated by heat; e.g., glutenin (wheat)
      d. Albuminoids—soluble in water; e.g., collagen (connective tissue), elastin (ligaments)
      e. Histone—water soluble; e.g., globin (hemoglobin)
      f. Prolamines—insoluble in water, soluble in 70% to 80% alcohol; e.g., gliadin (wheat), zein (corn)
      g. Protamines—water soluble; e.g., protamine (fish spermatozoa)
   2. Compound proteins—contain molecules other than amino acids
      a. Chromoproteins—proteins containing a colored molecule; e.g., hemoglobin, flavoproteins
      b. Glycoproteins—proteins containing carbohydrate molecule(s); e.g., mucopolysaccharide of synovial fluid
      c. Lipoproteins—simple proteins combined with lipid substances; e.g., lipovitellin in egg yolk
      d. Nucleoproteins—proteins complexed with nucleic acids; e.g., the DNA (genetic material) found in chromosomes in complexed with proteins; chromosomes are sometimes referred to as nucleoprotein structures

e. Metalloproteins—proteins containing metal ions; e.g., ferritin (iron transport compound of plasma)

f. Phosphoproteins—proteins containing phosphoric acid radical; e.g., casein of milk

3. Derived proteins—also called *denatured* proteins; treatment with acids, bases, heat, x-ray films, ultraviolet rays, and many other agents causes proteins to alter their molecular arrangements

B. Reactions of proteins

1. Amphoteric properties—like the amino acids forming them, proteins can act as acid or base in solutions; can act as buffers

2. Hydrolysis—acid, base, or enzyme hydrolysis splits peptide bond; yields proteose → peptones → peptides → amino acids

3. Denaturation—change in structure renders the protein less soluble, leads to coagulation of protein

a. Heat—protein and heat → coagulated protein; e.g., cooked egg white, cooked meat

b. Salts of heavy metals—silver, lead, mercury, etc.; taken internally, poison because they denature the enzymes of the cells, which are protein in nature

c. Acetone and alcohol—both harden skin proteins

d. Inorganic acids and bases—coagulate and hydrolyze proteins

e. Alkaloids and organic acids—tanning of hides, precipitation of blood proteins for clinical tests

f. Rays—x-ray films, infrared rays, ultraviolet rays—long exposure can cause cataracts (precipitation of lens protein in eye)

4. Salting out—concentrated salt solutions render soluble proteins insoluble

5. Color reactions

a. Xanthoproteic test—protein having benzene ring (as found in the amino acids tyrosine and phenylalanine) will turn yellow on addition of concentrated nitric acid; heat and a second addition of sodium hydroxide will turn the yellow to orange

b. Millon's test—protein having a phenolic ring (as found in the amino acid tyrosine) will form red precipitate on addition of a mixture of mercuric and mercurous nitrates

c. Biuret test—test for the peptide bond; violet appears on addition of a hydroxide and dilute copper sulfate solution; negative for free amino acids (no peptide bond)

d. Hopkins-Cole test—protein that contains the indole structure (amino acid tryptophan) shows violet on addition of glyoxylic acid and concentrated sulfuric acid

e. Ninhydrin test—test for free amino acids, ninhydrin reagent gives blue color

Nucleoproteins

A. Specific proteins found in cells, made of large and complex molecules having important functions

B. Composition of nucleoproteins

1. Hydrolysis of nucleoproteins results in nucleic acids and protein

2. Hydrolysis of nucleic acid yields

a. Phosphoric acid—H_3PO_4

b. Pentose sugars—ribose or deoxyribose

c. Purine or pyrimidine bases
(1) Purine bases—adenine, guanine
(2) Pyrimidine bases—cytosine, uracil, thymine

3. Combination of a purine or pyrimidine base with either ribose or deoxyribose forms a nucleoside

4. Addition of phosphoric acid to a nucleoside forms a nucleotide

5. Polymerization of nucleotide molecules via ester bonds yields a nucleic acid—the shape of DNA is that of a double helix

C. Two main forms of nucleic acid—RNA and DNA (ribonucleic acid and deoxyribonucleic acid)

1. RNA yields the following on hydrolysis: adenine, guanine, cytosine, uracil, ribose, phosphoric acid

2. DNA yields the following on hydrolysis: adenine, guanine, cytosine, thymine, deoxyribose, phosphoric acid

D. Role of DNA and RNA in protein synthesis

1. DNA is found chiefly in the chromatin material of interphase cells and in the chromosomes of cells in mitosis

a. Portions of DNA molecules are the genes of classic genetics; the genetic code consists of sequences of bases (adenine, guanine, cytosine, and thymine) linearly arranged along the DNA molecule; every 3 bases represent a code for 1 amino acid (a triplet code)

b. One enormous DNA molecule represents thousands of genes separated from each other by specific triplets (codons) representing periods or commas; i.e., the linear triplet code is punctuated so that it can be eventually translated correctly on the ribosome

c. DNA is also found in mitochondria, chloroplasts, and certain other cellular organelles (like centrioles) and is thought to play some role in their replication and metabolism

2. RNA is found both inside the nucleus and in the cytoplasm of cells

3. RNA occurs in three forms: messenger RNA (mRNA), transfer RNA (tRNA), and ribosomal RNA (rRNA)

a. DNA transcribes its coded message of how to make proteins into mRNA; the function of mRNA is to carry this coded genetic information from the DNA in the nucleus to the ribosome in the cytoplasm where proteins can be synthesized

b. The transcribed genetic code being carried by mRNA is translated into the synthesis of proteins on the ribosomes; these proteins then serve both structurally and enzymatically in the cell

c. tRNA molecules each carry an amino acid to the ribosome where protein synthesis is occurring; there is a specific tRNA molecule for each amino acid

d. rRNA is part of the structure of the ribosome

4. The protein difference between individuals is ultimately determined by differences in the genetic code carried by DNA; the DNA and RNA molecules are presently the only known molecules that store information and can result in the accurate transmission of genetic information from one generation of cell or organism to the next; the cellular mitotic and meiotic processes are elaborate and precise mechanisms for partitioning the genetic material appropriately between daughter cells

E. Other important related compounds

1. ATP and ADP (adenosine triphosphate and adenosine diphosphate) are energy-storing compounds in cells

2. NAD (nicotinamide adenine dinucleotide) and NADP (nicotinamide adenine dinucleotide phosphate) are important in hydrogen transport in the metabolism of foods

Enzymes

Hormones involved in regulating GI tract

A. Gastrin—stimulates flow of gastric juices

B. Enterogastrone—inhibits flow of gastric juices
C. Secretin—stimulates flow of sodium bicarbonate from the pancreas to the duodenum
D. Pancreozymin—stimulates the flow of pancreatic enzymes from the pancreas to the duodenum
E. Cholecystokinin—stimulates contraction of gallbladder
F. Enterocrinin—stimulates flow of intestinal juice

REVIEW OF MICROORGANISMS RELATED TO THE GASTROINTESTINAL SYSTEM

A. Bacterial pathogens

1. *Brucella*—*Brucella abortus*, *Brucella suis*, and *Brucella melitensis* are small, gram-negative bacilli that are somewhat pleomorphic (variable in shape); they cause brucellosis, an infection primarily of domestic animals (cattle, goats, swine, sheep), which humans acquire by drinking infected milk

2. *Escherichia coli*—small, gram-negative bacillus composing the major portion of the normal flora of the large intestine; certain strains are the most common cause of urinary tract infections and infantile diarrhea

3. *Leptospira icterohaemorrhagiae*—long, tightly-coiled spirochete similar in appearance to *Treponema pallidum;* causes infectious jaundice (Weil's disease)

4. *Shigella*—gram-negative bacilli, similar to *Salmonella; Shigella dysenteriae* and a number of other species cause an illness known as bacillary dysentery, dysentery, or shigellosis

5. *Vibrio cholerae* (formerly *V. comma*)—curved, gram-negative bacillus with a single polar flagellum; causes Asiatic cholera

B. Protozoal pathogens

1. *Balantidium coli*—ciliated protozoan; causes enteritis

2. *Entamoeba histolytica*—an ameba; causes amebiasis (amebic dysentery)

3. *Giardia lamblia*—flagellated protozoan; causes enteritis

C. Parasitic pathogens

1. Nematodes (roundworms)

a. *Ancylostoma duodenale* (hookworm)—intestinal parasite very similar to *Necator americanus*

b. *Ascaris lumbricoides* (roundworm)—intestinal parasite very much resembling the earthworm

c. *Enterobius vermicularis* (pinworm, seatworm)—small, white parasitic worm found in the upper part of the large intestine; the female lays eggs in perianal area causing irritation

d. *Necator americanus* (American hookworm)—intestinal parasite about ½ inch (1.2 cm) in length

e. *Trichuris trichiura* (whipworm)—intestinal parasite about 2 inches (5 cm) in length

2. Cestodes (tapeworm)

a. *Diphyllobothrium latum* (fish tapeworm)—large tapeworm (about 20 feet [6.1 m] in length) found in adult form in the intestine of cats, dogs, and humans (vertebrate and aquatic hosts in sequence)

b. *Echinococcus granulosa* (dog tapeworm)—small tapeworm of dogs; larval stage (hydatid) may develop in humans forming hydatid tumors or cysts in the liver, lungs, kidneys, and other organs

c. *Hymenolepsis nana* (dwarf tapeworm)—a species about 1 inch (2.5 cm) in length; found in the adult form in the intestine

d. *Taenia marginata* (beef tapeworm)—the common tapeworm of humans, a species from 12 to 25 feet (3.6 to 7.6 m) in length, found in the adult form in the human intestine

e. *Taenia solium* (pork tapeworm)—a species 3 to 6 feet (0.9 to 1.8 m) in length, found in the adult form in the intestine of humans

3. Trematodes (flukes)

a. *Clonorchis sinensis*—one of the most common liver flukes, especially in China and Japan

b. *Fasciola hepatica*—the common liver fluke of herbivorous animals; occasionally found in the human liver

c. *Fasciolopsis buski*—the largest of the intestinal flukes

d. *Paragonimus westermani*—the lung fluke; found in cysts in the lungs, liver, abdominal cavity, and elsewhere

PHARMACOLOGY RELATED TO GASTROINTESTINAL SYSTEM DISORDERS

A. Antiemetics
1. General implications for nurses
   a. Observe occurrence and characteristics of vomitus
   b. Eliminate noxious substances from diet and environment
   c. Provide oral hygiene
   d. Observe patient for adverse effects
      (1) Drowsiness
      (2) Hypotension
      (3) Dry mouth
      (4) Blurred vision
      (5) Uncoordination
2. Actions
   a. Diminish the sensitivity of the chemoreceptor trigger zone to irritants; e.g., drugs, radiation therapy
   b. Those drugs prescribed for motion sickness decrease labyrinthine excitability and the conduction of vestibular-cerebellar stimuli (motion sickness control)
3. Examples of antiemetics
   a. Promethazine hydrochloride (Fellozine, Ganphen, Phenergan)
   b. Trimethobenzamide hydrochloride (Tigan)
   c. Prochlorperazine (Compazine)
   d. Dimenhydrinate (Dramamine)
   e. Diphenidol hydrochloride (Vontrol)
   f. Hydroxyzine hydrochloride (Atarax, Vistaril)
   g. Meclizine hydrochloride (Bonine)
B. Anorexiants (drugs for appetite suppression)
1. General implications for nurses
   a. Educate patient regarding drug misuse
   b. Counsel concerning diet and exercise
   c. Observe patient for adverse effects
      (1) Constipation
      (2) Blurred vision
      (3) Nausea and vomiting
      (4) Metallic taste
      (5) Tachycardia
      (6) Irritability
2. Actions
   a. Primary drugs are amphetamines or drugs with comparable action, which act at hypothalamic appetite centers to suppress desire for food
   b. Amine oxidase inhibition in cerebrocortical and reticular-activating structures provides elevated mood and increased mental acuity
3. Examples
   a. Amphetamine sulfate (Benzedrine)
   b. Benzphetamine hydrochloride (Didrex)

c. Chlorphentermine hydrochloride (Pre-Sate)
d. Dextroamphetamine sulfate (Dexedrine)
e. Diethylpropion hydrochloride (Tenuate, Tepanil)
f. Fenfluramine hydrochloride (Pondimin)
g. Phenmetrazine hydrochloride (Preludin)
C. Antacids
1. General implications for nurses
a. Teach patient about overuse of antacids
b. Explain need for continued supervision
c. Attempt to eliminate the source of discomfort
d. Caution patients on sodium-restricted diets that many of the antacids contain sodium
e. Observe patient for adverse effects
(1) Constipation or diarrhea
(2) Systemic antacids (sodium bicarbonate) may lead to alkalosis and renal insufficiency
2. Actions
a. Provide a protective film on the stomach lining
b. Lower gastric acid level, which allows more rapid movement of stomach contents into the duodenum
c. Drugs containing aluminum, magnesium, and calcium have minimal absorptive tendency
3. Examples
a. Aluminum carbonate gel, basic (Basaljel)
b. Aluminum hydroxide gel (Amphojel)
c. Aluminum hydroxide with magnesium trisilicate (Gelusil)
d. Aluminum and magnesium hydroxides (Maalox)
e. Aluminum phosphate gel (Phosphaljel)
f. Magaldrate (Riopan)
g. Sodium bicarbonate (which is absorbed from the intestine and may cause alkalosis)
D. Anticholinergics
1. General implications for nurses
a. Provide dietary counseling with emphasis on bland foods
b. Observe patient for adverse effects
(1) Abdominal distention
(2) Constipation
(3) Urinary retention
2. Actions
a. Decrease production of glandular (salivary, gastric, pancreatic) secretions
b. Decrease the motility of the digestive tract
c. Used in the treatment of peptic ulcer

3. Examples
a. Atropine sulfate
b. Belladonna leaf, tincture
c. Isopropamide (Darbid)
d. Propantheline bromide (Pro-Banthine)
e. Dicyclomine hydrochloride (Bentyl)
E. Antidiarrheal agents
1. Absorbants
a. General implications for nurses
(1) Observe color, characteristics, and frequency of stool
(2) Observe for signs of electrolyte imbalance
(3) Assess and eliminate cause of diarrhea
(4) Give after each loose bowel movement
(5) Because these drugs are not absorbed, there are minimal side effects
b. Actions
(1) Absorb toxic substances as well as nutrients from digestive tract
(2) Given after each loose bowel movement, these drugs improve the consistency of stool but do not necessarily stop the diarrhea
c. Examples
(1) Bismuth subcarbonate
(2) Kaolin and pectin (Kaopectate)
2. Enteric bacteria replacements
a. General implications for nurses
(1) Store in refrigerator
(2) Contraindicated in children with high fever
(3) Observe patient for adverse effects
(a) Excessive flatulence
(b) Abdominal cramps
b. Actions
(1) Used when prolonged use of antibiotics has suppressed natural bacterial flora and overgrowth of pathogenic bacteria has occurred
(2) Enhance production of lactic acid from carbohydrates in intestinal lumen; acidity suppresses pathogenic bacterial overgrowth
c. Examples
(1) *Lactobacillus acidophilus* (Bacid)
(2) *Lactobacillus bulgaricus* (Novaflor and Lactinex)
3. Motility suppressants
a. General implications for nurses

(1) Warn patient of risk of physical dependence with long-term use
(2) Observe patient for adverse effects
  (a) Urinary retention
  (b) Tachycardia
  (c) Dry mucous membranes
  (d) Sedation
  (e) Paralytic ileus
  (f) Respiratory depression
b. Actions
(1) Increase tone of intestinal musculature, ileocecal valve, and anal sphincter to slow expulsion of intestinal content
(2) Decreased motility allows larger amounts of water to be absorbed from the intestine
c. Examples
(1) Diphenoxylate hydrochloride (Lomotil)
(2) Tincture of opium (Paregoric)
(3) Camphorated opium tincture (0.04% opium content)

F. Cathartics
  1. Intestinal lubricants
    a. General implications for nurses
      (1) Do not administer with meals or immediately following meals, since they delay entry of food into the intestines
      (2) Teach patient regarding overuse of cathartics
      (3) Teach patient to be aware of side effects of continued use
        (a) Inhibit absorption of fat-soluble vitamins from foods and drug sources
        (b) Anal leaking of oil with continued use
    b. Actions
      (1) Nonabsorbable oil that decreases dehydration of feces
      (2) Lubricates intestinal tract
    c. Examples
      (1) Mineral oil
      (2) Olive oil
  2. Fecal softeners
    a. General implications for nurses
      (1) Encourage increased roughage and fluid in diet
      (2) Increase patient's activity level
      (3) Observe consistency and frequency of stool
    b. Actions
      (1) Act in the colon to lower surface tension of feces
      (2) Allow water and fats to penetrate feces and ease evacuation of softer stool
    c. Examples
      (1) Dioctyl calcium sulfosuccinate (Surfak)
      (2) Dioctyl sodium sulfosuccinate (Colace, Doxinate)
      (3) Peri-Colace
  3. Bulk-forming cathartics
    a. General implications for nurses
      (1) Explain to patient that overuse leads to dependence
      (2) Encourage increased fluid and roughage in diet
      (3) Use with caution for patients on sodium-restricted diets if drug contains sodium
      (4) Observe consistency and frequency of stool
    b. Action—increased bulk in intestinal lumen stimulates propulsive movements by pressure on mucosal lining
    c. Examples
      (1) Methylcellulose (Cellothyl, Cologel, Hydrolose, Melozets, Methulose, Syncelose)
      (2) Sodium carboxymethylcellulose (Bu-Lax, C.M.C.)
      (3) Psyllium hydrophilic mucilloid (Metamucil, Mucilose)
      (4) Agar
  4. Colon irritants
    a. General implications for nurses
      (1) Explain to patient that prolonged use may lead to dependence
      (2) Observe for adverse effects
        (a) Nausea
        (b) Abdominal cramps
        (c) Diarrhea
      (3) Increase fluid and roughage in diet
      (4) Observe consistency and frequency of stool
    b. Action—stimulate peristalsis by reflex response to irritation caused by drug contacting the mucosa of the intestinal lumen
    c. Examples
      (1) Cascara sagrada (Peristim)
      (2) Senna (Senokot)
      (3) Castor oil
      (4) Bisacodyl (Dulcolax)
  5. Saline cathartics

a. General implications for nurses
   (1) Instruct patient to increase bulk in diet with bran, fresh fruit, cereals, vegetables
   (2) Observe patient for adverse effects
       (a) Nausea
       (b) Dehydration
       (c) Increased accumulation of sodium ions in blood
b. Actions
   (1) Increase osmotic pressure within the intestine, drawing fluid from the blood and bowel wall
   (2) This increases bulk and stimulates peristalsis
   (3) May be used to treat edema
c. Examples
   (1) Magnesium sulfate (Epsom salts)
   (2) Milk of magnesia
   (3) Magnesium citrate solution
   (4) Effervescent sodium phosphate (Fleet Phospho-Soda)

G. Intestinal antibiotics
1. General implications for nurses
   a. Know why the drug is being administered
   b. Observe characteristics of bowel movements
   c. Avoid use of drugs that are also ototoxic and nephrotoxic while patient is receiving these drugs
   d. Observe patient for adverse effects
      (1) Damage to auditory nerve and kidney
      (2) Nausea, vomiting, diarrhea
      (3) Fungal infections if therapy is prolonged
2. Actions
   a. Used in the treatment of bacterial diarrhea and as preparation for bowel surgery
   b. Neomycin also used in treatment of hepatic coma, since it suppresses growth of intestinal flora that will cause a secondary decrease in the blood ammonia level
3. Examples
   a. Neomycin sulfate
   b. Kanamycin sulfate (Kantrex)

H. Pancreatic enzymes
1. General implications for nurses
   a. Do not crush drugs that are enteric coated to avoid destruction by gastric juices
   b. Administer with meals
   c. Provide balanced diet to prevent indigestion
2. Action—supply digestive enzymes: lipase, protease, and amylase

3. Examples
   a. Pancrelipase (Cotazym)
   b. Pancreatin (Viokase)

RELATED PROCEDURES
Endoscopy

A. Definition—visualization of the esophagus, stomach, colon, or rectum using a hollow tube with a lighted end
   1. Gastroscopy—stomach
   2. Esophagoscopy—esophagus
   3. Sigmoidoscopy—sigmoid colon
   4. Proctoscopy—rectum
B. Nursing responsibilities
   1. Obtain informed consent for procedure
   2. If rectal examination is indicated, administer cleansing enemas prior to test
   3. Restrict diet (NPO) prior to procedure
   4. Following the procedure, observe patient for bleeding, changes in vital signs, or nausea
   5. If the throat is anesthetized (as for a gastroscopy or esophagoscopy), check for the return of gag reflex before offering oral fluids
C. Physical principle involved: light refraction

Gastrointestinal (GI) series

A. Definition—introduction of barium, an opaque medium, into the upper GI tract via the mouth, gastrostomy tube, or nasogastric tube to visualize area by x-ray methods
B. Nusing responsibilities
   1. Explain procedure to patient
   2. Maintain patient NPO prior to examination
   3. Inform patient that stool will be white or pink for 24 to 72 hours following the procedure
   4. Encourage fluids and administer cathartics as ordered
C. Physical principle involved: x rays

Barium enema

A. Definition—introduction of barium, an opaque medium, into the intestines for purpose of x-ray visualization of intestines for pathologic changes
B. Nursing responsibilities
   1. Explain procedure to patient
   2. Prepare patient for procedure by
      a. Administration of cathartics and/or enemas as ordered to evacuate the bowel
      b. Maintaining patient NPO for 8 to 10 hours prior to test

3. Observe bowel movements following procedure for presence of barium
4. Administer enemas and/or cathartics as ordered if stool does not return to normal

C. Physical principle involved: x rays

Gastric analysis

A. Definition
   1. Analysis of stomach contents for presence of abnormal constituents or lack of normal constituents such as hydrochloric acid, blood, acid-fast bacteria, and lactic acid
   2. Acid content is elevated in ulcers, decreased in malignant conditions of stomach, and absent in pernicious anemia

B. Nursing responsibilities
   1. Explain procedure to patient
   2. Maintain patient NPO prior to test and have a nasogastric tube passed at time of procedure
   3. Administer histamine or caffeine to stimulate hydrochloric acid secretion prior to procedure if ordered
   4. Obtain contents and secure in appropriate container and send to laboratory

C. Physical principle involved: Boyle's law

Stool specimens

A. Definitions
   1. Stool for guaiac (occult blood)—a specimen or smear of stool on a commercially prepared card is sent to the laboratory for analysis; positive results indicate the presence of blood in the stool and may suggest diverse diseases such as peptic ulcer, gastritis, gastric or colonic carcinoma, colitis, or diverticulitis
   2. Stools for O and P (ova and parasites)—must be sent to the laboratory while still warm for microscopic examination
   3. Stool culture—a specimen or swab of stool is sent in a sterile container for identification of abnormal bacterial growth

B. Nursing responsibilities
   1. Explain procedure to patient
   2. Collect specimen in appropriate container
   3. Label container with patient's name, identification number, physician and room number
   4. Chart that specimen was sent and any unusual assessment of stool

Enemas

A. Definitions
   1. Tap water enema (TWE)—introduction of water into the colon to stimulate evacuation
   2. Soapsuds enema (SSE)—introduction of soapy water into the colon to stimulate peristalsis by bowel irritation; contraindicated as a preparation for an endoscopic procedure because it may alter the appearance of the mucosa
   3. Harris flush or drip—introduction of water into the colon as tolerated and subsequent repeated drainage of that water through the same tubing to facilitate passage of flatus from the bowel
   4. High colonic irrigation—introduction of water into the upper portion of the colon to facilitate complete fecal evacuation
   5. Instillation—introduction of a liquid (usually mineral oil) into the colon to facilitate fecal activity through lubricating effect

B. Nursing responsibilities
   1. Explain procedure to patient
   2. Provide privacy for patient
   3. Obtain correct solution
   4. Lubricate tip of rectal catheter with water-soluble jelly
   5. Insert catheter 4 to 6 inches (10 to 15 cm) into rectum
   6. Allow solution to enter slowly; keep solution no more than 12 to 18 inches (30.5 to 45.7 cm) above rectum
   7. Allow ample time for patient to expel enema
   8. Observe and record amount and consistency of returns

C. Physical principle involved: gravity

Irrigation of nasogastric (Levin) tube

A. Definition
   1. The Levin tube is commonly used for gastric decompression
   2. Purposes of insertion of a nasogastric tube include emptying the stomach, obtaining a specimen for diagnostic purposes, or providing a means for nourishment
   3. Irrigation is the insertion of fluid (usually normal saline) to maintain patency

B. Nursing responsibilities
   1. Check that order for irrigations has been written by physician
   2. Ascertain patency of Levin tube attached to inter-

mittent suction by observing for drainage; nausea or abdominal discomfort may indicate the tube is occluded
3. Assemble equipment: 30-ml syringe or bulb syringe, irrigating solution, and basin for returning fluid
4. Instill approximately 30 ml of fluid into the tube
5. Gently withdraw the same volume of fluid as was instilled; if patient has had gastric surgery, the physician will generally order instillations; in this case, irrigation fluid is instilled but not withdrawn; the amount instilled must be subtracted from total gastric output
6. Chart amount, color, and consistency of drainage
C. Physical principle involved: Boyle's law

Paracentesis

A. Definition—the surgical puncture of the peritoneal membrane of the abdominal cavity for the purpose of removing fluid
B. Nursing responsibilities
  1. Explain procedure; obtain consent
  2. Have patient void prior to procedure
  3. Assist patient to a sitting position
  4. Observe patient for signs of shock; sudden fluid shifts can result in hypotension
  5. Chart amount and characteristics of fluid withdrawn
  6. Apply dry sterile dressing to puncture site
  7. Properly label specimen if required and send to laboratory
C. Physical principle involved: Boyle's law

Ileostomy care

A. Definition—physical care of the ileostomy stoma and surrounding skin
B. Nursing responsibilities
  1. Protect the skin from irritation, since the feces will be liquid because of the anatomical location of the stoma
  2. Explain procedure to patient and family and encourage self-care
  3. Do not irrigate the stoma
  4. Affix an appliance with an adequate seal (Karaya) to prevent accidental leakage around stoma; the appliance is generally worn for 2 to 4 days but emptied every 6 hours
  5. Skin care to the area around the stoma should be meticulous to prevent breakdown of the surrounding tissues

Colostomy care

A. Definition
  1. Instillation of fluid into the lower colon via a stoma on the abdominal wall to stimulate peristalsis and facilitate the expulsion of feces
  2. Cleansing the colostomy stoma and collection of feces (stool consistency will depend on location of ostomy; a colostomy of the sigmoid colon will tend to produce formed stools, whereas a transverse colostomy will result in those less formed; an ileostomy will constantly ooze liquid feces)
B. Nursing responsibilities
  1. Secure a physician's order
  2. Irrigate stoma at the same time each day to approximate normal bowel habits
  3. Insert well-lubricated catheter tip into the stoma approximately 7 cm in the direction of the remaining bowel (anatomy of ascending, transverse and descending colon should be considered); as solution is allowed to flow, the catheter may be advanced
  4. Hold the irrigating container approximately 20 inches (51 cm) above the colostomy; irrigating solution should be 40.5° C (105° F)
  5. Clamp tubing or temporarily lower the container if patient complains of cramping
  6. Provide privacy while waiting for fecal returns or permit patient to ambulate with collection bag in place to further stimulate peristalsis
  7. Cleanse stoma with soap and water; if excoriation occurs, a soothing ointment may be ordered
  8. Apply a colostomy bag or gauze dressing (if the colostomy is well regulated)
  9. Teach patient to control odor when necessary by placing two aspirin tablets or commercially available deodorizers in the colostomy bag or by taking bismuth subcarbonate tablets orally to control odor
C. Physical principle involved: gravity

Gastric gavage (tube feeding)

A. Definition—feeding a prepared liquid formula via a tube passed into the stomach
B. Nursing responsibilities
  1. Verify the placement of the tube before feedings
    a. Inject small amount of air into the tube and, with a stethoscope placed over the epigastric area, listen for the passage of air into the stomach

b. Aspirate for stomach contents
c. Place the end of the nasogastric tube in water; presence of bubbling indicates the tube is in the lungs (this method is the least reliable)
2. Place patient in a sitting position to prevent aspiration
3. Introduce a small amount of water first to verify the patency of the tube; the tube should not be allowed to empty during feeding so that excess air is not forced into the stomach
4. Administer the feeding (which may be the patient's normal foods blenderized) at room or body temperature slowly; observe and question patient to determine tolerance; the higher the feeding container and the larger the lumen of the feeding tube, the more rapid the flow
5. Administer a small amount of water to clear the tube at the completion of feeding
6. Clamp tubing and clean equipment
7. Provide special skin care if the patient has a gastrostomy tube; the skin may become irritated from gastric enzymes; wash and apply a protective ointment as necessary
8. Encourage patient to chew certain foods that will stimulate gastric secretions while providing psychologic comfort
C. Physical principle involved: Boyle's law

Hyperalimentation (total parenteral nutrition [T.P.N.])

A. Definition
1. Hyperalimentation is a high-protein, high-caloric intravenous feeding used for patients with disturbances of ingestion or digestion
2. One liter of the specially prepared solution may provide 70 to 80 g of protein in the form of amino acids, as well as vitamins, electrolytes, and 1000 to 2000 calories
B. Nursing responsibilities
1. Infuse fluid through a large vein such as the subclavian because of the high osmolarity of the solution
2. Ensure proper placement of tube by chest x-ray examination after insertion of catheter; accidental pneumothorax can occur during insertion
3. Precisely regulate fluid infusion rate; an intravenous pump should be used if available
a. Rapid infusion may result in movement of fluid from intravascular compartment; dehydration, circulatory overload, and hyperglycemia can occur
b. Slow infusion may result in hypoglycemia, since the body adapts to the high osmolarity of this fluid by secreting more insulin; for this reason, hyperalimentation is never terminated abruptly but is gradually discontinued
4. Use aseptic technique when handling infusion or changing dressing (in many institutions, only nurses specially trained are allowed to change the dressing because of the high risk of infection)
5. Record daily weights and monitor urinary sugar and acetone levels every 4 to 6 hours
6. Check laboratory reports daily, especially glucose, creatine, BUN, and electrolytes
7. Monitor temperature q 4 h, since infection is the most common complication of hyperalimentation; if the patient has a temperature elevation, order cultures of blood, urine, and sputum to rule out other sources of infection

MAJOR DISEASES
Stomatitis

A. Etiology and pathophysiology
1. Inflammation of buccal mucosa as the result of disease, trauma, irritants, nutritional deficiencies, or medications
2. Categories
a. Aphthous stomatitis—canker sore that can result from chronic cheek biting
b. Herpes simplex—virus that causes vesicle formation in mouth, on lips, or on nose
c. Vincent's angina—ulceration of buccal membrane due to *Borrelia vincentii* (trench mouth)
d. Thrush—fungal invasion of mouth by *Candida albicans,* characterized by white patches
B. Signs and symptoms
1. Subjective
a. Foul taste in mouth
b. Pain in mouth
2. Objective
a. Erythema of mucous membranes
b. Changes in salivation
c. Unpleasant odor to breath
d. Bleeding gums in Vincent's angina
e. White patches in thrush
C. Treatment
1. Adequate nutrition and hydration
2. Alkaline mouthwashes

3. Antifungal agents for thrush
4. Antibiotics for Vincent's angina
D. Nursing care
 1. Provide mouth washes every 2 hours
 2. Encourage foods that can be tolerated, such as soft foods, cool drinks, eggnogs
 3. Promote oral hygiene; use soft toothbrush or padded tongue blade

Fracture of the jaw

A. Etiology and pathophysiology—the bones in the jaw are generally broken as the result of trauma such as motor vehicle accidents or physical combat
B. Signs and symptoms
 1. Subjective
  a. History of trauma to face
  b. Pain in face and jaw
 2. Objective
  a. Bloody discharge from mouth
  b. Swelling of face on affected side
  c. Difficulty opening or closing the mouth
C. Treatment
 1. The separated fragments of broken bone are re-united and immobilized by the use of wires and rubber bands; usually placed without surgical incision
 2. Open reduction of the jaw is indicated for severely fractured or displaced bones; interosseous wiring is done
D. Nursing care
 1. Postoperatively control vomiting and reduce the chance of aspiration pneumonia by positioning patient on abdomen
 2. Keep wire cutters at the bedside to release the wires and rubber bands if emesis occurs
 3. Explain diet to patient and family; no solid foods are permitted; encourage high-protein liquids or blenderized soft foods
 4. Stress the importance of regular oral hygiene and institute it early in postoperative period

Cancer of the mouth

A. Etiology and pathophysiology
 1. Occurs primarily in patients who smoke and drink alcohol in large quantities
 2. Cancer of the lip is easily diagnosed, and prognosis is very good; incidence is highest in pipe smokers
 3. Cancer of the tongue usually occurs with cancer

of the floor of the mouth; metastasis to the neck is common
 4. Tumors of the submaxillary glands are highly malignant and grow rapidly
B. Signs and symptoms
 1. Subjective
  a. Pain is not an early symptom
  b. Alterations of taste sensation
 2. Objective
  a. Leukoplakia (white patches on mucosa, which are considered precancerous)
  b. Ulcerated areas are seen in the involved structure
C. Treatment
 1. Reconstructive surgery if indicated
 2. Radiation or implantation of radioactive material may arrest growth of tumor
D. Nursing care
 1. Maintain fluid and electrolyte balance
 2. Provide for a means of communication
 3. If radiation therapy is indicated, relieve dryness of the mouth by frequent mouthwashes and ample fluids
 4. Consider time and distance in relation to radioactive material when giving nursing care

Gastritis

A. Etiology and pathophysiology
 1. An inflammation of the stomach; either acute or chronic
 2. May be caused by
  a. Ingestion of irritating chemicals such as asprin and alcohol
  b. Bacterial or viral infections
  c. Allergic reactions
  d. Chronic uremia, which often leads to chronic gastritis
B. Signs and symptoms
 1. Subjective
  a. Anorexia
  b. Nausea and vomiting
  c. Epigastric fullness
 2. Objective
  a. Diarrhea and cramps if caused by an infection
  b. Dehydration
  c. Hemorrhage if aspirin or other chemicals are involved
C. Treatment
 1. Early treatment is aimed at correcting fluid and

electrolyte imbalance; patients are kept NPO during acute phase of illness and then progress to bland diet
2. If caused by infection, appropriate antibioics may be given
3. Other medications that may be prescribed include antispasmodics, anticholinergics, and antacids
D. Nursing care
1. Observe for signs of dehydration and electrolyte imbalance
2. Provide adequate fluid intake
3. Alert patient to possible causes
4. Teach patient the necessary dietary alterations such as omission of coffee, alcohol, and spices and maintaining a bland diet

Peptic ulcer

A. Etiology and pathophysiology
1. Ulcerations of the gastrointestinal mucosa and underlying tissues caused by gastric secretions that have a low pH (acid)
2. Causes include conditions that increase the secretion of hydrochloric acid by the gastric mucosa or that decrease the tissues' resistance to the acid
   a. Zollinger-Ellison syndrome—tumors secreting gastrin, which will stimulate the production of excess hydrochloric acid
   b. Certain drugs such as aspirin and indomethacin will decrease tissue resistance
   c. Many feel that psychosomatic causes are strongly related to peptic ulcers; a person who is considered a perfectionist may have an increased risk of developing a peptic ulcer
3. Peptic ulcers may be present in the esophagus, stomach, or duodenum (the most common site)
4. Complications include pyloric or duodenal obstruction, hemorrhage, and perforation
B. Signs and symptoms
1. Subjective
   a. Gnawing or burning epigastric pain that occurs 1 to 2 hours after eating and may be relieved by eructation, vomiting, food, or antacids
   b. Nausea
2. Objective
   a. If bleeding occurs, signs of anemia will be evident; passage of tarry stools (melena) may occur
   b. Vomiting (coffee ground to port wine color if bleeding has occurred)

C. Treatment
1. Institute measures to neutralize or buffer hydrochloric acid, inhibit acid secretion, and decrease the activity of pepsin and hydrochloric acid such as
   a. Radiation and gastric hypothermia to suppress gastric secretions
   b. Diet regulation through the use of bland foods, and restriction of irritating substances such as nicotine, caffeine, alcohol, spices, and gassy foods
   c. Antacids to reduce acidity
2. Type and cross match so that blood will be available if gastric hemorrhage occurs
3. Sedatives, tranquilizers, anticholinergics, and analgesics for pain and restlessness
4. Antiemetics for nausea and vomiting
5. Bed rest to reduce physical activity
6. Encourage patient to seek counseling or psychotherapy to explore the emotional components of the illness
7. If hemorrhage occurs, a nasogastric tube is inserted and iced saline lavages may be ordered; irrigations with medications that cause vasoconstriction to control bleeding are also used
8. Surgical intervention
   a. Vagotomy—the vagus nerve, which innervates the stomach, is cut to decrease the secretion of hydrochloric acid
   b. Bilroth I—the lower portion of the stomach is removed and the remaining portion attached to the duodenum
   c. Bilroth II—removal of the antrum and distal portion of the stomach and subsequent anastomosis of remaining section to the jejunum
   d. Antrectomy—removal of the antral portion of the stomach
   e. Gastrectomy—removal of 60% to 80% of the stomach
9. Common complications of partial or total gastric resection
   a. Dumping syndrome—involves the rapid passage of food from the stomach to the jejunum; the food, being hypertonic (especially if high in carbohydrates), will draw fluid from the circulating blood into the jejunum causing diaphoresis, faintness, and palpitations
   b. Hemorrhage
   c. Pneumonia
   d. Pernicious anemia

D. Nursing care
1. Allow ample time for patient to express feelings and concerns
2. Administer and assess effects of sedatives, antacids, anticholinergics, and dietary modifications
3. Encourage hydration to reduce anticholinergic side effects and dilute the HCl in the stomach
4. Refrain from administering drugs such as salicylates, phenylbutazone, steroids, and ACTH, which are normally contraindicated
5. Observe for complications such as gastric hemorrhage, perforation, and drug toxicity
6. Postoperative care after gastric resection
   a. Monitor vital signs; assess dressing for drainage
   b. Maintain patent nasogastric tube to suction to prevent stress on suture line
   c. Observe color and amount of nasogastric drainage; excessive bleeding or the presence of bright red blood after 12 hours should be reported immediately
   d. Cough, deep breathe, and change position frequently to prevent the occurrence of pulmonary complications
   e. Monitor intake and output
   f. Apply abdominal binder if ordered
   g. Apply antiembolism stockings and ambulate early to prevent vascular complications
   h. To prevent dumping syndrome, instruct the patient to
      (1) Eat smaller meals at more frequent intervals
      (2) Avoid high-carbohydrate intake
      (3) Limit amount of fluid ingested with meals
      (4) Lie down or rest after eating
7. Teach drug regimen and signs and symptoms of recurrence
8. Prevent recurrence by teaching patient to modify dietary, working, and living patterns; maintain regularity in activities of daily living; continue medical supervision

Carcinoma of the stomach

A. Etiology and pathophysiology
1. Carcinoma of the stomach is often not diagnosed until metastasis occurs because of the stomach's ability to accommodate the growth of a tumor and the fact that pain occurs late in the disease
2. May metastasize by direct extension, lymphatics, or blood to the esophagus, spleen, pancreas, liver, or bone
3. Heredity appears to be a factor in the development of carcinoma of the stomach, as is the presence of precursors such as ulcerative disease and pernicious anemia
4. Incidence is higher in men over 40 years of age; Japan has a 4 times greater rate of cancer of the stomach than the United States

B. Signs and symptoms
1. Subjective
   a. Anorexia
   b. Nausea
   c. Belching (eructation)
   d. Heartburn
2. Objective
   a. Weight loss
   b. Anemia
   c. Positive stools for guaiac (occult blood)
   d. Achlorhydria (absence of hydrochloric acid determined by gastric analysis)

C. Treatment
1. Subtotal or total gastrectomy
2. Radiation
3. Chemotherapy (fluorouracil is often used)

D. Nursing care
1. Offer patient every opportunity to verbalize fears (i.e., cancer, death, family problems, self-image)
2. Postoperative care the same as nursing care after a gastric resection (see Peptic ulcers); in addition, if a total gastrectomy is performed, the chest cavity is usually entered, so the patient will have chest tubes (see Pneumothorax for related nursing care)
3. Modify diet to include smaller, more frequent meals
4. If total gastrectomy has been performed, the patient will have a vitamin B_{12} deficiency (see Pernicious anemia)
5. Patient may require gavage feedings via nasogastric tube or gastrostomy tube (see section on procedures)

Hiatus hernia

A. Etiology and pathophysiology
1. A portion of the stomach protrudes through a hiatus (opening) in the diaphragm into the thoracic cavity
2. May result from a congenital weakness of diaphragm or from injury, pregnancy, or obesity

3. Function of the cardiac sphincter is lost, gastric juices enter the esophagus, and edema and hyperemia may result
B. Signs and symptoms
 1. Subjective
  a. Substernal burning pain
  b. Heartburn after eating, which increases in the recumbent position
  c. Nocturnal dyspnea
 2. Objective
  a. GI series and endoscopy show protrusion of stomach through diaphragm
  b. Regurgitation
C. Treatment
 1. Small, frequent, bland feedings
 2. Antacids
 3. Surgical repair (done infrequently)
D. Nursing care
 1. Teach patient and family about dietary regime
 2. Encourage attempts at weight loss
 3. Avoid constricting clothing
 4. Elevate head of bed after meals
 5. Encourage patient to eat slowly

Cancer of the esophagus

A. Etiology and pathophysiology
 1. Etiology unknown—occurs predominantly in persons with a history of alcohol abuse or hiatus hernia
 2. The tumor may develop anywhere in the esophagus, but most commonly in the middle and lower third
B. Signs and symptoms
 1. Subjective
  a. Dysphagia
  b. Substernal pain
  c. Substernal burning after drinking hot liquids
 2. Objective
  a. Regurgitation
  b. X-ray examination of esophagus reveals irregularities of the lumen
  c. Cytologic examination of cells obtained after esophageal lavage reveals malignant cells
C. Treatment
 1. Surgical removal of the esophagus is the treatment of choice
  a. Esophagogastrostomy—resection of a portion of the esophagus; a portion of the bowel may be grafted between esophagus and stomach, or

the stomach may be brought up to the proximal end of the esophagus
  b. Esophagectomy—removal of part or all of the esophagus, which is replaced by a Dacron graft
  c. Gastrostomy—opening directly into the stomach in which a feeding tube is usually inserted to bypass the esophagus
 2. Radiation and or chemotherapy may be used prior to or instead of surgery as a palliative measure
D. Nursing care
 1. Support patient and family emotionally
 2. Formulate realistic goals in planning patient care
 3. Observe for respiratory distress caused by pressure of tumor on the trachea; place in semi- or high Fowler's position to facilitate respirations
 4. Monitor vital signs, especially respirations
 5. Provide oral care, since dysphagia may result in increased accumulation of saliva in mouth
 6. Maintain nutritional status by providing high-protein liquids along with vitamin and mineral replacements

Cholecystitis

A. Etiology and pathophysiology
 1. An inflammation of the gallbladder that is usually caused by the presence of stones (cholelithiasis), which are composed of cholesterol, bile pigments, and calcium
 2. The diseased gallbladder is unable to contract in response to fatty foods entering the duodenum because of obstruction by calculi or edema
 3. When the common bile duct is completely obstructed, the bile is unable to pass into the duodenum and is absorbed into the blood
 4. Incidence is highest in obese women in the fourth decade
B. Signs and symptoms
 1. Subjective
  a. Indigestion after eating fatty or fried foods
  b. Pain, usually in the right upper quadrant of the abdomen, which may radiate to the back
  c. Nausea
 2. Objective
  a. Vomiting
  b. Elevated temperature and WBC
  c. Jaundice in approximately 25% of patients
  d. Diagnostic tests
   (1) Intravenous cholangiogram; patients who are allergic to the dye will complain of

sensation of warmth, urticaria, nausea, and vomiting
        (2) Serum bilirubin will be elevated
        (3) Gallbladder series; approximately 6 radiopaque tablets such as Telepaque or Bilopaque are taken with water the evening before so that the gallbladder will be visible on x-ray examination
C. Treatment
   1. Rest
   2. Low-fat diet to avoid stimulating gallbladder, which constricts to excrete bile with subsequent pain; calories principally from carbohydrate foods in acute phases; if weight loss is indicated, calories may be reduced to 1000 to 1200; postoperatively patients may be on fat-restricted diets initially but progress to regular diets
   3. Surgical intervention
      a. Cholecystotomy—incision into the gallbladder for the purpose of drainage
      b. Cholecystectomy—removal of the gallbladder
      c. Choledochotomy—incision into the common bile duct
D. Nursing care
   1. Teach dietary modification to limit fatty foods
   2. Relieve pain both preoperatively and postoperatively
   3. Observe for signs of bleeding (vitamin K is fat soluble and is not absorbed in the absence of bile); administer vitamin K preparations as ordered
   4. Postoperative care
      a. Patients will generally have a nasogastric tube to suction to prevent distention
         (1) Maintain patency
         (2) Assess and measure drainage
      b. Fluid and electrolytes are initially provided by IV route
         (1) Monitor intake and output
         (2) Check IV site for redness, swelling, heat, or pain
      c. Keep patient in low Fowler's position
      d. Cough and deep breathe; splint incision (incision is high and midline, making coughing extremely uncomfortable)
      e. Care of patients with a T tube to bile drainage (if the common bile duct has been explored a T-shaped tube is inserted to maintain patency)
         (1) Secure drainage bag; avoid kinking of tube

         (2) Measure drainage at least every shift; drainage during the first day may reach 500 to 1000 ml and then gradually decline
         (3) Apply protective ointments if ordered to prevent excoriation
         (4) When tube is removed, usually in 7 days, observe stool for normal brown color, which indicates bile is again entering the duodenum

Acute pancreatitis

A. Etiology and pathophysiology
   1. May result from gallstones, alcoholism, carcinoma, or acute trauma to the pancreas or abdomen
   2. Inflammation with or without edema of pancreatic tissues, suppuration, abscess formation, hemorrhage, or necrosis, depending on the severity of the disease and the cause
B. Signs and symptoms
   1. Subjective
      a. Abrupt onset of pain in the central epigastric area that may radiate to shoulder, chest, and back described as aching, burning, stabbing, or pressing
      b. Abdominal tenderness
      c. Nausea
   2. Objective
      a. Elevated temperature
      b. Vomiting
      c. Tachycardia
      d. Changes in character of stools
      e. Hypotension
      f. Shock
      g. Grossly elevated serum amylase and lipase
   3. Severity of symptoms depends on the cause of the problem; amount of fibrous replacement of normal duct tissue; degree of autodigestion of organ; type of associated biliary disease, if present; and the amount of interference in blood supply to the pancreas
   4. Symptoms may be exaggerated by the development of complications such as pseudocysts, abscesses, pancreatic fistulas, and hyperglycemia
C. Treatment
   1. Antacids to neutralize gastric secretions
   2. Barbiturates and tranquilizers to reduce emotional tension
   3. Narcotics to control pain

4. Cardiotonics to lessen strain on the heart caused by increased metabolic demands and altered circulatory volume
5. Bedrest to decrease metabolic demands and promote healing
6. Nasogastric decompression to control nausea and remove gastric hydrochloric acid
7. Diet regulated according to patient's condition: nothing by mouth; parenteral administration of fluid, electrolytes, and other nutrients; diet low in fats and proteins with restriction of stimulants such as caffeine and alcohol
8. Anticholinergics to supress vagal stimulation and decrease gastric motility and duodenal spasm
9. Antibiotics to prevent secondary infections and abscess formation
10. Surgical intervention if patient fails to respond to medical management, develops persistent jaundice, or bleeds; type of surgery is determined by the cause; e.g., biliary tract surgery, removal of gallstones, drainage of cysts

D. Nursing care
   1. If patient has a nasogastric tube
      a. Administer frequent, thorough mouth care
      b. Apply lubricant to external nares to prevent irritation and eventual breakdown of mucous membranes
      c. Observe for electrolyte imbalances manifested by symptoms such as tetany, irritability, jerking, muscular twitching, mental changes, and psychotic behavior
      d. Observe for signs of adynamic ileus; e.g., nausea and vomiting, abdominal distention
   2. Be alert for hyperglycemic states
   3. Monitor vital signs
   4. Teach importance of taking medications containing amylase, lipase, and trypsin in controlling pancreatic insufficiency
   5. Encourage adoption of a life-style that allows for emotional stability, rest, follow-up medical care
   6. Use semi-Fowler's position and encourage deep breathing and coughing to promote deeper respiration and prevent respiratory problems
   7. Maintain NPO during the acute stage of illness
   8. Closely monitor IV feedings until oral feedings can be tolerated
   9. Assist patient in ingestion of small feedings of low-fat, gaseous-free fluids, progressing to diet as tolerated and prescribed
   10. Teach patient and family the importance of dietary discretion, especially the avoidance of alcohol, coffee, spicy foods, and heavy meals, while recognizing religious and cultural factors
   11. Help patient set realistic goals for convalescent period
   12. Teach patient and family about prevention of recurrences and/or control of symptoms; e.g., diet therapy, drug therapy, avoiding foods and substances such as alcohol and caffeine, regular medical supervision, rest requirements

Cancer of the pancreas

A. Etiology and pathophysiology
   1. Malignant growth from the epithelium of the ductal system producing cells that block the ducts of the pancreas
   2. There is fibrosis, pancreatitis, and obstruction of the pancreas
   3. Lesion tends to metastasize by direct extension to duodenal wall, splenic flexure of colon, posterior stomach wall, and common bile duct
   4. Cause is unknown
B. Signs and symptoms
   1. Subjective
      a. More common in middle-age men than women
      b. History of chronic pancreatitis, diabetes mellitus, and alcoholism is common
      c. Weight loss, anxiety, depression, anorexia, and nausea
      d. Severe pain present in most patients
   2. Objective
      a. Jaundice
      b. Diarrhea and steatorrhea, clay-colored stools, and dark urine
      c. Physical examination usually demonstrates presence of right upper quadrant mass
      d. Decreased serum amylase and lipase levels due to decreased secretion of enzymes
      e. Increased serum bilirubin and alkaline phosphatase levels when biliary ducts are obstructed
C. Treatment
   1. Prepare for surgical intervention by ordering red blood cell and blood volume replacement and medications to correct coagulation problems and nutritional deficiencies

2. Chemotherapy and radiation when surgery is not possible to provide comfort, or in conjunction with surgery to limit metastasis
3. Medications to control diabetes if present
4. Drug therapy such as pancreatic enzymes, bile salts, and vitamin K to correct deficiencies
5. Analgesics and tranquilizers for pain
6. Intervene surgically (treatment of choice, although postsurgical prognosis is grim), Whipple's procedure (removal of head of the pancreas, duodenum, portion of stomach and the common bile duct), or a cholecystojejunostomy may be performed

D. Nursing care
1. Provide emotional support for patient and family and set realistic goals in planning care
2. Administer analgesics as ordered as soon as needed to promote rest and comfort
3. Use soapless bathing and antipruritic agents to relieve pruritus
4. Observe patient for complications such as peritonitis, gastrointestinal obstruction, jaundice, hyperglycemia, and hypotension if patient has had surgery
5. Observe stools for undigested fat
6. Frequently monitor vital signs observing for wound hemorrhage caused by coagulation deficiency
7. Administer vitamin K parenterally as ordered
8. Encourage coughing, turning, and deep breathing
9. Assist with IPPB therapy as required
10. Monitor urinary output
11. Observe for chemotherapeutic and radiation side effects; e.g., skin irritation, anorexia, nausea, and vomiting
12. Maintain skin markings of radiation therapist
13. Encourage frequent and supplemental feedings as tolerated
14. Control nausea and vomiting before feedings, if possible
15. Administer vitamin supplements, bile salts, and pancreatic enzymes, as ordered
16. Provide oral hygiene and maintain an esthetic environment especially at mealtime

Hepatitis

A. Etiology and pathophysiology
1. Type A hepatitis (infectious hepatitis)
   a. Caused by Type A hepatitis virus
   b. Transmitted via fecal-oral route, contact with blood or contaminated food (i.e.; shellfish)
   c. Incubation period 30 to 40 days
   d. Immune serum antigen (ISG) given after exposure is helpful in preventing disease
   e. Confers immunity on individual
2. Type B hepatitis (serum hepatitis)
   a. Caused by Type B hepatitis virus
   b. Transmitted by contact with contaminated blood or blood products (e.g., toothbrush, razors, needles)
   c. Incubation period 40 to 180 days
3. Phases of disease
   a. Prodromal or preicteric phase
   b. Icteric phase
   c. Recovery (may take 4 months)
4. Progression to cirrhosis, hepatic coma, and death may occur, although this is rare
5. Other causes of hepatitis include chemical agents such as halothane (an anesthetic agent), carbon tetrachloride, gold compounds, and arsenic

B. Signs and symptoms
1. Prodromal (preicteric) phase
   a. Malaise
   b. Weight loss
   c. Anorexia
   d. Symptoms of upper respiratory tract infection
   e. Intolerance for smoking
2. Icteric phase
   a. Jaundice
   b. Bile-colored urine that foams when shaken
   c. Acholic (clay-colored) stools
3. Recovery phase—easy fatiguability

C. Treatment
1. Rest
2. Diet therapy
   a. High protein—healing of liver tissue vital; daily intake should include 1 qt milk, 2 eggs, 8 oz lean meat, fish, or cheese; total should approximate 75 to 100 g protein
   b. High carbohydrate—energy needs, restore glycogen reserves; use daily 4 servings vegetables including potato, 4 servings fruit with frequent juices, 6 to 8 servings bread or cereal; total carbohydrate should be 300 to 400 g
   c. Moderate fat—2 to 4 tablespoons butter or fortified margarine, sufficient for making food palatable; a moderate amount of easily usable foods such as whole milk, cream, butter, mar-

garine, or vegetable oil is beneficial; total fat should be 100 to 150 g daily

d. High calorie—increased energy needs for disease process and tissue regeneration and to spare protein for healing; these food amounts should provide about 2500 to 3000 calories daily

D. Nursing care
1. Encourage quiet activities
2. Attempt to stimulate appetite
   a. Oral hygiene
   b. Selection of foods based on patient's preferences
   c. Provide pleasant, unhurried atmosphere for eating
3. Use special precautions to prevent spread of infectious hepatitis to others
   a. Special handling of needles
   b. Food and utensils should be isolated and sterilized; visitors should be taught how to handle this or to use disposable utensils
   c. Gloves should be worn when handling patient's bedpan

Hepatic cirrhosis

A. Etiology and pathophysiology
1. Refers to irreversible fibrosis and degeneration of the liver
2. There are several types of cirrhosis; Laënnec's cirrhosis (alcoholic cirrhosis, nutritional cirrhosis) is most common
3. Incidence is higher in alcoholics, who are often malnourished, and in those who have had hepatitis
4. Pressure rises in the portal system, which drains blood from the digestive organs
5. As liver failure progresses, there is increased secretion of aldosterone, decreased absorption and utilization of the fat-soluble vitamins (A, D, E, K), and ineffective detoxification of protein wastes
6. Hepatic coma may result from high blood ammonia levels when the liver is unable to convert the ammonia to urea

B. Signs and symptoms
1. Subjective
   a. Nausea
   b. Weakness, fatigue
   c. Anorexia
   d. Abdominal discomfort

2. Objective
   a. Weight loss
   b. Ascites
   c. Esophageal varices as a result of portal hypertension
   d. Hemorrhoids
   e. Edema of extremities
   f. Hematemesis
   g. Hemorrhage due to decreased formation of prothrombin
   h. Jaundice
   i. Delirium caused by rising blood ammonia levels
   j. Elevated liver enzymes (SGOT, SGPT, LDH)
   k. Decreased serum albumin

C. Treatment
1. Rest
2. Restriction of alcohol intake
3. Vitamin therapy; especially A, D, E, and K
4. Diuretics to control ascites and edema
5. Neomycin and lactulose may be prescribed for elevated blood ammonia levels
6. If respiratory distress occurs as a result of ascites, a paracentesis is done; slow removal of fluid from the peritoneal cavity will relieve acute symptoms
7. Surgical intervention for portal hypertension—a portal caval shunt in which the circulation from the portal vein bypasses the liver and enters the vena cava; usually decreases portal hypertension
8. Blakemore-Sengstaken tube is utilized in the treatment of bleeding esophageal varices to apply direct pressure to the varices
9. Dietary modification
   a. Cirrhosis
      (1) Protein according to tolerance—with increasing liver damage protein metabolism is hindered; hold to 80 to 100 g as long as tolerated; reduce as necessary
      (2) Continue high carbohydrate, moderate fat as in hepatitis to supply energy; vitamin supplements, especially B complex
      (3) Low sodium—usually restricted to 500 to 1000 mg daily by eliminating salt and controlling foods processed with salt or sodium-based preservatives; sodium restriction helps to control the increasing ascites
      (4) Soft foods—if esophageal varices are present, to prevent danger of rupture and bleeding

(5) Alcohol strictly forbidden to avoid continued irritation and malnutrition
  b. Hepatic coma
     (1) Low protein–reduced according to tolerance, 15 to 30 g
     (2) High calories and vitamins according to need—about 1500 to 2000 calories sufficient to prevent tissue catabolism and the liberation of additional nitrogen
     (3) Fluid carefully controlled according to output
D. Nursing care
   1. Observe patient for objective signs of disease
   2. Observe mental status, which may vary
   3. Observe for bleeding
   4. Provide special skin care and keep nails trimmed, since pruritus is associated with jaundice
   5. Maintain patient in a semi-Fowler's position to prevent ascites from causing dyspnea
   6. Monitor intake and output, abdominal girth, and daily weight to assess fluid and electrolyte balance
   7. Assist with paracentesis (see procedures)
   8. When a Blakemore-Sengstaken tube is in place
      a. Maintain traction once the tube is passed and the gastric balloon is inflated to ensure proper placement
      b. Maintain the esophageal balloon as it has been inflated to 30 to 35 mm Hg
      c. If ordered, deflate the balloon for a few minutes at specific intervals to prevent necrosis
      d. Irrigate with iced saline if ordered
      e. Suction orally as necessary, since the patient is unable to swallow saliva

Carcinoma of the liver

A. Etiology and pathophysiology
   1. May be primary or metastatic carcinoma; primary carcinoma of the liver is rare
   2. Generally lethal within a few months
B. Signs and symptoms
   1. Subjective
      a. Anorexia
      b. Ache in epigastric area
   2. Objective
      a. Weight loss
      b. Anemia
C. Treatment
   1. Generally palliative

2. Hepatic lobectomy if the tumor is confined (the liver has extraordinary regenerative capacity)
   3. Percutaneous infusions with cytotoxic agents
D. Nursing care
   1. Provide comfort
   2. Be available to both patient and family members to discuss their feelings
   3. Postoperatively
      a. Maintain fluid and electrolyte balance with IV therapy
      b. Monitor intake and output
      c. Observe for signs of bleeding, hypoglycemia, and other metabolic dysfunctions resulting from impaired liver function
      d. Cough and deep breathe; change position frequently to prevent pulmonary and circulatory complications
      e. Because the thoracic cavity may be entered during surgery, the nurse should also be aware of care of a patient with chest tubes (see Pneumothorax)

Regional enteritis

A. Etiology and pathophysiology
   1. Etiology is unknown
   2. Usually occurs in young adults but can occur at any age
   3. Inflammatory changes involving any part of the alimentary tract but usually involving demarcated segments of the small bowel
   4. Ulceration of the intestinal submucosa accompanied by congestion, thickening of the small bowel, and fissure formations
   5. Enlargement of regional lymph nodes
   6. Fibrosis and narrowing of intestinal wall
   7. Abscesses and fistulas to abdominal wall, bladder, and vagina
B. Signs and symptoms
   1. Subjective
      a. Pain in lower right quadrant, cramping, and spasms
      b. Nausea
      c. Exacerbations related to emotional upsets or dietary indiscretions with milk, milk products, and fried foods
   2. Objective
      a. Borborygmus, flatulence
      b. Weight loss
      c. Fever

d. Electrolyte disturbances

e. Diarrhea

f. Gastrointestinal x-ray series to detect and outline congested, thickened, fibrosed, and narrowed appearance of the intestinal wall; abscesses and fistulas; partial bowel obstruction; ulceration of mucosa

g. Proctosigmoidoscopy is performed to exclude other disease, such as ulcerative colitis and diverticulitis

h. Stools are examined to determine presence of blood, fat, protein, parasites, or ova

i. Fecal fat test is performed to determine fat content, an abnormal amount of which is significant in malabsorptive disorders or hypermotility

j. D-Xylose tolerance test is performed to determine absorptive ability of upper intestinal tract

C. Treatment

1. Nothing by mouth in presence of vomiting

2. Clear fluid diet progressing to bland low-residue, low-fat diet but increased in calories, proteins, vitamins (especially vitamin K), and carbohydrates

3. Hyperalimentation may be ordered when oral intake is inadequate

4. Medications such as

a. Antiemetics

b. Vitamins and minerals

c. Anticholinergics

d. Antidiarrheics

e. Anti-inflammatories

f. Anti-infectives

5. Intervene surgically (resection of diseased part) if patient does not respond to medical therapy or if complications such as obstruction, abscesses, or fistulas occur

D. Nursing care

1. Monitor intake and output

2. Offer clear liquids hourly as ordered once patient ceases to experience nausea and vomiting

3. Encourage high-caloric, high-protein, high-carbohydrate diet supplemented with vitamins and potassium as ordered

4. Assist with hyperalimentation therapy if ordered (see procedure)

5. Offer small, frequent feedings considering patient preference, types of foods allowed, and esthetic factors

6. Record weight daily

7. Observe for signs of complications such as elevated temperature, increasing nausea and vomiting, abdominal rigidity

8. Communicate concern and awareness regarding patient's discomfort and emotional lability during exacerbations of this chronic illness

9. Teach patient

a. To avoid taking laxatives and salicylates that irritate intestinal mucosa

b. How to effectively take antidiarrheics and mucilloid drugs and the observations to make during their use

c. Skin care if perineal area is irritated

d. The importance of seeking help early when exacerbations occur

Crohn's disease

A. Etiology and pathophysiology

1. Although the causative mechanisms are unknown, there are various theories involving genetic predisposition, autoimmune reaction, or environmental causes

2. Cobblestone ulcerations form along the mucosal wall of the terminal ileum, cecum, and ascending colon, which form scar tissue and inhibit food absorption in the area

3. The ulcerations may perforate through the intestinal wall and form fistulas with adjoining organs

B. Signs and symptoms

1. Subjective

a. Severe pain in right lower quadrant

b. Malaise

2. Objective

a. Moderate fever

b. Elevated WBC

c. Mild diarrhea with mucus but *no blood*

d. Anemia

C. Treatment

1. High-calorie, high-protein diet

2. Vitamin supplements, including B_{12}, if large portion of ileum is involved

3. Medications such as

a. Anticholinergics

b. Analgesics

c. Intestinal antibiotics

d. Immunosuppressives

4. Surgery is performed when fistulas or intestinal obstruction occurs; the involved area of intestine is removed and the ends are anastomosed, if pos-

sible; an ostomy is indicated if large areas of intestine are involved
D. Nursing care
1. Provide an emotionally therapeutic environment in which patient can communicate concerns and stresses resulting from this illness
2. Plan diet with patient and family, using sample menus to promote compliance
3. Observe patient for signs of fluid and electrolyte imbalances

Ulcerative colitis

A. Etiology and pathophysiology
1. May be caused by emotional stress, an autoimmune response, or a genetic predisposition
2. There is edema of the mucous membrane of the colon, which leads to bleeding and shallow ulcerations
3. Abscess formation occurs, and the bowel wall shortens and becomes thin and fragile
4. Due to the shortening of the intestinal wall, there is increased flow of contents, which leads to diarrhea
B. Signs and symptoms
1. Subjective
a. Weakness, debilitation
b. Anorexia
c. Nausea
2. Objective
a. Dehydration with poor skin turgor
b. Passage of bloody, purulent, mucoid, watery stools
c. Anemia
d. Low-grade fever
C. Treatment
1. Diet, if tolerated, includes unrestricted fluid intake; high-protein, high-calorie diet; avoidance of food allergens, especially milk
2. Medications such as
a. Antiemetics
b. Anticholinergics
c. Corticosteroids
d. Antibiotics
e. Sedatives, analgesics, and tranquilizers
f. Antidiarrheics
3. Replacement of fluids and electrolytes that are lost because of diarrhea
4. A temporary ileostomy, a partial colectomy, or a total colectomy with a permanent ileostomy may be performed when no response is evident to

medical treatment; when course of disease is downhill; when massive hemorrhage or colonic obstruction occurs; or when cancer is suspected
D. Nursing care
1. Serve small frequent feedings of a high-protein, high-calorie, low-residue, bland nature
2. Teach patient about importance of diet in controlling and/or minimizing symptoms
3. Involve patient in dietary selection, recognizing preferences as much as possible
4. Initiate accurate administration and recording of fluid, electrolyte, or blood replacements as ordered by the physician
5. Plan nursing care to allow for complete bed rest and maximum number of rest periods
6. Institute comfort measures such as use of warm, powdered bedpan; sheepskin under buttocks; and gentle, thorough perineal care as required
7. Observe for complications such as rectal hemorrhage, fever, dehydration
8. Allow patient and family time to verbalize feelings and participate in care
9. If an ileostomy is performed, help patient accept the changes of body image and function involved (see Ostomy care)

Intestinal obstruction

A. Etiology and pathophysiology
1. Interference with normal peristaltic movement of intestinal contents due to neurologic or mechanical impairments
2. Causes
a. Carcinoma of the bowel
b. Hernias
c. Adhesions (scar tissue that forms abnormal connections after surgery or inflammation)
d. Intussusception (telescoping of the bowel on itself)
e. Volvulus (twisting of the intestines)
f. Paralytic ileus (an interference with neural innervation of the intestines resulting in a decrease in or absence of peristalsis; may be caused by surgical manipulation, electrolyte imbalance, or infection)
B. Signs and symptoms
1. Subjective
a. Colicky abdominal pain
b. Constipation
2. Objective
a. Abdominal distention

  b. Vomiting; may contain fecal matter
  c. Decreased or absent bowel sounds
  d. Signs of dehydration and electrolyte imbalance
  e. Flat plate of abdomen shows bowel distended with air
C. Treatment
  1. Restriction of oral intake; administration of parenteral fluid and electrolytes
  2. Surgical correction of cause (i.e., hernias, adhesions)
  3. A colostomy, cecostomy, or ileostomy may be necessary
  4. Drugs such as pantothenyl alcohol (Ilopan) and neostigmine (Prostigmin) may be given to stimulate the passage of flatus
  5. Gastric decompression by means of nasogastric, Cantor, or Miller-Abbott tube
D. Nursing care
  1. Assess patient for dehydration and electrolyte imbalance
  2. Monitor intake and output
  3. Auscultate for bowel sounds; note passage of flatus
  4. Administer mouth care frequently
  5. Measure abdominal girth daily to assess distention
  6. Provide special care for patients with Miller-Abbott or Cantor tube
    a. Once lubricated tube is passed, position patient first on the right side, to facilitate passage of tube through pylorus, and then in semi-Fowler's position to continue the gradual advance into the intestines
    b. Coil and loosely attach extra tubing to the patient's gown to avoid tension against peristaltic action
    c. Irrigate as ordered to maintain patency
    d. Frequently assess placement of the tube; record level of advancement
    e. Remove tube gradually because it is being pulled against peristalsis

Cancer of the small and large intestines

A. Etiology and pathophysiology
  1. Carcinoma of the colon and rectum can cause a narrowing of the lumen of the bowel, ulcerations, necrosis, or perforation
  2. Predisposing factors include familial polyps,

chronic ulcerative colitis, and possibly bowel stasis or ingestion of food additives
  3. Cancer of the colon is more common in males, and incidence increases after 50 years of age
  4. Malignant tumors of the small intestine are usually adenocarcinomas
B. Signs and symptoms
  1. Subjective
    a. Abdominal discomfort
    b. Weakness
  2. Objective
    a. Alterations in usual bowel function (constipation or diarrhea or alternating constipation and diarrhea)
    b. Blood in stool
    c. Distention
    d. Changes in shape of stool (pencil shaped, ribbon)
    e. Weight loss
    f. Secondary anemia
C. Diagnosis and treatment
  1. Diagnostic measures
    a. Digital examination of rectum to detect any palpable masses
    b. Proctosigmoidoscopy to directly visualize bowel to determine presence of abnormalities and to perform a biopsy
    c. Stool examination to test for occult blood
    d. Cytologic examination to detect for malignant cells
    e. Hemoglobin level to detect anemia
    f. Alkaline phosphatase and SGOT levels to detect metastasis to liver
    g. Serum carcinoembryonic antigen (C.E.A.) measure to screen for carcinoma of colon
  2. After diagnosis is established, the physician may prepare the patient for surgery by
    a. Prescribing antibiotics to reduce bacteria in bowel
    b. Ordering type and cross match and blood transfusions to correct anemia
    c. Ordering vitamin supplements to improve nutritional status
    d. Inserting a Cantor or Miller-Abbott tube with suction to decompress the colon
  3. Surgical intervention to remove mass and restore bowel function; e.g., hemicolectomy, resection of transverse colon, or abdominal perineal resection

4. Radiation in nonsurgical situations in an attempt to relieve symptoms or postoperatively to limit metastases
5. Chemotherapy orally or parenterally in an attempt to reduce the lesion and limit metastases
6. Postoperatively
   a. Antibiotic therapy to reduce infection
   b. Parenteral fluids and electrolytes to maintain levels
   c. Cholinergics to stimulate peristalsis
   d. Cantor or Miller-Abbott tube clamped for regular, increasing periods and removed when patient is able to tolerate clamping and bowel sounds have returned
   e. Sips of water progressing to clear liquid diet and to low-residue diet as tolerated
7. If colostomy has been performed
   a. Colostomy irrigations as required
   b. Irrigations of perineal incision if present and the application of enzymes such as streptokinase to liquefy protein matter and promote drainage
D. Nursing care
   1. Observe vital signs, increasing abdominal pain, nausea and vomiting to detect early signs of complications
   2. Monitor patency of Cantor or Miller-Abbott tube to ensure that accumulated air and fluid are decreased and distention is minimized; instill or irrigate tube with normal saline as ordered
   3. Note character of drainage from decompression tube
   4. Implement measures for mechanical cleansing and intestinal antisepsis preoperatively; e.g., enemas, colonic irrigations, antibacterial therapy such as neomycin or sulfonamides
   5. Administer chemotherapeutic drugs if ordered and observe for significant side effects such as stomatitis (ulceration of mouth), dehydration, nausea and vomiting, diarrhea, leukopenia
   6. Administer electrolyte and parenteral fluid replacement as ordered in situations of bleeding, vomiting, and/or obstruction
   7. Carefully note patient's tolerance to introduction of oral fluids and foods while intestinal tube is clamped
   8. Teach patient and family dietary modifications, including low-residue, nongas-forming foods, avoidance of stimulants, adequate fluid intake; diet should be as close to patient's normal diet as possible
   9. Provide colostomy care using medically aseptic technique (see procedures)
   10. Recognize that the patient with a colostomy may experience sadness, withdrawal, depression, and suicidal thoughts as a result of body image changes
   11. Assess patient's reaction to the colostomy, recognizing that a great deal will depend on how patient sees it affecting life-style, patient's physical and emotional status, patient's social and cultural background, and patient's place and role in the family
   12. Encourage patient's involvement in colostomy care as soon as physical and emotional status permit
   13. Encourage visiting by family members, stressing patient's increased need for love and acceptance
   14. Recognize that the patient with a cecostomy or colostomy is especially sensitive to gestures, odors, facial expressions, and amount of attention given
   15. Teach patient and family care of colostomy, measures to facilitate acceptance and adjustment, resumption of activities, and the need for regular medical supervision
   16. Teach patient that colostomy drainage can be controlled by following a regular irrigation schedule and dietary modifications
   17. Arrange for follow-up care with community agencies as required; e.g., Public Health, Home Care Program, Cancer Society, ostomy resource person

Peritonitis
A. Etiology and pathophysiology
   1. An inflammation of the peritoneal cavity
   2. Generally caused by infection from perforation of GI tract or by chemical stress, as in pancreatitis
B. Signs and symptoms
   1. Subjective
      a. Abdominal pain, rebound tenderness
      b. Malaise
      c. Nausea
   2. Objective
      a. Muscle rigidity over area
      b. Elevated temperature and WBC
      c. Vomiting

C. Treatment
  1. Bed rest in semi-Fowler's position to drain area
  2. Nasogastric tube attached to suction and left in place until patient passes flatus
  3. Fluids and electrolytes replaced parenterally
  4. Antibiotic therapy
  5. Surgical intervention to correct cause of peritonitis (i.e., appendectomy, incision and drainage of abscesses, or closure of perforation)
D. Nursing care
  1. Maintain semi-Fowler's position to help localize infection in pelvic area
  2. Assess temperature, vital signs, and pain
  3. Monitor IV therapy and gastrointestinal decompression
  4. Monitor intake and output
  5. Auscultate for bowel sounds; note passage of flatus

Hemorrhoids

A. Etiology and pathophysiology
  1. Varicosities of the rectum that can be internal or external
  2. Constipation, prolonged sitting or standing, straining at defecation, and pregnancy increase the risk of developing hemorrhoids
B. Signs and symptoms
  1. Subjective
    a. Anal pain
    b. Pruritus
  2. Objective
    a. Protrusion of hemorrhoids
    b. Rectal bleeding and mucous discharge
C. Treatment
  1. Low-roughage diet (elimination of raw fruits and vegetables)
  2. Use of laxatives and stool softeners to regulate bowel habits
  3. Analgesic suppositories and ointments may be prescribed in addition to sitz baths to alleviate discomfort
  4. Internal hemorrhoids may be ligated with rubber bands; as necrosis occurs the tissue sloughs off
  5. Hemorrhoidectomy—surgical removal of hemorrhoids
D. Nursing care
  1. Administer medication as ordered to relieve discomfort
  2. Provide privacy and sufficient time for defecation
  3. Educate patient about the use of roughage, fluids, laxatives, an stool softeners
  4. Assist the patient with sitz baths
  5. Administer cleansing enemas and prepare the perineal area preoperatively
  6. Observe for rectal hemorrhage and urinary retention postoperatively
  7. Administer retention enema on the second or third postoperative day if ordered to stimulate defecation and soften stool
  8. Explain to patient that postoperatively a small amount of bleeding with a bowel movement is normal

Hernias

A. Etiology and pathophysiology
  1. A protrusion of an organ or structure through a weakening in the abdominal wall; the protrusion may contain fat, intestine, or an organ, such as the bladder
  2. The abdominal wall can become weakened due to a congenital or acquired defect
  3. If the protruding structure can be manipulated back in place, the hernia is said to be reducible; if it is not able to be replaced, it is considered incarcerated
  4. Strangulation occurs when blood supply to the tissues within the hernia is disrupted; this is an emergency situation, since gangrene occurs
  5. Hernias are named according to location
    a. Incisional—occurs due to failure of fascia or muscles to heal postoperatively; intra-abdominal pressure causes herniation through the scar tissue
    b. Umbilical—occurs due to failure of the umbilicus to close at birth or to a congenital weakness of the musculature in the area; increased intra-abdominal pressure due to obesity, pregnancy, or chronic cough causes herniation through the umbilicus
    c. Femoral—occurs when a loop of intestine herniates through the femoral canal due to a weakness in the femoral ring; more common in women than men; strangulation is a common complication
    d. Inguinal—occurs when a loop of intestine herniates through a weakened abdominal ring through the spermatic cord into the inguinal canal; more common in men than women

B. Signs and symptoms
   1. Subjective
      a. History of appearance of swelling after lifting, coughing, or vigorous exercise
      b. Pain may occur due to irritation or strangulation
      c. Nausea can accompany strangulation
   2. Objective
      a. A swelling or lump in the groin, umbilicus, or near an old surgical incision that may subside when patient is in recumbent position
      b. Vomiting and abdominal distention may develop when strangulation occurs
C. Treatment
   1. Manual reduction by gently pushing mass back into abdominal cavity
   2. When patient is a poor surgical risk, use of a truss (pad worn next to skin held in place under pressure by a belt)
   3. A herniorrhaphy may be performed (surgical repair of the defect in the abdominal musculature or fascia)
   4. A hernioplasty may be indicated to prevent recurrence (wire, mesh, or plastic may be inserted to strengthen abdominal wall)
D. Nursing care
   1. Teach patient using a truss that it should be applied prior to getting out of bed
   2. After surgery
      a. Observe patient for signs of respiratory infection; administer cough suppressants as ordered to prevent stress on incision
      b. Instruct patient to self splint when coughing and turning to provide incisional support
      c. When spinal anesthesia is used, peristalsis is not interfered with and postoperative diet can be normal; when general anesthesia is used, nasogastric decompression may be employed until peristalsis returns
      d. Administer mild cathartics as ordered to prevent straining and increased intra-abdominal pressure at defecation
      e. Apply ice bag and scrotal support with a rolled towel or suspensory if scrotum is edematous postoperatively to reduce edema and pain
      f. Administer medication for pain as ordered when necessary
      g. Instruct patient to avoid lifting or strenuous exercise on discharge until permitted by surgeon

Food poisoning

A. *Staphylococcus aureus*
   1. Etiology and pathophysiology
      a. Gram-positive *Staphylococcus* strain that clots plasma (coagulase positive); is the most virulent type and causes a variety of infections
      b. Most food poisoning resulting in GI upset occurs as a result of this bacterium
      c. Organism is found in unrefrigerated creams, mayonnaise, stuffing, meats, and fish
      d. Bacteria usually are transmitted to food on the hands of food handlers
      e. Incubation period is 1 to 6 hours after ingestion of contaminated food, with symptoms lasting 24 to 48 hours
   2. Signs and symptoms
      a. Subjective
         (1) Nausea
         (2) Malaise
         (3) Abdominal cramps and pain
      b. Objective
         (1) Diarrhea
         (2) Subnormal temperature
         (3) Vomiting
   3. Treatment
      a. Supply with adequate fluid and electrolytes orally or parenterally
      b. Bed rest
   4. Nursing care
      a. Offer fluids in small amounts as tolerated
      b. Teach patient the importance of eating foods that are properly prepared and stored
B. Botulism
   1. Etiology and pathophysiology
      a. *Clostridium botulinum*—large, gram-positive bacillus; an obligate anaerobe; its exotoxin, the most powerful biologic toxic known, is responsible for botulism
      b. This organism causes the most serious, often fatal, form of food poisoning
      c. Organism is found in improperly processed foods (mostly canned foods) that had been infected with the anaerobic bacillus *Clostridium botulinum*
      d. Toxins block neuromuscular transmission in cholinergic nerve fibers by possibly binding with acetylcholine
      e. Incubation period is usually 12 to 72 hours after ingestion of contaminated food but may be as long as 4 to 8 days

2. Signs and symptoms
   a. Subjective
      (1) Lassitude and fatigue
      (2) Diplopia
      (3) Weakness of muscles in extremities
      (4) Dysphasia
   b. Objective
      (1) Diminished visual acuity
      (2) Loss of pupillary light reflex
      (3) Diminished gag reflex
3. Treatment
   a. Keep patient in darkened room
   b. IV feedings to prevent aspiration
   c. Tracheostomy and other supportive measures as necessary
   d. Cathartics and cleansing enemas to remove toxins from the body
   e. Trivalent antitoxins as necessary
4. Nursing care
   a. Prevent aspiration pneumonia by proper positioning; keep suction equipment available at bedside
   b. Carefully observe neurologic status to determine progression of disease
   c. Prevent contractures and emboli formation by the use of ROM exercises
   d. Provide emotional support to patient and family in an attempt to reduce anxiety
C. Salmonellosis
   1. Etiology and pathophysiology
      a. A great many species of *Salmonella* cause a local GI infection in which organisms do not enter blood (unlike *S. typhosa* and *S. paratyphi*); such infections are referred to as salmonellosis or salmonella food poisoning
      b. Organism is found in inadequately cooked meats
      c. Organisms multiply in the intestines causing GI upset and infection
      d. Incubation period is usually 10 to 24 hours after ingestion of contaminated food, and symptoms usually last 2 to 3 days
   2. Signs and symptoms
      a. Subjective
         (1) Nausea
         (2) Malaise
         (3) Abdominal cramps and pain
      b. Objective
         (1) Chills and fever
         (2) Vomiting

3. Treatment
   a. Bed rest
   b. Fluid and electrolyte replacement
4. Nursing care
   a. Offer patient small amounts of fluids as tolerated
   b. Teach patient importance of eating foods that have been cooked properly

Genitourinary system

REVIEW OF ANATOMY AND PHYSIOLOGY OF THE GENITOURINARY SYSTEM
Urinary system

Functions
A. Secrete urine
B. Eliminate urine from body (urination, micturition, or voiding) to
   1. Excrete various normal and abnormal metabolic wastes
   2. Regulate composition and volume of blood and regulate blood pressure; especially important in maintenance of fluid and electrolyte balance and acid-base balance (see urinary mechanisms in Fluid, electrolyte, and acid-base balance section)

Organs
Kidneys
A. Gross anatomy
   1. Size, shape, and location—about $4 \times 2 \times 1$ inch ($10 \times 5 \times 2.5$ cm); shaped like lima beans; lie against posterior abdominal wall, behind peritoneum at level of last thoracic and first 3 lumbar vertebrae; right kidney slightly lower than left
   2. External structure
      a. Hilum—concave notch on mesial surface; blood vessels, nerves, lymphatics, and ureter enter kidney through this notch
      b. Renal capsule—protective capsule of fibrous tissue that envelops kidney
   3. Internal structure
      a. Cortex—outer layer of kidney substance; composed of renal corpuscles, convoluted tubules, and adjacent parts of loops of Henle
      b. Medulla—inner portion of kidney; composed of loops of Henle and collecting tubules
      c. Pyramids—triangular wedges of medullary substance that have striped appearance and are composed of collecting tubules

d. Columns—inward extensions of cortex between pyramids

e. Papillae—apices of pyramids; collecting tubules drain into minor calyces here

f. Calyces—bell-mouthed cups that drain papillae; 8 to 12 minor calyces open into 2 or 3 major calyces that form the pelvis

g. Pelvis—a small funnel tapering into ureter and formed by union of several calyces

B. Blood flow in kidney

1. Kidneys receive 20% of cardiac output during rest; reduced to 2% to 4% during physical or emotional stress

2. Abdominal aorta gives rise to renal artery, which enters the hilum of each kidney; renal artery branches into interlobar arteries, which fan out into kidney cortex; smaller arterial branches form afferent arterioles, which enter glomerular capillary beds

3. Efferent arterioles leave glomerular capillary bed, forming peritubular capillary network, which then converges into progressively larger veins until the renal vein leaves the kidney

C. The nephron—anatomic and functional unit of kidney; approximately one million per kidney

1. Anatomy

a. Glomerulus—cluster of capillaries invaginated in Bowman's capsule

b. Bowman's capsule—funnel-shaped upper end of urinary tubules

c. Renal corpuscle—composed of Bowman's capsule and the glomerulus invaginated in it

d. Proximal convoluted tubule—first portion of kidney tubules

e. Henle's loop—second portion of kidney tubules

f. Distal convoluted tubule—third portion of kidney tubules

2. Physiology—nephron functions via principles of filtration, reabsorption, and secretion (Fig. 6)

a. Glomerulus—urine formation starts with process of filtration; water and solutes (except cellular elements of blood, albumins, fibrinogen, and other blood proteins) filter out of capillaries through glomerular-capsular membrane and into Bowman's capsule

b. Bowman's capsule—filtrate collects here prior to flow to tubules

c. Tubular reabsorption and secretion—epithelial lining of tubules reabsorbs substances useful to body and excretes, dissolved in water, all excess and waste substances; secretes electrolytes essential to acid-base balance

(1) Proximal tubule

(a) Reabsorption of glucose and other nutrients (e.g., vitamins and amino acids) from tubular filtrate to blood in peritubular capillaries; mainly by active transport mechanisms in tubular epithelium

(b) Reabsorption of electrolytes from tubule filtrate to blood in peritubular capillaries; cations (notably sodium) are reabsorbed by active transport, stimulated by aldosterone; anions (notably chlorides and bicarbonate) are reabsorbed by diffusion following cation transport

(c) Reabsorption of about 80% of water from tubular filtrate to blood in peritubular capillaries by osmosis as result of electrolyte reabsorption

(2) Loop of Henle

(a) Establishes osmotic conditions that promote water reabsorption

(b) Actively transports chloride ions from filtrate thus passively removing sodium ions with the chloride; sodium chloride excretion results in increased osmotic force and promotes reabsorption of water in collecting tubules

(3) Distal tubule

(a) Reabsorption of electrolytes, particularly sodium, under influence of the mineralocorticoid aldosterone

(b) Reabsorption of water into blood by osmosis; ADH controls amount of water osmosing out of distal tubule, whereas amount of electrolytes reabsorbed controls amount of osmosis out of proximal tubule

(c) Secretion of hydrogen, potassium, ammonia, and some other substances from blood in peritubular capillaries to tubular filtrate; secretion accomplished by active transport mechanism

D. Collecting tubules

1. Each collecting tubule receives urine from several nephrons

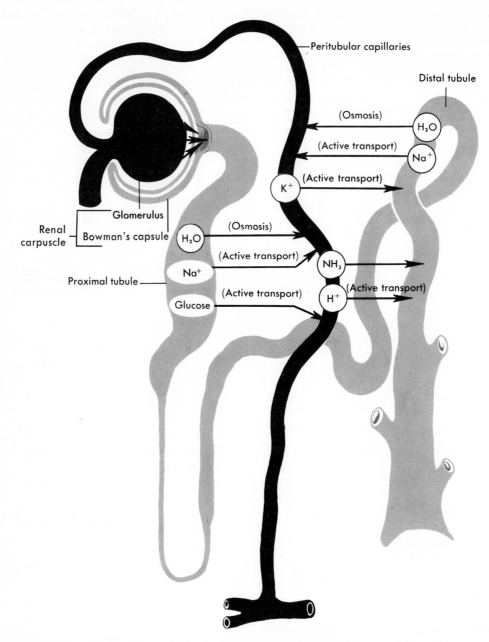

Fig. 6. Nephron showing glomerular filtration, tubular reabsorption, and tubular secretion—the three processes by which the kidneys secrete urine. In the proximal tubule, note that water is reabsorbed from the tubular filtrate into blood by osmosis, but sodium and glucose are reabsorbed mainly by active transport mechanisms. Note, too, that water and sodium are also reabsorbed from the distal tubule. Potassium and hydrogen ions and ammonia, in contrast, are secreted into the tubule from the blood. (From Anthony, C. P., and Kolthoff, N. J.: Textbook of anatomy and physiology, ed. 9, St. Louis, 1975, The C. V. Mosby Co.)

2. Under ADH influence, final osmotic reabsorption of most of remaining water in urine occurs
E. Urine composition
   1. Water—1.5 L per day average
   2. Urea—waste product of protein and amino acid metabolism
   3. Uric acid—waste product of metabolism of purines by liver
   4. Creatinine—waste product of muscle metabolism
   5. Ions (electrolytes); e.g., K^+, Na^+, Ca^{++}, Cl^-
   6. Hormones and their breakdown products—presence of chorionic gonadotropin is basis for pregnancy test
   7. Vitamins—particularly the water-soluble B vitamins and C
   8. Drugs excreted in the urine; e.g., aspirin, penicillin
   9. Other molecules, in low concentrations, have been identified
   10. Abnormal constituents; e.g., glucose, albumin, red blood cells, calculi
F. Urine volume is controlled normally by mechanisms that regulate the amount of water reabsorbed by the kidney tubules; only under abnormal conditions does the glomerular filtration rate influence urine volume
   1. The ADH mechanism—neurons in the hypothalamus (mainly in the supraoptic nucleus) produce the antidiuretic hormone, and the posterior pituitary gland secretes it into the blood; ADH secretion is stimulated by two conditions, an increase in the osmotic pressure of extracellular fluid or a decrease in the volume of extracellular fluid; ADH acts on distal and collecting tubules, causing more water to osmose from the tubular filtrate back into the blood; this increased water reabsorption tends to increase the total volume of body fluid by decreasing the urine volume; ADH has both a water-retaining and an antidiuretic effect
   2. The aldosterone mechanism—an increase in aldosterone secretion tends to decrease urine volume by stimulating kidney tubules to reabsorb primarily more sodium and secondarily more water; thus aldosterone tends to produce sodium retention, water retention, and a low urine volume
   3. Control by amount of solutes in tubular filtrate; in general, increase in tubular solutes causes decreased osmosis of water from proximal tubule back into blood and therefore an increase in urine volume; e.g., in diabetes, excess glucose in tubule filtrate leads to increased urine volume (polyuria, diuresis)
   4. Glomerular filtration rate normally is quite constant at about 125 ml per minute; it does not vary enough to alter volume of urine produced, but in certain pathologic conditions glomerular filtration rate may change markedly and alter urine volume; e.g., in shock, glomerular filtration decreases or even ceases, causing decreased urine volume (oliguria) or urinary suppression (anuria)
G. Control of amount of blood flow through kidneys
   1. Reduced renal blood flow results in renal excretion of the hormone renin
   2. Renin chemically interacts with blood proteins, producing angiotensin II
   3. Angiotensin II causes vasoconstriction and aldosterone secretion, resulting in an increase in blood pressure and renal blood flow

Ureters
A. Location—behind parietal peritoneum; extend from kidneys to posterior part of bladder floor
B. Structure—ureter expands as it enters kidney to form renal pelvis; subdivided into calyces, each of which contains renal papillae; ureter walls composed of smooth muscle with mucosa lining and fibrous outer coat
C. Function—collect urine secreted by kidney cells and propel it to bladder by peristaltic waves

Urinary bladder
A. Location—behind symphysis pubis, below parietal peritoneum
B. Structure—collapsible bag of smooth muscle lined with mucosa arranged in rugae, 3 openings—2 from ureters and 1 into the urethra
C. Functions
   1. Reservoir for urine until sufficient amount accumulated for elimination
   2. Expulsion of urine from body by way of urethra

Urethra
A. Location
   1. Female—behind symphysis pubis, in front of vagina
   2. Male—extends through prostate gland, fibrous sheet, and penis
B. Structure—musculomembranous tube lined with mucosa; opening to exterior called urinary meatus

C. Functions
   1. Female—passageway for expulsion of urine
   2. Male—passageway for expulsion of both urine and semen

Reproductive system
Male reproductive organs
Glands
A. Main male sex glands (gonads) are the testes
   1. Structure—fibrous capsule covers each testis and sends partitions into interior of gland, dividing it into lobules composed of tiny tubules called seminiferous tubules, embedded in connective tissue containing interstitial cells; ducts emerge from top of gland to enter head of epididymis
   2. Location—in scrotum, 1 testis in each of 2 compartments of scrotum
   3. Functions
      a. Seminiferous tubules carry on spermatogenesis; that is, they form spermatozoa, the male sex cells, or gametes
      b. Interstitial cells secrete testosterone, the main androgen, or male hormone
   4. Structure of spermatozoon—consists of head, middle piece, and whiplike tail that propels sperm; microscopic
B. Accessory glands
   1. Seminal vesicles
      a. Location—on posterior surface of bladder
      b. Structure—convoluted pouches, mucous lining
      c. Function—secrete nutrient-rich fluid estimated to constitute about 30% of semen
   2. Prostate gland
      a. Location—encircles urethra just below bladder
      b. Structure—walnut sized gland with ducts opening into urethra
      c. Function—secretes estimated 60% of semen; prostatic secretion is alkaline, which increases sperm motility; prostatic secretion contains abundance of enzyme, acid phosphatase; therefore blood level of this enzyme increases in metastasizing cancer of prostate
   3. Bulbourethral glands (Cowper's)
      a. Location—just below prostate gland
      b. Structure—small, pea-shaped structures with duct leading into urethra
      c. Function—secrete alkaline fluid that lubricates urethra prior to ejaculation

Ducts
A. Epididymis
   1. Location—lies along top and side of each testis
   2. Structure—each epididymis consists of single, tightly coiled tube enclosed in fibrous casing
   3. Function—conducts seminal fluid (semen) from testes to vas deferens; secretes small part of semen; stores semen prior to ejaculation, sperm mature during this period
B. Vas deferens (seminal ducts)
   1. Location—extend through inguinal canal into abdominal cavity, over top and down posterior surface of bladder to join ducts from seminal vesicles
   2. Structure—pair of tubes or ducts
   3. Function—conduct sperm and small amount of fluid from each epididymis to an ejaculatory duct
   4. Clinical application—vasectomy is the surgical procedure in which a short section of each vas is cut out and its separated ends tied off; as a result, sperm cannot enter the ejaculatory ducts and be ejaculated; semen from a vasectomized male contains no sperm; hence vasectomy sterilizes a man (makes him infertile); it does not render him impotent; it does, however, slightly decrease the amount of semen ejaculated
C. Ejaculatory ducts—formed by union of each vas with duct from seminal vesicle; pass through prostate gland to terminate in urethra; function—ejaculate semen into urethra
D. Urethra—described under Urinary system

Supporting structures
A. External—scrotum and penis
   1. Scrotum—skin-covered pouch suspended from perineal region; divided into 2 compartments, each one containing testis, epididymis, and first part of seminal duct; allows sperm to develop at 2° to 3° below the temperature of rest of body, which is ideal for sperm development
   2. Penis—made up of 3 cylindrical masses of erectile tissue that contain large vascular spaces; filling of these with blood causes erection of penis; 2 larger and upper cylinders named corpora cavernosa; smaller, lower one surrounding urethra called corpus cavernosum; glans penis—a bulging structure at distal end of penis, over which double fold of skin, prepuce or foreskin, fits loosely
B. Internal—spermatic cords are fibrous tubes located in each inguinal canal; serve as casing around each

vas deferens and its accompanying blood vessels, lymphatics, and nerves

Female reproductive organs

Ovaries—female gonads

A. Location—behind and below uterine tubes, anchored to uterus and broad ligaments
B. Size and shape of large almonds
C. Microscopic structure—each ovary of newborn female consists of several hundred thousand graafian follicles embedded in connective tissue; follicles are epithelial sacs in which ova develop; usually, between years of menarche and menopause, 1 follicle matures each month, ruptures surface of ovary, and expels its ovum into pelvic cavity
D. Functions
 1. Oogenesis—formation of mature ovum in graafian follicle
 2. Ovulation—expulsion of ovum from follicle into pelvic cavity
 3. Secretion of female hormones—maturing follicle secretes estrogens; corpus luteum secretes progesterone and estrogens

Uterine tubes (fallopian tubes, oviducts)

A. Location—attached to upper, outer angles of uterus
B. Structure—same 3 coats as uterus; distal ends fimbriated and open into pelvic cavity; mucosal lining of tubes and peritoneal lining of pelvis in direct contact here (facilitates spread of infection from tubes to peritoneum)
C. Function—serve as ducts through which ova travel from ovaries to uterus; fertilization normally occurs in tube

Uterus

A. Location—in pelvic cavity between bladder and rectum
B. Structure
 1. Shape and size—pear-shaped organ approximately the size of a clenched fist
 2. Divisions
  a. Body—upper and main part of uterus; fundus bulging upper surface of body
  b. Cervix—narrow, lower part of uterus; projects into vagina
 3. Walls—composed of smooth muscle (myometrium) lined with mucosa (endometrium)
 4. Cavities
  a. Body cavity—small and triangular with 3 openings into it; 2 from uterine tubes, 1 into cervical canal

  b. Cervical cavity—canal with constricted opening, internal os into body cavity and another, external os, into vagina
C. Position—flexed between body and cervix portions with body portion lying over bladder, pointing forward and slightly upward; cervix joins vagina at right angles; ligaments of uterus hold uterus in position
 1. Broad ligaments (2)—a double fold of parietal peritoneum that forms a kind of partition across pelvic cavity, suspending uterus between its folds
 2. Uterosacral ligaments (2)—foldlike extensions of peritoneum from posterior surface of uterus to sacrum, 1 on each side of rectum
 3. Posterior ligament (1)—fold of peritoneum between posterior surface of uterus and rectum; forms deep pouch, cul-de-sac of Douglas (or rectouterine pouch); this pouch lowest point in pelvic cavity and therefore the place where pus accumulates in pelvic inflammations; can be drained by posterior colpotomy (incision at top of posterior vaginal wall)
 4. Anterior ligament (1)—fold of peritoneum between uterus and bladder; forms shallow cul-de-sac
 5. Round ligaments (2)—fibromuscular cords from upper, outer angles of uterus, through inguinal canals, terminating in labia majora
D. Functions
 1. Menstruation
 2. Pregnancy
 3. Labor

Vagina

A. Location—between rectum and urethra
B. Structure—collapsible, musculomembranous tube, capable of great distention; outlet to exterior protected by fold of mucous membrane called hymen
C. Functions
 1. Receives semen from male
 2. Constitutes lower part of birth canal
 3. Acts as excretory duct for uterine secretions and menstrual flow

Vulva

 Consists of numerous structures that together constitute external genitals
A. Mons veneris—hairy, skin-covered pad of fat over symphysis pubis
B. Labia majora—hairy, skin-covered lips
C. Labia minora—small lips covered with modified skin

D. Clitoris—small mound of erectile tissue, below junction of two labia minora
E. Urinary meatus—just below clitoris; opening into urethra
F. Vaginal orifice—below urinary meatus; opening into vagina; hymen, fold of mucosa, partially closes orifice
G. Skene's glands—small mucous glands whose ducts open on either side of the urinary meatus
H. Bartholin's glands—2 small, bean-shaped glands; duct from each gland opens on either side of the vaginal orifice; both Bartholin's glands and Skene's glands have clinical interest because they frequently become infected (especially by the gonococci)

Breasts, or mammary glands
A. Location—just under skin, over pectoralis major muscles
B. Size—depends on deposits of adipose tissue rather than amount of glandular tissue (which is approximately same in all females)
C. Structure—divided into lobes and lobules that, in turn, are composed of racemose glands; excretory duct leads from each lobe to opening in nipple; circular pigmented area, the areola, borders nipples
D. Function—secrete milk (lactation)
   1. Shedding of placenta causes marked decrease in blood levels of estrogens and progesterone, which, in turn, stimulates anterior pituitary to increase prolactin secretion; high blood level of prolactin stimulates alveoli of breast to secrete milk
   2. Suckling controls lactation in 2 ways; by acting in some way to stimulate anterior pituitary secretion of prolactin and to stimulate posterior pituitary secretion of oxytocin, which stimulates release of milk out of alveoli into ducts from which infant can remove it by suckling (letdown reflex)

Menstrual cycle
A. Refers mainly to changes in the uterus and ovaries, which recur cyclically from the time of the menarche to the menopause
B. Length of cycle—usually 28 days, although considerable variations occur
C. Hormonal control of menstrual cycle
   1. Menses—brought on by marked decrease in blood levels of progesterone and estrogens at about cycle day 25
   2. Growth of new follicle and ovum—the low blood concentration of estrogens present for a few days before and during the menses stimulates the anterior pituitary gland to secrete follicle-stimulating hormone (FSH); the resulting high blood concentration of FSH stimulates 1 or more primitive graafian follicles and their ova to start growing and also stimulates the follicle cells to secrete estrogens; this leads to a high blood concentration of estrogens, which, in turn, has a negative feedback effect on FSH secretion by the anterior pituitary gland
   3. Endometrial thickening—in preovulatory phase is caused by proliferation of endometrial cells stimulated by the increasing concentration of estrogens in blood; the premenstrual phase is caused partly by endometrial cell proliferation and partly by fluid retention caused by increasing progesterone concentration
   4. Ovulation—brought on by high LH concentration
   5. Postovulatory phase—increased secretion of estrogen and progesterone from corpus luteum further prepares uterine endometrium in event of fertilization and implantation of ovulated egg
   6. Premenstrual phase—gradual drop in level of estrogen and progesterone, leading to menses
D. Clinical applications
   1. Contraceptive pills contain synthetic preparations of estrogen-like and/or progesterone-like compounds
   2. Most commonly used contraceptive pills prevent pregnancy by preventing ovulation—pituitary secretion of FSH inhibited
E. Progestogen replacement provides the stimulus for desquamation of the uterine lining required for completion of the menstrual cycle or for maintenance of the uterine lining during pregnancy
   1. Drugs
      a. Dydrogesterone (Duphaston, Gynorest)
      b. Ethisterone
      c. Hydroxyprogesterone caproate (Delalutin)
      d. Medroxyprogesterone acetate (Depo-Provera, Provera)
      e. Norethindrone (Norlutin)
      f. Norethindrone acetate (Norlutate)
      g. Progesterone (Gesterol, Lipo-Lutin, Proluton)
   2. Adverse effects—initial use causes profuse vaginal flow (shedding of accumulatioins of endometrial tissue), spotting, irregular bleeding, nausea, lethargy, jaundice

Development of the individual

Formation of gametes

A. The egg and spermatozoon each have 1 set of chromosomes (23); this is in contrast to other cells of the body that have 2 sets, or 46 chromosomes (23 pairs)

B. The production of ova (eggs) and spermatozoa (sperm) requires a special type of nuclear division (meiosis) in which the chromosome number is reduced from 2 sets (46 chromosomes) to 1 set (23 chromosomes)

Fertilization

A. Spermatozoa are deposited in the vagina

B. Fertilization usually occurs in the uterine tube when the egg is about one third of the way down the tube; usually this is about 24 hours after ovulation

C. Sperm must be in the genital tract 4 to 6 hours before they are able to fertilize an egg; during this period the enzyme hyaluronidase is activated; this enzyme is able to dissolve the cement substance (hyaluronic acid) that holds together the cells that surround the ovum

D. The male nucleus enters the cytoplasm of the egg and several events follow
  1. A fertilization membrane forms around the egg that prevents the entrance of other sperm
  2. The sperm tail is lost and the male nucleus (male pronucleus) moves toward the female nucleus (female pronucleus)

E. Fertilization proper occurs when the male pronucleus unites with the female pronucleus; thus the chromosome number is restored to 2 sets (46 chromosomes)

F. Contraception
  1. Contraceptive pill
  2. IUD—intrauterine device placed in uterus; irritates endometrium or in some other unidentified manner prevents implantation; does not prevent fertilization
  3. Diaphragm with spermicidal jelly—provides physical barrier to movement of sperm flow back of vagina into uterus; also provides acid conditions unfavorable to sperm
  4. Condom—most widely used method of contraception (cheapest); prevents entering of sperm into female genital tract; only form of contraception providing protection from venereal disease
  5. Tubal ligation—egg cannot be reached by sperm because fallopian tubes are blocked or severed; fertilization prevented
  6. Vasectomy—sperm cannot be ejected because vas deferens has been blocked or severed

Cleavage

A. In a short time after fertilization the zygote undergoes rapid division to produce a mass of cells (morula) that descends in the uterine tube

B. As it descends it also divides to form a hollow ball referred to as the blastocyst

Implantation

A. The blastocyst implants in the uterine wall
  1. The blastocyst is differentiated into an inner cell mass, a blastocoele (internal cavity)
  2. An outer covering of cells, the trophectoderm, which becomes trophoderm and will form the fetal portion of the placenta
  3. Implantation occurs 7 to 8 days after fertilization

B. During implantation, cells of trophoderm secrete enzymes that digest the endometrium and allow the embryo to sink below surface; endometrium heals over implantation site

Embryonic period

A. First 2 months, after this period it is called a fetus

B. The inner cell mass differentiates into germ layers
  1. Ectoderm—outer layer of skin and mouth cavity and nervous tissue
  2. Mesoderm—connective tissue, including blood and muscle tissue
  3. Endoderm—linings of the alimentary tract, respiratory system, and several glands

C. About the twelfth day after fertilization a fetal membrane, the amnion, forms around the embryo; another membrane, the yolk sac, develops beneath the embryo
  1. Amnion is fluid filled (amniotic fluid) and serves as a fetal shock absorber
  2. Yolk sac serves as an initial embryonic source of erythrocytes

D. Later an allantois develops that will supply placental blood vessels

E. A chorion surrounds the embryo; this will eventually form the major part of the placenta; fingerlike projections of the chorion called chorionic villi grow into the endometrium; chorionic villi project into placental blood sinuses; the combination of chorionic villi, placental blood sinuses, and placental blood constitutes the placenta

Umbilical cord

A. Consists of an outer layer of amnion

B. Contains 2 umbilical arteries and 1 umbilical vein

Fetal growth

A. Differentiation of cells occurs

B. Development of organs progresses from anterior to posterior in the growing fetus

Hormones

A. During pregnancy the chorion of the placenta secretes a hormone, chorionic gonadotropin, that maintains the corpus luteum; the continuation of progesterone and estrogen secretion from the corpus luteum maintains the pregnancy during the early weeks of development
B. Chorionic gonadotropin reaches a peak in the third month and then drops
C. Estrogen and progesterone increase and continue to be secreted from the placenta during the last 6 months of pregnancy; progesterone acts to inhibit uterine contractions, which might occur due to uterine stretching as the fetus grows
D. In the last month uterine contents shift downward so that the fetus is in contact with the cervix; this contact may induce oxytocin secretion by the posterior pituitary
E. The secretion of oxytocin, which stimulates uterine contractions, coupled with the drop in progesterone brings about labor; uterine contractions increase in frequency and intensity, culminating in fetal expulsion (birth)

Heredity

Chromosomes

A. Humans have 23 pairs of homologous chromosomes
B. In males the sex chromosomes (the X and Y) are not equal in size
C. Homologous chromosomes carry sets of matching genes (alleles) in which 1 may be dominant and the other recessive, or they may have blending expressions

Sex determination in humans

A. Genetic females have 2 sets of autosomes (nonsex chromosomes) and 2 X chromosomes, whereas genetic males have 2 sets of autosomes and 1 X chromosome and 1 Y chromosome
B. All eggs produced by females have 1 set of autosomes and 1 X chromosome; spermatozoa produced by a male have a set of autosomes and either an X or a Y chromosome
C. If an X-bearing spermatozoon fertilizes an egg, a female will result; if a Y-bearing spermatozoon fertilizes an egg, a male will result

Genes

A. Sex-linked genes—genes carried on the X chromosome are called sex-linked genes and are always expressed in the male, even though they may be recessive; examples of such genes cause hemophilia and color blindness
B. Multiple genes—many different genes may combine to produce cumulative effects, such as the degree of pigmentation or height
C. Multiple alleles—an example of human traits controlled by multiple alleles are the genes controlling normal blood types; the genes for type O are dominated by the genes for type A or type B; the genes for A and B are both expressed

Genes	Blood type
OO	O
AO	A
AA	A
BO	B
BB	B
AB	AB

D. Following are some other obvious human traits controlled by genes

Dominant	Recessive
Brown eyes	Blue eyes
Normal blood clotting	Hemophilia (sex-linked)
Normal color vision	Color blind (sex-linked)
Normal pigmentation	Albinism
Rh positive (multiple alleles)	Rh negative
Normal red blood cell development	Sickle cell trait

Chromosomal alterations

A. In rare cases additional sex chromosomes may appear and produce abnormal individuals
   1. X chromosome and no Y chromosome—Turner's syndrome
   2. Two or more X chromosomes and a Y chromosome—Klinefelter's syndrome
B. Translocation of chromosome—a cytogenetic abnormality such as trisomy 21 (Down's syndrome)
C. Mutations
   1. Changes in the DNA are mutations; there may also be chromosomal changes
   2. The frequency of mutations may be increased by certain agents such as ultraviolet radiation, x-ray films, radioactive radiation, and certain chemical substances

REVIEW OF PHYSICAL PRINCIPLES RELATED TO THE GENITOURINARY SYSTEM
Principles of mechanics

Law of motion
   Newton's law
   EXAMPLES
   1. The pumping action of the heart supplies hydro-

static force to filter blood in the glomerular capillary bed

2. The contraction of muscle is responsible for the force of propulsion of semen along and out of the male reproductive tract

Momentum

EXAMPLE: During micturition, the walls of the urinary bladder exert a force of prolonged duration that imparts great momentum to the urine being expelled from the body

Energy

EXAMPLE: The chemical energy of ATP is used to actively transport nutrients and electrolytes from glomerular filtrate into the tubular epithelium

Principles of physical properties of matter

Elasticity

EXAMPLES

1. The elastic properties of the bladder permit it to hold several hundred milliliters of urine before urination
2. Elastic properties of uterine connective tissue partly account for the tremendous increase in size of uterus during pregnancy

Surface area

EXAMPLE: The proximal convoluted tubules of the nephron have a brush border consisting of numerous microvilli that have very high surface-to-volume ratio; these tiny cellular extensions greatly increase the surface area of the tubule for reabsorption of materials from the glomerular filtrate

Liquids

Pascal's principle

EXAMPLE: In conditions resulting in the lack of micturition reflex, manual pressure over the bladder region will be transmitted to the urine, which results in the opening of the sphincters and the expulsion of urine from the bladder

REVIEW OF CHEMICAL PRINCIPLES RELATED TO THE GENITOURINARY SYSTEM
Urine

A. Water solution of inorganic salts and organic compounds
B. Important in excretion of wastes
C. Analysis yields information of physical condition in health and disease
D. Normal urine
   1. Amount—800 to 1800 ml/24 hours

2. Color—light yellow to dark brown, resulting from pigments (urobilin, urochrome, etc.)
3. Odor—aromatic (fresh); food and drugs alter odor
4. Sediment—varies; caused by diet and other normal changes
   a. Few blood cells
   b. Few epithelial cells
   c. Phosphates
   d. Urates
   e. Uric acid crystals
   f. Calcium oxalate
5. Specific gravity (1.005 to 1.025) varies greatly, depending on fluid intake and the quantity of solutes dissolved in the urine; the individual having diabetes insipidus may excrete 5 to 15 L of urine daily; this urine has a very low specific gravity (very close to that of pure water); an individual having diabetes mellitus may excrete urine of high specific gravity caused by excessive quantities of glucose dissolved in the urine
6. Reaction—usually acid (pH 4.5 to 7.5 is the normal range); alkaline immediately after a meal
7. Proteins—negative; protein in urine is usually associated with pathology although albumin traces may occasionally appear after heavy exercise or cold showers (these traces being of no consequence)
8. Sugar—trace to negative; presence of urinary carbohydrate usually pathologic
9. Ketone bodies—negative; ketone bodies in urine appear in metabolic disorders
10. Indican—negative; positive results indicate intestinal obstruction
11. Bile—negative; positive results indicate liver or gallbladder dysfunction
12. Blood—trace to negative; positive results indicate bleeding in organs of urinary system

Hormones

See Endocrine system

REVIEW OF MICROORGANISMS RELATED TO THE GENITOURINARY SYSTEM

A. Bacterial pathogens
   1. *Enterobacter aerogenes*—small, gram-negative bacillus (morphologically indistinguishable from *Escherichia coli*); causes urinary tract infections
   2. *Haemophilus ducreyi*—morphologically indistin-

guishable from *H. influenzae* and *H. aegyptius;* causes the venereal ulcer called chancroid (soft chancre)
3. *Neisseria gonorrhoeae*—gram-negative diplococcus; causes gonorrhea
4. *Pseudomonas aeruginosa*—gram-negative, motile bacillus; a common secondary invader of wounds, burns, outer ear, and urinary tract; the infection characterized by blue-green pus; may be transmitted by catheters and other hospital instruments
5. *Treponema pallidum*—a long, slender, highly motile spirochete; causes syphilis
B. Protozoal pathogen—*Trichomonas vaginalis*—flagellated protozoan; causes trichomonas vaginitis (a venereal disease)

PHARMACOLOGY RELATED TO URINARY SYSTEM DISORDERS

See kidney-specific drugs under section on controlling infection

RELATED PROCEDURES
Cystoscopy

A. Definition
1. The visualization of the bladder wall through a tube with a fiberoptic end
2. Indicated as a diagnostic measure or as a means to enter the bladder for therapy
B. Nursing responsibilities
1. Obtain an informed consent
2. Maintain patient NPO prior to procedure (may be done with or without general anesthesia)
3. Following procedure
a. Maintain patient in comfortable state
b. Observe patient's urine for clots of hemorrhage
c. Ascertain that patient has voided through observation and palpation of bladder

Intravenous pyelography (IVP)

A. Definition—x-ray examination of the kidneys, ureters, and bladder after the injection of a contrast medium into an antecubital vein
B. Nursing responsibilities
1. Explain procedure to patient
2. Obtain informed consent
3. Administer a cathartic as ordered the evening prior to test to remove feces and flatus

4. Allow patient a light supper prior to procedure and maintain NPO for 6 to 8 hours prior to test

Common urine tests

A. Definition
1. Urinalysis—microscopic examination of urine for cells, as well as chemical study for pH and specific gravity
2. Culture and sensitivity tests of urine—microscopic examination of urine for bacterial growth and determination of antibiotic appropriate to control growth
B. Nursing responsibilities
1. Explain procedure to patient
2. Obtain container for specimen
a. For urinalysis a urine container is used
b. For culture a sterile specimen jar is used
3. For urinalysis obtain a freshly voided specimen and place in container
4. For culture have patient
a. Cleanse outer urinary meatus with bacteriostatic solution
b. Instruct patient to void a small amount into bedpan, urinal, or toilet and then stop stream
c. Instruct patient to continue voiding in container without contaminating lid or inside of jar
d. Seal jar
5. Send specimen to laboratory with label indicating contents, patient's name, and date

MAJOR DISEASES
Cystitis

A. Etiology and pathophysiology
1. Inflammation of the bladder wall usually caused by an ascending bacterial infection *E. coli* most common)
2. More common in females due to
a. Shorter urethra
b. Childbirth
c. Anatomic position of urethra
B. Signs and symptoms
1. Subjective
a. Urgency, frequency, burning, and pain on urination
b. Nocturia
c. Bearing down on urination
2. Objective
a. Pyuria and hematuria
b. Bacterial growth evident on culture of urine

C. Treatment
   1. Chemotherapeutic and antibiotic agents; e.g., sulfonamides, penicillin, tetracycline
   2. Antispasmodics to soothe the irritable bladder; e.g., phenazopyridine (Pyridium)
   3. Diet directed toward maintaining an acid urine; e.g., cranberry juice
   4. Intake of additional fluids to dilute the urine
D. Nursing care
   1. Teach patient to seek medical attention at the first sign of symptoms
   2. Teach patient to take medications as directed
   3. Encourage patient to drink additional fluids
   4. Monitor intake and output with attention to character of urine
   5. Teach patient proper perineal care

Renal and ureteral calculi

A. Etiology and pathophysiology—the formation of stones in the urinary tract; stones may be composed of calcium phosphate, uric acid, or oxalate; they tend to recur and may cause obstruction, infection, and/or hydronephrosis
B. Signs and symptoms
   1. Subjective
      a. Severe pain in kidney area radiating down the flank to the pubic area
      b. Frequency and urgency of urination
      c. History of prior or associated health problems; e.g., gout, parathyroidism, immobility, dehydration, urinary tract infections
   2. Objective
      a. Diaphoresis, pallor, nausea and vomiting
      b. Hematuria; pyuria may occur if infection is present
C. Treatment
   1. Narcotics for pain
   2. Antispasmodics to reduce the renal colic
   3. Allopurinol or sulfinpyrazone to reduce uric acid excretion
   4. Antibiotics to reduce infection
   5. Monitor intake and output; forced fluids and straining of urine
   6. Diet therapy
      a. Large fluid intake to produce dilute urine
      b. Diet altered according to type of stone
         (1) Calcium stone—low calcium, low phosphate, or oxalate according to calcium compound, acid ash; calcium foods, mainly dairy products, are eliminated;

acid ash foods such as meat, egg, and grains are emphasized; alkaline foods such as milk, vegetables, fruits are controlled
         (2) Uric acid stones—low purine (uric acid is a metabolic product of purines in the body), controlling purine foods such as meat, especially organ meats, meat extractives, and to a lesser extent plant sources such as whole grains and legumes; alkaline ash as the stone composition is acid
         (3) Cystine stones—rare genetic type; diet is low methionine, since methionine is the essential amino acid from which the nonessential amino acid cystine is formed; controlling protein foods such as meat, milk, egg, cheese; alkaline ash, since the stone is an acid composition
   7. Surgical intervention if stone is not passed or complications are present; e.g., nephrolithotomy, litholapaxy
D. Nursing care
   1. Administer medications as ordered
   2. Permit patient to set own pattern of activity
   3. Plan care to provide patient with periods of undisturbed rest
   4. Strain all urine
   5. Monitor intake and output
   6. Force fluids
   7. Administer medication as ordered
   8. Encourage patient to accept medication for pain
   9. Provide as much privacy as possible
   10. Encourage patient to remain on diet
   11. Teach patient to read labels on food preparations for the presence of contraindicated additives such as calcium or phosphate

Hydronephrosis (renal colic)

A. Etiology and pathophysiology
   1. When there is an obstruction at any point in the urinary system, pressure occurs that can damage renal tissue
   2. Obstruction may be due to tumors, trauma, calculi, polycystic disease, congenital abnormalities, lymph enlargement, or nephrotosis (floating kidney)
B. Signs and symptoms
   1. Subjective
      a. Pain, local tenderness
      b. Dull pain in flank region or colicky pain

   2. Objective
     a. Nausea and vomiting
     b. Nocturia
C. Treatment
   1. Treat underlying cause
   2. Promote urinary drainage with catheter
   3. Urinary antiseptics
   4. Antispasmodics for colicky spasms
D. Nursing care
   1. Observe for signs of uremia
   2. Medicate as ordered
   3. Maintain patency of drainage tubes

Acute renal failure

A. Etiology and pathophysiology
   1. Usually follows direct trauma to the kidneys or overwhelming physiologic stress such as burns, septicemia, nephotoxic drugs and chemicals, hemolytic blood transfusion reaction, severe shock, or renal vascular occlusion
   2. Sudden and almost complete loss of glomerular and/or tubular function
   3. Acute renal failure may cause death from acidosis, potassium intoxication, pulmonary edema, or infection
   4. May progress from the anuric or oliguric phase through the diuretic phase to the convalescence phase (which can take 6 to 12 months) to recovery of function
   5. May progress to chronic renal failure; chronic renal failure may develop as a separate entity and does not have to be a sequela of acute failure
B. Signs and symptoms
   1. Subjective
     a. Lethargy and drowsiness than can progress from stupor to coma
     b. Irritability and headache
     c. Circumoral numbness
     d. Tingling extremities
     e. Anorexia
   2. Objective
     a. Sudden dramatic drop in urinary output appearing a few hours after the causative event
     b. Oliguria—urinary output less than 400 ml but more than 100 ml/24 hours; anuria—urinary output less than 100 ml/24 hours
     c. Restlessness, twitching, convulsions
     d. Nausea and vomiting
     e. Skin pallor, anemia, and increased bleeding time, which can progress to epistaxis and internal hemorrhage
     f. Ammonia (urine) odor to breath and perspiration, which can progress to uremic frost on skin and pruritis
     g. Generalized edema, hypervolemia, hypertension, and increased venous pressure, which can progress to pulmonary edema and congestive heart failure
     h. In addition, respirations are deep and rapid as a compensatory response to the developing metabolic acidosis
     i. Elevated serum levels of
       (1) BUN
       (2) Creatinine
       (3) Potassium
     j. Decreased serum levels of
       (1) Calcium
       (2) Sodium
       (3) pH
       (4) CO_2 combining power
     k. Anemia
     l. Albumin in urine
     m. Decreased specific gravity
C. Treatment
   1. Direct treatment toward correcting the underlying cause of renal failure; e.g., treat shock, eliminate drugs and toxins, treat transfusion reactions, restore integrity of urinary tract
   2. Maintain patient on complete bed rest
   3. Diet therapy
     a. Protein low to moderate according to tolerance: 30 to 50 g
     b. Carbohydrate relatively high for energy: 300 to 400 g
     c. Fat relatively moderate: 70 to 90 g
     d. Calories adequate for maintenance to prevent tissue breakdown: 2000 to 2500 daily
     e. Sodium controlled according to serum levels and excretion tolerance: varying from 400 to 2000 mg
     f. Potassium controlled according to serum levels and excretion capacities: varying from 1300 to 1900 mg
     g. Water controlled according to excretion: about 800 to 1000 ml; careful intake-output records vital
   4. Frequent monitoring of vital signs and intake and output

5. Packed cells, electrolytes, and glucose IV as necessary
6. Exchange resins to decrease serum potassium
7. Antibiotics to reduce possibility of infection
8. Peritoneal dialysis or hemodialysis
9. Surgical intervention if kidney transplant is a viable alternative

D. Nursing care
1. Monitor intake and output at frequent intervals
2. Limit fluid intake as ordered
3. Weigh patient daily
4. Observe for signs of overhydration; e.g., dependent, pitting, sacral, or periorbital edema; rales or dyspnea; headache, distended neck veins, and hypertension
5. Observe for signs of hyperkalemia and hyponatremia
6. Administer electrolytes as ordered
7. Provide periods of undisturbed rest to conserve energy and oxygen
8. Protect patient from injury caused by bleeding tendency, possibility of convulsions, and clouded sensorium
9. Protect patient from cross infection
10. Observe for early signs and symptoms of complications; e.g., hemorrhage, convulsions, cardiac problems, pulmonary edema
11. Provide special skin care frequently to prevent breakdown and remove uremic frost
12. Monitor vital signs and intake and output at frequent intervals; record and report any deviations immediately
13. Administer antibiotics as ordered
14. Encourage intake of diet as ordered and record amount consumed
15. Allow patient as much choice as possible in the selection of food while recognizing that little variation is possible
16. Provide mouth care before, after, and between meals
17. Administer dietary and electrolyte supplements as ordered
18. Administer antiemetics to control nausea and antacids to reduce GI irritation

Chronic renal failure

A. Etiology and pathophysiology
1. Chronic renal failure can occur as the result of chronic kidney infections, developmental abnormalities, and vascular disorders

2. The ongoing deterioration in renal function results in uremia

B. Signs and symptoms
1. Subjective
   a. Lethargy or drowsiness
   b. Headache
2. Objective
   a. Vomiting
   b. Mental clouding
   c. Kussmaul respirations
   d. Uremic frost (powdery substance on skin from urate wastes)
   e. Convulsions, coma, death

C. Treatment
1. Fluid and salt restrictions
2. Antihypertensive medications
3. Peritoneal dialysis—warmed dialyzing solution is introduced via trocar, which is in the peritoneal cavity; the peritoneal membrane is used as a dialyzing membrane to remove toxic substances, metabolic wastes, and excess fluid
4. Hemodialysis—the patient is attached (via surgically created arteriovenous fistula) directly to a machine that pumps patient's blood along a semipermeable membrane; dialyzing solution is on the other side of the membrane, and osmosis of wastes, toxins, and fluid from the patient occurs
5. Diet management
   a. General protein and electrolyte control
   b. The low-protein, essential amino acid diet (modified Giordano-Giovannetti regimen) to sustain patients with uremia and alleviate their difficult symptoms
      (1) Very low protein (20 g); minimal essential amino acids
      (2) Controlled potassium (1500 mg); feed only essential amino acids, causing the body to use its own excess urea nitrogen to synthesize the nonessential amino acids needed for tissue protein production; foods used include 1 egg, 6 oz milk, low-protein bread, 2 to 4 fruits, and 2 to 4 vegetables from special lists to control protein and potassium

D. Nursing care
1. Monitor intake and output
2. Provide skin care as needed
3. Monitor vital signs
4. When patient is undergoing dialysis

a. Explain procedure to patient and family; answer questions related to the procedure

b. Take vital signs and weigh patient before procedure is begun

c. Use surgical asepsis in preparation of site (abdomen or radial vessels)

d. Assure patient that a staff member will be present at all times

e. If indwelling catheter is not in place, have patient void before procedure is started

f. Once the procedure is instituted by the physician, monitor the patient's response and add dialysate as prescribed

g. Monitor vital signs every 15 minutes

h. During peritoneal dialysis keep an accurate flow chart

i. During hemodialysis observe site for clotting; check clotting time and administer heparin as prescribed by the physician

j. During both procedures check tubes for patency

k. Since both procedures are long, provide back care to promote comfort and diversional activities to help pass the time

Kidney transplantation

A. Etiology and pathophysiology

1. Patients with chronic renal failure who have no kidney function are candidates for transplantation

2. The least risk of rejection of the new kidney occurs if donor and recipient are identical twins

3. At the time of surgery, the patient's own kidney is not removed unless it is infected or enlarged

4. The new kidney is generally placed in the iliac fossa retroperitoneally, and the donor's ureter is attached to the bladder to prevent reflux of urine

B. Preoperative care

1. Prepare patient and family emotionally for the possible outcomes of surgery

2. Explain that, postoperatively, immunosuppressive drugs and dialysis may be indicated, as well as isolation to prevent infection

3. Explain routine properative procedures

C. Postoperative care

1. Maintain patency of drainage tubes, including Foley catheter; gross hematuria or clots are *not* expected postoperatively

2. Monitor fluid and electrolyte balance carefully, since no urine output may occur for several days or weeks

3. Monitor vital signs, weight, and temperature

4. Observe patient for signs of rejection

a. Increased serum creatinine

b. Decreasing urinary output

c. Malaise

d. Fever

e. Flank pain or tenderness

5. Administer steroids and immunosuppressives as ordered to prevent rejection

Adenocarcinoma of the kidneys

A. Etiology and pathophysiology

1. Adenocarcinoma is the most common cancer affecting the kidneys

2. Common sites of metastasis include lungs, liver, and long bones

3. Incidence is higher in males

B. Signs and symptoms

1. Subjective

a. There may be none until metastasis

b. Dull back pain

c. Weakness

2. Objective

a. Painless hematuria

b. Enlarged kidney palpable during physical examination

c. Elevated temperature

d. Weight loss

e. Anemia

C. Treatment

1. Nephrectomy

2. Radiation therapy if tumor is sensitive

3. Chemotherapy

4. Hormonal therapy with medroxyprogesterone (Provera)

D. Nursing care

1. Monitor intake and output

2. Increase oral fluid intake

3. Administer analgesics as ordered to alleviate postoperative pain

4. Encourage coughing and deep breathing while splinting incision

5. Examine dressing and linen under patient for drainage; a small amount of serosanguineous drainage is expected

6. Maintain integrity of urinary drainage system; avoid kinking of tubes

7. Observe urine for color, amount, and any abnormal components

Glomerulonephritis

A. Etiology and pathophysiology
   1. Glomerulonephritis involves damage to both kidneys resulting from filtration and trapping of antibody-antigen complexes within the glomeruli
   2. As a result, inflammatory and degenerative changes affect all renal tissue
   3. Often follows some form of streptococcal infection such as tonsillitis
   4. May be acute or chronic in nature; decreases life expectancy if progressive renal damage occurs
   5. Complications include hypertensive encephalopathy, heart failure, and infection
B. Signs and symptoms
   1. Subjective
      a. Flank pain, costovertebral tenderness
      b. Headache
      c. Malaise
      d. Dyspnea due to salt and fluid retention
      e. Weakness
      f. Visual disturbances
   2. Objective
      a. Hematuria
      b. Periorbital and facial edema
      c. Oliguria
      d. Fever
      e. Tachycardia
      f. Urine analysis reveals protein and casts
      g. Elevated plasma, BUN, and creatinine
      h. Anemia
C. Treatment
   1. Antibiotics such as penicillin to treat underlying infection
   2. Dietary restriction of sodium, fluids, and protein based on clinical status
   3. Diuretics and antihypertensives to control blood pressure
D. Nursing care
   1. Monitor intake and output
   2. Assess specific gravity of urine
   3. Weigh patient daily
   4. Monitor vital signs and temperature
   5. Special prophylactic skin care; these patients are prone to breakdown
   6. Protect patients from infection
   7. Observe for complications such as renal failure, cardiac failure, and hypertensive encephalopathy
   8. Evaluate laboratory results (BUN, creatinine, urinalysis)
   9. Encourage continued medical supervision
   10. Refer to social service as needed; the long-term nature of illness may create economic problems for the family

Bladder tumors

A. Etiology and pathophysiology
   1. Occur most frequently in men over 50 years of age
   2. Smoking, exposure to radiation, schistosomiasis, and exposure over prolonged periods to certain chemicals increase the risk of development of tumor
   3. Common sites of metastasis include lymph nodes, bone, liver, and lungs
B. Signs and symptoms
   1. Subjective
      a. Frequency and urgency of urination
      b. Dysuria
   2. Objective
      a. Direct visualization by cystoscopic examination
      b. Painless hematuria
C. Treatment
   1. Surgical intervention
      a. Resection of tumor
      b. Cystectomy (removal of bladder); requires urinary diversion
         (1) Ureterosigmoidostomy—the ureters are attached to the sigmoid colon, and urine is excreted through rectum; these patients have constant drainage and are usually troubled by recurrent infection of the urinary tract
         (2) Ileal conduit—a section of the ileum is resected and attached to the ureters; one end of this ileal conduit is sutured closed and the other brought to the skin as an ileostomy to drain urine; this is most widely used to divert urine
         (3) Nephrostomy—a catheter is inserted into the kidney through an incision
         (4) Ureterostomy—the ureters are implanted in the abdominal wall to drain urine
   2. Radiation therapy
   3. Chemotherapy
D. Nursing care
   1. Allow time for patient's verbalization of fears of surgery, cancer, death, and body image alterations

2. Preoperatively, in addition to routine care and explanations, prepare bowel by cleansing with laxatives, antibiotics, and enemas as ordered
3. Assess color and amount of urine frequently; maintain patency of drainage system
4. If the patient has a ureterosigmoidostomy, a drainage tube may be in the rectum for a few days; after removal, encourage the patient to void frequently via the rectum to prevent complications such as reflux and absorption of urine through intestinal wall
5. If the patient has an ileal conduit, a urinary drainage bag will be cemented around the stoma to collect urine; encourage self-care; teach patient gradually to change own appliance by using a mirror
   a. After equipment is collected, remove the collection bag; use water or commercial solvent to loosen cement
   b. Hold rolled gauze pad against the stoma to absorb urine during the procedure
   c. Cleanse the skin around the stoma and under the drainage bag with soap and water; inspect for excoriation
   d. After the skin is dry, apply skin cement to the area around the stoma and to the appliance
   e. Place the appliance over the stoma and secure in place by an adjustable belt
6. Expect a variety of psychologic manifestations such as anger or depression postoperatively
7. Arrange visit from a member of an ostomy club
8. Set realistic goals
9. Encourage fluids such as cranberry juice to keep the pH of the urine acidic and help prevent infection

Bladder trauma (rupture)

A. Etiology and pathophysiology
   1. Traumatic rupture of the bladder occurs following external crushing injury to the area, as in automobile accidents
   2. An overdistended bladder at time of trauma increases the risk of this occurrence
B. Signs and symptoms
   1. Subjective
      a. Pain
      b. Anxiety
   2. Objective
      a. Oliguria or anuria
      b. Hematuria

C. Treatment
   1. Exploration of bladder to aid in diagnosing rupture
   2. Surgical repair of laceration
   3. Insertion of suprapubic catheter to aid in urinary drainage (a tube inserted directly through the peritoneal cavity into the bladder to drain urine)
D. Nursing care
   1. Observe vital signs for changes indicative of shock or hemorrhage
   2. Observe urine for amount and color
   3. Promote rest and analgesia
   4. Maintain patency of catheters

Urethritis

A. Etiology and pathophysiology
   1. Inflammation of the urethra caused by staphylococci, *E. coli*, *Pseudomonas* species, and streptococci
   2. Although these inflammatory symptoms are similar to gonorrheal urethritis, sexual contact is not the cause
B. Signs and symptoms
   1. Subjective
      a. Burning on urination
      b. Urgency
      c. Frequency
   2. Objective
      a. Purulent drainage
      b. Bacteria in urine
C. Treatment
   1. Ascertain causative organism through a culture of urine
   2. Administer antibiotics
   3. Hot sitz baths
   4. Dilation of urethra and subsequent instillation of antiseptic solution
D. Nursing care
   1. Promote rest and comfort
   2. Encourage fluid intake
   3. Observe urine for clarity and hemorrhage

PHARMACOLOGY RELATED TO REPRODUCTIVE SYSTEM DISORDERS

A. Estrogens
   1. General implications for nurses
      a. Instruct patient to report unusual vaginal bleeding
      b. Observe patient for edema; teach patient to

observe for this at home, especially by weighing at least twice per week

  c. If ointments are used, explain how to apply; if vaginal suppositories are used, explain how to insert
  d. Reassure male patients that feminizing side effects will subside when therapy is completed
  e. Observe patient for adverse effects
    (1) Purpura
    (2) Thrombophlebitis
    (3) Decreased glucose tolerance
    (4) In males, gynecomastia, loss of libido, testicular atrophy
  2. Actions
  a. Estrogens are secreted by ovarian follicles in women and trigger the proliferation phase of the menstrual cycle
  b. Estrogen can be used to regulate menstrual disorders, uterine bleeding, and menopausal problems
  c. Estrogen may be used for inoperable prostatic cancer, postpartum breast engorgement, and breast cancer
  d. Estrogens are also used as contraceptives
  3. Examples
  a. Chlorotrianisene (Tace)
  b. Diethylstilbestrol (DES)
  c. Esterified estrogens
  d. Estradiol cypionate
  e. Estradiol valerate
  f. Estrone (Theelin, Menformon)
  g. Ethinyl estradiol (Estinyl)
B. Progesterone and progestins
  1. General implications for nurses
  a. Observe patient for edema and instruct patient to observe for this by recording weight and reporting increases
  b. Inform patient's family that drug may result in psychiatric depression
  c. Observe patient for adverse effects
    (1) Scleral jaundice
    (2) Blurred vision or decreased vision
    (3) Thrombophlebitis
  2. Actions
  a. Progesterone is a female ovarian hormone that acts on the uterus to prepare for implantation of a fertilized ovum and is essential for the maintenance of pregnancy
  b. Progesterone aids in the treatment of endo-

metriosis, infertility, dysmenorrhea, and threatened abortion; aids in suppression of ovulation
  3. Examples
  a. Hydroxyprogesterone caproate (Delalutin)
  b. Medroxyprogesterone acetate (Provera)
  c. Megestrol acetate (Megace)
  d. Progesterone (Proluton, Progestin, Lipo-Lutin)
C. Androgens
  1. General implications for nurses
  a. Use drug with a diet high in calories and proteins to aid in building body tissues
  b. Observe for signs of virilization in females
  c. Observe patient for side effects
    (1) Weight gain
    (2) Acne
    (3) Changes in libido
    (4) Hoarseness; deep voice
  2. Actions
  a. Androgens aid in the development of secondary sex characteristics in men and have anabolic properties, which stimulate the building and repair of body tissue
  b. Used in debilitating conditions and to restore hormone levels
  3. Examples
  a. Fluoxymesterone (Halotestin, Ultandren)
  b. Nandrolone phenpropionate (Durabolin)
  c. Norethandrolone (Nilevar)
  d. Testosterones (Testosterone, Oreton, Delatestryl, Andronate)
D. Oral contraceptives
  1. General implications for nurses
  a. Assist patient in choosing best method of birth control by providing an accepting atmosphere
  b. Discuss the importance of follow-up care with gynecologist
  c. Observe patient for adverse effects
    (1) Thrombophlebitis
    (2) Hypertension
    (3) Libido changes
    (4) Hyperglycemia
  2. Actions
  a. Cause thickening of cervical mucus to inhibit sperm travel
  b. Inhibit ovulation
  c. Cause atrophic changes in endometrium to prevent implantation

3. Examples
    a. Estrogen and progesterone tablets (Demulen, Enovid, Norlestrin, Ortho-Novum, Ovral, Provest)
    b. Sequential contraceptives were also used but have been removed from the market because of adverse effects

RELATED PROCEDURES
Bilateral vasectomy

A. Definition
    1. A surgical procedure to produce sterilization in men; often performed on an outpatient basis
    2. A small incision is made into the scrotum, and the vas deferens is ligated
B. Nursing responsibilities
    1. Explain possible complications to patient, such as bruising, edema, mild discomfort
    2. Explain the possibility of residual fertility; sterility is not achieved until semen is sperm free (there will be sperm in semen past the point of ligation following a vasectomy)

Tubal ligation

A. Definition
    1. A surgical procedure to produce sterilization in women; generally performed in the hospital
    2. A laparoscope is introduced through a small incision in the abdominal wall; an electric current is passed through forceps grasping the tubes to cause coagulation of the tissue
B. Nursing responsibilities
    1. Observe incision for signs of swelling or hemorrhage and report to physician
    2. Explain to patient that effects of procedure are immediate and that hormonal function is not altered

MAJOR DISEASES
Prostatitis

A. Etiology and pathophysiology
    1. Generally the result of urethritis
    2. The prostate gland becomes swollen and tender
B. Signs and symptoms
    1. Subjective
        a. Difficult urination
        b. Pain
    2. Objective
        a. Fever
        b. Hematuria

C. Treatment
    1. Antibiotics or chemotherapeutics
    2. Application of heat
D. Nursing care
    1. Administer antibiotics
    2. Apply heat as ordered
        a. Sitz baths
        b. Rectal irrigations
    3. Encourage fluids

Cancer of the prostate

A. Etiology and pathophysiology
    1. Slow, malignant change in the prostate gland
    2. Tends to spread by direct invasion of surrounding tissues and metastases to the bony pelvis and spine
B. Signs and symptoms
    1. Subjective
        a. Frequency and urgency
        b. Difficulty initiating stream
    2. Objective
        a. Decreased force of stream
        b. Urinary retention
        c. Elevated serum acid phosphatase
C. Treatment
    1. The type of surgical intervention depends on the extent of the lesion, the physical condition of the patient, and the patient's full awareness of the outcome (impotency follows radical prostatectomy)
    2. Radical prostatectomy, done by perineal or retropubic approach, removing the seminal vesicles and a portion of the bladder neck
    3. Radiation therapy alone or in conjunction with surgery may be ordered preoperatively or postoperatively to reduce the lesion and limit metastases
    4. Diethylstilbestrol (estrogen) may be ordered to reduce the size of inoperable lesions or postoperatively to limit metastases
    5. Orchiectomy may be done to limit production of testosterone
D. Nursing care
    1. Nursing care is similar to care of patient with a prostatectomy for benign prostatic hypertrophy
    2. Explain to patient that development of secondary female sexual characteristics will occur and is a result of the medication and not the surgery
    3. Allow time and opportunity for patient to express feelings about impotence

4. Support patient's male image
5. Explain situation to patient's family and include them in planning
6. Assist patient and family in dealing with diagnosis of cancer

Epididymitis

A. Etiology and pathophysiology
1. An acute or chronic inflammation of the epididymis
2. Occurs as a sequela of urinary tract infections, venereal disease, prostatitis
B. Signs and symptoms
1. Subjective
   a. Chills
   b. Scrotal pain
   c. Groin pain
2. Objective
   a. Fever
   b. Edema
   c. Elevated WBC
   d. Pyuria and bacteriuria
C. Treatment
1. Medication to control pain, fever, and infection
2. Scrotal support to facilitate drainage
3. Notification of the Department of Health if venereal disease is present
D. Nursing care
1. Maintain patient in restful state
2. Explain to patient the importance of good hygiene practices
3. Encourage fluid intake
4. Ascertain contacts if due to venereal disease
5. Teach to protect self from contracting venereal disease by use of a condom

Benign prostatic hypertrophy

A. Etiology and pathophysiology
1. Slow enlargement of the prostate gland common in men over 40 years of age
2. Constriction of urethra and subsequent interference in urination
B. Signs and symptoms
1. Subjective
   a. Frequency and urgency
   b. Difficulty initiating stream
2. Objective
   a. Decreased force of stream
   b. Nocturia
   c. Total urinary retention

C. Treatment
1. Reestablish emptying of bladder by ordering a hot bath to induce voiding or by inserting an indwelling catheter or a cystotomy tube
2. Urinary antiseptics and medications for reduction of pain and anxiety
3. Have patient prepared for surgical removal of prostate gland by means of a suprapubic, transurethral, perineal, or retropubic prostatectomy
4. Postoperatively, maintain drainage; force fluids; medicate for pain; antibiotics and stool softeners
D. Nursing care
1. Observe for or initiate measures to maintain patency of catheters
2. Irrigate catheters as ordered
3. Encourage increased fluid intake (2400 to 3000 ml/day)
4. Use sterile technique when necessary; e.g., insertion of urinary catheter, irrigations, dressing changes
5. Maintain integrity of closed drainage systems
6. Administer antiseptics, bacteriostatics, and antibiotics as ordered
7. In acute urinary retention, decompress the bladder slowly via Foley catheter (not more than 800 to 1200 ml at a time) to prevent shock and hematuria
8. Observe for signs of hemorrhage; e.g., change in vital signs, nature of drainage, pain, symptoms of shock, frank bleeding
9. Avoid postoperative complications by encouraging patient to deep breathe and cough and to exercise muscles in lower extremities
10. Teach patient preoperatively what can be expected postoperatively; e.g., presence of catheters, bloody drainage, bladder spasms, pain
11. Accept and encourage patient to express concerns about sexual functioning
12. Provide patient as much privacy as possible
13. Administer medication for pain as ordered

Cancer of the cervix

A. Etiology and pathophysiology
1. Slow, malignant change in the tissue forming the neck of the uterus (cervix)
2. Most common form of genital tract malignancy in women
3. High cure rate when diagnosed early
4. Tends to spread by direct invasion of surrounding

tissues and metastases to the lungs, bones, and liver

B. Signs and symptoms
1. Subjective
   a. Back pain
   b. Leg pain
2. Objective
   a. Spotting after intercourse
   b. Vaginal discharge
   c. Lengthening of menstrual period
   d. Papanicolaou cytologic finding of Class V is considered conclusive of cervical cancer; Papanicolaou cytologic findings of Class I, II, III, or IV require further studies before a conclusive diagnosis can be determined

C. Treatment
1. The type of surgical intervention depends on the extent of lesion and the physical condition of the patient
2. Hysterosalpingo-oophorectomy (panhysterectomy) to remove total uterus, fallopian tubes, and ovaries is usually done; in advanced lesions the parametrial tissue and lymph nodes may also be removed
3. A simple hysterectomy is done when preserving ovarian function is desirable
4. Radiation therapy alone or in conjunction with surgery may be ordered to reduce the lesion and limit metastases

D. Nursing care
1. Assist patient and family in dealing with diagnosis of cancer
2. Allow and encourage patient to express feelings and concerns about change in self-image and sexual functioning
3. Support patient's feminine image
4. If patient is receiving or is to receive internal radiation therapy
   a. Explain the side effects that may occur and the procedures involved, especially the need for isolation during treatment
   b. Instruct patient in maintaining proper positioning (supine and side-lying)
   c. Inspect implant for proper position
   d. Provide low-residue diet and prevent bowel and urinary distention to avoid displacement of radioactive substance and irradiation of adjacent tissues
   e. Explain to patient and family that visitors and

staff will be limited in the amount of time they can spend in the room to avoid their overexposure to radiation
5. If patient has surgical intervention
   a. Maintain patency of urinary catheter that has been inserted prior to surgery to decompress bladder and reduce stress on operative site
   b. Observe for reestablishment of bowel sounds
   c. Maintain accurate intake and output
   d. Following removal of urinary catheter, note amount of output and pattern of voiding; catheterize for residual urine if ordered and whenever necessary for urinary retention
   e. For additional nursing responsibilities, see postoperative care

Vaginitis

A. Etiology and pathophysiology
1. Trichomoniasis—an overgrowth of *Trichomonas vaginalis,* which normally is present in the vagina
2. Candidiasis (moniliasis)—caused by *Candida albicans,* a fungus; incidence is high in patients with diabetes mellitus and those receiving antibiotic therapy because of change in normal flora
3. Atrophic vaginitis—common in women in the postmenopausal period because the atrophied vaginal mucosa is prone to infection

B. Signs and symptoms
1. Subjective
   a. Pruritus, burning
   b. Dyspareunia (pain during intercourse)
2. Objective
   a. Vaginal discharge
      (1) Malodorous, thin yellow discharge (trichomoniasis)
      (2) White "cheesy" discharge (moniliasis)
   b. Vaginal smear can indicate *Trichomonas vaginalis, Candida albicans,* or other microorganisms

C. Treatment
1. Douches (acetic acid may be added)
2. Antifungal preparations for candidiasis
   a. Nystatin (Mycostatin) vaginal suppositories
   b. Propionic acid gel inserted vaginally
   c. Gentian violet applied to vaginal mucosa and cervix
3. Antiprotozoan preparations for trichomoniasis
   a. Metronidazole (Flagyl) tablets taken orally

b. Furazolidone-nifuroxime (Tricofuron) vaginal suppositories

4. Estrogen therapy prescribed for atrophic vaginitis

D. Nursing care

1. Advise patient to have sexual partner use condom during coitus until vaginitis is resolved

2. Explain to patient that frequent douching will alter the normal pH environment of the vagina, predisposing the individual to vaginitis

3. Instruct patient to use tampons to prevent discharge from irritating vulvar area

4. Administer douche if ordered

a. Explain procedure to patient; provide privacy

b. Assemble equipment, including douche can, tip, bedpan, gloves, waterproof pads, and solution at 45° C (110° F) (30 ml of vinegar may be added to a liter of solution for acetic solution; alkaline solutions should never be utilized)

c. Assist patient onto bedpan while maintaining privacy

d. Wearing gloves, separate the labia and insert the tip into the vagina

e. Rotate the douche tip gently so that the solution reaches all vaginal folds

f. When all solution is used, instruct the patient to bear down to expel as much remaining solution as possible; solution returns during entire procedure

g. Dry the perineal area gently

h. Resterilize nondisposable equipment

Endometriosis

A. Etiology and pathophysiology

1. Refers to the growth of endometrial cells in areas outside the uterus

2. Generally affects young nulliparous women

3. The endometrial cells are stimulated by the ovarian hormones and will cause bleeding during the normal menstrual cycle

4. Adhesions are common and may be the cause of sterility

5. Adenomyosis is a similar condition affecting women 40 to 50 years old in which the endometrial cells invade the muscles of the uterus

B. Signs and symptoms

1. Subjective

a. Lower abdominal pain beginning 2 to 7 days prior to menstruation becoming progressively worse and then diminishing as the menstrual flow decreases

b. Dyspareunia

c. Pain associated with defecation

2. Objective

a. Abnormal uterine bleeding (metrorrhagia, menorrhagia)

b. Infertility

C. Treatment

1. Hormone therapy to suppress ovulation; young married women are advised not to delay pregnancy if children are desired

2. Surgical intervention

a. Resection of lesions

b. Oophorectomy, salpingectomy, and total hysterectomy if condition is severe

D. Nursing care

1. Provide patient with as much privacy as possible

2. Explain procedures to patient

3. Ascertain patient's understanding of risks of sterility

4. Provide patient time to talk about feelings

5. Administer analgesics as ordered

6. Observe for hemorrhage; e.g., check for signs of shock, vaginal bleeding; check vaginal packing

7. Check patient's output; make certain patient is emptying bladder

8. Routine preoperative and postoperative care if surgery is necessary

Pelvic inflammatory disease (PID)

A. Etiology and pathophysiology

1. An inflammatory disease within the female pelvic cavity that can affect the fallopian tubes (salpingitis), the ovaries (oophoritis), and peritoneum, surrounding connective tissue, and pelvic veins

2. May be acute or chronic, bilateral or unilateral

3. Caused by introduction of bacteria (usually through the cervical opening) such as gonococci, streptococci, or tubercle bacillus that are transported by the blood from the lungs

4. If untreated, can lead to adhesions and sterility

B. Signs and symptoms

1. Subjective

a. Severe cramping pain in lower abdomen

b. Nausea

c. Malaise

d. Dysmenorrhea, dypareunia

2. Objective

a. Temperature elevation
b. Foul-smelling, purulent vaginal discharge
c. Elevated WBC
d. Cultures of vaginal discharge reveal causative organism

C. Treatment
1. Medication to control pain and fever
2. Specific antibiotics depending on the organism identified
3. Identify and notify sexual contacts and Department of Health if venereal disease is present

D. Nursing care
1. Maintain the patient on bed rest in semi-Fowler's position to localize the infection and prevent the fomation of abscesses within the abdominal cavity
2. Apply heat if ordered to abdomen or via douche to improve circulation
3. Observe and record amount and character of vaginal discharge
4. Change perineal pads frequently using gloves; tampons should not be used
5. Explain safety measures to prevent reinfection to patient or others; during acute phase patient should abstain from intercourse
6. Provide psychologic support because of the social aspects of venereal disease

Vaginal fistula

A. Etiology and pathophysiology
1. An abnormal opening between two organs
2. May be congenital or occur as a result of carcinoma or radiation therapy
3. Types
   a. Rectovaginal fistula is an opening between the vagina and uterus
   b. Vesicovaginal fistula refers to an opening between the vagina and bladder
   c. Ureterovaginal fistula is an opening between the vagina and a ureter

B. Signs and symptoms
1. Subjective
   a. Burning sensation
   b. Frequency of urination (if secondary urinary tract infection)
2. Objective
   a. Discharge of urine, feces, or flatus from the vagina
   b. Excoriation of vaginal mucosa
   c. Odor

C. Treatment
1. Dietary modification including high-protein, low-residue diet with vitamin supplement
2. Enemas, bladder irrigations, and douches using antibiotic solutions
3. Fistulas may be repaired surgically

D. Nursing care
1. Provide psychologic support, since patient may be embarrassed by odor and drainage and become withdrawn
2. Provide privacy during any treatments
3. Change pads frequently; sitz baths and irrigations to maintain cleanliness of area
4. Observe drainage and perineum for signs of inflammation
5. Assess urine for signs of infection; maintain patency of drainage tubes
6. Monitor temperature as indication of secondary infection

Cystocele and rectocele

A. Etiology and pathophysiology
1. Cystocele is the herniation of the bladder into the vagina
2. Rectocele refers to herniation of the rectum into the vagina
3. Both conditions may be present at the same time and are generally associated with relaxation or injury of the pelvic muscles during childbirth

B. Signs and symptoms
1. Subjective
   a. Feeling of fullness in vagina
   b. Constant urge to defecate
   c. Dysuria
2. Objective
   a. Soft reducible mass evident during vaginal examination that increases when patient is asked to bear down
   b. Stress incontinence
   c. Residual urine (60 ml or more after voiding)

C. Treatment
1. Anterior colporrhaphy to correct a cystocele
2. Posterior colporrhaphy to correct a rectocele

D. Nursing care
1. Encourage voiding every 4 hours to prevent strain on suture line from a distended bladder (no more than 150 ml should accumulate)
2. If patient has difficulty voiding, insert a Foley catheter if ordered
3. After each bowel movement and voiding, cleanse

the perineum with warm normal saline and sterile cotton balls; always cleanse away from the vagina and toward the rectum
4. Administer douches if ordered; include patient instruction
5. Apply heat lamp, anesthetic spray, or ice packs if ordered to relieve discomfort
6. Limit diet to liquids for first 5 days to avoid defecation and prevent strain on suture line
7. Administer medications to decrease GI motility if ordered
8. Administer cathartics and an oil-retention enema using a thin rectal tube if prescribed

Prolapsed uterus

A. Etiology and pathophysiology
   1. As a result of weakness of the pelvic floor, the uterus descends into the vagina; most often associated with childbirth
   2. If the prolapse is severe, the entire uterus may protrude outside the vaginal orifice; in this case, the vagina is actually inverted; referred to as procidentia
   3. Ulcerations in procidentia increase risk of cancer
B. Signs and symptoms
   1. Subjective
      a. Heaviness within the pelvis
      b. Low back pain
      c. Incontinence
   2. Objective
      a. Mass in lower vagina or outside orifice
      b. Elongated cervix
      c. Urinary retention
C. Treatment
   1. A vaginal pessary to maintain the uterus in correct position
   2. Surgical intervention
      a. Suspension of the uterus and correction of retroversion
      b. Hysterectomy (if postmenopausal)
D. Nursing care
   1. Encourage women to seek medical assistance if there is a prolapsed uterus
   2. If procidentia is present, observe for ulcerations; apply warm saline compresses or protective ointment to prevent ulceration
   3. Explain to patient that if pessary is used, it must be taken out by the physician frequently and cleaned

4. Observe color, amount, and frequency of urination
5. See section on cancer of the cervix for postoperative care

Carcinoma of the breast

A. Etiology and pathophysiology
   1. The tumor frequently begins as a hard, nontender, relatively fixed nodule found most often in the upper outer quadrant of the breast
   2. Metastasis by direct extension to surrounding tissue and via lymph and blood to axillary nodes, lungs, bone, brain, and liver
   3. Incidence increases with age and is influenced by heredity and the number of menstrual cycles a woman has had; multiparas and women with early menopause have a lower incidence, as do Japanese women
   4. Paget's carcinoma is a type of breast cancer that invades the nipple and milk ducts
B. Signs and symptoms
   1. Subjective
      a. Lesion is generally *non*tender
      b. Malaise in later stages
   2. Objective
      a. Dimpling of skin by lesion
      b. Inversion and discharge from nipple
      c. Changes in color of breast over lesion; in late stages skin has orange peel appearance
      d. Enlarged axillary lymph nodes
      e. Positive findings in following tests
         (1) Mammography, an x-ray examination of of the breast, is indicated when there is an increased risk of developing breast cancer
         (2) Thermography uses a heat-sensing device to evaluate abnormal circulatory signs
         (3) Xerography, in which a special x-ray plate subjected to an electric charge images all breast tissue
         (4) Biopsy for microscopic evaluation
            (a) Aspiration of tissue by syringe
            (b) Excised tissue may be sent to the laboratory for a frozen section from which thin slices are examined
C. Treatment
   1. The type of surgical and medical intervention depends on the extent of the lesion and the physical condition of the patient

2. Surgical intervention
   a. Lumpectomy—removal of lump and a fourth to a third of breast (only used for early, minute, peripheral lesions)
   b. Simple mastectomy—removal of breast only
   c. Radical mastectomy—removal of breast, pectoral muscles, pectoral fascia, and nodes (pectoral, subclavicular, apical, and axillary); this procedure may be modified
   d. An oophorectomy, adrenalectomy, and/or a hypophysectomy may be done to control metastases
3. Radiation therapy alone or in conjunction with surgery may be ordered preoperatively or postoperatively to reduce the lesion and limit metastases
4. Estrogen may be ordered for postmenopausal women; androgens for premenopausal women; corticosteroids (prednisone) used for those patients with metastases to brain or liver
5. Chemotherapy
   a. Alkylating agents
      (1) Cyclophosphamide (Cytoxan)
      (2) Chlorambucil (Leukeran)
      (3) Triethylenethiophosphoramide (Thio-TEPA)
   b. Antimetabolites
      (1) 5-fluorouracil (5-FU, Fluorouracil)
      (2) Methotrexate (Amethopterin, MTX)
   c. Other drugs
      (1) Adriamycin (Doxorubicin)
      (2) Vincristine (Oncovin)

D. Nursing care
1. Encourage and instruct concerning monthly breast examination
   a. Inspect while patient is setting with hand at sides and then overhead for retraction of nipple, dimpling of skin, color change, and asymmetry
   b. Palpate axillary and supraclavicular nodes
   c. Palpate breast tissue using circular pattern when patient is lying down with arm abducted
   d. Examine after each menstrual cycle because premenstrual hormones can cause harmless nodules that will disappear after menses
2. Assist patient and family to cope with diagnosis of cancer and altered body image by encouraging them to talk with staff and with each other
3. Administer medication for pain as ordered

4. Listen and accept patient's anger and depression and do not attempt to minimize it
5. Assist patient to identify feelings and encourage discussion of them
6. Support patient's feminine image
7. If patient is receiving cobalt therapy or antineoplastic drugs, inform, explain, and assist the patient to accept the side effects that may occur; e.g., nausea, vomiting, hair loss, anorexia, diarrhea, stomatitis, malaise, itching
8. If surgery is performed
   a. Observe for hemorrhage by checking all areas of the dressing, the drainage unit, and vital signs
   b. Maintain functioning of portable vacuum drainage unit by ensuring patency of tube, emptying when necessary, and supporting to avoid tension at site of insertion
   c. Encourage good posture and provide assistance with ambulation until patient adjusts to altered balance
   d. Prevent or reduce lymphedema by elevating and supporting hand above elbow and elbow above shoulder
   e. Instruct patient with radical mastectomy to avoid carrying heavy articles with affected arm and to avoid cuts or bruises, having blood drawn, injections, or blood pressure readings in affected arm because of impaired lymphatic drainage
   f. Encourage active exercises of affected arm beginning gradually the day after surgery if approved by physician
      (1) Wall hand climbing
      (2) Brushing hair
      (3) Turning rope
   g. Instruct patient as to types of prostheses and where to obtain them; cotton covered by gauze may be used to fill a patient's bra until she is seen by a professional fitter
   h. Use agencies such as Reach for Recovery to help patient with physical and emotional readjustment
9. If patient is receiving radiation therapy
   a. Observe for signs of radiation burns (erythema, desquamation)
   b. Avoid removal of skin markings drawn by the radiologist
   c. Instruct patient to use only ointments or emollients prescribed by physician

Venereal disease

A. Etiology and pathophysiology
1. Venereal diseases are transmitted by sexual contact
2. As a result of changing sexual habits, incidence of these diseases has increased and infections of the rectum and pharynx are common
3. Examples
   a. Syphilis, caused by the spirochete *Treponema pallidum*
   b. Gonorrhea, caused by the bacterium *Neisseria gonorrhoeae*
   c. Herpesvirus type 2 may also cause genital infections
4. During childbirth, infant may acquire gonococcal ophthalmia neonatorum; 1% silver nitrate solution is instilled into the infant's eyes at birth to prevent blindness
5. The organisms are inactivated easily if exposed to dryness, refrigeration, or other harsh environments

B. Signs and symptoms
1. Syphilis
   a. Primary (10 days to 3 months)
      (1) Chancre on genitalia, mouth, or anal canal
      (2) Serous drainage from chancre
      (3) Enlarged lymph nodes
      (4) Positive tests for syphilis (VDRL, Kolmer, or Wasserman can be used)
   b. Secondary (2 weeks to 6 months after chancre heals)
      (1) Skin lesions on palms and feet
      (2) Erosions of oral mucous membrane
      (3) Condylomata lata, which are wartlike growths, may appear on the genitalia
      (4) Alopecia
      (5) Enlarged lymph nodes
   c. Latent
      (1) May remain asymptomatic for life
      (2) Positive laboratory tests for syphilis
   d. Tertiary (affects approximately one fourth of cases)
      (1) Gummas, which are granulomas, attack almost any organ and cause cardiovascular syphilis (aortitis and thoracic aortic aneurysms) and neurosyphilis (personality changes, ataxia, strokes, and blindness)
      (2) During this stage it is rare for an individual to infect another; a fetus can be infected

2. Gonorrhea
   a. Males
      (1) Symptoms begin within a few days after exposure
      (2) Discharge from penis, initially clear mucus progressing to purulent drainage
      (3) Dysuria
      (4) Urethral smear positive for gonococcus
      (5) If untreated, complications such as sterility, urethral stricture, prostatitis, and epididymitis
   b. Females
      (1) Purulent yellow vaginal discharge
      (2) Dysuria, urgency
      (3) Endocervical smear positive for gonococcus
      (4) May be asymptomatic
3. Herpes genitalia
   a. Subjective
      (1) Anorexia
      (2) Genital pain
      (3) Dysuria
   b. Objective
      (1) Vesicles and papules on genitalia
      (2) Leukorrhea
      (3) Vaginal bleeding
      (4) Cultures reveal herpesvirus type 2
      (5) Increased risk of neonatal death and spontaneous abortion
      (6) Possible carcinogen

C. Treatment
1. Identification of patient contacts; report all cases to Health Department
2. Antibiotics (in particular penicillin) used to cure syphilis and gonorrhea; herpes genitalia is treated only by supportive therapy
3. Abstention from sexual contact until determined to be noninfectious

D. Nursing care
1. Provide supportive nonjudgmental environment
2. Encourage use of early screening and educational program such as V.D. clinics, hot lines, and workshops
3. Explain to patient that careful cleansing of the genitals as well as the use of condoms helps prevent the transmission of venereal disease
4. Teach about the diseases and their transmission
5. Encourage fluids
6. Assess any genital discharge for color, amount, and consistency

Endocrine system

REVIEW OF ANATOMY AND PHYSIOLOGY OF THE ENDOCRINE SYSTEM
Functions

Endocrine glands secrete products called hormones, which are chemical messengers that deliver stimulatory or inhibitory signals to target cells (Table 2-4)

Glands

Thyroid gland
A. Anatomy
1. Soft, red-brown mass having right and left pear-shaped lobes joined by narrow isthmus
2. Extends from sides of cricoid and thyroid cartilages to sixth tracheal cartilage
3. Half of glands observed have a pyramidal lobe extending upward from the isthmus
B. Actions of thyroid hormones (Table 2-5)
1. Accelerate cellular reactions in most body cells
   a. Increase BMR
   b. Accelerate growth
   c. Metabolic rate of over 100 enzyme systems altered due to profound stimulatory effect of thyroid hormone on cellular protein synthesis
2. Thyroid hormones bind to nuclear and cytoplasmic receptor sites
   a. Intranuclear chromatin protein binds thyroid hormones; this stimulates cellular protein synthesis and influences growth, development, and cell differentiation
   b. Mitochondrial membranes bind thyroid hormones, which regulate energy metabolism
C. Metabolism (inactivation) of thyroid hormones
1. Liver is principal organ regulating blood concentration of thyroid hormones; thyroxine and triiodothyronine and deaminated, deiodinated, and conjugated; conjugates excreted in bile
2. Skeletal muscle, kidney, liver, and heart tissues deiodinate thyroid hormones; this mechanism of hormone inactivation not as important as conjugation in liver

Parathyroid glands
A. Anatomy—generally, 4 small yellow glands (but varies between 2 and 12) ¼ inch (0.6 cm) in diameter at their widest part, usually embedded in the capsule of the posterior part of the thyroid (but may be behind the pharynx or in the thorax with the thymus)

B. Actions of parathyroid hormones
1. Parathormone—major sites of action are skeleton, kidneys, and intestine
   a. Bone tissue releases Ca^{++} into blood (requires active form of vitamin D)
      (1) Osteoclastic osteolysis stimulated
      (2) Osteocytic osteolysis stimulated
      (3) Enhanced rate of maturation of precursor cells into osteoclasts and osteoblasts
      (4) Inhibition of osteoblastic collagen synthesis
   b. Kidney tubule reabsortion of Ca^{++} and Mg^{++} is enhanced which helps to prevent further decreases in serum Ca^{++} levels; enhanced excretion of K^+, P^{+++} and HCO_3^-; decreased excretion of H^+ and NH_4^+
   c. Parathormone, through adenylate cyclase activation, stimulates kidney's production of the enzyme that converts 25-dihydroxycholecalciferol into 1,25-hydroxycholecalciferol, which is the active form of vitamin D that works with parathormone in bone to mobilize Ca^{++}
   d. The intestinal mucosa increases its absorption of Ca^{++} and P^{+++} with subsequent release into the blood
2. Calcitonin
   a. Decreases loss of Ca^{++} from bone through inhibition of osteocytic and osteoclastic osteolysis (cAMP mechanism)
      (1) Action is opposite to that of parathormone
      (2) Some bone cells specifically respond to calcitonin; others specifically respond to parathormone
   b. Decreases loss of Ca^{++} from bone and promotes hypocalcemia; this effect offsets postprandial hypercalcemia

Testes
A. Anatomy—see Genitourinary system
B. Actions of testicular (androgenic) hormones
1. Major androgenic action in target tissues is stimulation of protein synthesis through enhancement of nuclear DNA and RNA
2. Increased protein synthesis manifests itself as increased tissue growth, particularly in younger individuals; at puberty, rise in androgen level induces growth of long bones, muscular development, enlargement of the external genitalia, increased sex drive, laryngeal growth, and growth of body hair

Table 2-4. Location and hormones of endocrine glands

Endocrine gland	Location	Hormones
Anterior pituitary (adenohypophysis)	Cranial cavity, in sella turcica of sphenoid bone	Growth hormone (GH, somatotropin, somatropic hormone, STH)* Thyrotropin (thyroid-stimulating hormone, or TSH) Adrenocorticotropic hormone (ACTH, corticotropin)* Follicle-stimulating hormone (FSH) Luteinizing hormone (LH) in female; interstitial cell–stimulating hormone (ICSH) in male Prolactin (lactogenic hormone, luteotropin) Melanocyte-stimulating hormone (MSH) Alpha and beta lipotropins
Posterior pituitary (neurohypophysis)	In sella turcica of sphenoid bone	Antidiuretic hormone (ADH, vasopressin [Pitressin])† Oxytocin
Pineal	Midbrain	Melatonin
Thyroid	Overlays the thyroid cartilage below the larynx	Thyroid hormones (thyroxine and triiodothyronine) Calcitonin
Parathyroids	Usually 4 beads on posterior wall of the thyroid	Parathormone Calcitonin
Thymus	Root of neck and anterior thorax	Thymosin‡
Adrenal cortex	Rest upon the medial anterior surface of the kidney	Glucocorticoids (mainly cortisol and corticosterone) Mineralocorticoids (mainly aldosterone) Sex hormones (small amounts of androgens and estrogens)
Adrenal medulla		Epinephrine (mainly) Norepinephrine
Pancreas (islets of Langerhans)	Retroperitoneal in abdominal cavity	Insulin (secreted by beta cells) Glucagon (secreted by alpha cells) Somatostatin Pancreatic polypeptide

Ovaries
   Graafian follicles
   Corpus luteum
 Testes
   Interstitial cells of testes
	Pelvic cavity (female)
	
	 Scrotum (male)
		
		 Estrogens (estradiol, estrone)
		 Progesterone
		
		 Testosterone

*Also present in placenta along with estrogens and progesterone.
†ADH and oxytocin are synthesized in the hypothalamus but are secreted by the posterior pituitary gland. Synthesis occurs in cell bodies of neurons of the supraoptic and paraventricular nuclei. From here they migrate down the neurons' axons into the posterior pituitary gland, which secretes them into the blood.
‡One of several active thymic hormones.

Table 2-5. Functions of thyroid and parathyroid hormones

Hormones	Functions	Hypofunction effects	Hyperfunction effects
Thyroid hormones Thyroxine Triiodothyronine	Stimulate metabolic rate; therefore essential for normal physical and mental development Inhibit anterior pituitary secretion of TSH	Cretinism, if occurs early in life; myxedema, if occurs in older children or adults	Hyperthyroidism
Thyrocalcitonin	Quickly decreases blood calcium concentration if it increases about 20% above normal level; presumably accelerates calcium movement from blood into bone		
Parathyroid hormone Parathormone	Increases blood calcium concentration by accelerating following three processes:	Decreased blood calcium (hypocalcemia), which causes increased neural excitability and tetany	Increased blood calcium (hypercalcemia), which causes decreased neural excitability and muscle weakness Bone "softening"—decalcification
	1. Breakdown of bone with release of calcium into blood 2. Calcium absorption from intestine into blood 3. Kidney tubule reabsorption of calcium from tubular urine into blood, thereby decreasing calcium loss in urine		
	Decreases blood phosphate concentration by slowing its reabsorption by kidney tubules and thereby increasing phosphate loss in urine	Increased blood phosphorus (hyperphosphatemia)	Hypophosphatemia

3. Androgens influence fetal brain development through contributing to establishment of neural pathways that help to regulate adult brain functions and behavior

C. Metabolism of androgens
  1. Liver is major site for adrogen metabolism: testosterone and other androgenic steroids are enzymatically converted into other less androgenic steroids and then conjugated with glucuronic acid or sulfate
  2. The generally biologically inactive conjugates are excreted in bile and urine

Ovaries

A. Anatomy—see Genitourinary system
B. Actions of ovarian hormones
  1. Estrogens
    a. Enter target cells, bind cycloplasmic receptors, and enter nucleus; estrogen receptor complex regulates mRNA synthesis with overall effect of stimulating cellular RNA and protien synthesis
    b. Stimulate uterine and liver lipid metabolism
    c. Stimulate long bone calcification
    d. Play major role in ovulatory—menstrual cycle
    e. Increased protein and lipid synthesis are manifested in the reproductive system as uterine growth
    f. Other estrogenic effects associated with secondary sexual characteristics—growth of pubic and axillary hair, pelvic enlargement, subcutaneous lipid distribution, growth of mammary glands, and maturation of skin (increased glandular activity)
  2. Progesterone
    a. Increases mucus secretory activity of endometrium; such action required for implantation of young embryo
    b. Promotes growth of breasts
    c. Keeps uterine smooth muscle quiescent during pregnancy
    d. Inhibits oxytocin release by neurohypophysis (otherwise released in response to vaginal distention)

C. Metabolism of estrogens and progesterone

Table 2-6. Sex hormones (ovarian and testicular)

Hormones	Functions
Estrogens (secreted by graafian follicle and corpus luteum) 　Estradiol 　Estrone 　Estriol	Stimulate proliferation of epithelial cells of female reproductive organs; e.g., thickening of endometrium, breast development Stimulate uterine contractions Accelerate protein anabolism (including bone matrix synthesis) so promote growth; but also promote epiphyseal closure so limit height Mildly accelerate sodium and water reabsorption by kidney tubules; increase water content of uterus High blood estrogen concentration inhibits anterior pituitary secretion of FSH and prolactin but stimulates its secretion of LH Low blood estrogen concentration after delivery of baby stimulates anterior pituitary secretion of prolactin
Progesterone (secreted by corpus luteum and placenta)	Name "progesterone" indicates hormone's general function, "favoring pregnancy," e.g.: 　Stimulates secretion by endometrial glands, thereby preparing endometrium for implantation of fertilized ovum 　Inhibits uterine contractions, thereby favoring retention of implanted embryo 　Promotes development of alveoli (secreting cells) of estrogen-primed breasts; necessary for lactation 　Protein-catabolic and salt- and water-retaining effects similar to corticoids but milder; increases water content of endometrium
Testosterone (secreted by interstitial cells of testes)	Growth and development of male reproductive organs; promotes "maleness" Marked stimulating effect on protein anabolism, including synthesis of bone matrix and muscular development, hence, promotes growth; however, it also tends to limit height by promoting epiphyseal closure Mild acceleration of kidney tubule reabsorption of sodium chloride and water Inhibits secretion of ICSH by anterior pituitary

1. Liver conjugates estrogens with glucuronic and sulfuric acids; conjugates are excreted chiefly in urine
2. Conversion of estradiol to the less active estrone in the liver; placenta also carries out this conversion
3. Liver converts progesterone, synthesized from cholesterol in corpus luteum, placenta, and adrenals, to pregnanediol, which is then conjugated with glucuronic acid or sulfate; conjugates are excreted in urine

Adrenal glands
A. Anatomy
　1. Wedge-shaped, flattened, yellowish structures positioned like caps at the kidney's superior border
　2. Each adrenal gland actually two closely associated structures—the inner adrenal medulla and outer adrenal cortex; medulla and cortex each produce hormones with distinct effects on distant target structures
　3. Adrenal medulla produces two catecholamines, D-epinephrine and D-norepinephrine, in approximate ratio of 80% to 20%, respectively
　4. Adrenal cortex secretes three steroid hormones in relatively large amounts; aldosterone, a mineralocorticoid, and cortisol (hydrocortisone) and corticosterone, both glucocorticoids; also small amounts of several androgenic steroids; adrenocortical secretion is circadian with higher levels produced during daytime; aldosterone secretion increases as Na^+ decreases or K^+ increases
B. Actions of adrenal hormones
　1. Epinephrine and norepinephrine
　　a. Stimulate liver and skeletal muscle to break down glycogen
　　b. Increase O_2 utilization and increase CO_2 production

Table 2-7. Functions of adrenal cortex hormones

Hormones	Functions	Hypofunction effects (e.g., in Addison's disease)	Hyperfunction effects (e.g., in Cushing's syndrome)
Glucocorticoids, mainly cortisol (hydrocortisone) and corticosterone	In general, a normal blood concentration of glucocorticoids promotes normal metabolism of all three kinds of foods and a high blood concentration produces various stress responses, e.g.: Accelerates mobilization and catabolism of fats; i.e., causes shift from usual utilization of carbohydrates for energy to fat utilization		
	Accelerates tissue protein mobilization and catabolism (tissue proteins hydrolyzed to amino acids, which enter blood and are carried to liver for deamination and gluconeogenesis)		Muscle atrophy and weakness; osteoporosis
	Accelerates liver gluconeogenesis; i.e., formation of glucose from mobilized proteins (hyperglycemic effect)		Hyperglycemia
	Causes atrophy of lymphatic tissues, notably thymus and lymph nodes		Lymphocytopenia
	Decreases antibody formation (immunosuppressive, antiallergic effect)		Decreased immunity Decreased allergy
	Slows the proliferation of fibroblasts characteristic of inflammation (antiinflammatory effect)		Spread of infections; slower wound healing
	Mild acceleration of sodium and water reabsorption and potassium excretion by kidney tubules		High blood sodium (hypernatremia; sodium retention); also water retention; low blood potassium (hypokalemia)
	Decreases ACTH secretion		
Mineralocorticoids, mainly aldosterone	Marked acceleration of sodium and water reabsorption by kidney tubules	Low blood sodium (hyponatremia); dehydration	High blood sodium (hypernatremia); water retention, edema
	Marked acceleration of potassium excretion by kidney tubules	High blood potassium (hyperkalemia)	Low blood potassium (hypokalemia)

c. Increase blood concentration of free fatty acids through stimulation of lipolysis in adipose tissue
d. Cause constriction of nearly all blood vessels of body, thereby greatly increasing total peripheral resistance and arterial pressure
e. Increase heart rate and force of contraction and thereby raise cardiac output
f. Epinephrine significantly dilates bronchial smooth muscle

g. Inhibit contractions of gastrointestinal and uterine smooth muscle
2. Glucocorticoids and mineralocorticoids (Table 2-7)
C. Metabolism of adrenocortical steroids
1. Liver is major organ metabolizing adrenal steroids
2. Conjugation of steroids with glucuronic acid or sulfate produces inactive products primarily excreted in urine
3. In liver disease, adrenal steroids rise in concentration in blood due to decreased inactivation

Table 2-8. Functions of anterior pituitary hormones

Hormones	Functions	Hyposecretion effects	Hypersecretion effects
Growth hormone (GH)	Promotes protein anabolism (hence essential for normal growth) Promotes fat mobilization and catabolism; i.e., causes shift from carbohydrate catabolism to fat catabolism Slows carbohydrate metabolism; has anti-insulin, hyperglycemic, diabetogenic effect (promotes glucagon secretion)	Dwarfism (well-formed type) if it occurs before skeletal growth is completed Simmonds' disease after skeletal maturity	Giantism if it occurs before skeletal growth is completed) Acromegaly (if occurs after skeletal maturity) Hyperglycemia; chronic excess GH may cause diabetes mellitus
TSH	Stimulates synthesis and secretion of thyroid hormones	Hypothyroidism: cretinism in early life, myxedema in adults	Hyperthyroidism (exophthalmic goiter, various other names)
ACTH	Stimulates adrenal cortex growth and secretion of glucocorticoids; slight mineralocorticoid stimulation	Atrophy of adrenal cortex and hyposecretion (e.g., Addison's disease) Increased skin pigmentation	Hypertrophy of adrenal cortex and hypersecretion (Cushing's syndrome)
FSH	Stimulates primary graafian follicle to start growing and to develop to maturity Stimulates follicle cells to secrete estrogens In male, FSH stimulates development of seminiferous tubules and spermatogenesis by them	Failure of follicle and ovum to grow and mature; sterility	
LH	Essential for bringing about complete maturation of follicle and ovum Required for ovulation Causes formation of corpus luteum in ruptured follicle following ovulation; hence the name luteinizing hormone Stimulates corpus luteum to secrete progesterone In male, LH is called ICSH (interstitial cell–stimulating hormone) because it stimulates interstitial cells of testes to secrete testosterone		
Prolactin	Promotes breast development during pregnancy Initiates milk secretion after delivery of baby Stimulates progesterone secretion by corpus luteum	Failure to lactate	
Alpha and beta lipoproteins	Cause release of lipid from adipose cells		

Table 2-9. Functions of posterior pituitary hormones

Hormones	Functions	Hyposecretion effects	Hypersecretion effects
ADH (antidiuretic hormone; vasopressin)	Increases water reabsorption by kidney's distal and collecting tubules, thereby producing antidiuresis (less urine volume; name based on this effect) Stimulates vasoconstriction; raises blood pressure	Diuresis (polyuria); diabetes insipidus	Antidiuresis (oliguria)
Oxytocin	Stimulates powerful contractions by pregnant uterus Stimulates milk ejection from alveoli (milk-secreting cells) of lactating breasts into ducts; essential before milk can be removed by suckling		
Coherin	Regulates peristaltic rhythmicity in intestinal smooth muscle		
MSH (melanocyte-stimulating hormone)	Stimulates synthesis and dispersion of melanin in skin, causing darkening		

Pancreas
A. Anatomy (see Gastrointestinal system)
B. Actions of pancreatic hormones
 1. Regulate glucose homeostasis through action of insulin and glucagon; also secrete somatostatin and pancreatic polypeptide
 2. Insulin stimulates intracellular macromolecular syntheses, such as glycogen synthesis, protein synthesis, and lipogenesis
 3. Insulin stimulates cellular uptake of Na^+ and K^+ (latter is significant in that treatment of diabetic coma with insulin, and glucose also requires K^+ supplement to offset hypokalemia)
 4. Glucagon induces liver glycogenolysis similar to that produced by epinephrine, but glucagon functions at lower concentration and also does not raise blood pressure; antagonizes glycogen synthesis stimulated by insulin
 5. Glucagon inhibits hepatic protein synthesis; this makes amino acids available for gluconeogenesis and also increases urea production
 6. Glucagon stimulates hepatic ketogenesis and release of glycerol and fatty acids from adipose tissue
 7. Primary target organs are muscle, liver, and adipose cells, but other tissues also affected
 8. Somatostatin inhibits release of both insulin and glucagon
 9. Pancreatic polypeptide increases pancreatic and

gastric secretions; secreted into blood after a protein-rich meal; secretion inhibited by somatostatin

Thymus
A. Anatomy
 1. Soft, pink mass extending from lower border of thyroid to the fourth costal cartilages; great variation in size with its 2 lobes asymmetric
 2. Large at birth; decreases in size after puberty; hardly visible beyond middle age
B. Actions of thymic hormones
 1. Regulate immunologic processes possibly through regulation of the numbers and types of lymphoid cells; decrease in immune response; with aging, parallels thymus involution and decreasing blood concentrations of thymic hormones
 2. Just after birth, thymus produces specific lymphocytes that migrate to peripheral regions (e.g., lymph nodes, spleen) to provide immunologic potential
 3. Thymus synthesizes hormones that regulate the rate of development of lymphoid cells, particularly T cells

Pineal gland
A. Anatomy
 1. A firm, reddish, conical structure lying in the midbrain between the superior colliculi and attached by a short stalk to the roof of the third ventricle

2. Composed of cords of pinealocytes (or chief cells) separated by connective tissue; septa continuous with the pia mater covering the organ; cells accumulate calcareous granules (brain sand) by age 18 clearly visible by x-ray examination

B. Actions of pineal hormone
  1. Secretes melatonin
  2. Melatonin may regulate diurnal fluctuations of hypothalamic-hypophyseal hormones

Pituitary gland

A. Anatomy
  1. A rounded body ½ inch (1.2 cm) in diameter extending downward from the floor of the brain's third ventricle by a stalk (infundibulum); supported and protected by the sella turcica of the sphenoid bone; located near the optic chiasm
  2. Composed of anterior lobe (adenohypophysis) and posterior lobe (neurohypophysis)

B. Actions of pituitary hormones (Tables 2-8 and 2-9)

PHARMACOLOGY RELATED TO ENDOCRINE SYSTEM DISORDERS

A. Drugs that affect glucose assimilation
  1. General implications for nurses
    a. Administer all forms of insulin subcutaneously
    b. Use only regular insulin for intravenous administration
    c. When mixing insulins, draw regular insulin into the syringe first
    d. Rotate sites of administration
    e. Observe for adverse effects of each medication
  2. Insulin
    a. Action and types (Table 2-10)
      (1) Enables all tissues to utilize carbohydrates
      (2) Aids in metabolism of fat and protein
    b. Adverse effects
      (1) Irritability
      (2) Confusion
      (3) Convulsions
      (4) Tachycardia
      (5) Tremor
      (6) Moist skin
      (7) Headache
      (8) Hunger
  3. Oral hypoglycemic agents
    a. Action—stimulate pancreatic beta cells to pro-
duce insulin in adults with residual functioning cells
    b. Examples
      (1) Acetohexamide (Dymelor)
      (2) Chlorpropamide (Diabinese)
      (3) Tolazamide (Tolinase)
      (4) Tolbutamide (Orinase)
      (5) Phenformin hydrochloride (DBI)
    c. Adverse effects
      (1) Skin reactions
      (2) Jaundice
      (3) Pruritus
      (4) Possible arteriosclerotic disease
  4. Insulin antagonist
    a. Actions
      (1) Mobilizes glucose, which is stored in the liver
      (2) Stimulates gluconeogenesis from fats
    b. Example—glucagon
    c. Adverse effects
      (1) Nausea and vomiting
      (2) Circulatory collapse

B. Drugs that affect the thyroid gland
  1. General implications for nurses
    a. Anticipate that treatment is started in small doses and increased slowly
    b. Teach patient the importance of medical follow-up
    c. Observe patient for changes in weight, increased mental alertness, and improved condition of skin and hair
  2. Thyroid hormone substitutes
    a. Actions
      (1) Regulate the rate of metabolism in most cells
      (2) Aid in growth and development of bones and teeth
      (3) Affect protein, fat, and carbohydrate metabolism
    b. Examples
      (1) Levothyroxine sodium (Letter, Levoid, Synthroid)
      (2) Liothyronine sodium (Cytomel)
      (3) Thyroglobulin (Endothyrin, Proloid)
      (4) Thyroid (Thyrar)
    c. Adverse effects
      (1) Hyperactivity
      (2) Accelerated metabolism
  3. Antithyroid drugs

Table 2-10. Types of insulin

Insulin	Onset	Peak	Duration
Rapid acting			
Insulin injection (regular insulin)	½ to 1 hr	2 to 6 hr	5 to 8 hr
Prompt insulin zinc suspension (Semilente)	½ to 1 hr	3 to 9 hr	12 to 16 hr
Intermediate acting			
Globin zinc insulin injection	1 to 4 hr	6 to 16 hr	16 to 24 hr
Insulin zinc suspension (Lente)	1 to 4 hr	7 to 12 hr	24 to 30 hr
Isophane insulin suspension (NPH)	1 to 2 hr	7 to 12 hr	24 to 30 hr
Long acting			
Extended insulin zinc suspension (Ultralente)	4 to 8 hr	10 to 30 hr	34 to 46 hr
Protamine zinc insulin suspension (PZI)	1 to 8 hr	12 to 24 hr	30 to 36 hr

a. Inhibit oxidation of iodides to prevent their combination with tyrosine in formation of thyroxine
b. Examples
   (1) Methylthiouracil (Methiacil, Muracil)
   (2) Propylthiouracil
   (3) Methimazole (Tapazole)
c. Adverse effects
   (1) Hypothyroidism in fetus
   (2) Urticaria
   (3) Agranulocytosis
4. Strong Iodine Solution
  a. Actions
    (1) Makes the gland less vascular by producing an involution of an enlarged thyroid gland
    (2) Used preoperatively to decrease the risk of hemorrhage
  b. Example—Lugol's solution
  c. Adverse effects
    (1) Laryngeal edema
    (2) Hypersecretion of glands
    (3) Discoloration of teeth (administer diluted through straw)
C. Adrenocorticosteroids
  1. General implications for nurses
   a. Avoid infections
   b. Check patient for signs of other illnesses, since symptoms may be masked
   c. Monitor vital signs and weight

   d. Instruct patient to carry a card indicating medication prescribed
   e. Report symptoms of gastric distress
   f. Administer with antacids or milk
  2. Actions
   a. Play an important role in most of the metabolic processes in the body
   b. Anti-inflammatory effect aids the individual in coping with stress
   c. Alterations in the metabolism of protein, fat, and carbohydrates, as well as in fluid and electrolyte balance
  3. Examples
   a. Betamethasone valerate (Valisone)
   b. Corticotropin (ACTH, Cortigel)
   c. Dexamethasone (Decadron, Hexadrol)
   d. Fludrocortisone acetate (Florinef Acetate)
   e. Hydrocortisone (Cortef, Hydrocortone)
   f. Hydrocortisone succinate (Solu-Cortef)
   g. Methylprednisolone sodium succinate (Solu-Medrol)
   h. Prednisone
  4. Adverse effects
   a. Cushinglike symptoms
   b. Osteoporosis
   c. Hypertension
   d. Peptic ulcer
   e. Cataracts
   f. Delayed wound healing
   g. Euphoria, psychosis

D. Antidiuretic hormones from posterior pituitary
  1. General implications for nurses
    a. Observe for signs of dehydration
    b. Monitor intake and output
    c. If drug is administered to improve bladder or bowel tone, observe for continence or the passage of flatus
  2. Actions
    a. In general, this classification of medications is used in the treatment of diabetes insipidus, since it promotes water reabsorption by the distal renal tubules
    b. Vasopressin also causes vasoconstriction and increased muscle tone of the bladder, GI tract, uterus, and blood vessels
  3. Examples
    a. Lypressin (Diapid)—intranasal administration
    b. Vasopressin (Pitressin)
    c. Vasopressin tannate (Pitressin Tannate)
  4. Adverse effects
    a. Increased intestinal activity
    b. Hyponatremia
    c. Pallor
    d. Water intoxication

MAJOR DISEASES
Hyperpituitarism

A. Etiology and pathophysiology
  1. May occur due to overactivity of gland or as the result of an adenoma of the gland
  2. Characterized by an excessive concentration of pituitary hormones in the blood, overactivity, and changes in the anterior lobe of the pituitary gland
  3. There are two classifications of hyperpituitarism
    a. Giantism—generalized increase in size, especially in children; involves the long bones
    b. Acromegaly—occurs after epiphyseal closing with subsequent enlargement of cartilage, bone, and soft tissues of body
B. Signs and symptoms
  1. Subjective
    a. Headaches
    b. Depression
    c. Weakness
  2. Objective
    a. Increased soft tissue and bone thickness
    b. Facial features become coarse and heavy with enlargement of lower jaw, lips, and tongue
    c. Enlarged hands and feet

    d. Increased somatotropin serum levels
    e. X-ray films of long bones, skull (sella turcica area), and jaw demonstrate change in structure
    f. Amenorrhea
    g. Glycosuria
    h. Diabetes and hyperthyroidism may also occur
C. Treatment
  1. Medications to relieve symptoms of other endocrine imbalances resulting from pituitary hyperfunctioning
  2. Surgical intervention (hypophysectomy) or irradiation of the pituitary
D. Nursing care
  1. Assist patient to accept the altered body image that is irreversible
  2. Assist family to understand what the patient is experiencing
  3. Help patient to recognize that medical supervision will be required for duration of life
  4. Help patient to understand the basis for the change in sexual functioning
  5. Assist patient to express feelings
  6. If patient has hypophysectomy
    a. Encourage patient to follow established medical regimen
    b. Protect patient from stress situations
    c. Protect patient from infection
    d. Follow and maintain established schedule for hormone replacement
    e. Follow nursing care for patient undergoing intracranial surgery

Hypopituitarism (Simmonds' disease)

A. Etiology and pathophysiology
  1. Simmonds' disease is the total absence of pituitary hormones
  2. Hypopituitarism occurs when there is destruction of the anterior lobe of the gland by trauma, tumor, or hemorrhage
B. Signs and symptoms
  1. Subjective
    a. Lethargy
    b. Loss of strength
    c. Decreased tolerance for cold
  2. Objective
    a. Decreased temperature
    b. Decreased blood pressure
    c. Emaciation
    d. Diminished axillary and pubic hair

C. Treatment
  1. Replace hormones
  2. If tumor is present, surgical intervention is indicated
D. Nursing care
  1. Discuss the importance of adhering to medical regimen on long-term basis
  2. Allow patient ample time to verbalize feelings regarding the long-term nature of the disease

Diabetes insipidus

A. Etiology and pathophysiology
  1. Etiology is unknown, but it may occur as a result of head trauma, surgical ablation, or irradiation of gland and tumors
  2. Occurs when there is a deficiency of vasopressin (ADH), which is secreted by posterior pituitary
B. Signs and symptoms
  1. Subjective
     a. Polydipsia
     b. Craving for cold water
  2. Objective
     a. Polyuria (5 to 25 L/24 hours)
     b. Dilute urine; specific gravity 1.001 to 1.005
     c. Signs of dehydration (poor skin turgor, dry mucous membranes, elevated temperature)
C. Treatment
  1. Administer Pitressin Tannate, antidiuretic hormone
  2. Determine underlying cause and attempt to treat it
D. Nursing care
  1. Weigh patient daily
  2. Carefully monitor intake and output
  3. Replace fluid by mouth or parenteral route
  4. Check results of serum electrolytes evaluation
  5. Monitor specific gravity of urine

Hypothyroidism

A. Etiology and pathophysiology
  1. Absence or decreased production of thyroid hormone
  2. Classified according to the time of life in which it occurs
     a. Cretinism—hypothyroidism in infants and young children
     b. Hypothyroidism without myxedema—mild degree of thyroid failure in older children and adults
     c. Hypothyroidism with myxedema—severe degree of thyroid failure in older individuals
B. Signs and symptoms
  1. Subjective
     a. Dull mental processes
     b. Apathy
     c. Lethargy
     d. Intolerance to cold
  2. Objective
     a. Stolid masklike facies
     b. Increase in weight
     c. Constipation
     d. Subnormal temperature and pulse
     e. Dry brittle hair
     f. Thickened skin
     g. Enlarged tongue; drooling
     h. Decreased BMR
     i. Decreased T_4 and radioactive iodine uptake
C. Treatment
  1. Administer thyroid hormones
  2. Maintain vital functions
D. Nursing care
  1. Explain to patient and family the importance of continued use of medication
  2. Have patience with lethargic patient
  3. Teach patient and family to be alert for signs of complications: angina pectoris—chest pain, feeling of indigestion; cardiac failure—dyspnea, palpitations; myxedema coma—weakness, syncope, slow pulse rate, subnormal temperature, slow respirations, lethargy
  4. Teach patient to seek medical supervision on a regular basis and when any signs of illness develop
  5. Help patient and family to recognize that patient's inability to adapt to cold temperature requires the use of additional protection and modification of outdoor activity in cold weather
  6. Teach patient to avoid constipation by the use of adequate hydration and roughage in the diet

Hyperthyroidism (Graves' disease)

A. Etiology and pathophysiology
  1. An excessive concentration of thyroid hormones in the blood
  2. Overactivity and changes in the thyroid gland may be present
  3. May occur at periods of high physiologic and psychologic stress, although considered by some to be an autoimmune reaction

4. The gland may also enlarge (goiter) due to decreased iodine intake; no increase in secretion of thyroid is present

B. Signs and symptoms
  1. Subjective
    a. Polyphagia
    b. Emotional lability and apprehension
    c. Heat intolerance
  2. Objective
    a. Weight loss
    b. Increased systolic blood pressure and pulse
    c. Tremors
    d. Hyperhidrosis
    e. Increased respiratory rate
    f. Exophthalmos
    g. Increased BMR
    h. Increased radioactive thyroid uptake
    i. Increased T_3, T_4, and protein-bound iodine (PBI)
    j. Loose stools

C. Treatment
  1. Antithyroid medications such as propylthiouracil and methimazole (Tapazole) to block the synthesis of thyroid hormone
  2. Antithyroid medications such as iodine to reduce the vascularity of the thyroid gland
  3. Radioactive iodine to destroy thyroid gland cells, thereby decreasing the production of thyroid hormone (atomic cocktail)
  4. Medications to relieve the symptoms related to the increased metabolic rate; e.g., digitalis, propranolol (Inderal), phenobarbital
  5. Well-balanced, high-calorie diet with vitamin supplements
  6. Surgical intervention involves a subtotal or total thyroidectomy

D. Nursing care
  1. Assign patient to private room with means for temperature control
  2. Provide for periods of uninterrupted rest
  3. Administer medications to promote sleep
  4. Use nursing measures such as warm milk, warm bath, and back rub to establish a climate for rest
  5. Protect patient from stress-producing visitors
  6. Provide diet high in calories, vitamins, carbohydrates, and proteins with supplementary feedings between meals and at bedtime
  7. Understand that patient is upset by lability of mood and exaggerated response to environmental stimuli; take time to explain disease processes involved

  8. If the patient has thyroid surgery
    a. Observe for signs of respiratory distress and laryengeal stridor caused by tracheal edema (keep tracheotomy set available)
    b. Provide humidity with cold steam nebulizer to keep secretions moist
    c. Keep patient's bed in semi-Fowler's position without pillows and teach patient to support head
    d. Use soft cervical collar if ordered to prevent unnecessary neck movement
    e. Observe dressings at operative site and at back of neck and shoulders for signs of hemorrhage
    f. Observe for signs of thyroid storm; may occur due to manipulation of gland during surgery, which releases thyroid hormone into bloodstream
      (1) High fever
      (2) Tachycardia
      (3) Irritability; delirium
      (4) Coma
    g. Symptomatic treatment is indicated if thyroid storm occurs
    h. Observe for signs of tetany, which can occur after accidental trauma or removal of the parathyroid glands
      (1) Numbness of extremities
      (2) Spasm of glottis
    i. If tetany occurs, give calcium gluconate IV

Hyperparathyroidism

A. Etiology and pathophysiology
  1. Hyperfunction of the parathyroid glands is usually caused by adenoma; hypertrophy and hyperplasia of the glands may also be responsible
  2. As a result of hyperparathyroidism, the kidneys excrete excess calcium and phosphorus
  3. If dietary intake is not enough to meet calcium levels demanded by high levels of parathormone, demineralization of the bone occurs

B. Signs and symptoms
  1. Subjective
    a. Apathy
    b. Fatigue
    c. Muscular weakness
    d. Anorexia
    e. Emotional irritability

      f. Deep bone pain (if demineralization occurs)

      g. Constipation

  2. Objective

      a. Bone cysts, pathologic fractures

      b. Renal calculi composed of calcium

      c. Pyelonephritis, renal damage, uremia

      d. Vomiting

      e. Elevated serum calcium

      f. Decreased serum phosphorus

      g. Cardiac arrhythmias

C. Treatment

  1. Surgical excision of parathyroid tumor

  2. Increased fluid intake

  3. Activity is encouraged

  4. Calcium intake is restricted

D. Nursing care

  1. Observe for signs of skeletal (deep bone pain, skeletal deformities) and renal (lower back pain, hematuria) involvement

  2. Strain urine, observing for stones

  3. Encourage fluid intake, especially those, such as cranberry juice, which acidify the urine

  4. Assist patient to ambulate to help prevent demineralization

  5. Monitor intake and output

  6. Encourage foods such as prune juice and roughage to combat the problem of constipation

  7. Instruct the patient to limit intake of foods high in calcium, especially milk products

  8. Provide cardiac monitoring if hypercalcemia is severe

  9. If surgery is performed, postoperative care is the same as for patients undergoing thyroid surgery (see Hyperthyroidism)

Hypoparathyroidism

A. Etiology and pathophysiology

  1. The parathyroids may not secrete a sufficient amount of parathormone after thyroid surgery, parathyroid surgery, or x-ray therapy of neck; idiopathic hypoparathyroidism is rare

  2. As levels of parathormone drop, the serum calcium also drops, causing signs of tetany; a concomittant rise in serum phosphate occurs

B. Signs and symptoms

  1. Subjective

      a. Photophobia

      b. Diplopia

      c. Muscle cramps

      d. Irritability

      e. Dyspnea

  2. Objective

      a. Trousseau's sign (carpopedal spasm)

      b. Chvostek's sign (contraction of the facial muscle in response to tapping near the angle of the jaw)

      c. Decreased serum calcium

      d. Elevated serum phosphate

      e. Stridor, wheezing as a result of laryngeal spasm

      f. Convulsions

      g. Cataracts if the disease is chronic

      h. X-ray examination reveals increased bone density

      i. Cardiac arrhythmias

C. Treatment

  1. Calcium chloride or calcium gluconate is given IV for emergency treatment

  2. Calcium salts administered orally (calcium carbonate, calcium gluconate)

  3. Dihydrotachysterol to increase absorption of calcium from the GI tract

  4. Calciferol (vitamin D) to help raise serum calcium levels

  5. Parathormone injections

  6. High-calcium, low-phosphate diet

D. Nursing care

  1. Observe respiratory status and have emergency equipment available to perform a tracheostomy

  2. Observe seizure precautions

  3. Monitor serum calcium and phosphate levels

  4. Check vital signs frequently if a history of cardiac problems is present; place on a monitor

  5. Provide calm environment free of harsh stimuli

  6. Provide dietary instruction including elimination of milk, cheese, and egg yolks because of high phosphorus content

Diabetes mellitus

A. Etiology and pathophysiology

  1. Diabetes mellitus occurs when there is insufficient supply of insulin; may be due to

      a. Failure in body's production

      b. Blockage of insulin supply

      c. Autoimmune response wherein the insulin may bind to an immune serum globulin fraction, preventing utilization

  2. Incidence increases with obesity, aging, and familial predisposition

3. Juvenile type has a rapid onset and requires insulin administration, whereas adult onset type has a gradual onset and sometimes may be controlled by diet
4. The body does not have adequate insulin to convert glucose to glycogen
   a. Glucose levels in blood remain high
   b. Body attempts to rid itself of excess glucose by excreting some via kidneys
   c. An osmotic force is created within the kidneys due to glucose excretion, and body fluid is lost
   d. The body is unable to utilize carbohydrates properly, and fat is oxidized as a compensatory mechanism; oxidation of fats gives off ketone bodies
B. Signs and symptoms
   1. Subjective
      a. Polydipsia
      b. Polyphagia
      c. Fatigue
      d. Blurred vision from retinopathy
      e. Peripheral neuropathy
   2. Objective
      a. Polyuria
      b. Weight loss
      c. Hyperglycemia
      d. Glycosuria
      e. Peripheral vascular changes and gangrene
C. Treatment
   1. Attempt to manage mild uncomplicated diabetes by the use of diet, considering individual nutritional needs, maintenance of ideal weight, calories, and situational adaptations; a planned follow-up program according to need
      a. Characteristics of diet
         (1) Calories as needed to maintain ideal weight
         (2) Protein—optimum normal age group needs; usually 65 to 85 g for average adult
         (3) Carbohydrate—adequate for need but not excessive; usually about 100 to 250 g for an adult
         (4) Fat—moderation is the guideline; substitution of vegetable fats for some of the animal fats; usually about 70 to 100 g for adult
         (5) Dietary ratio—carbohydrate to protein to fat usually about 2:1:1
         (6) Distribution—fairly even distribution of food throughout the day in 3 meals, with snacks added between as needed from the day's total food allowances according to need and therapy with insulin or oral hypoglycemics
      b. Basic tools for planning diet—food exchange groups, using the exchange system of dietary control
   2. Insulin should be adjusted after considering the patient's physical and emotional stresses, selecting a specific type of insulin depending on the condition and needs of the patient (see Pharmacology section for discussion of insulin)
   3. Oral hypoglycemics for some patients; however, these patients must have some functioning beta cells in the islets of Langerhans; more commonly prescribed for the adult with late developing mild diabetes (see Pharmacology section)
D. Nursing care
   1. Assist patient to accept diagnosis
   2. Encourage patient to express feelings about illness and the necessary changes in life-style and self-image
   3. Assist patient and family to develop an understanding of the disease process
   4. Help patient with the administration of medication until self-administration is both physically and psychologically possible
   5. Assist patient to recognize the need for continuing health supervision
   6. Assist patient to recognize the need for activities and diet that promote and maintain health
   7. Patient teaching should include
      a. Testing urine and interpreting results; inaccurate readings may be obtained when patient is taking chephalosporins, aspirins, and ascorbic acid
      b. Selection of correct testing method based on patient's medication
      c. Avoidance of infection
      d. Proper care of legs, feet, and toenails
      e. Method of administration of insulin—use of sterile technique; rotation of injection sites; measurement of dosage; types and strengths of insulin; peak action periods
      f. Proper use of dietary chart and how to make substitutions
   8. Encourage patient to continue medical supervision and follow-up care, including visits to an eye care specialist and podiatrist

9. Teach patients who are receiving insulin and their families the signs of impending hypoglycemia (headache, nervousness, diaphoresis, rapid thready pulse, slurred speech)
10. Teach patient and family the signs of impending diabetic coma (restlessness; hot, dry, flushed skin; thirst; rapid pulse; nausea; fruity odor to breath)

Diabetic coma (ketoacidosis)

A. Etiology and pathophysiology
 1. Occurs when there is insufficient insulin available, a systemic infection, diarrhea and vomiting, overindulgence in eating, emotional stress, injury, surgery, or pregnancy
 2. Lack of insulin results in alterations of metabolism; proteins and fats are utilized; dehydration and electrolyte imbalance occur; and ketone bodies appear in the urine
B. Signs and symptoms
 1. Subjective
  a. Thirst
  b. Anorexia
  c. Drowsiness
  d. Headache
 2. Objective
  a. Vomiting
  b. Flushed appearance
  c. Lowered blood pressure
  d. Coma
  e. Sweet odor to breath
  f. Kussmaul breathing due to acidosis; very deep respirations as body attempts to blow off CO_2
  g. Hyperglycemia
  h. Glycosuria and ketonuria
C. Treatment
 1. Insert IV to provide direct access to circulatory system and a Foley catheter to obtain urine samples at frequent intervals
 2. Administer rapid-acting insulin
 3. Replace lost fluids and electrolytes, using blood studies to determine dosage
 4. Cardiac monitoring may be indicated if circulatory collapse is imminent
 5. Establish cause of acidosis and treat appropriately
D. Nursing care
 1. Stress adherence to dietary and therapeutic regimen to prevent occurrence
 2. Administer insulin as ordered

3. Keep accurate records of urine tests, vital signs, and fluid balance
4. Teach patient regarding dietary habits, prevention of infection, and signs of ketoacidosis

Hypoglycemia, or insulin shock

A. Etiology and pathophysiology
 1. Hypoglycemia may result when a diabetic patient receiving insulin therapy omits a meal, makes an error in insulin dosage, or vomits a meal; the majority of attacks occur in morning or late afternoon
 2. Hypoglycemia occurs when blood sugar falls below 60 mg/100 ml
B. Signs and symptoms
 1. Subjective
  a. Muscular weakness
  b. Diplopia
  c. Faintness
  d. Numbness and tingling in fingers, tongue, lips
 2. Objective
  a. Diaphoresis
  b. Trembling
  c. Tachycardia
  d. Disorientation
C. Treatment
 1. Oral glucose administration if patient is alert
 2. Administration of glucagon parenterally to stimulate glucogenolysis
 3. Administration of IV to provide access to vein for emergency
 4. Administration of 50% dextrose
D. Nursing care
 1. Administer medications as ordered
 2. Keep accurate record of intake and output, vital signs, and fractional urine tests
 3. If ordered, give patient protein or fat feeding after an easily absorbed carbohydrate meal is given

Primary aldosteronism (Conn's syndrome)

A. Etiology and pathophysiology
 1. Aldosterone, a mineralocorticoid, causes the kidneys to retain sodium and excrete potassium
 2. Hypersecretion of aldosterone is usually caused by an adenoma of the adrenal cortex but may also be caused by hyperplasia or carcinoma
 3. The disease is more common in females
B. Signs and symptoms
 1. Subjective

a. Muscle weakness

b. Polydipsia, polyuria

c. Paresthesia

2. Objective

a. Hypertension

b. Hypokalemia

c. Hypernatremia

d. Elevated urinary aldosterone levels

e. Renal damage

(1) Proteinuria

(2) Alkaline urine

(3) Decreased specific gravity of urine

(4) Pyelonephritis

C. Treatment

1. Surgical removal of tumor

2. Temporary management with spironolactone

3. Occasionally a bilateral adrenalectomy involving life-long corticosteroid therapy is necessary

D. Nursing care

1. Monitor vital signs

2. Observe for signs of electrolyte imbalance

3. Provide fluids to meet excessive thirst

4. Encourage continued medical supervision

5. Monitor intake and output and specific gravity of urine

6. If bilateral adrenalectomy is performed

a. Administer steroids with milk or antacid

b. Protect patient from infection

c. Explain drug and side effects to patient

d. Instruct patient to carry medical alert identification card

7. Provide dietary instruction; include foods high in potassium such as orange juice and bananas while avoiding or limiting intake of foods that contain sodium

Cushing's syndrome

A. Etiology and pathophysiology

1. Results from excess secretion of adrenocortical hormones

2. The hypersecretion is caused by hyperplasia or by a tumor of the adrenal cortex; however, the primary lesion may occur in the pituitary gland, causing excess production of ACTH

3. Administration of excess glucocorticoids or ACTH will also cause Cushing's syndrome

B. Signs and symptoms

1. Subjective

a. Weakness

b. Decreased libido

c. Mood swings to psychosis

2. Objective

a. Obese trunk with relatively thin arms and legs

b. Hypertension

c. Moon face

d. Buffalo hump

e. Acne

f. Increased susceptibility to infections

g. Hirsutism (increased hair on face and body)

h. Ecchymotic areas (easily bruised)

i. Purple striae on breast and abdomen

j. Amenorrhea

k. Hyperglycemia

l. Hypokalemia

m. Elevated 17-hydroxysteroids

n. Osteoporosis may be evident on x-ray examination

C. Treatment (aimed at correcting cause)

1. Reduce dosage of externally administered corticoids

2. If lesion on pituitary is causing hypersecretion of ACTH, a hypophysectomy or irradiation of the pituitary may be done

3. Surgical excision of adrenal tumors (adrenalectomy)

4. Potassium supplements

5. High-protein diet with sodium restriction

D. Nursing care

1. Monitor vital signs

2. Protect patient from exposure to infections

3. Collect 24-hour urine specimens for diagnostic purposes (17-ketosteroids and 17-hydroxysteroids)

4. Encourage ventilation of feelings by patient and spouse, since changes in body image and sex drives can alter support system

5. Attempt to minimize stress in the environment by measures such as limiting visitors and explaining procedures carefully

6. Monitor sugar and acetone

Addison's disease

A. Etiology and pathophysiology

1. Addison's disease is a hyposecretion of adrenocortical hormones

2. Generally caused by destruction of the cortex or by idiopathic atrophy

B. Signs and symptoms

1. Subjective
   a. Weakness
   b. Easy fatigue
   c. Nausea
2. Objective
   a. Increased bronze pigmentation of skin
   b. Vomiting
   c. Diarrhea
   d. Hypotension
   e. Hypoglycemia
   f. Small heart
   g. Increased plasma ACTH
   h. Decreased 17-ketosteroids and 17-hydroxy-steroids in 24-hour urines
   i. Hyponatremia
C. Treatment
   1. Replacement of hormones
      a. Glucocorticoids to correct metabolic imbalance
      b. Mineralocorticoids to correct electrolyte imbalance and hypotension
   2. High-carbohydrate, high-protein diet
   3. Special diagnostic tests to determine whether disease is caused by primary adrenocortical insufficiency or is secondary to pituitary insufficiency
      a. Eight-hour IV ACTH test to measure urinary steroid output after administration of ACTH; if output fails to rise, problem is primary adrenocortical insufficiency (Addison's); if output rises slowly (normal response is rapid rise), problem is secondary to pituitary insufficiency
      b. Plasma cortisol ACTH test to measure plasma cortisol level before and 30 minutes after administration of ACTH; if level fails to rise, problem is primary adrenocortical insufficiency (Addison's); if level rises (which is also the normal response), problem is secondary to pituitary insufficiency
      c. Thorn test to measure eosinophil count before and after administration of ACTH; if count remains the same, problem is primary adrenocortical insufficiency (Addison's)
D. Nursing care
   1. Administer steroids as ordered
   2. Administer steroids with milk or an antacid to limit ulcerogenic factor of the drug
   3. Put patient in a quiet room to prevent contact with patients having infectious diseases

4. Limit the number of visitors
5. Monitor vital signs 4 times a day; be alert for elevation in temperature (infection, dehydration), alterations in pulse rate (hyperkalemia), and alterations in blood pressure
6. Observe for signs of sodium and potassium imbalance
7. Monitor intake and output and weigh daily
8. Encourage adequate diet and fluid intake
9. Administer antiemetics to prevent fluid and electrolyte loss by vomiting

Pheochromocytoma

A. Etiology and pathophysiology
   1. Pheochromocytoma is a tumor of the adrenal medulla; usually benign
   2. Results in increased secretion of epinephrine and norepinephrine
   3. Heredity is believed to be involved in the development of the tumor
B. Signs and symptoms
   1. Subjective
      a. Headache
      b. Visual disturbances
      c. Nausea
   2. Objective
      a. Hypertension and orthostatic hypotension
      b. Tachycardia
      c. Diaphoresis
      d. Increased BMR
      e. Increased urinary catecholamines
      f. Hyperglycemia
C. Treatment
   1. Surgical removal of tumor
   2. Antihypertensive and antiarrhythmic drugs
D. Nursing care
   1. Monitor blood pressure frequently in both upright and horizontal positions
   2. Administer parenteral fluids and blood as ordered preoperatively and postoperatively to maintain blood volume
   3. Collect 24-hour urine to evaluate urinary catecholamines
   4. If bilateral adrenalectomy is performed, instruct patient regarding maintainance doses of steroids
   5. Emphasize importance of continued medical supervision and screening for other family members

Neuromusculoskeletal systems

REVIEW OF ANATOMY AND PHYSIOLOGY OF THE NEUROMUSCULOSKELETAL SYSTEMS
Nervous system

Cells

Neurons (nerve cells) are basic structural and functional unit; about 10 billion in human brain
A. General properties and functions
   1. Irritability—response to stimulus
   2. Conductivity—conduct electrical energy (nerve impulse); basis for body's rapid communication and integration network
   3. Types
      a. Sensory (afferent) neurons—transmit impulses to spinal cord or brain
      b. Motoneurons (motor or efferent neurons)—transmit impulses away from brain or spinal cord toward or to muscles or glands
         (1) Somatic motoneurons—transmit impulses from cord or brain stem to skeletal muscle
         (2) Visceral or autonomic motoneurons—transmit impulses from cord or brain stem to smooth muscle, cardiac muscle, or glands
      c. Interneurons (internuncial or intercalated neurons)—transmit impulses from sensory neurons to motoneurons
   4. Neurons cannot be replaced if lost; but neuronal contents constantly replenish; system of axonal flow distributes neural components to all regions from cell body where most synthesis occurs
B. Structure—well suited to transmitting impulses over distances
   1. Cell body contains nucleus and other cytoplasmic organelles
   2. Axon and dendrites—cellular extensions; single axon or dendrite referred to as nerve fiber
      a. Axon—one per neuron; carries impulse away from cell body; longer and thinner than dendrites; travels only at end where it communicates with other neurons, muscles, or glands; may be over 1 m (39 inches) in length and may communicate with 1000 other neurons
      b. Dendrites—delicate cellular extensions carry impulses toward cell body; several per neuron; each repeatedly branches, forming complex, bushlike network around cell body; increases surface area for reception by neuron of incoming electric signals; dendrite of sensory neurons exceptional in being extremely long, extending to periphery from ganglia near brain and spinal cord
   3. Supportive coverings and sheaths
      a. Myelin—multiple, dense layers of membrane wrapped around axon or dendrite; gaps in myelin every millimeter or so along fiber called nodes of Ranvier; myelinated nerve fibers transmit nerve impulses more rapidly than nonmyelinated fibers of same diameter
      b. Neurilemma—a sheath of Schwann cells forming an envelope around axons and some dendrites
         (1) Responsible for effective regeneration of nerve fiber after injury in peripheral nervous system; neurilemma forms cellular tube down which regenerating fiber travels
         (2) Forms the myelin sheath
   4. Neuronal cell membrane—similar in lipid content to cell membranes of all other body cells; however, specific proteins embedded in and attached to the surface of the lipid provide special characteristics; membrane proteins can be grouped into five classes
      a. Pumps—actively transport ions (notably Na^+ and K^+) between intracellular and interstitial fluid; establish ionic conditions for resting potential and nerve impulse
      b. Channels—provide selective pathways for diffusion of specific ions, as in neuronal depolarization and repolarization; channels open and close (gating mechanisms) in response to voltage changes and chemicals
      c. Receptors—depolarization and repolarization; channels provide specific binding sites for various naturally occurring transmitters and drugs
      d. Enzymes—catalyze chemical reactions on the membrane surface
      e. Structural proteins—interconnect cells to form tissues and organs; hold cell parts together
   5. Synapse—point of contact between 1 neuron and another
      a. Typical neuron may have between 1000 and 10,000 synapses
      b. Most often occurs between axon of 1 cell and dendrite of another, also commonly between axon and cell body of another

c. Physical gap (synaptic cleft) separates terminal axonal branches and dendrite or cell body of next neuron

d. At synapse, axon terminals enlarge to form terminal button, which is the information-delivering part of synapse; some synapses are excitatory and others inhibitory

6. Neuroglia take up most of space in nervous system not occupied by neurons; support, defend, and nourish neurons; chief source of CNS tumors; unlike neurons, neuroglia retain ability to divide; astrocytes, a type of neuroglial cell, provide framework of cells and fibers that suspend neurons and help to provide the blood-brain barrier

Nerve impulse

A. General considerations
1. Nerve impulse is a wave of electrical energy that flows over the surface of neurons and permits communication and integration between distant body regions
2. The larger the nerve fiber and the thicker the myelin sheath, the greater the velocity of the nerve impulse
3. Based on concentration differences between ions in the intracellular fluid of neuron and surrounding interstitial fluid
4. Ionic differences depend on ion pumps—most often studied is called sodium pump
   a. Requires ATP to work
   b. Pumps 3 sodium ions out of cell in exchange for 2 potassium ions taken into cell
   c. Due to action of sodium pump, intracellular fluid is about 10 times richer in potassium than is interstitial fluid, and interstitial fluid is about 10 times richer in sodium than is intracellular fluid

B. Impulse generation
1. Resting potential—after sodium pump establishes ionic gradients, some potassium diffuses out of cell through permanently open potassium channels; such potassium flow results in an excess of positive charge on the membrane's outer surface and a deficit of positive charge on the membrane's inner surface; the result is a voltage difference of 70 millivolts (mV) with the cell interior being negative; this is the resting potential
2. Action potential—a change in voltage across the neuronal membrane activates (opens) specific sodium ion channels in the membrane, allowing sodium ions to enter the cell and reverse the membrane's charge (inside becomes positive and outside becomes negative); as depolarization proceeds, the sodium channel closes and a voltage-gated potassium channel opens so that repolarization occurs with the voltage difference returning to the resting potential
3. Nerve impulse—the action potential, composed of depolarization and repolarization, propagates itself down the axon or dendrite and is known as the nerve impulse

C. Basic route of impulse conduction—the reflex arc
1. Description—impulse conduction
   a. Starts in receptors
   b. Continues over reflex arc(s)
   c. Terminates in effectors (muscles and glands)
   d. Results in a reflex—a response by muscles or glands in which impulse terminates; a reflex, therefore, is either contraction of muscle or secretion by gland
   e. Not all impulses result in reflexes; many are inhibited at some point along the reflex arc
2. Types of reflex arcs
   a. Two-neuron (monosynaptic) reflex arc—simplest arc possible; consists of at least 1 sensory neuron, 1 synapse, and 1 motoneuron; synapse is region of contact between axon terminals of one neuron and dendrites or cell body of another neuron
   b. Three-neuron arc (Fig. 7)—consists of at least 1 sensory neuron, 1 synapse, 1 interneuron, 1 synapse, and 1 motoneuron
   c. Complex multisynaptic neural pathways also exist; many not yet clearly mapped

D. Conduction across synapses
1. A given synapse can only transmit 1 type of transmitter substance
2. There are 30 different types of transmitters, including
   a. Monoamines (norepinephrine, dopamine, serotonin, acetylcholine); axons that release acetylcholine are called cholinergic, and axons that release norepinephrine are called adrenergic
   b. Amino acids (gamma-aminobutyric acid [GABA], glutamic acid, glycine, taurine); GABA is most common inhibitory transmitter in brain
   c. Neuropeptides (hormone-releasing hormones,

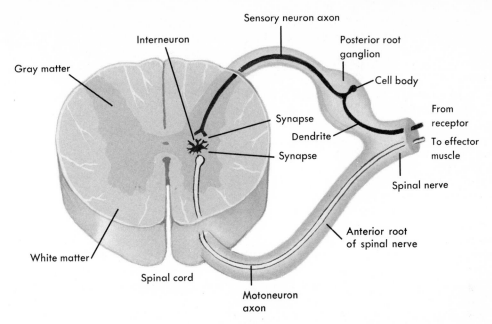

Fig. 7. Three-neuron ipsilateral reflex arc, consisting of a sensory neuron, an interneuron, and a motoneuron. Note the presence of two synapses in this arc: (1) between sensory neuron axon terminals and interneuron dendrites and (2) between interneuron axon terminals and motoneuron dendrites and cell bodies (located in anterior gray matter). Nerve impulses traversing such arcs produce many spinal reflexes. Example: withdrawing the hand from a hot object. (From Anthony, C. P., and Kolthoff, N. J.: Textbook of anatomy and physiology, ed. 9, St. Louis, 1975, The C. V. Mosby Co.)

enkephalins, and endorphins); some influence hormone levels and some influence perception and integration of pain and emotional experience

    d. Prostaglandins—high levels in brain tissue; some inhibit and some excite; may moderate action of other transmitters by influencing the neuronal membrane

3. Overall response of neuron—the sum or average of excitatory and inhibitory inputs determines whether cell will fire and rate at which it will fire; the neuron is seen to be an evaluator of signals, not just a passive transmitter; the result of its evaluation is its individual rate of impulse transmission

Organs of nervous system

A. Central nervous system (CNS)—spinal cord and brain

B. Peripheral nervous system (PNS)—nerves and ganglia

C. Definitions

    1. White matter—bundles of myelinated nerve fibers

    2. Gray matter—clusters of mainly neuron cell bodies

    3. Nerves—bundles of myelinated nerve fibers located outside CNS

    4. Tracts—bundles of myelinated nerve fibers located within CNS

    5. Ganglia (singular: ganglion)—microscopic structures consisting of neuron cell bodies; mainly located outside CNS

Spinal cord

A. Location—in spinal cavity, from foramen magnum to first lumbar vertebra

B. Structure

    1. Deep groove (anterior median fissure) and more shallow groove (posterior median sulcus) incompletely divide cord into right and left symmetric halves

    2. Inner core of cord consists of gray matter shaped like a 3-dimensional **H**

    3. Long columns of white matter surround the cord's inner core of gray matter; namely, right and left anterior, lateral, and posterior columns;

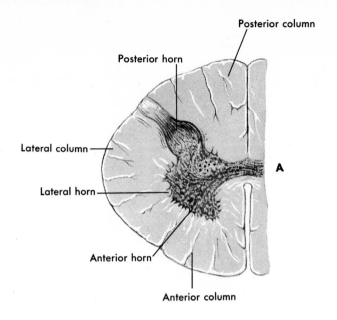

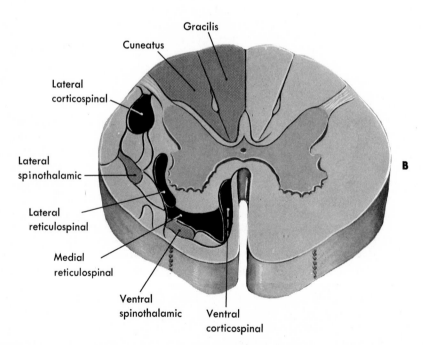

Fig. 8. A, Distribution of gray matter (horns) and white matter (columns) in a section of the spinal cord at the thoracic level. **B,** Location in the spinal cord of some major projection tracts. Black areas, descending motor tracts. Shaded areas, ascending sensory tracts. (From Anthony, C. P., and Kolthoff, N. J.: Textbook of anatomy and physiology, ed. 9, St. Louis, 1975, The C. V. Mosby Co.)

composed of numerous sensory and motor tracts (Fig. 8)

C. Functions
1. Sensory tracts conduct impulses up cord to brain; motor tracts conduct impulses down cord from brain
2. Gray matter of cord contains reflex centers for all spinal cord reflexes

Brain

A. General considerations
1. Most active of all body organs in energy consumption; has large blood supply and high oxygen consumption, which increases even further during dreaming stage of sleep
2. Unlike other cells of body, neurons can only utilize glucose for energy metabolism; therefore hypoglycemia can seriously alter brain function and lead to coma
3. Brain cells protected by blood-brain barrier, a selective filtration system that isolates brain from substances in general circulation; barrier based on relative impermeability of blood vessels in brain and to tight wrapping of neuroglial cells around neurons and blood vessels of brain; only selected brain regions designed to monitor the chemical composition of blood are not protected by blood-brain barrier
4. Ease of drug entry into the brain depends on size and fat solubility; the smaller the molecule and the greater the fat solubility, the more easily the drug enters brain tissue
5. Overall function of brain and spinal cord is to channel sensory input to a variety of neural structures whose analysis culminates in the convergence of impulses on various motor neurons, which effect movements of all types of muscles and activity of glands

B. Regions of brain and their functions
1. Basic tissue types
   a. Gray matter—aggregations of neuron cell bodies
   b. White matter—composed primarily of tracts of fibers (axons) interconnecting neurons in different regions of the CNS
2. Basic cellular types in CNS
   a. Association (intercolated) neurons—about 99.9% of all the neurons in CNS
   b. Motor neurons—several million found in CNS

3. Gross anatomic regions
   a. Hindbrain (brain stem)—lowermost brain division; formed by enlargement of spinal cord as it enters cranial cavity
      (1) Medulla—lowest portion of hindbrain
         (a) Consists mainly of white matter (sensory and motor tracts); also contains reticular formation (mixture of gray and white matter); some important reflex centers located in reticular formation: cardiac, vasomotor, respiratory, and swallowing centers
         (b) Functions—contains centers for vital heart, blood vessel diameter (blood pressure), and respiratory reflexes; also centers for vomiting, coughing, swallowing, etc.; conducts impulses between cord and brain (both sensory and motor)
      (2) Pons
         (a) Part of brain located just above medulla; consists mainly of white matter (sensory and motor tracts) interspersed with gray matter (reflex centers)
         (b) Conducts impulses between cord and various parts of brain and contains reflex centers for cranial nerves V, VI, VII, and VIII
   b. Cerebellum—dorsal appendage of hindbrain
      (1) Structure—second largest part of human brain; surface marked with sulci (grooves) and very slightly raised, slender convolutions; internal white matter forms pattern suggestive of veins of leaf
      (2) Functions
         (a) The cerebellum exerts synergic control over skeletal muscles; this means that impulses conducted by cerebellar neurons regulate and modulate output of somatomotor region of neocortex; this results in coordination of skeletal muscle contractions to produce smooth, steady, and precise movements
         (b) Because it coordinates skeletal muscle contractions, the cerebellum plays an essential part in producing normal postures and maintaining equilibrium

c. Midbrain—part of brain located between the pons, which lies below it, and the diencephalon and cerebrum, which lie above it; consists mainly of white matter (cerebral peduncles) with scattered bits of gray matter
  (1) Superior and inferior colliculi (corpora quadrigemina)—integrate and analyze sensory input from the ears, eyes, and various regions of the cerebral cortex; puts out motor information to lower motor system
  (2) Reflex centers for cranial nerves III and IV; pupillary reflexes and eye movements
  (3) Pineal body—precise function unknown; may be part of endocrine system helping to regulate gonadotrophic hormone secretion from hypophysis
d. Forebrain
  (1) Optic vesicles—develop into retinas connected to base of forebrain by their stalks, the optic nerves
  (2) Diencephalon—unpaired division of forebrain; cerebral hemispheres diverge from this structure
    (a) Thalamus—mass of gray matter in each cerebral hemisphere
      [1] Processes incoming sensory information prior to distribution to somatosensory cortex; crudely translates sensory impulses into sensations but does not localize them on a body region
      [2] Ventral nucleus of thalamus processes motor information from cerebral cortex and cerebellum and projects its analysis back to motor cortex
      [3] Contributes to concentrating ability by filtering out distracting sensory input
      [4] Contributes to emotional component of sensations (pleasant or unpleasant)
    (b) Hypothalamus—gray matter that forms floor of third ventricle and lower part of its lateral walls
      [1] Contains many higher autonomic reflex centers; these centers integrate autonomic functions by sending impulses to each other and to lower autonomic centers; they form a crucial part of the neural path by which emotions and other cerebral functions can alter vital, automatic functions such as the heartbeat, blood pressure, peristalsis, and secretion by glands and thereby produce psychosomatic diseases; neural path for psychosomatic disease—impulses from cerebral cortex to autonomic centers in hypothalamus, to lower autonomic centers in brain stem and cord, to visceral effectors; e.g., heart, smooth muscle, glands
      [2] Helps control the anterior pituitary gland; certain neurons in hypothalamus secrete neuropeptides into pituitary portal veins, which transport them to the anterior pituitary gland where they influence secretion of various important hormones; e.g., TRH and LHRH regulate pituitary secretions of TSH and gonadotrophic hormones, respectively
      [3] Neurons in the supraoptic nucleus of the hypothalamus synthesize ADH (antidiuretic hormone) and oxytocin; from the cell bodies of these neurons, ADH and oxytocin are transmitted down their axons into the posterior pituitary gland, from which they are released into the blood; in short, hypothalamic neurons make ADH and oxytocin, but the posterior pituitary gland secretes them
      [4] Certain hypothalamic neurons serve as an appetite center and others function as a satiety center; together these centers regulate appetite and food intake
      [5] Certain hypothalamic neurons serve as heat-regulating centers by relaying impulses to lower au-

tonomic centers for vasoconstriction, vasodilation, and sweating, and to somatic centers for shivering

[6] Maintains waking state; constitutes part of the arousal or alerting neural pathway

(c) Corpus callosum—mass of white matter (nerve tracts) that interconnects the two cerebral hemispheres

(d) Optic chiasm—point of crossing over (decussation) of optic nerve fibers from nasal half of each retina to opposite side where they join optic nerve fibers from lateral half of other eye's retina to form the optic tracts

(3) Paired cerebral hemisphere (telencephalon)—longitudinal fissure divides cerebrum into 2 hemispheres connected only by corpus callosum; each cerebral hemisphere divided by fissures into 4 major lobes: frontal, parietal, temporal, occipital; also contains deeper regions of gray matter and fiber tracts

(a) Cerebral cortex is outer layer of gray matter forming folds (convolutions) composed of hills (gyri) and valleys (sulci)

(b) Frontal lobes

[1] Abstract thinking, sense of humor, and uniqueness of personality

[2] Contraction of skeletal muscles and synchronization of muscular movements

[3] Exert control over hypothalamus; influences basic biorhythms

[4] Control muscular movements necessary for speech; only found in 1 cerebral hemisphere

(c) Parietal lobes

[1] Translate nerve impulses into sensations; e.g., touch, temperature

[2] Interpret sensations; provide appreciation of size, shape, texture, and weight

[3] Sense of taste

(d) Temporal lobes

[1] Translate nerve impulses into sensations of sound and interpret sounds

[2] Sense of smell

[3] Control of behavior patterns

(e) Occipital area

[1] Translates nerve impulse into sights and interprets sights

[2] Provides appreciation of size, shape, and color

(f) Angular gyrus—analysis and integration of sights, sounds, and somatic sensations

(g) Amygdala—controls patterns of emotional behavior

(h) Corpus striatum—helps to regulate muscle contraction and emotional reactions

(i) Cerebral tracts—bundles of axons compose white matter in interior of cerebrum; ascending projection tracts transmit impulses toward cerebral cortex; descending projection tracts transmit impulses from cerebral cortex; commissural tracts transmit from 1 hemisphere to the other; association tracts transmit from 1 convolution to another in same hemisphere

4. Brain and spinal cord coverings

a. Bony—vertebrae around cord; cranial bones around brain

b. Membranous—called meninges; consist of 3 layers

(1) Dura mater—white fibrous tissue, outer layer

(2) Arachnoid membrane—cobwebby middle layer

(3) Pia mater—innermost layer of meninges; adheres to outer surface of cord and brain; contains blood vessels

5. Cord and brain fluid spaces

a. Subarachnoid space around cord and extending beyond the cord into the fourth and fifth lumbar vertebrae

b. Subarachnoid space around brain

c. Central canal inside cord

d. Ventricles and cerebral aqueduct inside brain; 4 cavities within brain

(1) First and second (lateral ventricles)—large cavities, one in each cerebral hemisphere

(2) Third ventricle—vertical slit in cerebrum beneath corpus callosum and longitudinal fissure

(3) Fourth ventricle—diamond-shaped space between cerebellum and medulla and pons; is expansion of central canal of cord

6. Formation and circulation of cerebrospinal fluid (CSF)

a. Formed by plasma filtering from network of capillaries (choroid plexus) in each ventricle; active transport process also involved

b. Circulates from lateral ventricles to third ventricle, cerebral aqueduct, fourth ventricle, central canal of cord, subarachnoid space of cord and brain; returns to blood via venous sinuses of brain

Cranial nerves—12 pairs

See Table 2-11

Spinal nerves—31 pairs

A. Each nerve attaches to cord by 2 short roots, anterior and posterior; posterior roots marked by swelling, namely, spinal ganglion

B. Branches of spinal nerves form plexuses or intricate networks of fibers; e.g., brachial plexus from which nerves emerge to supply various parts of skin, mucosa, and skeletal muscles

C. All spinal nerves are mixed nerves composed of both sensory dendrites and motor axons and function in both sensations and movements

D. A nerve consists of bundles of nerve fibers (axons and dendrites) supported by connective tissue

Sensory neural pathways—conduction

A. Sensory pathways to the cerebral cortex from the periphery consist of relays of at least 3 neurons, which are identified by Roman numerals

1. Sensory neuron I—conducts from the periphery to the cord or to the brain stem

2. Sensory neuron II—conducts from the cord or brain stem to the thalamus

3. Sensory neuron III—conducts from the thalamus to the somatosensory area of the cerebral cortex

B. Crude awareness of sensations occurs when impulses reach the thalamus

C. Full consciousness of sensations with accurate localization and discrimination of fine details occurs when impulses reach the cerebral cortex

D. Most sensory neuron II axons decussate; so one side of the brain registers most of the sensations for the opposite side of the body

E. The principle of divergence applies to sensory neural pathways; each sensory neuron synapses with many neurons, and therefore impulses may diverge from any sensory neuron and be conducted to many brain regions, including cerebellum, reticular formation, and also more directly to motor neurons

F. Impulses that produce pain and temperature are conducted up the cord to the thalamus by the lateral spinothalamic tracts

G. Impulses that produce touch and pressure sensations are conducted up the cord to the thalamus by the following 2 pathways

1. Impulses that result in discriminating touch and pressure sensations (such as stereognosis, precise localization, and vibratory sense) are conducted by the tracts of the posterior white columns of the cord to the medulla and from there are transferred to the thalamus

2. Impulses that result in crude touch and pressure sensations are conducted up the cord to the thalamus by fibers of the ventral spinothalamic tracts

H. Sensory impulses that result in conscious proprioception or kinesthesia (sense of position or movement of body parts) are conducted over the same pathway as are impulses that result in discriminating touch and pressure sensations

I. Sensory impulses, in addition, are also conducted to the cerebral cortex via complex multineuron pathways known as the reticular activating system; spinoreticular tracts relay sensory impulses up the cord to the brain stem reticular gray matter, and from there other neurons relay them to the hypothalamus, thalamus, and probably other parts of the brain, then finally to the cerebral cortex; conduction by the reticular activating system is essential for producing and maintaining consciousness; presumably, general anesthetics produce unconsciousness by inhibiting conduction by the reticular activating system; conversely, amphetamines and norepinephrine are thought to produce wakefulness by stimulating the reticular activating system

Motoneural pathways to skeletal muscles

A. Principle of the final common path—the final common path for impulse conduction to skeletal muscles consists of anterior horn neurons (i.e., motoneurons whose dendrites and cell bodies lie in the anterior gray columns of the cord and whose axons extend out through the anterior roots of spinal nerves and their

Table 2-11. Distribution and function of cranial nerve pairs

Name and number	Distribution	Function
Olfactory (I)	Nasal mucosa, high up along the septum especially	Sense of smell (sensory only)
Optic (II)	Retina of eyeball	Vision (sensory only)
Oculomotor (III)	Extrinsic muscles of eyeball, except superior oblique and external rectus; also intrinsic eye muscles (iris and ciliary)	Eye movements; constriction of pupil and bulging of lens, which together produce accommodation for near vision
Trochlear (IV), smallest cranial nerve	Superior oblique muscle of eye	Eye movements
Trifacial (V) (or trigeminal), largest cranial nerve	Sensory fibers to skin and mucosa of head and to teeth; muscles of mastication (sensory and motor fibers)	Sensation in head and face; chewing movements
Abducens (VI)	External rectus muscle of eye	Abduction of eye
Facial (VII)	Muscles of facial expression; taste buds of anterior two thirds of tongue; motor fibers to submaxillary and sublingual salivary glands	Facial expressions; taste; secretion of saliva
Auditory (VIII) (acoustic)	Inner ear	Hearing and equilibrium (sensory only)
Glossopharyngeal (IX)	Posterior one third of tongue; mucosa and muscles of pharynx; parotid gland; carotid sinus and body	Taste and other sensations of tongue; secretion of saliva; swallowing movements; functions in reflex arcs for control of blood pressure and respiration
Vagus (X) (or pneumogastric)	Mucosa and muscles of pharynx, larynx, trachea, bronchi, esophagus; thoracic and abdominal viscera	Sensations and movements of organs supplied; for example, slows heart, increases peristalsis and gastric and pancreatic secretion; voice production
Spinal accessory (XI)	Certain neck and shoulder muscles (muscles of larynx, sternocleidomastoid, trapezius)	Shoulder movements; turns head; voice production; muscle sense
Hypoglossal (XII)	Tongue muscles	Tongue movements, as in talking; muscle sense

Note: The first letters of the words in the following sentence are the first letters of the names of the cranial nerves, and many generations of anatomy students have used it as an aid to memorizing the names: "On Old Olympus Tiny Tops, A Finn and German Viewed Some Hops." (There are several slightly different versions of this sentence.)

branches to terminate in skeletal muscles); besides being referred to as the final common path and as anterior horn cells, these neurons are also called lower motoneurons, somatic motoneurons, and lower motor system

B. Principle of convergence—axons of many neurons converge on (i.e., synapse with) each anterior horn motoneuron

C. Motor pathways from the cerebral cortex to anterior horn cells are classified according to the route by which the fibers enter the cord
  1. Pyramidal tracts (corticospinal tracts)—axons of neurons whose dendrites and cell bodies lie in the cerebral cortex; axons descend from cortex through internal capsule, pyramids of medulla, and spinal cord; a few of these axons synapse with anterior horn cells, but most of them synapse with internuncial neurons that synapse with anterior horn cells; conduction by pyramidal tracts is necessary for willed movements to occur; hence 1 cause of paralysis is interruption of pyramidal tract conduction
  2. Extrapyramidal tracts—all tracts that conduct between the motor cortex and the anterior horn cells, except the pyramidal tracts; upper extrapyramidal tracts relay impulses between the cortex, basal ganglia, thalamus, and brain stem; reticulospinal tracts (the main lower extrapyramidal tracts) relay impulses from the brain stem to the anterior horn cells in the cord; impulse conduction via extrapyramidal tracts is essential for producing large, automatic movements (e.g.,

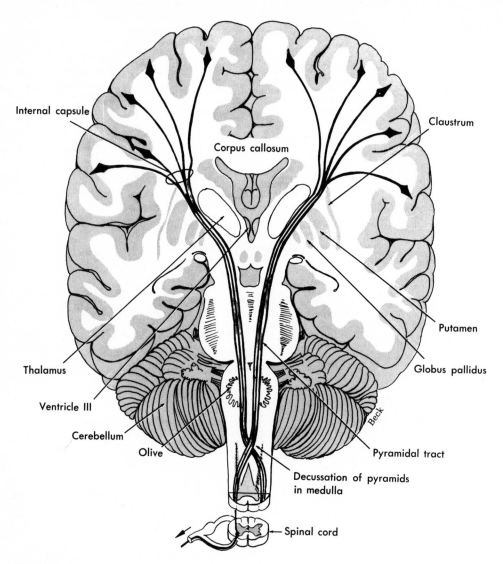

Fig. 9. The crossed pyramidal tracts (lateral corticospinal), the main motor tracts of the body. Axons that compose pyramidal tracts come from neuron cell bodies in the cerebral cortex. After they descend through the internal capsule of the cerebrum and the white matter of the brainstem, about ¾ of the fibers decussate—cross over from one side to the other—in the medulla, as shown here. Then they continue downward in the lateral corticospinal tract on the opposite side of the cord. Each lateral corticospinal tract, therefore, conducts motor impulses from one side of the brain to skeletal muscles on the opposite side of the body. (From Anthony, C. P., and Kolthoff, N. J.: Textbook of anatomy and physiology, ed. 9, St. Louis, 1975, The C. V. Mosby Co.)

walking, swimming) and for producing facial expressions and movements that characterize many emotions

D. The motor conduction pathway from the primary motor area of the cerebral cortex to skeletal muscles via pyramidal tracts consists of a 2-neuron relay; an upper motoneuron conducts impulses from cerebrum to cord and a lower motoneuron (anterior horn cell) conducts from cord to skeletal muscle (Fig. 9)

E. The motor conduction pathway from the cerebral cortex via extrapyramidal tracts consists of complex multineuron relays; several upper motoneurons relay impulses through basal ganglia, thalamus, brain stem, and down the cord to the lower motoneuron

F. Motor pathways from the cerebral cortex to anterior horn cells are classified according to their influence on anterior horn cells as follows
1. Facilitatory tracts—conduct impulses that have a facilitating or stimulating effect on anterior horn cells; main facilitatory tracts are the pyramidal tracts and the facilitatory reticulospinal tracts
2. Inhibitory tracts—conduct impulses that have an inhibiting effect on anterior horn cells; main inhibitory tracts are the inhibitory reticulospinal tracts; interruption of inhibitory reticulospinal tracts results in spasticity and rigidity

G. The ratio of facilitatory and inhibitory impulses impinging on anterior horn cells determines their activity (whether they are facilitated, stimulated, or inhibited)

Autonomic nervous system

A. Definition—the division of the nervous system that conducts impulses from the brain stem or cord out to visceral effectors; visceral effectors are cardiac muscle, smooth muscle, and glandular tissue

B. Divisions—autonomic nervous system consists of 2 divisions: the sympathetic (thoracolumbar) system and the parasympathetic (craniosacral) system
1. Sympathetic system
   a. Sympathetic ganglia—2 chains of 21 or 22 ganglia located immediately in front of the spinal column, 1 chain to the right, 1 to the left
   b. Collateral ganglia—located a short distance from the cord; e.g., celiac ganglia (solar plexus), superior and inferior mesenteric ganglia
   c. Sympathetic nerves—e.g., splanchnic nerves, cardiac nerves

2. Parasympathetic system
   a. Parasympathetic ganglia—located at a distance from the spinal column, in or near visceral effectors; e.g., ciliary ganglion in posterior part of the orbit, near the iris and ciliary muscle
   b. Parasympathetic nerves—e.g., vagus nerve, called the great parasympathetic nerve of the body

C. Neurons
1. Preganglionic sympathetic neurons—dendrites and cell bodies lie in lateral gray columns of thoracic and lumbar segments of cord; axons conduct from cord to sympathetic ganglia or to collateral ganglia
2. Postganglionic sympathetic neurons—dendrites and cell bodies lie in sympathetic ganglia or in collateral ganglia; axons conduct to visceral effectors
3. Preganglionic parasympathetic neurons—dendrites and cell bodies of some of these neurons lie in gray matter of brain stem, and other preganglionic fibers exit at the sacral segments of cord; conduct impulses from brain stem or cord to parasympathetic ganglia
4. Postganglionic parasympathetic neurons—dendrites and cell bodies lie in parasympathetic ganglia; axons conduct to visceral effectors

D. Some principles about the autonomic nervous system
1. Dual autonomic innervation—both sympathetic and parasympathetic fibers supply most visceral effectors
2. Single autonomic innervation—only sympathetic fibers supply sweat glands and probably the smooth muscles of hairs and of most blood vessels; preganglionic sympathetic fibers terminate in adrenal medulla (not postganglionic fibers as in other glands)
3. Autonomic chemical transmitters—all preganglionic axons are cholinergic fibers, as are most (or perhaps all) parasympathetic postganglionic axons and a few sympathetic postganglionic axons (to sweat glands, external genitalia, and smooth muscle in walls of blood vessels located in skeletal muscles); sympathetic postganglionic axons are the only adrenergic (i.e., norepinephrine-releasing) fibers; but, as just mentioned, a few of them are cholinergic

Table 2-12. Autonomic functions*

Visceral effectors	Parasympathetic (cholinergic) effects	Sympathetic (adrenergic or cholinergic) effects
Cardiac muscle	Slows heart rate; decreases strength of contraction	Accelerates heart rate; increases strength of contraction
Smooth muscle of blood vessels		
Skin blood vessels	No parasympathetic fibers	Adrenergic sympathetic fibers → stimulate → constrict skin vessels
Skeletal muscle blood vessels	No parasympathetic fibers	Adrenergic sympathetic fibers → stimulate → constrict skeletal muscle vessels Cholinergic sympathetic fibers → inhibit → dilate skeletal muscle vessels
Blood vessels in cerebrum, abdominal viscera, and genitalia	Parasympathetic fibers → inhibit → dilate vessels in cerebrum, abdominal viscera, and genitalia	Adrenergic sympathetic fibers → stimulate → constrict vessels in cerebrum and abdominal viscera Cholinergic sympathetic fibers → inhibit → dilate vessels in external genitalia
Smooth muscle of hollow organs and sphincters		
Bronchi	Stimulates → bronchial constriction	Inhibits → bronchial dilation
Digestive tract	Stimulates → increased peristalsis	Inhibits → decreased peristalsis
Anal sphincter	Inhibits → opens sphincter for defecation	Stimulates → closes sphincter
Urinary bladder	Stimulates → contracts bladder	Inhibits → relaxes bladder
Urinary sphincters	Inhibits → opens sphincters for urination	Stimulates → closes sphincters
Eye		
Iris	Stimulates circular fibers → constriction of pupil	Stimulates radial fibers → dilation of pupil
Ciliary	Stimulates → accommodation for near vision (bulging of lens)	Inhibits → accommodation for far vision (flattening of lens)
Hairs (pilomotor muscles)	No parasympathetic fibers	Stimulates → "goose pimples" (piloerection)
Glands		
Sweat	No parasympathetic fibers	Cholinergic sympathetic fibers stimulate sweat glands
Digestive (salivary, gastric, etc.)	Stimulates secretion of saliva and gastric juice	Decreases secretion of saliva and gastric juice
Pancreas, including islets	Stimulates secretion of pancreatic juice and insulin	Decreases secretion of pancreatic juice and insulin
Liver	No parasympathetic fibers	Stimulates glycogenolysis, which tends to increase blood sugar
Adrenal medulla	No parasympathetic fibers	Stimulates epinephrine (and some norepinephrine) secretion, which tends to increase blood sugar, blood pressure, and heart rate and to produce many other sympathetic effects

*From Anthony, C. P., and Kolthoff, N. J.: Textbook of anatomy and physiology, ed. 9, St. Louis, 1975, The C. V. Mosby Co.

4. Autonomic antagonism and summation—sympathetic and parasympathetic impulses tend to produce opposite effects; algebraic sum of 2 opposing tendencies determines response made by doubly innervated visceral effector

5. The principle of parasympathetic dominance of the digestive tract—normally, parasympathetic impulses to digestive tract glands and smooth muscle dominate over sympathetic impulses to them; dominance of parasympathetic impulses

Table 2-13. Receptors

Kinds	Locations	Stimulated by	Functions
Exteroceptors	Skin, mucosa, ear, eye	Changes in external environment (e.g., pressure, heat, cold, light waves, sound waves)	Initiate reflexes Initiate sensations of many kinds (e.g., pressure, heat, cold, pain, vision, hearing)
Visceroceptors (interoceptors)	Viscera	Changes in internal environment (e.g., pressure, chemical)	Initiate reflexes Initiate sensations of many kinds (e.g., hunger, sex, nausea, pressure)
Proprioceptors	Muscles, tendons, joints, semicircular canals of inner ear	Pressure changes	Initiate reflexes Initiate muscle sense, or sense of position and movement of parts; also called kinesthesia

promotes digestive gland secretion, peristalsis, and defecation

6. The principle of sympathetic dominance in stress—under the condition of stress, sympathetic impulses to visceral effectors usually increase greatly and dominate over parasympathetic impulses; however, in some individuals under stress, parasympathetic impulses via the vagus nerve to glands and smooth muscle of the stomach greatly increase, causing increased hydrochloric acid secretion and increased gastric motility that may eventually cause peptic ulcer, a condition that may aptly be called the great parasympathetic stress disease

7. In general, when the sympathetic system dominates control of visceral effectors, it causes them to function in ways that enable the body to expend maximum energy as is necessary in strenuous exercise and other types of stress; see Table 2-12 for sympathetic effects on specific effectors

8. Principle of nonautonomy—autonomic nervous system is neither anatomically nor physiologically independent of rest of nervous system; all parts of nervous system work together as single functional unit; e.g., dendrites and cells of all preganglionic neurons located in gray matter of brain stem or cord (lower autonomic centers) and influenced by impulses conducted to them from higher autonomic centers, notably in hypothalamus

9. Importance of autonomic nervous system—autonomic system plays major role in maintaining physiologic balance; under usual conditions, autonomic impulses regulate activities of visceral effectors so that they maintain or quickly restore this balance; under highly stressful conditions, problems may occur

Sense organs

Millions of receptors distributed widely throughout skin and mucosa; muscles, tendons, joints, and viscera are sense organs of body (Table 2-13)

A. General considerations

1. Receptors monitor internal and external environment

2. Stimuli are interpreted and converted to nerve impulses, which are conducted through sensory neurons to the brain

3. The receptors' degree of depolarization depends on the strength of the stimulus; the variable degree of depolarization is called the generator potential

4. The generator potential determines the frequency of nerve impulses sent to CNS by afferent nerve fibers attached to receptors

5. Most receptors display sensory adaptation—steady and prolonged stimulus of a receptor results in a steady decrease in strength of generator potential

B. Types of receptors

1. Exteroceptors of skin and mucosa—consist of receptors for spinal or cranial nerve branches; different types of receptors for different sensations such as heat, cold, pain, touch, and pressure

2. Proprioceptors of muscles, tendons, and joints—stretching of muscles or tendons during movements initiates stretch reflexes

3. Visceroceptors—pressoreceptors (baroreceptors) respond to stretch in walls of aorta and carotids, providing brain with measure of blood pressure;

O_2 chemoreceptors in aorta and carotid bodies monitor O_2 levels; CO_2 chemoreceptors in respiratory center in medulla help to control rate and depth of respirations

4. Taste
   a. Taste buds consist of groups of receptor cells bundled together with sensory hairs protruding from a pore in the taste bud and connected to cranial nerves VII and IX
   b. Respond to chemicals—sweet at tongue tip; sour and salt at tip and sides; bitter at back of tongue; receptors for bitter most sensitive
   c. Olfaction is intimately involved in sense of taste
5. Olfaction
   a. Receptors in epithelium of nasal mucosa
   b. Odors sensed as chemicals interact with receptor sites on sensory hairs of olfactory cells
   c. Olfactory neural pathways utilize cranial nerve I
6. Sight—the eye
   a. Coats of eyeball
      (1) Outer coat—sclera proper and cornea
      (2) Middle coat—choroid proper, ciliary body, suspensory ligament holding lens, and iris
      (3) Inner coat—retina
   b. Cavities and humors of eyeball
      (1) Anterior cavity with an anterior and posterior chamber; both chambers contain aqueous humor
      (2) Posterior cavity has no divisions and contains vitreous humor
   c. Muscles of the eye (Table 2-14)
   d. Refractory media of eye
      (1) Cornea
      (2) Aqueous humor
      (3) Crystalline lens (has greatest refractive power)
      (4) Vitreous humor
   e. Accessory structures of eye
      (1) Eyebrows and lashes
      (2) Eyelids or palpebrae—lined with mucous membrane (conjunctiva) that continues over surface of eyeball; corners of eyes, where upper and lower lids join, called inner and outer canthus
      (3) Lacrimal apparatus—lacrimal glands, ducts, sacs, and nasolacrimal ducts
   f. Physiology of vision
      (1) Formation of image on retina accomplished by
         (a) Refraction—bending of light rays as they pass through eye
         (b) Accommodation—bulging of lens for viewing near objects
         (c) Constriction of pupils—occurs simultaneously with accommodation and in bright light
         (d) Convergence of eyes for near objects in order that light rays from object may fall on corresponding points of 2 retinas; necessary for single binocular vision
      (2) Stimulation of retina—dim light causes breakdown of chemical rhodopsin present in rods, thereby initiating impulse conduction by rods; bright light causes breakdown of chemicals in cones; rods considered receptors for night vision and cones for daylight and color vision

Table 2-14. Eye muscles

Location	Kind of muscle	Names	Functions
Extrinsic—attached to outside of eyeball and to bones of orbit	Skeletal (voluntary, striated)	Superior rectus Inferior rectus Lateral rectus Mesial rectus Superior oblique Inferior oblique	Move eyeball in various directions
Intrinsic—within eyeball	Visceral (involuntary, smooth)	Iris Ciliary muscle	Regulate size of pupil Control shape of lens, making possible accommodation for near and far objects

(3) Most cones concentrated in small region of retina called fovea centralis; provides sharpest color vision

(4) Conduction to visual area in occipital lobe of cerebral cortex by fibers of optic nerves and optic tracts

7. Hearing—the ear
   a. External ear—consists of auricle (or pinna), external acoustic meatus (ear opening), and external auditory canal
   b. Middle ear—separated from external ear by tympanic membrane; middle ear contains auditory ossicles (malleus, incus, stapes) and openings from auditory (eustachian) tubes, mastoid cells, external ear, and internal ear; auditory tube is collapsible and lined with mucosa and extends from nasopharynx to middle ear; equalizes pressure on both sides of eardrum, as when tubes open during yawning, swallowing, or sucking
   c. Inner ear (or labyrinth)—composed of a bony labyrinth that has a membranous labyrinth inside it; parts of the inner ear
      (1) Bony vestibule that contains the membranous utricle and saccule, each of which, in turn, contains a sense organ called the macula; vestibular nerve (branch of eighth cranial nerve) supplies the maculae; maculae are sense organs for 3 sensations: equilibrium, position of the head, and acceleration and deceleration
      (2) Bony semicircular canals that contain the membranous semicircular canals in which are located the crista ampullaris, the sense organ for sensations of equilibrium and head movements; vestibular nerve supplies the crista as well as the macula
      (3) Bony cochlea that contains the membranous cochlear duct in which is located the organ of Corti, the hearing sense organ; cochlear nerve (branch of eighth cranial nerve) supplies the organ of Corti
   d. Physiology of hearing
      (1) Sound waves moving through air enter ear canal and move down it to strike against the tympanic membrane, causing it to vibrate
      (2) Vibrations of tympanic membrane move the malleus, whose handle is attached to the membrane
      (3) Movement of the malleus moves the incus, to which the head of the malleus attaches
      (4) Incus attaches to the stapes; so as the incus moves, it moves the stapes against the oval window into which it fits; as the stapes presses inwardly on the perilymph around the cochlear duct, it starts a ripple in the perilymph
      (5) Movement of the perilymph is transmitted to the endolymph inside the cochlear duct and stimulates the organ of Corti, which projects into the endolymph
      (6) Cochlear nerve conducts impulses from the organ of Corti to the brain; hearing occurs when impulses reach the auditory area in the temporal lobe of the cerebral cortex

Muscular system

A. Functions
   1. Movement
   2. Posture
   3. Heat production—metabolism in muscle cells produces relatively large share of body heat
B. Types of muscles and neural control
   1. Striated—controlled by voluntary nervous system via somatic motoneurons in spinal and some cranial nerves
   2. Smooth—controlled by autonomic nervous system via autonomic motoneurons in autonomic, spinal, and some cranial nerves; not under voluntary control (with rare exceptions)
   3. Cardiac—control is identical to that of smooth muscle
C. Anatomy of skeletal muscle as a whole
   1. Typically spindle shaped; composed of long muscle cells referred to as muscle fibers; invested by coating of fibrous connective tissue (fascia), which binds muscle to surrounding tissues
   2. Arranged in bundles or fasciculi; each muscle contains several fasciculi
   3. Contains rich blood supply; numerous capillary beds provide nutrients to and remove wastes from muscle
   4. Characteristics of individual skeletal muscle fibers
      a. Generally long and spindle shaped
      b. Multinucleate; called a syncytium

   c. Cell membrane called sarcolemma; endoplasmic reticulum called sarcoplasmic reticulum; mitochondria may be referred to as sarcosomes
   d. Contain myofibrils specialized for contraction; composed of two types of protein myofilaments, actin and myosin
D. Neuromuscular junction
   1. Axon terminal forms junction with sarcolemma of muscle fiber; tiny synaptic cleft separates presynaptic membrane (axon) from postsynaptic membrane (sarcolemma)
   2. Axon terminals contain tiny sacs, synaptic vesicles, that contain the neurotransmitter acetylcholine
   3. When nerve impulse reaches axon terminal, acetylcholine is released from synaptic vesicles into synaptic cleft; acetylcholine diffuses across synaptic cleft and attaches to receptor sites on sarcolemma; receptor sites are attached to channels in membrane; when acetylcholine binds to receptor site, channel opens and sodium and potassium ions flow down their concentration gradients; the sarcolemma is depolarized, and electrical energy flows into muscle fiber
   4. The enzyme cholinesterase, found in the synaptic cleft, inactivates acetylcholine; additional stimulation of muscle requires release of more acetylcholine
E. Muscle fiber contraction
   1. Electrical energy flows deep into muscle fiber along T tubules associated with sarcoplasmic reticulum
   2. Calcium ions released by flow of electrical energy inactivate troponin, which normally blocks interaction between actin and myosin
   3. Myosin releases and uses energy from ATP to cause actin to slide along myosin filaments (contraction); cessation of impulses leaves actin and myosin in a relaxed unassociated phase
   4. Energy for contraction—immediate energy is ATP; creatine phosphate, a high-energy molecule stored in abundance in muscle, replenishes supply of ATP as needed; ultimate source of energy is glucose and fatty acids oxidized aerobically to CO_2 and H_2O with release of energy
   5. Anaerobic breakdown of glucose during prolonged and vigorous muscle contraction results in lactic acid buildup associated with fatigue and an aching feeling; this oxygen debt is paid off during rest, when oxygen is plentiful

F. Basic principles of skeletal muscle action
   1. Skeletal muscles contract only if stimulated; a skeletal muscle and its motor nerve function as a physiologic (motor unit) unit; either is useless without the other's functioning; for this reason anything that prevents impulse conduction to a skeletal muscle paralyzes the muscle
   2. Most skeletal muscles attach to at least 2 bones; as a muscle contracts and pulls on its bones, it mobilizes the bone that moves most easily; the bone that moves is called the muscle's insertion bone, and the bone that remains stationary is its origin bone
   3. Bones serve as levers and joints as fulcrums of these levers; a muscle's contraction exerts a pulling force on its insertion bone at the point where the muscle inserts, pulling that point nearer the muscle's origin bone
   4. Skeletal muscles almost always act in groups rather than singly; members of groups are classified as follows
      a. Prime movers—the muscle or muscles whose contraction actually produces the movement
      b. Synergists—muscles that contract at the same time as the prime mover, helping it produce the movement or stabilizing the part; i.e., holding it steady, so the prime mover can produce a more effective movement
      c. Antagonists—muscles that relax while the prime mover is contracting (exception: antagonist contracts at the same time as the prime mover when a part needs to be held rigid, as the knee joint does in standing); antagonists are usually located directly opposite the bones they move; e.g., muscle that flexes lower arm lies on anterior surface of upper arm bone, whereas that which extends lower arm lies on posterior surface of upper arm
   5. The body of a muscle usually does not lie over the part moved by the muscle; instead it lies above or below, or anterior or posterior to, the part; thus the body of a muscle that moves the lower arm will not be located in the lower arm but in the upper arm; e.g., biceps and triceps brachii muscles
   6. Contraction of a skeletal muscle either shortens the muscle, producing movement, or increases

the tension (tone) in the muscle; contractions are classified according to whether they produce movement or increase muscle tone as follows

   a. Tonic contractions—produce muscle tone; do not shorten the muscle so do not produce movements; only a few fibers contract at one time, and this produces a moderate degree of muscle tone; in the healthy, awake body all muscles exhibit tone

   b. Isometric contractions—increase the degree of muscle tone; do not shorten the muscle so do not produce movements; daily repetition of isometric contractions gradually increases muscle strength

   c. Isotonic contractions—muscle shortens, thereby producing movement; all movements are produced by isotonic contractions

G. Origins, insertions, and functions of main skeletal muscles grouped according to functions (Table 2-15)

H. Weak places in abdominal wall where hernias may occur
1. Inguinal rings—right and left internal, right and left external
2. Femoral rings—right and left
3. Umbilicus

I. Metabolism of skeletal muscle
1. Hypertrophy is physical enlargement of muscle due to addition of more myofibrils to muscle fibers, making them swell; muscle fibers do not divide to produce new fibers
2. Atrophy is reduction in size of muscle due to decrease in number of myofibrils in muscle fiber
3. Treppe—when muscles have contracted a few times, subsequent contractions are more powerful; may be related to release of increased quantities of calcium ions from sarcoplasmic reticulum after the first few contractions
4. Shivering—rapid, repeating, involuntary skeletal muscle contractions; shivering contractions caused by hypothalamic temperature regulating center; makes use of inefficiency of muscle contraction; i.e., most of energy of ATP is converted to heat; smaller part of energy goes into the mechanical motion of contraction
5. Rigor mortis—ATP must combine with myosin to effect release of actin from myosin, which permits relaxation; after death, ATP is depleted from muscle fibers, and actin and myosin strongly associate, producing rigor mortis; subsequent

bacterial decomposition of muscle proteins brings about relaxation; body enters rigor state about 24 hours after death and comes out of rigor about 24 hours later

J. Bursae
1. Definition—small sacs lined with synovial membrane and containing synovial fluid
2. Locations—wherever pressure is exerted over moving parts
   a. Between skin and bone
   b. Between tendons and bone
   c. Between muscles or ligaments and bone
3. Names of bursae that frequently become inflamed (bursitis)
   a. Subacromial—between deltoid muscle and head of humerus and acromion process
   b. Olecranon—between olecranon process and skin; inflammation called student's elbow
   c. Prepatellar—between patella and skin; inflammation called housemaid's knee
4. Function—act as cushions, relieving pressure between moving parts

K. Tendon sheaths
1. Definition and location—tube-shaped structures that enclose certain tendons, notably those of wrist and ankle; made of connective tissue lined with synovial membrane
2. Function—facilitate gliding movements of tendon

Skeletal system

A. Functions
1. Furnishes supporting framework
2. Affords protection for viscera, brain, hemopoietic system
3. Provides levers for muscles to pull on to produce movements
4. Hemopoiesis by red bone marrow—formation of all kinds of blood cells; note that some lymphocytes and monocytes are formed in lymphatic tissue
5. Mineral storage—calcium, phosphorus in the form of phosphates, and sodium are stored in bone

B. Nature of bone substance
1. Organic matter—makes up about 33% of bone by weight
   a. Cells
     (1) Osteoblasts—bone-producing cells

Table 2-15. Origins, insertions, and functions of main skeletal muscles

Part of body moved	Movement	Muscle	Origin	Insertion
Upper arm	Flexion	Pectoralis major	Clavicle (medial half) Sternum Costal cartilages of true ribs	Humerus (greater tubercle)
	Extension	Latissimus dorsi	Vertebrae (lower thoracic, lumbar, and sacral) Ilium (crest) Lumbodorsal fascia	Humerus (intertubercular groove)
	Abduction	Deltoid	Clavicle Scapula (spine and acromion)	Humerus (lateral side on deltoid tubercle)
	Adduction	Latissimus dorsi contracting with pectoralis major	See above See above	See above See above
Shoulder	Shrugging, elevating	Trapezius	Occipital bone Vertebrae (cervical and thoracic)	Scapula (spine and acromion) Clavicle
	Lowering	Pectoralis minor Serratus anterior	Ribs (second to fifth) Ribs (upper 8 or 9)	Scapula (coracoid) Scapula (anterior surface)
Lower arm	Flexion (With forearm supinated)	Biceps brachii	Scapula (supraglenoid tuberosity) Scapula (coracoid)	Radius (tubercle at proximal end)
	(With forearm pronated)	Brachialis	Humerus (distal half, anterior surface)	Ulna (front of coronoid process)
	(With forearm semi-supinated or semi-pronated)	Brachioradialis	Humerus (above lateral epicondyle)	Radius (styloid process)
	Extension	Triceps brachii	Scapula (infraglenoid tuberosity) Humerus (posterior surface—lateral head above radial groove; medial head, below)	Ulna (olecranon process)
Thigh	Flexion	Iliopsoas (iliacus and psoas major)	Ilium (iliac fossa) Vertebrae (bodies of twelfth thoracic to fifth lumbar)	Femur (small trochanter)
		Rectus femoris	Ilium and anterior inferior iliac spine	Tibia (by way of patellar tendon)
	Extension	Gluteus maximus	Ilium (crest and posterior surface) Sacrum and coccyx (posterior surface) Sacrotuberous ligament	Femur (gluteal tuberosity) Iliotibial tract
		Hamstring group (see below)	Ischium (Tuberosity) Femur (linea aspera)	Fibula (head of) Tibia (lateral condyle, medial condyle, and medial surface)
	Abduction	Gluteus medius and minimus	Ilium (lateral surface)	Femur (greater trochanter)
		Tensor fasciae latae	Ilium (anterior part of crest)	Iliotibial tract

Table 2-15. Origins, insertions, and functions of main skeletal muscles—cont'd

Part of body moved	Movement	Muscle	Origin	Insertion
Thigh—cont'd	Adduction	Adductor group Brevis Longus Magnus	Pubic bone	Femur (linea aspera)
Lower leg	Flexion	Hamstring group Biceps femoris Semitendinosus Semimembranosus	Ischium (tuberosity) Femur (linea aspera)	Fibula (head of) Tibia (lateral condyle, medial condyle, and medial surface)
		Gastrocnemius	Femur (condyles)	Tarsal bone (calcaneus by way of tendo calcaneus)
	Extension	Quadriceps femoris group	Ilium (anterior inferior spine)	Tibia (by way of patellar tendon)
		Rectus femoris Vastus lateralis Vastus medialis Vastus intermedius	Femur (linea aspera and anterior surface)	
Foot	Flexion (dorsiflexion)	Tibialis anterior	Tibia (lateral condyle)	First cuneiform tarsal Base of first metatarsal
	Extension (plantar flexion)	Gastrocnemius	Femur (condyles)	Calcaneus, by way of tendo calcaneus
		Soleus	Tibia	Same as gastrocnemius, but underneath
Head	Flexion	Sternocleidomastoid	Sternum Clavicle	Temporal bone (mastoid process)
	Extension	Trapezius	Vertebrae (cervical) Scapula (spine and acromion) Clavicle	Occiput
Abdominal wall	Compress abdominal cavity; therefore assists in staining, defecation, forced expiration, childbirth, posture, etc.	External oblique	Ribs (lower 8)	Innominate bone (iliac crest and pubis by way of inguinal ligament) Linea alba
		Internal oblique	Innominate bone (iliac crest, inguinal ligament) Lumbodorsal fascia	Ribs (lower 3) Pubic bone Linea alba
		Transversus	Ribs (lower 6) Innominate bone (iliac crest, inguinal ligament) Lumbodorsal fascia	Pubic bone Linea alba
		Rectus abdominis	Innominate bone (pubic bone and symphysis pubis)	Ribs (costal cartilage of fifth, sixth, seventh)
Chest wall	Elevate ribs, thereby enlarging anteroposterior and anterolateral dimensions of chest and causing inspiration	External intercostals	Ribs (lower border of all but twelfth)	Ribs (upper border of rib below origin)

Table 2-15. Origins, insertions, and functions of main skeletal muscles—cont'd

Part of body moved	Movement	Muscle	Origin	Insertion
Chest wall—cont'd	Depress ribs	Internal intercostals	Ribs (inner surface, upper border of all except first)	Ribs (lower border of rib above origin)
	Pull floor of thorax downward, thereby enlarging vertical dimension of chest and causing inspiration	Diaphragm	Lower circumference of rib cage	Central tendon of diaphragm
Trunk	Flexion	Iliopsoas	Femur (small trochanter)	Ilium Vertebrae (bodies of twelfth thoracic to fifth lumbar)
	Extension	Sacrospinalis Iliocostalis (lateral) Longissimus (medial)	Vertebrae (posterior surface of sacrum, spinous processes of lumbar, and last 2 thoracic)	Ribs (lower 6) Vertebrae (transverse processes of thoracic) Ribs
			Ilium (posterior part of crest)	Vertebrae (spines of thoracic)
		Quadratus lumborum	Ilium (posterior part of crest) Vertebrae (lower 3 lumbar)	Ribs (twelfth) Vertebrae (transverse processes of first 4 lumbar)

(2) Osteoclasts—bone-dissolving cells

(3) Osteocytes—former osteoblasts embedded in and maintaining bone substance

b. Collagen—collagen fibers make up about 97% of organic matter of bone; gives bone tough and somewhat flexible quality; responsible for high tensile strength of bone

c. Polysaccharides—part of ground substance of bone consists of polysaccharides such as hyaluronic acid and sialic acid

d. Protein—polysaccharide complexes such as chondroitin sulfate are part of ground substance of bone

2. Inorganic matter—makes up about 67% of bone by weight

a. Apatite salts—apatite, a complex ion composed of calcium and phosphates, forms hydroxyapatite, carbonate apatite, and fluoride apatite; makes bone hard and is responsible for the high compressional strength of bone

b. Magnesium and sodium ions are part of bone matrix

c. Certain radioactive isotopes accumulate in bone; e.g., strontium 90, calcium 45, phosphorus 32, and plutonium 259; may increase likelihood of bone tumors and leukemia

C. Bone formation

1. Intramembranous ossification—fibrous membranes composing certain parts of fetal skeleton, such as skull bones and lower jaw, are converted to bone

2. Endochondral ossification—conversion of cartilage bone models into actual bone in fetus; most of fetal skeletal system ossifies by endochondral ossification

3. Ossification—end result of either intramembranous or endochondral ossification is the same, cancellous (spongy) bone; the denser type of bone substance, compact bone, forms later in development through conversion of selected regions of cancellous bone into compact bone

a. Distribution of cancellous and compact bone

(1) Outer surface of all bones, except at joints, composed of compact bone

(2) Interior of short, flat, and irregular bones (all bones except long bones) composed

of cancellous bone; epiphyses of long bones composed of cancellous bone in their interior

    (3) Diaphyses of long bones hollow; walls of diaphysis composed of compact bone

  b. Ossification process

    (1) Formation of bone matrix (the intercellular substance of bone), made up of collagen fibers and a cementlike ground substance composed of polysaccharides and protein-polysaccharide complexes; osteoblasts (bone-forming cells) synthesize collagen and cement substance from proteins provided by the diet; vitamin C promotes formation of bone matrix; exercise and estrogens act to stimulate osteoblasts to form bone matrix

    (2) Calcification of bone matrix—calcium salts deposited in the bone matrix; vitamin D promotes calcification by stimulating calcium uptake in small intestine

  c. Bone growth

    (1) In length—by continual thickening of epiphyseal cartilage followed by ossification; as long as bone growth continues, epiphyseal cartilage grows faster than it can be replaced by bone; therefore line of cartilage persists between diaphysis and epiphyses and can be seen on x-ray film; during adolescence cartilage is completely transformed into bone, at which time bone growth is complete

    (2) In diameter—osteoclasts destroy bone surrounding medullary cavity, thereby enlarging the cavity; at the same time, osteoblasts add new bone around outer surface of the bone; bones may thicken throughout life, depending on the stresses placed on the bone; the more prolonged the stress (walking, running, weight lifting), the thicker the bones become within physiologic limits

D. Structure of long bones (Fig. 10)

E. Names and numbers of bones (Table 2-16)

F. Joints

  1. Synarthrotic—generally nonmovable joints; also called fibrous joints—no joint cavity or capsule; joining bones held together by fibrous tissue

    a. Sutures—bind skull bones together

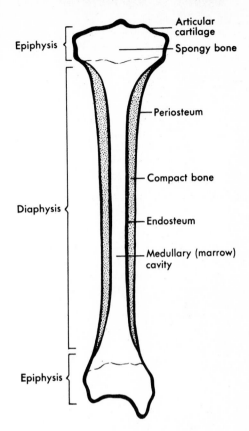

Fig. 10. Diagram to show structure of long bone as seen in longitudinal section. (From Anthony, C. P., and Kolthoff, N. J.: Textbook of anatomy and physiology, ed. 9, St. Louis, 1975, The C. V. Mosby Co.)

    b. Syndesmoses—bind tibia and fibula; bind diaphyses of radius and ulna

  2. Amphiarthrotic—slightly movable joints; also called cartilagenous joints—no joint cavity or capsule; joining bones held together by cartilage and ligaments

    a. Symphyses—disc of cartilage between bones, as between vertebrae or at pubic symphysis

    b. Synchondroses—costal cartilages bind ribs to sternum

  3. Diarthrotic—freely movable joint; joint cavity or space between articular surfaces of two bones united by joint, thin layer of hyaline cartilage covering articular surfaces of joining bones;

Table 2-16. Bones of the body

Part of body	Name of bone	Number	Description
1. Axial skeleton			
a. Skull*			
(1) Cranium	1. Frontal	1	1. Forehead bone
	2. Parietal	2	2. Bulging bones that form top sides of cranium
	3. Temporal	2	3. Form lower sides of cranium and part of cranial floor
	4. Occipital	1	4. Forms posterior part of cranial floor and walls
	5. Sphenoid	1	5. Forms mid portion of cranial floor
	6. Ethmoid	1	6. Composes part of anterior portion of cranial floor; lies anterior to sphenoid, posterior to nasal bones
(2) Face	1. Nasal	2	1. Form upper part of bridge of nose
	2. Maxillary	2	2. Upper jaw bones
	3. Zygomatic (malar)	2	3. Cheek bones
	4. Mandible	1	4. Lower jaw bone
	5. Lacrimal	2	5. Fingernail-shaped bones posterior and lateral to nasal bones, in medial wall of orbit
	6. Palatine	2	6. Form posterior part of hard palate
	7. Inferior conchae (turbinates)	2	7. Thin scroll of bone along inner surface of side wall of nasal cavity
	8. Vomer	1	8. Lower, posterior part of nasal septum
(3) Ear ossicles	1. Malleus (hammer)	2	Tiny bones in middle ear cavity in temporal bone; resemble, respectively, miniature hammer, anvil, and stirrups
	2. Incus (anvil)	2	
	3. Stapes (stirrups)	2	
b. Hyoid bone		1	U-shaped bone in neck between mandible and upper part of larynx; only bone in body that forms no joints with any other bones
c. Vertebral column	1. Cervical vertebrae	7	1. Upper 7 vertebrae
	2. Thoracic vertebrae	12	2. Next 12 vertebrae; ribs attached to these
	3. Lumbar vertebrae	5	3. Next 5 vertebrae, located in "small" of back
	4. Sacrum	1	4. In embryo, 5 separate vertebrae, but fused in adult into 1 wedge-shaped bone
	5. Coccyx	1	5. In embryo, 4 or 5 separate vertebrae, but fused in adult into 1 bone
d. Ribs and sternum	1. True ribs	7 pairs	1. Upper 7 pairs fastened to sternum by costal cartilages
	2. False ribs	5 pairs	2. Do not attach to sternum directly; upper 3 pairs of false ribs attached by means of costal cartilage of seventh ribs; last 2 pairs not attached at all and therefore called "floating" ribs
	3. Sternum	1	3. Breast bone
2. Appendicular skeleton			
a. Upper extremities	1. Clavicle	2	1. Collar bone; shoulder girdle fastened to axial skeleton by articulation of clavicle with sternum

*Paranasal sinuses—holes in frontal, sphenoidal, maxillary, and ethmoid bones reduce weight of skull, serve as resonating chambers in speech, produce mucus, and often become inflamed due to allergic responses and viral or bacterial infection.

†Sesamoid bones (rounded bones found in various tendons) have not been counted except for patellae, which are largest sesamoid bones; number of these bones varies greatly between individuals. Wormian bones (small islets of bones in some cranial sutures) have not been counted because of variability of occurrence.

Table 2-16. Bones of the body—cont'd

Part of body	Name of bone	Number	Description
2. Appendicular skeleton—cont'd			
a. Upper extremities—cont'd	2. Scapula	2	2. Shoulder blade
	3. Humerus	2	3. Long bone of upper arm
	4. Radius	2	4. Thumb side of forearm
	5. Ulna	2	5. Little finger side of forearm
	6. Carpals	16	6. Wrist bones; arranged in 2 rows at proximal end of hand
	7. Metacarpals	10	7. Long bones; form framework of palm of hand
	8. Phalanges	28	8. Miniature long bones of fingers; 3 in each finger, 2 in each thumb
b. Lower extremities	1. Os coxae, or pelvic bone	2	1. Large hip bones; lower extremities attached to axial skeleton by articulation of pelvic bones with sacrum
	2. Femur	2	2. Thigh bone
	3. Patella	2	3. Kneecap
	4. Tibia	2	4. Shin bone
	5. Fibula	2	5. Long, slender bone of lateral side of lower leg
	6. Tarsals	14	6. "Ankle" bones; form heel and proximal end of foot
	7. Metatarsals	10	7. Long bones of feet
	8. Phalanges	28	8. Miniature long bones of toes
	TOTAL	206†	

bones held together by fibrous capsule lined with synovial membrane and ligaments; may be ball and socket (as in hip), hinge (as in elbow), condyloid (as at wrist), pivot, gliding, or saddle

a. Kinds of movement possible at diarthrotic joints

(1) Flexion—bending one bone on another; e.g., bending forearm on upper arm

(2) Extension—stretching one bone away from another; e.g., straightening lower arm out from flexed position

(3) Abduction—moving bone away from body's midline; e.g., moving arms straight out from sides

(4) Adduction—moving bone back toward body's midline; e.g., bringing arms back to sides of body from outstretched, or abducted, position

(5) Rotation—pivoting bone on its axis; e.g., partial rotation such as turning head from side to side

(6) Circumduction—describing surface of cone with moving part; e.g., moving arm around so that hand describes circle

(7) Supination—forearm movement turning palm forward

(8) Pronation—forearm movement turning back of hand foreward

(9) Inversion—ankle movement turning sole of foot inward

(10) Eversion—ankle movement turning sole of foot outward

(11) Protraction—moving part, such as lower jaw, forward

(12) Retraction—pulling part back; opposite of protraction

(13) Plantar flexion—pointing toes (as a ballerina) away from body

(14) Dorsiflextion—pointing toes toward the body

G. Differences between male and female skeletons

1. Male skeleton larger and heavier than that of female

2. Male pelvis deep and funnel shaped with narrow pubic arch; female pelvis shallow, broad, and flaring with wider pubic arch

H. Age changes in skeleton

1. From infancy to adulthood, not only do bones

grow, but also their relative sizes change; head becomes proportionately smaller, pelvis relatively larger, legs proportionately longer, etc.

2. From young adulthood to old age, bone margins and projections change gradually; bone piles up along them (marginal lipping and spurs), thereby restricting movement; such continuing growth is due, in part, to stimulation of somatotrophic hormone

I. Repair of skeleton
   1. When bone is fractured, connective tissue called a callus grows into and around broken region
   2. Macrophages reabsorb dead and damaged cells
   3. Osteoclasts dissolve bone fragments
   4. Osteoblasts produce new bone substance and fuse bone together
   5. Final bone shape slowly remodeled; complete process takes several months; much slower than epithelial tissue, which has a higher metabolic rate and richer blood supply

REVIEW OF PHYSICAL PRINCIPLES RELATED TO THE NEUROMUSCULOSKELETAL SYSTEMS
Principles of mechanics

A. Applications of energy laws—machines
   Apart from friction, the work output of a machine is equal to the work input to the machine; the first law of thermodynamics indicates that energy cannot be created or destroyed; a machine can multiply force, that is, provide a mechanical advantage, but at the expense of distance
   1. Lever—a rigid bar that moves about a fixed point known as the fulcrum; a small force is applied through a large distance and the other end of the lever exerts a large force over a small distance; the musculoskeletal system operates through lever systems
      a. First-class lever—fulcrum between resistance and effort; e.g., scissors, hemostat, bending head backward or forward
      b. Second-class levers—resistance between fulcrum and effort; e.g., wheelbarrow, oxygen tank carrier
      c. Third-class lever—effort between resistance and fulcrum; e.g., forceps, bending over and using your back muscles to lift an object with your hips acting as the fulcrum; swinging the arm when using a tennis racquet

   2. Pulleys—this machine can also multiply force at the expense of distance; the use of a number of pulleys together, as in a block and tackle, provides a mechanical advantage equal to the number of ropes excluding the pull rope; thus a block and tackle with 2 ropes gives a mechanical advantage of 2; a 100-lb weight can be lifted by application of a force of 50 lb; e.g., traction, lifting heavy objects like engines; pulleys used to change direction of a force—used in traction to apply tension in back injuries

B. Center of gravity
   1. Position in a body where all the weight may be considered to be located; sphere, such as a rubber ball, has its center of gravity in its center
   2. An object is stable (will not topple over) as long as a line dropped from its center of gravity to the ground is within the base of the object; in a human the center of gravity is in the pelvic cavity, and for upright balance the line drawn from this point to the ground must fall somewhere between the legs
      a. When lifting a patient, the back should be kept straight to keep torque at a minimum; in addition, when bending over, the body's center of gravity shifts from a stable position between the legs to an unstable position outside the legs; the back muscles must then work even harder to prevent the body from toppling over
      b. When walking and carrying a load, the load should be carried as close to the body (center of gravity) as possible to maintain balance and to avoid strain

Principles of physical properties of matter

A. Pascal's principle—when pressure is applied to a fluid in a closed, nonflexible container, that pressure is transmitted undiminished throughout all parts of the fluid and the pressure acts in all directions
   EXAMPLE: Cerebrospinal fluid—an abnormal increase of pressure on this fluid is transmitted to all parts of the central nervous system containing the fluid
   1. Brain tumor—a mass of tissue displaces fluid and increases the pressure of the cerebrospinal fluid
   2. Hydrocephalus—blockage in the canal of Sylvius or overactivity of the choroid plexuses results in a tremendous collection of fluid and increased pressure

B. Electromagnetic radiation
1. X rays
EXAMPLE: Pneumoencephalogram—the ventricles of the brain can be imaged radiographically if the cerebrospinal fluid of the ventricles is temporarily replaced by air; as x rays pass through the brain, the ventricles are outlined; the picture obtained is called a pneumoencephalogram
2. Radiation hazards—individuals working with x rays should leave the room, stand behind a lead shield, or wear a lead apron when activating the x-ray machine, since there is some scattering of radiation in all directions even though the x-ray beam is aimed at a particular area; film badges (photographic film) should be worn when working near sources of radiation to provide a record of the individual's overall exposure to the radiation
C. Sound—mechanical vibration; cannot occur in vacuum; propagated best through solids and through liquids better than gases; travels in waves from vibrating source such as vocal cords, loudspeaker, or dropped object
1. Properties of waves
a. Transverse waves—if the particles of the medium vibrate at right angles to the direction of the wave, the wave is transverse; waves on the surface of liquids and all electromagnetic waves (light, infrared, and ultraviolet) are transverse waves
b. Longitudinal waves—the particles of the medium vibrate back and forth along the same direction as the wave; sound waves are longitudinal waves
c. Frequency—the number of complete vibrations (or waves) generated or moving along per second; referred to as cycles per second or as a hertz (Hz)
d. The passage of a wave through a medium (either gas, liquid, solid, or plasma) is actually the passage of a disturbance in the medium, not a flowing of the medium itself; the wave represents sequential vibration or swinging of the molecules of the medium from the vibrating source to the ears
e. Refraction of sound waves—sound travels faster in warm air than cool air; in warm air the average kinetic energy of the air molecules is higher than in cooler air and the wave can be propagated more quickly

f. Reflection of sound waves—many solid objects reflect sound waves from their surfaces resulting in an echo; a reverberation is a series of echoes
g. The energy of sound waves—all waves possess energy but to differing degrees; ultraviolet waves and gamma radiation possess high energy, whereas sound waves possess little energy; the structure of the ear reflects the need to amplify the relatively weak energy of sound waves into more energetic waves capable of stimulating the liquid-filled organ of hearing, the cochlea in the inner ear
h. The velocity of sound—the frequency of the wave times the length of the wave; the velocity of sound waves varies with the nature and temperature of the medium; since light travels much faster than sound, lightning is seen before thunder is heard
2. Interpretation of sounds
a. Loudness—a neurologic or psychologic interpretation of intensity; although the exact relationship is complex, one could say that the greater the intensity of the sound waves stimulating the organ of Corti, the greater the frequency of nerve impulses reaching the auditory centers of the brain and the louder the sound seems to be
(1) Noise level is measured in decibels (dB); a normal conversation is about 65 dB, amplified rock music about 120 dB, and the sound of a nearby jet airplane about 140 dB; the decibel scale is logarithmic so that 120 dB is 1 million times more intense than 60 dB
(2) Excessive noise can result in hearing loss at certain frequencies of sound; noise levels of about 85 dB and over can damage the organ of Corti; damage increases with the length and intensity of noise and is irreversible
(3) The Doppler effect—when a vibrating source and a receiver of sound move toward each other, the pitch or frequency of the sound produced by the source becomes higher; as the vibrating source and the receiver move away from each other, the frequency of the sound becomes lower
(4) Speech audiometry—this technique de-

tects the threshold of hearing of actual speech for individuals by presenting groups of 2-syllable words at successively lower levels until the person fails to hear; these data are presented as a speech reception threshold (SRT) in decibels; phonetically balanced single-syllable words can also be presented; these words represent a frequency of sounds of speech that approximates a typical conversation; the percentage of words repeated correctly is the Davis Social Adequacy Index (SAI); a score of 94% to 100% is considered normal

b. Pitch—corresponds to frequency; the higher the frequency, the higher the pitch of the sound
   (1) The human ear can potentially hear sounds whose frequencies range from 16 to 20,000 Hz; with increasing age, the upper range decreases slightly, which presents no problem in hearing speech, since speech falls in the range of 85 to 1050 Hz
   (2) The audiometer electronically produces sounds at a variety of frequencies as well as intensities and is used to measure hearing loss

c. Quality—people have different and distinct qualities or timbres to their voices; similarly, the sounds of different musical instruments are easily recognized; a musical sound or a voice rarely represents a pure tone but usually many frequencies occurring simultaneously

d. Ultrasonic sound—vibrational frequencies exceeding the upper level of human hearing (20,000 Hz)
   (1) Can be used in cleaning metal parts; the high-frequency vibrations shake the solution and produce bubbles that help in the cleaning process; ultrasonic cleaners are available for hospital use in cleaning syringes and needles
   (2) Low-intensity ultrasonic waves have been used to treat arthritis and bursitis, to break kidney stones, and to help dissolve scars
   (3) Ultrasonic dental drills can quickly drill into teeth without the pain associated with tooth vibrations, which stimulate the nerve of the tooth

(4) Sonograms are pictures of the body derived through differential reflection or transmission of sound waves

e. Deafness—the condition wherein sound vibrations are not transmitted to the brain for interpretation
   (1) Perforation or tear of the tympanic membrane
   (2) Inflexibility of the 3 middle ear bones or ossicles; vibrations are now only poorly transmitted to the oval window
   (3) Otosclerosis—abnormal bone formation over the oval window immobilizes the stapes
      (a) Surgery can remove the abnormal bony tissue in the early stages of the disease
      (b) In later stages, the stapes can be removed and a prosthesis can be implanted
      (c) If the oval window is ossified, a new opening in the cochlea is made to replace the oval window (fenestration)
      (d) Bone-conduction hearing aids can essentially bypass the middle ear
   (4) Deafness caused by auditory nerve damage; the nerve cannot be regenerated nor can hearing be helped by hearing aids

f. Hearing aids—electronic devices that amplify sounds and assist partially deaf persons to hear; a miniature microphone picks up the sound, sends it to an amplifier and then to a miniature loudspeaker fitted in or behind the ear
   (1) Air-conduction type sends an amplified sound wave into the ear, thus utilizing the person's own middle ear
   (2) Bone-conduction type bypasses the middle ear and transmits amplified vibrations to the skull bones, which in turn produce vibrations in the inner ear

D. Light
   1. Basic concepts
      a. Visible light is a type of electromagnetic radiation; all electromagnetic radiation consists of moving electric and magnetic energy fields that come into existence because of the vibrations of electrically charged particles
      b. All types of electromagnetic radiation have

the same electric and magnetic nature and travel at the same constant velocity:186,000 miles per second (speed of light)

   c. The electromagnetic spectrum varies from extremely long AM and FM radio waves measured in miles to very short gamma and cosmic rays measured in millimeters

   d. The product of the frequency of vibration and the wavelength is constant (the velocity of light); the lower the frequency of vibration of the wave, the longer the wavelength, and the higher the frequency, the shorter the wavelength

   e. The higher the frequency (or the shorter the wavelength) of electromagnetic radiation, the greater the energy content of the radiation

2. Wavelengths of electromagnetic radiation

   a. Wavelengths are measured in either millimicra or Angstrom units

      (1) A millimicron is one thousandth of a micron; a micron is one millionth of a meter (39 inches)

      (2) An Angstrom unit is one tenth of a millimicron

   b. The wavelength of visible light possesses just the right amount of vibrational energy to excite the photoreceptor cells (rods and cones) of the retina

   c. Different wavelengths of light are bent or refracted to slightly different degrees and appear to the eyes and brain as different colors; this principle of dispersion is responsible for a rainbow

   d. Emission of light—atoms can be excited by absorbing energy that causes orbiting electrons to jump to higher energy levels within the atom; as the electrons fall back to their lower, more stable energy levels (deexcitation) the energy of excitation is released and may appear as visible light; e.g., advertising signs and mercury vapor street lamps

      (1) A characteristic pattern of wavelengths of light (a discontinuous spectrum) is emitted from every element in the vapor state; this pattern is best seen using a spectroscope

      (2) Fluorescence—the property of absorbing radiation of one frequency and reemitting radiation of a lower frequency and energy;

a substance is said to be fluorescent if it emits visible light when energized or bombarded with ultraviolet (UV) light; high-intensity fluorescent light bulbs have been used to treat jaundice in newborn infants; the excess bilirubin in the blood, which is responsible for the jaundice, is oxidized by exposure to the bright light as blood passes through the vessels of the thin skin

      (3) Phosphorescence—the atoms of a phosphorescent substance become deexcited a relatively long period of time after being excited; the phosphorescent atoms in the dial of a luminous clock are excited during the day by the visible light striking it; it glows throughout the night as billions of excited atoms gradually become deexcited, releasing their energy as visible light

3. Lasers

   a. Laser is an acronym for **l**ight **a**mplification by **s**timulated **e**mission of **r**adiation; a laser produces coherent light, which means that the light waves are all of the same frequency, are all in phase with each other (peak with peak, trough with trough), and are all traveling in the same direction; in coherent light, millions of light waves become additive and form a single, concentrated beam of light that travels in a straight line without spreading out and that can be precisely focused on minute areas

   b. As coherent light leaves the laser (ruby crystal) it can be utilized for a variety of purposes

      (1) Eye surgery—the energy in the coherent light produced by a laser is used to fuse minute areas of the retina to the surrounding choroid coat; an ophthalmoscope is used to precisely focus the coherent light on specific, tiny areas of the retina; a detached retina can in this way be reattached, and the fusion points are so tiny that there is no apparent loss of light-sensitive retinal tissue; the machine used in this type of surgery is called a photocoagulator and uses a ruby laser

      (2) Cancer therapy—the laser has been used to selectively treat pigmented skin cancers, which apparently absorb the light

more readily than the surrounding, less pigmented normal tissue

4. Color
   a. The perception of color is the result of the translation and interpretation of certain nerve impulses in the brain that come from the retina; the frequency of light determines the color that is seen; the lowest frequency stimulating the retina is red, the highest is violet, in between are all the colors of nature
   b. An object may appear to be colored because it emits electromagnetic radiation that falls within the visible range; an object may also appear colored not because it emits light, but because of selective reflection
   c. Color mixing
      (1) Red, green, and blue are the additive primaries; any color in the spectrum can be obtained with the proper blend of these 3 colors; equal amounts of the 3 of them produce white light
      (2) Magenta, yellow, and cyan (turquoise) are the subtractive primaries; any color in the spectrum can be obtained using the proper blend of these 3 colors; they are sometimes loosely called, respectively, red, yellow, and blue
      (3) Complementary colors are any 2 colors that, when added together, produce white: red and cyan, magenta and green, and yellow and blue
   d. Perception of color is believed to depend on the cones of the retina that are located most densely at the part of the retina called the fovea centralis; one type of cone detects red, another detects green, and another detects blue; it is generally believed that the brain blends nerve impulses from these three types of cones to produce all the colors of nature
      (1) Faulty color vision is thought to be caused by cones that are either missing or not functioning properly; red-green color blindness is the most common type and is a genetically inherited trait resulting in individuals seeing red and green objects as shades of gray; more men are affected than women, since the trait appears to be sex linked
      (2) Color and emotion—even though red light has a lower frequency and therefore less energy than a quantum of blue light, the human mind generally associates red with warmth, excitement, and mental stimulation, and blue with coolness and calmness; for many individuals, the color of an object or a room determines to a great extent whether they will keep and use the object or stay in the room; thus color has a physical basis in the electromagnetic radiation but involves complex interpretation by the human mind

5. Reflection and refraction
   a. General principles
      (1) Source of light—the sun is the primary outdoor source; incandescent and fluorescent bulbs are indoor light sources
      (2) Most objects are visible because they reflect light emitted from various sources
      (3) An object such as a pane of glass is transparent if it allows light to pass through it in straight lines
      (4) An object such as a thin cloth window shade or a piece of paper is translucent if it allows light to pass through it in a diffused manner so that objects cannot be seen; in hospitals, use of shades or blinds diffuses light and cuts down on harsh glare
      (5) An object such as a heavy pair of drapes is opaque if light cannot pass through it
      (6) Light traveling in any single given medium travels in straight lines; each straight line is called a ray
   b. Reflection
      (1) When light strikes a surface off which it can reflect, the angle of incidence equals the angle of reflection as measured from the normal (a line perpendicular to the plane of the reflecting surface)
         (a) When successive elevations of any surface are less than about one fourth the wavelength of the incident light, the light reflected from the surface travels mainly in one direction and the surface is polished
         (b) Light reflected from rougher surfaces travels in many directions and is diffusely reflected; it is easier to read a

page of text that is printed on paper that provides more diffuse than polished reflection, since glare is eliminated

(c) The word *ambulance* is often printed backward on the front of small ambulances so that motorists seeing the lettering via reflected light through their rearview mirrors will read the lettering correctly

(2) Virtual images—as light reflects off a mirror, the angles of incidence and reflection are equal; the reflected rays of light appear to come from a point behind the mirror; because the light rays do not actually come from this point, the image is referred to as a virtual image as opposed to a real image; the virtual image of a mirror is as far behind the mirror as the object is in front of the mirror

c. Refraction

(1) Refraction—the bending of an oblique ray of light as it travels from one transparent medium into another; refraction is caused by the change in average velocity of light as it passes through the medium

(2) Index of refraction—the average speed of light varies in different, transparent media; the average speed of light in water is only 75% of its average speed in a vacuum; the average speed of light in a diamond is 41% of its average speed in a vacuum; the index of refraction is a measure of how much the average speed of light differs from the speed of light in a vacuum; index of refraction equals the speed of light in vacuum divided by the speed of light in medium; the higher the index of refraction, the slower the average speed of light through the medium

EXAMPLES

1. A thermometer or syringe half immersed in a beaker of water appears to be bent at the point of immersion in the water

2. An object in water appears to be nearer to the surface than it actually is; thus the object seems larger because it is magnified

3. A mirage—the average speed of light is slightly greater in hot air than cool air; on a hot paved road or a desert the light reflected from an object is refracted upward, away from the hot surface and may then produce an upside-down virtual image to an individual some distance away; the wet shimmering look of a hot road is refracted light from the sky reaching a motorist's eye after passing through hot air layers

4. Total internal reflection—at a certain critical angle, light between 2 media is not refracted (or bent) through the 2 media, but reflected back into the first medium

a. This phenomenon permits viewing of the interior walls of the stomach, intestines, and blood vessels

b. A dentist's flashlight will "curve" the light (via total internal reflection) to the appropriate part of an individual's mouth

c. Total internal reflection via the paired prisms in a pair of binoculars permits higher magnifications in a short optic tube

6. Diffraction

a. The bending of light or any type of electromagnetic wave around corners is called diffraction; the longer the wavelength of electromagnetic radiation, the larger the object that it can be bent around

EXAMPLES

1. AM radio waves, some of which are over 3 miles long, easily bend around objects, thereby allowing AM radio broadcasts to come in clearly even in cities having many tall buildings and mountainous regions

2. FM radio waves, which are from 9 to 12 feet long, cannot easily bend around large objects; consequently, a specific location in a city or suburban area with large obstructing objects can determine the quality of the reception of FM broadcasts

3. Some spectrophotometers used in certain laboratory analyses of blood and urine rely

on diffraction gradings to disperse white light into its component wavelengths and to utilize these specific wavelengths in the analytic procedure

4. X-ray diffraction—because of their very short wavelengths, x rays diffract around the atoms in large molecules and produce diffraction patterns on photographic plates; analyses of these patterns can reveal the details of the arrangement of the atoms in a molecule; used in DNA analysis

7. Polarization
   a. Certain naturally occurring crystals, like tourmaline and herapathite, absorb light waves striking them in all planes but one; the light transmitted through and emerging from the crystal vibrates in only one plane; this light is called plane polarized light

   EXAMPLES

   1. Polaroid filters contain a material, like herapathite or certain synthetic molecules, that will only permit light vibrating in a single plane to pass through; when used in sunglasses, they cut down on glare and eye strain; much of the light reflected from nonmetallic surfaces, such as water, glass, or roadways, is already polarized because these surfaces tend to absorb light waves perpendicular to their surfaces and to reflect light waves parallel to their surfaces; when this polarized light strikes the Polaroid filters in the sunglasses, many of the light waves are absorbed; thus fewer waves are transmitted and the harsh glare is reduced

   2. Polarizing filters for cameras cut down on glare in photographs and also have the effect of deepening the blue color of the sky

   3. Polarizing microscopes are used in research laboratories to analyze the molecular structure of many substances

8. Lenses
   a. The refraction of light through transparent glass (or quartz or fluorite) lenses is of great practical importance; magnification of objects is possible using simple lenses as well as groups of lenses arranged in telescopes and microscopes; the principal axis of a lens is the line joining the 2 points that represent the centers of curvature of the curved surfaces of a given lens

   b. Convex lenses (converging or positive lenses) converge light rays passing through them; concave lenses (diverging or negative lenses) diverge light rays passing through them

   c. When light rays parallel to the principal axis pass through a converging lens, they converge on a point called the focal point; light rays not parallel to the principal axis converge in a series of points above and below the focal point, making up the focal plane

      (1) A converging lens will magnify an object (acting as a simple magnifying glass) if it is held inside the focal point of the lens; the image is enlarged, right side up and virtual; this means that the image only appears to exist but has no physical reality

      (2) When an object is placed outside the focal point of a converging lens, a real, inverted image is obtained that can be focused on a screen; whenever a real image is formed, the object and image are on opposite sides of the lens

   EXAMPLES

   1. Motion pictures utilize converging lenses, and the movie screen is the plane where light rays are converged; slide projectors also operate under the same principle

   2. In cameras the film is flattened out and placed in the focal plane of the camera's lens; in popular single-lens reflex (SLR) cameras, a mirror diverts the light to a prism, which erects the image, allowing the viewer to see exactly what will be focused on the film; when the shutter button is pushed and the mirror flips out of the way, light is focused on and exposes the photographic film

   3. Diverging lenses used alone produce smaller, virtual images; they are used on some cameras (not SLR cameras) as "finders," since the virtual image seen approximates the proportions of the photograph; whenever a virtual image is formed, the object and the image are on the same side of the lens

   4. Lens defects—the distortions in an image

produced by a given lens are called aberrations; combining a number of lenses as a system can usually minimize aberrations; this is the reason that microscopes and telescopes employ compound lenses in their construction

a. Spherical aberration—an unsharp (uncrisp) image is formed because light refracted from the outer edges of the lens is focused at a slightly different point than light refracted from more central areas of the lens

   (1) In cameras and microscopes this is corrected by using more than one lens and also by using diaphragms to cover the outer regions of the lens

   (2) In the human eye the iris is generally contracted to varying degrees and acts, in effect, like a diaphragm to block light from being refracted through the outer regions of the lens

b. Chromatic aberration—each wavelength of visible light refracts through lenses at different angles; thus each wavelength (color) of white light is brought to focus at a slightly different point; the result of this is that objects take on colors that they do not possess; this is corrected in cameras, microscopes, and telescopes by using combinations of simple lenses made of different types of glass called achromatic lenses; in the human eye, vision is sharpest when the pupil is the smallest; cutting down on light moving through the periphery of the lens minimizes chromatic as well as spherical aberration

c. Astigmatism—the human eye astigmatism is a type of aberration caused by the surface of the cornea possessing irregular curves; since the cornea in addition to the lens is important in refracting (focusing) light on the retina, the result of astigmatism is blurred vision, which can be corrected by using lenses that have vari-

able curvature to compensate for the irregular curvature of the cornea

5. Focusing—the camera focuses on objects at varying distances by changing the distance between the lens and the film; the human eye focuses on objects at varying distances by changing the degree of curvature of the lens; this ability of the human eye to change the focal length of the lens is called accommodation; whereas the cornea, aqueous humor, and vitreous humor all help to focus light on the retina, only the crystalline lens can be accommodated; the muscle responsible for accommodation is the ciliary body; when the ciliary body contracts, the suspensory ligaments loosen and the lens rounds out and is in position for focusing on near objects; when the ciliary body relaxes, the suspensory ligaments pull the lens into a flattened position, which allows for focusing on distant objects; the limit for accommodation is represented by the near point; objects closer to the eye than the near point (about 6 inches [15 cm] from the surface of a normal eye) cannot be clearly focused on the retina

a. Emmetropia—the normal refractive state of the eye

b. Ametropia—any abnormality in refractive ability of the eye

   (1) Myopia—the eye focuses light anterior to the retina (somewhere in the vitreous humor); from this abnormal focal point, light rays diverge and produce a blurred image on the retina; however, if objects are held about 1 inch (2.5 cm) from the eye, they will focus on the retina; for this reason, myopia is also called near-sightedness; glasses containing diverting lenses correct this condition

   (2) Hyperopia—the eye focuses light posterior to the retina; thus a circle of not-yet-conveyed light strikes the retina, producing a blurred image; hyperopia is also called far-sightedness and can be

corrected using glasses containing converging lenses

c. Contact lenses—thin lenses that are molded to the shape of the outer surface of the cornea; this can correct near-sightedness, far-sightedness, and astigmatism; the lens is applied to the surface of the eye using a saline solution that helps adhere the lens to the eye's surface

6. Eye examination with the ophthalmoscope and the retinoscope

a. Ophthalmoscope—the interior of the eye as well as the vision can be studied with this instrument; light is shone into the eye, and, if the eye has normal refractive ability, the light will be focused on the retina and will be reflected back to the observer's eye; persons with myopia or hyperopia will not converge the light on the retina, and the observer will not clearly see the eye's interior; then by using lenses of varying refractive abilities the observer can compensate for the person's abnormal refraction and study the interior of the eye and determine the state of vision

b. Retinoscope—permits diagnosis and evaluation of the refractive state of the eye; a beam of light is shone into the eye, and the observer watches the red glow of reflected light from the retina as it leaves the pupil; by observing the distribution of the light as it leaves the pupil, the observer can determine the refractive error in the eye

7. Binocular vision—the visual fields of the 2 human eyes overlap; while each eye sees some areas of the environment that the other eye cannot see, both eyes see large areas in common; the human brain interprets these overlapping fields in terms of depth; the environment appears in 3 dimensions as opposed to the visual effect of a movie projected on a flat screen; the blind spot of the right eye can be seen by the left eye and vice versa; therefore there are no visual gaps in the field of vision

REVIEW OF CHEMICAL PRINCIPLES RELATED TO THE NEUROMUSCULOSKELETAL SYSTEMS
Amines

A. Organic compounds containing an NH_2 group that can be considered derivatives of ammonia
B. Reactions of the amines
1. Amines give a basic reaction in water solution
2. Amines react like a base with acids, forming complex ions
C. Important amines
1. Monoamines such as norepinephrine, dopamine, serotonin, acetylcholine, and histamine serve as transmitter chemicals in the nervous system
2. Amino acids such as gamma-aminobutyric acid (GABA) and glycine act as inhibitors; glutamic acid has an excitatory influence on the nervous system

Lipids

The phospholipids, lecithin, cephalins, and sphingomyelins are important components of nerve membranes and sheaths

Proteins

The proteins actin, myosin, and troponin are important in muscle contraction

Group I A alkali metals

A. Sodium—sodium ions of the extracellular fluid are responsible for action potentials of nervous and muscular tissues; after some stimulus, it is the diffusion of Na^+ from the interstitial fluid into the intracellular fluid of neurons and muscle fibers that brings about depolarization; thus sodium ions are basic to the functioning of the body's communication system, the nervous system, and all muscular movements
B. Potassium
1. The resting polarization of neurons, all types of muscle fibers (smooth, cardiac, and striated), and most cells of the body is caused by the continual diffusion of K^+ from the intracellular fluid to the interstitial fluid; similarly, repolarization of neurons and muscle fibers is caused by the outward diffusion of K^+ to the interstitial fluid from the intracellular fluid
2. A number of important cellular enzymes functioning in glucose and amino acid metabolism require K^+ as a cofactor

Group II A alkali earth metals

A. Magnesium
1. Activator for many enzymes
2. Present in bones
B. Calcium
1. Gives hardness to bones and teeth by forming phosphate, carbonate, and fluoride salts
2. Important in muscle contraction; ATP must combine with CA^{++} before its energy can be used to slide actin and myosin filaments together
3. Extracellular Ca^{++} concentration must be precisely regulated (through the parathyroid glands) for normal body functioning; hypocalcemia can result in tetany; hypercalcemia can result in depression of the nervous system
C. Strontium
1. May substitute for calcium in body
2. Radioactive isotope (strontium 90) can be a health hazard, forming pockets of radiation in tissues

Group VII A halogens

Fluorine prevents tooth decay when added to water supply

Group I B

A. Silver—filling for teeth, surgical mending of bone, photography
B. Gold—filling for teeth

REVIEW OF MICROORGANISMS RELATED TO THE NEUROMUSCULOSKELETAL SYSTEMS

A. Bacterial pathogens
1. *Clostridium tetani*—large, gram-positive, motile bacillus forming large terminal spores; like all clostridia, it is an obligate anaerobe; causes tetanus (lockjaw)
2. *Haemophilus aegyptius* (Koch-Weeks bacillus)—indistinguishable morphologically from *Haemophilus influenzae;* causes a common conjunctivitis called pinkeye
3. *Neisseria meningitidis*—gram-negative diplococcus; causes epidemic (meningococcic) meningitis
B. DNA viruses—herpesviruses—spherical and 150 to 200 nm in diameter; cause herpes simplex, varicella (chickenpox), herpes zoster (shingles), infectious mononucleosis, and cytomegalic inclusion disease
C. RNA viruses—togaviruses—spherical and 40 to 60 nm in diameter; mostly borne by mosquitoes and ticks; cause eastern equine encephalomyelitis, western equine encephalomyelitis, Venezuelan equine encephalomyelitis, and a number of other infections
D. Fungal pathogen—*Cryptococcus neoformans*—pathogenic yeast with a characteristic large capsule around the cell; causes cryptococcosis (torulosis, European blastomycosis), a serious infection involving the lungs and central nervous system
E. Protozoa—*Trypanosoma*—flagellated ribbonlike protozoa; *T. gambienese* and *T. rhodesience* cause African sleeping sickness (transmitted by tsetse flies) and *T. cruzi* causes South American trypanosomiasis or Chagas' disease (transmitted by reduviid bugs)
F. Worm—*Trichinella spiralis*—one of smallest parasitic nematodes (about 1.5 mm in length), causes trichinosis (muscle infestation with trichina)

PHARMACOLOGY RELATED TO NEUROMUSCULOSKELETAL SYSTEM DISORDERS

A. Anticonvulsant drugs
1. General implications for nurses
   a. Teach patient regarding maintaining therapeutic blood level of drug as well as continued medical supervision
   b. Instruct family about treatment and how to care for patient during a seizure
   c. Suggest medical alert card or other form of identification be carried by patient
   d. If seizure occurs
      (1) Maintain airway
      (2) Protect patient from injury
      (3) Observe type and duration of seizure
   e. Observe for adverse effects
      (1) Dizziness, drowsiness
      (2) Nausea and vomiting
      (3) The hydantoins (phenytoin and mephenytoin) cause
         (a) Respiratory and cardiovascular depression
         (b) Ataxia
         (c) Gingivitis and hyperplasia of gums
         (d) Hirsutism
         (e) Inhibition of the action of corticosteroids, digitalis, and folic acid
   f. Anticoagulants potentiate the action of phenytoin

g. Depression of cardiac and respiratory centers can be caused by magnesium sulfate 50% and diazepam

2. Actions
   a. Modify bioelectric activity at subcortical and cortical sites
   b. Raise the threshold response to stimuli precipitating seizure control

3. Examples
   a. Grand mal seizure control
      (1) Carbamazepine (Tegretol)—also used for control of psychomotor seizure and trigeminal neuralgia
      (2) Phenytoin (Dihycon, Di-Lan, Dilantin)—also used for psychomotor seizure control
      (3) Magnesium sulfate 50%
      (4) Mephobarbital (Mebaral)
      (5) Mephenytoin (Mesantoin)
      (6) Primidone (Mysoline)—also used for psychomotor seizure control
      (7) Diazepam (Valium)—given intravenously in instances of status epilepticus
   b. Petit mal seizure control
      (1) Ethosuximide (Zarontin)
      (2) Methsuximide (Celontin)
      (3) Paramethadione (Paradione)
      (4) Trimethadione (Tridione)

B. Osmotic diuretics for increased intracranial pressure (mannitol)
   1. General implications for nurses
      a. Observe for signs of increased intracranial pressure; e.g., decreasing pulse rate, increasing blood pressure, unequal pupils, or change in level of consciousness
      b. Monitor intake and output
      c. Mannitol is contraindicated in patients with congestive heart failure or impaired renal function
      d. Generally, the head of the bed should be elevated
      e. Observe for adverse effects
         (1) Headache
         (2) Nausea
         (3) Chills
         (4) Hyponatremia and hypochloremia
   2. Actions
      a. Increase osmotic pressure within the glomerulus, causing more fluid to be excreted in the urine

b. Used to reduce cerebral edema and intraocular pressure

C. Drugs used to increase calcium ion balance
   1. General implications for nurses
      a. Observe for signs of tetany and hypercalcemia
      b. Increase fluid intake
      c. Check patient's electrolytes
      d. Increase amounts of calcium and vitamin D in the diet
      e. Recognize that parathyroid hormone may be given to increase osteoclastic activity, which would raise serum calcium
   2. Actions
      a. Vitamin D improves the absorption of calcium from the intestines
      b. Observe for adverse effects
         (1) Nausea and vomiting
         (2) Constipation
         (3) Possible renal calculi
         (4) Muscle flaccidity
   3. Examples
      a. Calcium ion replacement
         (1) Calcium chloride
         (2) Calcium gluconate
         (3) Calcium carbonate (Os-Cal)
      b. Vitamin D replacement
         (1) Dihydrotachysterol (Hytakerol)
         (2) Calciferol

D. Antiparkinsonism drugs
   1. General implications for nurses
      a. Understand that treatment controls symptoms but is not a cure
      b. Provide emotional support
      c. Eliminate vitamin B_6 from diet if L-dopa is prescribed
      d. Observe for adverse effects
         (1) Levodopa and amantadine hydrochloride
            (a) Orthostatic hypotension
            (b) Ataxia
            (c) Depression, psychic disturbances
         (2) Anticholinergic drugs (ethopropazine, benztropine mesylate, and trihexyphenidyl)
            (a) Dry mouth
            (b) Blurred vision
   2. Actions
      a. Anticholinergic drugs act at central sites to inhibit cerebral motor impulses and to block efferent impulses that cause rigidity of the musculature

b. Supplies or causes the release of dopamine required for norepinephrine synthesis and maintenance of the neurohormonal balance at subcortical, cortical, and reticular sites that control motor function

3. Examples
   a. Levodopa (Dopar, Larodopa)
   b. Amantadine hydrochloride (Symmetrel)
   c. Ethopropazine hydrochloride (Parsidol)
   d. Benztropine mesylate (Cogentin)
   e. Trihexyphenidyl hydrochloride (Artane, Tremin)

E. Cholinesterase inhibitors
1. General implications for nurses
   a. Observe patient closely because dosage is adjusted according to needs
   b. Be aware of signs of drug toxicity, which can mimic myasthenia gravis
   c. Observe patient for adverse effects
      (1) Intestinal colic, diarrhea
      (2) Excess salivary secretion
      (3) Weak rapid pulse
      (4) Acute toxicity—pulmonary edema and respiratory failure
   d. Atropine sulfate may be given for treatment of overdose

2. Actions
   a. Prevent enzymatic breakdown of acetylcholine at nerve endings, which allows accumulation of the neurotransmitter
   b. Improves strength of contraction in all muscles, but a primary concern is maintaining contractile strength of respiratory muscles

3. Examples
   a. Neostigmine bromide (Prostigmin Bromide)—also used for stimulation of smooth muscle contraction in abdominal viscera (uterus, bladder)
   b. Ambenonium chloride (Mytelase)
   c. Pyridostigmine bromide (Mestinon Bromide)
   d. Edrophonium chloride (Tensilon)—because of its short-lived action, this drug is primarily used for diagnostic purposes

F. Skeletal muscle relaxants
1. General implications for nurses
   a. Caution patients to avoid activity requiring mental alertness
   b. Avoid giving to patients with a history of liver disease, since it may cause jaundice
   c. Provide for safety because of depression of CNS
   d. Advise patients not to take other CNS depressants

2. Actions
   a. Cause a relaxation of voluntary muscles by depressing the central nervous system
   b. Decrease effects of muscle spasms, trauma, arthritis, etc.

3. Examples
   a. Carisoprodol (Rela, Soma)
   b. Chlormezanone (Trancopal)
   c. Chlorphenesin carbamate (Maolate)
   d. Chlorzoxazone (Paraflex)
   e. Mephenesin (Mephson, Romeph, Tolax, Tolserol)
   f. Metaxalone (Skelaxin)
   g. Methocarbamol (Robaxin)
   h. Parafon Forte (which contains both chlorzoxazone and acetaminophen)
   i. Diazepam (Valium)

G. Drugs used in the treatment of arthritis
1. General implications for nurses
   a. Teach patient the serious nature of side effects, especially blood dyscrasias
   b. Encourage patient to remain under medical supervision even when relief of pain occurs
   c. Observe for diminishing signs of inflammation
   d. Administer with milk, meals, or antacids
   e. Alters effects of other drugs, especially anticoagulants
   f. Observe for adverse effects
      (1) Salicylates
         (a) Tinnitus, dizziness
         (b) Gastric irritation
         (c) Prolonged bleeding time
      (2) Gold compounds
         (a) Pruritus
         (b) Stomatitis
         (c) Albuminuria, hematuria
         (d) Thrombocytopenia, agranulocytosis
      (3) Phenylbutazone
         (a) Edema
         (b) Gastric distress
         (c) Vertigo
         (d) Hepatitis
         (e) Psychosis
         (f) Leukopenia, thrombocytopenia, agranulocytosis

(4) Indomethacin
  (a) Peptic ulcer
  (b) Light-headedness
  (c) Skin rashes
  (d) Bone marrow depression
(5) Ibuprofen
  (a) Gastric irritation
  (b) Dizziness
  (c) Skin rash
2. Actions
  a. The analgesic action is thought to be caused by action at peripheral nerve endings; therefore these drugs are effective in the treatment of musculoskeletal pain but not visceral pain
  b. Interfere with the normal inflammatory process
3. Examples
  a. Salicylates (aspirin, sodium salicylate)
  b. Gold compounds (usually given with salicylates)
  c. Phenylbutazone (Butazolidin, Butazolidin Alka)
  d. Indomethacin (Indocin)
  e. Steroids
  f. Ibuprofen (Motrin)
H. Drugs used in the treatment of gout
  1. General implications for nurses
    a. Administer anti-inflammatory drugs, such as corticosteroids and indomethacin, in addition to drugs that will lower serum uric acid during acute phase
    b. Increase fluids to discourage the formation of renal calculi
    c. Encourage weight reduction
    d. Monitor serum urate levels to determine effectiveness of treatment
    e. Observe for adverse effects
      (1) Nausea, vomiting
      (2) Blood dyscrasias
      (3) Liver damage
  2. Actions and examples
    a. Colchicine is thought to decrease urate crystal deposits by inhibiting lactic acid production by leukocytes
    b. Probenecid (Benemid) prevents the formation of tophi by inhibiting the reabsorption of urate by the kidneys
    c. Allopurinol (Zyloprim) actually blocks the formation of uric acid within the body
I. Drugs that affect the eyes

1. General implications for nurses
  a. Observe for adverse effects (see specific drug)
  b. Minimize side effects by administering drugs at bedtime
  c. Stress the need for medical supervision while on medications
2. Ophthalmic cholinergics (miotics)
  a. Actions
    (1) Used in the treatment of glaucoma
    (2) Constrict the pupil, pull the iris away from the filtration angle, and improve outflow of aqueous humor
  b. Examples
    (1) Timolol maleate (Timoptic)
    (2) Pilocarpine hydrochloride (or nitrate)
    (3) Carbachol
    (4) Methacholine chloride (Mecholyl)
    (5) Physostigmine
    (6) Neostigmine bromide (Prostigmin)
    (7) Demecarium (Humorsol)
    (8) Isoflurophate (Floropryl)
    (9) Echothiophate (Phospholine)
  c. Adverse effects
    (1) Twitching of eyelids
    (2) Brow ache
    (3) Headache
    (4) Conjunctival pain
    (5) Contact dermatitis
3. Anticholinergic drugs
  a. Actions
    (1) Paralyze accommodation (cycloplegia)
    (2) Dilate the pupil (mydriasis) by relaxing the ciliary muscle and the sphincter muscle of the iris
    (3) Facilitate examination of eye interior
  b. Examples
    (1) Atropine
    (2) Scopolamine
    (3) Homatropine hydrobromide
    (4) Cyclopentolate (Cyclogyl)
    (5) Eucatropine
    (6) Tropicamide (Mydriacyl)
  c. Adverse effects
    (1) Dry mouth and skin
    (2) Flushing
    (3) Fever
    (4) Rash
    (5) Tachycardia
    (6) Ataxia
4. Mydriatics

a. Action—dilate pupil (mydriasis) by causing contraction of dilator muscle of the iris with minimal effect on ciliary muscle, which lessens effect on accommodation

b. Examples
(1) Tropicamide (Mydriacil)
(2) Phenylephrine hydrochloride (Neo-Synephrine)
(3) Hydroxyamphetamine (Paredrine)

c. Adverse effects
(1) Brow ache
(2) Headache
(3) Blurred vision
(4) Tachycardia
(5) Hypertension

5. Carbonic anhydrase inhibitors
a. Action—decrease inflow of aqueous humor in control of intraocular pressure (administered orally or parenterally)

b. Examples
(1) Acetazolamide (Diamox)
(2) Dichlorphenamide (Daranide, Oratrol)
(3) Ethoxzolamide (Cardrase, Ethamide)
(4) Methazolamide (Neptazane)

c. Adverse effects
(1) Diuresis
(2) Paresthesia
(3) Nausea, vomiting
(4) Depression
(5) Confusion
(6) Destruction of the angle

6. Osmotic agents
a. Actions
(1) Reduce volume of intraocular fluids
(2) Administered systemically to decrease blood osmolality, which mobilizes fluid from the eye

b. Examples
(1) Glycerin (Glyrol, Osmoglyn)
(2) Urea (Urevert, Ureaphil)
(3) Mannitol (Osmitrol)

c. Adverse effects
(1) Headache
(2) Nausea
(3) Vomiting

RELATED PROCEDURES
Transfer of patients

A. Definitions
1. Transfer refers to methods of movement of the patient from one surface to another; e.g., bed to wheelchair, wheelchair to commode
2. Weight-bearing transfers—carried out by patients who have at least one stable lower extremity; e.g., hemiplegia, unilateral lower extremity amputation, patients with fractured hips
3. Nonweight-bearing transfers—carried out by patients who do not have a stable lower extremity; e.g., paraplegics not wearing braces, patients with double lower extremity amputations

B. Nursing responsibilities
1. Assess patient's abilities; e.g., sitting tolerance, balance, weight-bearing potential, strength, motivation, understanding of principles of transfer
2. Identify need for and selection of assistive devices; e.g., slide board, trapeze, wheelchair with a removable arm, hydraulic lift
3. Select most appropriate transfer method and teach and assist the patient with this new technique
4. Provide for patient safety; e.g., encourage use of low-heeled shoes; lock wheelchair brakes during transfer; remove hazards—scatter rugs, slippery floors, stepstools; ensure adequate assistance
5. Communicate individualized transfer techniques by instructing the patient and family and informing the entire health team
6. Consider the patient's abilities and disabilities when deciding appropriate transfer technique and need for assistive devices; e.g., hemiplegia—place wheelchair on side opposite affected extremities; paraplegia—may use trapeze, slide board, wheelchair with removable arm
7. Maintain correct proximity and visual relationship of wheelchair to bed; e.g., paraplegia—place wheelchair lateral or perpendicular to bed; hemiplegia—place wheelchair at a 30-degree angle to the bed on the unaffected side

Use of assistive devices for passive positioning

A. Devices and their purposes
1. Stryker or Foster frames—allow for horizontal turning of patient
2. Circ-O-lectric bed—allows for vertical turning of patient; the patient can be placed in a variety of positions (Trendelenburg, prone, standing, and supine); one nurse can turn the patient with the electric motor providing the power; attachments permit application of traction and other accessories

3. Purposes
   a. Hyperextension
   b. Immobilization
   c. Correction of deformities
   d. Facilitation of turning
   e. Relief of pressure
   f. Promotion of body functions (circulation, respiration, elimination)
B. Nursing responsibilities
   1. Turn all in one piece
   2. Since frames are narrow, for safety purposes do not permit patient to sit up, roll over, or reach out to the side; do not place extremely obese and disoriented patients on a frame
   3. Since only the prone and supine and, on the Circ-O-lectric bed, the vertical position, can be used, strict attention must be paid to prevention of decubiti
   4. Before releasing pivot pins, secure all bolts and straps to ensure patient safety
   5. When turning the Circ-O-lectric bed, do so slowly so that the patient's cerebral circulation can adjust to the new position; observe for signs of hypotension

Walking with a cane

A. Purposes
   1. Improve stability of patient with lower limb disability
   2. Maintain balance
   3. Prevent further injury
   4. Provide security while developing confidence in ambulating
   5. Relieve pressure on weight-bearing joints
   6. Assist in increasing speed of ambulation with less fatigue
   7. Provide for greater mobility and independence
B. Nursing responsibilities
   1. Ascertain that patient is able to bear weight on the affected extremity
   2. Ensure that patient is able to use upper extremity opposite the affected lower extremity
   3. Measure to determine length of cane
      a. The highest point of the cane should be about level with the great trochanter
      b. The handpiece should allow 30 degrees of flexion at the elbow with the wrist held in extension
   4. Explain the proper techniques in using cane

a. Hold in the hand opposite to the affected extremity
b. The cane and the affected extremity should be advanced simultaneously, and then the unaffected leg should be advanced
c. The cane should be kept close to the body
d. When climbing, the patient should step up with the unaffected extremity and then place the cane and the affected lower extremity on the step; when descending, the procedure is reversed
5. Observe patient for incorrect use of cane
   a. Leaning the body over the cane
   b. Shortening the stride on the unaffected side
   c. Inability to develop a normal walking pattern
   d. The abnormal gait pattern tends to persist after the cane is no longer needed

Locomotion on wheels

The patient is propelled or self-propelled on wheels or casters in a sitting position
A. Purposes
   1. Support the body
   2. Decrease cardiac workload
   3. Promote independence and stimulate activities
   4. Provide mobility for those who cannot ambulate or those who can ambulate but whose ambulation is unsteady, unsafe, or too strenuous
B. Nursing responsibilities
   1. Instruct the patient that prolonged sitting in one position can cause flexion contractures of the hips and knees and ischial decubiti (encourage the patient to change body positions and use padded cushions and exercise such as push-ups every hour to relieve pressure)
   2. Ensure that specific devices necessary for patient safety; e.g., wheel brakes, arm locks, seat belts, swing foot rests, are in operating condition
   3. Alert the wheelchair-bound patient to the accessories that meet the patient's specific needs; e.g., removable arms, lap boards, knobs on the hand-rims, extra long leg panels, battery or motor propulsion

Crutch walking

A. Purposes
   1. Support body weight, assist weak muscles, and provide joint stability
   2. Relieve pain

3. Prevent further injury and provide for improvement of function
4. Allow for greater patient independence
B. Nursing responsibilities
1. Ensure proper fit of crutches by measuring distance from anterior fold of axilla to point 6 inches (15 cm) out from heel
   a. Axillary bar must be 2 inches (5 cm) below axilla and may or may not be padded
   b. Hand bar should allow almost complete extension of arm with the elbow flexed about 30 degrees when the patient places weight on the hands
   c. Rubber crutch tip should be in good condition, about 5.1 to 7.6 cm (2 to 3 inches) in height, with a circumference of 3.8 to 4.4 cm (1½ to 1¾ inches)
2. Assist patient in use of proper technique, depending on ability to bear weight and to take steps with either one or both of the lower extremities
   a. Four-point alternate crutch gait
      (1) Right crutch, left foot, left crutch, right foot
      (2) Equal but partial weight-bearing on each limb
      (3) A slow but stable gait; there are always 3 points of support on the floor
      (4) The patient must be able to manipulate both extremities and get one foot ahead of the other; e.g., polio, arthritis, cerebral palsy
   b. Two-point alternate crutch gait
      (1) Right crutch and left foot simultaneously
      (2) There are always 2 points of support on the floor
      (3) This is a more rapid version of the 4-point gait and requires more balance and strength; e.g., bilateral amputation
   c. Three-point gait
      (1) Advance both crutches and the weaker lower extremity simultaneously, then the stronger lower extremity
      (2) A fairly rapid gait but requires more balance and strength in the arms and the good lower extremity
      (3) Used when one leg can support the whole body weight and the other lower extremity cannot take full weight-bearing; e.g., fractured hip

   d. Swing crutch gaits
      (1) Swing-to gait
         (a) Place both crutches forward, then lift and swing body *up to* crutches, place crutches in front of body and continue
         (b) There are always 2 points of support on the floor
         (c) This technique is indicated for any patient with adequate power in the upper arms
      (2) Swing-through gait
         (a) Place both crutches forward, then lift and swing body *through* crutches, place crutches in front of body and continue
         (b) A very difficult gait because as the patient swings through the crutches, it necessitates rolling the pelvis forward and arching the back to get the center of gravity in front of the hips
         (c) Indicated for the patient who has power in the trunk and upper extremities, excellent balance, self-confidence, and a dash of daring; e.g., bilateral amputation, paraplegic with braces
   e. Tripod crutch gaits
      (1) Tripod alternate gait
         (a) Right crutch, left crutch, drag the body and legs forward
         (b) The patient constantly maintains a tripod position—both crutches are held fairly widespread out front while both feet are held together in the back
         (c) Necessary for the individual who cannot place one extremity ahead of the other; e.g., flaccid paralysis from poliomyelitis, spinal cord injuries
      (2) Tripod simultaneous gait
         (a) Place both crutches forward, drag the body and legs forward
         (b) Because the tripod must have a large base, the patient's body must be inclined forward sufficiently to keep the center of gravity in front of the hips
3. Observe patient for incorrect use of crutches
   a. Using the body in poor mechanical fashion
   b. Hiking hips with abduction gait (common in amputee)

c. Lifting crutches while still bearing down on them
d. Walking on ball of foot with foot turned outward and flexion at hip or knee level
e. Hunching shoulders (crutches usually too long) or stooping with shoulders (crutches usually too short)
f. Looking downward while ambulating
g. Bearing weight under arms should be avoided to prevent injury to the nerves in the brachial plexus; damage to these nerves can cause paralysis and is known as crutch palsy

Ambulation with a walker

A. Purposes
  1. Maintain balance
  2. Provide additional support because of wide area of contact with floor
  3. Allow for some ambulatory independence
B. Nursing responsibilities
  1. Assist the patient in selecting a walker
    a. A walker should not be used unless the patient will never be able to ambulate with a cane or crutches
    b. Measurements for a walker are the same as for a cane
    c. The patient must have strong elbow extensors and shoulder depressors and partial strength in the hands and wrist muscles
    d. The patient needs maximum support to ensure security and enhance confidence
    e. Use is usually limited to the home because it cannot be used on steps
  2. Assist patient in ambulating with the walker
    a. Lift device off the floor and place forward a short distance, then advance between the walker
    b. Two-wheeled walkers—raise back legs of device off the floor, roll walker forward and then advance to it
    c. Four-wheeled walkers—push device forward on floor and then walk to it
  3. Observe patient for incorrect use of walker
    a. Keeping arms rigid and swinging through to counterbalance the position of the lower extremity
    b. Tending to lean forward with abnormal flexion at the hips
    c. Tending to step forward with good leg and shuffle affected leg up to the bar

Ambulation with braces or splints

A. Purposes
  1. Supports and protects weakened muscles
  2. Prevents and corrects anatomic deformities
  3. Aids in controlling involuntary muscle movements
  4. Immobilizes and protects a diseased or injured joint
  5. Provides for improvement of function
B. Nursing responsibilities
  1. Keep equipment in good repair; e.g., oil joints, replace straps when worn, wash with saddle soap
  2. Provide adequate shoes; e.g., keep in good repair, heels low and wide, high top to hold the heel in the shoe
  3. Examine skin daily for evidence of breakdown at pressure points
  4. Check alignment of braces; e.g., leg braces—joints should coincide with body joints; back brace—upright bars in center of back, brace should grip pelvis and trocanter firmly, lacing should begin from the bottom

Lumbar puncture

A. Definition—involves the introduction of a needle into the subarachnoid space, usually between L_3 and L_4 or L_4 and L_5 to prevent injury to the spinal cord above this level
B. Purposes
  1. Withdrawal of spinal fluid for diagnostic purposes or to reduce spinal pressure (normal is 70 to 200 mm of water)
  2. Measurement of spinal pressure (Queckenstedt's test involves compression of the jugular veins; normally pressure will rise, but if blockage exists, pressure will not change)
  3. Injection of air or dye for diagnostic x-ray examination
  4. Injection of medication such as anesthetics
C. Nursing responsibilities
  1. Explain procedure to patient and obtain signed consent
  2. Set up sterile field
  3. Assist patient into position that will enlarge the opening between the vertebrae
    a. Lying on side with feet drawn up and head lowered to chest; back near edge of mattress
    b. Sitting over side of bed, leaning on overbed table, and feet supported on stool

4. Observe patient for signs of shock, such as tachycardia, diaphoresis, and pallor
5. After procedure assist patient into recumbent position; patient should remain recumbent up to 24 hours, depending on physician's orders
6. Label specimens and send to laboratory
7. Note color and amount of spinal fluid, patient's condition, and record
8. Administer fluids unless contraindicated

Ear irrigations
A. Definition
 1. The introduction of fluid into the external auditory canal
 2. This is usually done for cleansing purposes but can be used to apply antiseptic solutions
B. Nursing responsibilities
 1. Explain procedure to patient
 2. Assemble equipment: irrigating solution, sterile irrigating syringe, cotton balls, cotton-tipped applicators, towel
 3. Assist patient to sitting position with head tilted to affected side to facilitate drainage
 4. Gently pull up and back on the external ear of an adult and down and forward on a child to straighten the canal
 5. Direct solution into the canal without exerting excessive force; collect returns in basin
 6. Dry the outer ear and have patient lie on affected side
 7. Record procedure, type of drainage, etc.

Bárány's caloric test
A. Definition
 1. Test used to assess vestibular labyrinthine function
 2. Warm or cold water is instilled rapidly into the auditory canal, causing motion of the endolymph within the semicircular canals and normally resulting in vertigo, nystagmus, and nausea
 3. Eyes deviate toward stimulated ear if cold water is used and away if warm water is used
B. Nursing responsibilities
 1. Explain procedure to patient
 2. Assemble equipment for procedure
 3. Assist physician and support patient during irrigation
 4. Observe and record reaction of patient

Instillation of eye medications
A. Purpose—to provide therapeutic effect of medication ordered
B. Nursing responsibilities
 1. Explain procedure to patient
 2. Position patient with head slightly backward
 3. Pull lower eyelid down and place ointment or solution in the center of the cul-de-sac of eye that is to be medicated (check order: O.D.—right eye, O.U.—both eyes, O.S.—left eye)
 4. Allow patient to gently close eyes and instruct not to rub eyes
 5. Record administration of medication appropriately

MAJOR DISEASES
Migraine headache
A. Etiology and pathophysiology
 1. Caused by constriction and then dilation of the cerebral arteries
 2. Individuals who have migraines are frequently described as perfectionists, inflexible, and ambitious
 3. Incidence is higher in females
B. Signs and symptoms
 1. Subjective
   a. Severe throbbing pain, often in temporal or supraorbital area, that lasts several hours to a day
   b. Fatigue and irritability may precede headache
   c. Nausea
   d. Visual disturbances
 2. Objective
   a. Pallor
   b. Vomiting
C. Treatment
 1. Methysergide maleate (Sansert) to prevent attacks; should not be continued for more than 6 to 12 months consecutively; then, should be omitted for a few months before it is resumed
 2. Ergotamine tartrate (Gynergen) or ergotamine with caffeine (Cafergot) to relieve migraines
 3. Elimination of factors (physical, psychologic, environmental) that precipitate illness
D. Nursing care
 1. Assist patient in identifying situations that seem to precipitate attacks
 2. Support patient in modification of life-style and development of insight

3. Provide dark, quiet environment when migraine begins
4. If patient is nauseated
   a. Administer antiemetic if ordered
   b. Offer small, frequent sips of fluid as tolerated
   c. Assist with mouth care

Head injuries

A. Etiology and pathophysiology
   1. Head injuries result from trauma and are frequently seen after motor vehicle accidents
   2. Fractures
      a. Linear—a simple break in the bone
      b. Depressed—a break that results in fragments of bone penetrating the brain tissue
   3. Hemorrhages
      a. Epidural—a hematoma forms between the dura and the skull; may result from a laceration of the middle meningeal artery
      b. Subdural—a hematoma forms between the dura and arachnoid layers; generally follows venous damage
   4. Concussion—a temporary disruption of synaptic activity
   5. Contusions—bruising of brain tissue with slight bleeding of small cerebral vessels into surrounding tissues
B. Signs and symptoms
   1. Subjective
      a. Lethargy
      b. Indifference to surroundings
   2. Objective
      a. Signs of increased intracranial pressure (see Brain surgery)
      b. Lack of orientation to time and place
      c. Paresthesia
      d. Labored respirations
      e. Positive Babinski sign (stroking bottom of foot causes dorsiflexion of foot)
      f. Coma
      g. Dilation and fixation of pupil
C. Treatment
   1. Control seizures with anticonvulsants
   2. Maintain adequate fluid and electrolyte balance
   3. Surgical intervention in cases of depressed skull fractures or hematomas
D. Nursing care
   1. Observe for signs of increased intracranial pressure (see Brain surgery); institute neural checks

every 15 minutes for several hours progressing to every hour and then every 4 hours
   2. Maintain airway
   3. If patient is unconscious, see Care of unconscious patient
   4. If surgery is indicated, see Care of patient undergoing brain surgery
   5. Institute seizure precautions; administer anticonvulsants if ordered

Brain tumor

A. Etiology and pathophysiology
   1. Tumors of the brain are either benign or malignant; they require intervention, since the skull can not accommodate the increasing size of the tumor, and intracranial pressure rises
   2. Classified according to tissue of origin
      a. Meningioma—occurs outside the brain from the covering meninges
      b. Acoustic neuroma and optic nerve spongioblastoma polare—occur from the cranial nerves
      c. Gliomas—originate in brain tissue
      d. Hemangioblastomas—occur from within blood vessels
B. Signs and symptoms
   1. Subjective
      a. Headache that increases with stooping
      b. Lethargy
   2. Objective
      a. Vomiting
      b. Papilledema (noted on ophthalmoscopy)
      c. Abnormal brain waves on EEG
   3. Symptoms may vary, depending on location of tumor
      a. Frontal lobe—personality changes, focal seizures, blurred vision, hemiparesis or aphasia
      b. Temporal lobe—seizures, headache, papilledema, aphasia
      c. Parietal lobe—jacksonian convulsions, visual loss
      d. Occipital region—focal seizures, visual hallucinations
      e. Cerebellar region—loss of coordination, papilledema
C. Treatment
   1. Radiation therapy or chemotherapy for inaccessible tumors
   2. Brain surgery for complete removal of lesion if

location and extension into surrounding tissues permit

3. Steroids, anticonvulsives, and osmotic diuretics to control symptoms

D. Nursing care
   1. Give emotional support to patient undergoing palliative procedures
   2. Maintain patient as comfortably as possible with analgesics and antiemetics as ordered
   3. If patient is having brain surgery
      a. Obtain consent for surgery and removal of hair (save hair)
      b. Following surgery keep patient's head elevated 12 inches (30 cm) to aid drainage
      c. Observe for return of cough and swallowing reflexes
      d. Assess patient's level of consciousness and neurologic status for changes
      e. Utilize hypothermia as ordered if patient is febrile; fever increases metabolic needs of the brain
      f. Observe dressings for CSF leakage or hemorrhage
      g. Maintain accurate intake and output records
      h. Observe for signs of increased intracranial pressure
         (1) Restlessness
         (2) Weakness or paralysis
         (3) Increased blood pressure
         (4) Decreased pulse
         (5) Pupillary dilation

Brain abscess

A. Etiology and pathophysiology
   1. Occurs when there is an infection in another region of the body that spreads to the brain or after a penetrating head wound
   2. The result of invasion of the brain is the formation and collection of exudate within the brain tissue

B. Signs and symptoms
   1. Subjective
      a. Malaise
      b. Headache
      c. Anorexia
   2. Objective
      a. Fever
      b. Vomiting
      c. Weight loss

C. Treatment
   1. Large doses of antibiotics
   2. In severe cases, a craniotomy may be performed to allow removal of the abscess

D. Nursing care
   1. Observe patient for changes in vital signs or neurologic responses
   2. See Care of patient undergoing brain surgery

Cerebral aneurysm

A. Etiology and pathophysiology
   1. A cerebral aneurysm is a sac formed by dilation of the walls of an artery within the cranial cavity
   2. This may occur due to a congenital weakness in the vessel, trauma, or arteriosclerosis
   3. Symptoms occur when the aneurysm compresses nearby nerves or when it ruptures

B. Signs and symptoms
   1. Subjective
      a. Unilateral headache
      b. Pain in the eye
      c. Diplopia
      d. Tinnitus
   2. Objective
      a. Rigidity of the back of the neck and spine
      b. Ptosis of the eyelid
      c. Hemiparesis

C. Treatment
   1. Attempt to keep patient hypotensive, usually with rauwolfia alkaloids
   2. If there is a stalk connecting the aneurysm, clips may be inserted surgically to cut off blood supply to the aneurysm permanently

D. Nursing care
   1. See Care of patient undergoing brain surgery
   2. See Care of patient with cerebral hemorrhage

Cerebral hemorrhage

A. Etiology and pathophysiology
   1. Occurs as the result of arteriosclerosis, trauma, hemorrhagic disorders, tumors of the brain, and ruptured aneurysms
   2. May occur in various areas of the brain
      a. Subarachnoid hemorrhage—generally occurs due to a congenital aneurysm near the circle of Willis
      b. Intracerebral hemorrhage—generally occurs due to hypertension, although may result from various disorders; the bleeding is usually located in the basal ganglia

c. Subdural hemorrhage—generally involves a bridging vein, and therefore a longer period of time may pass before a hematoma is formed

B. Signs and symptoms
1. Subjective
   a. Headache
   b. Dizziness
2. Objective
   a. Convulsions
   b. Hemiplegia
   c. Unconsciousness
   d. Right-sided hemiplegia usually accompanied by aphasia

C. Treatment
1. Complete bed rest
2. Steroids, stool softeners, anticonvulsants, analgesics, aminocaproic acid (Amicar) by continuous IV drip to inhibit fibrinolysis
3. Surgical intervention if indicated

D. Nursing care
1. Observe for changes in vital signs and neurologic status
2. Keep patient's head slightly elevated to reduce venous pressure within cranial cavity
3. If patient is unconscious
   a. Maintain airway by suctioning as necessary; use airway or endotracheal tube
   b. Provide sterile tracheostomy care; provide frequent oral hygiene
   c. Position patient to prevent pressure areas from forming decubiti
   d. Maintain adequate fluid balance
   e. Evaluate patient's level of consciousness at frequent intervals
   f. If patient's eyes remain open, protect corneas with moistened pads, mineral oil, or ointment as ordered
   g. Protect patient during seizures

Cerebral vascular accident (CVA or stroke)

A. Etiology and pathophysiology
1. CVA is a term applied to destruction (infarction) of brain cells caused by a reduction in the oxygen supply
2. This is caused by a sudden or gradual interruption in blood supply following an intracerebral hemorrhage, blockage of vessels by thrombi or emboli, or vascular insufficiency
3. Symptoms depend on the area of the brain involved and extent of damage

4. Conditions that predispose the individual to a CVA include cerebral arteriosclerosis, syphilis, dehydration, trauma, and hypertension
5. Transient ischemic attacks (TIA) may also occur without causing permanent damage; these usually last only a few minutes
6. Incidence increases with age

B. Signs and symptoms
1. Subjective
   a. Syncope
   b. Changes in level of consciousness
   c. Transient paresthesia
   d. Headache
   e. Mood swings
2. Objective
   a. Convulsions
   b. Nuchal rigidity (if caused by subarachnoid or intracerebral hemorrhage)
   c. Hemiplegia on side opposite lesion
   d. Aphasia—the brain is unable to fulfill its communicative functions because of damage to its input, integrative, or output centers; it is a disturbance of language function and may involve impairment of the ability to read, write, speak, or interpret messages
      (1) Expressive aphasia—the patient has difficulties making own thoughts known to others; speaking and writing are most affected
      (2) Receptive aphasia—the patient has difficulty understanding what others are trying to communicate; interpretation of speech and reading are most affected
      (3) Expressive-receptive aphasia—the patient has equal difficulty in speaking, writing, interpreting speech, and reading
   e. Alterations in reflexes
   f. Functional disorders of the bladder and bowel
   g. CSF is bloody if cerebral or subarachnoid hemorrhage is present
   h. Abnormal electroencephalogram
   i. Cerebral angiography may reveal vascular abnormalities such as aneurysms, narrowing, or occlusions
   j. If increased intracranial pressure exists, as with hemorrhage, elevated blood pressure and bounding pulse

C. Treatment
1. Complete bed rest with sedation as needed

2. Maintenance of nutrition by parenteral route or nasogastric feedings if patient is unable to swallow
3. Anticoagulant therapy
4. Antihypertensive agents if indicated
5. Surgical intervention
    a. To relieve pressure and control bleeding if hemorrhage is present
    b. Carotid endarterectomy to improve cerebral blood flow when carotid arteries are narrowed by arteriosclerotic patches may be done on a patient in stable condition
D. Nursing care
    1. Assess patient's respiratory functioning (vital signs, type and rate of respirations, color, blood gases, etc.)
    2. Observe for level of consciousness
    3. Monitor vital signs
    4. Observe for signs of increasing intracranial pressure
    5. Assess gag and swallowing reflexes
    6. Maintain patency of airway by positioning, suctioning, and inserting artificial airway
    7. Provide for drainage and expansion of lungs by placing patient in a low semi-Fowler's position with head turned to the side
    8. Provide oxygen as necessary
    9. Provide frequent oral hygiene
    10. Encourage patient to breathe deeply and cough; administer intermittent positive pressure if necessary
    11. Provide elastic stockings for both legs
    12. Provide for frequent nursing observations, since patient may be unable to signal for assistance
    13. Prevent decubiti
        a. Provide special care to back and bony prominences; keep patient clean and dry
        b. Relieve pressure by use of mechanical and supportive devices
        c. Turn patient every 2 hours
        d. Provide adequate hydration to maintain skin turgor
    14. Prevent muscle atrophy and contractures
        a. Provide for active and passive range of motion and other exercises
        b. Use footboards and other devices to prevent footdrop, flexion of fingers, abduction of hips, adduction of shoulders and arms
    15. Encourage the aphasic patient to communicate
        a. Be aware of own reactions to the speech difficulty

    b. Evaluate extent of patient's ability to understand and express self at a simple level
    c. Include health team, especially the speech therapist, in planning patient care
    d. Involve the family as much as possible
    e. Convey to the patient that there is a problem with communication, not with intelligence
    f. Try to eliminate anxiety and tension related to communication attempts; e.g., be consistent, give the patient time to respond, employ a calm, accepting, and deliberate manner
    g. Help the patient set attainable goals
    h. Stimulate patient's communication without pushing to point of frustration
    i. Keep distractions at a minimum, since they interfere with the reception and integration of messages; e.g., one-to-one conversations rather than group conversations, shut off radio when speaking
    j. Speak slowly, clearly, and in short sentences and do not raise voice
    k. Use alternate means of communication; e.g., gestures, writing, picture board
    l. Involve the patient in social interactions; e.g., encourage socialization, do not anticipate all needs, ask questions and expect answers, do not ignore patient in group conversations
    m. Make a definite transition between tasks to prevent or reduce confusion
    n. Be alert for clues and gestures when speech is garbled; e.g., continue to listen, nod, and make occasional neutral statements, let patient know when you cannot understand
    o. Provide for periodic reevaluation to demonstrate to the patient and health team the effect and nature of progress
    16. Attempt to prevent fecal impaction and/or urinary tract problems
        a. Provide adequate fluid intake
        b. Provide diet with enough roughage for sufficient quantity of bowel content and proper consistency for evacuation
        c. Avoid preoccupation with elimination
        d. Avoid overt encouragement of incontinence; e.g., routine use of diapers, Chux, and other depersonalizing devices
        e. Stimulate normal elimination by exercise and activity

f. Help patient develop regular bowel and bladder patterns

g. Respect the individual; e.g., provide for privacy, individuality of routine, avoidance of delay, encourage the patient to make decisions

h. Utilize physical and psychologic techniques to stimulate elimination; e.g., running water, place patient's hands in warm water, place patient in as normal a position as possible for elimination

i. Create an environment that keeps sensory monotony to a minimum; e.g., orient to time and place, use radio and television selectively, increase patient's social contacts, provide visual stimulus, extend environment beyond patient's room

j. Provide for self-esteem; e.g., encourage patient to wear own clothes, do self-care activities, make decisions

k. Accept and explore patient's feelings of fear, anger, and depression; a disabled person has few avenues by which to express anger; incontinence is often used in this manner

17. Keep side rails in place or use safety straps

18. Provide patient with tube feedings if gag and swallowing reflexes are depressed or absent

19. Provide foods in a form that is easily swallowed

20. Assist patient with feeding; e.g., use of padded spoon handle; feed on unaffected side of mouth; feed in as close to a sitting position as possible

21. Provide realistic encouragement and praise

22. Accept patient's mood swings and emotional outbursts

23. Assist patient and family to set realistic goals

24. Help patient to adjust to change in body image and altered self-concept

Epilepsy (convulsive disorders)

A. Etiology and pathophysiology

1. Epilepsy is characterized by the abnormal discharge of electric impulses from the nerve cells in the brain from idiopathic or secondary causes resulting in the typical manifestation of seizures

2. The onset of idiopathic epilepsy is generally before age 30

3. Other conditions associated with seizures include brain tumor, CVA, hypoglycemia, and head trauma

4. Types of seizures

a. Generalized motor seizures (grand mal seizures) characterized by an aura, loss of consciousness, tonic and clonic movements, interruption of respirations, loss of bladder and bowel control

b. Petit mal seizures characterized by brief transient loss of consciousness with or without minor motor movements of eyes, head, or extremities

c. Jacksonian seizures (focal-motor seizures) characterized by disturbed sensations and interrupted motor functioning, beginning in a somewhat localized area of the body and progressing to other parts of the body; the areas affected by the seizure usually reflect the area of the brain involved

d. Psychomotor seizures are characterized by a transient clouding of consciousness, behavioral alterations, and changes in affect and perception; may become violent and engage in antisocial activity

e. Status epilepticus is a continuous convulsion that may completely exhaust the patient and lead to death

B. Signs and symptoms (grand mal seizures)

1. Subjective

a. Aura or warning sensation such as seeing spots or feeling dizzy often precedes a grand mal seizure

b. Loss of consciousness during seizure

c. Lethargy often follows return to consciousness

d. Dyspnea

2. Objective

a. Pupils become fixed and dilated

b. Often patient cries out as seizure begins or as air is exhaled forcefully

c. Tonic and clonic movement of the muscles

d. Incontinence

e. Abnormal electroencephalogram; a test in which electrodes are applied to scalp to obtain a graphic record of brain activity

C. Treatment

1. Anticonvulsant therapy continued throughout life

a. Phenytoin sodium (Dilantin), mephenytoin (Mesantoin) and primidone (Mysoline) are often used to control grand mal seizures

b. Trimethadione (Tridione), phensuximide (Milontin), and ethosuximide (Zarontin) are drugs used to control petit mal seizures

   c. Diazepam (Valium) is given IV to treat status epilepticus

  2. Sedatives are used to reduce emotional stress; e.g., phenobarbital

D. Nursing care

  1. Assist patient to identify aura

  2. Help patient to prepare and provide some protection before the seizure develops

  3. Provide protection for patient during and after the seizure by maintaining and protecting from injury; a tongue blade should not be forced into a patient's mouth when teeth are firmly clenched, since this may cause the tongue to occlude the airway or may loosen teeth

  4. Encourage patient to carry and wear a medical alert tag

  5. Encourage patient to take medications even when seizure free

  6. Help the patient to plan a schedule that provides for adequate rest and a reduction of stress

  7. Instruct patient to refrain from excessive use of alcohol, since it is contraindicated with the medications

  8. The nurse should observe and teach patient and family to observe aura, initial point of seizure, type of seizure, level of consciousness, loss of control of bladder and bowel, progression of seizure, and postseizure condition

  9. Encourage patient to express feelings about illness and the necessary changes in life-style and self-image

  10. Assist patient and family to accept diagnosis and develop some understanding of the disease process

  11. Help patient to understand that medication must be taken continuously for the remainder of life

  12. Refer the patient for job counseling as needed

  13. Encourage patient and family to attend meetings of the local epilepsy association

  14. Refer the patient for genetic counseling if appropriate (age of patient, cause of seizures)

Mononeuritis and polyneuritis

A. Etiology and pathophysiology

  1. May involve only one nerve (mononeuritis) or several nerves (polyneuritis)

  2. Mononeuritis occurs when there is trauma to the trunk of a nerve, such as from pressure of a tumor, dislocation of a joint, or infection; the nerve involved near the area of injury becomes part of the scar tissue or callus of bone

  3. Polyneuritis occurs when there is a deficiency of thiamine (such as in alcoholism) and subsequent disturbances in metabolism of nerve tissue

B. Signs and symptoms

  1. Subjective

    a. Pain which increases after any body movement that stretches nerve involved

    b. Burning pain along injured nerve in mononeuritis

  2. Objective

    a. Swelling over affected nerve in mononeuritis

    b. Paresis or paralysis of affected limb in polyneuritis

C. Treatment

  1. Mononeuritis

    a. Sympathetic nerve block

    b. Physical therapy

    c. Analgesics

  2. Polyneuritis

    a. Thiamine replacement

    b. Bed rest

    c. Analgesics

D. Nursing care

  1. Administer pain medications as ordered

  2. Provide emotional support for patient during course of hospitalization

Bell's palsy

A. Etiology and pathophysiology

  1. A paralysis that occurs on one side of the face as a result of an inflamed seventh cranial nerve (facial); generally lasts only 2 to 8 weeks but may last longer in older patients

  2. May follow trauma or exposure to the elements

  3. Most common between ages 20 and 50 years

B. Signs and symptoms

  1. Subjective

    a. Facial pain

    b. Difficulty eating

  2. Objective

    a. Distortion of face

    b. Speech difficulty

    c. Diminished blink reflex

    d. Increased lacrimation

C. Treatment

1. Prednisone therapy
2. Heat, massage, and electric stimulation are used to maintain circulation and muscle tone
3. Prevention of corneal irritation with eyedrops and the use of a protective eye shield
D. Nursing care
   1. Explain to patient that in most cases recovery occurs within 2 to 8 weeks
   2. Assess blink reflex and patient's ability to close eye
   3. Keep the face warm
   4. Teach patient to gently massage face and perform simple exercises such as blowing
   5. Encourage ventilation of feelings, since self-image will be affected

Trigeminal neuralgia (tic douloureux)

A. Etiology and pathophysiology
   1. A disorder of the fifth cranial nerve characterized by excruciating knifelike pain along the branches of the nerve
   2. Etiology is unknown
   3. Incidence is higher in women of middle and older age
B. Signs and symptoms
   1. Subjective
      a. Burning or knifelike pain lasting 1 to 15 minutes, usually over the lip, chin, and in teeth
      b. Pain is precipitated by stimulation of trigger zones during activities such as brushing hair and eating or cold drafts
   2. Objective
      a. Sudden closure of eye
      b. Twitching of mouth
C. Treatment
   1. Carbamazepine (Tegretal) to relieve and prevent pain
   2. Antiepileptic drugs
   3. Injection of alcohol into the ganglion to relieve pain for several months or years until nerve regenerates
   4. Surgical intervention involves sectioning the sensory root of the nerve, which will cause loss of all sensation in the area supplied by the nerve
D. Nursing care
   1. Prevent factors that can trigger an attack
      a. Avoid foods that are too hot or cold
      b. Use cotton pads to gently wash the patient's face

c. Avoid jarring the bed
d. Keep room free from drafts
   2. Provide teaching to patients who have had surgery
      a. Inspection of the eye for foreign bodies, which the patient will not be able to feel, should be done several times a day
      b. Warm normal saline irrigation of the affected eye 2 or 3 times a day is helpful in preventing a corneal infection
      c. The need for dental checkups every 6 months, since dental caries will not produce pain

Paralysis agitans (Parkinson's disease)

A. Etiology and pathophysiology
   1. A progressive disorder in which there is a destruction of nerve cells in the basal ganglia of the brain, which results in a generalized degeneration of muscular function
   2. The suspected causes include neuromuscular imbalance (dopamine and acetylcholine), unknown virus, cerebral vascular disease, and chemical or physical trauma
B. Signs and symptoms
   1. Subjective
      a. Mild diffuse muscular pain
      b. Feelings of stiffness and rigidity, particularly of large joints
      c. Defects in judgment and emotional lability may be present, but intelligence is usually not impaired
      d. Sensitivity to heat
   2. Objective
      a. Increased difficulty in performing usual activities such as writing, dressing, and eating
      b. Generalized tremor commonly accompanied by "pill-rolling" movements of the thumb against the fingers; tremors are usually reduced by intentional movements
      c. Various disorders of locomotion; e.g., bent posture, difficulty in rising from a sitting position, shuffling propulsive gait, loss of rhythmic arm swing when walking
      d. Masklike facial expression with unblinking eyes
      e. Low-pitched, slow, poorly modulated, poorly articulated speech
      f. Drooling may be present because of difficulty in swallowing saliva

g. Various autonomic symptoms; e.g., lacrimation, constipation, incontinence, decreased sexual capacity, excessive perspiration
C. Treatment
1. Medical regimen is palliative rather than curative
2. Levodopa may be utilized to alleviate dopamine deficiency and decrease dyskinesia and rigidity
3. Anticholinergic agents that counteract the action of acetylcholine in the central nervous system
4. Medications to relieve related symptoms; e.g., antispasmodics, antihistamines, and analgesics to relieve muscular pains; sedatives to relieve restlessness or insomnia
5. Physiotherapy program designed to reduce rigidity of muscles and prevent contractures
6. Surgical intervention using alcohol, freezing (cryosurgery), electric cautery, ultrasound, etc. to destroy the globus pallidus (to relieve rigidity), and/or the thalamus (to relieve tremor) portions of the brain
D. Nursing care
1. Provide a safe environment
2. Teach patient or family to cut food into small bite-size pieces to prevent choking
3. Teach patient activities to limit postural deformities; e.g., use firm mattress without a pillow, periodically lie prone, keep head and neck as erect as possible, consciously think about posture when walking
4. Teach patient activities to maintain gait as normal as possible; e.g., clasp hands behind back when walking, exercise with stationary bicycle, use low-heeled shoes
5. Teach and encourage daily physical therapy program to limit rigidity and prevent contractures; e.g., warm baths, passive and active exercises
6. Attempt to administer care when patient is able to emotionally accept it and avoid rushing patient, since patient is unable to function under pressure
7. Encourage patient to continue taking medications even though results may be minimal
8. Limit foods high in pyridoxine (vitamin B_6), since it decreases the effectiveness of levodopa; e.g., dried beans, dry milk, salmon, tuna, pork, beef liver, and kidneys
9. Encourage small intake of alcohol, since it promotes relaxation and reduces rigidity
10. Encourage the intake of a well-balanced diet in small frequent amounts prepared so that it is easily masticated
11. Encourage an adequate intake of roughage and fluids to avoid constipation
12. Suction when necessary to maintain adequate airway (usually advanced stages)
13. Administer medications as ordered

Multiple sclerosis

A. Etiology and pathophysiology
1. Multiple sclerosis or disseminated sclerosis is a chronic, debilitating, progressive disease with periods of remission and exacerbation characterized by randomly scattered patches of demyelination in the brain stem, cerebrum, cerebellum, and spinal cord
2. Cause is unknown
3. Onset is in early adult life
B. Signs and symptoms
1. Subjective
a. Paresthesia
b. Altered position sense
c. Dysphagia
d. Ataxia
e. Weakness
f. Diplopia
g. Inappropriate emotional affect (euphoria occurs in later stages)
2. Objective
a. Nystagmus
b. Intention tremors
c. Slurred speech
d. Spastic paralysis
e. Increased deep tendon reflexes
f. Pallor of optic discs evident on examination with ophthalmoscope
g. Increased gamma globulin levels in the CSF
C. Treatment
1. Treatment is generally palliative
2. Corticosteroids
3. Physiotherapy, rehabilitation, and psychotherapy
D. Nursing care
1. Encourage patient to use supportive devices to maintain ambulation
2. Provide active and passive range of motion and other exercises
3. Teach patient to use assistive devices in carrying out activities of daily living

4. Assist family to understand why patient should be permitted and encouraged to be active
5. Assist patient and family to plan and implement a bowel and bladder regimen
6. Explain the disease process to both patient and family in understandable terms
7. Do not encourage false hopes during periods of remission
8. Spend time listening to both patient and family and encourage them to ventilate feelings
9. Attempt to refer patient and family to National Multiple Sclerosis Society
10. Encourage patient to seek counseling and rehabilitation
11. Explain to patient and family that mood swings and emotional alterations are part of the disease process
12. Help patient reestablish a realistic self-image
13. Teach patient to compensate for problems with gait (walk with feet farther apart to broaden base of support, use low-heeled shoes) and provide assistive devices when necessary (tripod cane, walker, wheelchair)
14. Teach patient to compensate for loss of sensation by using a thermometer to test water temperature, avoiding constricting stockings, using protective clothing in cold weather, changing position often
15. Teach patient to compensate for difficulty in swallowing by taking small bites, chewing well, using a straw with liquids, using foods of more solid consistency
16. If patient is immobilized
    a. Provide special skin care to prevent decubiti
    b. Provide special attention to joints and attempt to prevent dysfunctional contractures

Myasthenia gravis

A. Etiology and pathophysiology
1. A neuromuscular disorder in which there is a disturbance in the transmission of impulses at the myoneural junction
2. The dysfunction is thought to be caused by rapid breakdown or insufficient supply of acetylcholine at the junction
3. Highest incidence is in young adult females
4. Myasthenic crisis refers to the sudden inability to swallow or maintain respirations due to weakness of muscles of respiration

B. Signs and symptoms
1. Subjective
   a. Extreme muscle weakness, which becomes progressively worse as the muscle is used but disappears with rest
   b. Dysphagia (difficulty chewing)
   c. Diplopia
   d. Dysarthria (difficulty speaking)
2. Objective
   a. Ptosis of the lid
   b. Weak voice
   c. Myasthenic smile (snarling, nasal smile)
   d. Strabismus
   e. Diagnostic measures include administration of neostigmine (Prostigmin) subcutaneously or IV administration of edrophonium (Tensilon) to provide spontaneous relief of symptoms; edrophonium is also used to distinguish myasthenic crisis from toxic effects of neostigmine and similar drugs

C. Treatment
1. Specific medications that block the action of cholinesterase at the myoneural junction
   a. Neostigmine (Prostigmin)
   b. Pyridostigmine bromide (Mestinon)
   c. Ambenonium chloride (Mytelase)
2. X-ray therapy of thymus may cause partial remission
3. Corticosteroids or ACTH
4. Tracheostomy with mechanical ventilation is often necessary in myasthenic crisis

D. Nursing care
1. Administer medications on strict time schedule to prevent onset of symptoms; instruct patient and family to do same
2. Observe for signs of dyspnea, dysphagia, and dysarthria, which may indicate myasthenic crisis
3. Have emergency tracheostomy set at bedside
4. Plan activity to avoid fatigue based on individual's tolerance
5. Instruct patient to avoid people with upper respiratory tract infections, since pneumonia may develop as result of fatigued respiratory muscles
6. Encourage patient to carry a medical alert card or identification stating condition
7. Do not administer morphine to patients receiving anticholinesterases, since these drugs potentiate the effects of morphine and may cause respiratory depression

8. Provide emotional support and close contact with patient to allay anxiety
9. Administer tube feedings when necessary if patient has difficulty swallowing so that aspiration will not occur
10. In severe instances anticipate all needs, since patient is too weak to turn, drink, or even request assistance

Guillain-Barré syndrome

A. Etiology and pathophysiology
   1. The cause of this syndrome is unknown; thought to be a sequela to swine flu
   2. There are changes in the motor cells of the spinal cord and medulla with areas of demyelination
   3. Most common in young adults
B. Signs and symptoms
   1. Subjective
      a. Generalized weakness
      b. Paresthesia
   2. Objective
      a. Paralysis beginning in lower extremities
      b. The paralysis ascends the body, usually occurring within 24 to 27 hours
      c. Respiratory paralysis
      d. Hypertension, tachycardia, and low-grade fever
C. Treatment
   1. Steroids
   2. Support vital functions (similar to that for poliomyelitis)
D. Nursing care
   1. Carefully observe vital signs and vital capacity
   2. Suction, provide fluid replacement therapy, and monitor functioning of respirator as required
   3. Provide emotional support to patient and family due to the severity and lengthy convalescent period

Amyotrophic lateral sclerosis (ALS)

A. Etiology and pathophysiology
   1. The cause is unknown
   2. A progressive degenerative process involving the spinal, corticobulbar, and lower motor neurons, with subsequent atrophic and spastic changes in the cranial as well as the spinal muscles
   3. Occurs more frequently in men than women
B. Signs and symptoms
   1. Subjective

   a. Muscular weakness
   b. Malaise
   2. Objective
      a. Irregular spasmodic twitching in small muscle groups (fasciculations)
      b. Difficulty in chewing, swallowing, and speaking
      c. Outbursts of laughter or crying
C. Treatment
   1. Physiotherapy may be helpful in relieving spasticity
   2. Support respiratory functions
D. Nursing care
   1. Provide emotional support for patient and family
   2. Encourage range of motion
   3. Explain importance of maintaining good nutrition and preventing infection

Poliomyelitis

A. Etiology and pathophysiology
   1. Invasion of the lymph system by the polio virus occurs through the pharynx with eventual spread to lymph nodes, circulatory system, and the nervous system
   2. The virus causes inflammation and necrosis of the cells with resultant paralysis
   3. When it occurs in spinal cord, the anterior horn cells are affected; bulbar poliomyelitis involves the cranial nerves, and encephalitis cerebropoliomyelitis involves the cerebrum
   4. The incubation period is 5 to 12 days
B. Signs and symptoms
   1. Subjective
      a. Fatigue
      b. Headache
      c. Muscular pain, especially in head and back
   2. Objective
      a. Flaccid paralysis
      b. Absent deep tendon reflexes
      c. Increased spinal fluid pressure
      d. Polio virus in stool, throat secretions, blood, or spinal fluid
      e. Fever
      f. Respiratory paralysis may occur
C. Treatment
   1. Strict bed rest
   2. Support vital functions
      a. Tracheostomy

b. Fluid replacement
c. Urinary drainage
3. Antibiotics
D. Nursing care
1. Stress importance of immunizations as a way to prevent disease
2. Carefully observe vital signs and vital capacity
3. Maintain body alignment
4. Allow patient time to verbalize feelings; realize that paralysis may make this impossible, which can be frustrating for patient

Huntington's chorea

A. Etiology and pathophysiology
1. Inherited disorder that is considered autosomal dominant
2. There is progressive atrophy of the basal ganglia and some portions of the cerebral cortex
3. Appears during middle adult years
B. Signs and symptoms
1. Subjective
a. Memory loss
b. Disorientation
c. Eventual dementia
2. Objective
a. Uncontrolled jerky movements of the extremities or trunk
b. Disorganized gait
c. Uncontrolled periods of anger
d. Hesitant or explosive patterns of speech
e. Grimacing facial movements
C. Treatment
1. Control of jerky movements with haloperidol, fluphenazine, or levodopa
2. Symptoms are treated as they occur
D. Nursing care
1. Provide emotional support for patient and family
2. Provide for safety
3. Utilize community agencies to provide situational support

Rheumatoid arthritis

A. Etiology and pathophysiology
1. A chronic disease characterized by inflammatory changes in the body's connective tissue, particularly areas that have a cavity and easily moving surfaces
2. The cause is unknown, although theories include autoimmunity, heredity, and psychosomatic factors

B. Signs and symptoms
1. Subjective
a. Fatigue
b. Malaise
c. Joint pain
d. Muscle stiffness after periods of inactivity
e. Paresthesia
2. Objective
a. Anemia
b. Weight loss
c. Joint deformity as demonstrated by x-ray examination
d. Subcutaneous nodules
e. Elevated sedimentation rate
f. Presence of rheumatoid factors in serum through latex fixation test
C. Treatment
1. Corticosteroids, anti-inflammatories, analgesics, and immunosuppressive drugs may be indicated
2. Physiotherapy to minimize deformities
3. Surgical intervention to remove severely damaged joints; e.g., hip replacement
4. Paraffin dips of affected extremity for relief of joint pain by providing uniform heat
D. Nursing care
1. Administer analgesics and other medications as ordered
2. Teach patient to take medications as ordered
3. Apply heat and cold as ordered; heat paraffin to 52° to 54° C (125° to 129° F)
4. Promote rest and position to ease joint pains
5. Provide for range of motion exercises up to the point of pain, recognizing that some discomfort is always present
6. Encourage patient to verbalize feelings
7. Set realistic goals, focusing on strengths
8. Encourage use of supportive devices to help patient conserve energy and maintain independence
9. For nursing care of the patient following hip replacement see Fractured hip

Osteoarthritis

A. Etiology and pathophysiology
1. Etiology is unknown, but predisposing factors include obesity, aging, and joint trauma
2. A degeneration and atrophy of the cartilages and calcification of the ligaments
B. Signs and symptoms
1. Subjective
a. Pain after exercise

b. Stiffness of joints
2. Objective
   a. Heberden's nodes symmetrically occurring on fingers (bony extensions)
   b. Decreased range of motion
C. Treatment
1. Weight reduction in instances of obesity
2. Local heat to affected joints
3. Medications to reduce symptoms, such as analgesics, anti-inflammatory agents, and steroids
4. Exercise of affected extremities
5. Surgical intervention
   a. Synovectomy—removal of the enlarged synovial membrane before bone and cartilage destruction occurs
   b. Arthrodesis—fusion of joint performed when joint surfaces are severely damaged; this leaves patient with no range of motion of the affected joint
   c. Reconstructive surgery—replacement of badly damaged joint with a prosthetic device (see Hip replacement)
D. Nursing care
1. Assist patient in activities that require using affected joints; allow for rest periods
2. Attempt to relieve patient's discomfort by the use of medications or the application of heat as ordered
3. Allow patient ample time to verbalize feelings regarding limited motion and changes in life-style

Gouty arthritis (gout)

A. Etiology and pathophysiology
1. Gout is a disorder in purine metabolism that results in high levels of uric acid in the blood and the deposition of uric acid crystals (tophi) in tissues, especially joints, which is followed by an inflammatory response
2. Incidence is highest in males, and a familial tendency has been demonstrated
3. Renal urate lithiasis (kidney stones) may result from precipitation of uric acid in the presence of a low urinary pH
B. Signs and symptoms
1. Subjective
   a. Sudden onset of asymmetric joint pain usually in the metatarsophalangeal joint of the great toe
   b. Local pruritus
   c. Malaise

d. Headache
e. Anorexia
2. Objective
   a. Elevated serum uric acid
   b. Signs of inflammation of joint including swelling, heat, and redness
   c. Tophi in outer ear, hands, and feet
C. Treatment
1. Administration of anti-inflammatory and uricosuric agents (see Pharmacology)
2. Alkaline-ash diet to increase the pH of urine to discourage precipitation of uric acid and enhance the action of drugs such as probenicid (Benemid)
3. Elimination of foods high in purines
4. Weight loss is encouraged if indicated
D. Nursing care
1. Assess joint pain, motion, and appearance
2. Administer-anti-inflammatory agents such as phenylbutazone (Butazolidin), oxyphenbutazone (Tandearil), or indomethacin (Indocin) with antacids or milk to help prevent peptic ulcers; observe therapeutic response
3. Carefully align joints so they are slightly flexed during acute stage; encourage regular exercise, which is important for long-term management
4. Use a bed cradle during acute phase to keep pressure of sheets off joints
5. Increase fluid intake to 2000 to 3000 ml daily to prevent formation of calculi
6. Instruct patient to avoid foods such as brains, kidneys, liver, and sweetbreads, which have a high purine content
7. Provide education regarding drug therapy and avoidance of excess alcohol intake

Osteomyelitis

A. Etiology and pathophysiology
1. Occurs as the result of bacterial invasion of the bone by *Staphylococcus aureus*, streptococcal organisms, *E. coli,* and *Salmonella* organisms
2. Infection of the bone results from trauma or systemic infection and involves the entire bone and surrounding soft tissue
B. Signs and symptoms
1. Subjective
   a. Pain and tenderness of bone
   b. Malaise
   c. Difficulty in weight-bearing
2. Objective
   a. Fever

  b. Swelling over affected bone
  c. Signs of sepsis
C. Treatment
  1. Antibiotic therapy
  2. Incision and drainage of bone abscess
  3. Sequestrectomy—surgical removal of dead infected bone and cartilage
D. Nursing care
  1. Administer pain medications and antibiotics as ordered
  2. Use surgically aseptic technique when changing dressings
  3. Maintain good body alignment and promote comfort
  4. Utilize room deodorizer if foul odor is apparent
  5. Allow patient ample time to express feelings about long-term hospitalization

Osteoporosis

A. Etiology and pathophysiology
  1. Osteoporosis is a decrease in bone substance to the point where the bone can no longer maintain the skeletal structure
  2. Most commonly affects the vertebrae, pelvis, and femur
  3. Factors that seem to be related to osteoporosis include menopause, aging, inactivity, insufficient calcium intake or absorption, hyperparathyroidism, acromegaly, Cushing's syndrome, and hyperthyroidism
B. Signs and symptoms
  1. Subjective
    a. Backache
    b. Difficulty maintaining balance
  2. Objective
    a. Decreased height resulting from compression of vertebrae
    b. X-ray examination reveals a demineralization of bone and compression of the vertebrae
C. Treatment
  1. Planned program of exercise
  2. Estrogen therapy to decrease bone reabsorption
  3. High-protein, high-calcium diet with vitamin D supplement
  4. Support for spine; e.g., corset, Taylor brace
  5. Treatment of underlying disorder is vital to halt process
D. Nursing care
  1. Encourage active exercise, assist with passive exercises
  2. Instruct patient about proper body mechanics
  3. Provide diet that includes meats and milk products
  4. Consider safety factors associated with instability; a cane or walker may be necessary for ambulation
  5. Provide rest periods to prevent fatigue
  6. Encourage fluids in acute osteoporosis to discourage formation of renal calculi

Osteogenic sarcoma

A. Etiology and pathophysiology
  1. A malignant bone tumor that commonly begins in the long bones, especially around the knee
  2. Metastasis to the lungs is common and occurs early; prognosis is poor
  3. Highest incidence is between 20 and 30 years of age
B. Signs and symptoms
  1. Subjective
    a. Pain
    b. Limited motion
    c. Malaise
  2. Objective
    a. Local swelling
    b. Weight loss
    c. Anemia
    d. Elevated serum alkaline phosphatase
    e. Fever
    f. Microscopic evaluation of biopsy reveals neoplastic cells
C. Treatment
  1. Amputation of limb or resection of tumor
  2. Chemotherapy
  3. Radiation
D. Nursing care
  1. Be available for patient and family to discuss fears, concerns, and treatment
  2. Provide high-protein, high-calorie meals based on patient's preference
  3. Administer special nursing care following surgery (see Amputations)
  4. Administer analgesics and antiemetics as needed
  5. Provide special care if patient is receiving radiation therapy
    a. Observe skin for breakdown
    b. Do not wash off port marks
    c. Avoid use of powders and ointments that contain metals

Multiple myeloma

A. Etiology and pathophysiology
1. The cause is unknown, although genetic and viral factors are being closely considered
2. Malignant overgrowth of plasma cells and malignant tumor growth in bone and bone marrow
3. Occurs primarily in middle-aged men
B. Signs and symptoms
1. Subjective
   a. Bone pain
   b. Progressive weakness
   c. Low back pain
2. Objective
   a. Anemia
   b. Cachexia
   c. Idiopathic bone fractures
   d. Macroglobulinemia
   e. Platelet deficiency with resultant bleeding tendency
   f. Punched-out appearance of bones on x-ray examination
   g. Presence of Bence Jones protein in urine
C. Treatment
1. Chemotherapeutic agents, especially melphalan (Alkeran)
2. Radiation therapy
3. Analgesics and narcotics for pain
4. Supportive therapy such as transfusions as indicated
D. Nursing care
1. Carefully ambulate patient to prevent pneumonia and reduce pathologic fractures
2. Allow patient ample time to express feeling about disease and related therapies
3. Allow patient to participate in planning nursing care to aid in self-esteem and promote a feeling of self-control

Intractable pain

A. Etiology and pathophysiology
1. Refers to pain that is not relieved by conventional treatment
2. Causes include cancer, neuralgia, tic douloureux, and ischemic pain that cannot be controlled
B. Signs and symptoms
1. Subjective
   a. Pain
   b. Fatigue
   c. Irritability

2. Objective
   a. Evidence of malignancy
   b. Pallor
C. Treatment
1. Surgical intervention
   a. Rhizotomy—posterior spinal nerve root is resected between the ganglion and the cord, resulting in permanent loss of sensation; the anterior root may be cut to alleviate painful muscle spasm
   b. Cordotomy—to alleviate intractable pain in the trunk or lower extremeties; the transmission of pain and temperature sensation is interrupted by creating a lesion in the ascending tracts; this may be done by percutaneously using an electrode or surgically via laminectomy
   c. Sympathectomy—to control pain of vascular disturbances and phantom limb pain (see procedures related to gastrointestinal disorders)
2. Acupuncture therapy
3. Biofeedback helps the patient to develop control over anxiety and physiologic function
4. Electronic stimulation may alter the electric potential of the nerve to prevent complete depolarization or prevent transmission of pain sensations to brain
   a. Percutaneous stimulator—electrodes are applied over painful area or along nerve pathway
   b. Dorsal column stimulator and peripheral nerve implant involve direct attachment of electrode to sensory nerve; a transmitter attached to the electrode is carried by the patient so that electric stimulation can be administered as needed
D. Nursing care
1. Assess pain, including location, duration, type, and severity
2. Eliminate factors from environment that seem to intensify pain
3. Support patient and family, since patient frequently will withdraw
4. Educate patient and family about treatments available and the potential side effects
5. Provide postoperative care
   a. Nursing care for a patient having a cordotomy, rhizotomy, or dorsal column stimulator (see Ruptured nucleus pulposus)
   b. Neurologically assess extremities for movement, sensation, and skin temperature

c. Carefully inspect skin, since patient will not feel pain of ulceration

d. Instruct patient to avoid extreme environmental conditions and the use of heating pads and to check the temperature of bath water, since temperature sensitivity is absent

Ruptured nucleus pulposus (slipped disc, herniation of intervertebral disc)

A. Etiology and pathophysiology

1. A ruptured intervertebral disc involves the protrusion of the nucleus pulposus into the spinal canal and subsequent compression of the spinal cord or nerve roots, which usually occurs as a result of trauma

2. Most common site is lumbosacral area (between L_4 and L_5), but herniation can also occur in the cervical region (between C_5 and C_6 or C_6 and C_7)

B. Signs and symptoms

1. Subjective
   a. Lumbosacral disc
      (1) Acute pain in lower back, radiating across buttock and down leg (sciatic pain)
      (2) Pain when raising unflexed leg on affected side (Lasègue's sign)
      (3) Weakness of foot
   b. Cervical disc
      (1) Neck pain that may radiate down arm to hand
      (2) Weakness of affected upper extremity

2. Objective
   a. Straightening of normal lumbar curve with scoliosis away from the affected side (lumbosacral disc)
   b. Atrophy of the biceps and triceps may be present (cervical disc)
   c. Elevated CSF protein
   d. Myelogram shows impingement on spinal cord
   e. Electromyography (EMG) can help localize site of herniated disc

C. Treatment

1. Bed rest with traction to lower extremeties (lumbosacral disc) or cervical traction (cervical disc)
2. Back brace or support; cervical collar
3. Local application of heat
4. Muscle relaxant
5. Surgical intervention

a. Laminectomy—excision of the ruptured portion of the nucleus pulposus through opening created by removal of part of vertebra

b. Spinal fusion—if 3 or more discs are involved, the affected vertebrae will be permanently fused to stabilize the spine

D. Nursing care

1. Administer analgesics and other medications as ordered
2. Use a firm mattress and bed board under patient
3. Make certain traction and/or braces are correctly applied and maintained and that weights hang freely
4. Use fracture bedpan to avoid lifting of hips
5. Give frequent and extensive back care to relax muscles and promote circulation
6. Support patient's body alignment at all times
7. Use log-rolling method to turn patient (instruct patient to fold arms across chest, bend the knee on the opposite side to the direction of the turn and then roll over)
8. Increase fluid intake and roughage in diet to prevent constipation; use stool softeners to prevent straining
9. Keep patient flat for 24 hours and encourage fluids to limit headache after a myelogram is done
10. Provide special care for patient having laminectomy
    a. Explain to patient that pain may persist postoperatively for some time due to edema
    b. Place bedside table, phone, and call bell within reach to prevent twisting
    c. Observe dressing for hemorrhage and leakage of spinal fluid; notify physician immediately if either occurs
    d. Observe for inadequate ventilation, especially in patients undergoing a cervical laminectomy
    e. Assess patient for changes in neurologic functioning
11. Allow patient to be dependent, but foster independence
12. Encourage patient to express feelings about altered functioning and self-image
13. Encourage patient to verbalize fears about present condition and future disability
14. Teach patient to use proper body mechanics to prevent subsequent injury

Fractures

A. Etiology and pathophysiology
1. Fractures are breaks in the continuity of the bone, usually accompanied by localized tissue response and muscle spasm
2. The cause of fractures is usually trauma, but pathologic fractures may occur as a result of diseases such as osteoporosis, multiple myeloma, or bone tumors, which weaken the bone structure
3. Types of fractures
   a. Complete fracture—complete separation of the bone into 2 parts; may be transverse or spiral
   b. Incomplete fracture—only part of the bone is broken
   c. Comminuted fracture—bone is broken into several fragments
   d. Greenstick fracture—splintering on one side of the bone, with bending of the other side; occurs only in pliable bones, usually in children
   e. Simple, or closed, fracture—fracture is present, but there is no break in the skin
   f. Compound, or open, fracture—a break in the skin occurs at the time of fracture with or without protrusion of the bone
4. Stages of healing include formation of a hematoma followed by cellular proliferation and callus formation by the osteoblasts; finally ossification and remodeling of the callus

B. Signs and symptoms
1. Subjective
   a. Pain aggravated by motion
   b. Tenderness
2. Objective
   a. Loss of motion
   b. Edema
   c. Crepitus (grating sound heard when fractured limb is moved)
   d. Ecchymosis
   e. X-ray examination reveals break in continuity of bone

C. Treatment
1. Traction may be used to reduce the fracture or to maintain alignment of bone fragments until healing occurs
   a. Skin traction—weights are attached to adhesive, which is applied to the skin
      (1) Buck's extension—exerts a straight pull on a limb; often used temporarily to immobilize the leg when a patient fractures a hip
      (2) Bryants' traction—both lower limbs are extended vertically; used to align fractured femurs in young children
      (3) Russell traction—the lower leg is supported in a hammock, which is attached to rope and pulleys on a Balkan frame; used to treat fractures of the femur (the foot of the bed is usually elevated for countertraction)
   b. Skeletal traction is applied to the bone
      (1) Steinmann pin or Kirschner wire may be inserted through the bone and skin; weights are then attached to a spreader, which is attached to both ends of the pin or wire (this may be used in conjunction with a cast)
      (2) Crutchfield tongs are inserted into the skull and weights are attached to immobilize the patient with a cervical fracture in a position of hyperextension
2. Surgical intervention to align the bone (open reduction), often with plates and screws to hold fracture in alignment
3. Manipulation to reduce fracture (closed reduction)
4. Application of cast to maintain alignment and immobilize limb

D. Nursing care
1. Provide emergency nursing care
   a. Evaluate general physical condition
   b. Treat for shock
   c. Splint suspected fractures before moving patient; treat all suspected fractures as fractures until x-ray films are available
   d. Cover open wound with sterile dressing if available
2. Observe for signs of emboli (fat or blood clot); e.g., severe chest pain, dyspnea, pallor, and diaphoresis
3. Provide special care to a patient with a cast
   a. Observe for signs of circulatory impairment; e.g., change in skin temperature or color, numbness or tingling, unrelieved pain, decrease in pedal pulse, prolonged blanching of toes after compression
   b. Protect cast from damage until dry by elevat-

ing it on a pillow; handle with palms of hands only

c. Promote drying of cast by leaving uncovered; a hair dryer or light may be used with care to prevent burning

d. Maintain bed rest until cast is dry and ambulation is permitted

e. Observe for signs of hemorrhage and measure extent of drainage on cast when present

f. Observe for irritation caused by rough cast edges, and pad as necessary for comfort and to prevent soiling

g. Observe for swelling and notify physician if necessary

h. Administer analgesics judiciously and report unrelieved pain

i. Observe for signs of infection; e.g., elevated temperature, odor from cast, swelling

4. Provide special care to a patient in traction

a. Check that weights are hanging freely and that affected limb is not resting against the bed; countertraction may be necessary to prevent this by raising the foot of the bed (Russell traction and Buck's extension) or head of the bed (cervical traction)

b. Maintain patient in proper alignment

c. Observe for footdrop in patients with Russell traction or Buck's extension, since this may be indicative of nerve damage

d. Observe for signs of thrombophlebitis; this is a more common complication of Russell traction because there is pressure on the popliteal space in addition to the stress of immobility

e. Provide careful skin care

f. Observe skin for irritation and observe site of insertion of skeletal traction for signs of infection

g. Use aseptic technique when cleansing the site of insertion of skeletal traction (frequently an antiseptic ointment is also ordered)

5. Encourage high-protein, high-vitamin diet to promote healing; high-calcium diet is not recommended for the patient confined to prolonged bed rest, since decalcification of the bone will continue until activity is restored, and a high calcium intake could lead to formation of renal calculi

6. Encourage fluids to help prevent complications of constipation, renal calculi, and urinary tract infection

7. Teach patient isometric exercises to promote muscle tone

8. Teach patient appropriate crutch-walking technique; nonweight-bearing (3-point swing-through); weight-bearing (4-point) progressing to use of cane (see procedures)

Fractured hip

A. Etiology and pathophysiology

1. Fracture of hip refers to fractures of the head, neck (intracapsular fracture), or trochanteric area (extracapsular fracture) of the femur

2. Incidence is highest in elderly females due to osteoporosis

B. Signs and symptoms

1. Subjective

a. Pain

b. Changes in sensation

2. Objective

a. Affected leg appears shorter

b. External rotation of affected limb

c. X-ray examination reveals lack of continuity of bone

C. Treatment

1. Buck's extension or Russell traction may be used as a temporary measure to relieve the pain of muscle spasm or if surgery is contraindicated

2. Closed reduction with a hip spica cast may be used in the treatment of fractures of the intratrochanteric region

3. Open reduction and internal fixation

a. Austin Moore prosthesis

b. Thompson prosthesis

c. Smith-Petersen nail

d. Jewett nail

D. Nursing care

1. See Nursing care of patients with fractures

2. Encourage use of trapeze to facilitate movement

3. Use a fracture pan for elimination

4. Postoperative care

a. Inspect dressing and linen for bleeding

b. Use a trochanter roll to prevent external rotation of legs

c. Do not turn on operative side unless specifically ordered

d. Use pillows or abductor pillow to maintain legs in slight abduction; following a hip replacement it prevents displacement of the prosthesis

e. Encourage quadriceps setting exercises
f. Assist patient to ambulate first using walker, progressing to 3-point crutch walking, and then to total weight-bearing using a cane to provide stability
g. Avoid flexing the hips of patients with total-hip replacements; assist to a lounge chair position when permitted to sit

Spinal cord injury

A. Etiology and pathophysiology
1. Spinal cord injury refers to the sudden impingements on the integrity of the spinal cord as a result of trauma
2. Fractures of the vertebrae can cut, compress, or completely sever the spinal cord if the patient is not positioned and moved correctly at the scene of an accident; the symptoms depend on the location (lumbar, thoracic, cervical) and extent of the damage (complete transection, partial transection, compression) and may be temporary or permanent; the sensation and mobility of areas that are supplied by nerves below the level of the lesion are lost
B. Signs and symptoms
1. Subjective
a. Loss of sensation below level of injury
b. Inability to move
2. Objective
a. Early symptoms of spinal shock
(1) Absence of reflexes below level of lesion
(2) Flaccid paralysis (immobility accompanied by weak, soft, flabby muscles) below the level of injury
(3) Hypotonia caused by disruption of neural impulses results in bowel and bladder distention
(4) Inability to perspire in affected parts
(5) Hypotension
b. Later symptoms of spinal cord injury
(1) Reflex hyperexcitability (spastic paralysis)—the muscles below the site of injury becomes spastic and hyperreflexic
(2) A state of diminished reflex excitability (flaccid paralysis) below the site of injury follows the state of reflex hyperexcitability in all instances of total cord damage and may occur in some instances of partial cord damage

(3) In total cord damage, since both the upper and lower motoneurons are destroyed, the symptoms depend totally on the location of the injury; the loss of motor and sensory function present at this time is usually permanent
(a) Sacral region—paralysis (usually flaccid type) of lower extremities (paraplegia) accompanied by atonic (autonomous) bladder and bowel with impairment of sphincter control
(b) Lumbar region—paralysis of lower extremities that may extend to the pelvic region (usually flaccid type) accompanied by a spastic (automatic) bladder and loss of bladder and anal sphincter control
(c) Thoracic region—the same symptoms as in the lumbar region except the paralysis extends to the trunk below the level of the diaphragm
(d) Cervical region—the same symptoms as thoracic region except the paralysis extends from the neck down and includes paralysis of all extremities (quadriplegia); if injury is above C_4, respirations are depressed
(4) In partial cord damage either the upper or the lower motoneurons or both may be destroyed; therefore the symptoms depend not only on the location but also on the type of neurons involved; destruction of lower motoneurons will result in atrophy and flaccid paralysis of the involved muscles, whereas destruction of upper motoneurons causes spasticity
C. Treatment
1. Neurologic assessment
2. Maintain vertebral alignment by ordering
a. Bed rest with supportive devices (bed board, sand bags, etc.)
b. Bed rest with total immobilization (see procedures: Stryker frame, Circ-O-lectric bed)
c. Traction (skeletal or skin traction; e.g., Crutchfield tongs, Buck's extension)
d. Corsets, braces, and other devices when mobility is permitted
3. Surgery to reduce pain or pressure and/or stabilize the spine (i.e., laminectomy, spinal fusion)

4. Mechanical ventilation as needed
5. Temperature control via hypothermia or tepid baths
6. Extensive rehabilitation therapy

D. Nursing care
1. Maintain frequent observation of patient's respiratory and neurologic functioning
2. Maintain spinal alignment at all times; when turning patient use log-rolling method and make certain enough help is available to move patient as a single unit
3. Check safety locks on Stryker frames and Circ-O-lectric beds before turning patient
4. Maintain surgical asepsis for patient with Crutchfield tongs or spinal surgery
5. Provide special skin care to back and bony prominences
6. Maintain body parts in functional position; prevent dysfunctional contractures
7. Institute active and passive range of motion as soon as approved by physician
8. Provide patient with simple explanations
9. Encourage patient to verbalize and accept that hostility will surface
10. Stay with patient when possible to provide assurance
11. Allow patient to be independent when possible
12. Include patient in decision-making process
13. Help patient to adjust to change in body image and altered self-concept
14. Accept periods of depression that occur
15. Allow patient time to reorganize life-style
16. Set realistic short-term goals so that patient can achieve some success
17. Test temperature of bath water to avoid burns; teach patient to test water temperature in any water-related activity
18. Avoid bumps and bruises when involved in activities; utilize techniques to prevent pressure and examine skin for signs of pressure from positioning, braces, or splints
19. Use a footboard to stimulate pressure sensation and proprioception
20. Provide opportunity for patient to touch, grasp, and manipulate objects of different sizes, weights, and textures to stimulate tactile sensation
21. Encourage patient to be aware of all body segments; look at both extremities, comb both sides of hair, shave both sides of chin, put make-up on both sides of face
22. Protect affected limbs by proper positioning during transfer and using a sling when indicated
23. Teach the patient to use unaffected extremities to manipulate, move, and stabilize affected ones
24. Attempt to reestablish scheduled pattern of bowel function
    a. Understand what the individual's bowel functioning means to the patient and family
    b. Involve the patient, family, and entire health team in the development of a plan of care
    c. Review the patient's bowel habits prior to illness as well as the current pattern of elimination
    d. Supply diet adequate in bulk, roughage, and bowel-stimulating properties
    e. Encourage sufficient fluid intake—2000 to 3000 ml per day
    f. Encourage the patient to be as active as possible to develop the tone and strength of muscles that can be used
    g. Establish a specific and definite time for the bowel movement; regularity is the most important aspect of bowel reeducation
       (1) Exact time depends on patient's schedule
       (2) Depends on patient's past pattern
       (3) Consider scheduling evacuation after a meal to utilize the gastrocolic reflex (peristaltic wave in colon induced by entrance of food into fasting stomach)
    h. Determine if the patient is aware of need or act of defecation; e.g., feeling of fullness or pressure in rectum, flatus, rumbling in stomach
    i. Provide privacy for the patient during toileting activities
    j. Encourage the patient to assume a position most near the physiologic position for defecation (sitting the patient up frequently assists in preparing for this)
    k. Utilize assistive measures to induce defecation by
       (1) Teaching the patient to bear down and contract abdominal muscles (the Valsalva maneuver should be avoided by people with cardiac problems)
       (2) Teaching the patient to lean forward to

increase intra-abdominal pressure by compressing abdomen against the thighs

(3) Digital stimulation

(4) Using suppository if necessary

(5) Using enemas only as a last resort

l. Provide for adaptation of equipment as necessary; e.g., elevated toilet seat, grab bars, padded back rest

m. Teach the family the bowel training program

25. Attempt to reestablish bladder function

a. Determine type of bladder problem

(1) Neurogenic bladder—any disturbance in bladder functioning caused by a lesion of the nervous system

(2) Spastic (reflex or automatic) bladder—a bladder disorder caused by a lesion of the spinal cord above the bladder reflex center in the conus medullaris; there is a loss of conscious sensation and cerebral motor control; the bladder empties automatically when the detrusor muscle is sufficiently stretched (about 500 ml)

(3) Flaccid (atonic nonreflex or autonomous) bladder—a bladder disorder caused by a lesion of the spinal cord at the level of the sacral conus or below; the bladder continues to fill, becomes distended, and periodically overflows; the bladder muscle does not contract forcefully and therefore does not empty except with a conscious effort

b. Understand what the individual's bladder functioning means to the patient and family

c. Involve the patient, family, and entire health team in the development of a plan of care

d. Review the patient's bladder habits prior to illness as well as the current pattern of elimination

e. Encourage activity

f. Encourage sufficient fluid intake

(1) 3000 to 5000 ml per 24-hour period

(2) Drink a glass of water with each attempt to void

(3) Reduce amount of fluid as the day progresses and restrict fluid after 6 P.M. to limit amount of urine in bladder during the night

g. Provide for privacy during toileting activities

h. Encourage the patient to assume as normal a position as possible for voiding

i. Establish a voiding schedule

(1) Begin trial voiding at the time the patient is most often incontinent

(2) Attempt voiding every 2 hours all day and 2 to 3 times during the night

(3) Time intervals between voiding should be shorter in the morning than later in the day

(4) As the patient's ability to maintain control improves, lengthen time between attempts at voiding

(5) Time of intervals is not as important as regularity

j. Determine whether the patient is aware of need or act of urination; e.g., fullness or pressure, flushing, chilling, goose pimples, cold sweats

k. Utilize assistive measures to induce urination by teaching the patient to

(1) Use the Credé maneuver—manual expression of the urine from the bladder with moderate external pressure, downward and backward, from the umbilicus to over the suprapubic area

(2) Bend forward to increase intra-abdominal pressure

(3) Stimulate "trigger points"—those areas which, for the individual, will instigate urination; e.g., stroke thigh, pull pubic hair, touch meatus

l. Record intake, output, voiding times, and times of incontinence

m. Provide for adaptive equipment as necessary; e.g., elevated toilet seats, commode, urinals, drainage systems

n. Teach the family the bladder training program

Anterior segment disorders of the eye

A. Etiology and pathophysiology

1. Conjunctivitis—inflammation of the conjunctiva that can result from invasion by organisms, allergens, or irritants

2. Blepharitis—inflammation of the lid margins; classified as staphylococcal or seborrheic

3. Keratitis—inflammation of the cornea due to invasion of an organism
4. Uveitis—an inflammation of the iris, ciliary body, and/or the choroid
5. Pterygium—a segment of thickened conjunctiva that can extend over the cornea
6. Trachoma—viral infection of lids and conjunctiva that can result in corneal ulceration and blindness
7. Chalazion—a sterile cyst of the Meibomian gland that causes inflammation of the lid; the cyst remains when the inflammation subsides
8. Hordeolum—infection of a follicle of the eyelash commonly caused by staphyloccocal organisms

B. Signs and symptoms
1. Subjective
   a. Photophobia (keratitis, uveitis)
   b. Blurred vision (keratitis, uveitis, trachoma)
   c. Pain (keratitis, uveitis)
   d. Burning and itching of eyes (conjunctivitis, blepharitis, hordeola)
2. Objective
   a. Scaling and crust formation of lids (conjunctivitis, blepharitis, keratitis, uveitis)
   b. Swelling and redness (conjunctivitis, blepharitis, keratitis, uveitis, hordeola)
   c. Tearing (keratitis)
   d. Ciliary injection (uveitis)
   e. Purulent drainage (conjunctivitis)

C. Treatment
1. Conjunctivitis, blepharitis, hordeola
   a. Antibiotic ointments
   b. Warm compresses
2. Keratitis
   a. Culture analysis to determine causative organism
   b. Topical steroids and antibiotics
   c. If cornea is badly damaged, corneal transplant
3. Uveitis
   a. Mydriatics to keep iris at rest
   b. Topical steroids and antibiotics
   c. Dark glasses
4. Pterigium—surgical removal is indicated
5. Trachoma—oral antibiotics, usually tetracycline, for 3 to 5 weeks
6. Chalazion—surgical excision of cyst is generally indicated

D. Nursing care
1. Instruct patient on proper care of eyes (hand washing, avoidance of rubbing)

2. Administer antibiotic ointment and instruct patient in its use
3. Apply soaks as ordered
4. Prepare patient for surgery, if indicated
5. If patient has corneal transplant (keratoplasty)
   a. Maintain bed rest for 1 or 2 days with eyes bandaged
   b. Explain to patient the importance of avoiding Valsalva maneuver during healing process
   c. Explain to patient that healing may take up to 6 months due to the decreased circulatory supply of the cornea

Tumors of the eye

A. Etiology and pathophysiology
1. Tumors, either benign or malignant, may form in the eye or metastasize to the eye
2. Retinoblastoma is a congenital malignant neoplasm found in children; spreads easily by extension to the brain
3. Melanoma is common in the iris and choroid; grows slowly but metastasizes to the liver and lungs

B. Signs and symptoms
1. Subjective
   a. Headache
   b. A variety of visual complaints
2. Objective
   a. Increased injection of the conjunctiva
   b. Decreased vision
   c. In retinoblastoma, white pupillary reflex, strabismus, retinal detachment

C. Treatment
1. Chemotherapy
2. Radiation therapy
3. Enucleation (surgical removal of eye)

D. Nursing care
1. Support patient and family as they attempt to cope with diagnosis
2. Observe for side effects of medical therapy and attempt to limit their effects
3. If patient has an enucleation, care involves
   a. Maintaining pressure dressings on eye for 1 or 2 days to minimize hemorrhage
   b. Observing for signs of meningitis, which occurs as a complication, including headache or pain on operative side
   c. Explaining to patient that monocularity results in loss of depth perception, and activities that require this should be avoided

d. Explaining that artificial eye may be inserted when healing is complete, usually 6 to 8 weeks; support adaptation to changes in body image

Cataract

A. Etiology and pathophysiology
  1. A cataract is an opacity of the crystalline lens or its capsule
  2. Results from injury, exposure to heat, heredity, aging, or congenital factors that cause a diminution of sight
B. Signs and symptoms
  1. Subjective
    a. Distortion of vision; e.g., haziness, cloudiness, diplopia
    b. Photophobia
  2. Objective
    a. Progressive loss of vision
    b. The usual black pupil appears clouded and progresses to milky white appearance
C. Treatment
  1. Corrective lenses until cataract matures enough for removal
  2. Surgical intervention to remove opaque lens
    a. Preoperative preparation with mydriatics and ophthalmic antibiotics
    b. Antiemetics, analgesics, and stool softeners postoperatively
    c. Corrective lenses (contact lenses or glasses)
      (1) Contacts are fitted approximately 3 months postoperatively
      (2) Temporary eyeglasses are given soon after discharge, with the final prescription given several weeks later
  3. A lens implant is sometimes inserted at time of surgery
D. Nursing care
  1. Instruct patient to prevent pressure on eyes by
    a. Not touching or rubbing eyes
    b. Not closing eyes tightly
    c. Avoiding coughing, sneezing, or bending from waist (teach patient to open mouth when coughing)
    d. Lying on back or nonoperative side
    e. Avoiding rapid head movements
    f. Avoiding straining at stool
  2. Instruct patient to request prescribed analgesics and antiemetics as required
  3. Administer stool softeners

  4. Provide side rails to assist in turning and preventing falls
  5. Assist patient with ambulation because of distortions in depth perception and extremely blurred vision
  6. Provide an easily accessible call bell
  7. Reduce amount of light and encourage use of sunglasses when eye patch is removed
  8. Provide a quiet environment to promote rest
  9. Avoid substances that might precipitate coughing or sneezing; e.g., pepper, talcum powder
  10. Observe for signs of increased intraocular pressure; e.g., pain, restlessness, increased pulse rate
  11. Observe for signs of infection; e.g., pain, changes in vital signs
  12. Encourage deep breathing
  13. Explain to patient that depth perception will be altered but assure patient that the corrective lenses will help to compensate for this distortion

Acute angle glaucoma

A. Etiology and pathophysiology
  1. Glaucoma is a condition in which the pressure within the eyeball is higher than normal
  2. Closed angle of the drainage system of the canal of Schlemm prevents the aqueous from reaching the lymph drainage spaces called the trabecular meshwork
B. Signs and symptoms
  1. Subjective
    a. Nausea
    b. Halos around lights
    c. Malaise
  2. Objective
    a. Gradual loss of peripheral vision
    b. Increased intraocular pressure of 24 to 32 mm Hg as measured with a tonometer
    c. Steamy cornea
    d. Conjunctival injection
C. Treatment
  1. Lower intraocular pressure with miotics or carbonic anhydrase inhibitors
  2. Surgical intervention to facilitate drainage of the aqueous humor is called an iridectomy; a surgical incision is made through the cornea to remove a portion of the iris to facilitate aqueous drainage
D. Nursing care
  1. Explain the importance of continued use of eye medications as ordered

2. Explain the need for continued medical supervision for observation of intraocular eye pressure to ensure control of the disorder
3. Teach the patient to avoid exertion, stooping, heavy lifting, or wearing constricting clothing, since these increase intraocular pressure

Detached retina

A. Etiology and pathophysiology
   1. May occur due to trauma, the aging process, after cataract surgery, or in cases of myopia
   2. The retina separates from the choroid, and vitreous humor seeps behind the retina
B. Signs and symptoms
   1. Subjective
      a. Flashes of light
      b. Floaters
      c. Veil-like curtain sensation in line of sight
   2. Objective
      a. Retinal separation noted on ophthalmoscopy
      b. Assessment of visual loss
C. Treatment
   1. Bed rest, with area of detachment in a dependent position to promote healing
   2. Tranquilizers to promote rest and reduce anxiety
   3. Surgical intervention
      a. Cryosurgery—a supercooled probe causes retinal scarring and healing of area
      b. Photocoagulation—laser beam through pupil results in retinal burn, which causes scarring of involved area
      c. Scleral buckling—shortening of the sclera to force the choroid close to retina
D. Nursing care
   1. Keep patient on bed rest in position as ordered
   2. Provide patient with call bell and answer promptly
   3. Observe for signs of hemorrhage postoperatively (severe pain, restlessness)
   4. Diminish lights in room
   5. Explain to patient that return to a sedentary occupation may occur in approximately 3 weeks and to a more laborious job in 6 to 8 weeks

Chronic otitis media

A. Etiology and pathophysiology
   1. A chronic inflammatory disease of the middle ear that usually begins in childhood

2. Usually related to perforation of the eardrum and may be associated with mastoiditis
B. Signs and symptoms
   1. Subjective
      a. Hearing loss
      b. Feeling of fullness within ear
   2. Objective
      a. Drainage from ear that may be foul smelling
      b. Perforation of eardrum apparent during examination with otoscope
      c. Presence of cholesteatoma (epidermal inclusion cyst)
C. Treatment
   1. Systemic antibiotics
   2. Antibiotic eardrops
   3. Gentle irrigations to cleanse ear
   4. Treatment of upper respiratory tract infections
D. Nursing care
   1. Instill antibiotics as prescribed
   2. Instruct patient to report headache and stiff neck immediately, since this may indicate complication of meningitis

Mastoiditis

A. Etiology and pathophysiology
   1. A disease of the mastoid process that may be acute or chronic in nature
   2. Generally occurs secondary to otitis media
   3. There is disruption of the intercellular construction of the bone that may progress to necrosis or suppurative mastoiditis
B. Signs and symptoms
   1. Subjective
      a. Tenderness over mastoid process
      b. Headache and ear pain
   2. Objective
      a. Drainage from ear
      b. Elevated temperature
C. Treatment
   1. Antibiotic eardrops
   2. Systemic antibiotics
   3. Cleansing of ear
   4. Surgical intervention
      a. Mastoidectomy (radical or modified)
      b. Tympanoplasty
D. Nursing care
   1. Instruct patient to seek treatment for any ear infections
   2. Care of patient having mastoidectomy

a. Cleanse postauricular area preoperatively
b. Postoperatively reinforce dressing over drain site from mastoid
c. Observe for facial paralysis and report, since this may indicate damage to facial nerve
d. Utilize safety precautions such as side rails to pevent injury to patient who is experiencing vertigo

Otosclerosis

A. Etiology and pathophysiology
   1. Fixation of the stapes preventing transmission of auditory vibrations to the inner ear (conduction deafness)
   2. The cause of the disease is not known, but incidence is higher in females and heredity is a factor in its development
B. Signs and symptoms
   1. Subjective
      a. Loss of hearing reported by patient
      b. Ringing or buzzing in ears
   2. Objective
      a. Use of a tuning fork shows bone conduction is better than air conduction (Rinne test)
      b. Presence of spongy bone in labyrinth
C. Treatment
   1. Use of hearing aids to amplify sound
   2. Stapedectomy, which is the removal of the diseased portion of the stapes, and replacement with a prosthetic implant to conduct vibrations from the middle to inner ear
D. Nursing care
   1. Position postoperatively according to physician's preference
      a. Lying on the operative side facilitates drainage
      b. Lying on the nonoperative side helps prevent displacement of the graft
   2. Instruct patient to alter position gradually to prevent vertigo
   3. Question patient about pain, headache, vertigo, or unusual sensations in ear and report
   4. Instruct patient to avoid sneezing and blowing nose, swimming, showers, and flying until permitted by physician; if patient must sneeze, instruct to keep the mouth open to equalize the pressure on the ear
   5. Explain to patient that because of edema from surgery and presence of packing, hearing will be diminished but will improve

Meniere's disease

A. Etiology and pathophysiology
   1. A chronic disease of the inner ear causing severe vertigo
   2. Cause is unknown but follows infections of the middle ear or trauma
   3. Incidence is highest in males between the ages of 40 and 60 years
B. Signs and symptoms
   1. Subjective
      a. Vertigo
      b. Nausea
      c. Headache
      d. Sensitivity to loud sounds
      e. Sensory hearing loss, usually unilateral
      f. Tinnitus
   2. Objective
      a. Vomiting
      b. Diaphoresis
      c. Nystagmus during attacks
      d. Bárány's caloric test reveals diminished or absent response
      e. Weber test and auditory testing document hearing loss
C. Treatment
   1. Diuretics
   2. Antihistamines
   3. Surgical destruction of labyrinth or vestibular nerve, which will cause deafness in that ear
   4. Salt-free diet combined with administration of ammonium chloride
D. Nursing care
   1. Support patient emotionally
   2. Encourage patient not to move rapidly to prevent onset of symptoms
   3. Protect from injury during attack; use side rails; encourage patient to lie down during attack
   4. Instruct patient to pull off road if driving when an attack occurs
   5. Postoperative care for patient with total labyrinthectomy
      a. Bed rest may be necessary for up to 2 days due to severe vertigo
      b. Instruct patient to avoid sudden movements
      c. Explain that Bell's palsy may occur postoperatively but will subside within a few months
   6. Instruct patient to avoid foods such as salted meats and fish, cheese, condensed milk, carrots, and spinach

Integumentary system

REVIEW OF ANATOMY AND PHYSIOLOGY OF THE INTEGUMENTARY SYSTEM

Functions

A. Prevents loss of body fluids
B. Protects deeper tissues from pathogenic organisms
C. Protects deeper tissues from noxious chemicals and short wavelength ultraviolet radiation
D. Helps regulate body temperature
E. Provides location for sensory reception of touch, pressure, temperature, pain, wetness, tickle, etc.
F. Assists in vitamin D synthesis
G. Plays minor excretory role

Anatomy

A. Epidermis—contains no blood or lymphatic vessels; cells nourished by diffusion from underlying dermal papillae
  1. Layers from dermis outward
     a. Stratum germinatum—cell layers undergoing mitosis; progressive push of cells to surface to replace those exfoliated
     b. Stratum granulosum—granule-filled cells in several layers; contain keratohyalin, intermediate in keratin formation; most free nerve endings of epidermis are here; contains epidermal pigment
     c. Stratum lucidum—translucent layers; nails are outgrowths of this layer
     d. Stratum corneum—upper horny layer of flat, dead cells that exfoliate rapidly, taking bacterial flora with them; responsible for variations in skin thickness
  2. Melanocytes of lower epidermis produce melanin, which colors skin
  3. Exceptional epidermal regions
     a. Conjunctiva—epidermis so thin it is transparent
     b. Lips—epidermis very thin and highly vascular, which accounts for redness
B. Dermis
  1. Highly vascular fabric of collagen and elastic fibers woven to provide strength and flexibility
  2. Upper papillary layer joined to epidermis by upward projecting papillae; vascular loops in papillae nourish overlying epidermis; contain abundant touch receptors; double-row papillae in finger pads and palms and soles give great strength against shearing stress, provide fingerprint pattern as unique arrangement of ridges projected to epidermal surface, and allow hands and feet to grip surfaces
  3. Deeper reticular layer contains loose arrangement of connective tissue gradually merging with subcutaneous fatty layer (superficial fascia)
  4. Skin stretched beyond certain limits (e.g., during pregnancy) may rupture dermal collagen and elastic fibers; consequent scar tissue repair produces striae gravidarum
C. Glands
  1. Eccrine—tubular coiled glands deep in dermis; duct rises straight through dermis and spirals through epidermis, opening in sweat pore on crest of skin ridges; secretes clear fluid
  2. Apocrine—scent glands; very large branched tubular glands found in the axillary, mammary, and genital areas that produce an originally odorless secretion rapidly metabolized by bacteria to produce typical body odors
  3. Ceruminous glands—wax glands in external auditory canal; large branched glands frequently opening into hair sheaths along with sebaceous glands
  4. Sebaceous glands—small saclike glands lacking innervation, usually forming close to hairs and opening into upper portion of hair follicle; form independent of hairs at corners of mouth and in eyelids as Meibomian glands; absent on palms and soles, accounting for wrinkling of these areas after lengthy immersion in water
  5. Mammary glands—milk-secreting, compound tubular alveolar glands developing to full extent only during pregnancy
D. Hair
  1. Long strands of tightly compacted and cemented, dead and keratinized cells sheathed in hair follicles (tubes of epidermal cells plunged obliquely into dermis surrounded by dermal connective tissue sheath)
  2. Males and females have about the same number of follicles; hormones stimulate differential growth
  3. Hair shape determines appearance; round (straight hair); ribbon shaped (kinky hair); alternately round and oval (wavy hair)
  4. Arrector pili (smooth muscle) attached at one end to connective sheath in middle of hair follicle and

at other end to dermal papillary region of dermis; on contraction, elevates hair and surrounding skin but depresses skin overlying dermal papillary attachment point, result is "gooseflesh"; such contraction also stimulates sebaceous gland secretion

Tissue repair

A. Inflammation
1. Vascular changes—initial vasoconstriction (5 to 10 minutes) with vessel walls lined with leukocytes (margination); then vasodilation and increased blood flow and increased vessel permeability (effects of histamine from mast cells, kinins, and prostaglandins); lymphatics plugged with fibrin to wall off damaged area
2. Polymorphonuclear and mononuclear leukocytes leave vessels (diapedesis) and phagocytize foreign substances
3. In chronic inflammation, longer lived mononuclear leukocytes (macrophages) predominate, and fibroblasts deposit wall of collagen around each group of macrophages and foreign substances; stage of granuloma formation
B. Fibroplasia
1. Epithelization—epithelial cells of epidermis begin to cover tissue defect through migration of basal cells across wound defect with continued mitosis in intact epithelium
2. Deep in wound, fibroblasts synthesize collagen and ground substance; begins about fourth or fifth day and continues for 2 to 4 weeks
3. Capillaries regenerate by endothelial budding; tissue becomes red
4. Fibrin plugs are lysed
C. Scar maturation
1. Collagen fibers rearranged into a stronger, more organized pattern
2. Scar remodels, sometimes for months and years due to collagen turnover; if collagen synthesis exceeds breakdown, a hypertrophic scar or keloid forms; if collagen breakdown exceeds synthesis, scar gradually softens and fades
3. Wound contracture—contraction of wound margins begins about 5 days after injury due to fibroblast migration into wound along lines of fibrin strands initially deposited in wound; assists in closing the defect but may also result in contractures that can be debilitating

REVIEW OF PHYSICAL PRINCIPLES RELATED TO THE INTEGUMENTARY SYSTEM
Principles of mechanics

Friction—epidermal ridges due to upthrusting dermal papillae provide palms of hands, fingers, and soles of feet with friction surfaces for grasping and walking

Principles of physical properties of matter

Elasticity—molecular structure of elastin, a protein, permits stretching of skin under tension and the ability to snap back to original shape when tension is relieved; less elastic properties of collagen give skin its strength to resist tearing and shearing forces

Principles of heat

A. Radiation—heat brought to dermis by blood radiates through epidermis to dissipate excess body heat
B. Evaporation—evaporation of sweat cools body surface and acts to drain heat from body interior

Principle of light

Radiation absorption
A. Ultraviolet absorption by melanin protects skin and underlying structures from damage
B. Quantity and degree of dispersed melanin, which absorbs visible light wavelengths differently, produces different skin colors

REVIEW OF CHEMICAL PRINCIPLES RELATED TO THE INTEGUMENTARY SYSTEM
Solutions
Solubility

A. Fat-soluble substances have greater tendency to penetrate skin than do water-soluble substances
   EXAMPLE: Oleoresins of poison ivy, fat-soluble vitamins (A, D, E), and insecticides are absorbed, whereas water is repelled
B. Fat-soluble (oily) substances secreted by Meibomian glands (modified sebaceous glands) of eyelids, which are not capable of mixing with water; act as barriers to prevent tears from constantly flooding over lower eyelid

Water

Dehydration of epidermal cells leaves water-insoluble keratin impregnated in surface and corneum providing a water-resistant protective barrier

PHARMACOLOGY RELATED TO INTEGUMENTARY SYSTEM DISORDERS

A. Antibiotics and antifungals
1. General implications for nurses
   a. Assess lesion, including size, location, color, configuration, drainage, and any accompanying sensation such as pain or pruritus
   b. Thoroughly cleanse area before application of ointment, cream, or lotion
   c. Recognize that topical anti-infectives begin to act quickly after application, but systemic absorption is minimal
   d. Observe skin after application of anti-infective; if no improvement is noted, notify physician
   e. Obtain and check results of culture and sensitivity tests of drainage
   f. Observe for side effects
      (1) Erythema
      (2) Drying
      (3) Pruritus
      (4) Swelling
      (5) Vesicle formation
2. Actions
   a. Antibiotics generally interfere with one of the following cellular functions
      (1) Cell wall synthesis
      (2) Protein synthesis
      (3) Membrane permeability
   b. Antifungal agents usually act by altering the permeability of the cell membrane
   c. May be applied in form of ointment, lotion, cream, or powder
3. Examples
   a. Antibiotic preparations
      (1) Bacitracin (ototoxicity and nephrotoxicity have been reported as side effects)
      (2) Neomycin
      (3) Chloramphenicol (Chloromycetin)
      (4) Clotrimazole (Lotrimin)
      (5) Polysporin
      (6) Nitrofurazone (Furacin)
      (7) Silver sulfadiazine (Silvadene) (see drugs used in the treatment of burns)
   b. Antifungal preparations
      (1) Gentian violet
      (2) Nystatin (Mycostatin); may cause ototoxicity and nephrotoxicity with prolonged use
      (3) Potassium permanganate solution

B. Pediculicides and scabicides
1. General implications for nurses
   a. Inspect skin, particularly the scalp, for scabies and pediculosis before and after treatment
   b. Use gown, gloves, and cap to prevent spread of parasitic arthropods
   c. Keep linen of infected patient separate and sterilize to prevent reinfection
   d. Observe for irritation
   e. Assess source of infection; provide patient and family education
   f. Avoid contact with eyes and mucous membranes
2. Actions
   a. Exact mechanism for destruction of parasitic arthropods is not known
   b. May be absorbed through skin and mucous membranes; drugs then metabolized by the liver and excreted in the feces and urine
3. Examples
   a. Gamma benzene hexachloride (Gexane, Kwell)
   b. Benzyl benzoate lotion (Benylate, Albacide, Scabanca)

C. Topical drugs used in the treatment of burns
1. General implications for nurses
   a. Adhere to strict surgical asepsis
   b. Observe burns and patient's general condition
   c. See nursing care of burns
   d. Observe for side effects listed with each drug
2. Action—anti-infective agents act on bacterial cell wall or alter cellular function to produce bactericidal effects
3. Examples
   a. Silver sulfadiazine (Silvadene)
      (1) Apply to thickness of 1/16 inch
      (2) Cleanse burns and debride prior to application
      (3) Because hemolysis can occur in patients with deficiency of glucose-6-phosphate dehydrogenase, monitor G-6-PD level before initiation of treatment
      (4) Observe for other adverse effects
         (a) Rash
         (b) Pruritus
   b. Mafenide acetate (Sulfamylon)
      (1) Cleanse and debride prior to application
      (2) May cause burning sensation when first applied
      (3) Observe patient for acidosis, since medication acts as carbonic anhydrase inhib-

itor; if patient becomes dyspneic, the ointment should be removed
c. Silver nitrate 0.5% solution
   (1) Apply dressings soaked in silver nitrate and keep moist
   (2) Causes brown/black discoloration of anything it comes in contact with
   (3) May cause electrolyte imbalance if used on large area over long period because it is hypotonic; electrolyte levels should be evaluated frequently; observe for signs of electrolyte disturbance such as a change in behavior

D. Antipruritics
   1. General implications for nurses
      a. Assess lesion, including location and size
      b. Question patient regarding relief obtained from treatment
      c. Advise medical follow-up, since these medications only provide temporary relief of symptoms
      d. Observe for local irritation
      e. Discourage patient from scratching; keep nails well trimmed
   2. Actions
      a. Tars act as irritants, promoting circulation and decreasing inflammatory exudates
      b. Local anesthetics block the conduction of nerve impulses
      c. Anti-inflammatory agents decrease inflammation
   3. Examples
      a. Benzocaine (Anbesol, Dermoplast, Solarcaine)
      b. Lidocaine hydrochloride (Xylocaine jelly, ointment, or spray)
      c. Phenol
      d. Tars
      e. Calamine

E. Anti-inflammatory agents
   1. General implications for nurses
      a. Assess lesions for color, location, size, etc.
      b. Protect skin from scratching or rubbing
      c. Use appropriate topical agent
         (1) Use lotions in areas such as axilla and groin
         (2) Use creams if lesion is draining
         (3) Use ointments on dry lesions
      d. Avoid contact with eyes
      e. Cleanse skin before application
      f. Utilize occlusive dressings if ordered
      g. Observe for signs of sensitivity
         (1) Contact dermatitis
         (2) Irritation
         (3) Burning
         (4) Itching
         (5) Folliculitis
         (6) Adrenal insufficiency may occur if absorbed systemically
   2. Actions
      a. Reduce signs of inflammation; vasoconstriction decreases swelling and pruritus
      b. Absorbtion through skin is increased if a large area of skin is involved or if occlusive dressings are used
   3. Examples
      a. Betamethasone (Celestone)
      b. Betamethasone valerate (Valisone, Celestoderm)
      c. Fluocinolone acetonide (Fluonid, Synalar)
      d. Fluocinonide (Lidex)
      e. Flurandrenolone (Cordran, Drenison)
      f. Hydrocortisone (Acticort, Cortril, Hytone)
      g. Triamcinolone acetonide (Aristocort, Kenalog, Triamalone)

RELATED PROCEDURES
Skin grafts

A. Definition
   1. Covering of denuded tissue with skin to prevent infection and loss of body fluids, increase healing, and prevent contractures
   2. Applied between the fifth and twenty-first day, depending on extent of the burn
   3. Types of skin grafts
      a. Xenografts—utilize skin from animals, usually pigs (porcine xenograft)
      b. Homografts—utilize skin from another person
      c. Autografts—use skin from another part of patient's body
         (1) Mesh graft—a machine is used to mesh skin obtained from a donor site so it can be stretched to cover a larger area of burn
         (2) Postage stamp graft—an earlier method of accomplishing the same goal as that of a mesh graft; a small amount of skin is used to cover a larger area; the donor skin is cut into small pieces and applied to the burn
         (3) Sheet grafting—large strips of skin are placed over the burn as close together as possible

B. Nursing responsibilities
  1. Explain procedure to patient; obtain written consent
  2. Prepare donor site carefully
  3. Postoperatively keep donor sites (which are covered with a nonadherent dressing and wrapped in an absorbent gauze) dry using a heating lamp or hair dryer as ordered; remove absorbent gauze as ordered; nonadherent dressing will separate as healing occurs
  4. Grafts are generally left with a light pressure dressing for approximately 3 days; after the graft has ''taken,'' roll cotton-tipped applicators gently over the graft to remove underlying exudate; allowed to remain, exudate could promote infection, which could prevent the graft from adhering
  5. Observe for foul-smelling drainage, temperature elevation, and other signs of infection

MAJOR DISEASES
Primary skin lesions

A. Macule—flat circumscribed area from 1 to several centimeters in size, without elevation (freckle, flat pigmented moles)
B. Papule—raised circumscribed area less than 1 cm in size (acne)
C. Nodule—raised solid mass that extends into the dermis and is 1 to 2 cm in size (pigmented nevi)
D. Tumor—a solid raised mass that extends into the dermis and is over 2 cm in size (dermatofibroma)
E. Wheal—a flattened collection of fluid from 1 mm to several centimeters in size (mosquito bites)
F. Vesicle—raised collection of fluid less than 1 cm in size (chickenpox, herpes simplex)
G. Bulla—fluid-filled vesicle over 1 cm in size (second-degree burn, pemphigus)
H. Pustule—vesicle or bulla filled with pus and 1 mm to 1 cm in size (acne vulgaris)
I. Cyst—mass of fluid-filled tissue that extends to subcutaneous tissues or dermis and is over 1 cm in size (epidermoid cyst)

Burns

A. Etiology and pathophysiology
  1. Thermal burns that cause cell destruction and result in depletion of fluid and electrolytes
  2. The extent of the fluid and electrolyte loss in burns is directly related to the extent and degree of the burn

  a. First degree (also known as partial thickness)—erythema, edema, and pain; fluid loss is slight, especially if less than 15% of body surface is involved
  b. Second degree (also known as deep dermal)—erythema, pain, vesicles, with oozing; fluid loss is slight to moderate, especially if less than 15% of the body surface is involved
  c. Third degree (also known as full thickness)—charred or pearly white, dry skin, absence of pain; fluid loss is usually severe, especially if more than 2% of the body surface is involved
  3. Classification of second- and third-degree burns
    a. Minor burns—no burns involving hands, face, or genitalia; total burn area does not exceed 15%, and third-degree burns do not exceed 2% of body area
    b. Major burns—total burn area is between 15% and 30% of body, but third-degree burns do not exceed 10% of body area
    c. Critical burns—total burn area exceeds 30% of body surface; this classification is also used if patient has a preexisting chronic health problem, is under 18 months of age or over 50 years of age, or has additional injuries
  4. Pulmonary injury should be suspected if 2 of the following factors are present and expected if 3 or all 4 are present
    a. Hair in nostrils is singed
    b. The patient was trapped in a closed space
    c. The face, nose, and lips are burned
    d. The initial blood sample contains carboxyhemoglobin
  5. Extent of trauma can be estimated by rule of nines or other burn area chart
  6. Curling's ulcer may occur after a burn
    a. Patient may complain of gastric discomfort or there may be profuse bleeding
    b. Usually occurs by the end of the first week after a burn
    c. Treatment is essentially the same as for a gastric ulcer; however, mortality following surgical repair is high due to debilitated state of patient
B. Signs and symptoms
  1. Subjective
    a. Extreme anxiety
    b. Restlessness
    c. Pain, severity depending on type of burn

d. Tingling

e. Disorientation

2. Objective

a. Changes in appearance of skin indicate degree of burn (see etiology and pathophysiology)

b. Hematuria; blood hemolysis with subsequent rise in plasma hemoglobin may occur with third-degree burns

c. Elevated hematocrit as a result of fluid loss

d. Electrolyte imbalance

e. Presence of symptoms of hypovolemic shock caused by circulatory failure resulting from seepage of water, plasma, proteins, and electrolytes into burned area

f. Presence of symptoms of neurogenic shock (symptoms similar to hypovolemic shock) caused by the fright, terror, hysteria, and pain involved in the situation

g. Disorientation and confusion may be present

C. Treatment

1. Tetanus toxoid immediately

2. IV replacement therapy at a rate of 250 ml per hour to achieve an intake of between 6000 and 7000 ml for the first 24 hours (half of total IV solutions will be an electrolyte solution such as Ringer's lactate and half will be plasma or plasma substitute)

3. Reduction of total IV solutions during second 24 hours depending on patient's urinary output, blood work, and central venous pressure

4. Foley catheter; monitor hourly urinary output and specific gravity to observe kidney functioning and determine fluid replacement

5. Insert central venous pressure line and take hourly reading to monitor circulating fluid volume

6. Vital signs monitored every 15 minutes

7. Serum electrolytes and blood gases to observe for levels and to assist in deciding replacement therapy

8. IPPB and continuous oxygen to assist with respirations

9. A tracheostomy if laryngeal edema occurs

10. Reverse isolation

11. Permit patient nothing by mouth except mineral water for first 24 to 48 hours; allow clear liquids as tolerated after 2 days; after this period place patient on high-protein, high-carbohydrate, high-fat, high-vitamin diet as tolerated

12. Daily Hubbard tank baths after fifth day and dressings with antibiotic ointment and Kling dressing

13. Intervene surgically to perform debridement and skin grafts (see procedures), promote healing, and limit contractures

14. Debridement by mechanical means (wet to dry dressings) or by enzymatic debridement (such as Travase ointment)

15. IV and topical antibiotics to limit infection (Keflin and penicillin intravenously; Sulfamylon ointment; gentamicin; silver nitrate solution; and silver sulfadiazine)

16. Narcotics to reduce pain and sedatives to decrease anxiety, given IV or orally due to decreased muscle absorption

D. Nursing care

1. Observe vital signs, central venous pressure, intake and output, and specific gravity as ordered; notify physician if deviations occur or if output falls below 30 ml or rises above 50 ml per hour

2. Maintain patency of Foley catheter to ascertain correct information regarding fluid balance

3. Make certain blood electrolyte and gas tests are performed and results are available

4. Administer fluid and electrolytes as ordered

5. Observe for signs of electrolyte imbalance (calcium, potassium, and sodium) and metabolic acidosis

6. Observe for signs of tracheal edema (dyspnea, stridor)

7. Elevate head of bed

8. Encourage patient to cough and deep breathe

9. Maintain reverse isolation to prevent infection of burned areas

10. Use sterile technique (irrigating drainage tubes, dressings, and bed linens)

11. Administer tetanus toxoid as ordered

12. Administer IV and topical antibiotics as ordered

13. Observe for signs of infection (rising temperature and white blood cell count, odor)

14. Support joints and extremities in functional position

15. Support patient while turning

16. Keep room temperature as constant as possible

17. Observe for symptoms of Curling's (stress) ulcer

18. Give small, frequent high-protein, high-carbohydrate, high-fat, high-vitamin feedings

19. Give medication for pain as ordered and particularly before dressing change
20. Accept and expect patient to express negative feelings about burns
21. Explain need for staff wearing gowns and masks
22. Give realistic reassurance

Acne vulgaris

A. Etiology and pathophysiology
1. Hormonal activity produces hyperkeratosis of the follicular orifices, leading to blockage of secretions and the subsequent formation of fatty plugs known as blackheads
2. When a blackhead forms, the sebaceous gland involved becomes hypertrophic and infected
3. Cysts and nodules form, leaving scars
4. Acne vulgaris is most common among adolescents

B. Signs and symptoms
1. Subjective
   a. Pain when sebaceous glands become infected
   b. Depression
2. Objective
   a. Blackheads on skin (open comedo)
   b. Whiteheads on skin (closed comedo)

C. Treatment
1. Mechanical removal with comedo extractor
2. Use of abrasive cleaners, astringents, and bacteriostatic creams
3. Use of ultraviolet light as a peeling agent
4. Cryotherapy to produce desquamation of skin
5. Oral administration of antibiotics such as tetracycline
6. Intralesion injections of corticosteroids
7. Dermabrasion is performed to improve the scars but not to cure the condition
   a. The use of an instrument that functions at a high speed with a cylinder of wire or sandpaper at its end
   b. The epidermis and some of the dermis are removed at the high points of the scars so that they do not appear as deep
   c. Local anesthesia is used for treatment of small areas, and general is indicated for large areas

D. Nursing care
1. Promote good hygienic care when instructing patients how to wash areas and apply topical medications
2. Discuss the use of water-base cosmetics to prevent clogging of pores

3. Instruct patient on how to take medications
4. Emphasize importance of diet, especially vitamin A, and increased fluid intake
5. Postoperative care of the patient who has undergone dermabrasion
   a. Apply ointment to lubricate skin and remove crust from area
   b. Observe serum draining from the area and report copious amounts of drainage to the surgeon
   c. Explain to the patient that the feeling of being sunburned is normal after dermabrasion

Contact dermatitis

A. Etiology and pathophysiology
1. Contact dermatitis results from contact with a substance that reacts with the protein in the skin to form an antigen in a sensitized patient
2. The antigen causes proliferation of lymphocytes, and the interaction of these factors causes eczematous changes
3. Common causes of contact dermatitis include poison ivy, hair dye containing paraphenylenediamine, benzocaine, soaps, cements, insecticides, and rubber compounds

B. Signs and symptoms
1. Subjective
   a. Discomfort
   b. Pruritus
2. Objective
   a. Erythema at point of contact
   b. Vesicles and papules
   c. Edema
   d. Thickening of skin and scaling

C. Treatment
1. Identification of allergen through patch testing; a suspected allergen is applied to unbroken skin; the skin is observed for erythema, papules, and vesicles in 24 to 48 hours
2. Antihistamines, antipruritics
3. Topical corticosteroids

D. Nursing care
1. Instruct patient to avoid those situations or substances which involve identified allergen
2. Cool environment, provide tepid baths, and trim finger nails to help control injury from scratching
3. Provide diversional activities
4. If topical corticosteroids are ordered, apply occlusive plastic dressings (Saran Wrap) over the ointment or lotion as ordered

Psoriasis

A. Etiology and pathophysiology
   1. Psoriasis is an inflammatory disease that may be acute or chronic in nature
   2. Genetic predisposition is thought to be a factor in its development
   3. Uncommon in black individuals
   4. Injury to the skin and psychologic stress appear to be factors in flare-ups of the disease
B. Signs and symptoms
   1. Subjective
      a. Mild pruritus (severe if in skin folds)
      b. If psoriatic arthritis is present, joint pain and stiffness
   2. Objective
      a. Bright red, well-demarcated plaque covered with silvery scales, usually on knees, elbows, and scalp
      b. Stippling and thickening of the nails
      c. Inflammatory changes of joints if psoriatic arthritis is present
      d. Uric acid levels may be elevated
C. Treatment
   1. Exposure to solar or ultraviolet irradiation
   2. Application of coal tar ointment or anti-inflammatory topical agents
   3. Systemic corticosteroid therapy may be used in severe cases
   4. Methotrexate may also be used for severe psoriasis
   5. Exposure to black light combined with oral administration of methoxsalen has been useful in the treatment of intractable psoriasis
D. Nursing care
   1. Encourage ventilation of feelings about changes in body image; show acceptance of patient
   2. Assess lesions and response to therapy
   3. Determine factors linked to flare-ups of psoriasis; patient may need help coping with stressful situations
   4. Instruct patient to use a soft brush to remove scales when bathing
   5. If occlusive dressings are ordered with topical ointment, Saran Wrap, plastic bags, or rubber gloves may be used

Pemphigus

A. Etiology and pathophysiology
   1. A potentially fatal skin disease
   2. Occurs only in adults
   3. Cause is unknown
B. Signs and symptoms
   1. Subjective
      a. Debilitation
      b. Malaise
      c. Pain associated with lesions
   2. Objective
      a. Bullae on normal skin and mucosa
      b. Separation of epidermis caused by rubbing skin (Nikolsky's sign)
      c. Acantholysis (changes in intercellular connections of the epidermis) evident on microscopic examination
      d. Leukocytosis, eosinophilia
      e. Foul-smelling discharge
C. Treatment
   1. Oral corticosteroids
   2. Antibiotics for secondary infections
   3. Topical treatment for relief of symptoms
      a. Potassium permanganate baths
      b. Oatmeal baths
D. Nursing care
   1. Administer steroids with antacid or milk to prevent gastric irritation (see drugs)
   2. Monitor intake and output (NaCl and fluid are lost through skin)
   3. Test urinary sugar and acetone levels, since patient is receiving large doses of corticosteroids
   4. Protect patient from infection
   5. Monitor for signs of infection such as elevated temperature and WBC
   6. Provide oral hygiene and increased fluid intake to soothe oral lesions
   7. Encourage ventilation of feelings; patients are often discouraged and depressed

Cancer of the skin

A. Etiology and pathophysiology
   1. This is the most common cancer, but due to early detection and slow progression the cure rate is high
   2. Exposure to the sun, irritating chemicals, and chronic friction appear to be implicated as causes; more common in persons with fair complexions
   3. Types
      a. Squamous cell carcinoma develops rapidly and may metastasize through local lymph nodes; may develop secondarily to precan-

cerous lesions such as keratosis and leuko-plakia and is found most frequently on upper extremities and face, which are exposed to the sun; it appears as a small red nodular lesion
  b. Basal cell carcinoma is generally located on the face and appears as a waxy nodule that may have telangiectasias visible; the most common type of skin cancer, but metastasis is rare
  c. Malignant melanoma is the most serious type of skin cancer and arises from the pigment producing melanocytes; the color of the lesion may vary greatly (white, flesh, grey, brown, blue, black); changes in size, color, sensation, or characteristics of a mole suggest the possibility of malignant melanoma; metastasis via blood can be extensive
B. Signs and symptoms
  1. Subjective
    a. Pruritus may or may not be present
    b. Localized soreness
  2. Objective
    a. Change in color, size, or shape of preexisting lesion
    b. Oozing, bleeding, or crusting
    c. Biopsy of tumor reveals type of cancer
    d. Lymphadenopathy if metastasis has occurred
C. Treatment
  1. Surgical excision of lesion and surrounding tissue
  2. Chemosurgery, which involves the use of zinc chloride to fix the cells before they are dissected
  3. Cryosurgery utilizing liquid nitrogen to destroy the tumor cells by freezing
  4. Radiation; malignant melanoma does not respond well to this mode of treatment
  5. Chemotherapy
  6. Nonspecific immunostimulants such as BCG
D. Nursing care
  1. Assess skin lesions
  2. Instruct patients to examine moles for changes and have those subject to chronic irritation (bra or belt line) removed
  3. Encourage limitation of exposure to sun
  4. Emphasize continued medical supervision
  5. Use surgically aseptic technique when caring for surgical site
  6. Encourage verbalization; maintain therapeutic environment
  7. Provide care to patient receiving radiation

    a. Observe skin for local reaction
    b. Avoid use of ointments or powders containing metals
  8. Care related to specific chemotherapeutic agents (see pharmacology)

Herpes zoster (shingles)

A. Etiology and pathophysiology
  1. An acute viral infection of nerve structures caused by varicella-zoster virus
  2. Inflammation occurs along the pathway of one or more peripheral sensory nerves
  3. Occurs in patients who have not had chickenpox and are exposed to an affected individual
  4. May frequently occur in patients with other debilitating illness; e.g., tuberculosis, Hodgkin's disease
B. Signs and symptoms
  1. Subjective
    a. Malaise
    b. Headache
    c. Pain
    d. Paresthesia
  2. Objective
    a. Painful, pruritic vesicles arranged along the pathway of the involved nerves
    b. Stains made from lesion exudate isolate organism
C. Treatment
  1. Medications for pain, relaxation, itching, and preventing secondary infection
  2. Control of pain by blocking the nerve through injection of drugs such as lidocaine or applying medication such as triamcinolone (Kenalog)
  3. Anti-inflammatory drugs such as systemic steroids or Kenalog ointment to decrease inflammation
D. Nursing care
  1. Administer analgesics and other medications as ordered
  2. Reduce itching and protect lesions from air by the application of salves, ointments, lotions, and sterile dressings as ordered
  3. Protect from pressure by use of air mattress, bed cradle, and light loose clothing (avoid synthetic and woolen materials and use cotton fabrics)
  4. Use aseptic technique when caring for a patient with open lesions
  5. Administer antibiotics as ordered

6. Encourage patient to avoid scratching and use gloves at night to limit the possibility of accidental scratching
7. Assist patient to understand the basis for the rash and the itch
8. Allay fears that may be based on old wives' tales about shingles
9. Encourage patient to express feelings

Systemic lupus erythematosus (SLE)

A. Etiology and pathophysiology
1. SLE is a disease of unknown origin that affects the connective tissue and is thought to be due to a defect in the body's immunologic mechanisms or to genetic predisposition
2. Fibrinoid deposits are seen in blood vessels and among collagen fibers and on organs
3. There is necrosis of the glomerular capillaries, inflammation of cerebral and ocular blood vessels, necrosis of lymph nodes, vasculitis of the GI tract and pleura, and degeneration of the basal layer of skin
B. Signs and symptoms
1. Subjective
   a. Malaise
   b. Photosensitivity
   c. Joint pain
2. Objective
   a. Fever
   b. Butterfly erythema on face
   c. Erythema of palms
   d. Positive LE prep
C. Treatment
1. Corticosteroids and analgesics to reduce pain and inflammation
2. Supportive therapy as major organs become affected (heart, kidneys, CNS, GI tract)
D. Nursing care
1. Administer medications and observe for side effects
2. Help patient and family cope with severity of disease as well as poor prognosis

Polyarteritis nodosa

A. Etiology and pathophysiology
1. The cause is unknown; it occurs primarily in women in midlife
2. It is a collagen disease that causes inflammation and necrosis of the small and medium-sized arteries

3. When healing of the arteries occurs, there is a thickening of the walls with subsequent circulatory impairment
4. Common areas involved are the kidneys, heart, liver, and GI tract
B. Signs and symptoms
1. Subjective
   a. Malaise
   b. Weakness
   c. Severe abdominal pain, muscle aches
2. Objective
   a. Weight loss
   b. Low-grade fever
   c. Bloody diarrhea
   d. Proteinuria if kidneys are affected
   e. Positive rheumatoid factor (RF) and elevated sedimentation rate
C. Treatment
1. Corticosteroids and analgesics are given to control pain and inflammation
2. Balanced diet is indicated to combat weight loss
D. Nursing care
1. Provide relief of symptomatic pain
2. Provide emotional support for both patient and family due to poor prognosis

Progressive systemic sclerosis (scleroderma)

A. Etiology and pathophysiology
1. Thought to be caused by an autoimmune defect; occurs in women more frequently than men
2. It is a systemic disease that causes fibrotic changes in connective tissue throughout the body
3. May involve the skin, synovial membranes, esophagus, heart, lungs, kidneys, or GI tract
B. Signs and symptoms
1. Subjective
   a. Articular pain
   b. Muscle weakness
2. Objective
   a. Masklike hard skin that eventually adheres to underlying structures
   b. Telangiectases on the lips, fingers, face, and tongue
   c. Dysphagia
   d. Restriction of body motion as disease progresses
   e. Positive LE prep, elevated gamma globulin levels, false positive test for syphilis

C. Treatment
   1. Corticosteroids
   2. Salicylates or analgesics for joint pain
   3. Physical therapy
   4. Skin care to prevent decubitus formation
D. Nursing care

1. Support patient and family emotionally, since there is no cure at present
2. Administer medications as ordered
3. Encourage patients to actively exercise
4. Observe vital signs, urinary output, and vital capacity for changes in function of vital organs

MEDICAL-SURGICAL NURSING REVIEW QUESTIONS

1 A nursing hypothesis is a nurse's:
   1. Actual intervention
   2. Prescription
   3. Evaluation of data
   4. Evaluation of care
2 Where primary nursing is practiced, the nurse who plans for and delegates care with full authority to see that the plan is followed is the:
   1. Clinical specialist
   2. Head nurse
   3. Nurse clinician
   4. Primary nurse
3 The following is an example of primary health care by the nurse:
   1. Correction of dietary deficiencies
   2. Assisting in immunization programs
   3. Prevention of disabilities
   4. Rehabilitation
4 An objective method for data collection includes:
   1. Direct observation of the patient
   2. Speaking with the patient's family
   3. The patient's description of the illness
   4. Collection of specimens
5 The determining factor in the revision of a nursing care plan is the:
   1. Correctness of the original hypothesis
   2. Method for providing care
   3. Available time
   4. Effectiveness of implementation
6 Which of the following best defines the term "nursing process"? Nursing process is the:
   1. Activities a nurse employs to identify a nursing problem
   2. Process the nurse uses to determine nursing goals
   3. Steps the nurse employs in planning and giving nursing care
   4. Implementation of nursing care by the nurse
7 To begin the nursing process, the nurse must first:
   1. State the patient's nursing needs
   2. Identify goals for nursing care
   3. Obtain information about the patient
   4. Evaluate the effectiveness of nursing actions

8 The effectiveness of nurse-patient communication is validated by:
   1. Health team conferences
   2. Medical assessments
   3. Patient feedback
   4. Patient's physiologic adaptations

Situation: A small urban community in the western area of the country is flattened by a severe, widespread tornado. Questions 9 through 13 refer to this situation.

9 Immediately after the storm has passed the rescue team with which you are working is searching for injured people. You split up to search, and you find a man lying next to a broken natural gas main. He is not breathing and is bleeding heavily from a wound on the foot. Your first step would be to:
   1. Remove him from the immediate vicinity
   2. Apply surface pressure to the foot wound
   3. Start rescue breathing immediately
   4. Treat him for shock
10 You find a young boy under the wreckage of a frame house. He is conscious, breathing satisfactorily, and lying on his back. He complains of pain in his back and is unable to move his legs. First you would:
   1. Gently raise him to a sitting position to see if the pain either diminishes or increases in intensity
   2. Leave him lying on his back, give him instructions not to move, and seek additional help
   3. Roll him on his abdomen, place a pad under his head, and cover him
   4. Gently lift him onto a flat piece of lumber and, using any available transportation, rush him to medical help
11 You find another injured person, obviously in shock. You would keep him lying on his back and:
   1. Elevate the head higher than the rest of the body; give stimulants in small sips
   2. Surround the body with hot water bottles or chemical heating pads if available
   3. After evaluation, allow the patient to walk around if injuries permit
   4. Place the head lower than the rest of the body, prevent chilling, and give fluids if possible

12 When a disaster occurs, you may have to treat the mass hysteria first. The person or persons to be cared for immediately would be those in:
   1. Depression
   2. Euphoria
   3. Panic
   4. Comatose state

13 In any disaster concerning a number of people the function that contributes most to saving of lives is sorting, or triage. Assume that you are the nurse who has to determine this priority of patient needs. The patients who need immediate care are those with:
   1. Second-degree burns of 10% of the body
   2. Severe lacerations involving open fractures of major bones
   3. Closed fractures of major bones
   4. Significant penetrating or perforating abdominal wounds

14 A disease produced when a *Clostridium* organism enters wounds and produces a toxin causing crepitus is:
   1. Tetanus
   2. Gas gangrene
   3. Botulism
   4. Anthrax

15 The major benefit in using tetanus antitoxin is that it:
   1. Stimulates plasma cells directly
   2. Provides high titer of antibodies
   3. Provides immediate active immunity
   4. Stimulates long-lasting passive immunity

16 Antibodies are also produced by:
   1. Plasma cells
   2. Eosinophils
   3. Lymphocytes
   4. Erythrocytes

Situation: Mrs. Hollens, age 30 and a chemist, is the mother of 2 young children. For the past few months she has noticed that she tires easily, has painless swelling of the lymph nodes, and has been running a low-grade fever with excessive diaphoresis at night. She also has anorexia with loss of weight. She does not recall having any serious illness except that once during the winter she experienced what she believed was a viral infection. On her admission to the hospital the physician ordered a complete medical examination for Mrs. Hollens. On the basis of diagnostic tests, Mrs. Hollens is said to have Hodgkin's disease. Questions 17 through 21 refer to this situation.

17 The lymph nodes usually affected first are the:
   1. Inguinal
   2. Axillary
   3. Cervical
   4. Mediastinal

18 The highest incidence of Hodgkin's disease is in:
   1. Children

2. Young adults
   3. Middle-aged persons
   4. Elderly persons

19 Which of the following would you expect to develop as a result of whole-body irradiation? Increased:
   1. Red blood cell production
   2. Susceptibility to infection
   3. Tendency for pathologic fractures
   4. Blood viscosity

20 Whole-body irradiation injures or destroys bone marrow, making it unable to function normally. As a result, which of the following would you expect to develop?
   1. Anemia
   2. Decreased susceptibility to infections
   3. Increased tendency for bones to break
   4. Increased blood viscosity

21 The apparent paradox of radiation being a known cancer-inducing agent as well as a widely used therapy for cancer is clarified when one considers the:
   1. Extent of the body irradiated
   2. Nutritional environment of the cells
   3. Dosage of radiation utilized
   4. Physical condition of the patient

Situation: Mrs. Johnson, a 64-year-old housewife, is admitted to the hospital with a diagnosis of hypertension. Questions 22 through 27 refer to this situation.

22 Mrs. Johnson is receiving methyldopa hydrochloride (Aldomet) intravenously for control of hypertension. Her blood pressure, before the infusion started, was 150/90. Fifteen minutes after the infusion is started her blood pressure rises to 180/100. The response to the drug would be described as a(n):
   1. Synergistic response
   2. Individual hypersensitivity
   3. Allergic response
   4. Paradoxic response

23 To assess the effectiveness of Aldomet in lowering blood pressure levels, the nurse would take Mrs. Johnson's pulse and blood pressure:
   1. Thirty minutes after giving the drug
   2. Immediately after she gets out of bed
   3. After she has been supine for 5 minutes
   4. Prior to giving the drug

24 Mrs. Johnson's serum potassium level is low and she is placed on a cardiac monitor. She is to receive 40 mEq potassium chloride in 1000 ml of 5% dextrose in water IV. The nurse analyzes the monitor pattern to obtain a baseline for evaluating progress. The monitor pattern would show:
   1. Shortening of the QRS complex
   2. Elevation of the S-T segment
   3. Increased deflection of the Q wave
   4. Lowering of the T wave

25 Mrs. Johnson's IV medication inadvertently runs in rap-

idly. The physician prescribes insulin added to a 10% dextrose in water solution. The rationale for the prescription is:
1. Glucose and insulin increase the metabolic rate and accelerate potassium excretion
2. Potassium moves into body cells with glucose and insulin
3. Increased potassium causes a temporary slowing of pancreatic production of insulin
4. Increased insulin accelerates excretion of glucose and potassium

26 Mrs. Johnson's condition has improved, and Aldomet is being given orally. When explaining why orthostatic hypotension occurs, the nurse would base the response on knowledge that the drug causes vasodilation by:
1. Depleting acetylcholine
2. Decreasing adrenal release of epinephrine
3. Stimulating histamine release
4. Interrupting norepinephrine release

27 When discussing the plan for taking Aldomet at home, the nurse would tell Mrs. Johnson that orthostatic hypotension may be modified by:
1. Lying down for 30 minutes after taking the drug
2. Avoiding tasks that require high energy expenditures
3. Wearing support hose continuously
4. Sitting on the edge of the bed a short time before arising

---

28 The primary cause of essential hypertension is:
1. Generalized arteriosclerosis
2. Unresolved grief
3. Kidney failure
4. Unexpressed rage

29 Which mechanism mediates long-term (day to day, week to week) blood pressure regulation?
1. Fight or flight response
2. Adjustment of urinary output
3. Nervous system baroreceptors
4. Capillary fluid shifts

30 Patients receiving propranolol hydrochloride (Inderal) should be told they might:
1. Experience dizziness with strenuous activity
2. Have a flushing sensation for a few minutes after taking the drug
3. Notice acceleration of the heart rate after eating a heavy meal
4. Have pounding of the heart for a few minutes after taking the drug

Situation: Mr. Manning, a 48-year-old photographer, has developed fatigue and dyspnea on exertion. His ECG shows atrial fibrillation. The physician suspects mitral stenosis. Questions 31 through 38 refer to this situation.

31 Which health problem in Mr. Manning's past may be responsible for this disorder?

1. Rubella, age 6
2. Streptococcal throat infection, age 12
3. Pleurisy, age 20
4. Cystitis, age 28

32 After the initial workup, the physician orders a cardiac catheterization for Mr. Manning. In caring for the patient after the procedure, the nurse should:
1. Provide for rest
2. Check pulse in area distal to cutdown
3. Check ECG every 30 minutes
4. Administer oxygen

33 Mr. Manning requires surgery due to mitral incompetence. He is admitted to the hospital and states, "I need a new valve—and do an oil change too!!" The nurse replies "Welcome to our unit, Mr. Manning. . . .
1. "I'm glad to see you're handling the situation so well."
2. "I'm sure you have a great deal to ask about this procedure."
3. "You really don't need to hide your anxieties."
4. "You sure came to the right place for a valve job."

34 Postoperatively, Mr. Manning's peripheral pulses must be frequently checked. The chief purpose of this is to detect:
1. The existence of emboli
2. Arteriovenous shunting
3. Postsurgical bleeding
4. Atrial fibrillation

35 Mr. Manning develops a temperature of 102.8° F (39° C) The nurse notifies the physician because elevated temperatures:
1. May indicate cerebral edema
2. May be a forerunner of hemorrhage
3. Increase the cardiac output
4. Cause diaphoresis and possible chilling

36 One thousand milliliters of serosanguinous fluid drains from the chest tube during the first 24 hours postoperatively. The expected drainage during this time period is:
1. 800 to 1000 ml
2. 100 to 300 ml
3. 750 to 900 ml
4. 400 to 500 ml

37 During a blood transfusion Mr. Manning develops chills and headache. The nurse's best action is to:
1. Stop the transfusion immediately
2. Lightly cover the patient
3. Notify the physician STAT
4. Slow the blood flow to keep vein open

38 Mr. Manning's fever does not respond to A.S.A. He is placed on hypothermia blanket. One reaction to hypothermia that should be prevented is:
1. Venous stasis
2. Hypotension
3. Shivering
4. Dehydration

39 Mr. Evere, a 69-year-old retired musician, was admitted to the intensive care unit with a diagnosis of Adams-Stokes syndrome. Symptoms most likely include:
1. Syncope and low ventricular rate
2. Flushing and slurred speech
3. Cephalalgia and blurred vision
4. Nausea and vertigo

40 The lethal arrhythmia that often requires immediate intervention by the nurse is:
1. Atrial fibrillation
2. Auricular flutter
3. Second-degree heart block
4. Ventricular fibrillation

41 Pulse pressure is the:
1. Difference between the apical and radial rates
2. Force exerted against an arterial wall
3. Degree of ventricular contraction in relation to output
4. Difference between systolic and diastolic readings

Situation: Mr. Josh is admitted with a diagnosis of possible tuberculosis or pneumonia. Several diagnostic tests are performed. Questions 42 through 48 refer to this situation.

42 As a general rule, which of the following tests is most valuable in the selection of an antibiotic?
1. Susceptibility test
2. Tissue culture test
3. Serologic test
4. Sensitivity test of organism

43 Acid-fast rods found in sputum are presumed to be:
1. Influenza virus
2. *Bordetella pertussis*
3. Diphtheria bacillus
4. *Mycobacterium tuberculosis*

44 As a result of pulmonary tuberculosis, Mr. Josh has a decreased surface area for gaseous exchange in his lungs. Oxygen and carbon dioxide are exchanged in the lungs by:
1. Active transport mechanism
2. Diffusion
3. Filtration
4. Osmosis

45 Mr. Josh says the physician told him his tidal volume is slightly diminished and asks the nurse what this means. The nurse explains that tidal air is the amount of air:
1. Exhaled normally after a normal inspiration
2. Exhaled forcibly after a normal expiration
3. Forcibly inspired over and above a normal inspiration
4. Trapped in the alveoli that cannot be exhaled

46 Mr. Josh has been receiving streptomycin sulfate daily for 1 week. He is being discharged and the physician plans to have him come to the clinic for administration of the drug twice a week. The spaced dosage is planned to:
1. Increase compliance with the therapy plan
2. Lessen risk of adverse effects of the drug on neural tissue

3. Minimize disruption of the rest hours required for recovery
4. Lessen tissue trauma from injections while resistance is low

47 Vitamin B_6 is given with isoniazid (INH) because it:
1. Improves the nutritional status of the patient
2. Enhances tuberculostatic effect of isoniazid
3. Provides the vitamin when isoniazid is interfering with natural vitamin synthesis
4. Accelerates destruction of remaining organisms after inhibition of their reproduction by isoniazid

48 After Mrs. Josh has been receiving streptomycin sulfate for 2 weeks, he states that he is ''walking like a drunken seaman.'' The nurse withholds the drug and promptly reports the problem to the physician because the signs may be a result of drug effect on the:
1. Cerebellar tissue
2. Peripheral motor end-plates
3. Vestibular branch of the eighth cranial nerve
4. Internal capsule and pyramidal tracts

Situation: Mr. Arlo has come to the emergency room with shortness of breath, which occurred suddenly while he was getting dressed. He also has a history of emphysema. The physician diagnoses a spontaneous pneumothorax. Questions 49 to 56 refer to this situation.

49 The probable cause of a spontaneous pneumothorax is:
1. Rupture of a subpleural bleb
2. Pleural friction rub
3. Tracheoesophageal fistula
4. Puncture wound of the chest wall

50 Besides dyspnea, which of the following symptoms is generally associated with a spontaneous pneumothorax?
1. Increased chest motion
2. Unilateral chest pain
3. Hemoptysis
4. Mediastinal shift toward the involved side

51 Mr. Arlo questions the nurse as to what has happened to his lung. The nurse bases the explanation on the understanding that:
1. The heart and great vessels shift to the affected side
2. There is a greater negative pressure within the chest cavity
3. Inspired air will move from the lung into the pleural space
4. The other lung will collapse if not treated immediately

52 If Mr. Arlo has suffered a complete pneumothorax, there is danger of a mediastinal shift. If such a shift occurs, it may lead to:
1. Increased volume of the unaffected lung
2. Infection of the subpleural lining
3. Rupture of the pericardium or aorta
4. Decreased filling of the right heart

53 Mr. Arlo becomes extremely drowsy; his pulse and respirations increase. The nurse should suspect:
1. Elevated P_{O_2}
2. Respiratory alkalosis
3. Hypercapnia
4. Hypokalemia

54 In addition to calling the physician, the nurse should:
1. Place patient on his unaffected side
2. Administer 60% O_2 via Ventimask
3. Prepare for IV administration of electrolytes
4. Give 2 L O_2 per minute via nasal cannula

55 The physician inserts a chest tube in the right side and attaches it to a 2-bottle closed drainage system. In caring for Mr. Arlo, the nurse should:
1. Administer morphine sulfate, since the patient will be agitated
2. Apply a thoracic binder to prevent tension on the tube
3. Clamp the tubing to prevent a rapid decline in pressure
4. Observe for fluid fluctuations in the underwater glass tube

56 Complete lung expansion before the removal of chest tubes is evaluated by:
1. Absence of additional drainage
2. A decrease in adventitious sounds
3. Return of normal tidal volume
4. Comparison of chest radiographs

57 The poisonous nature of carbon monoxide results from:
1. Its preferential combination with hemoglobin
2. Its tendency to block CO_2 transport
3. Is inhibitory effect on vasodilation
4. The bubbles it tends to form in blood plasma

58 With an "oxygen debt" muscle shows:
1. High levels of calcium
2. Low levels of lactic acid
3. High levels of glycogen
4. Low levels of ATP

59 If breathing is deliberately stopped in a person:
1. The individual will soon die of suffocation
2. Rising oxygen concentrations will stimulate the breathing center
3. Accumulated CO_2 will force resumption of breathing
4. Increased N_2 concentration will have a toxic effect

60 Patients with fractured mandibles usually have them immobilized with wires. The life-threatening problem that can develop postoperatively is:
1. Vomiting
2. Infection
3. Osteomyelitis
4. Bronchospasm

61 A patient of yours has a temperature of 99.8° F. This is the same as a temperature of:
1. 37.7° C
2. 38.2° C
3. 37.0° C
4. 36.5° C

62 A patient with pyrexia will be expected to have:
1. Dyspnea
2. Elevated blood pressure
3. Increased pulse rate
4. Precordial pain

63 The chief complaint in a patient with Vincent's angina is:
1. Chest pain
2. Shortness of breath
3. Bleeding and ulcerations in mouth
4. Shoulder discomfort

64 After undergoing surgery for removal of impacted molars, the patient should be instructed to notify the physician if there is:
1. Pain and swelling after 1 week
2. Tenderness in the mouth when chewing
3. Pain associated with swallowing
4. Foul odor to the breath

65 A patient who undergoes a submucosal resection should be observed carefully for:
1. Occipital headache
2. Periorbital crepitus
3. Spitting up or vomiting of blood
4. White areas of healing sublingually

Situation: Mr. Fink, a soft drink vendor, enters the hospital with diarrhea, anorexia, weight loss, and abdominal cramps. A tentative diagnosis of colitis has been made. He is scheduled for a sigmoidoscopy and barium enema. Questions 66 through 73 refer to this situation.

66 In eliciting a healthy history, the nurse bases the interview on the knowledge that colitis is commonly associated with:
1. Chemical stress
2. Endocrine stress
3. Psychologic stress
4. Physiologic stress

67 Which of the following symptoms of fluid and electrolyte imbalance caused by Mr. Fink's symptoms should the nurse report immediately?
1. Extreme muscle weakness, tachycardia, and possible cardiac arrest
2. Development of tetany with muscle spasms
3. Nausea, vomiting, and leg and stomach cramps
4. Skin rash, diarrhea, and diplopia

68 Specific nursing responsibility in preparing Mr. Fink for his diagnostic procedures includes:
1. Administering soapsuds enemas till clear
2. Giving castor oil the afternoon before
3. Withholding food and fluid for 8 hours
4. Ensuring his understanding of what is to happen

69 Prior to the barium enema, Mr. Fink is to receive an enema. In what position should he be placed when receiving the enema?

1. Sims
2. Knee-chest
3. Mid-Fowler's
4. Back lying

70 What is the maximum safe height at which the container of fluid can be held?
 1. 12 inches (30.5 cm)
 2. 15 inches (37 cm)
 3. 18 inches (46 cm)
 4. 26 inches (66 cm)

71 During administration of the enema Mr. Fink complains of intestinal cramps. The nurse should:
 1. Give at a slower rate
 2. Lower the height of the container
 3. Stop until cramps are gone
 4. Discontinue the procedure

72 The visualization of the GI tract after a barium enema is made possible by:
 1. The high x-ray absorbing properties of barium
 2. Barium physically coloring the intestinal wall
 3. The high x-ray transmitting properties of barium
 4. The chemical interaction between barium and the electrolytes

73 To decrease GI irritability, the nurse should teach Mr. Fink to minimize use of:
 1. Triglycerides and amino acids
 2. Milk products and cola drinks
 3. Table salt and rice products
 4. Sugar products and proteins

Situation: Mr. Brown is admitted to the hospital with delirium tremens. His physician prescribes bed rest, and he is receiving paraldehyde, thiamine chloride, and nicotinic acid. Questions 74 through 78 refer to this situation.

74 On Mr. Brown's admission, the nurse should assign him to a:
 1. One-bed room next to the bathroom
 2. Two-bed room at the quiet end of the unit
 3. One-bed room next to the nurses' station
 4. Two-bed room next to the nurses' station

75 The nurse understands that paraldehyde is given to combat which of Mr. Brown's problems?
 1. Fluid and electrolyte
 2. Detoxification from alcohol
 3. Emotional
 4. Motor and sensory

76 When Mr. Brown is able to eat, the diet ordered for him is:
 1. High protein, low carbohydrate, low fat
 2. Protein to tolerance, moderate fat, high calorie, high vitamin, soft
 3. High carbohydrate, low saturated fat, 1800 calories
 4. Low protein, high carbohydrate, high fat, soft

77 A high-calorie diet fortified with vitamins will prevent damage to which organ that detoxifies alcohol?

1. Kidneys
2. Liver
3. Pancreas
4. Adrenals

78 Mr. Brown requires thiamine chloride and nicotinic acid because these vitamins are needed for the maintenance of:
 1. Good circulation
 2. The nervous system
 3. Prothrombin formation
 4. Elimination

Situation: Mrs. Smith is admitted to the hospital with an acute attack of ulcerative colitis. She has been very worried about her 2 small children and calls her mother frequently for help. She recently pleaded with her mother to come and live with them. Mr. Smith objects to this, goes out alone quite often, and does not seem to take an interest in the children. Questions 79 through 85 refer to this situation.

79 The nurse will understand the organic aspects of psychosomatic disease more readily if she recognizes the "stress" functions of the:
 1. Cerebral cortex and thyroid gland
 2. Sympathetic nervous system and the pancreas
 3. Autonomic nervous system and the adrenal glands
 4. Central nervous system and the hypothalamus

80 To give complete nursing care to Mrs. Smith, the nurse should:
 1. Understand the patient's emotional conflict
 2. Recognize her own feelings toward this patient
 3. Talk with the patient's husband and mother
 4. Develop rapport with the patient's physician

81 The nurse recognizes that the prognosis for Mrs. Smith will remain guarded until:
 1. A surgical procedure is performed to remove the somatic factor
 2. Her husband accepts her desire to have her mother move in with them
 3. Her emotional conflicts are resolved
 4. She reaches her 40s and endocrine activity is decreased

82 Which of the following symptoms should the nurse expect when assessing Mrs. Smith on admission?
 1. Diarrhea, anorexia, weight loss, abdominal cramps, anemia
 2. Anemia, nausea and vomiting, weight loss, abdominal cramps
 3. Fever, anemia, nausea and vomiting, leukopenia, diarrhea
 4. Leukocytosis, anorexia, weight loss

83 The physician orders daily stool examinations. Mrs. Smith is also scheduled for a sigmoidoscopy and barium enema. Stool examinations are ordered to determine:
 1. Culture and sensitivity
 2. Occult blood and organisms
 3. Ova and parasites
 4. Fat and undigested food

84 A serious complication of this disease is:
1. Hemorrhage
2. Perforation
3. Obstruction
4. Ileus

85 Mrs. Smith's initial hospital diet is residue free during the acute stage. Which food combination should the nurse indicate as the best choice for her?
1. Cream soup and crackers, omlet, mashed potatoes, roll orange juice, coffee
2. Stewed chicken, baked potato with butter, strained peas, white bread, plain cake, milk
3. Baked fish, macaroni with cheese, strained carrots, fruit gelatin, milk
4. Lean roast beef, buttered white rice with egg slices, white bread with butter and jelly, tea with sugar

---

86 An adult intolerance to milk, found mostly in black populations, is caused by a genetic deficiency of the enzyme:
1. Sucrase
2. Lactase
3. Maltase
4. Amylase

87 Mrs. Aster is diagnosed as having a hiatus hernia. She tells you she is having difficulty sleeping at night. Appropriate intervention is:
1. Suggesting a large glass of milk before retiring
2. Eliminating carbohydrates from the diet
3. Sleeping on 2 or 3 pillows
4. Administering antacids such as sodium bicarbonate

Situation: Dr. Kinsey was found in a coma in his room at the large hospital where he had begun his residency. There was a strong odor of acetone on his breath. He is married and 28 years of age. His wife, Jane, states he is a diabetic and recently switched to Orinase on his own instead of taking insulin as prescribed. Health records submitted did not reveal that Dr. Kinsey had diabetes mellitus. Emergency measures were instituted immediately. Questions 88 through 94 refer to this question.

88 Oral hypoglycemic agents may be used for diabetic patients with:
1. Ketosis or impending coma
2. Mature onset
3. Juvenile onset
4. Obesity

89 Dr. Kinsey has omitted pertinent information from his health record because:
1. Physicians with diabetes are not accepted for residency in many hospitals
2. He is unable to handle the psychologic stress related to alternation in body functioning
3. He needs assistance in developing a more favorable adaptation to this stress
4. Diabetics often have lapses of memory

90 Diabetic coma results from an excess accumulation in the blood of:
1. Nitrogen from protein catabolism, causing ammonia intoxication
2. Ketones from rapid fat breakdown, causing acidosis
3. Glucose from rapid carbohydrate metabolism, causing drowsiness
4. Sodium bicarbonate, causing alkalosis

91 The most common cause of diabetic ketoacidosis is:
1. Presence of infection
2. Failure to take prescribed insulin
3. Inadequate food and fluid intake
4. Additional stress

92 An independent nursing action in the care of this patient is:
1. Regulating insulin dosage according to the amount of ketones found in the urine
2. Withholding glucose in any form until the ketoacidosis is corrected
3. Observing for signs of hypoglycemia
4. Giving fruit juices, broth, and milk as soon as the patient is able to take fluids orally

93 The nurse suspected hypokalemia when she observed which of the following symptoms?
1. Edema, bounding pulse, confusion
2. Apathy, weakness, abdominal distention
3. Sunken eyeballs, Kussmaul breathing, hunger
4. Spasms, hypotension, convulsions

94 Important to both Dr. Kinsey and his wife Jane is an understanding that his diet for management of his diabetes:
1. Is based on nutritional requirements that are the same for all patients
2. Can be planned around a wide variety of commonly used foods
3. Should be rigidly controlled to avoid similar emergencies
4. Must not include combination dishes and processed foods, since they have too many variable seasonings

---

95 A basic concept of rehabilitation is defined by which of the following statements?
1. Rehabilitation is a specialty area with unique methods for meeting the patient's needs
2. Rehabilitation is not necessary for most patients because they will return to their usual activities following hospitalization
3. Rehabilitation needs, immediate or potential, are exhibited by all patients with a health problem
4. Rehabilitation needs are best met by the patient's family and community resources

96 Carbohydrates provide one of our main fuel sources for energy. Which of the following carbohydrate foods provides the quickest source of energy?

1. A slice of bread
2. A glass of orange juice
3. A glass of milk
4. Chocolate candy bar

97 An untreated diabetic may lapse into a coma because of acidosis. This acidosis is directly caused by an increased concentration in the blood of:
1. Glucose
2. Lactic acid
3. Glutamic acid
4. Alpha-keto acids

98 How should a fractional urine specimen be removed from a retention catheter?
1. Cleanse drainage valve and remove from collection bag
2. Disconnect and drain into clean catheter
3. Wipe catheter with alcohol and drain into sterile test tube
4. Use a sterile syringe to remove from a clamped, cleansed catheter

99 Which of the following secretes an antidiuretic substance important for maintaining fluid balance?
1. Anterior pituitary
2. Adrenal cortex
3. Adrenal medulla
4. Posterior pituitary

100 As the amount of antidiuretic hormone in blood increases:
1. Glomerular filtration tends to decrease
2. Tubular reabsorption of potassium and water increases
3. Tubular reabsorption of sodium and water increases
4. Urine concentration tends to decrease

101 The posterior pituitary gland secretes antidiuretic hormone (ADH), which influences normal kidney function by stimulating the:
1. Glomerulus to control the quantity of fluid passing through it
2. Glomerulus to withhold the proteins from the urine
3. Nephron tubules to reabsorb water
4. Nephron tubules to reabsorb glucose

102 Two body systems that interact with the bicarbonate buffer system to preserve the normal body fluid pH of 7.4 are the:
1. Respiratory and urinary systems
2. Muscular and endocrine systems
3. Skeletal and nervous systems
4. Circulatory and urinary systems

Situation: Mrs. Thompson, age 39, was admitted to the hospital with a diagnosis of Addison's disease. She exhibited the following signs and symptoms: muscular weakness, anorexia, emaciation, GI distress, generalized dark pigmentation, hypotension, hypoglycemia, low sodium and high potassium levels, and a loss of libido. Questions 103 through 110 refer to this situation.

103 The hypotension can be explained by the fact that Addison's disease involves a disturbance in the production of:

1. Glucocorticoids
2. Androgens
3. Mineralocorticoids
4. Estrogens

104 The nurse should observe Mrs. Thompson closely for signs of infectious complication because there is a disturbance of function in the:
1. Proinflammatory effect
2. Anti-inflammatory effect
3. Metabolic effect
4. Electrolytic effect

105 The emaciation, muscular weakness, and fatigue are due to disturbance of function in:
1. Protein anabolic effect
2. Electrolytic effect
3. Metabolic effect
4. Masculinizing effect

106 An important aspect of nursing care for Mrs. Thompson is:
1. Encouraging exercise
2. Providing a variety of diversional activities
3. Permitting as much activity as the patient desires
4. Protecting from exertion

107 Therapy for Mrs. Thompson is aimed chiefly at:
1. Restoring electrolyte balance
2. Improving carbohydrate metabolism
3. Increasing lymphoid tissue
4. Increasing eosinophils

108 Mrs. Thompson's treatment included a high-protein high-calorie diet with extra salt. As a means of encouraging her to eat, the nurse explained the reasons for this diet therapy as follows:
1. Extra salt is needed to replace the amount being lost due to lack of sufficient aldosterone to conserve sodium
2. Increased vitamins are needed to supply energy to help her regain lost weight
3. Increased protein is needed to heal the adrenal tissue and thus cure the disease
4. Increased amounts of potassium are needed to replace renal losses

109 Prior to discharge the physician prescribes hydrocortisone, 10 mg tid, and fludrocortisone, 0.1 mg qd. The nurse expects hydrocortisone to:
1. Prevent hypoglycemia and permit Mrs. Thompson to respond to stress
2. Increase amounts of angiotensin II to raise Mrs. Thompson's blood pressure
3. Control excessive loss of potassium salts
4. Decrease cardiac arrhythmias and dyspnea

110 The nurse teaches Mrs. Thompson to consult her physician immediately if she experiences which of these symptoms related to fludrocortisone therapy?
1. Fatigue, particularly in the afternoon
2. Increased frequency of urination

3. Rapid weight gain and dependent edema
4. Unpredictable changes in mood

---

111 A patient who is scheduled to have a bilateral adrenalectomy would most likely receive which of the following drugs on the day of surgery and in the immediate postoperative period?
1. Regular insulin
2. ACTH
3. Hydrocortisone succinate (Solu-Cortef)
4. Pituitary extract (Pituitrin)

112 Glucocorticoids and mineralocorticoids are secreted by the:
1. Pancreas
2. Hypophysis
3. Adrenal glands
4. Gonads

113 The most common cause of Cushing's syndrome is:
1. Deprivation of cortical hormones
2. Excess secretion of ACTH
3. Hyperplasia of adrenal cortex
4. Neoplasm of the pituitary gland

114 Cushing's syndrome is caused by functioning bilateral tumors of the adrenal cortex. Which of the following symptoms are commonly seen in Cushing's syndrome?
1. "Buffalo hump," and hypertension
2. Dehydration and menorrhagia
3. Pitting edema and frequent colds
4. Migraine headache and dysmenorrhea

115 An adrenalectomy is performed. Postoperatively, until regulated by steroid therapy, the patient may show symptoms of:
1. Hyperglycemia
2. Sodium retention
3. Potassium excretion
4. Hypotension

116 Rapid adjustments made by the body during an emergency are associated with the increased activity of which gland?
1. Pituitary
2. Thyroid
3. Adrenal
4. Pancreas

117 Prior to an adrenalectomy, steroids are administered to the patient. The nurse understands the reason for this is to:
1. Compensate for sudden lack of these hormones following surgery
2. Increase the inflammatory action to promote scar formation
3. Foster accumulation of glycogen in the liver
4. Facilitate urinary excretion of salt and water following surgery

Situation: Mrs. Dreck is admitted with a history of abdominal pain, chills, nausea, and a purulent vaginal discharge. She is diagnosed as having pelvic inflammatory disease. Questions 118 through 122 refer to this situation.

118 The nurse should place Mrs. Dreck in:
1. Sims' position
2. Fowler's position
3. Lithotomy position
4. Supine position with knees flexed

119 Mrs. Dreck menstruates regularly every 30 days. Her last menses started on January 1. When will she most probably ovulate next?
1. January 5 or 6
2. January 15
3. January 17
4. January 28

120 The incubation period for syphilis is about:
1. 72 hours
2. 1 week
3. 2 months
4. 2 to 6 weeks

121 A slide flocculation test for syphilis is the:
1. Wassermann test
2. Dick test
3. Kahn test
4. VDRL

122 At which stage is syphilis not considered contagious?
1. Primary
2. Tertiary
3. Secondary
4. Incubation

---

123 Condylomata acuminata refers to:
1. Veneral warts
2. Cancer of epididymis
3. Herpes zoster
4. Scabies

124 A disease produced by a gram-negative diplococcus that generally invades the urogenital tract is:
1. Cholera
2. Syphilis
3. Gonorrhea
4. Chancroid

125 Acute salpingitis is most commonly the result of:
1. Abortion
2. Gonorrhea
3. Hydatidiform mole
4. Syphilis

126 A disease that can arise from normal microbial flora, especially after prolonged antibiotic therapy, is:
1. Moniliasis or candidiasis
2. Scarlet fever
3. Q fever
4. Herpes zoster

127 Gram-negative diplococci found in a vaginal smear are presumed to be:

1. Gonococci
2. Meningococci
3. Pneumococci
4. *Treponema pallidum*

128 Which of the following tests might the physician perform to determine the underlying cause of uterine pain?
1. Endometrial smear
2. Laparoscopy
3. Tubal insufflation
4. Estradiol level

Situation: Mr. Saul, a 68-year-old retired civil service employee, is admitted to the hospital via the emergency service. He was found unconscious 30 minutes prior to admission. The physical examination reveals right hemiplegia. Tentative diagnosis is cerebral vascular accident. Questions 129 through 133 refer to this situation.

129 In observing Mr. Saul the nurse should check for signs of increased intracranial pressure. Which one of the following combinations of symptoms is indicative of increased intracranial pressure?
1. Slow bounding pulse, rising blood pressure, elevated temperature, stupor
2. Rapid weak pulse, fall in blood pressure, low temperature, restlessness
3. Weak rapid pulse, normal blood pressure, intermittent fever, lethargy
4. Slow bounding pulse, fall in blood pressure, temperature below 97° F (36° C), stupor

130 Since Mr. Saul is unconscious, the nurse should expect him to:
1. Be unable to react to painful stimuli
2. Be incontinent
3. Be capable of spontaneous motion
4. Demonstrate carphology

131 Mr. Saul regains consciousness and has expressive aphasia. As a part of the long-range planning, the nurse would:
1. Help the family to accept the fact that Mr. Saul cannot participate in verbal communication
2. Wait for Mr. Saul to verbalize his needs regardless of how long it may take
3. Begin associating words with physical objects
4. Help Mr. Saul accept this disability as permanent

132 Urinary retention and overflow, a frequent problem of the stroke patient, is evidenced by:
1. Decrease in total amount of urine voided
2. Frequency from inability to empty bladder
3. Continual incontinence
4. Oliguria and edema

133 Which of the following hospital methods is the most useful for the nurse to employ in encouraging patients to void?
1. Having patient listen to running water

2. Warming a bedpan
3. Placing patient's hands in warm water
4. Providing privacy

Situation: Ellen Smith, a 76-year-old woman, is admitted to the rehabilitation unit following a stroke. She is bedridden and aphasic. The morning following her admission the physician orders an indwelling catheter, since she has been incontinent during the night. Questions 134 through 140 refer to this situation.

134 It is learned from the daughter that her mother had not been incontinent while at home, and she insisted that the nurse had failed to communicate with her mother. This is an example of:
1. Treatment without consent of patient, which is an invasion of rights
2. A catheter inserted for the patient's benefit
3. Inability to obtain consent for treatment because the patient was aphasic
4. A treatment that does not need special consent

135 Mrs. Smith has left hemiplegia. The nurse contributes to her rehabilitation by:
1. Making a referral to the physical therapist
2. Not moving the affected arm and leg unless necessary
3. Beginning active exercises
4. Positioning Mrs. Smith to prevent deformity and decubiti

136 The nurse can best prevent footdrop in a patient for whom bed rest has been prescribed by the use of:
1. Boards
2. Blocks
3. Cradles
4. Sandbags

137 Mrs. Smith's emotional responses to her illness would probably be determined by:
1. Her premorbid personality
2. The location of her lesion
3. The care she is receiving
4. Her ability to understand her illness

138 Mrs. Smith's position should be changed:
1. Every hour
2. Every 2 hours
3. Every 4 hours
4. Every 6 hours

139 In aiding Mrs. Smith to develop independence, the nurse should:
1. Demonstrate ways she can regain independence in activities
2. Reinforce success in tasks accomplished
3. Establish long-range goals for the patient
4. Point out her errors in performance

140 For optimum nutrition the nurse may find that Mrs. Smith

needs assistance with her eating. To accomplish this goal, the nurse may:
1. Encourage her to participate in the feeding process to the extent of her capacity
2. Do all the feeding for her so Mrs. Smith can rest
3. Feed her rapidly to get in as much as possible before she tires
4. Leave the feeding entirely to a nursing aide

---

141 Arteriosclerosis of blood vessels leading to the brain may not become evident until there is an extremely severe blockage or until a stroke occurs because of collateral blood circulation supplied through the:
1. Hypothalamic-hypophyseal portal system
2. The bicarotid trunk
3. Circle of Willis
4. Jugular vessels

142 After undergoing an endarterectomy, the patient should be observed for changes in:
1. Bowel habits
2. Skin color
3. Tissue turgor
4. Appetite

143 The increased tendency toward coronary and cerebral thromboses seen in individuals with polycythemia vera is attributable to the:
1. Elevated blood pressure
2. Immaturity of red blood cells
3. Fragility of the cells
4. Increased viscosity

144 Vitamin C in human nutrition is related to tissue integrity and hemorrhagic disease. It controls such disorders by:
1. Preserving the structural integrity of tissue by protecting the lipid matrix of cell walls from peroxidation
2. Preventing tissue hemorrhage by providing essential blood clotting materials
3. Facilitating adequate absorption of calcium and phosphorus for bone formation to prevent bleeding in the joints
4. Strengthening capillary walls and structural tissue by depositing cementing material to build collagen from ground substance and thus prevent tissue hemorrhage

145 Mrs. Joyce, an elderly woman, was admitted to the surgical unit from a nursing home for treatment of decubitus ulcers. She was obviously dehydrated and her skin was dry and scaly. On admission the nurse immediately began to introduce fluids, applied emollients to the skin, and changed the dressings on the decubitus ulcers. Legally:
1. No treatment should have been instituted for Mrs. Joyce until a physician ordered it
2. The nurse should have instituted a plan for active range of motion exercise to all joints
3. The nurse provided supportive nursing care for the well-being of Mrs. Joyce

4. Debridement of the decubiti should have been done by the nurse before the dressing was applied

146 In general, the higher the red blood cell count:
1. The greater the blood viscosity
2. The higher the blood pH
3. The less it contributes to immunity
4. The lower the hematocrit

Situation: Mr. Ryan is admitted to the hospital with GI bleeding and a burning epigastric pain. The initial diagnosis is peptic ulcer or gastric carcinoma. Questions 147 through 153 refer to this situation.

147 The emotional response that most frequently contributes to psychosomatic illness is:
1. Anxiety
2. Depression
3. Fear
4. Rage

148 To differentiate between a gastric ulcer and gastric carcinoma, which one of the following diagnostic tests would provide conclusive evidence?
1. Gastric analysis
2. GI series
3. Gastroscopy
4. Stool examination

149 Mr. Ryan is placed on a stretcher and restrained with Velcro straps for his transport to the X-ray Department for a barium swallow. While coming out of the elevator, Mr. Ryan shifts his position, the Velcro strap breaks, and he falls to the floor and sustains a fractured arm. Mr. Ryan comments that "the Velcro strap was worn, just at the very spot where the strap snapped." The nurse is:
1. Completely exonerated, since only the hospital, as principal employer, is primarily responsible for the quality and maintenance of equipment
2. Exempt from any law suit because of the doctrine of *respondeat superior*
3. Normally liable, along with the employer, for misapplication of equipment or use of defective equipment that harms the patient
4. Totally and singly responsible for the obvious negligence because of her failure to report defective equipment

150 Barium salts in GI series and barium enemas serve to:
1. Give off visible light and illuminate the alimentary tract
2. Fluoresce and thus illuminate the alimentary tract
3. Dye the alimentary tract and thus give it color contrast
4. Absorb x rays and thus give contrast to the soft tissues of the alimentary tract

151 Peptic ulcer is diagnosed. This is considered to be a psychosomatic disorder about which it is believed that:
1. Structural changes have occurred as a result of psychologic conflicts

2. Illness is a defense against psychologic conflicts
3. Structural changes have occurred as a result of physiologic changes caused by psychologic conflict
4. Physiologic changes stimulated psychologic changes

152 The nurse should be aware that the most common complication of peptic ulcer is:
1. Perforation
2. Hemorrhage
3. Pyloric obstruction
4. Esophageal varices

153 Which of the following foods would be served to Mr. Ryan?
1. Sliced oranges, pancakes with syrup, coffee
2. Applesauce, cream of wheat, milk
3. Orange juice, fried eggs, sausage
4. Tomato juice, raisin bran cereal, tea

Situation: Mrs. Scully, a small 78-year-old woman, fell in her back yard. X-ray films were taken, and the attending surgeon told Mrs. Scully that she had fractured her hip (fractured neck of the femur). She was admitted to the hospital, and Buck's extension was applied to her limb. The following day she was given a general anesthetic, the fracture was reduced, and a Smith-Petersen nail inserted. Questions 154 through 159 refer to this situation.

154 When Mrs. Scully is helped from the bed to a chair after the nailing of her hip, the nurse encourages her to stand on her good leg before sitting in a chair (no weight-bearing on the involved limb). This is important because:
1. There is usually insufficient help to lift her from bed to chair
2. This will help maintain strength in her good limb
3. This is the quickest method of getting her to and from the bed
4. There is less danger of injuring her hip

155 When Mrs. Scully is in the side-lying position, the nurse ensures that she has a firm pillow placed between her thighs and that the entire length of her upper limb is supported. The most important reason for this is to:
1. Prevent strain on the fracture site
2. Make the patient more comfortable
3. Prevent flexion contractures of the hip joint
4. Prevent skin surfaces from rubbing together

156 When teaching crutch walking, the nurse instructs Mrs. Scully to place weight on:
1. The axillary region
2. Palms of the hands and axillary region
3. Palms of the hands
4. Both extremities, with partial weight-bearing

157 Aseptic necrosis of the head of the femur occurs. The nurse should be aware that this is caused by:
1. Wound infection
2. Immobilization following reduction of the fracture

3. Loss of blood supply to head of the femur
4. Weight-bearing before fracture is healed

158 Contractures that develop most frequently following fracture of the hip are:
1. Hyperextension of the knee joint with drop foot deformity
2. Internal rotation with abduction
3. Flexion and adduction of the hip, with flexion of the knee
4. External rotation with abduction

159 Intramedullary nailing is used in the treatment of:
1. Fracture of the shaft of the femur
2. Fracture of the neck of the femur
3. Slipped epiphysis
4. Intertrochanteric fracture of the femur

---

160 Postural changes immediately after spinal anesthesia may result in hypotension because there is:
1. Dilation of capacitance vessels
2. Decreased response of baroreceptors
3. Interruption of cardiac accelerator pathways
4. Decreased strength of cardiac contractions

161 When positioning a patient who is recovering from general anesthesia, it is important for the nurse to:
1. Keep the patient turned to the side
2. Place the patient in a Trendelenburg position
3. Elevate the head of the bed
4. Position the patient flat on the back

Situation: Mrs. Olin, a 38-year-old schoolteacher with rheumatoid arthritis, is admitted to the hospital with severe pain and swelling of the joints in both hands. Questions 162 through 167 refer to this situation.

162 Mrs. Olin's condition would indicate that a primary consideration in her care is:
1. Motivation
2. Education
3. Control of pain
4. Surgery

163 Which of the following laboratory tests or procedures would the nurse use in reference to the diagnosis of arthritis?
1. Latex agglutination
2. Lipase
3. Bence Jones protein
4. Phosphatase alkaline

164 A patient with rheumatoid arthritis must be protected against injury to the joints. Therefore therapeutic exercise by the nurse should be:
1. Only passive
2. Avoided
3. Preceded by heat
4. Active assistive

165 In helping Mrs. Olin toward self-reliance and independence the nurse should approach the problem with:
1. A positive attitude toward the eventual outcome
2. The understanding that little can be accomplished
3. A feeling that efforts should be made to place the patient in an extended care facility
4. Limited objectives

166 Through motivation and teaching, Mrs. Olin may:
1. Learn to perform most activities of daily living
2. Become vocationally employed
3. Ambulate with crutches
4. Be transferred to a halfway house

167 The nurse should expect that therapy for Mrs. Olin would not include:
1. Range of motion exercises
2. Braces
3. Massage
4. Conductive heat

---

168 A patient with degenerative arthritis may require a total-hip replacement. This surgery is done:
1. Using a ''laminar airflow room''
2. Using 3 separate stages
3. With the patient in lithotomy position
4. After the hip joint becomes ankylosed

169 A sprain accompanied by edema is treated with the application of compresses. What is the appropriate temperature range?
1. 65° to 80° F (18° to 26.6° C)
2. 80° to 93° F (26.6° to 34° C)
3. 93° to 98° F (34° to 36.6° C)
4. 98° to 105° F (36.6° to 40.5° C)

170 The temperature range for a tepid application is:
1. 80° to 93° F (26.6° to 34° C)
2. 70° to 78° F (21° to 25.5° C)
3. 60° to 68° F (15.5° to 20° C)
4. 55° to 65° F (12.8° to 18° C)

171 Local hot and cold applications transfer temperature to and from the body by:
1. Radiation
2. Convection
3. Insulation
4. Conduction

172 Short, cold applications produce:
1. Depression of vital signs
2. Peripheral vasodilation
3. Decreased viscosity of blood
4. Local anesthesia

Situation: Following a car accident Ed, an 18-year-old high school senior, is taken to the local hospital with a back injury. He did not lose consciousness and remembers that he was unable to move his legs following the accident. Questions 173 through 179 refer to this situation.

173 Following an accident when there is a questionable back injury, the individual involved:
1. May be transported in sitting position, if necessary, to secure immediate medical care
2. May be transported in any position because position is not important, since damage to the cord has already occurred
3. Should be protected from flexion and hyperextension of the spine
4. May be transported best when placed in the side-lying position

174 Following the examination the physician indicates that Ed is paraplegic. His family asks the nurse what this means. The nurse explains:
1. Both lower and upper extremities are paralyzed
2. Upper extremities are paralyzed
3. One side of the body is paralyzed
4. Lower extremities are paralyzed

175 If the anterior root of a spinal nerve were cut, what would be the result in the regions supplied by that spinal nerve?
1. Complete loss of sensation
2. Complete loss of movement
3. Complete loss of sensation and movement
4. Complete loss of sensation, movement, and autonomic control of blood vessels

176 When caring for a paraplegic, the nurse will remember that a high intake of fluid is necessary to help:
1. Prevent elevation of temperature
2. Maintain electrolyte balance
3. Prevent dehydration
4. Prevent urinary tract infection

177 Teaching Ed to care for himself while in the hospital:
1. Is not necessary, since he will be back to normal when he leaves the hospital
2. Is too complicated to be undertaken by a layperson
3. Is not necessary, since his family will not be able to care for him at home
4. Is an essential part of his nursing care

178 The paraplegic patient frequently loses calcium from the skeletal system. Which of the following factors contributes to this condition?
1. Inactivity
2. Decreased calcium intake
3. Inadequate kidney function
4. Inadequate fluid intake

179 Sympathetic hyperreflexia is a syndrome seen in patients with spinal cord injuries. The signs and symptoms include diaphoresis, pulsating headaches, and goose bumps. This syndrome may occur when:
1. The bowel and/or bladder is distended
2. The myelin sheath is deteriorating
3. The patient is upright on a tilt table
4. The spinal cord is crushed rather than severed

180 Following an accident, Mrs. Jean Boyhout is admitted unconscious to the medical unit with internal bleeding and head injuries. The physician orders a type and cross match for 1000 ml of whole blood to be administered within the next 6 hours. Mr. Boyhout arrives and refuses to allow his wife to be transfused with the whole blood, since they are Jehovah's Witnesses. As the nurse involved in this situation, you would:
1. Gently explain to the husband why the transfusion is necessary, emphasizing the implications of not having it
2. Institute the blood transfusion anyway, since the physician ordered it and the patient's survival depends on volume replacement
3. Phone the physician for a special administrative order to give the blood under these circumstances
4. Have the husband sign a treatment refusal form and notify the physician so a court order can be obtained

181 In caring for the confused or delirious patient, the nurse provides new information slowly and in small amounts. The principle underlying this care is:
1. Destruction of brain cells has occurred, interrupting mental activity
2. Confusion or delirium can be a defense against further stress
3. A minimum of information should be given, since the patient is unaware of his surroundings
4. Teaching is based on information progressing from the simple to the complex

Situation: Mr. Smith is a 60-year-old man who is admitted to the hospital with a diagnosis of idiopathic trigeminal neuralgia (tic douloureux). Questions 182 through 188 refer to this situation.

182 In planning the nursing care for Mr. Smith, the nurse would:
1. Emphasize the importance of mouth care
2. Be alert to prevent dehydration or starvation
3. Initiate exercises of the jaw and facial muscles
4. Apply iced compresses to the affected area

183 The nurse would expect Mr. Smith to exhibit:
1. Uncontrollable tremors of the eyelid
2. Excruciating facial and head pain
3. Unilateral muscle weakness
4. Multiple petechiae

184 Which of the following symptoms should the nurse also expect Mr. Smith to demonstrate?
1. Exhaustion and fatigue due to extreme pain
2. Excessive talkativeness due to apprehension
3. Hyperactivity due to medications received
4. Prolonged periods of sleep broken only by external stimuli

185 In planning care for Mr. Smith, the nurse must:
1. Avoid walking swiftly past the patient

2. Discontinue oral hygiene temporarily
3. Massage both sides of the face frequently
4. Keep the patient in the prone position

186 Mr. Smith tells the nurse he is taking all 4 of the medications listed. The nurse should be aware that the one used to treat trigeminal neuralgia is:
1. Carbamazepine (Tegretol)
2. Allopurinol (Zyloprim)
3. Morphine sulfate
4. Ascorbic acid

187 Surgery, with cutting of the nerve, is performed. Which of the following would be an unusual occurrence after surgery?
1. Development of a painless rash in the area
2. Recurrence of the pain, which will gradually decrease
3. Development of a crawling or tingling sensation in the area
4. Loss of muscle power in the area

188 In discharge planning for Mr. Smith, the nurse should counsel the patient to:
1. Perform facial exercises
2. Have regular dental checkups
3. Avoid stressful situations
4. Chew food on the affected side

189 Electric stimulation by the use of a peripheral nerve implant or dorsal column stimulator is used in intractable pain. The nurse should explain that after surgery:
1. The patient should not take tub baths
2. The device may interfere with the television remote control
3. Analgesics will no longer be necessary
4. The transmitter must be worn externally

190 A procedure done to relieve intractable pain in the upper torso is:
1. Chondrectomy
2. Cordotomy
3. Rhizotomy
4. Wolfgang's procedure

Situation: Mrs. Curran is admitted to the burn unit with second- and third-degree burns. Questions 191 through 196 refer to this situation.

191 Fluid shifts are a great danger to the patient with burns. Which of the following would be expected to occur?
1. Increased fluid shifts after 2 hours, which result in irreversible shock
2. Loss of sodium and increase in blood potassium
3. Decreased capillary permeability
4. Rise in blood volume

192 IV fluid replacement therapy is important. Which of the following would be expected in the first 24 hours?
1. Intake: 8000 ml; output: 480 ml
2. Intake: 12,000 ml; output: 4500 ml

3. Intake: 3000 ml; output: 2400 ml
4. Intake: 6000 ml; output: 1200 ml

193 The rate of fluid replacement for a patient with severe burns during the first 48 hours is considered satisfactory if the urinary output is approximately:
1. Half the intake
2. One tenth the intake
3. One third the intake
4. Equal to the intake

194 To maintain Mrs. Curran's nutrition during convalescence, which of the following measures would be most important?
1. Reduce protein intake to avoid overtaxing the kidneys
2. Limit caloric intake to decrease the work of the body
3. Encourage the intake of orange juice or other fluids containing vitamin C
4. Encourage excessive intake of sodium

195 Which of the following statements is true of the recovery and convalescent periods for the patient with extensive burns?
1. Death may still occur from septicemia
2. The danger of physical complications is past
3. Diversional therapy cannot be initiated as yet due to the need for rest
4. All mirrors should be removed from the room to decrease the patient's anxiety about appearance

196 An antacid is prescribed to prevent this condition, which tends to occur 2 weeks after the burn:
1. Curling's ulcer
2. Gastric ulcer
3. Colitis
4. Gastritis

---

197 When the fluid in a bottle is allowed to flow into a person intravenously:
1. Chemical energy is converted to kinetic energy
2. Potential energy is converted to kinetic energy
3. Potential energy is converted to chemical energy
4. Kinetic energy is converted to potential energy

198 An important function of the albumin of the blood is:
1. Red blood cell formation
2. The activation of white blood cells
3. Blood clotting
4. The development of the colloid osmotic pressure

199 The capillary endothelium is a selectively permeable membrane. Which of the following molecules cannot easily pass through it?
1. O_2 and CO_2
2. Plasma proteins
3. Glucose, O_2, and CO_2
4. Ions, amino acids, and water

200 The reabsorption of water from glomerular filtrate (in the kidney tubules), the flow of water between the intracellular and interstitial compartments, and the exchange of fluid between plasma and interstitial fluid spaces are caused by what important physical process?
1. Dialysis
2. Active transport
3. Osmosis
4. Diffusion

Situation: Mr. McGee, a 31-year-old private in the Marines, recently returned from Southeast Asia after a 13-month tour of duty. On the basis of the history and physical examination, the physician believes the most likely diagnosis is malaria. Questions 201 through 210 refer to this situation.

201 The most important diagnostic test in malaria is:
1. Smear of peripheral blood
2. Blood leukocyte count
3. Erythrocyte sedimentation rate
4. Splenic puncture

202 The nurse is reviewing Mr. McGee's physical examination and laboratory test. An important finding in malaria is:
1. Splenomegaly
2. Leukocytosis
3. Elevated sedimentation rate
4. Erythrocytosis

203 Mr. McGee asks the nurse how he could have prevented the disease. The nurse should explain that prophylaxis for the control of malaria includes:
1. Vaccination
2. Patient isolation
3. Prompt detection and effective treatment
4. Antibiotic therapy

204 Blackwater fever occurs in some cases of malaria. The nurse should observe Mr. McGee for:
1. Diarrhea
2. Coffee ground emesis
3. Low-grade fever
4. Dark red urine

205 A serious complication of acute malaria is:
1. Anemia and cachexia
2. Congested lungs
3. Changes in water and electrolyte balance
4. Impaired peristalsis

206 In caring for Mr. McGee, the nurse should know that:
1. Peritoneal dialysis is usually indicated
2. Patient should be awakened only for nourishment after a paroxysm
3. Attention should be focused on rest and nourishing food between paroxysms
4. Isolation is necessary to prevent cross infection

207 Because Mr. McGee is experiencing an acute attack of malaria, the physician orders 650 mg of quinine dihydrochloride to be given over an 8-hour period of time by IV drip in 1000 ml of normal saline. He further specifies that the drug must not be injected more rapidly than 50 mg per

minute. The IV equipment is calibrated at 20 drops per milliliter. To avoid exceeding a dosage of 50 mg per minute, the solution must never flow at the rate of:
1. 12 ml per minute
2. 80 ml per minute
3. 10 ml per minute
4. 5 ml per minute

208 Whenever quinine is used, the nurse should be alert to symptoms of severe cinchonism, which are:
1. Tinnitus, decreased auditory acuity, nausea
2. Deafness, vertigo, severe visual, GI, and central nervous system disturbances
3. Pruritus, urticaria, and difficulty in breathing
4. Leg cramps, fever, swollen and painful joints

209 When the danger of the acute attack has passed, the physician replaces the IV injection with quinine sulfate, 2 g per day in divided doses. The nurse should administer this medication after meals to:
1. Delay its absorption
2. Minimize gastric irritation
3. Decrease stimulation of appetite
4. Decrease its antiarrhythmic action

210 Which of the following statements is true concerning successful drug therapy against *P. falciparum* infections?
1. The infections can generally be eliminated
2. Transmission by the Anopheles mosquito can occur
3. The infections are controlled
4. Immunity will prevent reinfection

Situation: Walter Sams, a 75-year-old man, enters the hospital with benign prostatic hypertrophy for further tests and a prostatectomy. Questions 211 through 215 refer to this situation.

211 The nurse insists that a medication for sleep be taken at 9 P.M., even though the patient tells her he never went to sleep this early and would like the medication delayed. Later the patient awakens and is confused. He tries to get out of bed and in so doing falls, fracturing his hip. Legally:
1. Hospital policy requires that sleep medications be given at 9 P.M., and *respondeat superior* applies
2. Patient's rights have precedence over hospital policy or physician's orders
3. The time the medication was given has nothing to do with the confusion
4. When the physician orders a medication, it must be given at the scheduled time unless the nursing supervisor authorizes differently

212 The definitive diagnosis of benign prostatic hypertrophy is arrived at by:
1. Biopsy of prostatic tissue
2. Pap smear of prostatic fluid
3. Rectal examination
4. Serum phosphatase studies

213 Which of the following tests might be ordered to estimate the effect of Mr. Sams' illness on the kidneys?
1. PSP, urea clearance, urine concentration
2. Sulkowitch, catecholamines, urine dilution
3. Bence Jones protein, urine concentration, albumin
4. Microscopic porphyrins, urinalysis

214 While caring for Mr. Sams, the nurse is aware that benign prostatic hypertrophy:
1. Usually becomes malignant
2. Predisposes to hydronephrosis
3. Is a congenital abnormality
4. Causes an elevated acid phosphatase

215 Mr. Sams had a suprapubic prostatectomy with continuous bladder irrigations. The nurse, when caring for a patient with a continuous bladder irrigation, should:
1. Measure urinary specific gravity
2. Record hourly outputs
3. Include irrigating solution on intake and output records
4. Exclude irrigating solution from any 24-hour urine tests ordered

---

216 Ammonia is excreted by the kidney to help maintain:
1. Low bacterial levels in the urine
2. Osmotic pressure of the blood
3. Acid-base balance of the body
4. Normal red blood cell production

217 What structure encircles the male urethra?
1. Bulbourethral gland
2. Epididymis
3. Prostate gland
4. Seminal vesicle

Situation: Miss Jenner has chronic renal failure. Questions 218 through 222 refer to this situation.

218 Miss Jenner is not responding to treatment. Dialysis may be performed to remove waste products from the blood. The main indication for dialysis is:
1. Increase in blood pressure
2. High and rising potassium levels
3. Ascites
4. Acidosis

219 The artificial kidney machine primarily makes use of the physical principle of:
1. Filtration
2. Osmosis
3. Diffusion
4. Dialysis

220 Miss Jenner, who is on hemodialysis for chronic renal failure, is especially prone to develop:
1. Peritonitis
2. Renal calculi
3. Bladder infection
4. Serum hepatitis

221 In caring for Miss Jenner, who has had an arteriovenous shunt inserted for hemodialysis, the nurse would:
1. Notify the physician if a bruit is heard in the cannula
2. Use strict aseptic technique when giving shunt care
3. Cover the entire cannula with an elastic bandage
4. Take the blood pressure every 4 hours from the arm that contains the shunt

222 A nurse working in a hemodialysis unit runs a high risk of developing:
1. Type A viral hepatitis
2. Infectious hepatitis
3. Type B viral hepatitis
4. Hemolytic hepatitis

Situation: Mr. Carson is hospitalized with severe right flank pain, general weakness, and fever. He has a history of recurrent urinary tract infection, and the formation of renal calculi is suspected. The physician orders a 200-mg calcium diet for 3 days to be monitored with urinary calcium tests. Questions 223 through 228 refer to this situation.

223 In caring for patients with renal calculi, the most important nursing action is to:
1. Record blood pressure
2. Strain all urine
3. Limit fluids at night
4. Administer analgesics every 3 hours

224 What background knowledge helps the nurse understand the reasons for this strict 200-mg calcium diet?
1. Excessive calcium intake has little influence on renal stone formation
2. The thyroid hormone controls the serum levels of calcium and phosphorus
3. If calcium excretion is lowered on the test diet, hyperparathyroidism can be identified as the cause of the calculi
4. If calcium excretion is still elevated on the test diet, dietary influences can be ruled out

225 Mr. Carson's calcium balance studies following his test diet are negative. His diet order is increased to 400 mg calcium—a general low-calcium diet level. Which of the following foods would be allowed on his diet?
1. Vanilla ice cream with chocolate syrup and nuts
2. Salmon loaf with cheese sauce
3. Chocolate pudding
4. Roast beef with baked potato

226 The name of the procedure for the removal of a bladder stone is:
1. Cystolithiasis
2. Cystolithectomy
3. Cystometry
4. Cryoextraction

227 Diet therapy for renal calculi of calcium phosphate composition would probably be:

1. High calcium and phosphorus, alkaline ash
2. High calcium and phosphorus, acid ash
3. Low purine
4. Low calcium and phosphorus, acid ash

228 A patient with renal stones of calcium oxalate composition would need a diet:
1. Low in calcium and oxalate, acid ash
2. Low in calcium and oxalate, alkaline ash
3. Low in methionine, acid ash
4. Low in purines, alkaline ash

229 Mr. Andrews will be taking sulfisoxazole (Gantrisin) at home. The nurse instructs him to:
1. Measure and record urine output
2. Strain urine for crystals and stones
3. Maintain the exact time schedule for drugtaking
4. Stop the drug if his urinary output increases

Situation: Mrs. Harvey has an acute episode of right-sided heart failure and is receiving furosemide (Lasix). Questions 230 through 236 refer to this situation.

230 The physician has prescribed aspirin for her arthritic pain. When Mrs. Harvey asks why she is not receiving the same aspirin dosage she usually takes, the nurse's response would be based on knowledge that:
1. Aspirin in large doses after an acute stress episode increases the bleeding potential
2. Use of furosemide and aspirin concomitantly increases formation of uric acid crystals in the nephron
3. Competition for renal excretion sites by the drugs causes increased serum levels of aspirin
4. Aspirin accelerates metabolism of furosemide and decreases the diuretic effect

231 The symptoms that Mrs. Harvey most likely displayed on admission are:
1. Dyspnea, edema, fatigue
2. Weakness, palpitations, nausea
3. Fatigue, vertigo, and headache
4. A feeling of distress when breathing

232 Mrs. Harvey has edema during the day and it disappears at night. The patient states it is not painful and is located in the lower extremities. The nurse should suspect:
1. Pulmonary edema
2. Right-sided heart failure
3. Myocardial infarction
4. Lung disease

233 Pitting edema in the lower extremities occurs with right-sided heart failure because of the:
1. Increase in tissue colloid osmotic pressure
2. Increase in the tissue hydrostatic pressure at the arterial end of the capillary bed
3. Decrease in the plasma colloid osmotic pressure
4. Increase in the plasma hydrostatic pressure at the venous end of the capillary beds

234 The nurse can best assess the degree of edema in an extremity by:
1. Checking for pitting
2. Weighing the patient
3. Measuring the affected area
4. Observing intake and output

235 The nurse notes that Mrs. Harvey's abdomen is distended. The nurse should realize that the patient with congestive heart failure develops ascites because of:
1. Increased pressure within the circulatory system
2. Rapid diffusion of solutes and solvents into plasma
3. Rapid osmosis from tissue spaces to cells
4. Loss of cellular constituents in blood

236 Mrs. Harvey's condition worsens. The physician has ordered CVP readings q 2 h. Which of the following is true of CVP?
1. A high reading may be indicative of dehydration
2. A normal reading is 60 to 120 mm of water
3. The zero point of the manometer is level with the midaxilla
4. The patient must be kept flat in bed while the catheter is in place

237 Which of the following is most likely to occur in a patient with unresolved edema?
1. Thrombi formation
2. Tissue ischemia
3. Proteinemia
4. Contractures

238 The mercurial diuretics alter active transport systems in the kidney tubules, resulting in increased excretion of sodium and, secondarily, water. The principle explaining the secondary water loss (diuresis) is:
1. Osmosis
2. Diffusion
3. Filtration
4. Active transport

239 Mrs. Johnson has a urinary tract infection and is receiving chlorothiazide (Diuril). The planned therapeutic effect of the drug is to:
1. Decrease the amount of fluid reabsorption in Henle's loop
2. Increase the excretion of sodium and chloride
3. Decrease the reabsorption of potassium
4. Increase the glomerular filtration rate

240 Shock is:
1. Failure of peripheral circulation
2. An irreversible phenomenon
3. Always caused by decreased blood volume
4. A fleeting reaction to tissue injury

241 Common symptoms of Buerger's disease are:
1. Burning pain precipitated by cold exposure, fatigue, blanching of skin
2. Easy fatigue of part, continuous claudication

3. General blanching of skin, intermittent claudication
4. Intermittent claudication, burning pain after exposure to cold

242 Patients with peripheral vascular disease are instructed to stop smoking because the nicotine:
1. Dilates the peripheral vessels causing a reflex constriction of visceral vessels
2. Constricts the peripheral vessels and increases the force of flow
3. Constricts the collateral circulation, dilating the superficial vessels
4. Constricts the superficial vessels, dilating the deep vessels

243 In chronic occlusive arterial disease the precipitating cause for ulceration and gangrenous lesions often is:
1. Poor hygiene
2. Stimulants such as coffee, tea, or cola drinks
3. Emotions
4. Trauma from mechanical, chemical, or thermal sources

Situation: Mr. Wolfsmith, a 46-year-old executive, is admitted with chest pain and shortness of breath. A diagnosis of myocardial infarction is made. Questions 244 through 251 refer to this situation.

244 Mr. Wolfsmith is placed in the C.C.U., where the nurse will observe for one of the more common complications of myocardial infarction, which is:
1. Cardiac arrhythmia
2. Anaphylactic shock
3. Cardiac enlargement
4. Hypokalemia

245 To ascertain Mr. Wolfsmith's diagnosis, tests for which the nurse would prepare him include:
1. Paul-Bunnell test, serum potassium
2. LDH, CPK, SGOT
3. Sedimentation rate, SGPT
4. Serum calcium, APPT

246 Mr. Wolfsmith is in the coronary unit on a cardiac monitor. The nurse observes ventricular irritability on the screen. The medication the nurse might expect to administer is:
1. Digoxin (Lanoxin)
2. Lidocaine
3. Furosemide (Lasix)
4. Levarterenol bitartrate (Levophed)

247 The nurse observes Mr. Wolfsmith's monitor and identifies asystole. This arrhythmia requires nursing attention because the heart is:
1. Beating very rapidly
2. Not beating
3. Beating irregularly
4. Beating slowly

248 A cardiac arrest code is called for Mr. Wolfsmith. During

a cardiac arrest, the nurse and the arrest team must keep in mind the:
1. Time the patient is anoxic
2. Heart rate of the patient before arrest
3. Age of the patient
4. Emergency medications available

249 When it is discovered that Mr. Wolfsmith has no carotid pulse or respirations, the nurse:
1. Clears the airway
2. Gives 4 full lung inflations
3. Compresses the lower sternum 15 times
4. Checks for a radial pulse

250 There are 2 nurses performing CPR on Mr. Wolfsmith. During performance of cardiopulmonary resuscitation with 2 people, the rate of ventilation to cardiac compression is:
1. 1:5
2. 1:10
3. 2:15
4. 4:15

251 The nurse performing cardiac compression on Mr. Wolfsmith is aware that it is essential to exert a vertical downward pressure, which depresses the lower sternum at least:
1. ½ to ¾ inch (1.3 to 2 cm)
2. ¾ to 1 inch (2 to 2.5 cm)
3. 1 to 1½ inches (2.5 to 4 cm)
4. 1½ to 2 inches (4 to 5 cm)

252 Blood samples from the right atrium, right ventricle, and pulmonary artery are analyzed for their oxygen content during cardiac catheterization. Normally:
1. All contain about the same amount of oxygen
2. All contain less CO_2 than does pulmonary vein blood
3. Pulmonary artery blood contains more oxygen than the other samples
4. All contain more oxygen than does pulmonary vein blood

253 Many vitamins and minerals regulate the many chemical changes of cell metabolism by acting in a coenzyme role. This means that the vitamin or mineral:
1. May become a structural part of the enzyme controlling a particular reaction
2. May be a necessary catalyst present for the reaction to proceed
3. Forms a new compound by a series of complex changes
4. Prevents unnecessary reactions by neutralizing the controlling enzyme

254 Because fat is insoluble in water, it cannot travel freely in the blood. Therefore the main type of compound formed to serve as a vehicle of transport is:
1. Triglyceride
2. Plasma protein
3. Phospholipid
4. Lipoprotein

255 The food group lowest in natural sodium is:
1. Meat
2. Milk
3. Vegetables
4. Fruits

256 The terms *saturated* and *unsaturated,* when used in reference to fats, indicate degrees of:
1. Color
2. Taste
3. Hardness
4. Digestibility

257 When the transport fat compounds accumulate in abnormal levels in the blood, the diet may be modified as one effort to control them. The foods most affected by such diet therapy would be:
1. Vegetable oils
2. Fruits
3. Grains
4. Animal fats

258 The breakdown of triglyceride molecules can be expected to produce:
1. Urea nitrogen
2. Amino acids
3. Simple sugars
4. Fatty acids

259 Cholesterol is important in the human body for:
1. Bone formation
2. Blood clotting
3. Cellular membrane structure
4. Muscle contraction

260 Cholesterol is frequently discussed in relation to atherosclerosis. It is a substance that:
1. All persons would be better off without because it causes the disease process
2. Circulates in the blood, the level of which responds usually to dietary substitutions of unsaturated fats for saturated fats
3. Is found in many foods, both plant and animal sources
4. May be controlled entirely by eliminating food sources

Situation: Mrs. Smith is admitted to the hospital with a diagnosis of possible bronchogenic carcinoma. Questions 261 through 268 refer to this situation.

261 Which of the following is linked to a higher incidence of bronchogenic carcinoma?
1. Asbestos fibers
2. Carbon tetrachloride
3. Polyvinyl chloride
4. Ultraviolet radiation

262 To evaluate Mrs. Smith's lung capacity, the physician orders pulmonary function tests. The instrument used to measure this capacity is the:
1. Tenometer
2. Blow bottle

3. Ventilator
4. Spirometer

263 During the pulmonary function test the respiratory therapist asks Mrs. Smith to breathe normally. She is probably measuring Mrs. Smith's:
1. Vital capacity
2. Tidal volume
3. Inspiratory reserve
4. Expiratory reserve

264 When Mrs. Smith returns to the room following a bronchoscopy and biopsy, she is fully awake. The nurse should:
1. Advise her to stay flat in bed for 2 hours
2. Provide ice chips to reduce swelling
3. Encourage her to cough frequently
4. Evaluate the presence of a gag reflex

265 Mrs. Smith's diagnosis of bronchogenic carcinoma is confirmed and a right pneumonectomy is performed. During surgery the phrenic nerve is severed to:
1. Produce an atonic diaphragm
2. Limit the postoperative pain considerably
3. Allow the diaphragm to rise and partially fill the space
4. Permit greater excursion of the thoracic cavity

266 Mrs. Smith returns from surgery to the intensive care unit with an endotracheal tube in place. Which of the following would be the most effective way for the nurse to loosen Mrs. Smith's secretions?
1. Administration of fluids
2. Pulmonary toileting
3. Administration of humidified O_2
4. Instillation of SSKI into the endotracheal tube

267 When positioning Mrs. Smith postoperatively, which position would be most beneficial?
1. Right side with head slightly elevated
2. Left Sims with the head of the bed elevated 45 degrees
3. High Fowler's
4. Flat in bed with knees flexed slightly

268 The nurse should palpate Mrs. Smith's trachea at least once a day because:
1. Tracheal edema may lead to an obstructed airway
2. The position may indicate mediastinal shift
3. Nodular lesions may demonstrate metastasis
4. The cuff of the endotracheal tube may be overinflated

269 Cutting the left phrenic nerve:
1. Is done to relieve pain in the left side of the chest
2. Paralyzes the left side of the diaphragm
3. Collapses the right lung
4. Paralyzes the diaphragm on the opposite side

Situation: Mr. Psanka is admitted from the emergency room in acute respiratory distress resulting from an asthmatic attack. Questions 270 through 276 refer to this situation.

270 In which position should the nurse place Mr. Psanka to facilitate maximum air exchange?
1. High Fowler's
2. Semi-Fowler's
3. Orthopneic
4. Supine with pillows

271 Inhalation of isoproterenol (Isuprel), 1:200 prn, is prescribed for which of the following reasons?
1. To increase bronchial secretions
2. To decrease blood pressure
3. To produce sedation
4. To relax bronchial spasm

272 During therapy with isoproterenol Mr. Psanka complains of palpitation, chest pain, and a throbbing headache. In view of these symptoms, which of the following statements represents the most appropriate nursing action?
1. Reassure Mr. Psanka that these effects are temporary and will subside as he becomes accustomed to the drug
2. Withhold the drug until additional orders are obtained from the physician
3. Tell him not to worry; he is experiencing expected side effects from the medicine
4. Ask him to relax; then instruct him to breathe slowly and deeply for several minutes

273 Mr. Psanka's pulmonary function studies are abnormal. The nurse should realize that one of the most common complications of chronic asthma is:
1. Atelectasis
2. Emphysema
3. Pneumothorax
4. Pulmonary fibrosis

274 Emphysema causes a failure in oxygen supply because of:
1. Infectious obstructions
2. Respiratory muscle paralysis
3. Pleural effusion
4. Loss of aerating surface

275 When the alveoli lose their normal elasticity, the nurse teaches Mr. Psanka exercises that lead to effective use of the diaphragm because:
1. Mr. Psanka has an increase in the vital capacity of his lungs
2. The residual capacity of the lungs has been increased
3. Inspiration has been markedly prolonged and difficult
4. Abdominal breathing is an effective compensatory mechanism that is spontaneously initiated

276 Respiratory acidosis may occur as a result of a long-term problem in oxygen maintenance when:
1. The carbon dioxide is not excreted
2. Any localized tissue necrosis occurs as a result of poor oxygen supply to the area
3. Hyperventilation occurs, even if the cause is not physiologic
4. There is a loss of carbon dioxide from the body's buffer pool

277 Air rushes into the alveoli as a result of:
1. The rising pressure in the alveoli
2. The rising pressure in the pleura
3. The lowered pressure in the chest cavity
4. The relaxation of the diaphragm

278 A nurse will use an Ambu bag in the Intensive Care Unit when:
1. The patient is in ventricular fibrillation
2. A surgical incision with copious drainage is present
3. Respiratory output must be monitored at intervals
4. There is respiratory arrest

279 In suctioning a tracheostomy the nurse must remember that it is important to:
1. Initiate suction as the catheter is being withdrawn slowly
2. Insert catheter until cough reflex is stimulated
3. Untie the neck tapes while cleansing the skin edge of the wound
4. Remove the inner cannula before inserting the suction catheter

280 A patient has an anaphylactic reaction within the first half hour after an IV infusion containing penicillin is started. Problems occurring during an anaphylactic reaction are the result of:
1. Decreased cardiac output and dilation of major blood vessels
2. Bronchial constriction and decreased peripheral resistance
3. Respiratory depression and cardiac standstill
4. Constriction of capillaries and decreased cardiac output

281 Occurrence of an anaphylactic reaction after receiving penicillin indicates that a patient has:
1. An acquired atopic sensitization
2. Passive immunity to the penicillin allergen
3. Antibodies to penicillin acquired after prior use of the drug
4. Developed potent bivalent antibodies when the IV administration was started

282 A patient has an urticarial response after taking ampicillin (Polycillin) orally for 3 days. Diphenhydramine hydrochloride (Benadryl) is administered to:
1. Destroy histamine in tissues and reverse the urticarial response
2. Inhibit release of vasoactive substances and dilate tissue capillaries
3. Metabolize histamine and inhibit release of substances causing intense itching
4. Compete with histamine for receptors and interfere with vasodilation

283 This patient may also be given penicillinase (Neutrapen) to:
1. Displace penicillin from receptor sites
2. Counteract the effects of penicillin in tissues

3. Destroy the penicillin allergen
4. Maintain therapy with a nonallergenic form of penicillin

284 The most important aspect of hand washing is:
1. Water
2. Soap
3. Friction
4. Time

285 Vitamin K is essential for normal blood clotting because it promotes:
1. Ionization of blood calcium
2. Platelet aggregation
3. Fibrinogen formation by liver
4. Prothrombin formation by liver

286 Prophylaxis for serum hepatitis includes:
1. Enteric precautions applied to infected individuals
2. Screening of blood donors
3. Case finding and treatment of infection
4. Patient isolation

287 In the patient with serum hepatitis the earliest indication of parenchymal damage to the liver usually is:
1. Elevation in transaminase
2. Rise in bilirubin
3. Alteration in proteins
4. Rise in alkaline phosphatase

Situation: Mrs. Carter, the mother of 2 children, has infectious hepatitis. Questions 288 through 290 refer to this situation.

288 Mrs. Carter's children are being given gamma globulin to provide passive immunity, which:
1. Stimulates production of short-lived antibodies
2. Stimulates the lymphatic system to produce large numbers of antibodies
3. Provides antibodies that neutralize the antigen
4. Accelerates antigen-antibody union at hepatic sites

289 The physician has prescribed phenobarbital sodium (Luminal) for Mrs. Carter. The nurse tells Mrs. Carter to contact the physician if she notices:
1. Decreased tolerance to common foods, constipation
2. Diarrhea, rash on the upper part of her body
3. Anal pruritus, orthostatic hypotension
4. Loss of appetite, persistent lethargy

290 When caring for Mrs. Carter the nurse should take special precautions to:
1. Use caution when bringing food tray to patient
2. Wear mask and gown before entering the room
3. Use gloves when removing the patient's bedpan
4. Prevent droplet spread of infection

Situation: Mr. Bunger, age 45, has been aware of a mass in his right cheek and upper neck for several years. Although the mass had become increasingly noticeable, he did not seek medical attention. As a result of an extensive campaign in his community, he made an appointment at a local hospital for a cancer detection examination. Mr. Bunger was informed by the physician that he should be hospitalized for surgery immediately for a tumor involving the parotid gland. Questions 291 through 294 refer to this situation.

291 Although the physician has explained the possible extent of surgery, the patient is still quite anxious. Nursing intervention should be aimed at:
1. Attempting to discover what is bothering the patient
2. Elaborating on what the physician has already told the patient
3. Planning for postoperative communication, since a tracheotomy is likely to be performed
4. Teaching the patient to use the suction equipment preoperatively

292 On surgical intervention the tumor proves to be malignant, and right total parotidectomy is performed. The most distressing complication from the patient's point of view is:
1. Tracheostomy
2. Facial nerve dysfunction
3. Frey syndrome
4. Salivation

293 Postoperatively Mr. Bunger is kept in a high Fowler's position to:
1. Promote drainage of the wound
2. Prevent venous oozing from the incision
3. Prevent strain on the incision
4. Provide comfort for the patient

294 When Mr. Bunger complains of his dressings being too tight, the best nursing intervention involves:
1. Checking the dressings for signs of bleeding
2. Checking the dressings for signs of constriction
3. Informing the patient that the tight dressings serve a purpose
4. Altering the dressings to relieve this sensation

---

295 GI bleeding can be treated medically by infusing medication through an arterial line. The drug commonly used for this purpose is:
1. Phytonadione (Aquamephyton)
2. Neostigmine (Prostigmin)
3. Propantheline (Pro-Banthine)
4. Vasopressin (Pitressin)

296 A patient who may develop pernicious anemia is one who:
1. Has diabetes
2. Had a gastrectomy
3. Has hemorrhaged
4. Practices poor dietary habits

297 An antrectomy would most likely be done for a patient with a diagnosis of:
1. Trigeminal neuralgia
2. Otosclerosis
3. Gastric ulcers
4. Cataracts

Situation: Dr. Grove, a single, 25-year-old professor of mathematics at a major university, is hospitalized for bleeding gastric ulcers. A conservative regimen is being followed at present. At an early age it became apparent that Dr. Grove was a genius. His capabilities were encouraged to develop to their fullest potential by his mother. He graduated from high school summa cum laude at the age of 13 and at the age of 19 had received a Ph.D. in mathematics. Dr. Grove lives at home with his aging mother. Questions 298 through 302 refer to this situation.

298 Dr. Grove describes his pain as:
1. A dull ache radiating to the left side
2. An intermittent colicky flank pain
3. A generalized abdominal pain intensified by moving
4. A gnawing sensation relieved by food

299 Analysis of factors resulting in psychologic conflict for Dr. Grove reveals:
1. Unconscious concern with independence, success, and activity
2. The drive to excel in whatever he does
3. Conversion of emotional tension due to chronic repressed hostility
4. Many feelings that are unconscious but near the surface

300 Despite initiation of therapy, Dr. Grove continues to be apprehensive and restless. Nursing action will include:
1. Telling him everything will be all right
2. Administering antibiotics as ordered
3. Explaining the importance of rest
4. Administering sedatives as ordered

301 Dr. Grove's conservative dietary regimen has which basic goal?
1. To increase roughage and bulk
2. To eliminate chemical, mechanical, and thermal irritation
3. To provide optimum amounts of all nutrients
4. To provide psychologic support by offering a wide variety of foods

302 If Dr. Grove has lost enough blood to develop a mild anemia, which of the following drugs may be used in treatment of this condition?
1. Dextran
2. Carbacrylamine resins (Carbo-Resin)
3. Salts of iron
4. Vitamin B_{12}

---

303 Persons having prolonged anemia or polycythemia may eventually place a strain on their heart. The concept underlying this strain is:
1. Pressure
2. Surface tension
3. Viscosity
4. Temperature

304 In caring for the patient with an ileostomy the nurse would:
1. Expect the stoma to start draining on the third post-operative day
2. Explain that the drainage can be controlled with daily irrigations
3. Anticipate that emotional stress can increase intestinal peristalsis
4. Encourage the patient to eat foods high in residue

305 If the ileum is removed surgically, the individual may suffer from anemia because:
1. The hemopoietic factor is only absorbed in the terminal ileum
2. Folic acid is only absorbed in the terminal ileum
3. Iron absorption is dependent on simultaneous bile salt absorption in the terminal ileum
4. The trace elements copper, cobalt, and nickel, required for hemoglobin synthesis, only occur in the ileum

306 Which of the following types of sports should a patient with an ileostomy avoid?
1. Track events
2. Swimming
3. Skiing
4. Football

307 How far into the rectum should a rectal catheter be inserted?
1. 2 inches (5 cm)
2. 4 inches (10 cm)
3. 6 inches (15 cm)
4. 8 inches (20 cm)

308 A rectal tube is sometimes inserted for the relief of distention. What is the minimal time it should remain in place to be effective?
1. 15 minutes
2. 30 minutes
3. 45 minutes
4. 60 minutes

Situation: Mrs. Graham has a diagnosis of possible bowel obstruction. She complains of nausea, is vomiting dark bile material, and has severe crampy, intermittent, abdominal pain. Her physician suspects the bowel obstruction is caused by an intussusception. Questions 309 through 315 refer to this situation.

309 An intussusception is:
1. Kinking of the bowel onto itself
2. Telescoping of a proximal loop of bowel into a distal loop
3. A band of connective tissue compressing the bowel
4. A protrusion of an organ or part of an organ through the wall that contains it

310 A flat plate radiograph of the abdomen is ordered. The nurse recognizes that the patient should receive:
1. Nothing by mouth for 8 hours
2. A low soapsuds enema

3. No special preparation
4. A laxative the evening before the x-ray film is taken

311 Surgery is performed; Mrs. Graham is found to have a perforated appendix with localized peritonitis rather than an intussusception. In view of this finding, how would the nurse position Mrs. Graham postoperatively?
1. Semi-Fowler's
2. Trendelenburg
3. Sims
4. Dorsal recumbent

312 Four days after surgery Mrs. Graham has not passed any flatus and there are no bowel sounds. Despite the fact that her abdomen has become increasingly more distended, there is little discomfort. Paralytic ileus is suspected. In this condition there is an interference caused by:
1. Impaired blood supply
2. Impaired neural functioning
3. Perforation of the bowel wall
4. Obstruction of the bowel lumen

313 Mrs. Graham is convalescing from abdominal surgery when she develops thrombophlebitis. Which of the following signs would indicate this complication to the nurse?
1. Severe pain on extension of extremity
2. Pitting edema of lower extremities
3. Intermittent claudication
4. Warm, tender area on leg

314 Mrs. Graham is receiving Dicumarol, a coumarin derivative. Which of the following tests would be most specific for calculating daily dosage of anticoagulant?
1. Prothrombin time
2. Clotting time
3. Bleeding time
4. Sedimentation rate

315 Which of the following drugs would you expect the physician to order if symptoms of overdose of Dicumarol are observed?
1. Iron-dextran (Imferon)
2. Heparin
3. Vitamin K
4. Protamine sulfate

Situation: Alice, a 45-year-old college student, is admitted to the hospital for diabetic acidosis. Questions 316 through 322 refer to this situation.

316 The cause of Alice's symptoms is a:
1. Sudden increase in the concentration of cholesterol in the extracellular compartment
2. Physiologic phenomenon following the ingestion of too much highly acidic food
3. Rise in the pH of the blood to a point above 7.5
4. Decrease in the pH of the blood to a point below 7.3

317 Several laboratory tests are done. Alice's symptoms lead the nurse to expect the blood test to reveal:

1. Low sugar, decreased acidity, low CO_2 combining power
2. Elevated sugar, normal acidity, high CO_2 combining power
3. Elevated sugar, increased acidity, low CO_2 combining power
4. Low sugar, increased acidity, high CO_2 combining power

318 The type of insulin that will be used during the emergency treatment of the acidosis and until Alice is eating regularly is:
   1. Isophane insulin suspension (NPH insulin)
   2. Insulin injection (regular insulin)
   3. Insulin zinc suspension (lente insulin)
   4. Protamine zinc insulin suspension

319 After blood studies and observation of urinary volume, the physician orders potassium chloride, 20 mEq, to be added to the IV solution. The primary purpose for administering this drug to Alice is:
   1. Replacement of potassium deficit
   2. Treatment of hyperpnea
   3. Prevention of flaccid paralysis
   4. Treatment of cardiac arrhythmias

320 In the exchange system of dietary management, which of the following is not equivalent?
   1. 1 scoop ice milk = 1 slice bread
   2. 1 oz cheese = 1 cup milk
   3. 1 egg = 1 oz meat
   4. 1 slice bacon = 2 Tbsp cream

321 Alice and her family members should be taught the use of glucagon. The primary use of glucagon is to treat:
   1. Diabetic acidosis
   2. Insulin-induced hypoglycemia
   3. Idiosyncratic reactions to insulin
   4. Hyperinsulin secretion related to neoplasm

322 Alice's nursing plan includes that before discharge she will know how to give herself insulin, adjust the dosage, understand her diet, and test her urine. She progresses well and is discharged 10 days following admission. Legally:
   1. The physician was responsible and the nurse should have cleared her care with him
   2. The nurse was properly functioning as a health teacher
   3. The visiting nurse should do health teaching in the home
   4. A family member should have been taught also to administer the insulin

---

323 The main function of adipose tissue in fat metabolism is synthesizing:
   1. Lipoproteins for fat transport
   2. And storing triglycerides for energy reserves
   3. Cholesterol as needed
   4. And releasing glucose for energy

324 An individual with diabetes is brought to a hospital in a coma and is given an IV containing insulin, glucose, and potassium. Potassium in the extracellular fluid must be replenished because it:
   1. Is carried with glucose to the kidneys and excreted in the urine in increased amounts
   2. Enters the intracellular fluid due to the generalized anabolism induced by insulin and glucose
   3. Is rapidly lost from the body by copious diaphoresis present during coma
   4. Is quickly used up during the rapid series of catabolic reactions stimulated by insulin and glucose

325 When teaching a patient about an oral hypoglycemic medication, the nurse should emphasize the significance of:
   1. Manifestations of toxicity
   2. Untoward reactions
   3. Taking it regularly and on time
   4. Increasing dosage when necessary

326 Which of the following represents a normal pH for arterial blood?
   1. 7.0
   2. 7.30
   3. 7.42
   4. 7.50

Situation: Mr. Pierce, a patient who has acromegaly and diabetes mellitus, has had a hypophysectomy. Questions 327 through 331 refer to this situation.

327 An oversecretion of which hormone produces acromegaly?
   1. Growth hormone
   2. Thyroid hormone
   3. Thyroid-stimulating hormone
   4. Testosterone

328 Which of the following will not be true of Mr. Pierce following his hypophysectomy and should be included in his teaching plan by the nurse? He will:
   1. Be sterile for the rest of his life
   2. Have to take cortisone (or similar preparation) for the rest of his life
   3. Have to take thyroxin (or similar preparation) for the rest of his life
   4. Require larger doses of insulin than he did preoperatively

329 Increased blood concentration of cortisol (hydroxycortisone):
   1. Decreases anterior pituitary secretion of ACTH
   2. Makes the body less able to resist stress successfully
   3. Tends to accelerate wound healing
   4. Tends to decrease liver gluconeogenesis

330 Following the hypophysectomy the nurse should observe Mr. Pierce for signs of:
   1. Urinary retention

2. Bleeding at suture site
3. Increased intracranial pressure
4. Respiratory distress

331 The nurse knows that most of the hormones present in the body at any given time were secreted from the endocrine glands:
1. 24 hours ago
2. 4 to 6 hours ago
3. More than 72 hours ago
4. 8 to 12 hours ago

Situation: Mrs. Lamb is 39 years of age and has 3 children, ages 12, 9, and 5 years. She was admitted to the hospital with the diagnosis of severe metrorrhagia and menorrhagia of 1-year duration. She was found to have a submucous myoma that had grown over the past 6 months. Mrs. Lamb was told that a hysterectomy was necessary. Questions 332 through 336 refer to this situation.

332 The term metrorrhagia refers to:
1. Periods of bleeding between menstrual periods
2. Severe bleeding during each menstrual period
3. Presence of blood in vaginal discharge
4. Spotting or staining after intercourse

333 To provide preoperative teaching the nurse should know that after a hysterectomy:
1. Ovarian hormone secretion ceases, but the hypophysis continues secretion of gonadotrophic hormones
2. The cyclical oscillation of hormones between the hypophysis and ovaries continues
3. Menstruation ceases and ovarian hormone secretion decreases
4. Menopause begins immediately with the cessation of ovarian hormone production

334 Mrs. Lamb is recovering from the hysterectomy. Which of the following signs would be indicative of a developing thrombophlebitis?
1. Reddened area at ankle
2. Pruritus on calf and thigh
3. Pitting edema of the ankle
4. A tender, painful area on leg

335 As the nurse walks into Mrs. Lamb's room on the fifth postoperative day, the patient asks for sanitary pads because she feels like she is going to menstruate. The nurse's response is based on knowledge of which of the following statements?
1. Mrs. Lamb will have a surgical menopause
2. It will take several weeks before Mrs. Lamb will have a normal menstrual flow
3. Mrs. Lamb is showing signs of psychosomatic responses
4. The postoperative appearance of frank vaginal bleeding is expected

336 A patient with a hysterectomy and oophorectomy has an artificial onset of menopause. Estrogen therapy is often instituted to suppress symptoms. These include:
1. Heat intolerance
2. Flushing of the face
3. Premature aging
4. Dysmenorrhea

---

337 Mrs. Peters enters the hospital for exploratory abdominal surgery. She is 3 months pregnant and has been informed that there are many dangers involved. The nurse has her sign a consent form for an exploratory laparotomy. Cancer of the uterus is discovered and a hysterectomy is performed. On returning from surgery Mrs. Peters is informed that her uterus was removed. She sues the hospital, the surgeon, and the nurse. The decision in this case will be based on the fact that:
1. The patient received inadequate information to give consent
2. The surgeon has the legal right to do what was deemed necessary in surgery
3. General consent forms signed on admission are sufficient
4. Consent for exploratory surgery implies permission for removing organs if this is justified

338 Which one of the following operative procedures would result in surgical menopause?
1. Bilateral oophorectomy
2. Partial hysterectomy
3. Bilateral salpingectomy
4. Tubal ligation

339 Hot flashes are caused by:
1. Overstimulation of adrenal medulla
2. Accumulation of acetylcholine
3. Cessation of pituitary gonadotropins
4. Hormonal stimulation of sympathetic system

340 Menopause is the cessation of menstrual function. One of the reasons given is:
1. An increase in the secretion of progesterone from the follicles in the ovary
2. A decrease in the production of prostaglandins
3. The inability of the ovary to respond to gonadotropic hormones
4. A decrease in gonadotropin in the blood

341 Ovulation occurs when:
1. The blood levels of FSH and LH are high
2. The endometrial wall is sloughed off
3. Progesterone level is high
4. Oxytocin level is high

342 High concentration of estrogens in the blood:
1. Causes ovulation
2. Inhibits anterior pituitary secretions of FSH
3. Is one of the causes of osteoporosis
4. Stimulates lactation

Situation: Mr. Davis is a 55-year-old man who has suffered a cerebral vascular accident. He has right-sided paralysis and is dysphagic and dysphasic. His nursing care includes frequent monitoring of vital signs. Questions 343 through 349 refer to this situation.

343 Mr. Davis' temperature should be taken:
  1. Orally
  2. In the groin
  3. Rectally
  4. In the axilla

344 Mr. Davis is experiencing difficulty in:
  1. Swallowing
  2. Focusing
  3. Writing
  4. Understanding

345 Mr. Davis' dysphasia requires initial provision for:
  1. Routine hygienic needs
  2. Prevention of aspiration
  3. Effective communication
  4. Liquid formula diet

346 Blood pressure should not be taken on Mr. Davis' right arm because circulatory impairment may:
  1. Precipitate the formation of a thrombus
  2. Hinder restoration of function
  3. Produce inaccurate readings
  4. Cause excessive pressure on the brachial artery

347 Three days after admission Mr. Davis has a nasogastric tube inserted and is prescribed a liquid formula diet 6 times daily. For the first day the amount of liquid administered at one time should not exceed:
  1. 150 ml
  2. 350 ml
  3. 450 ml
  4. 250 ml

348 The formula temperature most compatible for administration is:
  1. Chilled
  2. Body
  3. Room
  4. 108° F (42° C)

349 The nurse should administer the tube feeding slowly to reduce the hazard of:
  1. Indigestion
  2. Regurgitation
  3. Flatulence
  4. Distention

350 The optic chiasm:
  1. Receives nerve impulses from the optic tracts
  2. Is the space posterior to the lens with the consistency of jelly
  3. Is a crossing of some optic nerves in the cranial cavity
  4. Is the cavity in which the eyeball is fixed

351 A feeling of pleasantness or unpleasantness, varying in degree from mild to intense, occurs when sensory impulses reach the:
  1. Basal ganglia
  2. Cerebral cortex
  3. Hypothalamus
  4. Thalamus

352 An arterial anastomosis present at the base of the brain is the:
  1. Volar arch
  2. Brachiocephalic sinus
  3. Circle of Willis
  4. Brachial plexus

353 Which part of the ear contains the receptors for hearing?
  1. Cochlea
  2. Middle ear
  3. Tympanic cavity
  4. Utricle

354 The ear bones that transmit vibrations to the oval window of the cochlea are found in the:
  1. Outer ear
  2. Inner ear
  3. Middle ear
  4. Eustachian tube

355 An injury or infection that would cause nerve deafness would most likely be to the:
  1. Cochlear nerve
  2. Vestibular nerve
  3. Trigeminal nerve
  4. Vagus nerve

356 The medulla has centers for:
  1. Control of sexual development
  2. Fat metabolism, temperature regulation, water balance
  3. Voluntary movements, taste, skin sensations
  4. Control of breathing, heart beat, blood vessel diameter

357 The part of the brain that exerts reflex control of respiration is the:
  1. Medulla
  2. Cerebral cortex
  3. Hypothalamus
  4. Cerebellum

358 A labyrinthectomy is frequently performed to treat Meniere's syndrome. The result of this procedure is:
  1. Absence of pain
  2. Permanent deafness
  3. Anosmia
  4. Reduction of tinnitus

359 Otosclerosis is the most common cause of conductive hearing loss. Which of the following statements is true?
  1. The patient is usually unable to hear bass tones
  2. Air conduction is more effective than bone conduction
  3. Hearing aids usually restore hearing
  4. Stapedectomy is the procedure of choice

Situation: Mr. Bloom, a 56-year-old baker, was admitted to the hospital 5 weeks ago with a fractured skull and concussion. Two weeks after admission he exhibited evidence of increasing intra-cranial pressure. Questions 360 through 365 refer to this situation.

360 Mr. Bloom has been receiving dexamethasone (Decadron) during the past 3 weeks for control of cerebral edema. The planned effect of the drug on his problem is to:
1. Increase fluid removal from tissues
2. Reduce CSF secretion by the choroid plexus
3. Increase elasticity of the ventricle walls
4. Suppress production of antibodies

361 While Mr. Bloom is receiving dexamethasone (Decadron) the nurse is testing his urine for sugar and acetone every 4 hours because the drug:
1. Lowers the renal threshold for glucose
2. Mobilizes liver stores of glycogen
3. Accelerates protein breakdown and liberates excess glycogen
4. Has a glucose component, which raises the blood sugar level

362 Mr. Bloom is receiving Maalox while he is receiving dex-amethasone. The antacid is prescribed because dexameth-asone is a drug that:
1. Is irritating to the gastric mucosa
2. Stimulates gastric production of hydrochloric acid
3. Increases acidity of the stomach and slows emptying time
4. Increases pepsin-induced erosion of the gastric mucosa

363 Mr. Bloom has several loose bowel movements and the physician changes his antacid prescription to Amphojel. The change is made because:
1. Maalox and dexamethasone act synergistically to in-crease fluid content of the intestine
2. Amphojel increases the bulk of feces and slows peri-stalsis
3. Amphojel neutralizes larger amounts of the hydro-chloric acid that causes diarrhea
4. Maalox contains a magnesium component that stimu-lates peristalsis

364 Mr. Bloom complains about the chalky taste of Amphojel. He states that he would rather take bicarbonate of soda that he takes at home. The nurse tells him it is not advisable to take bicarbonate of soda regularly. Her statement is based on knowledge that bicarbonate of soda:
1. Causes distention by producing carbon dioxide in the stomach
2. Is absorbed from the stomach, and the sodium com-ponent causes ankle edema
3. Is absorbed from the stomach and may cause alkalosis
4. Causes rebound hyperacidity after initial neutralization of hydrochloric acid

365 The physician states he plans to gradually reduce Mr.

Bloom's dexamethasone dosage and to continue him on a lower maintenance dosage during the next few weeks. The nurse explains to the patient that the reason for the gradual dosage reduction is to allow:
1. Production of adrenocorticotropic hormone (ACTH)
2. Return of cortisone production by the adrenal glands
3. Time to observe for return of increased intracranial pressure
4. Building of glycogen and protein stores in liver and muscle

Situation: Mary Jane Lee, age 33, is admitted from the emergency room of General Hospital to the neurologic service with a diagnosis of myasthenia gravis. Questions 366 through 372 refer to this situation.

366 Because of the involvement of the ocular muscles, a com-mon early symptom the nurse should observe for is:
1. Nystagmus
2. Diplopia
3. Blurring
4. Tearing

367 A test that might be performed on Ms. Lee in diagnosing this condition involves the use of which drug?
1. EDTA
2. Edrophonium (Tensilon)
3. Prednisolone
4. Phenytoin (Dilantin)

368 The prognosis of myasthenia gravis is most likely to be:
1. Poor, with termination in a few months
2. Chronic, with exacerbations and remissions
3. Slowly progressive without remissions
4. Excellent with proper treatment

369 The sex and age most frequently affected are:
1. Males ages 15 to 35
2. Females ages 10 to 30
3. Both sexes ages 20 to 40
4. Children ages 5 to 15

370 Ms. Lee is receiving neostigmine bromide (Prostigmin) for control of myasthenia gravis. In the middle of the night the nurse finds her weak, unable to move, and barely breathing. Signs that would identify the problems as being related to overactivity of neostigmine bromide are:
1. High-pitched, gurgling bowel sounds
2. Rapid pulse with occasional ectopic beats
3. Distention of the bladder
4. Fine tremor of the fingers and eyelids

371 Ms. Lee's husband asks the nurse whether his wife will be an invalid. Recognizing the individuality of responses to disease, the best answer would be:
1. ''The progression is slow, so she will spend her young life with few problems.''
2. ''Deformities will occur, but she will not be an in-valid.''

3. "With continuous treatment the disease progression can be controlled."
4. "There will be periods when she is confined to bed rest and times when she can have fairly normal activity."

372 Which one of the following diversional activities would meet the nursing objectives for Ms. Lee during remissions?
1. Watching selected television shows
2. Swimming with the family
3. Teaching sewing classes
4. Short hikes with the family

373 Energy stored as ATP, ADP, and other high-energy compounds is formed chiefly by:
1. Oxidation of glucose
2. Hydrolysis of fats
3. Respiration
4. Peptidation

374 Neostigmine bromide (Prostigmin) is used for the diagnosis of myasthenia gravis because this drug will cause a temporary:
1. Increase in symptoms
2. Drying of the mouth and throat
3. Decrease in blood pressure
4. Increase in muscle strength

Situation: Mrs. Pring, a 34-year-old mother of 5 children, has been diagnosed as having rheumatoid arthritis. Mrs. Pring is being admitted to the hospital because of a recent flare-up of symptoms. She has been taking aspirin and steroids for the past year. Questions 375 through 378 refer to this situation.

375 Daily blood work is ordered for Mrs. Pring during the first 3 days of her hospitalization. Which one of the following symptoms may be indicative of complications of the prolonged use of medications?
1. Elevated sedimentation rate
2. Leukepenia
3. Elevated C-reactive protein
4. Hypochromic, normocytic anemia

376 While taking a nursing history from Mrs. Pring, the nurse promotes communication by:
1. Asking questions that can be answered by a simple "yes" or "no"
2. Telling the patient there is no cause for alarm
3. Asking "why" and "how" questions
4. Using broad, open-ended statements

377 Mrs. Pring questions the nurse as to the source of her disease. The nurse is aware that this is a disease of:
1. Bones
2. Joints
3. Purine metabolism
4. Connective tissue

378 Gold salts may be used to treat rheumatoid arthritis. A serious side effect of this drug is:
1. Cardiac decompensation
2. Kidney damage
3. Persistent nausea
4. Pulmonary emboli

379 Allopurinol is used to treat gout. The objective of therapy is to:
1. Increase uric acid excretion
2. Decrease uric acid production
3. Prevent crystallization of uric acid
4. Decrease synovial swelling

380 One of the drugs that may be prescribed and that has long been known to be of value in the prevention and treatment of acute attacks of gout is:
1. Hydrocortisone
2. Colchicine
3. Phenylbutazone (Butazolidin)
4. Probenecid (Benemid)

381 Systemic lupus erythematous (SLE) is a collagen disease characterized by which of the following signs?
1. Butterfly rash
2. Painful erythema along peripheral nerves
3. Muscle mass degeneration
4. Hypotension and syncope

382 Mrs. Laukhardt is diagnosed as having scleroderma. Although no cause has been determined for this disorder, it is thought to be a defect in:
1. Amino acid metabolism
2. Sebaceous gland formation
3. Autoimmunity
4. Ocular motility

383 Mrs. Laukhardt discusses her prognosis with the nurse. She states, "I'm sure I'll live to a ripe old age. It's not too serious." In responding, the nurse should bear in mind that 50% of the patients with this disease:
1. Recover completely
2. Die within 6 months to 1 year
3. Succumb within 3 years
4. Have extended remissions

Situation: Mrs. Grey is a 45-year-old woman who has been admitted to the hospital with a diagnosis of open-angle chronic glaucoma. Questions 384 through 391 refer to this situation.

384 Which of the following symptoms is Mrs. Grey most likely to exhibit first?
1. A sudden, complete loss of vision
2. Impairment of peripheral vision
3. Sudden attacks of acute pain
4. Constant blurred vision

385 The nurse explains to Mrs. Grey that the chief aim of medical treatment in chronic glaucoma is:
1. Controlling intraocular pressure

2. Dilating the pupil to allow for an increase in the visual field
3. Allowing for healing process by resting the eye
4. Preventing secondary infections that may add to the visual problem

386 When the ciliary muscles contract:
1. They bring about convergence of both eyes
2. They close the eyelids
3. They focus the lens on distant objects
4. They focus the lens on near objects

387 Which of the following would not prove dangerous for Mrs. Grey?
1. Use of sedatives
2. Release of emotions by crying
3. Use of atropine in any form
4. Severe bouts of constipation

388 Mrs. Grey should be advised to:
1. Use eyewashes on a regular basis
2. Use laxatives daily
3. Keep an extra supply of eye medication on hand
4. Have prescriptions filled when necessary

389 Drugs instilled in the eye are said to be administered by which of the following methods?
1. Topical
2. Intraocular
3. Injection
4. Insufflation

390 A systemic drug that may be prescribed to produce diuresis and inhibit formation of aqueous humor is:
1. Acetazolamide (Diamox)
2. Bendroflumethiazide (Naturetin)
3. Chlorothiazide (Diuril)
4. Demecarium bromide (Humorsol)

391 Which one of the following drugs is likely to be prescribed to relieve symptoms if Mrs. Grey develops an inflammatory reaction in the eye?
1. Nitrofurazone (Furacin)
2. Sulfisoxazole (Gantrisin)
3. Neomycin
4. Cortisone

Situation: Miss Renee, 32 years old, is admitted to the emergency room with second-degree burns over 40% of her body and face, which she received when her nightgown caught fire. Questions 392 through 397 refer to this situation.

392 Her condition would be considered:
1. Good
2. Fair
3. Poor
4. Critical

393 Which of the following would not be a problem during the first few hours after the incident?

1. Edema of the larynx and trachea
2. Maintenance of blood volume
3. Rapid decrease in leukocyte count
4. Pain

394 In the immediate shock period after Miss Renee's injury, nutritional care is centered on replacement therapy by IV fluids. Which of the following would *not* be anticipated?
1. Colloid (protein) through blood or plasma transfusions or by use of plasma expanders such as dextran
2. Electrolytes sodium and chloride by use of a saline solution such as lactated Ringer's solution
3. Potassium added to replace losses
4. Water (dextrose solution) to cover additional insensible losses

395 It can be anticipated that the physician will wish to prevent tetanus from developing. If it is impossible to determine whether Miss Renee has been immunized against tetanus, which of the following preparations would produce passive immunization for several weeks with minimal danger of allergic reactions?
1. Tetanus antitoxin
2. Tetanus toxoid
3. Tetanus immune globulin
4. DPT vaccine

396 Sulfisoxazole (Gantrisin), which is often used to combat urinary tract infections, belongs to which of the following groups of drugs?
1. Antibiotics
2. Analgesics
3. Sulfones
4. Sulfonamides

397 When the urinary catheter is removed, Miss Renee continues to be unable to empty her bladder. Drugs used to relieve urinary retention include which of the following?
1. Bethanechol (Urecholine)
2. Pilocarpine hydrochloride
3. Carbachol injection
4. Neosporin

---

398 The best first-aid treatment for acid burns on the skin is to wash them with water and then apply a solution of:
1. Sodium hydroxide
2. Sodium chloride
3. Sodium bicarbonate
4. Sodium sulfate

399 A good first-aid treatment for an alkali (base) burn is to wash it with water and then flood it with:
1. A weak acid
2. A weak base
3. A solution of salt
4. Alcohol

400 The average adult human body has what percent of water?

1. 80
2. 60
3. 40
4. 20

401 The receptors for the regulation of body water through detection of osmotic pressure are located in the:
1. Hypothalamus
2. Neurohypophysis
3. Kidney tubules
4. Blood

402 Which play(s) the major role in maintaining fluid balance?
1. Heart
2. Kidneys
3. Liver
4. Lungs

403 The weight of extracellular body fluid is approximately 20% of the total body weight of an average individual. Which component of the extracellular fluid contributes the greatest portion to this amount?
1. Interstitial fluid
2. Plasma fluid
3. Fluid in body secretions
4. Fluid in dense tissue

404 The most important electrolyte of intracellular fluid is:
1. Calcium
2. Sodium
3. Potassium
4. Chloride

405 Which of the following body fluids make up 40% to 50% of the total body weight?
1. Intracellular
2. Extracellular
3. Intravascular
4. Interstitial

406 Which of the following correctly compares blood plasma and interstitial fluid?
1. Both contain the same kinds of ions
2. Plasma contains slightly more of each kind of ion than does interstitial fluid
3. Plasma exerts lower osmotic pressure than does interstitial fluid
4. The main cation in plasma is sodium, whereas the main cation in interstitial fluid is potassium

407 Which statement is true?
1. Glomeruli are small arteries present in the kidney
2. The volume of urine secreted is regulated mainly by mechanisms that control the glomerular filtration rate
3. An increase in the hydrostatic pressure in Bowman's capsule tends to increase the glomerular filtration rate
4. A decrease in blood protein concentration tends to increase the glomerular filtration rate

408 Which palliative method of urinary divergence is sometimes used for patients with advanced urinary disease?
1. Ileostomy
2. Nephrostomy
3. Cecostomy
4. Ureterostomy

409 The major disadvantage of an ileal conduit is that:
1. Stool continuously oozes from it
2. Absorption of nutrients is diminished
3. Peristalsis is greatly decreased
4. Urine drains from it continuously

410 Which of the following is the *least* accurate method used to estimate drainage postoperatively?
1. Counting saturated 4 × 4-inch gauze pads
2. Measuring drainage that has seeped through the dressing
3. Wringing saturated 4 × 4 pads into a graduated container
4. Weighing saturated dressings

411 Following a left nephrectomy Mrs. Wolfsmith arrives in the recovery room with a plastic airway in place. In observing the patient for signs of hemorrhage, the nurse must be certain to:
1. Keep the patient's nail beds in view at all times
2. Report any increase in blood pressure immediately
3. Observe for hemoptysis when suctioning
4. Turn patient to observe dressings

412 Which of the following nursing actions during the immediate postoperative period has the highest priority?
1. Checking vital signs every 15 minutes
2. Maintaining a patent airway
3. Recording intake and output
4. Observing for hemorrhage

413 In the recovery room, while caring for Mrs. Wolfsmith who has received a general anesthesia, the nurse should notify the physician if:
1. The patient pushes out the airway
2. The respirations are regular but shallow
3. The systolic blood pressure drops from 130 to 100 mm Hg
4. The patient has snoring respirations

414 The physician orders meperidine (Demerol), 50 mg, and atropine, gr 1/150 IM, preoperatively for Mrs. Wolfsmith, who is having a nephrectomy. Knowing that these 2 drugs are compatible and available in multidose vials, the nurse would *best* administer these medications by:
1. Drawing each up in separate syringes
2. Drawing saline to dilute both drugs
3. Drawing up the atropine and then Demerol in the same syringe
4. Drawing up Demerol and then atropine in the same syringe

Situation: Miss Stewart was admitted to the hospital with complaints of hematuria, frequency, urgency, and pain on urination. She stated she has had this problem for several days. Questions 415 through 418 refer to this situation.

415 The admitting diagnosis would most likely be:
1. Cystitis
2. Pyelitis
3. Nephrosis
4. Pyelonephritis

416 Women are more susceptible to this condition primarily because of:
1. Poor hygiene practices
2. Length of the urethra
3. Continuity of the mucous membrane
4. Inadequate fluid intake

417 Miss Stewart is receiving methenamine mandelate (Mandelamine) and ammonium chloride. The primary reason for administering the 2 drugs concurrently is that ammonium chloride:
1. Improves methanamine mandelate effect on bacteria by acidifying the urine
2. Promotes healing of irritated bladder mucosa
3. Interacts with methenamine mandelate to decrease crystal and stone formation
4. Decreases bladder irritation by acidifying the urine

418 Miss Stewart has a higher risk of developing cystitis than does a man. This is due to:
1. Hormonal secretions
2. Length of the urethra
3. Juxtaposition of the bladder
4. Altered urinary pH

Situation: Mr. Everett has been admitted to the C.C.U. with a tentative diagnosis of bundle branch block. Questions 419 through 423 refer to this situation.

419 When observing the patient's cardiac monitor the nurse would expect:
1. Absence of P waves
2. Widening of QRS complex to 0.12 second or greater
3. Inverted T waves
4. Sagging S-T segment

420 The physician has scheduled Mr. Everett for a pacemaker insertion. The pacing catheter will be inserted into a large vein such as the subclavian and advanced so that the electrode is positioned in the:
1. Superior vena cava
2. Left atrium
3. Right ventricle
4. SA node

421 The nurse realizes that a pacemaker is used in some individuals to perform the function normally performed by the:

1. Accelerator nerves to the heart
2. AV node
3. Bundle of His
4. SA node

422 While the pacemaker catheter is being inserted, Mr. Everett's heart rate drops to 38. Which of the following drugs might the nurse expect the physician to order?
1. Digoxin (Lanoxin)
2. Lidocaine
3. Atropine
4. Procainamide

423 The physician has inserted a permanent demand pacemaker. In doing patient teaching, the nurse should:
1. Instruct the patient to sleep on 2 pillows
2. Inform the patient that the pacemaker will function continuously at a set rate
3. Instruct the patient to take his pulse and keep a daily record
4. Encourage the patient to reduce his former level of activity indefinitely

424 Treatment should not be delayed for a patient with:
1. Head injury
2. Ventricular fibrillation
3. Penetrating abdominal wound
4. Fractured femur

425 In charting notes describing a patient's heart rate, the nurse uses the term bradycardia. This describes:
1. A grossly irregular heart rate
2. A heart rate of over 90 per minute
3. A heart beat that has regular "skipped" beats
4. A heart rate of under 60 per minute

Situation: Mr. McNabb, a 65-year-old self-employed grocer, is admitted to the hospital with congestive heart failure and pulmonary edema. His treatment includes oxygen by mask, digoxin, chlorothiazide (Diuril), and a low-sodium diet. He is dyspneic, apprehensive, and restless. Questions 426 through 432 refer to this situation.

426 Mr. McNabb would be most comfortable with the oxygen set at:
1. 12 to 14 L
2. 6 to 8 L
3. 2 to 4 L
4. 16 to 18 L

427 Safety precautions are especially important in Mr. McNabb's room because oxygen:
1. Is flammable
2. Has unstable properties
3. Increases apprehension
4. Supports combustion

428 The nurse attempts to allay Mr. McNabb's anxiety, since restlessness:
1. Decreases the amount of oxygen available

2. Interferes with normal respiration
3. Increases the cardiac workload
4. Produces elevation in temperature

429 When instituting oxygen therapy, the nurse recognizes that the method of oxygen administration least likely to increase apprehension in the patient is:
1. Catheter
2. Cannula
3. Tent
4. Mask

430 After receiving a sedative, Mr. McNabb says to the nurse, "I guess you are too busy to stay with me." The best response in this circumstance is:
1. "I have to see other patients."
2. "The medication will help you rest soon."
3. "I have to go now but I will come back in 10 minutes."
4. "You will feel better; I will adjust your oxygen mask."

431 Before giving Mr. McNabb digoxin, the nurse should measure the:
1. Radial pulse in one arm
2. Apical heart rate
3. Radial pulse in both arms
4. Difference between apical and raidal pulses

432 In addition to its cardiotonic action, the digitalis preparations also promote diuresis. As a result, Mr. McNabb can be seriously depleted of:
1. Calcium
2. Phosphates
3. Potassium
4. Sodium

---

433 Swan-Ganz catheters are inserted to give the medical team information on:
1. Stroke volume
2. Left-sided heart failure
3. Venous pressure
4. Cardiac output

434 Pulmonary edema is most likely to occur in an individual with:
1. Mitral stenosis
2. Calcification and incomplete closure of the tricuspid valve
3. Severe arteriosclerosis of the coronary arteries
4. Pulmonary valve stenosis

Situation: Mr. Singer, a patient with terminal cancer, is in the final stage of his illness. Questions 435 through 441 refer to this situation.

435 Mr. Singer is receiving prednisone and other chemotherapeutic agents and is placed in protective isolation. The administration of corticosteroids to control the symptoms of one disease can cause infections because of all the following except:

1. Interference with the inflammatory response of the body
2. Prevention of the production of leukocytes
3. Promotion of the growth and spread of enteric viruses
4. Stoppage of antibody production in lymphatic tissue

436 During Mr. Singer's chemotherapeutic course, he may develop soreness in the mouth and anus because:
1. The side effects of the chemotherapeutic agents tend to concentrate in these body areas
2. The entire GI tract is involved because of the direct irritating effects of chemotherapy
3. These tissue are poorly nourished because the patient is anorectic
4. These tissues normally divide rapidly and are damaged by the chemotherapeutic agent

437 In caring for Mr. Singer the nurse realizes that sink faucets in his room are considered contaminated because:
1. They are not in sterile areas
2. Water encourages bacterial growth
3. They are opened with dirty hands
4. Large numbers of people use them

438 On one occasion Mr. Singer says to the nurse, "If I could just be free of pain for a few days, I might be able to eat more and regain strength." In reference to the stages of dying, the patient indicates:
1. Rationalization
2. Frustration
3. Bargaining
4. Depression

439 When Mr. Singer reaches the point of acceptance in the stages of dying, it may be manifested in his behavior by:
1. Euphoria
2. Detachment
3. Apathy
4. Emotionalism

440 Mr. Singer drank 7½ oz of orange juice, 6 oz of tea, and 8 oz of eggnog. The calculated intake is:
1. 515 ml
2. 645 ml
3. 625 ml
4. 585 ml

441 The best nursing approach in dealing with Mr. Singer is to:
1. Ignore his behavior
2. Point out the reality of the situation
3. Join him, since denial is his only defense
4. Recognize and accept the behavior at this point

---

442 Characteristic behavior in the initial stage of a patient's coping with dying includes:
1. Asking for an additional medical consultation
2. Ringing a call light as soon as the nurse has left the room
3. Criticism of medical care
4. Sleeping for long periods

443 The family rather than the patient is likely to require more understanding during which stage of dying?
1. Denial
2. Anger
3. Depression
4. Acceptance

444 The nurse can best help a patient in the stage of acceptance by:
1. Allowing unrestricted visiting
2. Being around and not necessarily speaking
3. Explaining all that is being done
4. Allowing the patient to cry

445 A form of folic acid is being administered intramuscularly during intra-arterial chemotherapy with methotrexate. The drug is being administered intramuscularly to:
1. Provide levels of folic acid required by blood-forming organs
2. Provide the metabolite required for destruction of cancer cells
3. Provide folic acid, which acts synergistically with antineoplastic drugs to destroy cancer cells
4. Increase production of phagocytic cells required to remove debris liberated by disintegrating cancer cells

446 Antibiotic therapy is administered along with extensive and prolonged chemotherapy primarily because chemotherapeutic agents destroy rapidly growing cells in the:
1. Blood
2. Lymph
3. Liver
4. Bone marrow

Situation: Mr. Louis, a 36-year-old delicatessen clerk, is admitted with a pulmonary embolism. Questions 447 through 451 refer to this situation.

447 Mr. Louis is receiving an anticoagulant for pulmonary embolism. Which of the following drugs is contraindicated for patients receiving anticoagulants?
1. Isoxsuprine (Vasodilan)
2. Chloral hydrate
3. Chlorpromazine (Thorazine)
4. Aspirin

448 Which of the following actions would the nurse initiate with Mr. Louis as a measure to prevent further emboli?
1. Encourage deep breathing and coughing
2. Use of the knee gatch when positioning the patient
3. Limit the fluid intake of the immobilized patient
4. Encourage patient to move his legs while confined to bed

449 The nurse should observe Mr. Louis for:
1. Headache
2. Epistaxis
3. Nausea
4. Chest pain

450 Mr. Louis begins to expectorate blood. The nurse describes this episode as:

1. Hematuria
2. Hematemesis
3. Hematoma
4. Hemoptysis

451 Mr. Louis becomes dyspneic. In which position should the nurse place him?
1. Trendelenburg
2. Sims
3. Orthopneic
4. Supine

452 Which of the following postoperative patients has the least likelihood of developing pulmonary embolism? The patient with a(n):
1. Prostatectomy
2. Hysterectomy
3. Saphenous vein ligation
4. Appendectomy

453 A bilirubin level above 2 mg/100 ml blood volume could be indicative of:
1. Hemolytic anemia
2. Low oxygen-carrying capacity of erythrocytes
3. Pernicious anemia
4. Decreased rate of red cell destruction

454 One of the main functions of bile is to:
1. Produce an acid condition
2. Provide vitamins
3. Emulsify fats
4. Split protein

Situation: Mrs. Smith, a 45-year-old, rather obese mother of 5 children, is admitted to the emergency room complaining of nausea, belching, gas, and right upper quadrant pain that was not relieved by taking Alka-Seltzer. She states that she has had attacks for the past several years, especially after eating fatty or fried foods. After a series of diagnostic tests, the patient is prepared for surgery. A cholecystectomy and choledochotomy are performed. Mrs. Smith is reluctant to cough or move. Questions 455 through 461 refer to this situation.

455 Mrs. Smith experiences discomfort after ingesting fatty foods because:
1. The liver was manufacturing inadequate bile
2. Fatty foods are hard to digest
3. Obstruction of the common bile duct prevented emptying of the bile into the intestine
4. She did not eliminate fatty foods from her diet

456 A patient with obstruction of the common bile duct may show a prolonged bleeding and clotting time because:
1. The extrinsic factor is not absorbed
2. Vitamin K is not absorbed
3. The ionized calcium level falls
4. Bilirubin accumulates in the plasma

457 Cholecystography is performed to:
1. Detect obstruction at the ampulla of Vater

2. Observe patency of the common bile duct
3. Determine the concentration ability of the gallbladder
4. Distinguish stone formation from other types of obstruction

458 Mrs. Smith had an interference in bile utilization caused by cholecystitis. The ejection of bile into the alimentary tract is controlled by which of the following hormones?
1. Cholecystokinin
2. Secretin
3. Gastrin
4. Hepatokinin

459 Mrs. Smith has a Penrose drain inserted. The nurse caring for her in the recovery room notices that the dressing has become soiled with a brownish-red fluid. The nurse should:
1. Change the dressing
2. Reinforce the dressing
3. Apply an abdominal binder
4. Remove the tape and apply Montgomery straps

460 Postoperatively Mrs. Smith suddenly complains of numbness in the right leg and a ''funny feeling'' in the toes. The nurse should first:
1. Elevate the legs and tell her to stay in bed
2. Rub her legs to start circulation and place a warm blanket on her
3. Tell her she has been staying in bed too much and encourage ambulation
4. Tell her to remain in bed and notify the physician

461 When Mrs. Smith is able to eat solid food, which of the following special diets should be ordered?
1. High in protein and calories to help her regain her strength
2. Low in fat to avoid painful contractions in the wound area
3. Low in protein and carbohydrate to avoid excess calories and help her lose weight
4. High in fat and carbohydrate to meet energy demands

Situation: Mrs. Carpenter enters the hospital with esophageal strictures. She has not been able to eat solid food for many weeks. Nutritional edema does not mask the emaciation and malnourishment present. Questions 462 through 469 refer to this situation.

462 The nurse is aware that Mrs. Carpenter's nutritional edema is a result of the following primary homeostatic mechanism:
1. The capillary fluid shift mechanism
2. The aldosterone mechanism
3. The ADH mechanism
4. Nitrogen balance

463 The physician inserts a subclavian line for total parenteral nutrition. The nursing responsibilities include:
1. Measuring urinary specific gravity

2. Checking vital signs every 2 hours
3. Doing fractional urine tests
4. Checking for muscular cramps

464 The nurse can prevent a major reaction to hyperalimentation infusions by:
1. The slow administration of the fluid
2. Checking vital signs every 4 hours
3. Changing site every 24 hours
4. Recording intake and output

465 Later, a gastrostomy tube is inserted and Mrs. Carpenter is to be discharged with the tube in place. An advantage of gastrostomy tube feeding over nasogastric tube feeding is:
1. More tube feeding mixture can be given each time
2. Procedure does not require gravity
3. There is less chance of aspiration
4. Patient can self-administer feeding

466 The nurse administers the initial tube feeding. What nursing observation indicates that the patient is unable to tolerate further tube feeding?
1. Passage of flatus
2. Rapid flow of feeding
3. Epigastric tenderness
4. Rise of formula in tube

467 The nurse is teaching the tube feeding procedure to Mrs. Carpenter. She advises Mrs. Carpenter that when administering her tube feeding, she should:
1. Heat the feeding 10° above body temperature
2. Finish the feeding with water
3. Maintain supine position
4. Instill fluid prior to feeding to ascertain placement of tube in stomach

468 The nurse tells Mrs. Carpenter to heat her tube feeding to a temperature of:
1. 50° to 60° F (10° to 15.5° C)
2. 70° to 75° F (21° to 24° C)
3. 90° to 100° F (32° to 38° C)
4. 100° to 115° F (38° to 46° C)

469 Mrs. Carpenter must utilize a gastrostomy tube feeding as her only route of ingestion. To maintain the pleasure of eating, the nurse may advise her to:
1. Chew food prior to putting it in the gastrostomy tube
2. Use the blender to puree favorite foods
3. Feed via tube at normal meal times
4. Chew gum during gastrostomy tube feeding

Situation: Mrs. McCann, a 93-year-old widow, has been admitted to the hospital from a nursing home, complaining of severe lower abdominal pain, anorexia, nausea, and vomiting for the past 24 hours. History and physical examination reveal a thin, elderly white woman in remarkably good physical and mental condition except for the present complaints. The most likely cause of Mrs. McCann's illness is thought to be sigmoid diverticulitis. After the appropriate diagnostic work-up and preparation for surgery, an exploratory laparotomy is performed. Surgery confirms the admitting diagnosis but also reveals a large silent giant ulcer in the stomach, which requires a subtotal gastrectomy (Billroth I). Mrs. McCann does well after the surgery but on the fifth postoperative day develops severe abdominal pain with distended abdomen, a markedly elevated WBC, and temperature of 103° F (39.5° C) rectally. She is taken to the O.R. once again, where plication for a leak in the duodenostomy is performed. Questions 470 through 475 refer to this situation.

470 The primary reason for surgery being performed in the first instance is most likely because:
1. Diverticulitis in some instances is difficult to differentiate from carcinoma except surgically
2. Of the symptoms exhibited by the patient on admission
3. The complication—perforation—had occurred with resultant abscess formation or generalized peritonitis
4. Surgery is usually indicated for patients with a diagnosis of diverticulitis

471 One of the major problems after this type of surgery is the prevention of pulmonary complications. The nurse can best achieve this by:
1. Encouraging deep breathing and coughing to counteract voluntary diaphragm splinting
2. Promoting frequent turning, moving, and deep breathing to mobilize bronchial secretions
3. Ambulating to increase respiratory exchange
4. Administering IPPB q 4 h

472 A gastrectomy following severe stomach ulceration may eventually be associated with pernicious anemia because:
1. Vitamin B_{12} is only absorbed in the stomach
2. The stomach parietal cells secrete the intrinsic factor
3. The hemopoietic factor is secreted in the stomach
4. Chief cells in the stomach secrete the extrinsic factor

473 In caring for a patient with a nasogastric tube attached to suction, the nurse should:
1. Irrigate the tube frequently with physiologic saline
2. Allow the patient to have small chips of ice or sips of water unless nauseated
3. Use clean technique in irrigating the tube
4. Withdraw the tube quickly when decompression is terminated

474 Because Mrs. McCann's skin is extremely dry, flaky, wrinkled, sagging, and sallow, an important nursing measure is to:
1. Avoid daily bathing but use emollients
2. Bathe her once or twice a week and use emollients
3. Bathe when necessary and use emollients
4. Use emollients for skin care

475 The wisest guideline for Mrs. McCann's diet would be:
1. No oral feedings for a prolonged period
2. Gradual resumption of small, easily digested feedings
3. At her age allow anything she wants at any time
4. Give nothing by mouth and depend on IV feedings indefinitely

Situation: Mr. Gray is admitted to the hospital with carcinoma of the descending portion of the colon. Questions 476 through 483 refer to this situation.

476 The operative procedure that would probably be performed is a(an):
1. Cecostomy
2. Ileostomy
3. Colectomy
4. Colostomy

477 The nurse administers neomycin sulfate to Mr. Gray preoperatively to:
1. Decrease the possibility of postoperative urinary tract infection
2. Increase the production of vitamin K
3. Destroy intestinal bacteria
4. Decrease the incidence of any secondary infection

478 The nurse protects the skin surrounding the colostomy opening by using:
1. Petroleum jelly
2. Alcohol
3. Aluminum paste
4. Mineral oil

479 After surgery Mr. Gray asks what effect the surgery will have on his sexual relationships. The nurse should tell him that:
1. Sexual relationships must be curtailed
2. He should tell his partner about his surgery prior to sexual activity
3. He will be able to resume normal sexual relationships
4. The surgery will temporarily decrease his sexual impulses

480 In teaching Mr. Gray to care for the colostomy, the nurse should advise him to irrigate it at the same time every day and to choose a time:
1. When he can be assured of uninterrupted bathroom use at home
2. That approximates his usual daily time for elimination
3. About halfway between the 2 largest meals of the day
4. About 1 hour before breakfast

481 If, during the colostomy irrigation, Mr. Gray complains of abdominal cramps, the nurse should:
1. Lower the container of fluid
2. Discontinue the irrigation
3. Clamp the catheter for a few minutes
4. Advance the catheter about 1 inch

482 When performing the colostomy irrigation, the nurse inserts the catheter into the stoma:
1. 2 inches (5 cm)
2. 4 inches (10 cm)
3. 6 inches (15 cm)
4. 8 inches (20 cm)

483 When teaching Mr. Gray to irrigate his colostomy, the

nurse indicates that the distance of the container above the stoma should be no more than:
1. 18 inches (45 cm)
2. 6 inches (15 cm)
3. 10 inches (25 cm)
4. 12 inches (30 cm)

484 The 2 main sites for handling fat metabolism are the liver and adipose tissue. Of its several functions concerning fat, the main role of the liver is:
1. The production of phospholipids
2. Oxidizing fatty acids to produce energy
3. Converting fat to lipoproteins for rapid transport out into the body
4. Storing fat for energy reserves

485 A readily available form of energy, although limited in amount, is stored in the liver by conversion of glucose to:
1. Glycogen
2. Glycerol
3. Tissue fat
4. Amino acids

486 An important material produced in the liver and stored in the gallbladder is needed to prepare food fats for change to usable fuel forms. This material is:
1. Lipase
2. Amylase
3. Bile
4. Cholesterol

Situation: Mr. Weinberg is admitted to the hospital with cirrhosis of the liver and malnutrition. Questions 487 through 492 refer to this situation.

487 Mr. Weinberg begins to develop slurred speech, confusion, drowsiness, and tremors. With these symptoms his diet would be limited to:
1. 20 g protein, 2000 calories
2. 80 g protein, 1000 calories
3. 100 g protein, 2500 calories
4. 150 g protein, 1200 calories

488 Mr. Weinberg has a swollen appearance as a result of the edema and ascites. The ascites is caused by:
1. Portal hypertension
2. Kidney malfunction
3. Decreased production of potassium
4. Diminished plasma protein

489 The symptoms of portal hypertension are largely caused by:
1. Infection of the liver parenchyma
2. Fatty degeneration of Kupffer cells
3. Obstruction of the portal circulation
4. Obstruction of the cystic and hepatic ducts

490 What complication is most likely to occur when a patient has portal hypertension?
1. Perforation of the duodenum

2. Hemorrhage from esophageal varices
3. Liver abscess
4. Intestinal obstruction

491 Mr. Weinberg's long-standing poor nutrition, especially his deficiency of protein, has led to:
1. Fat accumulation in the liver tissue
2. Coagulation of blood in microcirculation
3. Tissue anabolism and positive nitrogen balance
4. Decreased bile in the blood

492 The nurse expects weight loss in a patient receiving IV administration of 5% dextrose in water due to:
1. Insufficient carbohydrate intake
2. Lack of protein supplementation
3. Insufficient intake of water-soluble vitamins
4. Increased concentration of electrolytes in cells

Situation: Mrs. Green, a known diabetic, has been admitted to the hospital in diabetic acidosis. Blood gases are determined immediately. Questions 493 through 499 refer to this situation.

493 In her state of uncompensated acidosis, which of the following might represent Mrs. Green's arterial blood pH?
1. 6.9
2. 7.2
3. 7.45
4. 7.48

494 Larger than normal amounts of acetoacetic acid have been entering Mrs. Green's blood as one of the indirect results of her insulin deficiency. Like lactic acid and other non-volatile acids, acetoacetic acid is buffered in the blood chiefly by:
1. Carbon dioxide
2. Potassium salt of hemoglobin
3. Sodium bicarbonate
4. Sodium chloride

495 As a result of excessive acetoacetic acid:
1. Mrs. Green's blood pH remains unchanged
2. Mrs. Green's blood pH increases slightly
3. The carbonic acid content of Mrs. Green's blood remains unchanged
4. The sodium bicarbonate content of Mrs. Green's blood necessarily decreases and its carbonic acid content increases

496 The insulin given to Mrs. Green in this emergency would be:
1. Protamine zinc
2. Globulin
3. NPH
4. Regular

497 Initially, when the acidosis is controlled, NPH insulin, 40 units each morning, is prescribed for Mrs. Green. NPH insulin (100 U = 1 ml) is available. To give 40 units, using a regular syringe, the nurse should withdraw:
1. 6 minims

2. 12 minims
3. 20 minims
4. 40 minims

498 The nurse knows that glucagon is given as a follow-up to 50% dextrose in the treatment of hypoglycemia because it:
1. Provides more storage of glucose
2. Increases blood sugar levels
3. Stimulates release of insulin
4. Inhibits glycogenesis

499 When Mrs. Green is discharged, she is receiving isophane insulin suspension (NPH) daily and also is receiving insulin injection (regular insulin) when her urine test is positive. In instructing Mrs. Green the nurse should teach her to:
1. Mix the insulins in any required dosage in the same syringe
2. Give the insulins separately unless the ratio of dosage is greater than 1:1
3. Give the insulins in the same syringe when the ratio is 1:1
4. Administer the insulins in separate syringes using different sites for injection

500 Glucose is an important molecule to a cell because this molecule is primarily used for:
1. The building of cell membranes
2. The synthesis of proteins
3. Extraction of energy
4. Building the genetic material

501 The source of glucose for maintaining blood glucose at normal levels at all times is:
1. Ingested food
2. Intestinal hydrolysis
3. Liver glycogen
4. Gluconeogenesis

502 Early treatment of diabetic acidosis will include administration of:
1. Potassium
2. IV fluids
3. NPH insulin
4. Sodium polystyrene sulfonate (Kayexalate)

503 As the patient recovers from diabetic acidosis:
1. The precipitating cause of the coma must be investigated to prevent a recurrence
2. The cause of his condition should be reviewed with him so that he understands how to avoid such a recurrence
3. Teaching will be necessary to help him accept his disease
4. He will need assistance in obtaining a clear conception of the general character of diabetes

504 When glucagon is administered for reversal of the hypoglycemic state, it acts by:
1. Liberating glucose from hepatic stores of glycogen

2. Competing for insulin and blocking its action at tissue sites
3. Providing a glucose substitute for rapid replacement of deficits
4. Supplying glycogen to the brain and other vital organs

505 The fuel glucose is delivered to the cells by the blood for production of energy. The hormone controlling the use of glucose by the cell is:
1. Thyroxine
2. Growth hormone
3. Adrenal steroids
4. Insulin

506 If a routine urine specimen cannot be sent immediately to the laboratory, the nurse should:
1. Discard and collect a new specimen later
2. Store on "dirty" side of utility room
3. Refrigerate the specimen
4. Take no special action

507 Which of the following nursing actions is most needed when collecting a 24-hour urine specimen?
1. Weighing the patient before starting
2. Checking if any preservatives are needed
3. Placing collection jar in ice
4. Checking intake and output

Situation: Mrs. Butler had a radical mastectomy and will start chemotherapy while hospitalized. Questions 508 through 510 refer to this situation.

508 The nurse is aware that many of the chemotherapeutic agents cause:
1. Increased Hgb and Hct
2. Bone marrow depression
3. Decreased sedimentation rate
4. Leukocytosis

509 Mrs. Butler's pathology report shows metastatic adenocarcinoma. She is to receive doxorubicin (Adriamycin), which modifies growth of cancer cells by:
1. Preventing folic acid synthesis
2. Changing the osmotic gradient in the cell
3. Inhibiting RNA synthesis by binding DNA
4. Increasing the permeability of the cell wall

510 Because of problems occurring in 80% of the patients receiving Adriamycin, the nurse will observe Mrs. Butler for evidence of:
1. Nausea or vomiting, tachycardia
2. Hair loss, erythema of the oral mucosa
3. Decreased appetite, necrosis at the IV site
4. Low blood pressure, decreased vital capacity

511 Tumors of connective tissue are classified as:
1. Osteoblastomas
2. Collagenomas
3. Sarcomas
4. Carcinomas

512 Which of the following is the most frequently occurring brain tumor?
1. Pituitary adenoma
2. Neurofibroma
3. Glioma
4. Meningioma

513 Teratomas are tumors that originate in:
1. Muscle cells
2. The embryo
3. The bone marrow
4. Multiple sites

514 When counseling a patient after a vasectomy, the nurse should advise the patient that:
1. It requires at least 10 ejaculations to clear the tract of sperm
2. Recanalization of the vas deferens is impossible
3. Unprotected coitus is possible within a week to 10 days
4. Some impotency is to be expected for several weeks

Situation: Mrs. O'Reilly, 62 years of age, has been admitted to the hospital after having had a cerebral vascular accident resulting in left hemiplegia. Questions 515 through 522 refer to this situation.

515 The nurse identifies left hemiplegia by the following observations:
1. Paralysis of the left lower extremity
2. Paralysis of the left arm, left leg, and left side of the face
3. Paralysis of the left arm and left side of the face
4. Paralysis of the left arm, left leg, and right side of the face

516 When the nurse brings in the dinner tray, Mrs. O'Reilly is staring blankly at the wall and states that she feels like half a person. Specific nursing care of Mrs. O'Reilly should be directed at:
1. Including her in all decisions
2. Helping her explore her feelings
3. Distracting her from self-pity
4. Preventing contractures and decubiti

517 Mrs. O'Reilly has been incontinent of feces. When establishing a bowel training program, the nurse must remember that the most important factor is the:
1. Patient's previous habits in the area of diet and use of laxatives
2. Timing of elimination to take advantage of the gastrocolic reflex
3. Use of medication to induce elimination
4. Planning with the patient a definite time for attempted evacuations

518 In aiding Mrs. O'Reilly to develop independence, the nurse can motivate the patient by:
1. Demonstrating ways she can regain independence
2. Establishing long-range goals for the patient
3. Reinforcing success in tasks accomplished
4. Pointing out her errors and helping her correct them

519 Mrs. O'Reilly's daughter threatens to sue when her mother develops a large decubitus ulcer after she insisted on lying on her back for long periods. She is very upset and blames the nurses. The decision in this suit would take into consideration the fact that:
1. The nurse should uphold the patient's right not to be moved
2. Decubitus ulcers frequently occur in immobilized patients
3. Patients should be turned at least every 2 hours
4. Nurses are not responsible to the patient's family

520 Which of the following drugs is likely to be used to treat Mrs. O'Reilly's decubitus ulcer?
1. Chymotrypsin
2. Hyaluronidase
3. Penicillinase
4. Dextranomer (Debrisan)

521 The nurse suspects Mrs. O'Reilly has become impacted when she states:
1. ''I don't have much of an appetite.''
2. ''I have a lot of gas pains.''
3. ''I feel like I have to go and just can't.''
4. ''I haven't had a bowel movement for 2 days.''

522 What assessment by the nurse is a further indication of the probable presence of a fecal impaction?
1. Tympanites
2. Decreased number of bowel movements
3. Fecal liquid seepage
4. Bright red blood in stool

---

523 What part of the cerebral cortex registers general sensations such as heat, cold, pain, and touch?
1. Frontal lobe
2. Occipital lobe
3. Parietal lobe
4. Temporal lobe

524 The relay center for sensory impulses is the:
1. Medulla oblongata
2. Hypothalamus
3. Cerebellum
4. Thalamus

525 The internal organs of humans, such as the bladder and the esophagus, are most directly under the control of the:
1. Peripheral nervous system
2. Central nervous system
3. Autonomic nervous system
4. Spinal cord

526 Stimulation of the vagus nerve results in:
1. Tachycardia
2. Dilation of the bronchioles
3. Slowing of the heart
4. Coronary artery vasodilatation

Situation: Mr. Ray, a 67-year-old retired plumber, falls and is unable to get up. His daughter calls an ambulance, and he is brought to the emergency room, where it is found that he has a fracture of the neck of the left femur. Mr. Ray is admitted to the orthopedic unit, put in Buck's extension, and prepared for surgery the next day. Questions 527 through 532 refer to this situation.

527 On examination of Mr. Ray, the nurse would expect to find:
 1. Shortening of the affected extremity with internal rotation
 2. Shortening of the affected extremity with external rotation
 3. Abduction with external rotation
 4. Adduction with internal rotation

528 The nurse should know that, following a fracture of the neck of the femur, the desirable position for the limb is:
 1. External rotation with flexion of the knee and hip
 2. External rotation with extension of the knee and hip
 3. Internal rotation with extension of the knee
 4. Internal rotation with flexion of the hip and knee

529 The nurse should explain to Mr. Ray that the chief reason for applying Buck's extension is to:
 1. Help reduce the fracture and to relieve muscle spasm and pain
 2. Keep him from turning and moving in bed
 3. Prevent contractures from developing
 4. Maintain the limb in a position of external rotation

530 Part of the nursing care of Mr. Ray is assessment of peripheral pulses. The important characteristics when assessing the peripheral pulse are:
 1. Contractility and rate
 2. Color of skin and type of spasms
 3. Amplitude, symmetry, and rhythm
 4. Local temperature and visible pulsations

531 When Mr. Ray is ready to walk with crutches after the hip pinning, he will probably be taught:
 1. Four-point crutch walking
 2. Two-point crutch walking
 3. Swing-through gait
 4. Three-point crutch walking

532 Which of the following principles should the nurse use in teaching Mr. Ray the 4-point gait once bone regrowth has occurred?
 1. Most of weight should be supported by the axillae
 2. Elbows should be maintained in rigid extension
 3. The patient must be able to bear weight on both legs
 4. The affected extremity should be kept about 6 inches (15 cm) off the ground

Situation: Mrs. Newt, a 35-year-old housewife and the mother of 5 young children, ages 6 months to 15 years, is involved in a serious auto accident on the highway when her car skids on the wet pavement, striking the concrete partition. She is taken to a hospital, where it is determined that she has multiple trauma,

possible fractured skull, fractures of the fifth and sixth cervical and the tenth, eleventh, and twelfth vertebrae, as well as a ruptured spleen and hematuria. Questions 533 through 539 refer to this situation.

533 A splenectomy was necessary because:
 1. The spleen is a highly vascular organ
 2. Rupture of the spleen is frequently associated with diseases of the liver and blood
 3. The spleen is the largest lymphoid organ in the body
 4. Enlarged spleen causes such discomfort or disability as to justify its removal

534 The nurse should observe Mrs. Newt for postoperative complications, such as:
 1. Hemorrhage, abdominal distention
 2. Peritonitis, pulmonary complications
 3. Shock, infection
 4. Intestinal obstruction, bleeding

535 When planning care for Mrs. Newt, the nurse should:
 1. Observe patient for signs of brain injury
 2. Place patient in Trendelenburg position if in shock
 3. Check for hemorrhaging from oral cavity
 4. Observe for decreased intracranial pressure and temperature

536 Following surgery the nurse should observe Mrs. Newt for the depletion of which of the following electrolytes?
 1. Sodium
 2. Calcium
 3. Chloride
 4. Potassium

537 The nurse can expect Mrs. Newt to complain of:
 1. Pain on expiration
 2. Pain on inspiration
 3. Difficulty in breathing
 4. Breathing rapidly and ineffectively

538 Since Mrs. Newt has hematuria, the nurse should observe for:
 1. Diarrhea
 2. Symptoms of peritonitis
 3. Gross or increasing hematuria
 4. Acetone in urine

539 Hematuria in this instance probably means that there has been injury to the:
 1. Kidneys
 2. Ureters
 3. Bladder
 4. Urethra

540 The protein of blood involved with immune responses is:
 1. Hemoglobin
 2. Albumin
 3. Globulin
 4. Thrombin

541 Fragments of cells in the bloodstream that break down on

exposure to injured tissue and begin the chain reaction leading to a blood clot are known as:
1. Red blood cells
2. Platelets
3. Leukocytes
4. Erythrocytes

542 With respect to human blood cells, sodium chloride solution of 0.85% strength is:
1. Isotonic
2. Hypertonic
3. Hypotonic
4. Isomeric

543 Which stage of sleep is associated with psychologic rest?
1. Stage 1
2. REM sleep
3. Stage 2
4. Stage 4

544 The action of bulk to promote defecation is a consequence of the:
1. Irritating effect of fiber on the bowel wall
2. Tendency of smooth muscle to contract when stretched
3. Direct chemical stimulation of the colonic musculature
4. Action of the multiflora of the large intestine

545 The physical law explaining the greatly increased venous return accompanying mild vasoconstriction underlies the use of:
1. Adrenaline in treating shock
2. Rotating tourniquets in pulmonary edema
3. Sympathectomy in treating hypertension
4. Digoxin to increase cardiac output

Situation: Mr. Anthony has second- and third-degree burns and is to receive a skin graft over the third-degree burn of his arm. Questions 546 through 551 refer to this situation.

546 The graft is taken from his left buttock. This is referred to as a(n):
1. Homograft
2. Autograft
3. Heterograft
4. Allograft

547 A pigskin graft is often applied to burned areas. This is known as a(n):
1. Homograft
2. Allograft
3. Heterograft
4. Isograft

548 Which of the following laboratory tests will best reflect loss of fluid due to burns?
1. Blood pH
2. Sedimentation rate
3. Hematocrit
4. BUN

549 In a burned patient the relationship between body surface area and fluid loss is:

1. Directly proportionate
2. Inversely proportionate
3. Equal
4. Unrelated

550 Which of the following medications should a burned patient receive as soon after admission as possible?
1. Phytonadione (Aquamephyton)
2. Gamma globulin
3. Tetanus toxoid
4. Isoproterenol (Isuprel)

551 Mr. Anthony is to have mafenide (Sulfamylon) cream applied to his burned areas. A serious side effect of Sulfamylon therapy is:
1. Renal shutdown
2. Hemolysis of RBCs
3. Metabolic acidosis
4. Curling's ulcer

Situation: Mr. Neil has a transurethral resection and returns to the unit with an indwelling urinary catheter. Questions 552 through 554 refer to this situation.

552 When irrigating the patient's catheter, the nurse would avoid which one of the following?
1. Using sterile aseptic technique
2. Allowing solution to flow in by gravity
3. Having irrigating solution at room temperature
4. Aspirating irrigating solution with a bulb syringe

553 The solution of choice for maintaining patency of an indwelling catheter is:
1. Isotonic saline
2. Hypotonic saline
3. Sterile water
4. Genitourinary irrigating solution

554 When irrigating Mr. Neil's catheter the nurse should:
1. Instill the fluid under pressure
2. Obtain and use sterile equipment
3. Aspirate to ensure return flow
4. Warm the solution to body temperature

Situation: Miss Fleming, a 35-year-old executive secretary, is hospitalized for treatment of hypertension. Her orders include bed rest with bathroom privileges, low-sodium diet, reserpine (Serpasil), and chlordiazepoxide (Librium). She has been active in both her business and social life, usually having a cocktail before dinner and smoking a pack of cigarettes daily. Miss Fleming expresses disgust for her regimen and dissatisfaction with the nursing care. Questions 555 through 561 refer to this situation.

555 Miss Fleming's behavior is probably a manifestation of her:
1. Denial of illness
2. Response to cerebral anoxia

3. Reaction to hypertensive medications
4. Fear of the health problem

556 The nurse should administer the Librium as ordered because it:
1. Promotes rest
2. Induces sleep
3. Produces hypotension
4. Reduces hostility

557 Miss Fleming has been receiving Librium, 10 mg qid, for the past 5 days. The nurse should question giving the medication if the patient exhibits:
1. Muscle twitching
2. Blurred vision
3. Hypotension
4. Extreme drowsiness

558 Miss Fleming is receiving Serpasil because it is an effective:
1. Diuretic
2. Hypnotic
3. Antihypertensive
4. Tranquilizer

559 To avoid an error of parallax when taking a patient's blood pressure, the nurse should:
1. Use a narrow cuff
2. Stand close to the manometer
3. Elevate the patient's arm on a pillow
4. Read at eye level

560 Miss Fleming has been told she must stop smoking and eliminate her predinner cocktail. The nurse discovers a pack of cigarettes in Miss Fleming's bathrobe. The best course of action to take at this time is to:
1. Report the situation to the head nurse
2. Let the patient know you found them
3. Discard them and say nothing to her
4. Call the physician and request directions

561 When Miss Fleming is being overtly verbally hostile, the most appropriate nursing response is:
1. Reasonable exploration of situations
2. Complete withdrawal from her behavior
3. Silent acceptance of her behavior
4. Verbal defense of your position

Situation: Mrs. Campenella, an 80-year-old widow, is admitted with congestive heart failure and pulmonary edema. Questions 562 through 566 refer to this situation.

562 To help alleviate Mrs. Campenella's distress, the nurse should:
1. Elevate the lower extremities
2. Place the patient in orthopneic position
3. Encourage frequent coughing
4. Prepare for modified postural drainage

563 When a patient is admitted to the coronary care unit with a diagnosis of acute pulmonary edema, the nurse should be prepared for:

1. Postural drainage
2. Inhalation therapy
3. Rotating tourniquets
4. Wet phlebotomy

564 Mrs. Campenella is receiving furosemide (Lasix) and digoxin. Nursing care for her includes observation for symptoms of electrolyte depletion caused by:
1. Sodium restriction
2. Inadequate oral intake
3. Continuous dyspnea
4. Diuretic therapy

565 To help assess Mrs. Campenella's condition, a CVP catheter is inserted. In taking a central venous pressure reading the nurse should place the patient:
1. Horizontal
2. In a low Fowler's position
3. Side lying, on affected side
4. Side lying, opposite to manometer

566 Since Mrs. Campenella will be staying with her daughter for the summer, the nurse suggests that her room be air conditioned. This is because:
1. The internal body temperature drops below 98.6° F (37° C)
2. The heart is relieved of the strain of pumping blood through many miles of blood vessels in the skin
3. The increased circulation in the skin causes excess body heat to radiate away
4. The increased circulation in the skin gives the heart the exercise it needs

Situation: Mr. Rogers, with a long history of emphysema, is now terminally ill with cancer of the esophagus. His plan of care includes a soft diet, modified postural drainage, and IPPB treatments bid. Mr. Rogers is weak, dyspneic, emaciated, and apathetic. Questions 567 through 573 refer to this situation.

567 Nursing care plans for Mr. Rogers should give priority to:
1. Diet and nutrition
2. Hygiene and comfort
3. Body mechanics and posture
4. Intake and output

568 Mr. Rogers expresses aversion to his meals and eats only small amounts. The nurse should provide:
1. Only foods he likes in small portions
2. Supplementary vitamins to stimulate appetite
3. Nourishment between meals
4. Small portions more frequently

569 The term used to describe Mr. Roger's response to food most accurately is:
1. Anorexia
2. Anoxia
3. Apathy
4. Dysphagia

570 To obtain maximum benefits after postural drainage, Mr. Rogers should be:

1. Placed in a sitting position to provide drainage
2. Encouraged to cough deeply
3. Placed on an IPPB machine
4. Encouraged to rest for 30 minutes before coughing

571 Mr. Roger's pain and dyspnea are increasing in severity. The physician has ordered 100 mg meperidine q 4 h and oxygen prn. In preparing Mr. Rogers's medication, the nurse should know that meperidine is commonly available for dispensation as:
1. Darvon
2. Doriden
3. Demerol
4. Narcan

572 The nurse administers nasal oxygen at 2 L/minute. The nurse would observe Mr. Rogers closely for:
1. Hyperemia and increased respirations
2. Cyanosis and lethargy
3. Anxiety and tachycardia
4. Drowsiness and decreased respirations

573 Mr. Rogers has a 44-year-old wife, a 16-year-old daughter in high school, and a 20-year-old son in college. They visit him frequently. In view of Mr. Rogers's extreme weakness and dyspnea, nursing care plans should include:
1. Limiting family visiting hours to the evening before sleep
2. Allowing self-activity whenever possible
3. Encouraging family to feed and assist him
4. Planning all necessary care at one time with long rests in between

Situation: Mr. Ergotano, 50 years old, recently came from Italy with his wife to visit with American relatives. While here, he is admitted to the hospital complaining of anorexia, loss of weight, abdominal distention, and passage of abnormal stools. The most likely diagnosis on the basis of history and physical examination is cancer of the stomach or malabsorption syndrome. Neither Mr. Ergotano nor his wife speaks any English. Their trip to America was sponsored by relatives. Questions 574 through 581 refer to this situation.

574 To determine the correct diagnosis, extensive diagnostic studies are performed. Tests in connection with cancer of the stomach include:
1. X-ray examination
2. CBC
3. Thorn test
4. Gastroscopy

575 Mr. Ergotano appears frightened and Mrs. Ergotano is near hysteria. Identifying their emotional state and being unable to communicate with only rudimentary sign language, the nurse should:
1. Give them a booklet with Italian translations of English medical terms
2. Call an Italian-speaking employee from another part of the hospital when necessary

3. Reduce communication to the bare essentials
4. Permit an American relative to stay with Mr. and Mrs. Erogotano at all times

576 An IV of 1000 ml 5% dextrose in water each shift is started on admission to correct fluid imbalance. The infusion set delivers 10 drops per milliliter. To regulate the rate of flow so that the solution would be infused over an 8-hour period, the nurse would select which of these rates of flow?
1. 160 gtt per minute
2. 60 gtt per minute
3. 20 gtt per minute
4. 40 gtt per minute

577 Later the physician changes the order to keep vein open. What is the longest possible period of time that 1 bottle of 1000 ml of 5% dextrose in water to keep a vein open can be infused without producing untoward effects?
1. 6 hours
2. 12 hours
3. 18 hours
4. 24 hours

578 Differential diagnosis establishes that Mr. Ergotano has nontropical sprue. Striking clinical improvement is noted after administration of:
1. A gluten-free diet
2. Folic acid
3. Corticotropin
4. Vitamin B_{12}

579 Because malabsorption syndrome seems to be present, a trial period on a gluten-free diet is ordered for Mr. Ergotano. He is not allowed to have:
1. Wheat, rye, or oats
2. Rice or corn
3. Milk or cheese
4. Fruit or fruit juices

580 A typical food combination served to Mr. Ergotano on his gluten-free diet would be:
1. Creamed turkey on toast, rice, green peas, milk
2. Roast beef, baked potato, carrots, tea
3. Cheese omlet, noodles, green beans, coffee
4. Baked chicken, mashed potatoes with gravy, zucchini, Postum

581 Since Mr. Ergotano's nutritional status is poor, the nurse should:
1. Encourage meats at mealtime to increase protein intake
2. Keep patient NPO, since he has diarrhea
3. Allow whatever foods he will eat from the diet
4. Institute IV therapy to improve hydration

582 What is the usual stimulant for the respiratory center?
1. Calcium ions
2. Carbon dioxide
3. Lactic acid
4. Oxygen

583 Oxygen dissociation from hemoglobin and therefore oxygen delivery to the tissues are accelerated by:
1. A decreasing oxygen pressure in the blood
2. A decreasing oxygen pressure and/or an increasing carbon dioxide pressure in the blood
3. An increasing oxygen pressure and/or a decreasing carbon dioxide pressure in the blood
4. An increasing carbon dioxide pressure in the blood

584 An anaerobic spore-forming rod that produces an exotoxin in canned food is:
1. *Salmonella typhosa*
2. *Clostridium botulinum*
3. *Clostridium tetani*
4. *Escherichia coli*

585 The most important method of preventing amebic dysentery is:
1. Proper pasteurization of milk
2. Killing biting gnats
3. Proper sewage disposal
4. Tick control

586 Ketone bodies appear in the blood and urine when fats are being oxidized in great amounts. This condition is associated with:
1. Starvation
2. Alcohol intoxication
3. Positive nitrogen balance
4. Bone healing

Situation: Mrs. Evans, a 60-year-old homemaker, is admitted because of possible intestinal obstruction. A Cantor tube has been inserted and attached to suction. Questions 587 through 592 refer to this situation.

587 A serious danger to which Mrs. Evans is exposed because of intestinal suction is excessive loss of:
1. Protein enzymes
2. Energy carbohydrates
3. Water and electrolytes
4. Vitamins and minerals

588 Critical assessment of Mrs. Evans includes observation of:
1. Dehydration
2. Nausea
3. Edema
4. Belching

589 The solution of choice used to maintain patency of the Cantor tube is:
1. Hypertonic glucose
2. Isotonic saline
3. Hypotonic saline
4. Sterile water

590 Mrs. Evans is scheduled for a colostomy after diagnostic workup. Her anxiety is overt and realistic. The most effective way to help Mrs. Evans at this point is to:
1. Encourage her to express her feelings

2. Reassure her that many people cope with this problem
3. Explain the procedure and postoperative course
4. Administer a sedative and tell her to rest

591 The primary step toward long-range goals in Mrs. Evans' rehabilitation is her:
1. Mastering techniques of colostomy care
2. Readiness to accept her altered body function
3. Knowledge of the necessary dietary modifications
4. Awareness of available community resources

592 Mrs. Evans has a transverse colostomy. When inserting the catheter, the nurse should:
1. Use an oil-base lubricant
2. Direct it toward patient's right side
3. Apply gentle but continuous force
4. Instruct the patient to bear down

593 Prolonged bed rest after surgery appears to promote hemostasis, particularly in the deep veins of the calves. The most likely pathologic result of such hemostasis may be thrombus formation and:
1. Cerebral embolism
2. Dry gangrene of a limb
3. Pulmonary embolism
4. Coronary occlusion

594 The absorption of fluids by gauze is explained by the principle of:
1. Diffusion
2. Osmosis
3. Capillarity
4. Dialysis

595 An attack of pancreatitis can be precipitated by heavy drinking because:
1. Alcohol directly inflames the pancreatic tissues
2. The pancreas is stimulated to secrete more insulin than it can immediately produce
3. The alcohol promotes pancreatic duct obstruction, which then induces backflow of pancreatic juice
4. Alcohol increases enzyme secretion and pancreatic duct pressure and causes backflow of enzymes into the pancreas

596 Surgery may be needed to excise a pseudocyst of the pancreas. A pseudocyst of the pancreas:
1. Is filled with pancreatic enzymes
2. Contains necrotic tissue and blood
3. Is a pouch of undigested food particles
4. Is generally a malignant growth

597 A hormone that stimulates the flow of pancreatic juice is:
1. Cholecystokinin
2. Enterocrinin
3. Enterogastrone
4. Pancreozymin

598 The major digestive changes in fat are accomplished in the small intestine by a lipase from the pancreas. This enzymatic activity:

1. Easily breaks down all the dietary fat to fatty acids and glycerol
2. Splits off all the fatty acids in only about 25% of the total dietary fat consumed
3. Synthesizes new triglycerides from the dietary fat consumed
4. Emulsifies the fat globules and reduces their surface tension

599 Secretin and pancreozymin are hormones secreted by the:
1. Duodenum
2. Pancreas
3. Adrenals
4. Liver

Situation: Mrs. Evad, with a history of upper abdominal pain, nausea, and vomiting, is admitted to the hospital for a diagnostic workup of cancer of the pancreas. She has a history of hypertension and is taking antihypertensive medication. Questions 600 through 606 refer to this situation.

600 As you are admitting Mrs. Evad to her room, she asks you, "Do you think I have anything serious—like cancer?" Your best reply is:
1. "Why don't you discuss this with your doctor."
2. "Don't worry, we won't know until all the test results are back."
3. "What makes you think you have cancer?"
4. "I don't know if you do, but let's talk about it."

601 A complete blood count, urinalysis, and x-ray film of the chest are ordered for Mrs. Evad prior to surgery. She asks why these tests are done. Your best answer would be:
1. "Don't worry, these tests are strictly routine."
2. "They are ordered for all patients having surgery."
3. "I don't know, but the doctor ordered them."
4. "They determine whether it is safe to proceed with surgery."

602 Mrs. Evad is to have an abdominal resection. Preoperative nursing care is mainly directed toward:
1. Teaching and answering all questions
2. Maintaining proper nutritional status
3. Recording accurate vital signs
4. Alleviating the patient's anxiety

603 A significant influence on Mrs. Evad's perception of pain is her:
1. Overall physical status
2. Intelligence and economic status
3. Previous experience and cultural values
4. Age and sex

604 A progressive ambulation schedule is to be instituted for Mrs. Evad the morning after surgery. Morphine sulfate, 10 mg, has been ordered q 4 h prn for pain. When the nurse helps Mrs. Evad out of bed, she should have her sit on the edge of the bed with her feet dangling first because her expected adaptation will be:
1. Postural hypotension

2. Respiratory distress
3. Initial hypertension
4. Abdominal pain

605 Early symptoms of morphine overdose are:
1. Profuse sweating, pinpoint pupils, and deep sleep
2. Slow respirations, dilated pupils, and restlessness
3. Slow pulse, slow respirations, stupor
4. Slow respirations, constricted pupils, and deep sleep

606 On the second postoperative day the patient complains of pain in her right calf. You should:
1. Elevate the extremity
2. Apply warm soaks
3. Notify the physician
4. Chart the symptoms

Situation: Mr. Smith, a 36-year-old father of 2 children, is admitted to the hospital after an episode of vomiting "coffee-ground" material. The tentative diagnosis is peptic ulcer. Questions 607 through 613 refer to this situation.

607 Most peptic ulcers occurring in the stomach are in the:
1. Pyloric portion
2. Body of the stomach
3. Cardiac portion
4. Esophageal junction

608 The physician orders propantheline (Pro-Banthine) for Mr. Smith. Pro-Banthine is an anticholinergic drug whose main action is to:
1. Neutralize gastric acidity
2. Increase gastric motility
3. Reduce the pH of gastric contents
4. Delay gastric emptying

609 Mr. Smith does not respond to conservative therapy, and a vagotomy and partial gastrectomy are scheduled. Mr. Smith is returned to the unit from the recovery room with IV solutions running and a nasogastric tube in place. Later that evening you note that there has been no nasogastric drainage for 1½ hours. Physician's orders state: "Irrigate nasogastric tube prn." Which of the following actions would you employ? Insert:
1. 30 ml of normal saline and withdraw slowly
2. 15 ml of distilled water and disconnect suction for 30 minutes
3. 20 ml of air and clamp off suction for 1 hour
4. 50 ml of saline and increase pressure of suction

610 A vagotomy:
1. Increases heart rate
2. Hastens gastric emptying
3. Eliminates pain sensation
4. Decreases secretions in the stomach

611 Intravenous orders for Mr. Smith state that he is to receive 1000 ml of fluid every 8 hours. If the equipment you are using delivers 15 gtt/ml, you would regulate the flow at:
1. Approximately 60 gtt/minute

2. Approximately 15 gtt/minute
3. Approximately 23 gtt/minute
4. Approximately 31 gtt/minute

612 When preparing an IV piggyback medication for Mr. Smith, the nurse is aware that it is essential to:
1. Rotate the bag after adding the medication
2. Use strict sterile technique
3. Use exactly 100 ml fluid to mix medication
4. Change needle prior to adding medication

613 During the convalescent period the nurse sets up a health teaching program designed specifically to meet Mr. Smith's needs. This plan would include:
1. A thorough explanation of the dumping syndrome and how to limit or prevent it
2. A warning to avoid all gas-forming foods
3. Encouragement to resume his previous eating habits as soon as possible
4. An explanation of the therapeutic effect of a high-roughage diet

---

Situation: Mrs. McNeil has been diagnosed as having Graves' disease. Radioactive iodine is prescribed to decrease the activity of the thyroid, but this therapy is unsuccessful. Questions 614 through 622 refer to this situation.

614 The nurse knows Mrs. McNeil is:
1. Not radioactive and can be handled as any other individual
2. Highly radioactive and should be isolated as much as possible
3. Mildly radioactive and should be treated with standard precautions
4. Not radioactive but may still transmit some dangerous radiations and must be treated with precautions

615 Mrs. McNeil would probably be placed on a:
1. High-calorie diet with supplementary feeding
2. High-protein diet with supplementary nourishment
3. Regular diet with nourishment between meals
4. Soft, easily digested, nourishing diet

616 The physician decides to do a thyroidectomy. Which medication can the nurse expect the physician to prescribe pior to surgery to decrease the size and vascularity of the thyroid gland?
1. Propylthiouracil
2. Liothyronine sodium (Cytomel)
3. Lugol's Iodine Solution
4. Potassium permanganate

617 To evaluate possible laryngeal nerve injury following a thyroidectomy, the nurse should, on an hourly basis:
1. Swab the patient's throat to test gag reflex
2. Ask the patient to swallow
3. Ask the patient to speak
4. Have the patient hum a familiar tune

618 While taking Mrs. McNeil's blood pressure the nurse notices she is pale and has spasms of her hand. The nurse prepares for replacement of:
1. Potassium chloride
2. Magnesium
3. Calcium
4. Bicarbonate

619 The nurse suspects accidental removal of the parathyroids, which causes:
1. Tetany and death
2. Adrenocortical stimulation
3. Myxedema
4. Hypovolemic shock

620 Calcium is required because parathormone is the hormone that tends to:
1. Accelerate bone breakdown with release of calcium into the blood
2. Decrease blood calcium concentration
3. Decrease blood phosphate concentration
4. Increase calcium absorption into bone

621 Overall calcium balance in the body is maintained between 2 sets of balances: (1) absorption-excretion, regulating the amount that will be absorbed; and (2) deposition-mobilization of bone tissue, regulating the amount for building of bone and withdrawing from bone. This dynamic homeostasis is controlled by which 2 interbalanced regulatory agents?
1. Vitamin A and thyroid hormone
2. Ascorbic acid and growth hormone
3. Phosphorus and ACTH
4. Vitamin D and parathyroid hormone

622 The hormone that tends to decrease calcium concentration in the blood is:
1. Aldosterone
2. Thyrocalcitonin
3. Parathyroid hormone
4. Thyroid hormone

---

623 Underproduction of thyroxin produces:
1. Myxedema
2. Acromegaly
3. Cushing's disease
4. Graves' disease

624 The rate of oxidation in all the body cells is regulated primarily by which gland?
1. Pituitary
2. Thyroid
3. Adrenal
4. Pancreas

Situation: Mrs. Garvin is admitted for treatment of cancer of the cervix. Questions 625 through 629 refer to this situation.

625 An early symptom of cancer of the cervix that should have brought Mrs. Garvin to the gynecologist is:

1. Bloody spotting after intercourse
2. Foul-smelling discharge
3. Abdominal heaviness
4. Pressure on the bladder

626 Mrs. Garvin is to have a radium implant. When caring for Mrs. Garvin, the nurse would:
1. Spend as much time with the patient as possible
2. Have the patient void q 2 h
3. Use rubber gloves when giving the patient a bath
4. Maintain the patient in isolation

627 Radium is stored in lead containers because:
1. Considerable heat is produced when radium disintegrates
2. The lead absorbs the harmful radiations
3. Radium is a heavy substance
4. Lead prevents disintegration of the radium

628 In caring for Mrs. Garvin after the radium implant, the nurse would:
1. Collect and store urine for examination by nuclear medicine methods
2. Wear a lead apron when giving care
3. Restrict visitors to a 10-minute stay
4. Avoid giving IM injections into the gluteal muscle

629 Before discharge the nurse would explain to Mrs. Garvin the importance of:
1. Eating a diet high in fat
2. Taking daily multivitamin supplements
3. Returning for medical follow-up care
4. Limiting daily fluid intake

---

630 During the ovulation phase of the menstrual cycle, ovulation is caused by secretion of:
1. Follicle-stimulating hormone
2. Luteinizing hormone
3. Estrogen
4. Progesterone

631 The large amount of progesterone secreted during the secretory phase of the menstrual cycle is responsible for:
1. Sustaining the thick endometrium of the uterus
2. The regulation of menstruation
3. The onset of ovulation
4. The incidence of capillary fragility

632 The hormones responsible for the proliferation phase of menstruation are:
1. Luteinizing hormone and progesterone
2. Follicle-stimulating hormone and estrogen
3. Lactogenic hormone and progesterone
4. Luteinizing hormone and estrogen

633 Eve is 15 years old and has complained of persistent dysmenorrhea. The nurse should encourage her to:
1. Practice relaxation of abdominal muscles
2. Have a gynecologic exam
3. Maintain daily activities
4. Eat a nutritious diet containing iron

634 When a young woman complains of especially severe abdominal cramps for a day or two each month at the time of menstruation, the nurse should suspect:
1. Hypocalcemia
2. Hyperglycemia
3. Hypernatremia
4. Hypokalemia

Situation: Mrs. Johns tells the nurse preparing her for surgery that she is "terribly scared." Questions 635 through 637 refer to this situation.

635 The nurse knows that which one of the following statements does not accurately describe the autonomic nervous system?
1. Both sympathetic and parasympathetic impulses continually play on most visceral effectors
2. Sympathetic impulses tend to stimulate and parasympathetic impulses tend to inhibit the functioning of any visceral effector
3. The autonomic nervous system does not function autonomously but is regulated by impulses from the hypothalamus and other parts of the brain
4. Visceral effectors (namely, cardiac muscle, smooth muscle, and glandular epithelial tissue) receive impulses only via autonomic neurons

636 In caring for Mrs. Johns, the nurse observes which of the following indications of sympathetic control:
1. Mrs. Johns' pupils appear no bigger than the head of a common pin
2. Her skin is very pale
3. Her skin feels very dry
4. She has a pulse rate of 60

637 Which of the following indicate(s) parasympathetic dominance?
1. Excess epinephrine secretion, causing vasoconstriction and leading to hypertension
2. Excess hydrochloric acid secretion, leading to stomach ulcer
3. Constipation
4. Goose pimples

---

638 Neural impulses travel in one direction because:
1. Polarization occurs laterally
2. Only axons secrete acetylcholine
3. Sodium pump does not work in reverse
4. Cholinesterase acts along the entire axon

639 The terminals of axons supplying skeletal muscle:
1. Release acetylcholine
2. Release ATP
3. Release cholinesterase
4. Release epinephrine

Situation: Mrs. Smith is admitted with a diagnosis of partial occlusion of the left common carotid artery. She is an epileptic and has been taking phenytoin (Dilantin) for 10 years. Questions 640 through 644 refer to this situation.

640 In planning her care the nurse would:
1. Place an airway, suction, and restraints at her bedside
2. Ask her to remove her dental bridge and eyeglasses
3. Obtain a history of seizure incidence
4. Observe her for evidence of increased restlessness and agitation

641 Mrs. Smith is scheduled for an arteriogram at 10 A.M. and is to have nothing by mouth before the test. Her phenytoin (Dilantin) is scheduled for administration at 9 A.M. The nurse would:
1. Administer the drug with 30 ml of water at 9 A.M.
2. Give the same dosage of the drug rectally
3. Omit the 9 A.M. dose of the drug
4. Ask the physician if the drug can be given IV

642 Mrs. Smith is scheduled to receive phenytoin (Dilantin), 100 mg, orally at 6 P.M. She is having difficulty swallowing capsules since the arteriogram. The nurse would:
1. Open the capsule and sprinkle the powder on pureed fruit
2. Give her 4 ml of phenytoin suspension containing 125 mg/5 ml
3. Obtain a change in the prescribed administration route to allow IM administration
4. Insert a rectal suppository containing 100 mg phenytoin

643 The nursing history indicates that Mrs. Smith neglects her personal hygiene. The nurse plans health teaching and emphasizes meticulous oral hygiene because phenytoin (Dilantin):
1. Causes hypertrophy of the gums
2. Irritates the gingiva and destroys tooth enamel
3. Increases alkalinity of the oral secretions
4. Increases plaque and bacterial growth at the gum lines

644 Mrs. Smith will receive folic acid at home. The reason for continuing the drug is:
1. Folic acid will prevent neuropathy caused by phenytoin
2. Folic acid improves absorption of iron from foods
3. Folic acid content of common foods is inadequate to meet her needs
4. Phenytoin inhibits folic acid absorption from foods

Situation: Mrs. Burt is unconscious when admitted to the hospital. Questions 645 through 651 refer to this situation.

645 Mrs. Burt's right eye stays open and its pupil appears dilated. Nonconduction by which cranial nerve would explain the fact that Mrs. Burt cannot close her right eye?
1. Second
2. Third
3. Fourth
4. Seventh

646 Nonconduction by which cranial nerve would explain Mrs. Burt's dilated right pupil?
1. Second
2. Third
3. Fourth
4. Seventh

647 Mrs. Burt's mouth is drawn over to the left, a fact suggesting nonconduction by which cranial nerve?
1. Left facial
2. Right facial
3. Left abducens
4. Right trigeminal

648 Tendon reflexes, for example, the knee-jerk on the right side of Mrs. Burt's body, are found to be exaggerated. Therefore which of the following structures must still be conducting impulses?
1. Anterior horn neurons
2. Basal ganglia
3. Pyramidal tracts
4. Upper motoneurons

649 When Mrs. Burt regains consciousness, she has a spastic paralysis of the right side of her body. Spasticity results from nonconduction by certain:
1. Extrapyramidal pathways
2. Lower motoneurons
3. Spinothalamic tract fibers
4. Pyramidal tract fibers

650 Mrs. Burt's physician performs a lumbar puncture. To do this procedure, he inserts a needle into the:
1. Aqueduct of Sylvius
2. Foramen ovale
3. Subarachnoid space
4. Pia mater

651 Which of the following conducts impulses initiated by stimulation of pain receptors?
1. Lateral spinothalamic tracts
2. Posterior white columns
3. Reticulospinal tracts
4. Ventral spinothalamic tracts

Situation: Mrs. Purcell is a 72-year-old woman with Parkinson's disease. Questions 652 through 656 refer to this situation.

652 This disease is caused by:
1. Disintegration of the myelin sheath
2. Degeneration of neurons of the basal ganglia
3. Decreased acetylcholine levels at synapses
4. Degeneration of the corpus quadrigeminus

653 Which of the following would the nurse expect Mrs. Purcell to exhibit?
1. Grand mal seizures
2. Decreased intelligence
3. A flattened affect
4. Changes in pain tolerance

654 Levodopa is prescribed for Mrs. Purcell. The nurse should know that this drug:
1. Causes severe side effects when wine or cheese is ingested
2. May cause a side effect of orthostatic hypotension
3. Must be monitored by weekly laboratory tests
4. Causes an initial euphoria followed by depression

655 L-Dopa appears to be useful in treating Parkinson's disease because it can:
1. Replace the dopamine in the brain cells
2. Cause regeneration of injured thalamic cells
3. Increase acetylcholine production
4. Cross the blood-brain barrier

656 Coordination of skeletal muscles and equilibrium are controlled by the:
1. Medulla oblongata
2. Hypothalamus
3. Cerebellum
4. Thalamus

657 Rehabilitating exercises carried out under water use:
1. Water pressure
2. Water vapor
3. Water's buoyant force
4. Water temperature

Situation: Mr. Brown is a 68-year-old retired widower who lives alone. He has a 10-year history of arthritis and has just been admitted to the hospital in an acute episode. Questions 658 through 662 refer to this situation.

658 In planning the nursing care for Mr. Brown, the nurse would take into consideration the fact that:
1. If redness and swelling of a joint occur, they signify irreversible damage
2. Bony ankylosis of the joint is irreversible and causes immobility
3. Inflammation of the synovial membrane will rarely occur
4. Complete immobility is desired during the acute phase of inflammation

659 A regimen of rest, exercise, and physical therapy will:
1. Help prevent the crippling effects of the disease
2. Prevent arthritic pain
3. Provide for the regaining of joint motion that has been lost for a prolonged period
4. Halt the inflammatory process

660 The occurrence of a chronic illness that limits major activity is:
1. Present to the same degree in every age group
2. Greatest in children because of the prevalence of congenital defects
3. Greatest in the older age group
4. Greatest in the middle years of life

661 Mr. Brown reports that over the years the following diet suggestions have been given him for his arthritis. Which of the following recommendations for his daily diet should the nurse reinforce?
1. Yogurt and blackstrap molasses
2. Wheat germ and yeast
3. A variety of meats, fruits, vegetables, milk, cereal grains
4. Multiple vitamin supplements in large doses

662 The nurse understands the joints that would most likely be involved in a patient with osteoarthritis are the:
1. Fingers and metacarpals
2. Hips and knees
3. Ankles and metatarsals
4. Cervical spine and shoulders

663 Psoriasis is characterized by:
1. Shiny, scaly lesions
2. Pruritic lesions
3. Multiple petechiae
4. Erythematous macules

664 Treatment of psoriasis usually involves:
1. Avoiding exposure to the sun
2. Potassium permanganate baths
3. Topical application of steroids
4. Debridement of necrotic placques

665 When caring for a patient with scabies, the nurse should be aware that scabies is:
1. Highly contagious
2. Caused by a fungus
3. Associated with other allergies
4. A chronic problem

666 Which system does the disease pemphigus vulgaris affect?
1. Gastrointestinal
2. Reproductive
3. Neuromuscular
4. Integumentary

Situation: Following a car accident Harry Martin, a 26-year-old high school math teacher, is diagnosed as having quadriplegia. He is critically ill and needs specific services and equipment; therefore he is admitted to the hospital's Intensive Care Unit. Questions 667 through 671 refer to this situation.

667 Harry is placed on a Stryker frame because it:
1. Allows horizontal turning of the patient
2. Promotes body functions
3. Allows vertical turning of the patient
4. Helps prevent deformities

668 Before releasing the pivot pins and turning the Stryker frame, the nurse should:
1. Tell the patient to hold on to the bottom part of the frame
2. Observe the patient for signs of hypotension

3. Secure all bolts and straps to ensure patient safety
4. Get another nurse, since this procedure requires 2 people

669 Two weeks after his accident Harry's physical condition has stabilized. He is overcoming his initial health crisis but still has special needs that could not be met on a general unit; therefore Harry is transferred to the Intermediate Care Unit. Progressive patient care means:
1. Providing specialized nursing care using an episodic approach
2. Utilizing a variety of services and facilities to provide specialized care, depending on a patient's individual needs
3. Transferring patients from an area of greater intensive care to an area of lesser intensive care
4. Providing total nursing care by using the latest techniques and technology

670 Three weeks after his injury Harry is placed on a tilt table for 1 hour while the head of the table is elevated to a 20-degree angle. Each day the angle is gradually increased. The tilt table is used to:
1. Facilitate turning
2. Prevent pressure sores
3. Promote hyperextension of the spine
4. Prevent loss of calcium from the bones

671 The majority of patients with quadriplegia are taught to use wheelchairs because:
1. They usually are not and never will be functional walkers
2. It assists them in overcoming orthostatic hypotension
3. Their lower extremities are paralyzed but they have the strength in the upper extremities for self-propulsion
4. It prepares them for bracing and crutch walking

Situation: Mr. Amond, age 84, is admitted to the hospital with the following signs and symptoms: severe dyspnea, marked generalized edema of lower extremities, penis, scrotum, back, and abdomen, confusion, irritability, and frequent complaint of low back pain. Three months earlier he had been hospitalized for acute urinary retention, at which time a transurethral prostatectomy (TURP) was done, followed by bilateral orchidectomy and radiation therapy when the pathology report revealed carcinoma of the prostate. Laboratory findings indicate markedly elevated chemistries. Corticosteroids are currently being administered. Questions 672 through 678 refer to this situation.

672 In cancer of the prostate it is possible to follow the course of the disease through the study of:
1. Serum acid phosphatase
2. Creatinine
3. Blood urea nitrogen
4. Nonprotein nitrogen

673 Bladder irritability may follow radiation therapy. A sign of this complication would probably be:

1. Polyuria
2. Dribbling
3. Hematuria
4. Dysuria

674 Mr. Amond requests the urinal at frequent intervals but either does not void or voids in very small amounts. This is most likely due to:
1. Renal failure
2. Edema
3. Retention
4. Suppression

675 A urinary retention catheter is inserted. If Mr. Amond had complained of persistent discomfort in the bladder and urethra, the nurse most likely would do which of the following first?
1. Check the patency of the catheter
2. Notify the physician at once
3. Milk the tubing gently
4. Irrigate the catheter with prescribed solutions

676 The nurse can best prevent the contamination from retention catheters by:
1. Forcing fluids
2. Cleansing around the meatus periodically
3. Perineal cleansing
4. Irrigating the catheter

677 A Foley catheter operates by the principle of:
1. Inertia
2. Diffusion
3. Osmosis
4. Gravity

678 Mr. Amond experiences difficulty in voiding after the catheter is removed because of:
1. Interruption in normal voiding habits
2. Nervous tension
3. Remaining effects of anesthetics
4. Toxic symptoms from chemotherapy

679 Torsion of the testes requires immediate surgical correction because:
1. Irreversible damage occurs after a few hours
2. There is no other way to control the pain
3. Swelling is excessive and the testicle may rupture
4. The reduction in testicular blood flow leads to rapid death of sperm

Situation: Mr. Arnold is admitted to the C.C.U. with a diagnosis of acute pulmonary edema. The physician has ordered rotating tourniquets. Questions 680 through 686 refer to this situation.

680 When rotating tourniquets are used, the nurse should remember that:
1. The automatic tourniquets occlude arterial blood flow
2. The tourniquets are simultaneously applied to all 4 limbs
3. The tourniquets are rotated every 15 minutes
4. The tourniquets are rotated 2 at a time

681 The rotating tourniquet technique is effective for:
1. Decreasing arterial flow of blood to the body
2. Restricting visceral flow in the internal body cavities
3. Decreasing venous flow of blood to the heart
4. Increasing the flow of blood through the capillaries

682 Mr. Arnold's respirations are rapid and he appears extremely anxious. The nurse should be aware that the medication most frequently used to relieve anxiety and apprehension in the patient with pulmonary edema is:
1. Hydroxyzine (Atarax)
2. Sodium phenobarbital
3. Chloral hydrate
4. Morphine sulfate

683 An example of a rapidly acting diuretic that can be administered intravenously to patients with acute pulmonary edema is:
1. Spironolactone
2. Ethacrynic acid
3. Chlorothiazide
4. Chlorthalidone

684 Mr. Arnold is receiving aminophylline intravenously to relieve pulmonary edema. The nurse should observe him for:
1. Decreased pulse rate
2. Decreased urinary output
3. Hypotension
4. Visual disturbances

685 Mr. Arnold's condition worsens; he is intubated and placed on a mechanical ventilator. Central venous pressure must be monitored. In caring for Mr. Arnold, the nurse understands that:
1. The patient should not be taken off the ventilator for the central venous pressure readings
2. The fluid level in the manometer fluctuates with each respiration
3. Blood should not be easily aspirated from the central venous pressure line
4. The zero mark on the manometer should be at the level of the diaphragm

686 The physician orders an IV digitalis preparation. Which of the following preparations is only administered intravenously?
1. Digoxin
2. Gitalin
3. Deslanoside
4. Digitalis leaf

Situation: Mr. Rush is admitted to the coronary care unit with atrial fibrillation and a rapid ventricular response. The nurse prepares for cardioversion. Questions 687 through 693 refer to this situation.

687 Cardioversion is a procedure that is used to convert certain arrhythmias to normal rhythm. In addition to atrial fibrillation, which of the following arrhythmias is an indication for cardioversion?
1. Ventricular fibrillation
2. Premature ventricular contractions
3. Ventricular tachycardia
4. Ventricular standstill

688 When ventricular fibrillation occurs in a coronary care unit, the first person reaching the patient should:
1. Initiate cardiopulmonary resuscitation
2. Defibrillate the patient
3. Administer sodium bicarbonate intravenously
4. Administer oxygen

689 To overcome the potential danger of inducing ventricular fibrillation during cardioversion, the nurse should ensure that:
1. The energy level is set at its maximum level
2. The synchronizer switch is in the "on" position
3. The skin electrodes are applied after the T wave
4. The alarm system of the cardiac monitor is functioning simultaneously

690 That portion of the cardiac monitor which sets an alarm if the heart rate goes above or below a certain predetermined setting is called the:
1. Oscilloscope
2. Voltmeter
3. Pacemaker
4. Synchronizer

691 Cardioversion is only temporarily successful. Mr. Rush again develops atrial fibrillation. The physician has prescribed quinidine sulfate (Quinicardine) and digoxin (Lanoxin). The nurse should understand that the goal of the drug therapy plan is to:
1. Decrease atrial irritability and slow transmission of impulses through the AV node
2. Stimulate SA node control of conduction and shorten the refractory period of atrial tissue
3. Suppress irritability of atrial and ventricular myocardial tissue
4. Slow SA node firing rate and decrease irritability of the atrial myocardial tissue

692 When taking Mr. Rush's apical pulse the nurse should place the stethoscope:
1. At the xiphoid process
2. Between the third and fourth ribs and to the left of the sternum
3. Slightly below the left nipple
4. Just to the left of the median point of the sternum

693 Mr. Rush is receiving digoxin (Lanoxin). Because he will continue taking the drug after discharge, the nurse should be primarily concerned with:
1. Taking his apical pulse before drug administration and teaching him how to count his pulse rate
2. Observing him for return of normal cardiac conduction patterns and for adverse effects of the drug

3. Observing him for changes in cardiac rhythm and planning activity at home based on his tolerance
4. Monitoring vital signs and encouraging gradual increase in activities of daily living

Situation: Mrs. Oliver is hospitalized with coronary heart disease. She is receiving IV fluids, vital signs are checked q 4 h, and bed rest and medications, including digitalis and a sedative, are prescribed. She does not seem to be acutely ill but her prognosis is guarded. Questions 694 through 700 refer to this situation.

694 The nurse who has been caring for Mrs. Oliver for several days notes a change in respiration and beginning cyanosis. The nurse starts oxygen administration immediately. Which of the following statements is correct?
1. Oxygen had not been ordered and therefore should not be administered
2. The physician should have been called for an order before oxygen was begun
3. The symptoms were too vague for the nurse to diagnose a need for oxygen
4. The nurse's observations were sufficient to begin administration of oxygen

695 Mrs. Oliver asks what the coronary arteries have to do with her angina. In determining her answer, the nurse should take into consideration that the coronary arteries:
1. Carry reduced oxygen–content blood to the lungs
2. Carry blood from the aorta to the myocardium
3. Supply blood to the endocardium
4. Carry high-oxygen–content blood from the lungs toward the heart

696 After activity Mrs. Oliver states she has anginal pain. The nurse should realize that angina pectoris is a sign of:
1. Myocardial ischemia
2. Myocardial infarction
3. Coronary thrombosis
4. Mitral insufficiency

697 Mrs. Oliver's condition improves. Nitroglycerin is prescribed for anginal pain prn. When teaching Mrs. Oliver how to use nitroglycerin, the nurse tells her to place 1 tablet under her tongue when she has pain and to repeat the dose in 5 minutes if pain persists. The nurse should also tell her to:
1. Place 2 tablets under her tongue when intense pain occurs
2. Place 1 tablet under her tongue 3 minutes before activity and repeat the dose in 5 minutes if pain occurs
3. Swallow 1 tablet and place 1 tablet under her tongue when pain is intense
4. Place 1 tablet under her tongue when pain occurs and use an additional tablet after the attack to prevent recurrence

698 The nurse would tell Mrs. Oliver that she should suspect her nitroglycerin tablets to have lost their potency when:

1. Slight tingling is absent when the tablet is placed under her tongue
2. Onset of relief is delayed but duration of relief is unchanged
3. Pain occurs even after taking the tablet prophylactically to prevent its onset
4. Pain is unrelieved but facial flushing is increased

699 In addition to a decreased apical rate, which one of the following symptoms would the nurse teach the patient to be alert for as an indication to withhold the digitalis?
1. Decreased urinary output
2. Singultus
3. Chest pain
4. Blurred vision

700 When discharged, Mrs. Oliver will continue to take a diuretic and digitalis. The nurse reviewing Mrs. Oliver's diet would be especially careful to look for adequate sources of potassium because:
1. Under conditions of hyperglycemia digitalis exerts toxic effects on the heart
2. Potassium is a necessary ion for normal body function
3. Under conditions of hypokalemia, digitalis exerts toxic effects on the heart
4. Potassium is a cofactor for several important enzymes

701 When cardiovascular disease is a concern, reduction of the saturated fat in an ulcer diet may be desired and substitutes made of polyunsaturated fat. In such a case which of the following foods should not be allowed?
1. Whole milk
2. Special soft margarine
3. Corn oil
4. Fish

702 If you were instructing a cardiac patient on a high–unsaturated fatty acid diet, which of the following foods should be increased in the diet?
1. Liver and other glandular organ meats
2. Enriched whole milk
3. Red meats, such as beef
4. Vegetable oils, such as corn oil

703 Thromboplastin is found in:
1. Plasma
2. Erythrocytes
3. Platelets
4. Bile

704 When blood clots, what soluble substance becomes an insoluble gel?
1. Fibrin
2. Fibrinogen
3. Prothrombin
4. Thrombin

705 An ion that acts as a catalyst in blood clotting is:
1. Fe^{+++}
2. Ca^{++}
3. F^-
4. Cl^-

706 A rocking bed promotes circulation and breathing through which of the following principles?
1. Centrifugal force
2. Inertia
3. Momentum
4. Gravity

707 The efficacy of the abdominal-thoracic thrust (Heimlich maneuver) to expel a foreign object in the larynx demonstrates the gas volume related to the individual's:
1. Vital capacity
2. Residual volume
3. Tidal volume
4. Inspiratory reserve volume

708 Mrs. Jesse has diminished urine output after cardiac surgery. Her serum potassium level is elevated and the physician has prescribed polystyrene sodium sulfonate (Kayexalate) and sorbitol orally. This drug combination will:
1. Remove potassium ions from serum and provide carbohydrate for nutrition
2. Stimulate transfer of potassium ions and increase coupling with the resin
3. Allow exchange of sodium ions for potassium ions and increase intestinal water content
4. Increase solubility of polystyrene sodium sulfonate and facilitate its absorption

Situation: Twenty-year-old Jimmy Barbino is involved in a motorcycle accident and sustains a cervical fracture. To maintain cervical immobilization, he is placed in Crutchfield tongs and on a Circ-O-lectric bed. Questions 709 through 713 refer to this situation:

709 In providing care the nurse should:
1. Keep a small roll behind the patient's neck to provide support
2. Provide for urinary elimination when in the prone position
3. Keep sandbags on either side of the head to keep it immobile
4. Take vital signs before and after turning patient

710 Which of the following is a true statement about Circ-O-lectric beds?
1. Two people must be present when turning the bed
2. The patient is rotated from side to side to prevent decubiti
3. A receptacle for elimination is easily accessible
4. Postural hypotension after prolonged bed rest can be prevented

711 In caring for Jimmy, the nurse should:
1. Avoid the cervical spine area when administering back care
2. Clean the area around the tongs daily and apply antibiotic ointment
3. Relieve tension on tongs for 5 minutes every hour

4. Remove the weights attached to the tongs prior to rotating the Circ-O-lectric bed

712 Nerve fibers of the brain or spinal cord that are destroyed do not regenerate because they lack:
1. A myelin sheath
2. A neurolemma
3. Nissl bodies
4. Nuclei

713 Crushing of the spinal cord above the level of the phrenic nerve origin will result in:
1. Ventricular fibrillation
2. Activity counter to that indicated by control of the vagus nerve
3. Spinal shock and paralysis of the lower extremities
4. Respiratory paralysis and cessation of diaphragmatic contractions

---

Situation: Mrs. Simone is admitted to the unit with a diagnosis of liver cirrhosis and hepatic coma. Questions 714 through 718 refer to this situation.

714 One classic sign of hepatic coma is:
1. Elevated cholesterol
2. Bile-colored stools
3. Flapping hand tremors
4. Depressed muscle reflexes

715 Which of the following skin characteristics might be exhibited by Mrs. Simone?
1. Uremic "frost"
2. Urticaria
3. Hemangioma
4. Icterus

716 The ascites seen in cirrhosis is in part due to:
1. Increased plasma colloid osmotic pressure due to excessive liver growth and metabolism
2. The escape of lymph into the abdominal cavity directly from the inflamed liver sinusoid
3. Compression of the portal veins with resultant increased backpressure in the portal venous system
4. The decreased levels of ADH and aldosterone due to increasing metabolic activity in the liver

717 Liver cirrhosis may promote varicose veins because of:
1. Toxic irritating products released into the blood from the diseased organs
2. Increased plasma hydrostatic pressure in veins of the extremities
3. Decreased plasma protein concentration resulting in pooling of blood in the venous system
4. Ballooning of the vein walls due to decreased venous pressure and incompetent valves

718 The physician's decision to order neomycin enemas for Mrs. Simone is based on the results of which of the following laboratory tests?
1. Culture and sensitivity

2. SGPT
3. White blood count
4. Ammonia level

719 The portal vein can be identified as the one that:
1. Brings blood away from the liver
2. Brings venous blood from the intestinal wall to the liver
3. Enters the superior vena cava from the cranium
4. Is located superficially on the anteromedial surface of the thigh

720 A vitamin necessary for the synthesis of prothrombin by the liver is:
1. Vitamin K
2. Vitamin B_{12}
3. Vitamin D
4. Vitamin C

721 Jaundiced patients are susceptible to postoperative hemorrhage because their blood does not clot normally. Why?
1. Excess bile salts in blood inactivate prothrombinase
2. Excess bile salts in blood inhibit liver synthesis of prothrombin
3. Excess bile salts in blood inhibit liver synthesis of vitamin K
4. Lack of bile in intestines causes inadequate vitamin K absorption, which causes inadequate prothrombin synthesis by liver

722 Miss McGill was admitted to the hospital for diagnostic tests, which included blood and stool. The blood samples were drawn by the laboratory technician. The patient was told that a stool specimen was necessary. However, she was not told a total specimen was necessary and saved only a small amount. When it was noted a whole specimen was not available, the test was cancelled. This necessitated an additional day in the hospital. The patient is very disturbed and insists on not paying for the additional day because of the error. In situations such as this:
1. The order for a total specimen should have been written by the physician
2. A full explanation of tests or treatments is the right of the patient, and the nurse was negligent
3. Tests do go wrong, and hospital personnel are not responsible unless there is gross negligence
4. The patient is responsible for the hospital bill and must pay

723 Which of the following statements are true about the sources of vitamin K?
1. Vitamin K is found in a wide variety of foods so there is no danger of a deficiency
2. Vitamin K can easily be absorbed without assistance so that all that is consumed is absorbed
3. Vitamin K is rarely found in dietary food sources so a natural deficiency can easily occur
4. Almost all vitamin K sufficient for metabolic needs is produced by intestinal bacteria

Situation: Mrs. Eve, a 40-year-old housewife, is admitted to the hospital with a history of vomiting, tarry stools, ascites, and long-standing poor nutrition due to excessive alcohol intake. Her admitting diagnosis is bleeding esophageal varices. After emergency treatment the plan of therapy involves preparing Mrs. Eve for a portal-caval anastomosis. Questions 724 through 731 refer to this situation.

724 The pathophysiologic problem in cirrhosis of the liver causing esophageal varices is:
1. Dilated veins and varicosities
2. Portal hypertension
3. Ascites and edema
4. Loss of regeneration

725 Medical management that may be used to control the hemorrhage includes:
1. Aminocaproic acid (Amicar)
2. Balloon tamponade
3. Gastric suctioning
4. Iced lavage

726 Neomycin may be administered to prevent formation of:
1. Urea
2. Ammonia
3. Bile
4. Hemoglobin

727 If intubation is favored, the type of tube most likely to be used is:
1. Sengstaken-Blakemore
2. Miller-Abbott
3. Andersen
4. Levin

728 Characteristic signs that are a direct result of liver insufficiency may include:
1. Anuria
2. Fetor hepaticus
3. Globus hystericus
4. Blepharospasm

729 In an effort to prevent hepatic coma, it may become necessary to:
1. Eliminate protein from diet
2. Eliminate carbohydrate from the diet
3. Give Fleet enemas
4. Prepare for emergency surgery

730 When Mrs. Eve is able to eat, the diet ordered for her is:
1. High protein, low carbohydrate, low fat
2. Low sodium, protein to tolerance, moderate fat, high calorie, high vitamin, soft
3. High carbohydrate, low saturated fat, 1200 calories
4. Low protein, low carbohydrate, high fat, soft

731 Mrs. Eve begins to develop slurred speech, confusion, drowsiness, and a flapping tremor. With these evidences of impending hepatic coma, her diet is changed to:
1. 20 g protein, 2000 calories
2. 80 g protein, 1000 calories

3. 100 g protein, 2500 calories
4. 150 g protein, 1200 calories

Situation: Mr. Greene, a 56-year-old married construction worker, has been in the hospital for 2 weeks with a diagnosis of cerebral thrombosis. His symptoms include aphasia, right-sided paresis, and loss of the gag reflex. Questions 732 through 737 refer to this situation.

732 Due to the location of the lesion, Mr. Greene has expressive aphasia. As part of the long-range planning, the nurse should:
   1. Help the family to accept the fact that Mr. Greene cannot be verbally communicated with
   2. Wait for Mr. Greene to verbalize his needs regardless of how long it may take
   3. Begin associating words with physical objects
   4. Help Mr. Greene accept this disability as permanent

733 Since Mr. Greene was comatose on admission, the nurse would expect him to:
   1. Not be able to react to painful stimuli
   2. Be incontinent
   3. Be capable of spontaneous motion
   4. Have twitching or picking motions

734 Since one of the primary nursing objectives is maintenance of the airway, the nurse should place Mr. Greene in which of the following positions initially?
   1. Sims' or semiprone
   2. Prone
   3. Semi-Fowler's
   4. Orthopneic or Fowler's

735 Mr. Greene is still confined to bed rest, and, even though his physician has not ordered physical therapy for him, the nurse may institute:
   1. Active exercises of all extremities
   2. Passive range of motion exercises
   3. Light weight-lifting exercises of the right side
   4. Exercises that would actively capitalize on returning muscle function

736 Mr. Greene's wife insists on doing everything for him when she visits. After she leaves, Mr. Greene seems to be quite depressed. The nurse could assume that:
   1. Mr. Greene feels guilty about being a burden to his wife
   2. This depression is a natural outcome of his illness
   3. Mr. Greene feels the loss of his independence
   4. Mr. Greene is losing faith in the future

737 Mrs. Greene seems unable to accept the idea that her husband must be encouraged to do things for himself. The nurse may be able to work around these feelings by:
   1. Telling Mrs. Greene to let her husband do things for himself
   2. Letting Mrs. Greene know that the nursing staff has full responsibility for the patient's activities

3. Letting Mrs. Greene assume the responsibility as she sees fit
4. Asking Mrs. Greene for her assistance in planning the activities most helpful to the patient

---

Situation: Mr. Brown suffered severe head injuries in an automobile accident. Questions 738 through 744 refer to this situation.

738 Because Mr. Brown is still unconscious when placed on a stretcher to move him from the emergency room to the Intensive Care Unit, the nurse makes sure his arms do not hang down over the edge of the cart. By taking this precaution the nurse prevents injury to which plexus?
   1. Basilic
   2. Brachial
   3. Celiac
   4. Solar

739 Injury to which of the following parts of the brain is particularly likely to cause death?
   1. Medulla
   2. Midbrain
   3. Pons
   4. Thalamus

740 Mr. Brown's temperature, soon after admission to the hospital, registered 102.2° F (39° C), a fact suggesting injury of the:
   1. Hypothalamus
   2. Pallidum
   3. Temporal lobe
   4. Thalamus

741 After Mr. Brown recovers consciousness, he complains of hearing ringing noises, a fact suggesting injury of:
   1. Cranial nerve VI
   2. Cranial nerve VIII
   3. Frontal lobe
   4. Occipital lobe

742 Mr. Brown has a grand mal seizure. The physician prescribes phenytoin (Dilantin) to control the seizures. The expected effect of this drug is to:
   1. Alter the permeability of the cell membrane to potassium
   2. Control nerve impulses to the skeletal muscles
   3. Prevent depression of the central nervous system
   4. Produce an antispasmodic action on the muscles

743 Mr. Brown's condition has stablized and he is transferred out of the Intensive Care Unit. The nurse should automatically place at the bedside:
   1. A sphygmomanometer
   2. Oxygen equipment
   3. A padded tongue blade
   4. A rubber or plastic airway

744 Mr. Brown questions the nurse regarding the scheduling of his medication. The nurse informs him that the medications:

1. Can usually be stopped after a year's absence of seizures
2. Need to be taken only in periods of emotional stress
3. Will probably have to be continued for life
4. Will prevent the occurrence of seizures

Situation: Mrs. Crane, a 32-year-old woman who has intermittently been having painful, swollen knee and wrist joints during the past 3 months, is being admitted to the hospital for treatment of rheumatoid arthritis. Questions 745 through 748 refer to this situation.

745 One would expect the physician to order the following diet for Mrs. Crane:
1. High protein
2. Salt free
3. General diet, supplemented with vitamins and iron
4. Bland diet

746 Which of the following medications would the nurse expect to be prescribed to relieve the pain in Mrs. Crane's knees?
1. Codeine, 30 mg, every 4 hours
2. Aspirin, 0.6 g, every 4 hours
3. Codeine, 30 mg, every 4 hours prn
4. Nembutal, 90 mg, every hour

747 To prevent deformity of the knee joint, the physician will:
1. Immobilize the joint in a cylinder cast for a period of several weeks
2. Discourage use of the knee joint
3. Encourage motion of the joint within limits of pain
4. Put patient on bed rest regimen

748 Mrs. Crane asks the nurse why the physician may inject hydrocortisone into the knee joint. The nurse explains that the most important reason for doing this is to:
1. Prevent ankylosis of the joint
2. Reduce inflammation
3. Provide psychotherapy
4. Relieve pain

749 Which of the following terms does not refer to hypertrophic arthritis?
1. Degenerative
2. Nonankylosing
3. Herberden's nodes
4. Marie-Strumpell

750 The synovial fluid of the joints minimizes:
1. Velocity of movements
2. Friction in the joints
3. Efficiency
4. Work output

751 Mrs. Paul was hospitalized for an acute exacerbation of rheumatoid arthritis. In talking with the nurse, Mrs. Paul states she does not want cortisone even if it is prescribed by the physician. Later the nurse attempts to administer

cortisone that had been ordered by the physician. When Mrs. Paul asks what the medication is, the nurse gives an evasive answer. The patient takes the medication and later finds that she had been given cortisone. She states she intends to sue. The decision in this suit would take into consideration the fact that:
1. A physician's order takes precedence over a patient's preference
2. The patient has insufficient knowledge to make such a decision
3. The nurse is required to answer the patient truthfully
4. The nurse should have notified the physician

752 The type of membrane that lines the knee joint is called the:
1. Serous
2. Synovial
3. Mucous
4. Epithelial

753 If the nurse finds the supply of Darvon Compound-65 is depleted, but the patient needs this medication urgently, the nurse should most appropriately:
1. Give two capsules of Darvon Compound
2. Borrow a capsule of Darvon Compound-65 from the supply belonging to another patient
3. Ask the pharmacist to refill the prescription immediately
4. Ask the patient if he can wait another hour until the next delivery from the pharmacy is scheduled

Situation: Mr. Fritz, a 32-year-old car salesman, suffered a spinal cord injury in an auto accident, resulting in paraplegia. Questions 754 through 760 refer to this situation.

754 Good nursing care of Mr. Fritz will provide that he be turned every 2 hours. This is necessary mainly to:
1. Keep the patient comfortable
2. Prevent pressure sores
3. Improve circulation in the lower extremities
4. Prevent flexion contractures of all the extremities

755 Which measure would *not* prevent contractures of the joints of Mr. Fritz's lower extremities?
1. Changing bed position every 2 hours
2. Maintaining proper bed positions
3. Passively moving the extremities through a full range of motion several times daily
4. Providing the patient with active exercise instructions

756 Mr. Fritz questions the need for a tilt table. The nurse explains that the tilt table is used to help:
1. Prevent hypertension
2. Prevent pressure sores
3. Prevent loss of calcium from long bones
4. Encourage increased activity

757 Formation of urinary calculi is a complication that may be encountered by the paraplegic patient. A factor that contributes to this condition is:

1. High fluid intake
2. Increased intake of calcium
3. Inadequate kidney function
4. Increased loss of calcium from the skeletal system

758 Rehabilitation plans for Mr. Fritz:
1. Should be considered and planned for early in his care
2. Are not necessary, since he will return to his usual activities following hospitalization
3. Should be left up to the patient and his family
4. Are not necessary, since he will not be able to work again

759 Since Mr. Fritz has paraplegia, the nurse recognizes that one major early problem will be:
1. Use of mechanical aids for ambulation
2. Patient education
3. Quadriceps setting
4. Bladder control

760 The nurse may expect that Mr. Fritz will have some spasticity of the lower extremities. To prevent the development of contractures, careful consideration must be given to:
1. Proper positioning
2. Use of a tilt board
3. Active exercise
4. Deep massage

761 Mr. Brown had no paralysis after his accident, a fact suggesting no injury to the:
1. Basal ganglia
2. Parietal lobe
3. Precentral gyrus
4. Postcentral gyrus

Situation: Mr. Wilson has a herniated lumbar disc. Questions 762 through 766 refer to this situation.

762 Mrs. Wilson generally experiences a sudden increase in pain when he:
1. Sits on cold surfaces
2. Lies prone with knees flexed
3. Sneezes
4. Stands for extended periods

763 He is to undergo a myelogram before surgery. Which of the following will *not* be necessary when caring for Mr. Wilson postoperatively?
1. A thorough neurologic watch
2. Maintenance of a prone position for 24 hours
3. Encouragement of fluids to replace CSF
4. Application of cold compresses distal to the puncture

764 In caring for Mr. Wilson after the laminectomy, the nurse should be least concerned with which patient need?
1. Keeping the patient flat in bed
2. Turning the patient from side to side
3. Ambulating the patient with a back brace
4. Assessing for symmetry of movement

765 The main postoperative complication that the nurse should observe for following the laminectomy is:
1. Atony of the bladder
2. Pain referred to the flanks
3. Compression of the cord
4. Cerebral edema

766 When caring for a patient with a cervical laminectomy, in contrast to caring for a patient with a lumbar laminectomy, the nurse:
1. Should provide range of motion exercise early during the postoperative period
2. Has the added responsibility of removing oral secretions
3. Should maintain the patient's head in a flexed position
4. Must keep the patient's head at a 45-degree angle from the spine

Situation: Mrs. Elliot is a 52-year-old woman admitted to the hospital with the diagnosis of cancer of the cervix. She is scheduled for a hysterectomy and insertion of radium. She returns to the floor from the recovery room with a Foley catheter in place and vaginal packing. The packing is to be removed in 24 hours. Questions 767 through 770 refer to this situation.

767 The nurse checking the perineum found the packing protruding from the vagina. The immediate action to take is to report this situation to the physician at once because the:
1. Packing is radioactive
2. Purpose of the packing is to increase the distance between the insert and the rectum and/or bladder
3. Packing must be removed
4. Purpose of the packing is to prevent bleeding

768 In caring for Mrs. Elliot the nurse would do all of the following *except:*
1. Plan the care to limit the time spent at or close to the bedside
2. Keep Mrs. Elliot as quiet as possible so as not to dislodge the radium insert
3. Check all bed linen carefully before discarding
4. Spend as much time as possible in close contact with Mrs. Elliot to alleviate her anxiety

769 Which symptoms observed by the nurse following radium insertion are indicative of a radium reaction?
1. Nausea and vomiting
2. Pain and elevation of temperature
3. Restlessness and irritability
4. Vaginal discharge

770 Which of the following should the nurse avoid when assisting with radium removal?
1. Handle radium carefully with long forceps
2. Cleanse radium carefully in ether or alcohol using long forceps

3. Chart date and hour of removal and total time of treatment
4. Handle radium carefully wearing foil-lined rubber gloves

Situation: Mr. Piter has developed acute renal failure and uremia. Questions 771 through 776 refer to this situation.

771 Metabolic acidosis develops in renal failure as a result of:
1. Depression of respiratory rate by metabolic wastes causing carbon dioxide retention
2. Inability of renal tubules to secrete hydrogen ions and conserve bicarbonate
3. Inability of renal tubules to reabsorb water to achieve dilution of the acid contents of the blood
4. Impaired glomerular filtration causing retention of sodium and metabolic waste products

772 Of the following, which is most important in maintaining the fluid and electrolyte balance of the body?
1. Urinary system
2. Respiratory system
3. Antidiuretic hormone (ADH)
4. Aldosterone

773 Mr. Piter is to receive a modified Giordano-Giovannetti dietary regimen. This diet is based on which of the following principles?
1. A high-protein intake ensures an adequate daily supply of all amino acids to compensate for losses
2. Essential and nonessential amino acids are necessary in the diet to supply materials for tissue protein synthesis
3. Urea nitrogen cannot be used to synthesize amino acids in the body, so all the nitrogen for amino acid synthesis must come from the dietary protein
4. If the diet is low in protein and supplies only essential amino acids, the body will use the excess urea nitrogen to synthesize the nonessential amino acids needed for tissue protein production

774 Mr. Piter complains of tingling of the fingers and toes and muscle twitching. This is caused by:
1. Acidosis
2. Potassium retention
3. Calcium depletion
4. Sodium chloride depletion

775 Mr. Piter becomes confused and irritable. The nurse realizes that this behavior may be caused by:
1. A consistently elevated BUN
2. Hypernatremia
3. Limited fluid intake
4. Hyperkalemia

776 Patients who require hemodialysis may have an external shunt to gain access to a vein and an artery. The most serious problem with an external shunt is:
1. Clot formation
2. Septicemia

3. Sclerosis of vessels
4. Exsanguination

---

777 Which statement is false?
1. When renal blood pressure increases above normal, the kidneys release a substance called renin into the blood
2. The substance renin from the kidneys changes a normal blood protein to a substance that tends to constrict blood vessels
3. Glucose is reabsorbed into the blood only in the proximal tubules
4. Urine always has an acid reaction

778 Severe glomerulonephritis and albuminuria may cause edema because of the:
1. Rise in plasma hydrostatic pressure
2. Fall in plasma colloid osmotic pressure
3. Fall in tissue hydrostatic pressure
4. Rise in tissue colloid osmotic pressure

Situation: Mrs. Green had a cholecystectomy. Questions 779 through 783 refer to this situation.

779 When changing Mrs. Green's dressing, the nurse is careful not to introduce microorganisms into the surgical incision. This is an example of what kind of asepsis?
1. Concurrent
2. Medical
3. Wound
4. Surgical

780 Symptoms of obstructive jaundice include:
1. Dark-colored urine, clay-colored stools, itchy skin
2. Straw-colored urine, putty-colored stools, yellow sclera
3. Inadequate absorption of fat-soluble vitamin K
4. Light amber urine, dark brown stools, yellow skin

781 To promote healing of the large incision, Mrs. Green's physician would order daily doses of which of these vitamins?
1. Ascorbic acid
2. Mephyton
3. Vitamin B_{12} complex
4. Vitamin A

782 Mrs. Green is prone to upper respiratory tract complications because of:
1. Lowering of resistance due to bile in the blood
2. Invasion of the bloodstream by infection from the biliary tract
3. Proximity of the incision to the diaphragm
4. Length of time required for the surgery

783 Because vitamin A is fat soluble, it requires a helping agent for absorption. This agent is:
1. Lipase
2. Amylase
3. Hydrochloric acid
4. Bile

784 Advocating megadoses of vitamin A must be questioned because:
1. The vitamin cannot be stored, and the excess amount would saturate the general body tissues
2. The vitamin is highly toxic even in small amounts
3. The liver has a great storage capacity for the vitamin, even to toxic amounts
4. Although the body's requirement for the vitamin is very large, the cells can synthesize more as needed

785 Most of the work of changing raw fuel forms of carbohydrates to the refined usable fuel glucose is accomplished by enzymes located in the:
1. Mouth
2. Stomach mucosa
3. Small intestine
4. Large intestine

786 Calculate the intake-output of the following patient for an 8-hour period:
8 A.M.: IV with 5% D/W running and 900 ml left in bottle
8:30 A.M.: 150 ml urine voided
9 A.M. to 3 P.M.: q 3 h intervals 200 ml gastric tube formula and 50 ml H_2O; no aspirate obtained until final feeding; 25 ml at this time
8 A.M. to 4 P.M.: vitamin solution, 10 ml q 4 h
1 P.M.: 220 ml voided
3:15 P.M.: 235 ml voided
4 P.M.: IV with 550 ml left in bottle
1. Intake: 930 ml; output: 650 ml
2. Intake: 1050 ml; output: 680 ml
3. Intake: 1080 ml; output: 595 ml
4. Intake: 1130 ml; output: 630 ml

787 Excessive loss of gastric juice caused by gastric lavage or pernicious vomiting can lead to:
1. Acidosis
2. Alkalosis
3. Loss of osmotic pressure of the blood
4. Loss of oxygen from the blood

788 The correct patient position for the insertion of a gavage tube is:
1. High Fowler's
2. Mid-Fowler's
3. Low Fowler's
4. Supine

Situation: Mrs. Gorham, a 56-year-old woman, is admitted for repair of a cystocele and rectocele. She has 9 children: 3 are married, 2 are away at college, and 4 are still at home. The youngest child is 17 years old. Her husband is a Civil Service worker. Questions 789 through 792 refer to this situation.

789 In taking the health history, which of the following symptoms should the nurse expect Mrs. Gorham to experience?
1. Sporadic bleeding accompanied by abdominal pain
2. Stress incontinence, feeling of low abdominal pressure
3. Heavy leukorrhea, pruritus
4. Change in acidity level of vagina, leukorrhea, spotting

790 Rectocele and cystocele:
1. Are usually due to relaxation of musculature of the pelvic floor
2. Are usually due to injury during childbirth
3. Are usually due to infection of the bladder
4. Are usually due to trauma in repair of an episiotomy or laceration

791 Based on Mrs. Gorham's age and parity, the nurse expects the surgery done will most likely be:
1. Insertion of a pessary
2. Abdominal hysterectomy
3. Vaginal hysterectomy
4. Vaginoplasty

792 Mrs. Gorham returned from the operating room with a Foley catheter in place. The reason for this procedure was to prevent all the following *except:*
1. Retention with overflow
2. Bleeding following surgery
3. Discomfort due to bladder distention
4. Loss of bladder tone

793 The main blood supply to the uterus is directly from the:
1. Uterine and ovarian arteries
2. Uterine and hypogastric arteries
3. Ovarian arteries and the aorta
4. Aorta and the hypogastric arteries

794 The following hormones are responsible for the menstrual cycle:
1. Estrogen and progesterone
2. Gonadotropins
3. Gonadotropins and estrogen
4. Gonadotropins, estrogen, and progesterone

Situation: Mrs. Thomas, 62 years of age, is admitted to the hospital complaining of nausea, vomiting, weight loss of 20 pounds in 2 months, and periods of constipation and diarrhea. A diagnosis of carcinoma of the colon is made. Questions 795 through 801 refer to this situation.

795 A sigmoidoscopy is performed as a diagnostic measure. The nurse should place Mrs. Thomas in which position for this examination?
1. Prone
2. Lithotomy
3. Sims
4. Knee-chest

796 As part of the preparation of Mrs. Thomas for the sigmoidoscopy, the nurse:
1. Should withhold all fluids and foods for 24 hours before the examination
2. Should explain to the patient that she will have to swallow a chalklike substance

3. Will have to administer an enema the morning of the examination
4. Will have a container available for collection of a stool specimen

797 During the preoperative shaving preparation Mrs. Thomas starts to cry and says, "I'm sorry you have to do this messy thing for me." The choice response for a nurse at this time is:
1. "I don't mind it."
2. "Nurses get used to this."
3. "This is part of my job."
4. "You are upset."

798 For which of the following reasons is neomycin especially useful prior to colon surgery?
1. It is effective against many organisms
2. It acts systemically without delay
3. It will not affect the kidneys
4. It is poorly absorbed from the GI tract

799 The physician performs a colostomy. Postoperative nursing care should include:
1. Having the patient change her own dressing
2. Keeping the skin around the stoma clean and dry
3. Limiting fluid intake
4. Withholding all fluids for 72 hours

800 A person who has a permanent colostomy:
1. Needs special clothing
2. Has to limit her activities
3. Will have to dilate the stoma periodically
4. Needs to be on a bland, low-residue diet

801 Mrs. Thomas' diet should be:
1. As close to normal as possible
2. Rich in protein
3. Low in fiber content
4. High in carbohydrate

Situation: Mr. and Mrs. Lund, a retired couple who spent the winter in Florida, flew back to New York to see their newest grandson. On returning to their apartment after a family dinner, Mrs. Lund, age 72, tripped over a rug in the foyer. X-ray films at the hospital reveal a fracture of the acetabulum of the femur. Mrs. Lund's general state of health appears good except for the necessity to take enemas periodically. Questions 802 through 807 refer to this situation.

802 A fracture of the acetabulum most likely involves which of the following parts of the femur?
1. Head
2. Shaft
3. Neck
4. Trochanteric region

803 Mrs. Lund expresses concern about the treatment she will need. The nurse should be aware that the treatment of choice in this instance will probably be:
1. Insertion of hip prosthesis with traction

2. Hip pinning or nailing
3. Application of spica cast
4. Skeletal traction

804 To prevent pulmonary and circulatory complications, the nurse should make sure that Mrs. Lund is:
1. Turned from side to side every 5 hours
2. Ambulated as soon as the effects of anesthesia are gone
3. Turned on the unaffected side every 2 hours
4. Permitted to be up in a chair as soon as the effects of anesthesia are gone

805 Mrs. Lund has an Austin-Moore prosthesis inserted. After surgery the nurse should *not* routinely place Mrs. Lund:
1. On her affected side
2. On her unaffected side
3. In semi-Fowler's position
4. In supine position

806 Since Mrs. Lund is accustomed to taking enemas periodically to avoid constipation, the nurse should:
1. Arrange to have enemas ordered
2. Realize that enemas will be necessary because the normal conditioned reflex has been lost
3. Offer Mrs. Lund a large glass of prune juice in warm water each morning
4. Arrange to have laxatives ordered

807 Elderly patients have a high incidence of hip fractures because of:
1. Carelessness
2. Fragility of bone
3. Associated medical diseases
4. Sedentary existence and disease

Situation: Joan Yeats, 16 years of age, comes to the clinic because of severe burning on urination, persistent vaginal discharge, and irritation of the vulva. On examination, the vulva and vagina appear red and irritated and there is profuse greenish yellow discharge. A cervical culture and smear are taken. The smear reveals a gonorrheal infection. Questions 808 through 812 refer to this situation.

808 The causative organism of gonorrhea is:
1. *Treponema pallidum*
2. Gonococcus
3. *Staphylococcus* organism
4. Döderlein's bacillus

809 The nurse understands that gonorrhea is a highly infectious disease and that it:
1. Is easily cured
2. Can produce sterility
3. Occurs very rarely
4. Is limited to the external genitalia

810 In relation to the public health implications of this condition, the nurse would be most interested in:
1. The reasons for Joan's promiscuity
2. Interviewing Joan's parents to find out how she got this infection

3. Finding Joan's contacts
4. Instructing Joan in birth control measures

811 The drug of choice for the treatment of gonorrhea is:
1. Penicillin
2. Actinomycin
3. Chloramphenicol (Chloromycetin)
4. Colistin

812 The nurse tells Joan that the drug therapy can be expected to:
1. Cure the infection
2. Prevent complications
3. Control its transmission
4. Reverse pathologic changes

Situation: Mrs. Bond, 35 years of age, has had a midthigh amputation following injury in an automobile accident. Questions 813 through 818 refer to this situation.

813 To promote early and efficient ambulation, the nurse would:
1. Place pillows under the stump
2. Encourage the patient to lie supine
3. Turn the patient to the prone position frequently
4. Keep backrest elevated

814 When Mrs. Bond is allowed to be up, the nurse should teach her to:
1. Keep her hip in extension and adduction
2. Keep her hip raised with stump elevated
3. Lift her shoulder and hip of affected side when taking a step
4. Walk with crutches until stump is completely healed

815 Before ambulation is started, which of the following activities will make walking with crutches easier?
1. Frequent use of the trapeze to strengthen the biceps muscles
2. Push-up exercises with sawed-off crutches to strengthen the triceps, finger flexors, wrist extensors, and elbow extensors
3. Sitting in a chair until circulatory status is stable
4. Keeping limb in extension and abduction to prevent contractures

816 Which crutch gait should the nurse teach to the patient with a single leg amputation and wearing a prosthesis?
1. Tripod crutch gait
2. Four-point gait
3. Three-point gait
4. Swing-through type of crutch gait

817 In preparing Mrs. Bond for ambulation with crutches, the nurse should *not* instruct her to:
1. Stand and maintain balance
2. Ambulate several hours a day for practice
3. Do active exercises for muscle strengthening
4. Sit down and stand up

818 Rehabilitation of Mrs. Bond should begin:
1. Before the surgery

2. During the convalescent phase
3. On discharge from the hospital
4. When she is ready for a prosthesis

Situation: Mrs. Uri is 45 years old. She has 3 children ages 12, 9, and 5 years. She is admitted to the hospital with complaints of severe metorrhagia and menorrhagia of 1 year's duration. She was found to have a submucous myoma 6 months ago and has been carefully examined monthly. On the last examination, a week ago, the myoma was found to have grown appreciably, and she was told that a hysterectomy was necessary. Questions 819 through 822 refer to this situation.

819 The term *metrorrhagia* refers to:
1. Periods of severe bleeding in between menstrual periods
2. Severe bleeding during each menstrual period
3. Presence of occult blood in vaginal discharge
4. Spotting or staining at time of ovulation

820 Mrs. Uri expresses concern about having a hysterectomy done at her age because she has heard from friends that she will undergo severe symptoms of menopause after surgery. Based on her knowledge, the most appropriate response for the nurse to make should be:
1. "This is something that does occur in older women on occasion, but you don't have to worry about it."
2. "It's too bad you did not discuss this with your doctor. I really can't give you any kind of information about this."
3. "You were misinformed. This never happens following this type of surgery. Your friend probably had a different diagnosis."
4. "Some women occasionally experience exaggerated symptoms of menopause. This is usually transitory, since the ovaries are mainly responsible for maintenance of the hormone balance."

821 Mrs. Uri wants to know if it would be wise for her to take hormones right away to prevent symptoms. The most appropriate response should be:
1. "It is best to wait; you may not have any symptoms at all."
2. "You have to wait until symptoms are severe; otherwise, hormones will have no effect."
3. "This is something you should discuss with your physician, since it is important for him to know how you feel and what your concerns are."
4. "Isn't it comforting to know that hormones are available if you should need them?"

822 Mrs. Uri, when being prepared for the night, starts to sob a little and says, "I told my husband today that after this operation I will only be half a woman. He reassured me, but I know that was just a front." The most appropriate response would be:
1. "You feel this operation will have an effect on how your husband feels about you as his wife?"

2. "You know of course that this is silly. I wish you would not worry about such irrelevant things. The main thing is that you have to get well quickly."
3. "It must be frightening to know that your husband rejects you as a woman."
4. "I think I'll call your physician. He might want to postpone the operation until you and your husband have adjusted better to the outcomes of a hysterectomy."

---

823 Which of the following indicates the need for oral contraceptives?
1. A history of hypertension
2. A diagnosis of cardiac insufficiency
3. A history of repeated abortions
4. An irregular menstrual cycle

824 Compact bone is stronger than cancellous bone because of its greater:
1. Volume
2. Size
3. Weight
4. Density

825 An overexercised muscle that has an insufficient oxygen supply may become sore from a buildup of:
1. Butyric acid
2. Lactic acid
3. Acetoacetic acid
4. Acetone

Situation: Mr. Styles is brought to the ophthalmologist's office by his wife. He has minimum vision in his left eye and tells the nurse, "I'm sure it's a cataract; my brother just had cataract surgery." Questions 826 through 829 refer to this situation.

826 A cataract is:
1. A thin film over the cornea
2. A crystallinization of the pupil
3. An opacity of the lens
4. An increase in the density of the conjunctiva

827 After a patient has cataract surgery, the nurse should:
1. Encourage coughing and deep breathing
2. Discourage the patient from vigorously brushing teeth and hair
3. Keep the patient in the supine position with sand bags on either side of the head
4. Encourage eye exercises to strengthen ocular musculature

828 After examination the physician informs Mr. Styles that he has a detached retina. Retinal detachment is a:
1. Separation between the photoreceptor and neural layers of the retina
2. Separation between the sensory portion of the retina and the pigment layer
3. Consequence of optic-retinal atrophy
4. Separation of the choroid and optic chiasm

829 The goal of surgery for the treatment of a detached retina is to:
1. Create a scar that aids in healing retinal holes
2. Graft a healthy piece of retina in place
3. Promote growth of new retinal cells
4. Adhere the sclera to the choroid layer

---

830 The vision cycle in the eye requires vitamin A. Here the vitamin functions as:
1. A necessary component of rhodopsin (visual purple), which controls light-dark adaptations
2. A part of the rods and cones that controls color blindness
3. The material in the cornea that prevents cataract formation
4. An integral part of the retina's pigment—melanin

831 Vitamin A is a fat-soluble vitamin produced by humans and other animals from its precursor carotene-provitamin A. One of the main sources of this vitamin is:
1. Skim milk
2. Leafy greens
3. Oranges
4. Tomatoes

832 The preferred treatment for malignant melanoma of the eye is:
1. Chemotherapy
2. Radiation
3. Cryosurgery
4. Enucleation

Situation: Mrs. Prior, 35 years of age, had her third baby 6 months ago and is returning for a routine gynecologic examination. The doctor finds a small erosion of the cervix. He cauterizes the area with silver nitrate and tells her to douche once daily with 3 tablespoons of vinegar to 2 quarts of water. Questions 833 through 837 refer to this situation.

833 Erosions of the cervix are common when:
1. There has been a long labor
2. The cervix stretches during delivery and there is an unhealed laceration
3. The cervix is not dilated completely and delivery occurs
4. The normal acidity of the vagina is altered

834 Douches are ordered for Mrs. Prior to:
1. Keep the vaginal canal clean and free of bacteria
2. Promote healing by heat and elimination of sloughed tissue
3. Promote healing by altering the pH of the vagina
4. Make her comfortable

835 In administering a douche the best position for Mrs. Prior to assume would be the:
1. Knee-chest
2. Sims
3. Dorsal
4. Fowler's

836 Mrs. Prior should be instructed to direct the douche nozzle:
1. Downward
2. Upward
3. Downward and backward
4. Backward and upward

837 Early treatment of cervical erosions prevents:
1. Infections of the reproductive system
2. Cancer of the cervix
3. Metrorrhagia
4. Further erosions from occurring

838 When giving oral tetracycline to a patient, the nurse should:
1. Provide orange or other citrus fruit juice with the medication
2. Offer antacids 30 minutes after administration if GI side effects occur
3. Provide medication an hour before or after milk products have been ingested
4. Carefully monitor the total dosage to pregnant women and children

839 The primary reason for the ease of penetration of the needle through the tissue when administering an IM injection is:
1. The force used by the nurse when inserting the needle
2. The extremely high pressure developed at the tip of the needle due to its very small area
3. The softness of the tissue compared with the hardness of the needle
4. The long, slender shape of the needle

840 The end products of protein digestion—amino acids (the ''building blocks'')—are absorbed from the small intestine by:
1. Simple diffusion because of their small size
2. Active transport with aid of vitamin B_6 (pyridoxine)
3. Osmosis caused by their greater concentration in the intestinal lumen
4. Filtration according to the osmotic pressure direction

841 A complete protein, a food protein of high biologic value, is one that contains:
1. All 22 of the amino acids in sufficient quantity to meet human requirements
2. All 8 of the essential amino acids in correct proportion to meet human needs
3. The 8 essential amino acids in any proportion, since the body can always fill in the difference needed
4. Most of the 22 amino acids from which the body will make additional amounts of the 8 essential amino acids needed

842 Twenty-two amino acids are involved in total body metabolism, building and rebuilding various tissues. Of these, 8 are essential amino acids. This means that:
1. The body cannot synthesize these 8 amino acids and thus they must be obtained in the diet
2. These 8 amino acids are essential in body processes and the remaining 14 are not
3. These 8 amino acids can be made by the body because they are essential to life
4. After synthesizing these 8 amino acids the body uses them in key processes essential for growth

843 Phospho-Soda is classified as which of the following types of cathartics?
1. Drastic purgative
2. Saline cathartic
3. Emollient cathartic
4. Surface tension–lowering agent

844 Infection with Group A beta-hemolytic streptococci is associated with:
1. Rheumatoid arthritis
2. Infectious hepatitis
3. Spinal meningitis
4. Rheumatic fever

845 The common factor of puerperal sepsis, scarlet fever, otitis media, bacterial endocarditis, rheumatic fever, and glomerulonephritis is that all:
1. Can be easily controlled through childhood vaccination
2. Result from streptococcal infections that enter via the upper respiratory tract
3. Are noncontagious, self-limiting infections by spirilla
4. Are caused by parasitic bacteria that normally live outside the body

846 The darkening of tissue seen in the various forms of gangrene is due to the breakdown of hemoglobin with subsequent formation of:
1. Ferrous sulfide
2. Ferric chloride
3. Heme
4. Insoluble proteins

847 A solution containing 1 gram-equivalent weight of solute in 1 L of solution is called:
1. An isotonic solution
2. A normal solution
3. A molar solution
4. A saturated solution

848 Noble Manor, a 21-year-old patient, admits himself to the psychiatric unit for help in coping with the realities of life and activities of daily living. He develops severe pain in the right lower quadrant and is diagnosed as having acute appendicitis. In preparing Noble for an appendectomy, you will:
1. Ask Noble to sign his own preoperative consent after he is informed of the procedure and required care
2. Phone his next of kin to come in to sign his consent because he is on a psychiatric unit
3. Have 2 physicians, the surgeon and psychiatrist, sign for the surgery, since it is an emergency procedure
4. Have 2 nurses witness the operative consent as the patient signs it

849 The best definition of a tort is:
1. Doing something that a reasonable person under ordinary circumstances would not do
2. The application of force to the person of another by a reasonable individual
3. An illegality committed by one person against the property or person of another
4. An illegality committed against the public and punishable by the law through the courts

850 Intentional torts are:
1. Malpractice and assault
2. False imprisonment and battery
3. Negligence and invasion of privacy
4. Malpractice and negligence

851 Nurses are protected from all legal action when they:
1. Report incidences of suspected child abuse to the appropriate authorities identified in legislation and policies
2. Administer C.P.R. measures on an unconscious child pulled from a swimming pool
3. Offer first aid at the scene of an automobile-bus accident
4. Offer health teaching regarding family planning

852 The hospital in which you are employed as a nurse hires only registered or licensed nurses. Regulating the practice of nursing has its primary purpose the protection of:
1. The public
2. Practicing nurses
3. Professional standards
4. The employing agency

Situation: Mrs. Franklin, a known epileptic whose seizures are controlled by phenytoin, is receiving IV heparin sodium and oral warfarin sodium (Coumadin) concurrently for a partial occlusion of the left common carotid artery. Questions 853 through 857 refer to this situation.

853 Mrs. Franklin expresses concern about why she needs both drugs. The nurse's explanation is based on knowledge that the plan:
1. Immediately provides maximum protection against clot formation
2. Allows clot dissolution and prevents new clot formation
3. Maintains levels of circulating anticoagulant during the periods when the oral drug is being absorbed
4. Provides anticoagulant intravenously until the oral drug reaches its peak effect

854 After Mrs. Franklin has received IV heparin sodium for 3 days, the drug is discontinued. The nurse continues to observe her closely during the early days of treatment with Coumadin because:
1. Coumadin action is greater in patients with epilepsy
2. Seizures increase the metabolic degradation rate of coumadin

3. Coumadin affects the metabolism of phenytoin
4. Phenytoin increases the clotting potential

855 Mrs. Franklin is being discharged from the hospital at the end of the week. When discussing problems that relate to adverse effects of Coumadin, the nurse will tell her to consult with the physician if which one of the following problems occurs?
1. Increased incidence of transient ischemic attacks
2. Excess menstrual flow
3. Swelling of ankles
4. Decreased ability to concentrate

856 Mrs. Franklin's prothrombin levels have been somewhat unstable when checked in the clinic laboratory. The nurse interviews the patient to identify factors contributing to the problem. She first asks her about:
1. Intake of vitamin tablets or capsules
2. Use of sleeping medications
3. Use of analgesics
4. Compliance with the plan for taking Coumadin

857 Mrs. Franklin calls the clinic nurse after her weekly prothrombin test to find out if her oral anticoagulant dosage is to be changed. She mentions that her sleeping medication, secobarbital sodium (Seconal), is gone, but she plans to get more when she comes for her appointment in 3 days. The nurse tells her to come for a refill today because:
1. Absence of sleep may precipitate seizures
2. Discontinuance of the drug may affect the prothrombin level
3. She may have withdrawal symptoms because she has been taking the drug for 3 weeks
4. Her seizure control is dependent on the combined action of phenytoin (Dilantin) and the barbiturate

858 A patient who complains of tinnitus is describing a symptom that is:
1. Functional
2. Prodromal
3. Objective
4. Subjective

859 Patients with general paresis are usually treated by:
1. Behavior modification
2. Major tranquillizers
3. Penicillin
4. Electroconvulsive therapy

860 Comprehension of which of the following principles is most beneficial in establishing routine patterns of defecation?
1. Gastrocolic reflex
2. Inactivity produces muscle atonia
3. Increased fluid promotes ease of evacuation
4. Increased potassium is needed for normal neuromuscular irritability

Situation: Mrs. Row is seen at the gynecology clinic because of profuse vaginal discharge, pruritus, and burning. A smear for microscopic examination is done and reveals presence of *Trichomonas vaginalis*. Questions 861 through 863 refer to this situation.

861 A trichomonal infection is caused by which organism?
1. Fungus
2. Yeast
3. Spirochete
4. Protozoa

862 Mrs. Row would be treated by medication and douches with:
1. Physiologic saline to decrease the pH of the vagina
2. Vinegar to decrease the pH of the vagina
3. Sodium bicarbonate to increase the pH of the vagina
4. Tap water to increase the pH of the vagina

863 It is most likely that which drug will be prescribed orally for treatment of *Trichomonas vaginalis*?
1. Gentian violet
2. Fumagillin (Fugillin)
3. Metronidazole (Flagyl)
4. Nystatin

864 Spermatogenesis occurs:
1. During embryonic development
2. Immediately following birth
3. At the time of puberty
4. At any time following birth

865 The testes are suspended in the scrotum to:
1. Facilitate the passage of sperm through the urethra
2. Protect the sperm from the acidity of urine
3. Protect the sperm from high abdominal temperatures
4. Facilitate their maturation during embryonic development

Situation: Mrs. Vale is 42 years old and the mother of 2 children, ages 3 and 7. She is admitted to the hospital because of spotting between menstrual periods. The bleeding increases during intercourse and when straining on defecation. Her admission diagnosis is possible cervical polyps, and she is scheduled for a dilation and curettage (D and C) and polypectomy. The nurse admitting her notes that she is pale, wringing her hands, and unable to sit still, but not speaking unless asked a direct question. From these observations the nurse deduces that Mrs. Vale is very anxious. Questions 866 through 871 refer to this situation.

866 To help Mrs. Vale express her anxieties, the best approach for the nurse to use would be to:
1. Tell Mrs. Vale that there is no need to worry; a polypectomy and a D and C are considered minor surgery

2. Say, "I can tell that something is troubling you. It might help to talk about it."
3. Tell Mrs. Vale that it is normal for her to be anxious; everybody is fearful, even though there is no reason to worry
4. Ask, "What are you really upset about, Mrs. Vale?"

867 Mrs. Vale finally tells the nurse that she believes she has cancer because the physician told her that he would have to remove the polyps and wait for laboratory reports. The best response of the nurse would be:
1. "No operation is done without specimens being sent to the laboratory; that's strictly routine."
2. "Of course you don't have cancer; polyps are always benign. The laboratory report is simple routine."
3. "Worrying today is not going to help you at all. It will only interfere with your rest, and you need to be relaxed for the surgery."
4. "It is very upsetting to have to wait for a laboratory report. It might help you to know that most of the time polyps are not cancerous."

868 The nurse knows that cervical polyps:
1. Are usually benign, but curettage of the uterus is always done to rule out malignancy
2. Are usually malignant, and curettage is always done
3. Do not cause bleeding until they are malignant
4. Are frequently the precursors of uterine cancer

869 Following surgery the laboratory reports reveal a stage O lesion. According to the International Federation of Gynecology and Obstetrics, stage O is indicative of:
1. Carcinoma in situ
2. Carcinoma strictly confined to cervix
3. Early stromal invasion
4. Parametrial involvement

870 The most common site for cancer cell growth in the cervix is at the:
1. Internal os
2. External os
3. Junction of the columnar and squamous epithelium of the internal and external ossa
4. Junction of the cervix and lower uterine segment

871 Following discharge Mrs. Vale is asked to return in 3 months for an excisional conization of the cervix or a hysterectomy. This is done because:
1. Mrs. Vale is anxious about her condition and needs time to make her decision
2. Cervical cancer is slow growing so there is no need to hurry
3. In the preevasive stage prognosis is excellent if treatment is performed
4. This period of time is needed to rule out pregnancy

3 PSYCHIATRIC NURSING

Since nursing is concerned with the basic needs of people, the nurse, to understand and assist the individual, must be constantly aware of the many factors that influence a person's behavioral response. Individuals are constantly interacting with both the internal and the external environments and at any given moment stand as a conglomerate of their own and their forebears' experiences. The individual is continuously faced with emotional stress from the moment of birth until the moment of death. How people adapt to this stress and the problems resulting from the adaptations are the focus of psychiatric nursing. Psychiatric nursing is therefore the care of patients with emotional problems. However, the principles used in the care of psychiatric patients are applicable to all patients regardless of their diagnosis. Nursing, which is concerned with total care, must provide for the individual's physical (soma) as well as emotional (psyche) needs.

Background information from the behavioral sciences

BASIC CONCEPTS FROM ANTHROPOLOGY

A. All people are influenced by the culture into which they are born
B. Cultural factors include race, nationality, and religion
C. Groups that share a common race, nationality, religion, or language are known as ethnic groups
D. Society as a whole frequently develops a fixed set of expected responses for certain ethnic groups
E. When each member of an ethnic group is expected to respond in a specific manner, the expected responses are called stereotypes
F. Cultural variability occurs in all stages of the life cycle: child rearing, marriage patterns, health maintenance, etc.

Cultural influences

Race
A. Race is defined as a certain combination of physical traits that are transmitted by lineage or heredity
B. Physical traits of a race include skin color; texture and/or color of hair; eye shapes and folds; shape of nose, lips, and cheekbones; contour of the head; and body build
C. Of all the factors involved in ethnic group membership, race, which is given a great deal of emphasis, appears to be a biologic phenomenon that seems to contribute few specifics to the cultural background

Nationality
A. Nationality is defined as original or acquired membership in a particular nation
B. The culture of nationalities is passed down through generations in the form of
   1. Beliefs and superstitions
   2. Foods and national dishes
   3. Festivals and feast days
   4. Language and the meanings of certain words
C. Nationality and the culture it imparts frequently become even more important when a group of people immigrate to a new country when the members tend to join together to form a subculture of the new national culture
D. The subculture provides its members with a sense of security by furnishing a collective identity and maintaining the familiar

Religion

A. Religion is defined as the quest for values of the ideal life usually embodied in a particular set of beliefs practiced individually or within an organized system

B. Religious beliefs in some form have existed in every group during every period of history

C. Organized religions have been instrumental in developing an ethical and moral system that has frequently been based on a society's needs

D. Most of the world's religions have developed many rituals as part of their worship, and these rituals form the basis of the religious culture that is passed down from generation to generation

E. In contrast to traditional religion there exist numerous religious cults; persons seeking a sense of belonging and purpose join a religious cult that gives them a group identity through communal living and rigorous rituals

Culture and health

A. General influences
  1. Cultural background influences the way in which people view both health and disease
  2. The cultural influences seem to be derived from the areas of nationality and religion rather than race

B. Specific influences
  1. National culture may influence an individual's
     a. Response to illness
     b. Response to pain and even the tolerance of pain
     c. Need for superstitions and rituals
     d. Acceptance of dietary change both in type or in consistency of food
     e. Need for support and comfort from the family
     f. Ability to communicate in understandable terms
     g. Response to loss of independence
     h. Feelings about loss of privacy and exposure of parts of the body
     i. Feelings about loss of body parts
     j. Need for specific rites and rituals associated with dying
  2. Religious culture may influence an individual's
     a. Views on conception, birth, and child care
     b. Views about the meaning of pain and suffering
     c. Feelings about the meaning of death
     d. Desire for guidance from the clergy

     e. Acceptance of certain treatments such as immunizations and blood transfusions
     f. Concept of illness as a punishment
     g. Dietary restrictions including the types of food and their preparation
     h. Need for specific rites and rituals associated with dying

BASIC CONCEPTS FROM SOCIOLOGY

A. Every human society has institutions for the socialization of its members
  1. Process by which individuals are compelled or induced to conform to the customs of the group
     a. Group establishes rules and codes of conduct governing its members, and these become the norms, values, and mores of the group
     b. Role of members includes specified rights, duties, attitudes, and actions
  2. Controls established through a system of rewards and punishment
     a. Reward leads to acceptance as a member of the group
     b. Punishment for antisocial behavior leads to rejection and separation from the group

B. Development of society requires sanction of group members
  1. Growth takes place in social space
     a. Social boundaries separate one group from another
     b. Barriers to participation are established through mores and customs
  2. Leader's influence is always limited to conditions placed on it by the total group
  3. Behavioral roles are established by members of the group

C. A society is a reflection of all the functional relationships that occur between its individual members
  1. Products of group life are a major determinant in an individual's intellect, creativity, memory, thinking, and feeling
     a. Human beings have no memory, thought, or feeling that does not include society
     b. Intellect and creativity can be enhanced or hampered by society
  2. Members of a society have functional and rewarding social contact
     a. Members are accepted and approved and then participate in establishing rules, norms, and values

b. The nonmembers have, at best, limited social contacts with the members; this causes a segmentation of relationships and provides few rewarding experiences for the nonmembers

D. A society or a group can change because of conflict among members
1. This conflict is greatest when there is an absence of certain members, an introduction of new members, or a change in leadership
2. The resulting reorganization goes through 3 stages
   a. Tension stage caused by the conflict
   b. Integration stage, during which members learn about "the other's" problem
   c. Resolution of tension stage, during which a reconstruction of the group's norms and values takes place
3. The resolution of conflict and the restoring of equilibrium
   a. This takes place when people interact with one another and the group is dynamic
   b. Conflicts are not resolved when groups are rigid with fixed membership and ideas

E. The family is the primary group
1. Helps society to establish and maintain its code of behavior
2. Provides individual members with
   a. Strong emotional ties
      (1) Much sensory contact is present
      (2) Members learn to care about the emotional and physical well-being of each other
      (3) Members are responsive to one another's feelings, acts, and opinions
      (4) Members learn empathy by vicariously living the experiences of others
      (5) Members view selves through the eyes of others
   b. A feeling of security by meeting dependent needs
   c. A system of communication
      (1) Overt—words
      (2) Covert—body language
   d. Role identification and intimacy that help to internalize the acceptable behavioral patterns of the group
   e. A spirit of cooperation and competition through sibling interaction
3. Changes that have influenced the family's ability to indoctrinate children with the norms of society

a. The Industrial Revolution changed an agrarian society into an industrial one
   (1) Families became nuclear rather than extended
   (2) Families depended more on secondary groups for survival
   (3) New social groups were established to replace the extended family
   (4) Labor unions replaced patriarchal management
      (a) Laws enacted to protect the rights of children and other dependent people of society
      (b) Laws enacted to establish minimum wage and hour benefits
   (5) There was increased mobility of individuals
b. The altered male and female role patterns
   (1) The changing status of women
      (a) More women go outside the home to work
      (b) Women have an increased role in decision making and are better educated
   (2) The changing status of men
      (a) More men are willing to assume homemaking responsibilities
      (b) Men share decision making with women, thus decreasing dominance
   (3) Increased partnership in home and financial management has resulted in less stereotyped sex roles
c. Factors resulting in a reduction in the size of families
   (1) Increase in financial cost involved in raising and educating children
   (2) Emphasis on limited population growth
   (3) Wide dissemination of birth control information
   (4) Legalization of abortions
   (5) Persons choosing to marry in later adulthood

F. Peer groups help youth to establish norms of behavior and assist in the rites of passage from the family group to society
1. Youth learns about society through contact with the peer group
2. Youth develops further self-concept in contact with other youths

3. Peer group interaction can produce change in its individual members

4. Members have a strong loyalty to the peer group because of the reciprocal relationships and other rewards the group offers

5. Peer group norms may conflict with family or society's norms

G. Group membership helps individuals achieve goals that are not attainable through individual effort

1. Types of groups are task oriented, therapy, self-awareness, social

2. Group functional roles include task roles, group building or maintenance roles, individual or self-serving roles

3. Group content refers to the subject matter or task being worked on

4. Group process refers to what is happening between and to group members while working; it deals with morale, feeling tones, influence, competition, conflict

H. The type of leadership in a group depends on the needs of the group members as well as the personality of the leader

1. Authoritarian leader—is rigid and uses leadership role as an instrument of power; the leader makes all the decisions, which are then handed down to the membership; little communication and interrelating between leader and group

2. Democratic leader—is fair and logical, uses the leadership role to stimulate others to achieve a collective goal; the leader encourages interrelating among members by relating to all members; weaknesses as well as strengths are accepted; the contributions of all members are fostered and utilized

3. Emotional leader—reflects the feeling tones, norms, and values of the group

4. Laissez-faire leader—is passive and unproductive; usually assumes the role of a participant-observer and exerts little control or guidance over group behavior

5. Bureaucratic leader—is rigid and assumes a role that is determined by formal criteria or rules that are inherent in the organization and frequently unrelated to the present group; the leader is not emotionally involved and avoids interrelating with the group members

6. Charismatic leader—can assume any of the above behaviors, since the group attributes supernatural power to this person or the office and frequently follows directions without question

I. The community is a social organization that is considered the individual's secondary group

1. Relationships among members are usually more impersonal

2. Individuals participate in a more delimited manner or in a specific capacity

3. The group frequently functions as a means to an end

a. The group enables diversified groups to communicate

b. The group helps other groups to identify community problems and possible solutions

4. The secondary group is usually rather large and meets on an intermittent basis; contacts are usually maintained through correspondence

5. Leaders of the community facilitate group interaction

a. They have a knowledge of the community and its needs

b. They have the skill to stimulate others to act

6. Secondary groups help establish laws that are necessary to limit antisocial behavior

a. Laws provide diversified groups with a common base of acceptable behavior

b. Some laws may favor and protect the vested interests of specific groups within the society

Sociology and health

A. The role of society

1. Traditionally societies have placed great emphasis on caring for their members when they are ill

2. Recently society's role in health maintenance and the prevention of disease has been given an increased priority

3. Society's provision for health maintenance includes

a. Protection of food, water, and drug supplies

b. Establishment of public health agencies for the supervision, prevention, and control of disease and illness

c. Development of public education programs

d. Awarding scholarship grants for health education and research

e. Development of unemployment insurance programs

f. Establishment of Workmen's Compensation insurance

g. Establishment of Social Security and Medicare programs

h. Establishment of social welfare services and Medicaid programs

i. Supervision of medical and hospital insurance programs

B. The health agency as a social institution has
   1. A bureaucratic structure
   2. Policies, rules, and regulations governing behavior of its members
   3. An impersonal viewpoint
   4. A status hierarchy
   5. An increasingly specialized subculture

C. The hospital as a subculture of society
   1. The employees develop both written and unwritten hospital policies that
      a. Set standards of acceptable behavior for both patients and staff
      b. Regulate the patient's contact with the primary group by limiting visitors
      c. Force both patients and staff to relate to the secondary group
      d. Punish unacceptable behavior by any members of the group, including the patient
   2. The folklores and folkways of the hospital serve to
      a. Maintain the mystique of medicine by fostering the use of a unique language and system of symbols
      b. Attach stigmas to various social illnesses such as venereal disease, mental illness, drug addiction, and alcoholism, which are associated with certain patterns of living and acting that are not acceptable to the group
      c. Perpetuate the roles and values of the health team members and maintain the status quo
   3. The hospital has several functions
      a. The primary functions of the hospital are to help the patient regain health and resume a role in society by providing services directed toward
         (1) The treatment of illness
         (2) Rehabilitation
         (3) The maintenance of health
         (4) Protecting the patient's legal rights
      b. The secondary functions of the hospital are to help society by providing services directed toward
         (1) The education of health professionals
         (2) The education of the general public
         (3) Research

D. The delivery of health services—a responsibility of the community
   1. Members of society become active participants in prevention of illness
   2. Community health centers care for the ill in the home rather than in the hospital
   3. Extended care facilities are established with more community and homelike atmosphere
   4. Nonmedical community leaders take an active role in establishing health policy for society
   5. Lay members of the community become involved with health agencies' policies and decisions
   6. Health maintenance and treatment are no longer considered a privilege but the right of all members of society

BASIC CONCEPTS FROM PSYCHOLOGY

A. Human beings must be able to perceive and interpret stimuli to interact with the environment
   1. Perception and cognitive functioning are influenced by
      a. The nature of the stimuli
      b. Culture, beliefs, attitudes, and age
      c. Past experiences
      d. Present physical and emotional needs
   2. An individual's personality development is influenced by the ability to perceive and interpret stimuli
      a. Through these processes the external world is internalized
      b. The external world may in turn be distorted by the individual's perceptions

B. Humans have to communicate to be able to interact with the environment
   1. Communication is a behavior that is learned through the process of acculturation
   2. People have to communicate with others to make needs known
      a. The infant uses the cry to bring attention to needs
      b. Hearing is essential to the development of good speech, since one learns to form words by hearing the words of others
      c. The written word usually replaces the spoken word when face-to-face encounters are impractical or supplements the spoken word when further clarification is necessary

3. Productive communication depends on the consensual validation of all involved
   a. To understand the intent of the message, each person must be aware of the meaning of the spoken word as well as the inflections in the speaker's voice (verbal and nonverbal communication)
   b. Validation can best be accomplished when participants are empathetic
   c. The language and channel of communication must be adapted to the person and the purpose for which it is intended
   d. Feedback is necessary to evaluate the effectiveness of the words and guide the communication
   e. Satisfaction is enhanced for all involved when lines of communication are kept open
4. Barriers to effective communication include
   a. Variations in culture, language, and education
   b. Problems in hearing, speech, or comprehension—poor perception
   c. A refusal to listen to another point of view—inability to evaluate
   d. The use of selective inattention, which may cause an interruption or distortion of the message
5. Nonverbal behavior communicates the inner feelings of the individual performing the behavior
   a. Facial expression, posture, and body movement may express the anxiety, pain, tension, fear, happiness, joy, or satisfaction the individual is experiencing
   b. Nonverbal communication may transmit a different message than the individual's verbal communication (covert, overt messages)
   c. Confusion arises when there is a difference in the verbal and nonverbal message received
C. Psychologic experiences provide the energy that is transformed into behavior
   1. Anxiety frequently provides the push that moves people to action because it
      a. Develops when 2 goals or needs are in conflict
      b. Is a state of apprehension or tension aroused by impulses from within
      c. Prepares one for action or completely overwhelms and inhibits action
   2. Anxiety develops in stages that progress from increased alertness to panic

3. The sympathetic nervous system prepares the body's physiologic defense for fight or flight by stimulating the adrenal medulla to secrete epinephrine and norepinephrine
   a. The heart beat is accelerated to pump more blood to the muscles
   b. The peripheral blood vessels constrict to provide more blood to the vital organs
   c. The bronchioles dilate, and breathing becomes rapid and deep to supply more oxygen to the cells
   d. The pupils dilate to provide increased vision
   e. The liver releases glucose for quick energy
   f. The prothrombin time is lowered to protect the body from loss of blood in the event of injury
4. Selye's general adaptation syndrome (GAS) is the body's physiologic adaptation to stress (anxiety)
   a. The adrenal cortex secretes cortisone during the emergency stage
   b. When stress continues, the increased secretion of cortisone causes the body to go through a resistive stage
   c. If the process continues, the last stage is exhaustion and death
5. Defense mechanisms serve to protect the personality by controlling anxiety and reducing emotional pressures

The development of the personality

Factors involved in personality development
A. Behavior is a learned response that develops as a result of past experiences
B. To protect the individual's emotional well-being, these experiences are organized in the psyche on 3 different levels
   1. The conscious level is composed of post experiences easily recalled to mind that create little, if any, emotional discomfort
   2. The subconscious level of awareness has been deliberately pushed out of consciousness but can be recalled with some effort
   3. The unconscious level of awareness contains the largest body of material and greatly influences behavior
      a. This material cannot be deliberately brought back into awareness, since it is usually unacceptable to the individual
      b. If recalled, this material is usually disguised

or distorted, as in dreams; however, it is still capable of producing a good deal of anxiety
C. According to Freud the personality consists of 3 parts—the id, the ego, and the superego
  1. The id is that part of the personality which contains the instincts, impulses, and urges; it is totally self-centered and unconscious
  2. The ego is the conscious self; the ''I'' that deals with reality; the part of the personality that is shown to the environment
  3. The superego is that part of the personality that controls, inhibits, and regulates those impulses and instincts whose uncontrolled expression would endanger the emotional well-being of the individual and the stability of the society

Critical periods in the formation of the personality
A. The personality of an individual develops in overlapping stages that shade and merge together
  1. Certain goals must be accomplished during each stage in the development from infancy to maturity
  2. If these goals are not accomplished at specific periods, the basic structure of the personality will be weakened
  3. Factors in each stage persist as a permanent part of the personality
  4. Each stage has particular frustrations and major traumas that must be overcome
  5. Successful resolution of the conflicts associated with each stage is essential to development
  6. Unresolved conflicts remain in the unconscious and may, at times, result in maladaptive behavior
B. The tasks related to personality development during infancy
  1. Freud: oral stage—the infant obtains gratification by taking everything in; begins to develop self-concept from the responses of others
  2. Erikson: trust versus mistrust—trust develops from the inner feeling of self-worth that is transmitted through maternal care; the child learns to depend on the satisfaction that is derived from this care, and when the need is met, trust develops
  3. Sullivan: need for security—the infant learns to rely on others to gratify needs and satisfy wishes; develops a sense of basic trust, security, and self-worth when this occurs
C. The tasks related to personality development during early childhood
  1. Freud: anal stage—the struggle of giving of self

and breaking the symbiotic ties to mother; as the ties are broken, the child learns independence
  2. Erikson: autonomy versus shame and doubt—the struggle of holding on to or letting go; an internal struggle for self-identity; love versus hate
  3. Sullivan: learning to communicate needs through the use of words and the acceptance of delayed gratification and interference with wish fulfillment
D. The tasks related to personality development during preschool period
  1. Freud: oedipal stage—love for and desire to possess parent of the opposite sex creates fear and guilt feelings; desires are repressed and role identification with parent of the same sex occurs
  2. Erikson: initiative versus guilt—stage of intensive activity, play, and consuming fantasies where the child interjects parents' social consciousness
  3. Sullivan: development of body image and self-perception—organizes and uses experiences in terms of approval and disapproval received; begins using selective inattention and disassociating those experiences which cause physical or emotional discomfort and pain
E. The tasks related to personality development during school age or preadolescence
  1. Freud: latency stage—the period of low sexual activity and identification with peer groups
  2. Erikson: industry versus inferiority—the child wants to learn how to make things with others and strives to achieve success
  3. Sullivan: the period of learning to form satisfying relationships with peers by using competition, compromise, and cooperation; in this period the preadolescent learns to relate to peers of the same sex
F. The tasks related to personality development during adolescence
  1. Freud: genital stage—time when sexual activity increases and sexual identity is strengthened or attacked
  2. Erikson: identity versus identity diffusion—the developmental task involves integrating childhood identifications with the basic drives, native endowments, and opportunities offered in social roles
  3. Sullivan: learning to be independent and to establish satisfactory relationships with members of the opposite sex

G. The tasks related to personality development during young adulthood
   1. Erikson: intimacy versus isolation—the developmental task involves moving from the relative security of self-identity to the relative insecurity involved in establishing intimacy with another
   2. Sullivan: becoming economically, intellectually, and emotionally self-sufficient
H. The tasks related to personality development during later adulthood
   1. Erikson: generativity versus self-absorption—the mature person is interested in establishing and guiding the next generation
   2. Sullivan: learning to be interdependent and assuming responsibility for others
I. The tasks related to personality development during senescence
   1. Erikson: the older person adapts to triumphs and disappointments with a certain ego integrity
   2. Sullivan: the older person has an acceptance of responsibility for what life is and was and of its place in the flow of history

The influence of basic needs on the development of the personality

A. Humanity has certain basic needs that must be satisfied
   1. The need to communicate
      a. Through communication, humans maintain contact with reality
         (1) The individual needs to validate findings with others to correctly interpret reality
         (2) Validation is enhanced when communication conveys an understanding of feelings
      b. Through communication, the individual develops a concept of self in relation to others
   2. The need for security
      a. The need to feel secure as an assurance of survival is fundamental
      b. Fear emerges when survival is threatened
      c. Initially the infant's security is related to the satisfaction of physical needs
      d. Security is enhanced when the same individual meets the infant's physical needs in a consistent manner
      e. The infant must also perceive love to feel secure
      f. Security is derived from the individual's perception of self in relation to others

g. How the individual handles these perceptions influences personality development
   3. The need to move from dependence to independence
      a. The infant is dependent on the parents but through learning acquires faculties for independence
      b. There is no real security or deep assurance of survival in being dependent on others, since uncertainties develop if one's security is totally derived from this source
      c. The infant must feel love and security before reaching out to struggle with the problems in the environment
      d. When the need for love and security is met, the child is sustained in the failures and hurts associated with learning and independence
      e. Denial of the opportunity to learn or frustration in the drive for independence will produce emotional problems
   4. The need to develop a self-concept
      a. Self-concept begins to develop early in infancy
      b. The determination of the self-concept develops primarily through interaction with significant persons in the environment
      c. An integral part of the self-concept is the body image
      d. The first and most deeply learned perception of body image develops from the attitudes of significant others, since children view themselves as others view them
      e. The concept of self is the root of security and future developmental needs
      f. Communication enhances the development of self
      g. A person's self-concept is the basis for emotional stability or instability; a secure person has strength and capacity for independence and becomes less anxious when circumstances require the help of others
   5. The need to find relief from organic discomfort
      a. Through experience, one learns the most satisfying ways of relieving discomfort
      b. Adjustment to illness depends on how the individual adjusts to life
B. The needs of a specific individual at a given time will vary according to internal and external environmental factors

C. To attain psychologic equilibrium and achieve need satisfaction, the individual attempts to maintain a feeling of safety and comfort in adapting to life's situations; this is often achieved by maintaining a feeling of worth and a feeling of being needed by others

Anxiety and behavior

A. Anxiety
1. Is a state of apprehension, tension, or uneasiness
2. Is an internal phenomenon aroused by impulses
3. Occurs when the ego is threatened
4. Frequently stems from an anticipation of danger
5. May arise from known, unknown, or unrecognized sources

B. Levels of anxiety
1. Alertness level—an automatic response of the central nervous system that
   a. Prepares the body for danger by regulating internal processes
   b. Concentrates all energies for internal activity
2. Apprehension level—a response to anticipation of short-term danger that
   a. Prepares the individual for efficient performance
   b. Occurs when facing new situations
   c. Creates some conscious awareness of discomfort
3. Free-floating level—a response to generalized anxiety that
   a. Creates a feeling of impending doom
   b. Produces an acute feeling of discomfort
4. Panic level—a total response to anxiety characterized by uncontrolled, unrealistic behavior that
   a. Lessens perception of the environment to protect the ego from awareness
   b. Increases the danger to the entire system

C. Defenses
1. Conscious defenses—first-line defenses against anxiety that are used by all people in times of stress; they comprise the individual's deliberate effort to maintain control, reduce tension, and limit anxiety (individual may be aware of behavior but is not always aware of underlying reason)
   a. Remove self from source of anxiety
   b. Escape through bodily satisfactions
   c. Focus psychic energy on other more pleasant activities

d. Use of substitute gratifications
e. Consciously avoid painful subjects
f. Give socially acceptable reasons for behavior
g. Release tensions by acting out impulsively
2. Unconscious defenses—include the second-, third-, and fourth-line defenses against anxiety; these defenses may be used by all people in extremely stressful situations; however, if these defenses are used consistently, the individual is considered emotionally ill
   a. Second-line defenses are the personality traits developed to handle interpersonal relationships and protect the ego
      (1) Exaggerated dependency and immaturity
      (2) Passive submission
      (3) Domination of others
      (4) Aggression toward others
      (5) Withdrawal from others
      (6) Compulsive ambition
      (7) Perfectionism and grandiosity
   b. Third-line defenses are the neurotic traits developed to handle interpersonal relationships and protect the ego
      (1) Repudiation and opposition of inner drives by the use of reaction formation
      (2) Avoidance of emotional or feeling level by placing complete emphasis on intellectual reasoning
      (3) Inhibition of affective, autonomic, and visceral functions to deaden actual awareness of repressed impulses
      (4) Displacement of impulses to an external object, which is then feared and avoided
      (5) Use of compulsive rituals to magically neutralize inner impulses
   c. Fourth-line defenses are the psychotic traits developed to handle interpersonal relationships and protect the ego
      (1) Regression to dependency level of development frequently accompanied by the attitudes and behavior of the child
      (2) Denial and withdrawal from others and reality
      (3) Internalization of hostility
      (4) Excited, uncontrolled acting out
3. As anxiety and the threat to the ego are increased or decreased, shifts in the lines of defense will occur; the individual's behavior is altered by these shifts

D. Major sources of anxiety
   1. Threat to one's biologic integrity; interference with one's basic physiologic needs
   2. Threat to one's self system—self-esteem, self-worth, self-respect

Personality defenses

Defense mechanisms provide initial protection for the personality

A. Commonly used normal defense mechanisms that help an individual to deal with reality are
   1. Identification—the individual internalizes the characteristics of an idealized person
   2. Substitution—the individual replaces one goal for another
   3. Compensation—the individual makes up for a perceived lack in one area by emphasizing capabilities in another
   4. Sublimation—a socially acceptable behavior is substituted for an unacceptable instinct; this mechanism is used when the expression of these instincts would prove a threat to the self
   5. Compromise—the reciprocal give-and-take necessary in many relationships to salvage some part of the situation or the goal
   6. Rationalization—the individual makes acceptable excuses for behavior and feelings; attempts to explain behavior by logical reasoning
B. In addition to the normal defenses, all individuals may use compensatory type defenses in times of stress; these defenses, when used in moderation, are adaptive; if used to excess, they frequently create greater emotional problems
   1. Conversion—the emotional conflict is unconsciously changed into a physical symptom that can be expressed openly and without anxiety
   2. Denial—the emotional conflict is blocked from the conscious mind and the individual refuses to recognize its existence
   3. Displacement—the emotions related to an emotionally charged situation or object are shifted to a relatively safe substitute situation or object
   4. Fantasy—the conscious distortion of unconscious wishes and needs to obtain gratification and satisfaction
   5. Projection—the unconscious denial of unacceptable feelings and emotions in oneself while attributing them to others
   6. Reaction formation—the individual unconsciously reverses unacceptable feelings and behaves in the exact opposite manner
   7. Regression—the return to an earlier stage of behavior when stress creates problems at the present stage
   8. Repression—the involuntary exclusion from consciousness of those ideas, feelings, and situations which are creating conflict and causing discomfort
   9. Suppression—the voluntary exclusion from consciousness of those ideas, feelings, and situations which are creating conflict and causing discomfort
   10. Transference—feelings and emotions that were previously present toward important figures are applied and attributed to another person in the present
   11. Intellectualization—use of thinking, ideas, or intellect to avoid emotions
   12. Introjection—complete acceptance of another's opinions and values as one's own
C. As the use of these compensatory defenses increases and encompasses more of the individual's life, contact with reality is interrupted and distortions begin
D. Identifiable patterns of response begin to form when individuals respond to most situations they encounter with the same type of behavior
E. These patterns of behavior are considered deviations and are usually looked on as symptoms of emotional problems
F. Although all individuals may, in times of severe emotional stress, use many of the behaviors listed, it is their repetitive use in most situations that is indicative of problems

Motivation, learning, and behavior

A. All behavior is motivated
   1. A motive always implies some purpose
   2. Social motives are often changed through learning
   3. Symbolic rewards are the major factors in learning
   4. Social approval is an important form of symbolic reward
B. Behavior and emotions
   1. Emotions act as motives for behavior, since they often involve a reaction to some external situation
   2. Behavior is always accompanied and often controlled by the emotions

3. Emotions may facilitate or hinder the learning process
4. Emotions exert a strong influence on the thinking process

C. Automatic behavior
1. Is the predetermined or repetitive type behavior that has been used successfully in prior situations
2. Requires little effort or thought
3. Is adapted to definite situations and can be difficult to alter if the situation changes
4. Is integrated with cognition in the functioning of a mature and independent adult

D. Life is a continually changing process, and when these changes occur in areas of significance they often produce rather distinct emotional responses; these changes include
1. Resistance to change—the individual hesitates to accept or adapt to the change and may attempt to deny its occurrence or reject its outcome
2. Regression—the individual returns to an earlier type of behavior that, at the time, provided some satisfaction and gratification and now provides an escape from the unacceptable or anxiety-producing situation
3. Acceptance and progression—the individual adapts to the change and expends energy on outside objects rather than self-centered aims

Nursing in psychiatry

BASIC PRINCIPLES OF PSYCHIATRIC NURSING

A. These principles
1. Are by necessity general in nature
2. Form the guidelines for the emotional care of all patients

B. In caring for patients, the nurse should attempt to
1. Accept and respect people as individuals regardless of their behavior
2. Limit or reject the individual's inappropriate behavior without rejecting the individual
3. Recognize that all behavior has meaning and is meeting the needs of the performer regardless of how distorted or meaningless it appears to others
4. Accept the dependency needs of individuals while supporting and encouraging moves toward independence

5. Help individuals set appropriate limits for themselves or set limits for them when they are unable to do so
6. Encourage individuals to express their feelings in an atmosphere free of reprisal or judgment
7. Recognize that individuals need to use their defenses until other defenses can be substituted
8. Recognize how feelings affect behavior and influence relationships
9. Recognize that individuals frequently respond to the behavioral expectations of others—family, peers, staff
10. Recognize that all individuals have a potential for movement toward higher levels of emotional health

THE THERAPEUTIC NURSING RELATIONSHIP

A. Fundamental requirements of a therapeutic relationship
1. The ability to communicate therapeutically requires a basic understanding and use of interviewing techniques in developing a trusting relationship through
   a. Open-ended rather than probing questions
   b. Reflection of words and feelings and paraphrasing
   c. Acceptance of the patient's behavior
   d. Nonjudgmental objective attitude
   e. Focusing on the emotional needs of the patient
   f. Having a therapeutic goal for the interview
2. The recognition that an individual has a potential for growth
   a. Individuals need to learn about their own behavior in relation to others
   b. Exchanging experiences with others provides the reassurance that reactions are valid and feelings shared
   c. Participating with groups increases knowledge of interpersonal relationships and helps individuals to identify their strengths and resources
   d. The identification of the individual's strengths and resources helps to convey the expectation of growth
3. The recognition that an individual needs to be accepted
   a. Acceptance is an active process designed to convey respect for another through empathetic understanding

b. Acceptance of others implies and requires acceptance of self

c. To be nonjudgmental, one has to become aware of one's own attitudes and feelings and their effect on perception

d. Acceptance requires that individuals be permitted and even encouraged to express their feelings and attitudes even though they may be divergent from the general viewpoint
  (1) Individuals should be encouraged to express both positive and negative feelings
  (2) This encouragement must occur on both the verbal and nonverbal level

e. Acceptance means showing interest in another person; interest requires
  (1) Face-to-face contact and really listening to what the other person has to say
  (2) Developing an awareness of the other person's likes and dislikes
  (3) Attempting to understand another's point of view
  (4) Using nonverbal as well as verbal expressions of acceptance

f. Acceptance requires the development of interpersonal techniques that encourage others to express problems; the listener's
  (1) Reflection of feelings, attitudes, and words helps the speaker to identify feelings
  (2) Open-ended questions permit the speaker to focus on problems
  (3) Paraphrasing assists the speaker in clarifying statements
  (4) Use of silence provides both the listener and the speaker with the necessary time for thinking over what is being discussed

g. Acceptance requires the recognition of factors that block communication, including
  (1) Any overt or covert response that conveys a judgmental or superior attitude
  (2) Direct questions that convey an invasive or probing attitude
  (3) Ridicule that conveys a hostile attitude
  (4) Talking about one's own problems and not listening, which conveys a self-serving attitude and loss of interest in the speaker

B. The recognition of behavioral changes that result from physical illness

1. Anxiety, fear, and depression occur whenever there is a health problem
  a. Body image and feelings of being in control of one's body have their basis in the early developmental period
  b. Anxiety develops whenever a real or imagined threat to the body image occurs

2. Signs of the anxiety, fear, and depression associated with illness are variable and include
  a. Indifference to symptoms—usually related to failure to accept the occurrence of a health problem
  b. Denial of reality—usually related to attempts to maintain stability and integrity of the personality
  c. Reaction formation—usually related to attempts to block the reality from consciousness and acting as if nothing is wrong
  d. Failure to keep appointments and follow physician's or nurse's directions—usually related to fear of finding additional problems or admitting there is something wrong
  e. Overconcern with body functions and symptoms—usually related to fear of death
  f. Asking many questions and offering many complaints—usually related to attempts at keeping a staff member by the bedside because of fears associated with illness; fear of abandonment
  g. Opportunity to ventilate feelings

3. Emotional needs of the ill person include
  a. The security of continuous relationships with friends and members of their families
  b. Some way of achieving the feeling of self-worth and self-esteem
  c. Assistance in accepting the dependent role of the patient
  d. Assistance in resolving conflicts while maintaining security
  e. Assistance in refocusing inner resources
  f. Contact with the reality of the external world

4. To help the individual maintain the self-concept during illness, the nurse must understand the normal stages of illness
  a. Denial—the individual cannot believe it is happening
  b. Anger—something has happened that one cannot control
  c. Bargaining—promising to be a better person if something occurs

d. Depression—one grieves for loss or expected loss

e. Acceptance of the illness and learning how to adapt—this stage can only be reached when the individual has resolved the conflicts that develop during the earlier stages

5. Common reactions occur to the change in body image associated with many health problems

a. Attitudes toward one's body and self-concept greatly influence response

b. Fear is a universal response; individual may focus on fear of
(1) Pain
(2) Incapacitation
(3) Disfigurement
(4) Altered self-concept
(5) Rejection by loved ones
(6) Death

c. Questioning is a universal response; individual may focus on
(1) This can't be happening to me
(2) Is this really happening to me?
(3) What did I do to deserve this?
(4) Why am I being punished?

d. Grief and mourning are universal responses; individual may focus on
(1) What was in the past
(2) What could have been for the future
(3) Loss of missed opportunities
(4) A magnified view of the loss
(5) Avoiding interpersonal contacts

DEVIATE PATTERNS OF BEHAVIOR
Withdrawn behavior

A. Definition—a pathologic retreat from or an avoidance of people and the world of reality

B. Developmental factors
1. Unhappy childhood caused by conflict, tension, and anxiety in the home
2. Inconsistent relationships with parents
   a. Lack of firm standards for reward or punishment
   b. Variations between verbal and nonverbal communications
3. Failure to develop a sense of security
4. Failure to develop positive self-image
5. Interpersonal relationships create a continuous source of anxiety

6. Chronic anxiety results in loss of interest in interpersonal relationships and reality testing
7. Extreme sensitivity, narcissism, and introversion develop

C. Compensatory mechanisms used to reduce and avoid stress include
1. Fixation
2. Rigidity and compulsiveness
3. Reaction formation
4. Sublimation
5. Rationalization
6. Regression

D. Effects of compensatory mechanisms on behavior
1. Isolation and failure to test reality result in greater distortions of reality situations
2. Behavior can progress until loss of contact with reality develops and individual retreats into the psychosis usually identified as schizophrenia

Projective behavior

A. Definition—a pathologic denial of one's own feelings, faults, failures, and emotions while continually attributing them to others

B. Developmental factors
1. Parents set extremely high demands and continually raise expected standards of performance
2. Expectations of failure are fostered, creating feelings of inadequacy and feelings of inferiority
3. Childhood experiences continue to reinforce these feelings and, chronic insecurity, suspiciousness, and extreme sensitivity develop
4. Feelings of hostility develop and cannot be expressed
5. Inability to establish interpersonal relationships with others interferes with reality testing
6. Individual develops a rigid, structured, narcissistic personality
7. Competitive society fosters and supports projective patterns of behavior

C. Compensatory mechanisms used to reduce and avoid stress include
1. Displacement
2. Projection
3. Rigidity
4. Denial
5. Rationalization
6. Delusions
7. Ideas of reference

D. Effects of compensatory mechanisms on behavior
1. Unable to tolerate suspense, prolonged anxiety, or tension
2. Unacceptable impulses and wishes are denied and faults and failures are disclaimed for self and attributed to others
3. Delusional ideas develop and begin to dominate behavior
4. Ideas of reference result in continual misinterpretation of events
5. Delusions become more systemized and spread out
6. Behavior can progress until loss of contact with reality is complete and the individual retreats into the psychosis usually identified as paranoid schizophrenia or paranoid states

Aggressive behavior

A. Definition—pathologic anger and hostility that are turned outward onto others or inward on oneself
B. Developmental factors
1. Security is chronically threatened, resulting in a continual struggle to maintain it
2. Strong need for approval
3. Failure to develop self-concept and self-esteem
4. Chronic anxiety and tension, which are often increased by the real or imagined loss of a love object
5. Demands and responsibilities are high
C. Compensatory mechanisms used to reduce and avoid stress include
1. Displacement
2. Rigidity
3. Denial
4. Rationalization
5. Repression
6. Hostility that can be directed on
   a. Self
   b. Environment
D. Effects of compensatory mechanisms on behavior
1. Need for approval results in compliance to demands
2. Necessary compliance creates resentment
3. Hostility develops and fosters feeling of guilt
4. Self-doubt increases anxiety and tension
5. Increased anxiety and tension reduce interpersonal relationships and reality testing
6. Behavior can progress until there is a complete

loss of contact with reality and the individual retreats into the psychosis usually identified as an affective disorder

Psychoneurotic behavior

Includes anxiety reactions, conversion reactions, phobic reactions, and obsessive-compulsive reactions
A. Definition—a maladjustive type of response, characterized by many fears, anxieties, and/or physical symptoms
B. Developmental factors
1. Usually lack a stable family life and effective guidance
2. Frequently overprotected and fail to acquire the necessary skills to cope with problems
3. Experience chronic insecurity, anxiety, and tension
4. Goals are set for them by the parents, and acceptance depends on achieving the goals
5. Constant struggle to gain reassurance and security
6. Gains satisfaction from behavior and substitutes this satisfaction for the satisfaction desired but not obtained through interpersonal relations
C. Compensatory mechanisms used to reduce anxiety and avoid stress include
1. Displacement
2. Rationalization
3. Regression
4. Rigidity and compulsiveness
5. Conversion
6. Denial
D. Effects of compensatory mechanisms on behavior
1. Behavior is purposeful and is unconsciously resorted to when the person feels threatened
2. Continued use of behavior can
   a. Create new problems for the individual
   b. Be out of proportion to the degree of stress, impair social effectiveness, and dominate the individual's total life
3. When impairment of functioning occurs, the individual is usually considered to be deviating from the normal and is usually classified as psychoneurotic

Socially aggressive behavior

A. Definition—a maladjustive response resulting from a defect in the development of the personality that is characterized by peculiar actions or misbehavior

B. Developmental factors
1. Approval and disapproval do not appear sufficiently strong in childhood to influence the behavior along accepted patterns
2. Long history of maladjustment that creates more problems as child matures and standards for acceptable behavior are increased
3. May show a history of severe emotional trauma in early life that interferes with emotional development
4. Parents frequently provide a cold, emotionally sterile environment
C. Compensatory mechanisms used to reduce anxiety and avoid stress include
1. Displacement
2. Repression
3. Denial
4. Regression
5. Hostility
6. Rejection
D. Effects of compensatory mechanisms on behavior
1. Appear competent but are usually unreliable and lack a sense of responsibility
2. Have the potential to succeed but show a history of repeated failure
3. Lack perseverance, honesty, and sincerity
4. Completely egocentric and incapable of emotional investment in others
5. Experience no remorse or shame
6. Explosive under pressure
7. Unable to tolerate criticism
8. Fail to profit from past experiences and care little about the consequences for present acts
9. Impairment of judgment usually creates problems and brings individual into conflict with society; usually classified as personality disturbances

Addictive behavior

A. Definition—the repeated or chronic use of alcohol or drugs with a resulting dependency on these substances
B. Developmental factors
1. Feelings of loneliness and isolation develop
2. Chronic anxiety, fears, and low tension tolerance develop as a result of early relationships
3. Feelings of inadequacy in interpersonal relationships serve to increase anxiety
4. Inability to delay satisfaction
5. Struggle for independence yet unconscious desire to be dependent

6. Impulsiveness and resentment of responsibility
7. Peer pressure and drug availability
8. Sexual conflict
9. Family factors
C. Compensatory mechanisms used to reduce anxiety and avoid stress include
1. Denial
2. Regression
3. Rationalization
4. Addiction
5. Displacement
6. Fantasy
7. Repression
8. Intellecutalization
D. Effects of compensatory mechanisms on behavior
1. Drug or alcohol reduces inhibitory self-control
2. Drug or alcohol allows for expression of inner feelings but increases the guilt and requires more of the substance to relieve the guilt
3. Alcohol and drugs decrease feelings of inferiority and reduce anxiety
4. Alcohol and drugs increase social isolation and cause deterioration of personal habits
5. Individual becomes increasingly less efficient and devotes less energy to goals and ambitions
6. Dependency and tolerance develop and the substances are needed in increasing amounts to achieve the same dulling of reality
7. Securing the alcohol or drug becomes the main objective in life, and functioning is totally impaired; these individuals are then classified as drug addicts or alcoholics

CLASSIFICATION OF MENTAL DISORDERS

The following is the Standard Nomenclature of Mental Disorders*
A. Organic brain syndromes
1. Psychoses
a. Senile and presenile dementia
b. Alcoholic psychosis
c. Psychosis associated with intracranial infection
d. Psychosis associated with other cerebral conditions
e. Psychosis associated with other physical conditions

---

*Adapted from Diagnostic and statistical manual of mental disorders, ed. 3, Washington, D.C., 1978, American Psychiatric Association.

2. Nonpsychotic organic brain syndromes
B. Psychoses not attributed to physical condition
  1. Major affective disorders
  2. Schizophrenia
  3. Paranoid states
  4. Other psychoses
C. Neuroses
D. Personality disorders and certain other nonpsychotic mental disorders
  1. Personality disorders
  2. Sexual deviations
  3. Alcoholism
  4. Drug dependence
E. Psychophysiologic disorders
F. Special symptoms
G. Transient situational disturbances
H. Behavioral disorders of childhood and adolescence
I. Mental retardation
J. Conditions without manifest psychiatric disorders and nonspecific conditions
  1. Social maladjustment without manifest psychiatric disorder
  2. Nonspecific conditions

PATHOLOGY, SYMPTOMS, THERAPIES, AND NURSING APPROACHES FOR THE MAJOR DIAGNOSTIC ENTITIES IN PSYCHIATRY
Organic brain syndromes

Associated with actual changes in the tissue of the brain

Psychoses

A. Acute brain syndrome—syndromes from which patient usually recovers, since the situation is often reversible and temporary
  1. Pathology
    a. Infection
      (1) Intracranial or nervous system; e.g., meningitis or encephalitis
      (2) Systemic or toxic; e.g., pneumonia or typhoid
    b. Trauma to the head
    c. Circulatory disturbances resulting in impairment of blood flow to the brain
    d. Metabolic disorders—electrolyte imbalance; e.g., dehydration, diarrhea, vomiting
    e. Drug intoxication or poisoning
    f. Alcoholic intoxication
  2. Symptoms
    a. Delirium and its accompanying confusion, hallucinations, and delusions

b. Disorientation and confusion as to time, place, identity
    c. Memory defects for both recent and remote facts
    d. Slurring of speech may occur along with an indistinct pronunciation or use of words
    e. Tremors, incoordination, imbalance, and incontinence may develop
  3. Therapy
    a. Reduce causative agent such as fever, toxins, drugs, or alcohol
    b. Prevent further damage
    c. Provide diet high in calories, protein, and vitamins
    d. Provide mild sedative if necessary
  4. Nursing approach
    a. Provide quiet environment, reduce stimuli
    b. Provide assurance to patient and family
    c. Since lability of mood is common, plan care so that the staff approaches these patients when they appear receptive
    d. Ensure adequate intake and output
    e. Observe for changing physiologic and neurologic symptoms
B. Chronic brain syndrome—syndromes from which patient does not recover, since the damage is irreversible and permanent; there may be some improvement with treatment of the underlying cause, but disturbances in memory and judgment will remain
  1. Pathology
    a. Prenatal injury or malformation; e.g., hydrocephalus, microcephalus, neurosyphilis
    b. Infections such as general paresis
    c. Alcohol; e.g., alcoholic encephalopathy, Korsakoff's syndrome
    d. Trauma in which head injury results in permanent brain damage
    e. Circulatory disturbances causing anoxia and permanent brain damage; e.g., cerebral arteriosclerosis, cerebral vascular accidents
    f. Deterioration and death of brain cells; e.g., senile psychosis
    g. Loss of brain tissue in presenile psychosis; e.g., Alzheimer's disease and Pick's disease
    h. Nutritional deprivation of brain cells; e.g., pellagra
    i. Damage resulting from generalized diseases; e.g., multiple sclerosis, hepatolenticular dis-

ease, Huntington's chorea, Parkinson's disease
   j. Damage resulting from pressures of brain tumors
2. Symptoms—same as those resulting from acute brain syndrome
3. Therapy—same as those for acute brain syndrome with greater emphasis placed on preventing further damage
4. Nursing approach
   a. Provide a safe environment
   b. Continually orient the patient to time, date, and place
   c. Keep schedule of activities flexible to make use of patient's lability of moods and easy distractability
   d. Provide adequate nutrition
   e. Provide exercise
   f. Provide diversional activities that the patient enjoys and can handle
   g. Provide emotional support for family

Nonpsychotic organic brain syndromes

Included in this classification are all the acute and chronic brain syndromes in which there is a demonstrable organic change in the brain, but where psychotic behavior is not a major problem

Psychoses not attributed to physical condition

Classified as functional psychoses, since there is no organic basis or change in the structure of the brain

Major affective disorders

A. Manic-depressive psychosis
   1. Pathology
      a. Premorbid personality utilizes the compensatory mechanisms associated with the aggressive patterns of behavior
      b. Occurs between 20 and 49 years of age
   2. Symptoms
      a. Cyclic, periodic episodes of acute self-limiting mood swings; can be all manic, all depressed, or mixed manic and depressed; occurring before 40 years of age but after 20 years of age
      b. Individual is able to function at usual activity between episodes
      c. Obesity is frequent precursor of attack, and onset can be slowed or modified by dieting
      d. Depression most common form

      (1) Triad of symptoms is present: lowering of mood tone—dejection, slowing of thinking and speech, and decrease in psychomotor activity
      (2) Insomnia—difficulty in falling asleep and staying asleep, tend to wake early
      (3) Decreased appetite
      (4) Feelings of guilt and worthlessness
      (5) Difficulty in performing daily tasks
      (6) Tearful with a great deal of suicidal rumination
      (7) Speaks slowly and uses monosyllabic words
      (8) Orientation and logic are unaffected
      (9) Sex drive is decreased
      (10) Constipation and urinary retention may occur
      e. Manic phase occurs less frequently
      (1) Difficulty sleeping
      (2) Extremely active—always in a hurry
      (3) Humor good, although remarks can be caustic
      (4) Monopolizes conversations, and irritability is only superficially covered
      (5) Orientation is clear but judgment is poor
      (6) Always planning and scheming
      (7) Increased sex drive
   3. Therapy
      a. Electroconvulsive therapy is the treatment of choice; succinylcholine chloride (Anectine), a depolarizing muscle relaxant causing paralysis, is used to reduce the intensity of muscle contractions during the convulsive stage
      b. Lithium carbonate, mood-elevating psychotherapeutic drugs, and sedatives are used
      c. High-protein, high-carbohydrate diet is provided for energy, especially in manic phase
      d. Psychotherapy is useful between attacks
   4. Nursing approach
      a. Monitor patient's intake and output
      b. Keep environment nonchallenging and nonstimulating
      c. Avoid irritating routines as much as possible
      d. Protect patient against suicide during the entire episode
      e. Keep activities simple, uncomplicated, and repetitive in nature; they should be of short duration and require little concentration
      f. Overactive manic patients should be

    (1) Accepted by staff even though their behavior may be rejected

    (2) Permitted to express hostility and ambivalence without reinforcement of guilt feelings

    (3) Approached in a calm, collected manner by staff members that have good self-control

    (4) Given limits for their behavior

    (5) Responded to in a nonargumentative manner, using their easy distractibility

    (6) Approached in a consistent manner by all staff members

g. Depressed patients should

    (1) Be allowed time for their slowness

    (2) Be accepted even when they are unable to carry out daily routines

    (3) Be given demands they can meet

    (4) Be helped to express hostility and have their responses accepted without rejection

    (5) Have their self-esteem realistically built up

    (6) Be presented with simple rather than complex routines and activities

    (7) Have their feelings of worthlessness accepted as real to them; their feelings should not be denied, condoned, or approved, just accepted

    (8) Be protected against suicide attempts, especially when the depression begins to lift (suicide is a real and ever-present danger)

5. Pharmacologic approach—antidepressant drugs that increase the level of norepinephrine at subcortical neuroeffector sites

a. Monoamine oxidase (MAO) inhibitors—elevate norepinephrine levels in brain tissues by interference with the enzyme MAO; act as psychic energizers

    (1) Drugs

        (a) Isocarboxazid (Marplan)

        (b) Phenelzine sulfate (Nardil)

        (c) Tranylcypromine sulfate (Parnate)

    (2) Drug interactions—MAOI potentiate the effects of alcohol, barbiturates, anesthetic agents (cocaine), antihistamines, narcotics, corticoids, anticholinergics, sympathomimetic drugs

    (3) Drug-food interactions—hypertensive crisis with vascular rupture, occipital headache, palpitation, stiffness of neck muscles, emesis, sweating, photophobia, and cardiac arrhythmias may occur when neurohormonal levels are elevated by ingestion of foods with high tyramine content (pickled herring, beer, wine, chicken livers, aged or natural cheese, chocolate)

    (4) Adverse effects—central nervous system stimulation (headache, restlessness, insomnia), peripheral edema, orthostatic hypotension, dry mouth, constipation, urine retention, transient impotence, anorexia, nausea

b. Norepinephrine blockers provide elevated levels of the neurohormone by preventing reuptake and storage at the axon (tricyclic compounds)

    (1) Drugs

        (a) Amitriptyline hydrochloride (Elavil)

        (b) Desipramine hydrochloride (Norpramin, Pertofrane)

        (c) Doxepin hydrochloride (Adapin, Sinequan)

        (d) Imipramine hydrochloride (Presamine, Tofranil)

        (e) Nortriptyline hydrochloride (Aventyl)

        (f) Protriptyline hydrochloride (Vivactil)

    (2) Drug interactions—potentiate effects of anticholinergic drugs and central nervous system depressants; e.g., alcohol and sedatives

    (3) Adverse effects—orthostatic hypotension, skin rash, drowsiness, dry mouth, blurred vision, constipation, urine retention, tachycardia, central nervous system stimulation in elderly patients (excitement, restlessness, incoordination, fine tremor)

c. Norepinephrine release stimulators (cerebral stimulants)—improve productivity by decreasing psychomotor activity or response to environmental stimuli

    (1) Drugs

        (a) Methylphenidate hydrochloride (Ritalin)

        (b) Pipradrol hydrochloride (Meratran)

    (2) Adverse effects—hyperexcitability, irritability, restlessness

d. Norepinephrine uptake accelerator—alters sodium transport in nerve and muscle cells and affects a shift in intraneural metabolism of norepinephrine

    (1) Drug—lithium carbonate (Eskalith, Lithane, Lithonate)

    (2) Drug-food interaction—restriction of sodium intake increases drug substitution for sodium ions, which causes signs of hyponatremia (nausea, vomiting, diarrhea, muscle fasciculations, stupor, convulsions)

    (3) Adverse effects—excess voiding and extreme thirst caused by drug suppression of antidiuretic hormone (ADH) function, which causes dehydration

B. Psychotic depressive reactions

  1. Pathology—similar to manic-depressive psychosis except

    a. Occurs before 20 years of age or after 60 years of age

    b. Precipitating factor can always be identified

  2. Symptoms

    a. Severe depression

    b. Absence of history of repeated episodes

    c. Gross misinterpretations of reality

  3. Therapy—same as for manic-depressive psychosis

  4. Nursing approach—same as for manic-depressive psychosis

  5. Pharmacologic approach—same as for manic-depressive psychosis

C. Involutional depressive psychosis

  1. Pathology similar to manic-depressive psychosis except

    a. Depression is agitated rather than retarded

    b. Depression occurs after 40 years of age and before 60 years of age

    c. Precipitating factors such as the marriage of children, the loss of a job, the breakup of a marriage, the death of a partner can often be identified

    d. Depression is closely related to the menopause or climacteric, and hormonal and endocrine changes are considered by many to play an important role in this disorder

    e. Individual is usually rigid, inflexible, overassertive, overly meticulous, and worrisome

  2. Symptoms

    a. Wakes early after difficulty in falling asleep

    b. Feelings of unreality and sinfulness

    c. Complains of somatic delusions

    d. Extremely jumpy and agitated

    e. Pacing and wringing of hands as well as other increased motor activity

    f. Triad of symptoms present—delusions of sin and/or poverty, obsession with death, somatic delusions especially related to the GI tract

  3. Therapy—same as for manic-depressive psychosis

  4. Nursing approach—same as for manic-depressive psychosis

  5. Pharmacologic approach—same as for manic-depressive psychosis

Schizophrenia

This syndrome constitutes the largest group of behavioral disorders in our society; at the present time 1 person in 100 will spend some time in a hospital with this disorder, and this number is increasing

A. Pathology

  1. Premorbid personality—individuals use the compensatory mechanism of the withdrawn pattern of behavior; in addition, a paranoid schizophrenic uses the compensatory mechanism of the projective pattern of behavior

  2. Severe emotional problems, although unrecognized, begin early in life; however, the most common age for the break with reality is from 18 to 34 years of age

  3. There is chronic insecurity and an almost total failure in interpersonal relationships

  4. Etiology is still unknown, although some interesting findings in genetics, biochemistry, psychology, family therapy, and sociology present hope for a breakthrough

  5. Regardless of the ultimate etiology, there appears to be a close causal relationship with the environment

  6. Course of the disease is either acute or chronic; although it can stop or retrogress at any point, it does not appear to ever permit a full restoration of integrity to the personality

B. Symptoms

  1. Alterations in feeling, thinking, and relating to the external world are present

  2. Association defects occur, and association links weaken; the individual appears incoherent, bizarre, and unpredictable

  3. Distortions interfere with attention, perception, concentration, and memory

4. Affect and emotional expression are flattened
5. Ambivalence is common and frequently is so exaggerated that any action or decision becomes impossible
6. Detachment from reality results in autistic thinking and serves to further distort reality
7. Disturbance occurs in body image, since the undeveloped ego has few strengths and no boundaries (frequently refers to self in the second or third person instead of using the first person)
8. Secondary symptoms such as hallucinations, delusions, confusion, stupor, and catatonia may or may not be present

C. Types of schizophrenia—although historically a great deal of time and effort were directed toward identifying types of schizophrenia, it should be recognized that the classification is not static; there is a great deal of overlapping symptomatology; individuals diagnosed as being in one classification frequently are diagnosed at a later time in another classification

1. Simple schizophrenia—these individuals are rarely hospitalized, since they are the unattached, withdrawn, affectively and intellectually diminished individuals who are a part of the vagabond or transient groups of our society
2. Hebephrenic schizophrenia—picture of severe and pronounced mental incapacity; great mental and emotional deterioration occurs; behavior is retarded with sexual preoccupations, emotional dulling, infantile silliness; onset is usually between 12 and 25 years of age
3. Catatonic schizophrenia—picture of withdrawal and distortions in reality testing, accompanied by total ambivalence, which is frequently exhibited in rather unpredictable motor activity; the ambivalence makes movement and decision making impossible, since the individual cannot decide how or where to move; they can be literally frozen in their tracks—akinetic (stuporous)—or forced into the aimless hyperkinetic fugue (excited) movements
4. Paranoid schizophrenia—these individuals use the withdrawn compensatory mechanisms to distort reality and then develop a rather intricate delusional system by using the projective pattern of behavior; they are secretive, suspicious, use ideas of reference, and finally develop delusions of grandeur

5. Undifferentiated schizophrenia—these individuals demonstrate the primary thought, affect, and withdrawal defects of schizophrenia but cannot be classified under a specific type because of mixed symptoms
6. Schizoaffective schizophrenia—these individuals demonstrate a mixture of symptoms from both the schizophrenia and the affective reactions; the thought processes and bizarre behavior appears schizophrenic, but there is usually marked elation or depression; such individuals usually prove to be basically schizophrenic in nature
7. Pseudoneurotic schizophrenia—these individuals appear neurotic but cannot function as a neurotic; they present the autism, ambivalence, and thought disturbances of the schizophrenic while also demonstrating the all-pervading anxiety of the neurotic; such individuals are difficult to diagnose but usually prove to be basically schizophrenic in nature

D. Therapy
1. Administration of chlorpromazine and other major tranquilizers
2. Psychotherapy—individual, family, and group
3. Motivation therapy
4. Occupational and vocational therapy
5. Electroconvulsive therapy may be useful in some instances to modify behavior
6. Day care treatment programs in community settings
7. Pharmacologic approach—antipsychotic drugs (major tranquilizers)—control behavior when the patient's uncontrolled actions are destructive to self, others, or the environment
   a. Types of major tranquilizers
      (1) Phenothiazine derivatives
         (a) Acetophenazine maleate (Tindal)
         (b) Chlorpromazine hydrochloride (Thorazine)
         (c) Fluphenazine hydrochloride (Prolixin)
         (d) Perphenazine (Trilafon)
         (e) Prochlorperazine (Compazine)
         (f) Promazine hydrochloride (Sparine)
         (g) Thioridazine hydrochloride (Mellaril)
         (h) Trifluoperazine (Stelazine)
         (i) Triflupromazine hydrochloride (Vesprin)

(2) Butyrophenones
  (a) Droperidol (Inapsine)
  (b) Haloperidol (Haldol)
(3) Dihydroindolone
  (a) Molidone hydrochloride (Moban)
(4) Thioxanthenes
  (a) Chlorprothixene (Taractan)
  (b) Thiothixene (Navane)

b. Adverse effects of major tranquilizers—manifestations of extrapyramidal tract irritation, drowsiness (highest incidence in initial days of therapy), orthostatic hypotension, constipation, urinary retention, anorexia, hypersensitivity reactions (tissue fluid accumulation, photoallergic reaction, impotence, cessation of menses or ovulation), cardiac toxicity

(1) Extrapyramidal symptoms
  (a) Pseudoparkinsonism—resembles true parkinsonism (tremor, masklike facies, drooling, restlessness)
  (b) Akinesia—fatigue, weakness of arms and legs
  (c) Akathisia—motor restlessness
  (d) Persistent dyskinesia—protrusion of tongue, facial disturbances, opisthotonos; these symptoms can persist even after administration of an antiparkinsonian agent and cessation of the tranquilizer; cosmetically disturbing to patient and family

(2) Antiparkinsonian drugs—block the extrapyramidal symptoms
  (a) Benztropine (Cogentin)
  (b) Biperiden (Akineton)
  (c) Diphenhydramine (Benadryl)
  (d) Trihexyphenidyl (Artane)

(3) Tardive dyskinesias—symptoms seen in some patients receiving phenothiazine drugs; these include linguofacial hyperkinesias and bizarre movements of the neck and trunk; can occur after drug reduction or discontinuation; antiparkinsonian drugs are most often of no benefit in alleviating symptoms

E. Nursing approach
  1. Observe for adverse drug reactions in all patients receiving large doses of the major tranquilizers
  2. Encourage patients to follow a plan of organized activity and a prescribed drug regimen

3. Respect patients as human beings with both dignity and worth
4. Accept patients at their present level of functioning
5. Avoid trying to argue patients out of their delusions or hallucinations
6. Accept that the patients' hallucinations and delusions are real and frightening to them
7. Encourage the development of interpersonal relationships between patients and others
8. Point out reality to patients but do not force your reality on them

Paranoid states

Those individuals who demonstrate the suspiciousness and delusions common to paranoid conditions but who do not exhibit the thinking and behavioral disorganization or the personality disintegration found in the other psychoses

A. Pathology
  1. The premorbid personality uses the compensatory mechanism of the projective pattern of behavior
  2. Paranoid defenses are considered by some to be defenses against unconscious homosexuality or overt hostility
  3. Exact etiology is unknown

B. Symptoms
  1. Paranoia—these individuals exhibit a rather elaborate, highly organized paranoid delusional system while preserving the other functions of the personality; in spite of this system, thinking is not interfered with and personality function usually continues without interruption
  2. Involutional paranoid state—these individuals experience an onset of delusions during the involutional period; the thought and emotional disorganization of schizophrenia are absent; the depressive overtones present lead many to believe that this state is a manifestation of the involutional psychosis

C. Therapy
  1. Chemotherapy with major tranquilizers is the most helpful in treating these individuals
  2. Individual psychotherapy may provide some relief of symptoms
  3. Electroconvulsive therapy may prove helpful for some patients
  4. Paranoid patients are the most challenging to reach, since none of the present therapies appear to be helpful in breaking down the delusional system

D. Nursing approach
  1. Provide an environment with some intellectual challenge that does not threaten security
  2. Avoid counteraggression and retaliation against the patient
  3. Accept and recognize patient's need for superior attitude
  4. Meet sarcasm and ridicule in a matter-of-fact manner
  5. Guard patient's self-esteem from attack by other patients
  6. Accept patient's misinterpretations of events
  7. Point out reality but do not directly challenge patient's delusions

Neuroses

Common responses to emotional problems that are rarely treated in psychiatric settings; they are disturbances in personality but there is no great defect in reality testing or severe antisocial behavior
A. Pathology
  1. All 6 subgroups of the neuroses use the compensatory mechanisms of the psychoneurotic pattern of behavior
  2. The development of the symptoms usually permits some measure of social adjustment
  3. Usually begins in early 20s as a result of environmental factors in childhood
  4. Early life is rigid and orderly
  5. Pressures of decision making regarding life-style that occur in the early adult years seem to act as precipitating factors
B. Symptoms
  1. Anxiety reactions—anxiety is unconsciously expressed through physical means
    a. Pervasive, continuous feeling of free-floating anxiety, tension, and apprehension
    b. Episodes of dyspnea, palpitations, irritability, dizziness, insomnia, fainting, weakness, chest pain, trembling, and headaches
    c. Symptoms usually appear in relation to stress situations such as crowded rooms, public gatherings, pregnancy, military service, etc.
    d. Patient appears anxious and is often mildly depressed
  2. Conversion reactions—anxiety is unconsciously converted to physical symptoms
    a. Patient presents a history of loss of motor or sensory function without any adequate phys-

ical cause; e.g., paralysis, blindness, deafness
    b. There is a noticeable lack of concern about the problem; this lack of concern has been labeled *la belle indifférence*
    c. Impairment may vary over different episodes and does not follow anatomic structure; paralysis or numbness may circle the foot or arm instead of beginning at the joint and is known as stocking and glove anesthesia
    d. Patient appears relieved by symptoms and demonstrates little anxiety when observed
  3. Dissociative reactions—anxiety is unconsciously isolated from consciousness
    a. Alterations in state of consciousness
    b. Patient attempts to deal with anxiety by walling off certain areas of reality
    c. Frequently expressed as amnesia or somnambulism (sleepwalking)
    d. Patient escapes by isolating self from situation
    e. In very rare instances multiple personalities may develop; they result from the splitting off of certain mental processes from the main body of consciousness; the multiple personalities may be 2 or more organized systems of behavior that take turns in controlling the individual; coconscious personalities are usually aware of the conscious personality, but the conscious personality is usually unaware of the coconscious personalities
  4. Phobic reactions—anxiety is unconsciously transferred to an inanimate object, which then symbolically represents the neurotic conflict and can be avoided
    a. Anxiety appears when patients find themselves in places that threaten their sense of security
    b. Patients attempt to avoid these distressing situations
    c. Depending on the phobic object, the individual's life-style can be greatly limited
    d. Common phobias include
      (1) Acrophobia—high places
      (2) Astraphobia—thunder and lightening
      (3) Claustrophobia—closed places
      (4) Hydrophobia—water
      (5) Photophobia—strong lights
  5. Obsessive-compulsive reactions—unconscious control of anxiety by the use of rituals and thoughts

a. Patients complain about thoughts that persist and become repetitive and obsessive
b. These thoughts may be turned into compulsions that are repetitive acts of irrational behavior which the individual is emotionally forced to carry out although they serve no rational purpose
c. Patients are indecisive and demonstrate a striving for perfection and superiority
d. Intellectual and verbal defenses are used
e. Anxiety and depression may be present in various degrees particularly if rituals are prevented
6. Depressive reactions—guilt and depression are used unconsciously to relieve anxiety
a. Symptoms of depression, insomnia, anorexia, decreased sexual drive, weight loss, constipation, fatigue; closely resembles manic-depressive psychosis but differs in depth and awareness of reality
b. Depression is real and suicide can occur
C. Therapy
1. Complete medical workup to reassure patient and rule out medical problems
2. Psychotherapy, family therapy, group therapy
3. Sedatives and minor tranquilizers may be used if necessary
4. Pharmacologic approach—antianxiety drugs (minor tranquilizers)—used when individuals are incapable of coping with environmental stresses and accomplishing daily activities
a. Types of drugs
(1) Propanediol compounds
(a) Drugs
[1] Meprobamate (Equanil, Meprospan, Meprotabs)
[2] Phenaglycodol (Ultran)
[3] Tybamate (Solacen)
(b) Drugs have some effect on skeletal muscle relaxation by action on interneurons
(c) Adverse effects—hypotension (caused by depressive effect on vasomotor centers), headache, insomnia, hypersensitivity reactions
(2) Benzodiazepine group
(a) Drugs
[1] Chlordiazepoxide hydrochloride (Librium)

[2] Clorazepate dipotassium (Tranxene)
[3] Diazepam (Valium)
[4] Oxazepam (Serax)
(b) Produce significant relaxant effect on skeletal muscles by depression of polysynaptic reflex arcs of the spinal cord (useful in convulsions of alcohol withdrawal or status epilepticus)
(c) Adverse effects—hypotension incidence high with parenteral administration
(3) Nonphenothiazine compounds (resemble antihistamines)
(a) Drugs
[1] Hydroxyzine hydrochloride (Atarax)
[2] Hydroxyzine pamoate (Vistaril)
(b) Adverse effects—similar to antihistamines and atropine
b. General drug interactions—potentiation of depressant effects of alcohol or sedatives
c. General adverse effects of minor tranquilizers—drowsiness, hypotension, muscle relaxation, decreased ability to concentrate occur frequently in initial days of therapy; hypersensitivity reactions
D. Nursing approach
1. Establish a trusting relationship
2. Accept symptoms as real to patient
3. Attempt to limit use of defenses, but do not stop them until patient is ready to give them up
4. Encourage patient to develop a balance between work and play so that anxiety is lessened
5. Help patient develop better ways of handling anxiety-producing situations through problem solving
6. Accept physical symptoms, but do not emphasize or call attention to them
7. Reduce demands on the individual as much as possible

Personality disorders and certain other nonpsychotic mental disorders

Personality disorders
Borderline states falling between the neuroses and psychoses, characterized by defects in the development of the personality or by pathologic trends in its structure
A. Personality can be defined as

1. The sum of all traits, which differentiates one individual from another
2. The total behavior pattern of an individual through which the inner interests are expressed
3. The individual's unique and distinctive way of behaving and interacting with others
4. The constellation of defense mechanisms for dealing with inner and outer pressures
5. A functional role within a family system

B. Manifestations of personality disorders
1. Habitual attitudes and reaction patterns in human relationships develop early in life and form the character structure of the individual
2. In most instances these behaviors create little discomfort or stress
3. The personality disturbances are, in reality, the selection and utilization of specific defense mechanisms which are used so often that they form a lifelong pattern of action that, although not normal, is neither neurotic nor psychotic
4. The premorbid personality of individuals demonstrating any of the 10 classified personality disturbances resembles the compensatory mechanism associated with the psychotic or neurotic counterpart

C. Symptoms
1. Paranoid personality
   a. Frequent use of projective mechanisms
   b. Presence of suspiciousness, fear, irritability, and stubbornness
   c. Reality testing is not greatly impaired
2. Cyclothymic personality
   a. Alternating mood swings between elation and sadness, which seem unrelated to external environment
   b. Usually warm and friendly, approaching life with an obvious enthusiasm
   c. Mood swings do not demonstrate great emotional intensity
3. Schizoid personality
   a. Avoidance of meaningful interpersonal relationships
   b. Use of autistic thinking, emotional detachment, and daydreaming
   c. Although introverted since childhood, maintain fair contact with reality
4. Explosive personality
   a. Periodic outbursts of rage with verbal and/or physical acting out

b. These outbursts are intense and unable to be controlled
c. Outbursts are easily stimulated by environmental stresses
5. Obsessive-compulsive personality
   a. Characterized by rigidity, overconscientiousness, and an inordinate capacity for work
   b. Individuals are driven by obsessive concerns
   c. Behavior contains many rituals
6. Hysterical personality
   a. Characterized by emotional instability and great excitability
   b. Behavior is extroverted and directed toward gaining attention
   c. These individuals are vain and deliberately manipulative
7. Asthenic personality
   a. Characterized by lack of enthusiasm
   b. Overwhelmed by physical and emotional stress
   c. Appear unable to experience enjoyment
8. Antisocial personality (sociopathic personality disturbances)
   a. Chronic lifelong disturbances that conflict with society's laws and customs
   b. Unable to postpone gratification
   c. Randomly act out their aggressive egocentric impulses on society
   d. Do not profit from past experience or punishment and live only for the moment
   e. Have the ability to ingratiate themselves but they "do not wear well"
   f. Are in contact with reality but do not seem to care about it
9. Passive-aggressive personality
   a. Rather helpless and indecisive demonstrating passive obstructionism while clinging and pouting
   b. Frequent outbursts and temper tantrums when frustrated
   c. Frequently create many problems for others
10. Inadequate personality
    a. Limited intellectual, emotional, social, and physical response
    b. Appear to be mentally deficient but are not
    c. Demonstrate poor judgment and social ineptness

D. Therapy
1. Individual, group, family

2. Crisis intervention when necessary
3. Vocational and occupational therapy
E. Nursing approach
1. Maintain consistency and concern in approach
2. Accept patients as they are and do not retaliate if provoked
3. Protect them from other patients and other patients from them
4. Place realistic limits on behavior and let individual know what the limits are

Sexual deviations

Changing social and cultural mores have resulted in removing many of the sexual behaviors that were previously considered deviations from the list; sexual deviations today are considered those sexual activities directed toward objects other than people of the opposite sex and toward sexual acts not considered "normal" or not performed under usual circumstances

A. Pathology—may be symptomatic of other personality or psychiatric disorders or may occur as a behavior aberration of a disordered personality
B. Symptoms
1. Homosexuality—sexual relations between members of the same sex as the preferred method of gratification; when this relationship occurs between 2 consenting adults, some no longer consider it a sexual deviation
2. Fetishism—substitution of an inanimate object for the genitals
3. Transvestism—individual wears clothing of the opposite sex to achieve sexual pleasure
4. Exhibitionism—sexual pleasure is obtained by exposing the genitals
5. Pedophilia—attraction to children as sex objects
6. Voyeurism—sexual gratification obtained by watching the sexual play of others
7. Sadism—cruelty to others is substituted for or must accompany the sex act
8. Masochism—self-suffering is substituted for or must accompany the sex act
C. Therapy—rather unsuccessful with these individuals unless they really want to change; if change is desired, psychotherapy or psychoanalysis may be effective
D. Nursing approach
1. Accept patients as individuals in emotional pain
2. Avoid punitive remarks or responses
3. Protect patient from others
4. Set limits on patient's sexual acting out
5. Provide diversional activities

Alcoholism

Alcohol intake that interferes with normal functioning or is necessary as a prerequisite to normal functioning

A. Pathology—premorbid personality utilizes the compensatory mechanisms of the addictive pattern of behavior
B. Patterns of drinking and symptoms
1. Intoxication—a state in which coordination or speech is impaired and behavior is altered
2. Episodic excessive drinking—individual becomes intoxicated as infrequently as 4 times a year; episodes may vary in length from hours to days or weeks
3. Habitual excessive drinking—individual becomes intoxicated more than 12 times a year or is recognizably under the influence of alcohol more than once a week even though not considered intoxicated
4. Alcohol addiction—direct or strong presumptive evidence that individual is dependent on alcohol; evidence may be demonstrated by withdrawal symptoms or by the inability to go for a day without drinking; when there is a history of heavy drinking for 3 or more months, the individual is considered addicted to alcohol
5. Early symptoms of alcoholism include frequent drinking sprees, increase in intake, drinking alone or in the early morning, occurrence of blackouts
C. Therapy
1. Should be multifaceted social and medical; involves psychotherapy, both individual, family, and group, especially Alcoholics Anonymous
2. Negative conditioning with the use of disulfiram (Antabuse) appears to help
3. Patients can only be assisted when they admit they need help
4. Physical needs must be cared for, since dietary needs have often been ignored for long periods
D. Nursing approach
1. Provide well-controlled, alcohol-free environment
2. Plan a full program of activities but provide adequate rest periods
3. Meet patient's need for a great deal of support without criticism or judgment
4. Avoid trying to talk patient out of problem
5. Accept individual's smooth facade while approaching the lonely and fearful individual behind it

6. Accept failures without judgment or punishment
7. Accept hostility without criticism or retaliation
8. Recognize ambivalence and limit need for decision making
9. Maintain patient's interest in therapy program

Drug dependence

The misuse of drugs usually by self-administration

A. Pathology—premorbid personality utilizes the compensatory mechanisms of the addictive pattern of behavior
B. Definitions
1. Addiction—the condition of habituation and tolerance to drugs other than alcohol, tobacco, and ordinary caffeine-containing beverages; medically prescribed drugs are excluded if they are taken under medical direction; addiction can occur simultaneously to 2 or more drugs or to alcohol and drugs; lately, combined addiction to a multiplicity of drugs has become more common
2. Habituation—there may be both physical and psychological dependency
3. Tolerance—the condition of physical dependency to a drug in which the presence of the drug in increasingly higher dosage is needed to achieve the same effect; tolerance can exceed the usual lethal limits of a drug
C. Symptoms
1. Needle marks on limbs along path of veins may be present
2. Addicted individuals may tend to wear long-sleeved shirts, even in warm weather
3. Yawning, lacrimation, rhinorrhea, and perspiration appear 10 to 15 hours after last opiate injection
4. Severe abdominal cramps will develop if too much time elapses between injections
5. Physical examination may reveal an underweight, malnourished individual with multiple dental caries and depressed central nervous system functioning
6. Job or academic failure; marital conflicts; poor reality testing; personality change
D. Therapy
1. Methadone maintenance for opiate addiction—programs do not treat addiction but change the addiction from an illegal drug to a legal drug, which is administered under supervision; has only proved successful in individuals with long-standing addictions

2. High-calorie, high-protein, high-vitamin diet because of poor eating habits
3. Treatment in groups run by ex-addicts
4. Therapeutic community setting
5. Psychotherapy and family therapy on an outpatient basis
6. If patient is to be withdrawn from drugs, decreasing amounts of methadone and/or tranquilizers must be administered to reduce physiologic and psychologic discomfort
7. Vocational counseling
E. Nursing approach
1. Set firm controls and keep area drug free when patient is hospitalized
2. Keep atmosphere pleasant and cheerful but not overly stimulating
3. Contribute to patient's self-confidence, self-respect, and security in a realistic manner
4. Walk the fine line between a relatively permissive but firm attitude
5. Expect and accept evasion, manipulative behavior, and negativism, but require the patient to shoulder certain standards of responsibility
6. Accept the patient without approving the behavior
7. Do not permit patients to isolate themselves
8. Introduce patient to group activities as soon as possible
9. Protect patients from themselves and others

Psychophysiologic disorders

A. Physical illnesses where psychogenic factors are the predominant causative agents
B. Anxiety stimulates the autonomic nervous system, and the nervous and endocrine impulses appear to center on one particular organ, creating actual physical illness and changes in the tissue structure
C. The reason a certain organ is involved with one patient and a different organ with another is still undetermined
1. Pathology—premorbid personality appears to be one of unexpressed aggression resulting from the unresolved struggle between dependent need and independent striving; may be familial
2. Symptoms
a. Skin
(1) In neurodermatitis, dermatitis factitia, pruritus, and trichotillomania, psychic factors appear to dominate

(2) There appears to be a relationship between endocrine imbalance and disturbances in the autonomic regulation of skin physiology

(3) Stress seems to lead to rash, itching, and discomfort

b. Musculoskeletal

(1) Anxiety and fear often create a tightening of muscles

(2) This becomes an aggravating factor in arthritis, backache, tension headache, or any other musculoskeletal disorder in which increased tension and spasm are involved

c. Respiratory

(1) Hyperventilation syndrome

(a) Panting occurs with tension and excitement and this forced respiration can produce biochemical changes in the blood

(b) These changes can alter the cerebral circulation and cause a reduction in consciousness and syncope

(2) Bronchial asthma

(a) Stress and tension appear to create increased secretions and changes in the bronchi

(b) Individuals with asthma tend to exhibit a strong desire for protection and dependency yet fear rejection or engulfment

(c) The wheeze associated with asthma is considered by some to be a suppressed cry for this protection

d. Cardiovascular

(1) Essential hypertension

(a) Anxiety and other stresses are believed to play a role in releasing a pressor from the kidneys, which causes chronic vasoconstriction of the vessels

(b) All other primary causes for hypertension must be ruled out before this cause can be diagnosed

(c) Individuals with hypertension have difficulty handling hostile feelings, are less assertive, and have more obsessive-compulsive traits than nonhypertensive ones

(d) Hypertension may be considered a state of chronically unexpressed rage that arises from conflicts between passive-dependent longings and the struggle for independence

(2) Coronary occlusion and angina

(a) Coronary attacks frequently occur following periods of fatigue and anxiety

(b) These individuals place a high value on work and success; they become depressed when inactive

e. Hemolymphatic

(1) Certain blood dyscrasias and responses can be linked to emotional stress

(2) In some individuals the neutrophil count drops, the clotting time is decreased, both blood viscosity and erythrocyte sedimentation rate rise

(3) Nature of this response to stress is still controversial

f. Gastrointestinal

(1) Peptic ulcer

(a) Anxiety and other stress appear to create a condition of hyperactivity, hypersecretion, hyperacidity, and engorgement of the mucosa

(b) Related to stresses in life, particularly those concerned with conflicts between passivity and aggression

(c) Use reaction formation to cover the strong, somewhat irrational need to achieve security from others

(2) Ulcerative colitis

(a) Parasympathetic stimulation of the lower bowel produces an enzyme that interferes with the protective coating of the bowel

(b) May occur as a reaction to a variety of stresses but most often in situations that demand accomplishment and arouse fear of not succeeding

(c) Many patients are immature and have not gained any feelings of independence

g. Genitourinary

(1) Disturbances in genital and urinary problems may occur under stress

(2) Enuresis, amenorrhea, frigidity, and impotence appear to be related to psychologic factors

(3) Depression and feelings of helplessness may be related to urinary retention

(4) Fear may be related to urgency and frequency

h. Endocrine

(1) Eating patterns and dependency on food for satisfaction and reduction of stress appears related to both diabetes mellitus and obesity

(2) Feelings of insecurity and an unusual sense of responsibility appear associated with onset of hyperthyroidism

i. Organs of special sense—some evidence that certain neurologic disturbances, such as atypical facial neuralgia, are related to emotional conflict

3. Therapy—must be directed toward both the physical and emotional problems

4. Nursing approach

a. Reduce emotional stimulation when possible

b. Explain all procedures carefully and allow patient time for questions

c. Provide patient with talking time

d. Avoid material that appears to stimulate conflict for the patient

e. Accept patient's behavior and encourage expression of feelings

f. Remember patient is really physically ill and the symptoms have a physiologic basis

Other psychiatric problems

Special symptoms

Primary symptoms of emotional conflict rather than symptoms of other emotional disorders

A. Pathology—mainly unknown, does seem to relate to unresolved conflicts

B. Symptoms

1. Learning disturbances—appear in children of normal intelligence

2. Speech disturbances—stuttering and stammering

3. Somnambulism—sleepwalking

4. Enuresis that is not related to genitourinary problems

C. Therapy—determine the underlying cause of the conflict and work toward resolution

D. Nursing approach

1. Recognize and accept that a problem exists

2. Help the patient and/or parents identify the problem

3. Support and avoid humiliation of the patient

4. Provide empathic understanding

Transient situational disturbances

Acute reactions to overwhelming environmental stress

A. Pathology

1. No apparent underlying mental disorder in these individuals, although present behavior may be extremely disturbed

2. The individual seems to have the capacity to adapt to the overwhelming stress when given the time to do so

3. Problems with distortions or interruptions in thinking process and decision making tend to resolve themselves

B. Symptoms

1. Adjustment reaction of infancy—the infant is upset and demonstrates grief when separated from the mother

2. Adjustment reaction of childhood—the child regresses to an earlier level of development when a new sibling arrives or experiences intense anxiety on entering school

3. Adjustment reaction of adolescence—the adolescent's struggle for independence leads to hypersensitivity and frequent episodes of heightened anxiety

4. Adjustment reactions of adult life—the adult experiences heightened anxiety in response to the stresses associated with marriage, pregnancy, divorce, change of employment, purchase of a house, etc.

5. Adjustment reaction of later life—the menopause and climacteric, the plan for retirement, the "loss" of children to marriage, and the death of a mate all serve to produce extreme stress situations

Behavioral disorders of childhood and adolescence

A. Diagnosis is difficult, since pathology must be separated from the normal disturbances that occur during this period of life

B. The most common problems found in children are the personality disorders and the psychophysiologic disorders; the neuroses and the psychoses are less common

C. The American Psychiatric Association has classified these disorders under the behavior exhibited

1. Hyperkinetic reaction

2. Withdrawal reaction

3. Overanxious reaction

4. Runaway reaction

5. Unsocialized aggressive reaction
6. Group delinquent reaction
D. The symptoms exhibited by children so classified can arise from organic or environmental disease
E. Behavioral disorders can occur as a response to illness
   1. Pathology
     a. Can be responses to alterations in the central nervous system cells such as those created by
       (1) Infectious disorders such as high fevers
       (2) Communicable diseases such as viral, toxic, or postinfectious encephalitis
       (3) Anemias and blood dyscrasias
       (4) Brain lesions or tumors
     b. Can be responses to organic changes in other body tissues and cells such as those created by
       (1) Thyroid, adrenal, and pituitary glands
       (2) Any change in any part of the endocrine or autonomic nervous system
     c. Can be responses to the stress of being ill
       (1) Regression to earlier levels of development occurs with any illness
       (2) Restriction in activities, pain, and separation
   2. Symptoms—the symptoms of these disorders depend on the cells affected as well as the child's ability to contain or integrate the experience
   3. Therapy—therapy is directed at reducing the underlying cause of the problem
   4. Nursing approach—since the nursing approach for children and adolescents is similar for all types of behavioral disorders, it will be summarized at the end of this area
F. Behavioral disorders can occur as symptoms of neuroses
   1. To be classified as neurotic behavior, disorders should meet the following criteria; the behavior
     a. Is destructive to the child's own general aims
     b. Is repeated despite rational arguments to the contrary and despite punishment
     c. Involves the discharge of affects stemming from unconscious conflicts
     d. Leads to getting caught and punished
   2. Pathology—the same developmental factors listed under the psychoneurotic pattern of behavior are involved
   3. Symptoms—the more common types of neuroses found in childhood are
     a. Sleeping difficulties—somnambulism and insomnia

     b. Stealing—truancy and running away
     c. Learning difficulties—severe reading problems, underachievement, school phobias, reverse or backward reading (the reading from right to left rather than left to right)
     d. Enuresis—bedwetting
     e. Regressive reaction
     f. Physiologic disturbances
       (1) Eating problems—nausea and vomiting
       (2) Excretion problems—constipation or diarrhea
       (3) Respiratory and circulatory problems—asthma and tachycardia
       (4) Allergies—skin rashes and hives
     g. Excessive rebelliousness
     h. Excessive conformity
   4. Therapy
     a. Psychotherapy—in children, usually in the form of play therapy
     b. Medications—amphetamines and mild tranquilizers are quite effective with children
   5. Nursing approach—since the nursing approach for child and adolescents is similar for all types of behavioral disorders, it will be summarized at the end of this area
G. Behavioral disorders can occur as symptoms of psychoses
   1. The psychoses of children have 2 basic features
     a. An alienation or withdrawal from reality
     b. A severe disturbance in the child's feeling of self-identity
   2. Pathology
     a. As with adult psychoses, many theories are being studied as causes of child psychoses; however, no definitive cause has as yet been established
     b. Failure to develop satisfactory relationships with the significant adults, regardless of the cause, appears to be an underlying problem with all these children
   3. Symptoms
     a. General symptoms
       (1) Inability to differentiate between self and environment
       (2) Confusion in self-boundaries frequently characterized by speaking of self only in the third person
       (3) A defect in ego formation or an inadequately functioning ego system
       (4) A conflict between self and reality

(5) A defect in the adaptive, inhibitory, and steering mechanisms of the personality

(6) Interference with intellect may be so profound, child appears to be mentally retarded

b. Autistic psychosis
   (1) Lack of meaningful relationships with outside world
   (2) Use of autistic fantasy resulting in communication defects
   (3) Turning to inanimate objects and self-centered activity for security

c. Symbiotic psychosis
   (1) Intense though morbid relationship between mother and child
   (2) Child unable to separate identity from that of mother
   (3) Lacks adequate concept of reality
   (4) Inability to relate to peers or adults

d. Childhood schizophrenia
   (1) Profound apathy
   (2) Looseness of association
   (3) Autistic thinking
   (4) Ambivalence
   (5) Absence of communication skills
   (6) Poor grasp of reality
   (7) Bizarre, unpredictable, uncontrolled behavior
   (8) Inability to relate to others
   (9) Total interference with intellectual functioning

4. Therapy
   a. Psychotherapy directed toward the developmental level of the child—play, group, or individual therapy
   b. Medications—tranquilizers and amphetamines provide some reduction of symptoms
   c. Removal from the home situation may be necessary, although day school situations frequently provide enough relief so that hospitalization can be avoided

5. Nursing approach—these approaches are general and provide a guide that can be used for the care of all children with emotional problems; care should be directed toward helping the child grow up emotionally by
   a. Establishing a favorable environment in which the child can gain or regain a favorable equilibrium
   b. Establishing a constructive relationship
   c. Helping child to see self as a worthwhile person
   d. Recognizing that the behavior has meaning for the child
   e. Being as realistic and as truthful as possible in dealing with the child
   f. Attempting to establish trust
   g. Setting limits that are as realistic as possible but as firm as necessary
   h. Pointing out reality, but accepting the child's views of it while pointing it out
   i. Being consistent both in approach and in rules and regulations
   j. Making all explanations as clear as possible
   k. Supporting and encouraging the child's moves toward independence but allowing dependency when necessary

Mental retardation

The area of mental retardation is covered in Pediatric nursing

Conditions without manifest psychiatric disorders and nonspecific conditions

A. Individuals without diagnosable psychosis or other psychiatric illness who have problems that are severe enough to interfere with their usual level of functioning are included in this category

B. This category includes social maladjustment, marital maladjustment, occupational maladjustment, and the dissocial behavioral group

C. These individuals usually benefit from brief psychotherapy; some may progress to the other psychiatric disorders if help is not received

Community mental health services

A. Purposes
   1. To provide prevention, treatment, and rehabilitation services for individuals and families with emotional problems
   2. To maintain these individuals and families in the community
   3. To provide hospital care within the community in those instances when the individual cannot be maintained on an outpatient basis

B. Types of settings in which services are provided
   1. Outpatient services
      a. Storefront clinics
      b. Walk-in clinics in hospitals
      c. Emergency rooms

d. Crisis intervention centers including hot-line phone centers

e. Day-care centers

f. Private offices

2. Inpatient services
   a. Specialized psychiatric hospitals
   b. General hospital psychiatric units

3. After-care services
   a. Foster homes
   b. Halfway houses
   c. Sheltered workshops
   d. Day-care services

C. Types of services
   1. Observation and diagnosis
   2. Assessment of patient's needs
   3. Crisis intervention
   4. Provide direct care services to patients including
      a. Individual, family, and group therapy
      b. Medications
      c. Electroconvulsive therapy
      d. Occupational therapy
      e. Recreational therapy
   5. Provide a therapeutic milieu that
      a. Supports the individual during the period of crisis
      b. Helps the individual learn new ways of coping with problems
   6. Referral to proper community agencies for necessary services
   7. Provide educational setting for various professional groups in mental health concepts
   8. Vocational counseling
   9. Health screening

D. The nurse's role includes
   1. Case finding
   2. Assessment of patient's needs
   3. Establishment of the therapeutic milieu
   4. Consultation with other professionals; e.g., physicians, psychologists, social workers, school teachers, clergy
   5. Active participation with the health team including the patient and family
   6. Active involvement in individual, family, and group therapy
   7. Coordination of health services for the patient and family
   8. Education of groups within the community

ADDITIONAL PHARMACOLOGY
Drugs that produce sedation and sleep

A. Drugs that produce sedation and sleep (sedatives and hypnotics) can be used in addition to tranquilizers for psychiatric and other patients; as central nervous system depressants, they have antianxiety effects in low dosages; produce sleep in high dosages and general anesthetic-like states in very high dosages; all hypnotic drugs probably alter either the character or duration of REM sleep

B. Types of drugs
   1. Trichloroacetic acid—produces natural sleep
      a. Drugs
         (1) Chloral betaine (Beta-Chlor)
         (2) Chloral hydrate (Felsules, Lorinal, Noctec, Somnos)
         (3) Petrichloral (Periclor)
      b. Adverse effects—gastric irritation causing diarrhea
      c. Drug interactions—potentiates the effects of alcohol taken concurrently causing sudden loss of consciousness
      d. Considerations during therapy—drug metabolites cause false positive reaction for glycosuria when Benedict's reagent is used for testing
   2. Paraldehyde primarily is used to control hyperactivity of alcoholics or to control convulsions; drug has a pungent odor and taste, and elimination of drug from lungs maintains environmental odor
   3. Phenothiazine derivatives (act like antihistamines) used for sleep induction in anxious patients
      a. Drugs
         (1) Methotrimeprazine hydrochloride (Levoprome)
         (2) Promazine hydrochloride (Sparine)
         (3) Propiomazine hydrochloride (Largon)
      b. Adverse effects—hypotension, dizziness, dry mouth, cardiac palpitation, pseudoparkinsonism symptoms, cholestatic jaundice, agranulocytosis
   4. Barbiturate sedatives—most frequently used hypnotics
      a. Barbiturates with high lipoid tissue affinity producing rapid response; short acting
         (1) Hexobarbital (Sombucaps, Sombulex)

    (2) Pentobarbital sodium (Nembutal)
    (3) Secobarbital (Seconal)
  b. Barbiturates with moderate lipoid tissue affinity producing moderately slow response; intermediate-acting
    (1) Amobarbital (Amytal)
    (2) Aprobarbital (Alurate)
    (3) Butabarbital sodium (Bubartal Sodium, Butisol Sodium)
    (4) Probarbital calcium (Ipral)
    (5) Talbutal (Lotusate)
  c. Barbiturates with low lipoid tissue affinity producing slow response
    (1) Barbital (Neuronidia)
    (2) Phenobarbital (Luminal)
  d. Adverse effects—morning drowsiness, hypersensitivity reactions (photosensitivity, dermatologic reactions), respiratory depression, and hypotension (most frequent with parenteral use)
  e. Fatalities from overdosage are affected by differences in lipoid tissue affinity
    (1) High lipotropic group rapidly produces respiratory depression and marked hypotension after ingestion of excess drug
    (2) Moderate lipotropic group produces a protracted period of sedation but allows timelapse for resuscitation or reconsideration
    (3) Low lipotropic group allows excretion concurrent with slow action and is least popular for self-induced overdosage
  f. Drug interactions—barbiturates lower blood levels of orally administered griseofulvin and decrease the therapeutic effect; barbiturates increase activity of hepatic microsomal enzymes, and accelerated metabolism of oral anticoagulants lowers their hypoprothrombinenic effect
5. Other sedatives and hypnotics
  a. Ethchlorvynol (Placidyl)—adverse effects include morning drowsiness, blurring vision, transient hypotension
  b. Ethinamate (Valmid)—adverse effects include morning drowsiness

  c. Flurazepam hydrochloride (Dalmane)—adverse effects include dizziness, tachycardia, GI disturbances
  d. Methaqualone (Quaalude, Sopor)—adverse effects include morning drowsiness, GI disturbances
  e. Methyprylon (Noludar)—adverse effects include morning drowsiness, GI disturbances
  f. Sodium bromide used primarily for daytime sedation—adverse effects include gastric irritation, generalized rash, tremulousness of hands, lips, and tongue, impaired mental processes, auditory and visual hallucinations, or coma with long-term use allowing excess levels of drug
  g. Glutethimide (Doriden)
    (1) Adverse effects—morning drowsiness, transient hypotension, and infrequently produces pharyngeal and laryngeal reflex depression
    (2) Drug interactions—acts synergistically with oral anticoagulants to decrease their effectiveness
C. Excess ingestion
  1. Any of the sedative-hypnotics may cause unconsciousness, coma, death
  2. Addiction to these drugs alone or in combination has increased
  3. Removal of gastric content of drug by aspiration, resuscitative measures (assisted ventilation, cardiac massage), hemodialysis of diffusible drug, vasopressor administration to counteract vascular collapse, and correction of acidosis
  4. Follow-up supervision to avoid repetition of the problem
D. These drugs are habit forming, and withdrawal after long-term use may precipitate severe symptoms—anxiety, tremor, insomnia, confusion, perceptual distortions, agitation, delirium, GI disturbances, orthostatic hypotension, convulsions leading to cardiovascular collapse and death

PSYCHIATRIC NURSING REVIEW QUESTIONS

1 Mental experiences operate on different levels of awareness. Which level best portrays one's attitudes, feelings, and desires?
   1. Foreconscious
   2. Preconscious
   3. Conscious
   4. Unconscious

2 Which level of anxiety best enhances an individual's power of perception?
   1. Mild
   2. Moderate
   3. Severe
   4. Panic

3 Sublimation is a defense mechanism that helps the individual to:
   1. Act out in reverse something already done or thought
   2. Channel unacceptable sexual desires into socially approved behavior
   3. Return to an earlier, less mature stage of development
   4. Exclude from the conscious things that are psychologically disturbing

4 An example of displacement is:
   1. Ignoring unpleasant aspects of reality
   2. Imaginative activity to escape reality
   3. Pent-up emotions directed to other than the primary source
   4. Resisting any demands made by others

5 Personality is unique for every individual because it is the result of the person's:
   1. Genetic background, placement in family, and autoimmunity
   2. Biologic constitution, psychologic development, and cultural setting
   3. Childhood experiences, intellectual capacity, and socioeconomic status
   4. Intellectual capacity, race, and socioeconomic status

6 In the process of development the individual strives to maintain, protect, and enhance the integrity of the ego. This is normally accomplished through the use of:
   1. Ritualistic behavior
   2. Withdrawal patterns
   3. Defense mechanisms
   4. Affective reactions

7 Another term for the superego is:
   1. Self
   2. Ideal self
   3. Narcissism
   4. Conscience

8 Which relationship is of extreme importance in the formation of the personality?
   1. Parent-child
   2. Sibling
   3. Peer
   4. Heterosexual

9 Which part of the nervous system is primarily affected during a "fight or flight" reaction?
   1. Central
   2. Peripheral
   3. Parasympathetic
   4. Sympathetic

10 The superego is that part of the self which says:
   1. I want what I want
   2. I can wait for what I want
   3. I should not want that
   4. I like what I want

11 Groups are important in the emotional development of the individual because groups:
   1. Go through the same developmental phases
   2. Always protect their members
   3. Are easily identified by their members
   4. Identify acceptable behavior for their members

12 The family is important in the emotional development of the individual because the family:
   1. Gives rewards and punishment
   2. Helps one to learn identity and roles
   3. Provides support for the young
   4. Reflects the mores of a larger society

13 Communication ties people to their:
   1. Physical surroundings
   2. Environmental surroundings
   3. Social surroundings
   4. Materialistic surroundings

14 The primary emergence of the personality is demonstrated around the age of:
   1. 6 months
   2. 9 months
   3. 2 years
   4. 6 years

15 Problems with dependence versus independence develop during which stage of growth and development?
   1. Infancy
   2. Toddler
   3. Preschool
   4. School age

16 Strict toilet training before a child is ready will cause problems in personality development because at this stage a child is learning to:
   1. Identify own needs
   2. Satisfy parents' needs

3. Live up to society's expectations
4. Satisfy own needs

17 The basic emotional task for the toddler is:
1. Trust
2. Independence
3. Identification
4. Industry

18 The problem of separation anxiety initially occurs during the:
1. Oral stage
2. Anal stage
3. Phallic stage
4. Latency stage

19 For an emotional balance the individual always needs:
1. Family, work, and play
2. Biologic satisfaction and social acceptance
3. Individual recognition and group acceptance
4. Security and social recognition

20 A 5-year-old boy is constantly found slapping his little sister. This behavior is probably caused by:
1. Sibling rivalry
2. Unresolved oedipal conflicts
3. Negativistic id impulses
4. Overcompensation efforts of superego

21 Since people need some gratifying communication to learn, to grow, and to function in a group, all events that significantly curtail communication will eventually produce:
1. Some degree of mental deficiency
2. Severe disturbances
3. Further attempts to increase communication
4. Withdrawal

22 In applying mental health principles to the care of any person with children, the nurse should be aware that:
1. Many parents experience feelings of resentment toward their children
2. Every parent has inborn feelings of love and acceptance for children
3. It is pathologic to feel anger and resentment toward a child
4. It is easier to adjust to the first child than to later ones

23 In which stage of growth and development should surgery be delayed, if possible, because of the effects on personality development?
1. Oral
2. Anal
3. Oedipal
4. Latency

24 A person has a mature personality if the:
1. Ego acts as a balance between the id and the superego pressures
2. Ego responds to the demands of the superego
3. Ego responds to the demands of society
4. Superego has replaced and increased all the controls of the parents

25 Play for the preschool-age child is necessary for the emotional development of:
1. Projection
2. Competition
3. Introjection
4. Independence

26 During the oedipal stage of growth and development, the child:
1. Loves the parent of the same sex and hates the parent of the opposite sex
2. Loves the parent of the same sex and the parent of the opposite sex
3. Has ambivalence toward both parents
4. Loves the parent of the opposite sex and hates the parent of the same sex

27 Which stage of growth and development is basically concerned with role identification?
1. Oral
2. Oedipal
3. Latency
4. Genital

28 Which personality factor is the main problem for patients who need props to blur reality?
1. Dependency
2. Mistrust
3. Role blurring
4. Ego ideal

29 Many persons who are "well adjusted" in ordinary daily living become dependent and demanding when physically ill and hospitalized. This is probably an example of the mechanism of:
1. Denial
2. Compensation
3. Reaction formation
4. Regression

30 The defense mechanism in which emotional conflicts are expressed through motor, sensory, or somatic disability is identified as:
1. Dissociation
2. Psychosomatic
3. Compensation
4. Conversion

31 A college boy who is small in build and unable to participate in sports becomes the life of the party and a mod dresser. This is an example of the mechanism of:
1. Reaction formation
2. Compensation
3. Sublimation
4. Introjection

32 A person, seeing a design on the wallpaper, perceives it as an animal. This is an example of a:
1. Delusion
2. Hallucination
3. Illusion
4. Idea of reference

33 The ability to tolerate frustration is an example of one of the functions of the:
1. Id
2. Superego
3. Ego
4. Unconscious

34 An emotional experience in childhood becomes traumatic when:
1. The ego is overwhelmed by anxiety it cannot handle
2. The superego has not been internalized
3. The child is unable to verbalize own feelings
4. The parents are harsh and restrictive

35 Resolution of the oedipal complex takes place when the child overcomes the castration complex and:
1. Rejects the parent of the same sex
2. Identifies with the parent of the opposite sex
3. Identifies with the parent of the same sex
4. Introjects behaviors of both parents

36 Which of the following is a generally accepted concept of personality development?
1. The personality is capable of change and modification throughout life
2. By the end of the first 6 years, the personality has reached its adult parameters
3. The capacity for personality change decreases rapidly after adolescence
4. The basic personality is rather firmly set by 2 years of age

37 The superego is that part of the psyche which:
1. Is the source of creative energy
2. Develops from internalizing the concepts of parents and significant others
3. Contains the instinctual drives
4. Operates on the pleasure principle and demands immediate gratification

38 Evidence of the existence of the unconscious is demonstrated by:
1. Déjà vu experiences
2. Slips of the tongue
3. The ease of recall
4. Free-floating anxiety

39 Which one of the following is most characteristic of the emotionally disturbed child?
1. Responds to any stimulus
2. Totally involved with the environment
3. Responds to little external stimulus
4. Seems unresponsive to the environment

40 The nurse should observe the autistic child for signs of:
1. Not wanting to eat
2. Crying for attention
3. Catatonic-like rigidity
4. Enjoying being with people

41 Hyperkinesis in children is usually treated with:
1. Chlorpromazine (Thorazine)
2. Haloperidol (Haldol)
3. Methylpenidate (Ritalin)
4. Methocarbamol (Robaxin)

42 A person who deliberately pretends an illness is usually:
1. Psychotic
2. Neurotic
3. Malingering
4. Using conversion defenses

Situation: Mrs. Avery, age 29, was a capable librarian before her marriage. However, she was always very sensitive, aloof, withdrawn, and lacking in the ability to feel warm toward others; she rarely joined any organizations and distrusted people in general. Shortly after the birth of her last child she was admitted to a psychiatric hospital for care. At this time she is convinced that the neighbors are accusing her of indiscretions and that they have her home "bugged" so that they may overhear any conversations taking place there. Since her admission she has remained aloof from the other patients, paces the floor, and believes that the hospital is a house of torture and the food poisoned. Questions 43 through 51 refer to this situation.

43 Mrs. Avery's prepsychotic personality might be described as:
1. Suspicious and socially inadequate
2. Rigid and controlling
3. Dependent and immature
4. Schizoid and introverted

44 Nursing interventions for Mrs. Avery should appropriately be directed toward:
1. Convincing her that the hospital staff is trying to help
2. Helping her enter into group recreational activities
3. Arranging the hospital environment so that her contact with other patients is limited
4. Helping her learn to trust the staff through selected experiences

45 Mrs. Avery frequently refuses to eat because she believes that the food is poisoned. One of the most appropriate ways in which the nurse might initially handle this situation is to:
1. Simply state that the food is not poisoned
2. Suggest that food be brought in from home
3. Taste the food in her presence
4. Tell her that she will have to be tube fed if she does not eat

46 After the initial intervention the nurse should pursue the matter of Mrs. Avery's belief by saying:
1. "Why do you think the food is poisoned?"
2. "You feel someone wants to poison you?"
3. "Your feeling is a symptom of your illness."
4. "You'll be safe with me. I won't let anyone poison you."

47 Mrs. Avery has refused to eat for 36 hours. She states that the voice of her dead father has commanded her to

atone for her sins by fasting for 40 days. What initial intervention on the part of the nurse might interrupt the delusional system?
1. Asking the physician to write an order for tube feeding
2. Asking Mrs. Avery exactly what the voice said
3. Telling Mrs. Avery that she has nothing to atone for
4. Suggesting other means of atonement that may be less damaging

48 Mrs. Avery remains aloof from all other patients. What might the nurse, with whom she has developed a friendly relationship, do to help her participate in some ward activity?
1. Invite another patient to take part in a joint activity with the nurse and Mrs. Avery
2. Ask the physician to speak to Mrs. Avery about entering into ward activities
3. Find solitary pursuits that Mrs. Avery can enjoy on the ward
4. Speak to Mrs. Avery about the importance of entering into activities

49 Mrs. Avery has been assigned to a 4-bed room. The night nurse reports that she has been awake for several nights. What may be the cause of her sleeplessness? She may be:
1. Fearful of the other patients
2. Worrying about her family
3. Trying to work out her problems
4. Watching for an opportunity to escape

50 The nurse could most appropriately begin to help Mrs. Avery with her sleep problem by saying:
1. "Don't worry, you'll sleep when you're tired."
2. "I'm going to move you to a private room."
3. "I'll get you the sedative your doctor ordered."
4. "You seem unable to sleep at night."

51 While talking with the nurse about her problem of not being able to make friends with any of the other patients, Mrs. Avery begins to cry. What action on the part of the nurse would be most therapeutic at this time?
1. Suggest that they play a game of Scrabble
2. Tell her that her crying isn't going to help
3. Sit quietly with her
4. Point out how she can change this

Situation: Mr. Frank, 21 years of age, is an only child who has never earned his own living and has always been pampered and coddled by his domineering mother and ignored by his quiet retiring father. When he started dating, his mother chose the girls he took out. Recently Mr. Frank married a woman several years older than he, even though his mother seriously disapproved of her. Despite this, he brought his wife to his home to live. Both the mother and the wife were unhappy with this arrangement. Mr. Frank had many guilt feelings about his marriage and soon began to complain of pain in his right arm, which progressed to the point of paralysis. After seeking help from competent orthopedic specialists, he was referred for psychiatric evaluation. Questions 52 through 54 refer to this situation.

52 Mr. Frank's symptoms may be an unconscious attempt to solve a conflict evolving from:
1. Hostile feelings toward his home
2. Ambivalent feelings toward his wife
3. Inadequate feelings in regard to assuming the role of husband
4. Needs to be a dependent child and an independent adult

53 What could be said about Mr. Frank's prognosis after appropriate treatment?
1. His symptoms of paralysis may spread to other parts of his body
2. Continuous psychiatric treatment will be required to maintain him as a functioning individual
3. Recovery of the use of the arm can be expected, but under stress he may utilize similar symptoms
4. It is not possible to predict what the future for this patient holds

54 In dealing with Mr. Frank the nurse should realize that:
1. This symptom is necessary for him to cope with his present situation
2. This symptom is an unconscious method of getting attention
3. He can get well if he is helped to focus on other things
4. His problems will be solved when he learns to deal with his mother and wife

Situation: Mrs. Sam, a 45-year-old homemaker, was recently admitted to the psychiatric hospital because of a history of hopelessness, anxiety, and suicide attempts. In the hospital she paces the halls, cries, and says that the terrible condition of the world is her fault. She believes that her insides are decayed, that her husband and children are dead, and that the food she eats is of no nutritional value to her. Mrs. Sam has 3 daughters, all of whom are away at college. Her life has always centered about her family and her meticulously kept home. She has never had any hobbies or outside interests, and her moral standards have been strict and unbending. Questions 55 through 60 refer to this situation.

55 Mrs. Sam's prepsychotic personality can best be described as:
1. Withdrawn and seclusive, with an active fantasy life
2. Rigid, narrow, overly conscientious
3. Suspicious, sensitive, aloof
4. Dependent, immature, insecure

56 One of the nurse's primary responsibilities in caring for Mrs. Sam is to:
1. Help her realize that her children are not dead
2. Protect her against her suicidal impulses
3. Reassure her that she is a good woman
4. Keep up her interest in the outside world

57 One of the nursing responsibilities is to help Mrs. Sam

pace the halls less frequently, since this wears her out physically. This can best be accomplished by:
1. Supplying her with simple monotonous tasks
2. Restraining her in a chair so she is unable to pace
3. Requesting a sedative order from her physician
4. Placing her in a single room so she can pace in a smaller area

58 In reassuring Mrs. Sam concerning the many fears that are upsetting to her, it would be helpful to say:
1. "Your daughters and your husband love you very much."
2. "You know that you are not a bad woman."
3. "Mrs. Sam, those ideas of yours are in your imagination."
4. "Those ideas are part of your illness and will change as you improve."

59 The nurse continues to sit with Mrs. Sam, although there is little verbal communication. One day, Mrs. Sam asks her, "Do you think they'll ever let me out of here?" The nurse's best response is:
1. "Why, do you think you are ready to leave?"
2. "You have the feeling that you might not leave?"
3. "Everyone says you're doing just fine."
4. "Why don't you ask your doctor?"

60 Mrs. Sam confides to the nurse that she has been thinking about suicide. Which statement best explains her action?
1. She feels safe with the nurse and can share her feelings with her
2. She wishes to frighten the nurse
3. She is fearful of her own impulses and is seeking protection from them
4. She wants attention from the staff

Situation: Mrs. Jones, a young female patient, believes that doorknobs are contaminated and refuses to touch them, except with the aid of a paper tissue. Questions 61 through 63 refer to this situation.

61 What response should the nurse use in dealing with this behavior?
1. Force her to touch doorknobs by removing all available paper tissue until she learns to deal with the situation
2. Explain to her that her idea about doorknobs is part of her illness and is not necessary
3. Encourage her to scrub the doorknobs with a strong antiseptic so she does not need to use tissues
4. Supply her with paper tissues to help her function until her anxiety is reduced

62 Symptoms such as using tissues to touch doorknobs develop because the patient is:
1. Consciously using this method of punishing herself
2. Unconsciously controlling unacceptable impulses or feelings

3. Listening to voices that tell her the doorknobs are unclean
4. Fulfilling a need to punish others by carrying out an annoying procedure

63 Therapeutic treatment for Mrs. Jones should be directed toward helping her to:
1. Forget her fears by administering antianxiety medications
2. Understand her behavior is caused by unconscious impulses that she fears
3. Redirect her energy into activities to help others
4. Learn that her behavior is not serving a realistic purpose

Situation: Mrs. Smith has been admitted to a psychiatric hospital with the diagnosis of senile psychotic reaction. Questions 64 through 69 refer to this situation.

64 Which of the following behaviors would the nurse find atypical for a patient like Mrs. Smith?
1. Resistance to change
2. Tendency to dwell on the past and ignore the present
3. Preoccupation with personal appearance
4. Inability to concentrate on new activities or interests

65 Senile psychosis is characterized by:
1. Areas of brain destruction called senile plaques
2. Periodic remissions and exacerbations
3. Aggressive acting out behavior
4. Hypoxia of selected areas of brain

66 Which of the following approaches would be most helpful in meeting Mrs. Smith's needs?
1. Simplifying the environment as much as possible while eliminating need for choices
2. Providing a nutritious diet high in carbohydrates and proteins
3. Developing a consistent nursing plan with fixed time schedules to provide for emotional and physical needs
4. Providing an opportunity for many alternative choices in the daily schedule, to stimulate interest

67 In attempting to understand Mrs. Smith's behavior the nurse recognizes that Mrs. Smith is probably:
1. Attempting to develop new defense mechanisms to meet her current life situation
2. Not capable of using any defense mechanisms at all
3. Making exaggerated use of old familiar mechanisms
4. Using one method of defense for all situations

68 The nursing care plan for the patient with senile brain deterioration should include:
1. An extensive reeducation program
2. Details for protective and supportive care
3. The introduction of new leisure time activities
4. Plans to involve the patient in group therapy sessions

69 In planning care for Mrs. Smith the nurse should appropriately:

1. Maintain the daily routine of living with which she is familiar
2. Discuss current events to keep her in contact with reality
3. Teach her new social skills to encourage participation
4. Encourage her to talk of her youth and early experiences

Situation: Dr. Kay, a 45-year-old physician, is admitted to the psychiatric unit of a general hospital. He is restless, loud, aggressive, and resistive during the admission procedure. Questions 70 through 72 refer to this situation.

70 Dr. Kay shouts at the nurse who is trying to take his admission blood pressure, ''I'm a physician. Do you think you're more qualified than I? I'll do it myself.'' The most therapeutic response by the nurse would be:
   1. ''Right now, doctor, you're just another patient.''
   2. ''If you'd rather, doctor; I'm sure you'll do it OK.''
   3. ''I'm sorry but I can't allow that. I must take it.''
   4. ''If you won't cooperate, I'll get the attendants in to hold you down.''

71 After the admission examination a nurse is assigned to introduce Dr. Kay to the other patients. He tells her that he wishes to be introduced as Dr. Kay. The nurse's response should be:
   1. ''I can't do that. It's better if they don't know you are a doctor.''
   2. ''That's fine, Dr. Kay; that's how I'll introduce you.''
   3. ''All the patients here call one another by their first names.''
   4. ''Why do you insist on being called Doctor?''

72 By the time Dr. Kay has been a patient on the service for 3 days he has questioned everyone's authority, has advised other patients that their treatments are wrong, and has talked 4 other patients into forming their own therapy group. The staff's most appropriate response would be to:
   1. Ignore him and hope he will stop trying to disrupt the ward
   2. Understand that he is unable to control his actions and that limits must be set for him
   3. Tell the other patients that he is just another patient and they should not pay attention to him
   4. Restrict his contact with other patients until he stops bothering everyone

---

Situation: The nurse is assigned to care for Mr. Bishop, a 39-year-old, hyperactive, elated patient who exhibits flight of ideas. Questions 73 through 76 refer to this situation.

73 The nursing care plan for Mr. Bishop should appropriately include plans to:
   1. Encourage him to talk as much as needed
   2. Arouse and focus his interest in reality
   3. Persuade him to complete any task that he begins

4. Provide constructive channels for redirecting his excess energy

74 In approaching Mr. Bishop during a period of great overactivity it is essential to:
   1. Use a firm, warm consistent approach
   2. Anticipate and physically control his hyperactivity
   3. Allow the patient to choose the activities in which he will participate
   4. Let him know you will not tolerate destructive behavior

75 Mr. Bishop is not eating. The nurse recognizes that this may be because he:
   1. Feels that he does not deserve the food
   2. Believes that he does not need the food
   3. Wishes to avoid the patients in the dining room
   4. Is so busy that he does not take time to eat

76 The nurse can best respond to Mr. Biship's eating problem by:
   1. Providing a tray for him in his room
   2. Assuring him that he is deserving of food
   3. Ordering foods that he can hold in his hand to eat while moving around
   4. Pointing out that the energy he is burning up must be replaced

---

Situation: Mrs. Virginia Rose, a 39-year-old married woman, is admitted to the psychiatric service with the diagnosis of anxiety reaction. Questions 77 through 81 refer to this situation.

77 The nurse and Mrs. Rose walk to a quiet corner of the unit. Mrs. Rose's anxiety mounts. She becomes increasingly restless, moving rapidly from one foot to the other, and wringing her hands. Her face is contorted as though she is in pain. The nurse suddenly feels uncomfortable and wishes she could leave the scene. The probable reason for her feeling is:
   1. The empathic communication of anxiety
   2. Her desire to go off duty after a busy day
   3. Her inability to tolerate any more bizarre behavior
   4. Her fear of the patient becoming assaultive

78 Mrs. Rose is crying and states that she has never been in in the hospital except to have children. The nurse realizes that an environment conducive to reducing emotional stress and providing psychologic safety is one in which:
   1. Needs are a primary concern
   2. All the patient's needs are met
   3. Realistic limits and controls are set
   4. Physical environment is kept in order

79 Mrs. Rose attempts to manipulate the staff and control situations. Just before the nurse is to go off duty she is confronted by Mrs. Rose who says ''That feeling, it may come back. I'm so afraid that the evening staff won't like me like this. They'll seclude me.'' The nurse can best assist the patient by saying:
   1. ''Don't worry, I told you that you'd be all right.''

2. ''Mrs. Rose, you know I leave at this time. Can we talk about this in the morning?''
3. ''Tell me more about what you're feeling now.''
4. ''I'll ask the staff not to lock you up.''

80 The next afternoon Mrs. Rose meets the nurse in the hallway. She says, ''That was a terrible feeling I had yesterday. I'm so afraid to talk about it.'' The nurse's most useful response would be:
1. ''Okay, let's not talk about it.''
2. ''It's best that you try to talk about it.''
3. ''What were you doing yesterday when you first noticed the feeling?''
4. ''Don't worry; that feeling probably won't come back.''

81 Mrs. Rose cries bitterly after a conference with her psychiatrist. She pounds the bed in frustration and threatens to kill herself. What response by the nurse would be most helpful?
1. Pat her reassuringly on the back and say, ''I know it is hard to bear.''
2. Sit beside her and listen attentively if she wishes to talk about the situation
3. Ask her to talk about her troubles and point out that other people also have problems
4. Leave her for a short period until she regains control

82 Two 20-year-old female patients have become very much attached to one another and were recently found in bed together. They became angry and sarcastic when the nurse asked one of them to return to her own bed. How can this situation best be handled by the nurse?
1. Ask the physician to transfer one of the patients to another unit
2. Supervise them carefully and separate them when possible throughout the day and especially at night
3. Restrict both their privileges for several days because their behavior is undesirable and immature
4. Adopt a matter-of-fact, noncondemning attitude toward these patients while setting limits on their behavior

83 Which of the following factors is one of the most frequent findings concerning adult homosexuality?
1. Inadequate physical development of the sexual organs
2. Deficiency of gonadal and pituitary hormones
3. Failure to progress normally through the stages of psychosexual development
4. Poor adjustment due to association with homosexual companions

Situation: Mrs. Lord, 23 years old, has been married 3 months. She was admitted to a psychiatric hospital after a month of unusual behavior that included eating and sleeping very little, talking or singing constantly, charging hundreds of dollars' worth of furniture to her father-in-law, and picking up dates on the street. In the hospital, Mrs. Lord monopolizes conversation, insists on unusual privileges, and frequently becomes demanding, bossy, and sarcastic. She has periods of great overactivity and sometimes is destructive. She frequently uses vulgar and profane language. Mrs. Lord was formerly witty, gay, and the ''life of the party.'' Questions 84 through 89 refer to this situation.

84 The symptoms that Mrs. Lord exhibits are usually found in patients experiencing:
1. Affective disorders
2. Schizophrenic reactions
3. Personality disorders
4. Involutional reactions

85 When Mrs. Lord's language becomes vulgar and profane, the nurse should:
1. State: ''We don't like that kind of talk around here.''
2. State: ''When you can talk in an acceptable way, we will talk to you.''
3. Recognize it as part of her illness but set limits on it
4. Ignore it, since the patient is using it only to get attention

86 During Mrs. Lord's phase of extreme elation and hyperactivity the nursing staff should consider her nutritional needs by:
1. Following her around the dining room with her tray
2. Providing her with frequent high-calorie feedings that can be held in the hand
3. Accepting the fact that she will eat when she is hungry
4. Allowing her to prepare her own meals and eat when she pleases

87 Mrs. Lord's hyperactivity might be redirected therapeutically in which one of the following ways?
1. Give her cleaning equipment and suggest that she assist with the ward work
2. Ask her to guide other patients as they clean their rooms
3. Suggest that she initiate social activities on the ward for the patient group
4. Give her a pencil and paper and encourage her to write

88 In helping Mrs. Lord with personal hygiene the nurse would:
1. Keep makeup away from her because she will apply it too freely
2. Suggest that she wear hospital clothing to avoid confrontations
3. Allow her to apply makeup in whatever manner she chooses
4. Encourage her to dress attractively and in her own clothing

89 Three new staff members are assigned to the floor on which Mrs. Lord is a patient. During their orientation tour, Mrs. Lord greets them by saying, ''Welcome to the funny farm. I'm Jo-Jo the head yo-yo.'' This comment might mean that the patient is:

1. Looking for attention from the new staff
2. Unable to distinguish fantasy from reality
3. Anxious over the arrival of the new staff members
4. Trying to fill her role as "life of the party"

90 Projection, rationalization, denial, and distortion by hallucinations and delusions are examples of a disturbance in:
1. Thought process
2. Association
3. Logic
4. Reality testing

91 A patient expresses the belief that the F.B.I. is out to kill him. This is an example of a(n):
1. Hallucination
2. Self-accusatory delusion
3. Delusion of persecution
4. Error in judgment

92 Mr. James is withdrawn and noncommunicative; to encourage him to talk, the best plan of nursing intervention would be to:
1. Ask simple questions that require an answer
2. Focus on nonthreatening subjects
3. Try to get him to discuss his feelings
4. Sit and look through magazines with him

93 When caring for patients exhibiting withdrawn patterns of behavior, an important aspect of nursing care is to:
1. Help the patient understand that it is harmful to withdraw from situations
2. Involve the patient in activities throughout the day
3. Help keep the patient oriented to reality
4. Encourage the patient to discuss why he does not mix with the other patients

94 Observation is an important aspect of nursing care. It is especially important in the care of the withdrawn patient because it:
1. Helps in understanding the patient's feelings
2. Is useful in making a diagnosis
3. Indicates the degree of psychic depression
4. Tells the staff how ill the patient is

95 The best approach in helping a very withdrawn patient is to provide an environment with:
1. A large variety of activities
2. A specific routine
3. A trusting relationship
4. Group involvement

96 The most accurate definition of "depression," as used in psychiatry, is:
1. A disturbance in mood as a reaction to the loss of a love object
2. A total loss of control over emotional impulses
3. An inability to make decisions or function
4. A disturbance in mood as a result of frustration of instinctual strivings

97 Schizophrenia is classified as a functional psychosis. This means that the:
1. Genes of the child may carry the schizophrenic factor
2. Brain itself undergoes actual physical change that produces the symptoms of schizophrenia
3. Brain itself undergoes no physical change, but the operation of the organ is disturbed, producing the symptoms of schizophrenia
4. Individual is predisposed to schizophrenia because of poor housing and living conditions during childhood

98 The affect most commonly found in the schizophrenic patient is one of:
1. Happiness and elation
2. Apathy and flatness
3. Sadness and depression
4. Anger and hostility

99 Mental illness is evidenced when an individual:
1. Has difficulty relating to others
2. Experiences frequent periods of high anxiety
3. Expresses little desire for work or social activities
4. Has difficulty completing activities

100 Carolyn Demarke has been a patient on the Psychiatric Unit for several days. She arouses anxiety and frustration in the ward staff and manipulates so well that she intimidates any nurse who comes near her. One morning, Carolyn yells out at the nurse, "You've worked it so that I can't go out with the group today to bowl. You're as cunning as a fox—I hate you! Get out or I'll hit you." When a nurse is threatened this way, the best response would be:
1. "You are being rude and I don't like it. Your behavior is stopping me from wanting to stay with you."
2. "Go ahead and hit me if you have a need to."
3. "Tell me what I did to hurt you."
4. "I don't really like to hear your threats and insults. Can you tell me why you feel this way?"

101 Functional mental illnesses are mainly the result of:
1. Genetic endowment
2. Social environment
3. Infection and inflammation
4. Deterioration of brain tissue

102 When there is nothing organically wrong with the organs of comunication and yet the individual is unable to communicate, the condition is referred to as:
1. Organic psychosis
2. Mental deficiency
3. Functional psychosis
4. Chronic brain pathology

103 Mrs. Ray is hospitalized because of a severe depression. While at home she refused to eat, stayed in bed most of the time, and did not talk with family members. Finally, unable to cope with the problem, the husband took her to the hospital. Here the symptoms persist and she will not leave her room. The nurse caring for her attempts to talk

to her, asking questions but receiving no answers. Finally, in exasperation, the nurse tells the patient that if she does not respond she will be left alone. The nurse:

1. Attempts to use reward and punishment to motivate the patient
2. Is really assaulting the patient and should have refrained from this
3. Recognizes that the patient has the right to make the decision
4. Should get her involved in group therapy rather than attempting one-to-one therapy

104 Mr. James, a patient on the psychiatric unit, becomes upset in the day room. In attempting to deal with the situation the nurse should:
1. Lead the patient from the room by taking him by his arm
2. Allow the patient to act out until he tires
3. Give directions in a firm low-pitched voice
4. Instruct the patient to be quiet

105 Susan is your patient. As you are talking to another patient, Susan comes up to you and yells, "I hate you. You're talking about me again," and throws a glass of juice at you. Your nursing approach would be to:
1. Remove Susan to an isolation room because she needs to have limits placed on her behavior
2. Say to yourself, "She's very sick. I must understand her behavior"; then say, "You hate me? Tell me about that."
3. Say to yourself, "She's acting this way because she's sick"; then, ignore both the behavior and Susan, clean up the juice, and promise yourself you'll talk to her when she is better
4. Verbalize your own feelings of annoyance as an example to Susan that it is more acceptable to verbalize feelings than to act out

Situation: Mr. Long, age 35, has been admitted to the Mental Health Unit of a general hospital. Over the past month he has had difficulty in sleeping and has lost his appetite. Although very anxious and tense, he appears sad and has lost all initiative. He has difficulty in concentrating, and most of his thoughts center on his unworthiness and his failures. Questions 106 to 115 refer to this situation.

106 Mr. Long is being interviewed by the admitting nurse. Which question is the most appropriate at this time?
1. "Tell me what has been bothering you?"
2. "Why do you feel so bad about yourself?"
3. "Tell me how you feel about yourself."
4. "What can we do to help you during your stay with us?"

107 Which of the following behaviors best portrays Mr. Long's feelings of self-effacement?
1. Voice is quiet and monotonous
2. Lack of initiative

3. Gestures and affect are inappropriate
4. Attitude is one of "don't listen to me"

108 The nurse needs to evaluate Mr. Long's potential for suicide. Which approach would best gain this information?
1. Ask his family if he has ever attempted suicide
2. Ask him if he has ever thought of suicide
3. In a group discussion, direct patients to talk of suicide
4. Ask him what his plans are for the future

109 Which action by the nurse would be most therapeutic when Mr. Long states, "I am no good. I'm better off dead."
1. Unobtrusively removing those articles which could be used in a suicide attempt
2. Stating, "I think you are good; you should think of living."
3. Stating, "I will stay with you until you are less depressed."
4. Alerting the staff to provide 24-hour observation of the patient

110 In making a nursing care plan for Mr. Long, which approach would be most therapeutic?
1. Allow time for his slowness when planning activities
2. Encourage patient to perform menial tasks to meet the need for punishment
3. Help Mr. Long focus on family strengths and support systems
4. Reassure him that he is worthwhile and important

111 Mr. Long refuses to cooperate with the staff. All planned activities are rejected, since he is "just too tired." Which nursing approach best expresses an understanding of his needs?
1. Explain why the activities are therapeutic for him
2. Accept his behavior calmly, and without excessive comment set firm limits
3. Help him express his feelings of hostility toward the activities
4. Plan a rest period for him during activity time

112 The nurse understands that one of the most difficult tasks for Mr. Long is to express his:
1. Feelings of low self-esteem
2. Remorse and guilt
3. Anger toward others
4. Need for comforting

113 Mr. Long is to have electroconvulsive therapy (ECT). What information should the nurse give him about this treatment?
1. He will be put to sleep and will have no pain
2. With new methods of administration treatment is totally safe
3. Answer only those questions asked by him
4. He will have complete memory loss as a result of the treatment

114 The physician has ordered imipramine (Tofranil), 75 mg tid, for Mr. Long. Which of the following is an appropriate nursing action in giving this drug?

1. Warn him not to eat cheese, fermenting products, and chicken liver
2. Do not give any barbiturates or steroids with this drug
3. Have him checked for intraocular pressure and instruct him to watch for symptoms of glaucoma
4. Observe him for increased tolerance so that therapeutic dosage is maintained

115 Mr. Long is to be discharged from the hospital. Which statement by the nurse gives the most understanding at this time?
   1. "I am going to miss you; we have become good friends."
   2. "Call the unit night or day if you have problems."
   3. "This is my phone number; call me and let me know how your doing."
   4. "I know you are going to be all right when you go home."

116 An individual with a psychoneurotic disorder usually handles anxiety *in all but one* of the following ways:
   1. Converting anxiety into a physical symptom
   2. Acting out the anxiety with antisocial behavior
   3. Displacing anxiety onto less threatening objects
   4. Regressing to earlier levels of adjustment

117 A phobic reaction will rarely occur unless the person:
   1. Thinks about the feared object
   2. Absolves the guilt of the feared object
   3. Introjects the feared object into the body
   4. Comes into contact with the feared object

118 School phobia is usually treated by:
   1. Calmly explaining why attendance at school is necessary
   2. Returning the child to school immediately
   3. Allowing the parent to accompany child to classroom
   4. Allowing the child to enter classroom before other children

119 The person with socially aggressive behavior needs an environment that:
   1. Allows freedom of expression
   2. Is mainly group oriented
   3. Provides controls by setting limits
   4. Can be manipulated

120 The patient who has obsessive-compulsive behavior can best be treated by:
   1. Calling attention to the behavior
   2. Restricting his movements
   3. Supporting but limiting the behavior
   4. Keeping him busy to distract him

121 Many people control anxiety by ritualistic behavior. When taking care of these patients it is important to:
   1. Allow time to carry out the ritual
   2. Prevent patient from carrying out the ritual
   3. Explain the meaning of the ritual
   4. Avoid mentioning the ritual

122 Sally, age 16, is admitted to the psychiatric service. She has lost 20 pounds in 6 weeks. She is very thin but concerned about being overweight. Her daily intake is 10 cups of coffee. The most important initial nursing intervention would be to:
   1. Compliment her on her lovely figure
   2. Explain the value of good nutrition
   3. Explore the reasons why she does not eat
   4. Try to establish a relationship of trust

123 Shortly after admission, Sally falls to the floor and has tonic and clonic movements. She does not respond verbally but you note that she is still chewing gum. Which of the following is your best response?
   1. Remove the chewing gum
   2. Send another patient for help
   3. Report and record all observations
   4. Insert a tongue blade between her teeth

124 A young handsome man with a diagnosis of sociopathic personality is being discharged from the hospital next week. He asks you for your phone number so he can call you for a date. Your best response would be:
   1. "No, you are a patient and I am a nurse."
   2. "We are not permitted to date patients."
   3. "I like you, but our relationship is professional."
   4. "It is against my professional ethics to date patients."

125 The patient with a sociopathic personality disorder:
   1. Is generally unable to postpone gratification
   2. Suffers from a great deal of anxiety
   3. Has a great sense of responsibility toward others
   4. Rapidly learns by experience and punishment

126 The sociopath has difficulty in relating to others because of never having learned to:
   1. Count on others
   2. Be dependent on others
   3. Communicate with others socially
   4. Empathize with others

Situation: Mr. James has been admitted to the Psychiatric Unit for psychologic testing. He is a 43-year-old, well-dressed male, whom you find sitting with his face in his hands. He is charged with molesting a 7-year-old child. Questions 127 and 128 refer to this situation.

127 When you ask Mr. James to come to dinner, he refuses, stating "I don't want anyone to see me. Leave me alone." Your best response would be:
   1. "Certainly, Mr. James. I respect your wishes."
   2. "It will be easier to face other people right away."
   3. "Only the staff knows why you are here."
   4. "You are the hardest judge you must face, Mr. James."

128 Mr. James looks intently at you without saying anything else. You could best respond by stating:
   1. "I'll be at the desk if you need me."
   2. "Pull yourself together, Mr. James. I'll walk you to dinner."

3. "Tell me what you are feeling now, Mr. James."
4. "It must be difficult to be on a psychiatric unit."

Situation: Mrs. Jordon is admitted with a severe anxiety reaction. She is crying, wringing her hands, and pacing. Questions 129 through 134 refer to this situation.

129 The first nursing intervention should be to:
1. Ask the patient what is bothering her
2. Tell the patient to sit down and try to relax
3. Stay physically close to her
4. Try to get her involved in some nonthreatening activity

130 Unsatisfied needs create anxiety that motivates an individual to action. This action is brought about mainly to:
1. Relieve physical discomfort
2. Reduce tension
3. Remove the problem
4. Deny the situation

131 The nurse should teach Mrs. Jordon's family that anxiety can be recognized as:
1. Fears that are related to the total environment
2. A behavior pattern observable in ourselves and others
3. A totally unique experience and feeling
4. Consciously motivated thoughts and wishes

132 The nurse can minimize Mrs. Jordon's psychologic stress by:
1. Learning what is of particular importance to the patient
2. Explaining in fine detail all procedures and therapies
3. Confidently advising the patient that the nurse is in charge of the situation
4. Avoiding the discussion of any areas that may be emotionally charged

133 Physiologically, the nurse would expect Mrs. Jordon's anxiety to be manifested by:
1. Dilated pupils, dilated bronchioles, increased pulse rate, hyperglycemia, and peripheral vasoconstriction
2. Constricted pupils, constricted bronchioles, increased pulse rate, hypoglycemia, and peripheral vasodilation
3. Dilated pupils, constricted bronchioles, decreased pulse rate, hypoglycemia, and peripheral vasoconstriction
4. Constricted pupils, dilated bronchioles, increased pulse rate, hypoglycemia, and peripheral vasodilation

134 The most appropriate way to decrease Mrs. Jordon's anxiety is by:
1. Prolonged exposure to fearful situations
2. Introducing an element of pleasure into fearful situations
3. Avoiding unpleasant objects and events
4. Acquiring skills with which to face emergencies

Situation: Mrs. Queen, 28 years old, is admitted to the hospital with a diagnosis of hysterical conversion neurosis. Questions 135 through 138 refer to this situation.

135 Mrs. Queen states that she is unable to move her legs. Which of the following behaviors would you expect to observe in Mrs. Queen? She:
1. Appears greatly depressed
2. Exhibits free-floating anxiety
3. Appears calm and composed
4. Demonstrates anxiety when discussing symptoms

136 When caring for Mrs. Queen, a positive nursing intervention would be to:
1. Encourage her to try to walk
2. Avoid focusing on her physical symptoms
3. Tell her there is nothing wrong
4. Help her follow through with the physical therapy plan

137 In a patient such as Mrs. Queen, anxiety is:
1. Diffuse and free floating
2. Localized and relieved by the symptom
3. Consciously felt by the patient
4. Projected onto the environment

138 In planning nursing care for Mrs. Queen, the nurse recognizes that:
1. It is best to ignore her complaints
2. Her behavior indicates a lack of willpower
3. Her symptoms are evidence of a disturbed personality
4. If additional stress is added she will become psychotic

Situation: The staff and patients have just learned that, while on a weekend pass from the hospital, Sally Finn has committed suicide. A meeting is called to attempt to deal with the feelings this incident has aroused among staff and patients alike. The collective mood of the group is tense and restless. Questions 139 through 141 refer to this situation.

139 The nurse sitting beside Mrs. Smith observes that she is sobbing and rocking back and forth in a sitting position while she hugs her arms around herself. The nurse hears her moaning softly, "I'm next. Oh, my God, I'm next. They couldn't stop Sally and they can't protect me." The nurse could best respond by saying:
1. "Sally was a lot sicker than you are, Mrs. Smith."
2. "It's different, Mrs. Smith. Sally was home; you're here."
3. "You are afraid you will hurt yourself, Mrs. Smith?"
4. "Don't worry. All passes will be canceled for a while."

140 Jim May, a friend of Sally's, stands up and shouts, "Oh! I know what you're all thinking, you think that I should have known that she was going to kill herself. You think that I helped her plan this." The group leader's response should be:
1. "Oh no, Jim, we all know you liked Sally."
2. "You feel we're blaming you for Sally's death, Jim?"
3. "It'll help if you tell us the truth, Jim."
4. "Helping her plan her suicide would not be healthy."

141 During the group discussion it is learned that Sally had not shared her strong suicidal feelings and had successfully masked her depression. The group leader should be prepared primarily to deal with:

1. The guilt that the group feels because it could not prevent Sally's suicide
2. The fear and anxiety which some members of the group may have that their own suicidal urges may go unnoticed and unprotected
3. The guilt, fear, and anger of the staff, that they have failed to anticipate and prevent Sally's suicide
4. The lack of concern over Sally's suicide expressed by some of the group

---

Situation: Miss Hayes, 19 years of age, came to the psychiatric hospital from a girl's dormitory on a nearby college campus where she was a freshman. Throughout high school she had always been an excellent student who was interested in modern art, ballet, dancing, symphony concerts, and good literature. She played the violin very well. She had no close friends and was considered a lone wolf. Her family states that she always has been sensitive and different from other girls. She was admitted to the psychiatric hospital when she refused to get out of bed and go to classes. Her personal appearance deteriorated steadily during the past month, and recently she did not bother to comb her hair or put on makeup. In the hospital she talks to unseen people, voids on the floor, sometimes masturbates openly, occasionally eats with her hands, and refuses to shower or wear her own clothes. Questions 142 through 150 refer to this situation.

142 The nurse's efforts should be directed especially toward which aspect of Miss Hayes' care?
1. Frequent rest periods to avoid exhaustion
2. Appropriate attempts to establish a meaningful relationship with her
3. Reduction of environmental stimuli and maintenance of dietary intake
4. Improving social relationships with her peer group

143 The most appropriate way to begin to help Miss Hayes accept the realities of daily living would be to:
1. Encourage her to join the other patients in group singing
2. Assist her to care for her own personal hygiene
3. Encourage her to take up playing the violin again
4. Leave her alone when she is disinterested in the activity at hand

144 When Miss Hayes openly masturbates, the nurse should most appropriately:
1. Restrain her hands
2. Not react to the behavior
3. Put her in seclusion
4. Simply state that such behavior is not acceptable

145 Miss Hayes starts to repeat phrases that others have just said. This type of speech is known as:
1. Autism
2. Echopraxia

3. Echolalia
4. Neologism

146 The nurse could best handle the problem of Miss Hayes voiding on the floor by:
1. Making the patient mop the floor
2. Restricting the patient's fluids throughout the day
3. More frequent toileting with supervision
4. Withholding privileges each time the patient voids on the floor

147 When Miss Hayes eats with her hands, the nurse can handle this problem by:
1. Placing the spoon in her hand and suggesting that she use it
2. Commenting, ''I thought college girls had better manners than that.''
3. Removing the food and saying, ''You can't have any more until you can use your spoon.''
4. Saying in a joking way, ''Well, fingers were made before forks.''

148 While watching TV in the day room Miss Hayes suddenly screams, bursts into tears, and runs out of the room to the far end of the hallway. What would be the most therapeutic action for the nurse to take?
1. Write up the incident on the patient's chart while it is still fresh in her memory
2. Ask another patient what made Miss Hayes act as she did
3. Walk to the end of the hallway where Miss Hayes is standing
4. Accept the action as just being the impulsive behavior of a sick person

149 Miss Hayes feels that ''a man on television'' is responsible for her being sick. This is an example of:
1. Autistic thinking
2. Illusion
3. Hallucination
4. Delusion

150 Miss Hayes has been observed watching the nurse for a few days. She suddenly walks up to her and shouts, ''You think you're so damned perfect and pure and good. I think you stink.'' What would be the most appropriate response for the nurse to make?
1. ''I can't be all that bad can I?''
2. ''You seem angry with me.''
3. ''Stink? I don't understand.''
4. ''Boy, you're in a bad mood.''

Situation: Mrs. Ohream is a 46-year-old woman who was admitted to the psychiatric hospital because she drank poison and slashed her wrists. She cries a great deal, refuses food, and says that she is not fit to live. The physician has ordered electroconvulsive treatment for her. Questions 151 through 156 refer to this situation.

151 Which of the following physical problems occur when succinylcholine (Anectine) is administered before electroconvulsive therapy?
1. Dislocation of jaw
2. Compression fracture of vertebrae
3. Respiratory arrest
4. Electrocution

152 Mrs. Ohream has just awakened from her first electroconvulsive therapy treatment. The most appropriate nursing intervention would be to:
1. Get Mrs. Ohream up and out of bed as soon as possible and back into her normal routine
2. Orient Mrs. Ohream to time and place and tell her that she has just had a treatment
3. Arrange for the attendant to bring Mrs. Ohream a lunch tray
4. Take Mrs. Ohream's blood pressure and pulse rate every 15 minutes until she is fully awake

153 Which of the following factors is most important in helping to evaluate the risk of suicide in a depressed patient such as Mrs. Ohream?
1. Length of time the depression has existed
2. Impending anniversary of the loss of a loved one
3. Development of plans for discharge from hospital or program
4. Presence of multiple personal problems

154 A positive nursing action in caring for Mrs. Ohream is to:
1. Allow her to make decisions for herself
2. Provide her with frequent periods of thinking time
3. Hold her hand while sitting with her
4. Playing a game of chess with her

155 You are caring for Mrs. Ohream on a day she seems more withdrawn and depressed. An appropriate nursing action would be to:
1. Ask her if you may sit with her
2. Tell her you will spend some time with her
3. Remain visible to her
4. Get her involved in group activities

156 Depressed patients such as Mrs. Ohream seen to do best in settings where they have:
1. Many varied activities
2. A great deal of stimuli
3. A simple daily schedule
4. To make only simple decisions

157 When pouring liquid Thorazine, the nurse should:
1. Keep it away from the face during inspiration
2. Mix it with fruit juice
3. Administer immediately after pouring
4. Avoid contact with skin

158 Mrs. Somers is an elderly patient who has been taking chlorpromazine hydrochloride (Thorazine) for several months. After observing that the patient sits rigidly in her chair, the nurse observes her closely for other evidence of adverse effects of the drug, including:

1. Inability to concentrate, excess salivation
2. Minimal use of nonverbal expression, rambling speech
3. Incoordinated movement of extremities, tremors
4. Reluctance to converse, nonverbal clues indicating fear

159 In assessing the patient for adverse effects, the nurse would also:
1. Examine her eyeballs and question her about the color of her stools
2. Take her temperature and ask her if she has any symptoms of a cold
3. Take her blood pressure and ask if she has frequent headaches
4. Examine her skin and ask if she has numbness or coldness of her feet

160 A patient on a high dosage of Thorazine has developed tremors of the hands. The appropriate action of the nurse would be to:
1. Report the symptoms to the physician
2. Withhold the medication
3. Tell the patient it is transitory
4. Give the patient finger exercises

161 An extrapyramidal symptom that is a potentially irreversible side effect of chlorpromazine and other antipsychotic drugs is:
1. Pseudoparkinsonism
2. Torticollis
3. Tardive dyskinesia
4. Occulogyric crisis

162 Lithium carbonate is used for the:
1. Acute agitation of schizophrenia
2. Agitated phase of involutional melancholia
3. Modification of depressive phase of affective disorders
4. Control of manic episode of manic-depressive psychosis

163 A common manageable side effect of the major tranquilizers is:
1. Jaundice
2. Unintentional tremors
3. Ptosis
4. Melanocytosis

164 When monoamine oxidase (MAO) inhibitors are prescribed, the patient should be cautioned against:
1. The use of medications with an elixir base
2. Prolonged exposure to the sun
3. Ingesting wines and cheeses
4. Engaging in active physical exercise

165 Photosensitization is a side effect associated with the use of:
1. Chlorpromazine
2. Thioridazine
3. Methylphenidate (Ritalin)
4. Trifluoperazine (Stelazine)

166 The major tranquilizers are the drugs of choice to relieve symptoms of:

1. Narcotic withdrawal
2. Depression
3. Hyperkinesis
4. Psychosis

167 Drugs such as trihexyphenidyl (Artane), biperiden (Akineton), and benztropine (Cogentin) are often prescribed in conjunction with:
1. Major tranquilizers
2. Minor tranquilizers
3. Barbiturates
4. Antidepressants

168 Many psychiatric patients are given the drugs Cogentin or Artane in conjunction with the phenothiazine derivatives to:
1. Potentiate the effect of the drug
2. Reduce postural hypotension
3. Combat extrapyramidal side effects
4. Modify depression that often accompanies schizophrenia

Situation: Mr. Daniels, 19 years old and a known heroin addict, is unconscious when admitted to the emergency room with the diagnosis of narcotic (heroin) overdose. Questions 169 through 171 refer to this situation.

169 The medication used to combat an overdose of narcotics is:
1. Amphetamine sulfate (Benzedrine)
2. Naloxone hydrochloride (Narcan)
3. Dextroamphetamine (Dexedrine)
4. Caffeine sodium benzoate

170 The planned effect of this drug is to:
1. Stimulate cortical sites controlling consciousness and cardiovascular function
2. Accelerate metabolism of heroin and stimulate respiratory centers
3. Compete with narcotics for receptors controlling respiration
4. Decrease analgesia and the comatose state induced by heroin

171 Within an hour Mr. Daniels is responding. Close observation of his status is indicated because:
1. The combined action of naloxone hydrochloride and heroin causes cardiac depression
2. Naloxone hydrochloride may cause neuropathy and convulsions
3. Narcotic effect may cause return of symptoms after the naloxone chloride is metabolized
4. Hyperexcitability and amnesia may cause the patient to thrash about and become abusive

Situation: James Cote is a narcotic addict who had surgery to repair a laceration of his heart caused by a bullet. Postoperatively he is receiving methadone hydrochloride orally. Questions 172 through 177 refer to this situation.

172 Methadone hydrochloride:
1. Provides postoperative pain control without causing narcotic dependence
2. Counteracts the depressive effects of long-term opiate usage on cardiac and thoracic muscles
3. Allows symptom-free termination of narcotic addiction
4. Converts narcotic use from an illicit to a legally controlled drug

173 Drug abuse is best defined as:
1. A physiologic need for a drug
2. A psychic dependence on a drug
3. An excessive drug use inconsistent with acceptable medical practice
4. A compulsion to take a drug on either a continuous or periodic basis

174 Hard drugs easily cause dependence because of their ability to:
1. Ease pain
2. Clear sensorium
3. Blur reality
4. Decrease motor activity

175 How many hours after the last dose would the nurse expect Mr. Cote's withdrawal symptoms to reach a peak?
1. 8 to 24
2. 24 to 48
3. 48 to 72
4. 72 to 96

176 The nurse would expect Mr. Cote's basic personality to be marked by insecurity and:
1. Infantile passion for self-gratification
2. The need to delay gratification
3. The use of psychosomatic mechanisms
4. Weak id drives

177 When methadone hydrochloride dosage is lowered, Mr. Cote must be observed closely for evidence of:
1. Agitation, attempts to escape from the hospital
2. Piloerection, lack of interest in surroundings
3. Skin dryness, scratching under incisional dressing
4. Lethargy, refusal to participate in therapeutic exercise

Situation: Mr. Winford, a 42-year-old executive, is admitted for treatment of his alcoholism. Questions 178 through 183 refer to this situation.

178 Mr. Winford is suspicious of others and blames others for his difficulty. The nurse understands that the patient uses this behavior because he has problems:
1. In identifying who bothers him
2. With dependence and independence
3. In telling the truth
4. Meeting his ego ideal

179 Mr. Winford asks if you can see the bugs that are crawling on his bed. Your best reply would be:
1. "I will get rid of them for you."
2. "No, I don't see any bugs."

3. ''I will stay with you until you are calmer.''
4. ''Those bugs are a part of your sickness.''

180 Mr. Winford often makes up stories to fill in the blank spaces of his memory. This is said to be:
1. Denying
2. Confabulating
3. Lying
4. Rationalizing

181 As Mr. Winford begins to feel better, he denies excessive use of alcohol. The nurse understands that denial is meeting Mr. Winford's need to:
1. Make him look better in the eyes of others
2. Live up to other's expectations
3. Make him seem more independent
4. Reduce his feelings of guilt

182 Mr. Winford asks if it is required that he attend Alcoholics Anonymous. Your best reply would be:
1. ''No, it is best to wait until you feel you really need them.''
2. ''Yes, because you will learn how to cope with your problem.''
3. ''Do you have feelings about going to these meetings?''
4. ''You'll find you'll need their support.''

183 Groups such as Alcoholics Anonymous help people like Mr. Winford because in a group the person learns that:
1. He does not need a crutch
2. His problems are not unique
3. His problems are caused by alcohol
4. People stand stronger together

---

184 Mrs. Jane, a 45-year-old woman, is hospitalized because of chronic alcoholism. She is irritable with the nurses and seems only to wait for a friend who visits daily. After such visits Mrs. Jane seems happier and more relaxed. One day the nurse sees the visitor give her a package, which she puts away quickly. Later Mrs. Jane, obviously intoxicated, tells the staff that her friend has brought gin regularly. Mrs. Jane's husband is very upset and threatens to sue. The decision is this suit would take into consideration the fact that:
1. Patients may have gifts brought to them without prior inspection
2. Mrs. Jane's response to her friend's visit was a clue the nurse missed
3. The nurse is responsible for observing the patient's behavior
4. Psychotic patients need close supervision

185 Chronic alcoholic patients with Wernicke encephalopathy associated with Korsakoff's syndrome are treated initially by:
1. Oral administration of paraldehyde
2. Judicious use of tranquilizers
3. Providing a high-protein diet
4. Intramuscular injections of thiamine

186 Which of the following statements regarding alcohol and drug use is correct?
1. Most polydrug abusers also abuse alcohol
2. Most alcoholics become polydrug abusers
3. An unhappy childhood is a causative factor in addictions
4. Addictive individuals tend to use hostile abusive behavior

Situation: Mr. Ray, a 32-year-old salesman, is attending his first meeting of Alcoholics Anonymous because he finally realized and admitted that he is an alcoholic. Questions 187 through 191 refer to this situation.

187 The most effective treatment of alcoholism is accomplished by:
1. Admission to an alcoholic unit in a hospital
2. Individual or group psychotherapy
3. The daily administration of disulfiram (Antabuse)
4. Active membership in Alcoholics Anonymous

188 Self-help groups such as Alcoholics Anonymous are successful because they meet the patient's need to:
1. Be trusted
2. Grow
3. Be independent
4. Belong

189 Self-help groups assist their members to:
1. Deal with present behavior and changes in behavior
2. Identify with their peers
3. Set long-term goals
4. Identify the underlying cause of their behavior

190 For patients with alcoholism, the primary rehabilitator is the:
1. Nurse
2. Physician
3. Entire health team
4. Patient

191 The most important factor in Mr. Ray's rehabilitation is:
1. His emotional or motivational readiness
2. The qualitative level of his physical state
3. His family's accepting attitude
4. The availability of community resources

Situation: Donald Raye, a 19-year-old college sophomore, has been admitted through the university health service. He had become increasingly withdrawn, unkempt, isolated, and depressed. The referring psychiatrist notes strong suicidal tendencies. A contributing factor appears to be an abrupt ending of a relationship with a 22-year-old senior. His grades have fallen to the extent that he is in danger of failing all his courses. Questions 192 through 195 refer to this situation.

192 Donald's prognosis for reasonably rapid recovery is:
1. Poor, since he has suicidal tendencies
2. Bad, since he is failing in all sectors of his life

3. Fair, since he is intelligent enough to pull himself together

4. Good, since the onset is fairly sudden and no previous emotional problems existed

193 On the second day after his admission Donald asks the nurse why he is being observed around the clock and has his freedom of movement restricted. The nurse's most appropriate reply would be:

1. "Your doctor has ordered it. He's the one you should ask."

2. "Why do you think we are observing you?"

3. "We are concerned that you might try to harm yourself."

4. "What makes you think that, Donald?"

194 On the fourth day Donald tells the nurse, "Hey look! I was feeling pretty depressed for a while, but I'm certainly not going to kill myself." Which comment by the nurse best responds to the patient's communication?

1. "Kill yourself? I don't understand."

2. "We have to observe you until your doctor tells us to stop."

3. "Suppose we talk some more about this?"

4. "You do seem to be feeling better."

195 With treatment Donald progresses satisfactorily and is to be discharged within a day or 2. He appears to be responsible for his actions and the staff is pleased with his progress. The day before discharge the nurse leaves the door to the unit unlocked. On her return a few minutes later Donald is gone. He is found in a bathroom where he has hanged himself. In this situation:

1. Determined patients almost always succeed at suicide, even with constant supervision

2. The lifting of the depression demonstrated Donald's recovery, so supervision was unnecessary

3. Suicidal patients should be observed until all symptoms of depression have disappeared

4. Donald's actions should have been anticipated by the nurse

---

196 For most nurses the most difficult part of the nurse-patient relationship is:

1. Developing an awareness of self and the professional role in the relationship

2. Being able to understand and accept the patient's behavior

3. Accepting responsibility in identifying and evaluating the real needs of the patient

4. Remaining therapeutic and professional at all times

197 The goal of the therapeutic psychiatric environment is to:

1. Help the patient become popular in a controlled setting

2. Improve the patient's ability to relate to others

3. Help the staff to help the patient

4. Make the hospital atmosphere more homelike

198 During a group meeting a patient, Mr. Thomas, tells everyone of his fear of his impending discharge from the hospital. Which response by the group leader would be most appropriate?

1. "Maybe you're not ready to be discharged yet, Mr. Thomas."

2. "Maybe others in the group have similar feelings that they would share."

3. "You ought to be happy that you're leaving Mr. Thomas."

4. "How many in the group feel that Mr. Thomas is ready to be discharged?"

199 The emotional leader of a group is one who:

1. Reflects the feeling tone of the group

2. Has an authoritarian role within the group

3. Designates the roles within the group

4. Selects those who are to be members of the group

200 Group therapy can best help those who:

1. Are emotionally ill

2. Are dependent on others

3. Feel they have a problem

4. Have no one to listen to them

201 The group setting is especially conducive to therapy, since it:

1. Creates a new learning environment

2. Fosters one-to-one relationships

3. Decreases the focus on the individual

4. Confronts individual members with their shortcomings

202 When providing group therapy, the nurse must focus on:

1. Behavior of individual members

2. Personal feelings affecting behavior

3. Jointly experienced stress

4. Confrontation between members

203 Which of the following interventions is most important in helping to resolve a crisis situation: The nurse should:

1. Meet all dependency needs

2. Encourage socialization

3. Support ego strengths

4. Involve patient in new group

204 The current trend in the treatment of the emotionally ill is to:

1. Medicate during stressful periods

2. Maintain them in the community

3. Encourage assumption of responsibility

4. Provide occupational therapy

205 The referral of discharged psychiatric patients to a psychiatric day hospital facility in their own community is done primarily to assist them to:

1. Maintain goals attained during hospitalization

2. Increase social skills and awareness

3. Avoid direct confrontation with the community

4. Get out of the house for a few hours daily

4 MATERNITY NURSING

This section, maternity nursing, includes reproductive problems and emphasizes the pubertal changes of adolescence; the normal processes of conception, embryologic development, pregnancy, labor, delivery, and postpartum developments; and family planning. In addition, the newborn and the mother are discussed in relation to prematurity, birth injuries, and complications of labor and delivery. Current topics such as abortion, infant narcotic addiction, venereal disease, and sterility are included.

Childbirth is a family experience. Humanity's basic needs for survival are centered in the family because without continuous love, physical contact, food, and stimulation of the senses, the infant would never survive. As each new member becomes a part of the family unit, interactions with the environment and other human beings become a part of early physical and emotional development. What is learned is determined by the kinds of stimulation received from the interactions occurring within the family. It is through this reciprocal give-and-take between the newborn and the family that each person becomes an individual, unique self.

Although childbearing patterns differ the world over, there are constants. In order of priority, they are: immediate physical contact between the infant and the parents; ability of the parents to give the infant love, food, and protection from the environment; the biologic need in men and women to reproduce; and the maturation and growth process that occurs in males and females in their changing roles as parents.

The unique and changing responsibilities in the life cycle event of parenthood can be a real crisis. The changes occurring in society, whether social, economic, technical, or political, directly affect the patterns of childbearing and childrearing. Parenthood today is given serious thought, since it concerns both the family and society with the emphasis on quality rather than quantity.

PUBERTY

A period during which the organs of reproduction mature and are prepared for their reproductive function
A. Physical and physiologic changes
  1. In male
    a. Occur between 10 and 14 years of age—less dramatic than in female
    b. Heralded by deepening of voice and growth of body hair on face, axillae, and genitalia
    c. Second year after onset—increased activity of sweat glands, spermatogenesis occurs with periodic erections and emissions of mature sperm
    d. Dramatic body growth spurt
    e. Ejaculation is beginning of fertility and end of puberty
  2. In female
    a. Occurs between 9 and 13 years of age
    b. Sudden enlargement of breasts, growth of body hair on axillae and genitalia—changes in size and vascularity of internal reproductive organs
    c. Heralded by first menstrual flow called *menarche* (unlike male's first ejaculation, many first menstrual cycles are anovulatory and infertile)
    d. Dramatic body growth more evident than in male
B. Psychologic changes
  1. Age differences in maturation
  2. Heterosexual interests—girls earlier than boys, girls interested in older boys

3. Emancipation struggles with parents—independence versus dependence
4. Need for belonging to a peer group

C. Menstrual cycle
1. A rhythmic reproductive cycle in females extending from the onset of a period of uterine bleeding to the onset of the next period of bleeding; mean cycle length is 28 days; normal range is 20 to 45 days per cycle
2. During each cycle several (about 20) follicles commence maturation, but usually only one reaches full maturity and ruptures its contained ovum (and some surrounding granulosa cells) into the abdominal cavity
3. The rhythmic menstrual cycles begin at puberty and cease at menopause
4. Menstrual cycle divided into 3 stages based on endometrial histologic makeup and may be correlated with concentration fluctuations in hypothalamic, hypophyseal, and ovarian hormones (which cause the endometrial and other reproductive tract histologic changes)
   a. First stage—menstruation or menses—lasts 4 to 6 days; characterized by endometrial hemorrhage with the discharge exiting through the vagina; estrogen and progesterone blood levels are relatively low; FSH level is elevated and, combined with a steady low level of LH secretion, initiates ovarian estrogen secretion, leading to second stage
   b. Second stage—follicular or proliferative—lasts 8 to 10 days culminating in ovulation; endometrium repairs and proliferates in preparation for possible implantation, and a single ovarian follicle approaches full maturation as estradiol (principle estrogenic hormone) blood concentration rises; estradiol exerts a negative feedback on FSH secretion and a positive feedback on LH secretion (the latter hormone induces ovulation); estradiol's feedback effects are exerted on the hypothalamic secretion of FSH-LH–releasing hormone, whose secretion controls hypophyseal FSH and LH secretion
   c. Third stage—luteal or secretory—final stage is 9 to 13 days and begins after ovulation; LH promotes formation of a temporary endocrine gland, the corpus luteum, from the ruptured follicle: granulosa and theca interna cells of follicle enlarge, divide into and occupy the cavity (antrum) of the follicle, and secrete progesterone and estrogen; progesterone stimulates the already proliferated endometrium to become glandular with a high glycogen-secreting potential (uterus now prepared for implantation); if fertilization does not occur, corpus luteum functions for 7 to 8 days after ovulation and then involutes, becoming nonfunctional (corpus albicans) 10 to 12 days after ovulation; progesterone and estrogen blood levels drop, the negative feedback effect of estradiol on FSH is released, and the first stage begins again

MATERNITY CYCLE
Antepartal period

A. Maturation, fertilization, and implantation
1. Maturation of ovum and sperm by mitosis and meiosis; reduction in chromosome number from 46 to 23
2. Fertilization occurs when ovum and sperm unite in distal portion of fallopian tube
3. Rapid division by cleavage without increase in cell size in 6 days (morula stage)
4. Implantation within 6 to 9 days generally in upper fundal portion of uterus; in this blastocyst stage cells are arranged into 3 layers: ectoderm, mesoderm, endoderm
5. Trophoblastic stage—projection of villi into maternal tissue, later to become placenta, vehicle for exchange of nutrients and wastes

B. Growth and development of baby (cephalocaudal)
1. 14 days—heart begins to beat, brain, early spinal cord, and muscle segments present
2. 26 days—tiny buds for arms appear
3. 28 days—tiny buds for legs appear
4. 30 days—embryo ¼ to ½ inch (0.6 to 1.2 cm) in length, definite form, beginning of umbilical cord is visible
5. 31 days—arm buds develop into hands, arms, and shoulders
6. 33 days—finger outlines present
7. 46 to 48 days—cartilage in upper arms replaced by first bone cells, amniotic fluid surrounds fetus (amniotic fluid is a protective cushion, equalizes pressures, and facilitates baby's movements for adequate growth and development)
8. 3 months (12 weeks)—fetus moves body parts,

swallows, practices inhaling and exhaling, weighs 1 oz (28 g)

9. 4 to 5 months (16 to 20 weeks)—fetal movements felt by mother (known as quickening), weighs 6 oz (170 g), is 8 to 10 inches (20 to 25 cm) in length

10. 5 to 6 months (20 to 24 weeks)—hair growth on head, eyelashes and brow, skeleton hardens, eyelids closed, weighs 1 lb (0.45 kg), is 12 inches (30.5 cm) in length, fetal heart audible with fetoscope

11. 6 to 7 months (24 to 28 weeks)—eyelids open, amniotic fluid increases to 1 quart with a daily exchange of 6 gallons, weighs 1¼ lb (0.5 kg)

12. 7 to 8 months (28 to 32 weeks)—many fat deposits, weighs 1 to 1½ lb (0.45 to 0.7 kg)

13. 8 to 9 months (32 to 36 weeks)—stores protein for extrauterine life, gains 4 lb (1.81 kg)

C. Fetal circulation—differs from adult because of following accessory structures

1. Placenta
   a. Organ of dual origin (maternal and embryonic portions) serving interchange of food and wastes between mother and embryo (or fetus) during pregnancy
   b. Villous portion of chorion (chorion frondosum) and the portion of the uterine endometrium (called the decidua during pregnancy) directly underlying the implanted embryo (decidua basalis) constitute the placenta: chorionic villi project into placental sinuses (in decidua basalis) filled with maternal blood
   c. Placenta functions as fetal digestive tract and also as fetal lungs, kidneys, and as a major endocrine gland (producing estrogens, progesterone, ACTH, growth hormone, and gonadotropic hormones HCG and HPL) (see Endocrine system)

2. Umbilical cord
   a. Inserted close to the central portion of the placenta and attached to fetus
   b. Umbilical cord has 1 vein (transports nourishment) and 2 arteries (transports wastes) between mother and baby
   c. Wharton's jelly is a protective covering surrounding the entire cord

3. Foramen ovale is an opening between the right and left atria during fetal life, bypassing fetal lungs

4. Ductus arteriosus is a connection between pulmonary trunk and aorta, also bypassing fetal lungs

5. Ductus venosus is a connection between umbilical vein and ascending vena cava, bypassing fetal liver

6. As a result of previously mentioned structures all blood in fetal heart is mixed blood; less than maximal O_2 saturation

7. Only oxygenated blood in the fetus is at the immediate entrance of the umbilical vessel on entering the liver

D. Physical and physiologic changes in mother during pregnancy; pregnancy is a normal physiologic process that affects all body systems and results in both objective and subjective changes; it is a stressful time requiring many adaptations

1. Endocrine and reproductive systems
   a. Fatigue is a result of increased hormonal levels causing sodium and water retention and relaxation of smooth muscles
   b. Amenorrhea occurs, since the corpus luteum persists and ovulation is inhibited due to high levels of circulating estrogens and progesterones
   c. Breast changes such as fullness, tingling, soreness, darkening of areola and nipple occur along with an increase in hormonal levels
   d. Leukorrhea is increased as hormonal levels rise, and the increased acidity is a protection from bacterial invasion
   e. Changes in uterus are circulatory, hormonal, and related to fetal growth
      (1) Softening of cervix—Goodell's sign
      (2) Softening of lower uterine segment—Hegar's sign
      (3) Purplish hue to vaginal mucosa—Chadwick's sign
      (4) Changes in position of uterus—first trimester uterus is in pelvic cavity, second and third trimester uterus is in abdominal cavity before lightening occurs

2. Digestive system
   a. Reduction in hydrochloric acid interferes with gastric motility, causing nausea and vomiting
   b. Constipation is secondary to hypoperistalsis, lack of fluids, poor dietary habits, pressure of enlarged uterus on internal organs, and effects of progesterone on smooth muscle

3. Excretory system
   a. Proximity of uterus and bladder in early and late pregnancy causes urinary frequency

b. Bladder tone is reduced by effects of hormones on smooth muscle

c. Bladder capacity increases gradually to 1500 ml

d. Increased urinary output results in lowered specific gravity

e. Increased excretion of sugar caused by lowered renal threshold

f. Presence of gonadotropic hormones in the urine (used as basis for pregnancy tests)

4. Circulatory system

a. Physiologic anemia occurs as a result of increased blood volume with no proportional increase in red blood cells

b. Cardiac output increases 25% to 50% during pregnancy, peaking at 7 or 8 months

c. Heart rate increases 10 beats per minute in the latter half of pregnancy—approximately 14,000 extra beats in 24 hours

d. Edema of extremities common in last 6 weeks of pregnancy because of stasis of blood

e. Leg cramps are believed to result from an imbalance of the calcium/phosphorus ratio in the body and from pressure of the gravid uterus on nerves supplying lower extremities

5. Respiratory system

a. At 36 to 38 weeks, pressure of enlarged uterus on diaphragm and lungs may cause dyspnea that subsides when lightening occurs

b. Oxygen consumption is increased by about 15% between the sixteenth and fortieth weeks, although there may be only a slight increase in vital capacity during pregnancy

6. Integumentary system

a. Excretion of wastes through skin causes diaphoresis

b. Skin changes—darkening of areola of breasts, darkening patches on face (chloasma), linea alba becomes nigra on abdomen, striae on abdomen and legs caused by skin stretching as pregnancy advances, erythematous changes on palms of hands and face in some women

7. Skeletal system—a softening of all ligaments and joints (especially pubic symphysis and sacroiliac joint) caused by increased hormonal action of estrogens and relaxin

8. Nervous system—no specific changes unless related to nonpregnant state or stress of pregnancy

E. Course, signs, and diagnosis of pregnancy

1. Estimated date of delivery—Nagele's rule—count back 3 months from the first day of the last normal menstrual period and add 7 days (9 calendar months, 270 days or 10 lunar months, 290 days)

2. Estimated gestational age—noninvasive techniques

a. Fundal height

b. Estriol levels in maternal urine

3. Estimated gestational age—direct invasive techniques

a. Ultrasonography—term pregnancy can be diagnosed if biparietal diameter is greater than 9.8 cm

b. Radiography—presence of distal femoral ossification centers indicate fetal age of 36 weeks; if proximal tibial centers are present, fetal age is 40 weeks

c. Amniocentesis—L/S ratio that is greater than 2 indicates adequate lung maturity for extrauterine life; if optical density of bilirubinoid pigments is 450 mm < 0.01, gestational age is greater than 38 weeks

4. Positive signs of pregnancy are auscultation of fetal heart tones (fetoscope or Doppler ultrasound), palpation of fetal parts, roentgenogram of fetal skeleton, and ultrasound scanning of fetus

5. Diagnostic pregnancy tests—urine of pregnant women used to detect chorionic gonadotropin

a. Animal tests—Friedman's, Aschheim-Zondek

b. Chemical—Pregnosticon, Gravindex, radioimmunoassay for chronic gonadotropin

Prenatal period

A. Medical supervision during pregnancy

1. History, including medical, surgical, gynecologic and obstetric data; family history of hereditary and transmittable diseases such as diabetes, tuberculosis, heart disease

2. Physical examination of skin, thyroid, teeth, lungs, heart, and breasts, abdominal palpation, auscultation, height of fundus, vaginal examination, and pelvic evaluation (prior to last 4 weeks of pregnancy)

3. Smears taken for monilial and trichomonal infections, Papanicolaou test done for cancer

4. Blood pressure; weight; and urinalysis for acetone, albumin, and sugar done at intervals

5. Blood determination for typing, cross matching, Rh factor, serologic test for syphilis, and a sickle-cell test for black women are done

B. Nutritional needs during pregnancy

1. Consideration of preconceptional nutritional status; age and parity of mother; biologic interactions between mother, fetus, and placenta; and individual needs such as in times of stress
2. Weight gain should be evaluated with regard to quality of gain (Is weight gain caused by edema or fat deposition?)
3. Severe caloric restriction during pregnancy is contraindicated, since it is a potential hazard to mother and fetus
4. Weight reduction should never be started as a regimen during pregnancy
5. Restriction of sodium and administration of diuretics are potentially dangerous to mother and fetus during pregnancy
6. Nausea and vomiting—limited fluids with meals, small frequent feedings, restricted fats, high carbohydrate
7. Constipation—increased fluids and residue or fiber; appropriate activity level
8. Consideration of the demands of pregnancy related to growth and development of the fetus during the various trimesters; provide adequate nutrition to meet increased maternal and fetal nutrient demands
   a. Increased calories to meet increased basal metabolic needs and spare protein for growth, to promote weight gain to support pregnancy (averages 11.4 kg, or 25 lb, but is individual according to need), and for lactation
   b. Increased protein to provide for growth demands
   c. Increased vitamins, especially folic acid supplement to prevent anemia
   d. Increased minerals with supplement of iron to prevent anemia
   e. Iodized salt to provide needed sodium and iodine
9. The lactating mother needs additional caloric requirements
10. Dietary assessment should be an integral part of prenatal care for every pregnant woman
11. Changes in dietary regimen should consider cultural, economic, and psychologic implications of food habits
12. Food guide may be based on basic 4 groups with
    a. Increased protein foods—1 qt milk, 2 eggs, 2 servings of meat, added cheese

b. Additional servings from each of the remaining food groups—grains, vegetables, fruits
c. Additional calories, protein, and fluids during lactation

C. Nursing goals to prepare parents for childbirth
   1. Assist parents to understand the anatomy and physiology of pregnancy, labor, and delivery
   2. Help parents to discuss and explore feelings related to childbearing and childrearing in attempting to alleviate fears
   3. Prepare the mother for the physical work of labor through the use of muscle and breathing exercises for the various phases of labor
   4. Identify parents' situational support systems
   5. Prepare the father for coaching and supporting role during pregnancy, labor, and delivery
   6. Introduce families to health facilities available for continued health care of the family

Intrapartal period

A. Labor—a physiologic and mechanical process in which the baby, placenta, and fetal membranes are expelled through the pelvis and birth canal
B. Anatomy of bony pelvis
   1. Parts—ischium, ilium, sacrum, coccyx
   2. Joints—sacroiliacs, sacrococcygeal, symphysis pubis (all soften during pregnancy)
   3. Divisions—false pelvis supports the enlarged uterus in the abdominal cavity; true pelvis is the bony inner pelvis through which the baby must pass
   4. Diameters at inlet—true conjugate (anteroposterior diameter), transverse (widest diameter at inlet), right and left oblique diameters; at outlet—conjugate diagonal (anteroposterior is widest diameter), transverse (one ischial tuberosity to other)
   5. Classification of pelvis—gynecoid (normal female pelvis), android (male pelvis), anthropoid, and platypelloid
   6. Normal female pelvis has an ample pubic arch, curved sacrum, curved side walls, blunt ischial spines, and a movable coccyx
C. Attitude—relationship of fetal parts to each other
D. Presentation—baby's body part that engages into true pelvis
   1. Cephalic (head)—vertex, brow, or face
   2. Breech—frank, complete, single, or double footling
   3. Shoulder—must be turned for delivery

E. Position—relationship of presenting parts to 4 quadrants of mother's pelvis (the letters L and R are used for left or right; the letters A and P are used for anterior or posterior; the letter O signifies occiput; the letter M signifies mentum or face; the letter S signifies sacrum)
   1. Vertex—occiput, L.O.A., L.O.P., R.O.A., R.O.P.
   2. Face—chin (mentum), L.M.A., L.M.P., R.M.A., R.M.P.
   3. Breech—sacrum, L.S.A., L.S.P., R.S.A., R.S.P.
F. Station—relationship of presenting part to false and true pelvis
   1. Floating—presenting part movable above true pelvic inlet
   2. Engaged—suboccipitobregmatic diameter fixed into pelvic inlet
   3. Station O—presenting part at level of ischial spines—levels below spines $+1$, $+2$, $+3$; levels above spines -1, -2, -3
G. Signs and symptoms prior to true labor
   1. Lightening—baby drops down into true pelvis
   2. Mother experiences Braxton Hicks contractions—painless tryout contractions in preparation for true labor
   3. Increased vaginal secretions
   4. Softening of cervix
H. Signs and symptoms of true labor
   1. Uterine contractions that increase in frequency, strength, and duration
   2. Bloody show—pressure of presenting part on the cervix causes effacement and dilation of the cervix
   3. Rupture of the membranes
I. Mechanisms of labor—rotation of vertex presentation through true pelvis
   1. Engagement, descent with flexion—at onset of labor, head descends and chin flexes on chest
   2. Internal rotation—as labor contractions and uterine forces move baby downward, head internally rotates to pass through ischial spines
   3. Extension—occiput emerges under symphysis pubis and head is delivered by extension
   4. External rotation—to allow for rotation of shoulders to anteroposterior position
   5. Lateral flexion—allows for delivery of shoulders and body
J. Stages of labor

1. First stage—encompasses period from onset of true labor to complete effacement and dilation of cervix
2. Second stage—from complete effacement and dilation of cervix to birth of the baby
3. Third stage—from birth of the baby through expulsion of the placenta
4. Fourth stage—first hour following delivery
K. Changes in mother during labor
   1. First stage
      a. Latent phase—irregular contractions, cervix dilated 0 to 2 cm, mother excited and happy labor has started, some apprehension
      b. Relaxation phase—moderate to strong contractions 5 to 8 minutes apart, cervix dilates from 2 to 6 cm, bloody show, membranes may rupture, breathing techniques help in relaxing, medication may be necessary for discomfort, supportive measures by husband or nurse (such as encouragement, praise, reassurance, keeping mother informed of progress, providing rest between contractions, and presence of a supporting person) help
      c. Transition phase—strong contractions 1 to 2 minutes apart (often last 60 to 90 seconds each with little or no rest in between), bloody show, mother becomes irritable, restless, agitated, highly emotional, belches, has leg tremors, perspires, pale white ring around mouth (circumoral pallor), flushed face, sudden nausea, and vomiting; generally lasts less than an hour
   2. Second stage—beginning with full dilation of cervix and ending with birth of baby, perineum bulges, pushing with contractions, grunting sounds, behavior changes from great irritability to great involvement and work, sleep and relaxation occur between contractions, leg cramps are common
L. Nursing care during labor and delivery
   1. Emotional support by husband, nurse, or significant others
   2. Maintenance of asepsis
   3. Timing frequency, duration, and strength of contractions
   4. Auscultation or monitoring of fetal heart sounds as to rate, regularity, and tone
   5. Frequent observation of perineum for show, rupture of membranes, and presenting part

6. Check vital signs at frequent intervals
7. Emergency equipment available for safe care of mother and baby such as oxygen, blood, drugs
8. Assessment of basic needs such as body fluids, bladder and bowel function
9. Assist mother with breathing techniques throughout labor

M. Induction and control of uterine contractions by pharmacologic agents
1. Oxytocin (Pitocin, Syntocinon, Uteracon)
   a. Used to induce labor by stimulation of characteristic rhythmic contraction and relaxation of uterine muscles
   b. Administered IM after delivery of the anterior shoulder or IV after delivery of the baby to provide uterine contractions that complete expulsion of uterine contents and decrease bleeding from endometrial sites
2. Sparteine sulfate (Spartocin, Tocosamine)
   a. Used to stimulate uterine muscle contraction when inertia occurs during labor
   b. Adverse effects—lengthens refractory period of cardiac muscle and may cause bradycardia

N. Danger signs and symptoms during labor
1. Tonic, strong, continuous contractions with sharp abdominal pain and, on palpation, abdomen taut and boardlike
2. Variations in rate, regularity, and tone of fetal heart sounds
3. Meconium-stained or excessive amount of amniotic fluid
4. Elevation or drop in blood pressure
5. Increase in pulse or temperature
6. Sudden excessive fetal movements
7. Bleeding, protrusion of umbilical cord or placenta

O. Nursing care immediately following delivery
1. Mother
   a. Palpate fundus frequently for firmness and height in relation to umbilicus
   b. Keep airway open if inhalation anesthesia has been given
   c. Monitor blood pressure and pulse; report fluctuations
   d. Check perineum for vaginal and suture line bleeding
   e. Administer oxytocic drug as ordered
   f. Administer lactogenic inhibitor as ordered if bottle feeding preferred

g. Administer RhoGAM as ordered if mother is Rh negative
2. Baby
   a. Clear airway of mucus
   b. Observe frequently
   c. Use Apgar scoring to determine respiratory effort
   d. Maintain body heat
   e. Assess the newborn for visible anomalies
   f. Instill silver nitrate or other medication into each eye to prevent ophthalmia neonatorum
   g. Identify mother and baby prior to leaving delivery room by use of prints and application of bands
   h. In Leboyer technique, newborn immersed in warm water bath in room with lights dimmed; mother, father, and newborn spend extra time together

Postpartal period

Puerperium—a 6-week period following delivery in which the reproductive organs undergo physical and physiologic changes, a process called *involution;* because of the many physiologic and psychologic stresses of the postpartum period, there is a current trend to increase this period to 3 months following delivery and call it the fourth trimester of pregnancy

A. Systemic changes during puerperium
1. Reproductive system
   a. Uterus—intermittent contractions bring about involution, after-contractions may cause discomfort necessitating analgesics
   b. Lochia—vaginal flow following delivery, changes from rubra to serosa in 1 week then becomes alba (uterine lining regenerates with new epithelium in 2 or 3 days)
   c. Vagina practically returns to its prepregnant state through a healing of soft tissue and cicatrization
   d. Abdominal wall soft and flabby but eventually regains tone
   e. Breasts
      (1) As placenta is delivered, there is activation of luteinizing hormone in the anterior pituitary—secretion of prolactin also stimulates milk production
      (2) Posterior pituitary secretes pitocin, an oxytocic that initiates the letdown reflex with milk ejection as the baby suckles
      (3) Breast engorgement occurs on second or

third day because of vasodilation prior to lactation

2. Digestive system
   a. Added proteins and calories to replenish those lost with the process of involution
   b. Lactating mother needs added calories and fluids
   c. Roughage and exercise relieve constipation and distention
3. Circulatory system
   a. Blood volume usually back to normal by third week after delivery
   b. Blood fibrinogen levels increase during first week
   c. Increase in leukocytes especially if labor was lengthy
   d. Drop in hemoglobin and red blood count on fourth postpartal day
4. Excretory system
   a. Increased urinary output second to fifth postpartal day
   b. Bladder tone altered during pregnancy—retention with overflow may occur
   c. Activation of lactogenic hormone may result in lactose in urine
   d. Excretion of nitrogen as involution occurs
5. Integumentary system—profuse diaphoresis as wastes are being excreted

B. Nursing care during puerperium—the nurse should
   1. Use aseptic techniques in giving perineal care
   2. Inspect breasts for tissue and nipple breakdown, palpate to rule out growths (teach breast self-examination for continued health), support breasts with well-fitted brassiere
   3. Teach importance of handwashing in caring for self and baby (important for personnel to avoid cross contamination)
   4. Observe vital signs—temperature of 100.4° F (38° C) or above for 2 consecutive days (excluding first 24 hours after delivery) considered sign of beginning puerperal infection—bradycardia is a normal phenomenon following delivery
   5. Palpate fundus for firmness and descent below umbilical level (involution normally follows a 1-finger breadth descent daily, by fifth or sixth day fundus cannot be felt)—a fundus that is boggy indicates poor contractile power of uterus and results in bleeding
   6. Administer oxytocic medication as ordered to promote involution

   a. Ergonovine maleate (Ergotrate Maleate)
   b. Methylergonovine maleate (Methergine)
   c. Maintain the uterus in slightly contracted state that controls bleeding from intrauterine sites and maintains tone, rate, and amplitude of rhythmic contractions required for involution of the uterus
   7. Check lochia for color, amount, odor (foul odor indicates beginning infection); observe suture line for redness, ecchymosis, edema, or gapping
   8. Promote bladder and bowel function
   9. Provide diet high in proteins and calories to restore body tissues
   10. Ambulate early to prevent blood stasis
   11. Observe for postpartal blues that may be caused by a drop in hormonal levels on fourth or fifth day
   12. Meet mother's needs to enable her to meet the baby's needs
   13. Assist mother with self-care and care of baby as need arises
   14. Provide for group discussions on breast-feeding, infant care, etc.

C. Concepts basic to parent-infant relationships
   1. Early and frequent parent-infant contact is essential for survival
   2. Parenting abilities can be fostered and developed
   3. Biologic changes that occur at puberty and during pregnancy influence the development of nurturance
   4. Interaction between mother and child begins from the moment of conception and can be shared with the father
   5. Love for the infant grows as the parent interacts and cares for the infant
   6. As the parent gives to the infant and the infant receives, the parent in turn receives satisfaction from parenting tasks
   7. Any disturbance in the give-and-take cycle sets up frustrations in both the parent and the infant
   8. Parent behavior is learned and frequent parent-infant contact enhances the development of parenting abilities

THE NEWBORN
Family history

A. Chronic illness in mother's or father's family
B. Previous medical-surgical illnesses of mother and father

C. Age and present health status of mother and father
D. History of previous pregnancies
E. Prenatal history
1. Medical supervision during pregnancy
2. Nutrition during pregnancy
3. Course of pregnancy—illnesses, medications taken or treatments required
4. Duration of gestation
5. Course and amount of sedation and anesthesia required
6. Type of delivery and significant events during immediate period following delivery
7. Immediate response of newborn (Apgar score at 1 and 5 minutes following birth)

Parent-child relationships

A. Infant
1. Before birth
   a. First 8 weeks is a period of rapid growth and development for fetus
   b. Any interference with maternal physiology may cause irreparable damage to fetus; no drugs should be taken during this period if possible
   c. Increased maternal hormonal action is necessary for continued implantation of fetus in the uterus
2. Following birth, baby has need for
   a. Contact with one person on a consistent basis
   b. Food, fondling, caressing, rocking, speaking, clothing, bathing, comfort, and protection from environment
B. Mothering and fathering are
1. Based on a biologic inborn desire to reproduce
2. Role concepts that begin with own childhood experiences
3. Primitive emotional relationships
4. Maturing processes
5. Conceptualizations of the physiologic and psychologic processes following infant's birth
6. Fostered by the parent-infant interaction that constantly reinforces gratification as needs are met and security develops
7. Abilities that are learned rather than innate
C. Parent-child relationships are affected by
1. Readiness for pregnancy
   a. Planned or unplanned
   b. Health status prior to pregnancy
   c. Financial status

d. Determinants such as age, cultural backgrounds, number in family unit
e. Political forces
2. Nature of pregnancy
   a. Health status during pregnancy
   b. Preparation for parenthood
   c. Support from family members and members of health team
3. Character of labor and delivery
   a. Length and pattern of labor
   b. Type and amount of analgesia received
   c. Support from family and health team
   d. Anesthesia during delivery
   e. Type of delivery
4. Period immediately after birth
   a. Early parent-infant contact
      (1) Allow mother to touch, fondle, and hold
      (2) Give mother ample time to inspect and begin to identify with baby
      (3) Early give-and-take between parents and infant—rooming-in arrangement
      (4) Supportive nursing care in these beginning relationships
      (5) Identification of beginning disturbed relationships with nursing intervention
   b. Significant phases
      (1) Taking-in phase—mother's needs have to be met before she can meet baby's; behavior—talks about self rather than baby, doesn't seem too interested in baby, doesn't touch infant, cries easily
      (2) Transition phase—characterized by mother starting to take hold, looking at and reaching for baby, touching with fingertips, talking about baby, etc.
      (3) Taking-hold phase—kisses, embraces, gives care to infant, eye contact, uses whole hand to make contact, calls baby by name, etc.

Adaptation to extrauterine life

A. Immediate needs at time of delivery
1. Aspiration of mucus to provide an open airway
2. Evaluation by use of Apgar score 1 and 5 minutes following birth (Table 4-1)
3. Maintenance of body temperature to prevent acidosis
4. Constant observation of physical condition
5. Eye care—prophylactic instillation of silver ni-

Table 4-1. Apgar score chart*

Adaptation	0	1	2
Heart rate	Absent	Slow, below 100	Over 100
Respiratory effort	Absent	Weak cry	Strong cry
Muscle tone	Limp	Some flexion of extremities	Active motion
Reflex irritability	No response	Grimace	Cry
Color	Cyanotic, pale	Body pink, extremities cyanotic	Completely pink

*Scores: 7 to 10, good condition; 3 to 6, moderately depressed; 0 to 2, severely depressed.

trate or other medication in each eye to prevent ophthalmia neonatorum

B. Appraisal of newborn after delivery
1. Skin
   a. Body is normally pink with slight cyanosis of hands and feet for 24 hours (jaundice is abnormal during the first 24 to 48 hours of life)
   b. Check for abrasions, rashes, crackling, and elasticity, which indicates status of tissue hydration; at times, milia (white pinpoint spots over nose caused by retained sebaceous secretions), birthmarks, forceps marks, ecchymosis, or papules are present
2. Respirations are abdominal and irregular, with a rate of 30 to 50 per minute (retractions—depression of sternum—are abnormal)
3. Head and sensory organs
   a. Head and chest circumference nearly equal to the crown-rump length; chest slightly smaller than head
   b. Symmetry of face—as baby cries sides of face move equally
   c. Check head for molding, abrasions, or skin breakdowns; observe for caput succedaneum—edema of soft tissue of the scalp; cephalohematoma—edema of scalp caused by effusion of blood between the bone and periosteum; extend head fully in all directions for adequacy in range of motion
   d. Observe eyes for discharge or irritation, check pupils for reaction to light, equality of eye movements (normally there is some ocular incoordination); check sclera for clarity, jaundice, or hemorrhages
   e. Nose—observe for patency of both nostrils
   f. Mouth—observe gums and hard and soft palates for any openings—mucosa of mouth normally clear (white patches that bleed on rubbing indicate thrush, a monilial infection)
   g. Ears—auricles open; vernix covers tympanic membrane making otoscopic examination useless (ring bell close to ear—baby should stir); both eyes should be same level as ears; upper earlobes normally curved (flatness indicative of kidney anomaly)
4. Chest and abdomen
   a. Chest auscultation—only respiratory sounds should be audible (noisy crackling sounds abnormal); heart rate—regular 120 to 160 per minute (rubbing or unusual sounds abnormal)
   b. Abdomen
      (1) Listen to bowel sounds over abdomen
      (2) Palpate spleen with fingertips under left costal margin—tip should be palpable
      (3) Palpate liver on right side—normally 1 cm below costal margin
      (4) Observe umbilical cord for redness, odor, or discharge
      (5) Palpate femoral pulses gently at inner aspect of groin, which indicates intact circulation to extremities
5. Genitalia
   a. Boy
      (1) Palpate scrotum for testes, at times undescended at birth, which is normal (must descend by puberty or sperm destroyed by high temperature within the abdominal cavity)
      (2) Enlargement of scrotum indicates hydrocele (diagnosis affirmed by transparent appearance of scrotum when flashlight is held close to scrotal sac)
      (3) Observe tip of penis for urinary meatus

(epispadias—meatus on upper surface of penis; hypospadias—meatus on lower surface of penis)
  b. Girl—observe genitalia for labia and vaginal opening; edema of labia and bloody mucoid discharge normal, resulting from transfer of maternal hormones
6. Extremities
  a. Hands and arms—thumbs clenched in fist
    (1) Check for number and variation of fingers
    (2) Check clavicle and scapula while putting arm through normal range of motion (clicking or resistance indicates dislocation or fracture)
    (3) Palpate for fractures (crepitation is indicative)
  b. Feet and legs
    (1) Check toes, pattern and number
    (2) Adduct and abduct feet through range of motion; there should be no resistance or tightness
    (3) Flex both legs onto lower abdomen; there should be no resistance or tightness
    (4) Place both feet on flat surface and bend knees—both knees should be at same height (when unequal, hip dislocation is present)
7. Back—turn baby on abdomen, run finger along vertebral column (any separations or swellings indicative of spina bifida)
8. Anus—patency confirmed with passage of meconium (inability to insert rectal thermometer may be indicative of imperforate anus)
9. Neuromuscular development—check reflexes
  a. Rooting—touch baby's cheek, baby should root for finger
  b. Sucking—place an object close to baby's mouth; baby should make an attempt to suck
  c. Grasp—place fingers in palm of baby's hand and encircle palm with your hand; lift infant off a firm surface, baby will grasp; infant's head will lag as baby is raised
  d. Babinski—run thumb up middle undersurface of infant's foot; toes will separate and flare out
  e. Plantar—run thumb up lateral undersurface of infant's foot and toes will curl downward
  f. Moro—making a loud, sharp noise close to the baby will result in the baby bringing both arms and legs close to the body as if in an embrace (disappears by 4 months of age)

  g. Crawl—when the baby is on a firm surface and turned on the abdomen crawling movements will follow
  h. Step or dance—by supporting the infant under both arms, stepping movements will occur when feet are placed on a firm surface
C. Changes in newborn during the first week of life
  1. Circulatory
    a. Tying of cord at birth brings changes in fetal circulation—closure of foramen ovale and ductus arteriosus and obliteration of umbilical arteries produce an adultlike circulation within 1 hour following birth
    b. Heart rate regular—120 to 180, but variable depending on infant's activity—soft heart murmur common for first month of life
    c. Clotting mechanism poor because of low prothrombin concentration
    d. Liver immature (although large), cannot destroy excessive red cells in newborn, resulting in physiologic jaundice by third day
    e. Hemoglobin level high—14 to 20 g/100 ml of blood
    f. White blood count high—6000 to 22,000
  2. Respiratory—respirations diaphragmatic, irregular, abdominal—30 to 50 per minute, quiet with periods of apnea
  3. Excretory
    a. Kidneys immature—newborn should void during first 24 hours (2 weeks of age voids 20 times daily), albumin and urates (brick red staining on diaper) common during first week because of dehydration
    b. Stools—first stool, black-green and tenacious, called *meconium*, by third day, becomes mixed with light yellow, called *transitional*
  4. Integumentary
    a. Lanugo—fine downy hair growth over entire body
    b. Milia—small, whitish, pinpoint spots over nose caused by retained sebaceous secretions
    c. Mongolian spots—blue-black discolorations on back, buttocks, and sacral region that disappear by first year
  5. Digestive
    a. Has stores of nutrients from intrauterine existence, therefore needs very little nourishment first few days
    b. Roots and sucks when anything is brought to mouth

c. Digests simple carbohydrates, fats, and proteins readily

d. Cardiac sphincter of stomach not well developed, therefore regurgitates if stomach is overfull

e. Needs to be bubbled frequently to get rid of air bubbles in stomach

6. Endocrine
   a. Metabolic—all newborns normally lose 10% of their body weight by first week of life
   b. Hormonal—enlargement of breasts in boys and girls is normal as a result of hormones transmitted to baby by mother

7. Neural
   a. Central nervous system and brain not well developed—infant needs constant supply of oxygen
   b. Breathing, sucking, and crying are early neural activities necessary for the infant's survival

D. Needs of newborn
   1. Air for survival
      a. Suctioning of mucus as needed to maintain an open airway
      b. Positioning—side lying to facilitate drainage of mucus
      c. Observing any signs of air hunger such as cyanosis, flaring of nostrils, noisy respirations, sternal retractions would warrant aspiration and administration of oxygen by inhalation

   2. Warmth, comfort, and protection from the environment
      a. Keep in heated crib until body temperature is stabilized to prevent chilling
      b. Clothing should be loose, soft
      c. Crib should be firm and provide protection
      d. Skin should be kept clean and dry to maintain integrity

   3. Human contact—body contact with another human is paramount for the newborn's survival; ministrations in giving care should be carried out with purpose and awareness of the importance of these early beginning relationships (talking, rocking, singing are an essential part of body contact with a newborn)

   4. Food
      a. Initial weight loss of 10% of birth weight is normal and usually regained by tenth day of life

b. Infant feeding usually delayed immediately after birth because of
   (1) General weakness and danger of aspiration
   (2) Reduced calorie requirement because of inactivity and low heat production of infant

c. Newborn needs to ingest simple proteins, carbohydrates, fats, vitamins, and minerals for continued cell growth

d. Fluid (130 to 200 ml per kilogram or 2 to 3 oz fluid per pound of body weight)

e. Calories (110 to 130 calories per kilogram or 50 to 60 calories per pound of body weight)

f. Protein (2.2 to 2.0 g per kilogram of body weight from birth to 6 months of age; 1.8 g per kilogram of body weight from 6 to 12 months of age)

5. Sleep—since sleep lowers body metabolism, it helps restore energy and assimilate nutriments for growth

Breast-feeding

A. Advantages
   1. Psychologic value of closeness and satisfaction in beginning mother-child relationship
   2. Optimum nutritional value for infant
   3. Economical and readily accessible
   4. Greater immunity to infection
   5. Infant is less likely to be allergic to mother's milk
   6. Develops facial muscles, jaw, and nasal passages of infant, since stronger sucking is necessary
   7. Assists in involution of uterus
   8. Reduces chances of infection because of maternal antibodies present in colostrum and milk

B. Prerequisites
   1. Psychologic readiness of mother is a major factor in successful breast-feeding
   2. Adequate diet must be available prenatally and postnatally to ensure high quality milk
   3. Suitable rest, exercise, and freedom from tension for mother will provide increased satisfaction for both her and the infant
   4. Infant's sucking at breast stimulates the maternal posterior pituitary to produce pitocin whose properties in the blood system constrict the lactiferous sinuses to move the milk down through the nipple ducts—known as the letdown reflex; a poor sucking reflex of the child will inhibit the

letdown of milk; sucking also stimulates prolactin secretion

5. Absence of emotional stress in the mother, since anxiety inhibits the letdown reflex

C. Length of nursing period
   1. Self-demand schedule is desirable
   2. Length of feeding time is usually 20 minutes with greatest quantity of milk consumed in first 5 to 10 minutes

D. Feeding techniques
   1. Mother and infant in comfortable position, such as semireclining or in rocking chair
   2. Initiate feeding by stimulating rooting reflex (stroking cheek toward breast, being careful not to stroke other cheek, since this will confuse infant)
   3. Burp or bubble baby during and after feeding to allow for escape of air by
      a. Placing baby over shoulder
      b. Sitting baby on lap, flexed forward
      c. Rubbing or patting back (avoid jarring baby)
   4. Breast milk intake similar to formula intake
      a. 130 to 200 ml of milk per kilogram (2 to 3 oz of milk per pound) of body weight
      b. From $1/6$ to $1/7$ of baby's weight per day
   5. After lactation has been established, occasional bottle-feeding can be substituted
   6. Length of time for continuing breast-feeding is variable (may be discontinued when teeth erupt, since this can be uncomfortable for mother)

E. Care of breasts
   1. Cleanse with plain water once daily (soap or alcohol can cause irritation and dryness)
   2. Support breasts day and night with properly fitting brassiere
   3. Nursing pads should be placed inside bra cup to absorb any milk leaking between feedings
   4. Plastic bra liners should be avoided because they increase heat and perspiration and decrease air circulation necessary for drying of the nipple area

F. Contraindications
   1. In mother
      a. Active tuberculosis
      b. Acute contagious disease
      c. Chronic disease such as cancer, advanced nephritis, cardiac disease
      d. Extensive surgery
      e. Mastitis (temporary cessation)
      f. Narcotic addiction

   2. In infant—cleft lip or palate or any other condition that interferes or prevents grasp of the nipple is the only real contraindication

Bottle-feeding

A. Advantages
   1. Provides an alternative to breast-feeding
   2. Less restrictive than breast-feeding; may meet needs of working mothers
   3. Allows a more accurate assessment of intake
   4. May be indicated in the presence of a congenital anomaly such as cleft palate
   5. May be necessary for infants who require special formulas due to allergies or inborn errors of metabolism

B. Factors affecting success
   1. Pasteurization of milk
   2. Tuberculin testing of cows
   3. Sanitation in milk handling
   4. Adequate refrigeration and storage
   5. Preparation under clean conditions and sterilization to prevent contamination
   6. Formula designed to match nutrient ratio of breast milk composition: water dilution to reduce protein and mineral concentration; added carbohydrate to increase energy value

C. Types of formulas
   1. Fresh whole or skimmed milk
   2. Evaporated milk
   3. Dried milks (whole or skimmed)
   4. Commercial formulas

D. Preparation for bottle-feeding
   1. Calculation of formula to yield 110 to 130 calories and 130 to 200 ml of fluid per kilogram of body weight
   2. Proper preparation of formula by terminal heat method and feeding utensils (full 25 minutes of boiling)
   3. Proper refrigeration of formula
   4. Warming of formula before feeding by immersing bottle into warm water until approximately equal to body temperature (keep level of water in warmer below cap)

E. Feeding techniques
   1. Always hold infant during feeding to provide warm body contact (bottle propping may contribute to aspiration of formula)
   2. Hold bottle so nipple is always filled with milk to prevent excessive air ingestion

3. Adjust size of nipple hole to needs of baby (a premature infant needs a larger hole that requires less sucking)
4. After feeding and burping infant, place child on abdomen or side to aid digestion and prevent aspiration
5. Feeding should be offered on demand to meet the infant's needs

F. Comparison of breast milk and cow's milk

	Human milk	Cow's milk (whole)
Water	88%	88%
Protein	1.0% to 1.5%	3.5% to 4.0%
Sugar (lactose)	6.5% to 7.5%	4.5% to 5.0%
Fat	3.5% to 4.0%	3.5% to 5.0%
Minerals	0.15% to 0.25%	0.7% to 0.75%
Calories (per fluid ounce)	20	20

Self-regulation schedule

A. Each infant born with different degree of maturity and rhythm of needs
B. Superior to rigid schedule, but should be modified to meet needs of infant and parents
C. Usually fed every 4 hours, with a nighttime feeding for first month, although schedule and amount are highly variable
D. Feeding behavior and degree of satisfaction reflect psychologic development of child
E. Close mother-infant relationship in feeding process meets basic need of trust (Erikson's stage of trust)

DEVIATIONS FROM THE NORMAL MATERNITY CYCLE IN THE MOTHER
Toxemias of pregnancy

Characterized by a triad of symptoms: edema, elevation of blood pressure, and proteinuria

A. Classification (American Committee on Maternal Welfare)
1. Acute toxemia of pregnancy—onset after twenty-fourth week
   a. Preeclampsia—mild, severe
   b. Eclampsia—convulsions and/or coma associated with hypertension, proteinuria, and edema
2. Chronic hypertensive vascular disease with pregnancy
   a. Without superimposed acute toxemia (no exacerbation of hypertension or development of proteinuria occurs)

(1) Hypertension known to have antedated pregnancy
(2) Hypertension discovered in pregnancy (before the twenty-fourth week and with postpartal persistence)
   b. With superimposed acute toxemia
3. Unclassified toxemia (data insufficient to differentiate the diagnosis)

B. Guidelines for prevention of toxemia
1. Sound nutrition counseling during pregnancy and lactation—vitamins and minerals should complement a nutritious, protein-rich diet
2. An additional 30 to 60 mg of supplemental iron daily in the second and third trimester (continue for 2 to 3 months postpartally in breast-feeding mother)
3. Caloric intake should be increased 10% during pregnancy; severe calorie restriction is harmful during pregnancy
4. Restriction of sodium is harmful during pregnancy and can result in electrolyte imbalance and the elimination of essential nutritional components
5. Diuretics are contraindicated during pregnancy, since they cause hypovolemia and deplete essential nutrients for mother and fetus

C. Treatment and nursing care in preeclampsia
1. High-protein diet
2. Ambulatory care—frequent visits to obstetrician
3. Instructions to report headaches, dizziness, blurring of vision, and scotoma
4. Sedatives to ensure rest and sleep
5. Blood chemistry—rise in hematocrit, uric acid, blood urea nitrogen, and decrease in CO_2 combining power indicate worsening of toxemia
6. Qualitative urinalysis—increase in albumin output and/or decrease in urinary output indicates worsening of toxemia
7. Administration of albumin concentrate increases renal flow by correcting the hypovolemia
8. Conserve energy to decrease metabolic rate
9. Assess anxieties and concerns
10. Monitor to protect mother and fetus (includes respiratory rate, pulse, fetal heart rate, weight, intake and output, blood pressure)

D. Treatment and nursing care for eclampsia
1. Hospitalization and complete bed rest
2. Check vital signs, fetal heart, irritability, restlessness, signs of labor

3. When patient is receiving magnesium sulfate therapy, check frequently for depression of patellar reflexes and respirations (these side effects can be treated with the administration of calcium gluconate to the mother and levallorphan [Lorfan] to the newborn if respiratory depression occurs); magnesium sulfate also causes dizziness, diaphoresis, and vomiting

4. Emergency equipment for possible convulsion, equipment to maintain an open airway, suction and oxygen, sedatives such as morphine sulfate and sodium luminal, tracheotomy set readily available on unit

5. Once symptoms are under control, labor may be induced or emergency cesarean section performed

6. Insertion of Foley catheter ensures accurate record of urinary output

7. Limitation of visitors and reduction of environmental stimuli

8. Daily blood chemistry testing

Bleeding during the maternity cycle

Bleeding is an abnormal sign indicating a possible interruption of pregnancy

A. First trimester bleeding
1. Abortion
   a. Interruption of pregnancy in which there is complete expulsion or partial expulsion (incomplete) of the products of conception
   b. May be sudden, spontaneous, or induced by some external mechanical force
   c. Treatment consists of bed rest, immediate blood count, blood typing, Rh incompatibility, and cross matching with availability of blood
   d. Vital signs and observing for signs of labor will indicate course of abortion and treatment
   e. Complete abortion—24 to 48 hours observation for bleeding is imperative
   f. Incomplete abortion—dilation and curettage performed to empty the uterus of retained products of conception; same observation as with complete abortion
2. Ectopic pregnancy
   a. Pregnancy in which implantation occurs outside the uterus (most frequent site is middle portion of fallopian tube, other sites are abdomen, ovaries, or cervix)

b. Early signs and symptoms are usually concealed
c. Pattern in tubal pregnancy is usually one in which spotting may occur after 1 or 2 missed menstrual periods, sharp lower right or left abdominal pain radiating to shoulder develops, concealed bleeding from site of rupture leads to sudden shock
d. Treatment is immediate blood replacement and surgical removal of ruptured fallopian tube

3. Hydatidiform mole
   a. An abnormal pregnancy in which there is a benign growth of the chorion
   b. Spontaneous expulsion usually occurs between the sixteenth and eighteenth weeks of pregnancy
   c. Toxemia symptoms are common
   d. Diagnosis—suspected when uterus is excessively large for period of gestation and fetal parts are not palpable
   e. Treatment—if spontaneous evacuation does not occur, evacuation by delicate curettage or hysterotomy is performed
   f. Dangers include uterine perforation, hemorrhage, and infection
   g. Continued follow-up of serum gonadotropin levels is imperative for 1 year to rule out metastasis from chorionic carcinoma (increased gonadotropin levels warrant immediate hysterectomy)
   h. Preventing a new pregnancy is essential for follow-up

B. Third trimester bleeding
1. Placenta previa
   a. Implantation of the embryo in the lower uterine segment
   b. Three types: marginal (placental edge is close to internal os), partial (placenta partially covers internal os), and central (placenta completely covers internal os)
   c. Painless bleeding in the latter part of pregnancy is only symptom
   d. Treatment is to control bleeding—cesarean section is usually performed
2. Abruptio placentae
   a. Premature separation of a normally implanted placenta
   b. Symptoms—with partially detached placenta

there is external vaginal bleeding; with totally detached placenta, there is concealed bleeding, excruciating abdominal pain, and a board-like abdominal wall

   c. Common in individuals with toxemia, essential hypertension, and an abnormally short umbilical cord

   d. Treatment

     (1) Replacement of blood loss

     (2) With fetal distress—emergency cesarean section

     (3) Without fetal distress and in the presence of some cervical effacement and dilation—induction of labor may be attempted

C. Postpartum hemorrhage

  1. Bleeding in excess of 500 ml within the first 24 hours following delivery

  2. Frequent causes are uterine atony, vaginal and cervical lacerations, and retained placental fragments (bleeding occurring after 24 hours is usually caused by retained placental fragments)

  3. Treatment for atony—massage fundal portion of uterus, administer oxytocics, and, with severe blood loss, blood replacement

  4. Bleeding caused by retained placental fragments necessitates manual removal

  5. Vaginal and cervical lacerations require surgical repair

D. Nursing care of mother with bleeding during maternity cycle—the nurse should

  1. Institute measures to alleviate fear and anxiety

  2. Check vital signs frequently

  3. Observe for signs of labor and imminent delivery

  4. Monitor fetal heart if pregnancy is beyond twentieth week

  5. Explain the need for and maintain parenteral therapy

  6. Maintain asepsis to prevent infection

  7. Consider and provide for patient's spiritual needs

Dystocia (abnormal labor)

A. Dystocia, or difficult labor, may be mechanical (contracted pelvis, obstruction in pelvis, malpresentation or position of the fetus) or functional (caused by faulty uterine contractions)

  1. Treatment for mechanical dystocia is cesarean section

  2. Treatment for functional dystocia is oxytocics to stimulate labor or cesarean section—deciding

factors are length of labor, condition of mother and fetus, amount of cervical effacement and dilation, presentation, position, and station of presenting part

  3. Nursing care of mother in prolonged labor—the nurse should

   a. Observe for signs of maternal exhaustion such as elevation of body temperature, fruity odor to breath, diminished urinary output with positive acetone reaction

   b. Observe for signs of fetal distress

   c. Have oxygen suction and resuscitation equipment readily available

   d. Constantly monitor contractions, fetal heart, and vital signs when patient is receiving oxytocic stimulation

B. Precipitate labor—a rapid labor and delivery of less than 2-hour duration

  1. Hazards to mother are perineal laceration and postpartum hemorrhage

  2. Hazards to baby are anoxia and intracranial hemorrhage

  3. At times, a safe anesthesia may help slow down labor process

C. Labor induction—initiation of labor contractions by medical (oxytocic drugs) or mechanical means (artificial rupture of membranes)

  1. Elective induction may be done for medical or obstetric reasons: medical—diabetes, pyelonephritis; obstetric—toxemia, Rh incompatibility, polyhydramnios, abruptio placentae, premature rupture of membranes at term without onset of labor

  2. Medical methods of induction

   a. Sparteine sulfate (Tocosamine)—75 to 150 mg IM (series given every ½ hour, every hour, or every 2 hours)

   b. Oxytocin (Pitocin)—5 units in 1000 ml of 5% glucose in Ringer's lactate IV at 5 to 10 drops per minute or buccal Pitocin, 200 unit tablets, given in an hourly series

   c. Prostaglandins given orally, intravenously, or vaginally

   d. Breast pumping can be used but is the least effective method

  3. Nursing care of mother undergoing induction of labor—the nurse should

   a. Prepare mother with explanation of treatment

b. Vigilantly time contractions and monitor vital signs and fetal heart

c. Constantly monitor IV flow rate

d. Remain with patient at all times during induction

e. Provide for blood typing, Rh incompatibility, cross matching, and availability of blood

f. Have oxygen, suction, and resuscitation equipment readily available

g. Prepare for emergency cesarean section if necessary

D. Abdominal delivery (cesarean section)—delivery of baby via abdominal incision

1. Indicated in cephalopelvic disproportion, dystocia, placenta previa and abruptio placentae, postmaturity, growths impeding birth canal, diabetes, toxemia, Rh incompatibility, malpresentation, fetal distress

2. Nursing care following cesarean section—the nurse should

a. Encourage early ambulation to prevent blood stasis

b. Check vital signs and fundus

c. Observe abdominal dressing for drainage

d. Encourage eating of solids to promote peristalsis (prevents distention)

e. Record intake and output

f. Give analgesics as ordered

Childbirth injuries

A. Episiotomy is an incision into the perineum to facilitate delivery and prevent lacerations and overstretching of the pelvic floor

1. Routine procedure—closed surgically

2. Nursing care

a. Keep area clean and dry

b. Analgesics as ordered for comfort

c. Heat and local spray medications

d. Perineal exercise

B. Lacerations are tears of the perineum or vulva resulting from a difficult or precipitate delivery—characterized as first, second, third, or fourth degree depending on the amount of involvement

1. Treatment—surgical repair

2. Nursing care—same as above; however, healing is slower following repair of a laceration

C. Relaxations of the vaginal outlet—an overstretching of the perineal supporting tissues resulting from childbirth

1. Cystocele—a herniation of anterior vaginal wall with the descent and protrusion of the bladder

2. Rectocele—a herniation of the pararectal fascia into the vagina

a. Signs and symptoms—backache, feeling of heaviness and bearing down in the lower abdomen, urinary stress incontinence, and constipation

b. Treatment—Kegel's exercises for stress incontinence (after childbearing period is completed, vaginoplasty is done)

c. Nursing care with vaginoplasty consists of keeping perineal area clean and dry with insertion of Foley catheter or suprapubic catheter, warm sitz baths once healing has begun, analgesics for discomfort, antibiotics to prevent infection, high-protein diet to promote tissue repair; ambulation may be delayed to promote healing but leg motion and deep breathing are essential

D. Uterine prolapse—a condition in which the uterus is found in a position lower than normal resulting from stretching and tearing of tissues during childbirth

1. Signs and symptoms—bearing-down sensation and a feeling of a dropping of the pelvic organs, leukorrhea with marked congestion of cervix or lacerations of exposed vaginal walls, frequency with retention, and eventually cystitis

2. Treatment—dependent on age, desire for more children, and severity of symptoms; pessaries may be used as temporary measure; surgical intervention is usually a vaginal hysterectomy

E. Displacement of uterus—results from lesions of the pelvic organs or stretching and relaxation of the ligaments supporting the uterus (may be congenital or result from the trauma of childbirth)

1. Signs and symptoms—backache, excessive bleeding during menstruation, sense of pressure or fullness

2. Treatment—insertion of a pessary to relieve symptoms; severe symptoms warrant surgical intervention

F. Rupture of uterus usually occurs after fetus reaches a viable size

1. Causes—perforation during attempted abortion, rupture of a previous uterine scar, spontaneous rupture of an intact uterus with abdominal overdistention, labor induction

2. Treatment—relieve symptoms of shock from hemorrhage and surgical intervention (the extent

of surgical intervention depends on degree of rupture)

Medical diseases during pregnancy

A. Heart disease—90% of rheumatic origin, 10% congenital lesions or syphilis
   1. Normal hemodynamics of pregnancy that adversely affect the pregnant woman with heart disease
      a. Growing fetus needs increase in oxygen supply
      b. Accelerated heart rate of mother in latter half of pregnancy puts extra workload on her heart
      c. Steady increase in mother's blood volume during the 36 weeks of pregnancy
      d. Rise in cardiac output from the tenth week through the twenty-eighth week of pregnancy
      e. The increase in oxygen consumption with contractions during labor makes length of labor a significant factor
      f. The sudden tachycardia during delivery or the sudden bradycardia and the normal increase in cardiac output following delivery may cause cardiac arrest
   2. Review functional and therapeutic classification of heart disease in a medical-surgical nursing text
   3. Management of mother with heart disease during pregnancy
      a. Extra rest and protection from infection
      b. Medical supervision by cardiologist
      c. Obstetric supervision by obstetrician
      d. Low-sodium, high-protein diet
      e. Immediate reporting of fatigue, dyspnea, hemoptysis, or edema
      f. Hospitalization for any cardiac embarrassment
      g. Minimal analgesia and anesthesia during labor and delivery
      h. Forceps should be used to limit pushing efforts of mother, since this increases cardiac workload
      i. Scopolamine is contraindicated, since it is a vasodilator that will affect hemodynamics
      j. Oxytocics are administered cautiously if needed in IV solutions
      k. Observation of vital signs during labor, delivery, and immediately following delivery
      l. Prophylactic antibiotics are administered to prevent infection
      m. Digitalis and diuretic therapy are instituted to prevent heart failure and pulmonary edema
      n. Longer hospital stay to provide continued health supervision
   4. Nursing care of the mother with heart disease
      a. Prenatal—health teaching, rest and diet counseling, referral to community agencies for family care, avoidance of stress, preparation for the stress of labor and delivery, teaching importance of preventing infection
      b. Intrapartal—early admission prior to start of labor, vital signs, observation for signs of heart failure and pulmonary edema, maintenance of Fowler's position, availability of oxygen, added support during labor, delivery in bed if necessary
      c. Postpartal—observation for respiratory distress, since there is an increase in cardiac output with tachycardia, monitoring of vital signs, rest and sedation to decrease heart action, referral to various agencies for family aid on discharge

B. Diabetes mellitus
   1. Normal physiology of pregnancy that affects the pregnant woman with diabetes
      a. Vomiting during pregnancy, especially in first trimester, decreases carbohydrate intake with resulting acidosis
      b. Increased activity of anterior pituitary decreases the tolerance for sugar
      c. Elevated basal metabolic rate and decrease in CO_2 combining power increase tendency toward acidosis
      d. Normal lowered renal threshold for glucose can result in glucosuria that might confuse diabetic picture
      e. Muscular activity during labor depletes glycogen; therefore carbohydrate intake must be increased
      f. During puerperium, hypoglycemia is common as involution and lactation occur
   2. Hazards of diabetes during pregnancy
      a. Often there is a history of repeated stillbirths and fetal deaths
      b. Babies are excessively large, weighing over 4000 g
      c. Neonatal deaths occur as a result of hypoxia, hypoglycemia, congenital anomalies, and premature labor
      d. Toxemia and hydramnios are common
   3. Nursing care of the mother with diabetes
      a. Early medical and prenatal supervision

    b. Prevention of acidosis

    c. Effective dietary regimen

    d. Awareness of signs and symptoms of acidosis and hypoglycemia

    e. Teaching hygiene and avoidance of stress

    f. Referral to public health nurse for continuity in care

    g. Identification card on person

  4. Nursing care of baby of a diabetic mother

    a. Keep infant warm because of poor temperature control mechanisms

    b. Observe respiration (stomach aspiration imperative at time of delivery, since hydramnios inflates stomach, which pushes up and interferes with diaphragm)

    c. Observe for signs of hypoglycemia such as lethargy, poor sucking reflex, cyanosis, or muscular twitching

    d. Provide glucose water feeding to prevent acidosis (with poor sucking reflex, glucose should be given parenterally)

C. Acute and chronic pyelonephritis

  1. Acute pyelonephritis is a diffuse inflammatory process of interstitial connective tissue of kidney (nephron involved when infection is extreme)

  2. Most common organism is *Escherichia coli;* occasionally *Staphylococcus* and *Streptococcus* organisms

  3. Signs and symptoms are chills, fever, severe backache, tenderness over kidney region, rise in nonprotein nitrogen, decrease in phenolsulfonphthalein excretion and dye excretion on pyelography

  4. Nursing care of mother with pyelonephritis

    a. Adequate diet and rest

    b. Force fluids

    c. Sulfonamides and antibiotics

    d. Intake and output monitoring

    e. Sims' position to relieve pressure on uterus

    f. Teaching importance of health supervision and follow-up care after delivery

    g. Family planning avoids risk of early recurrence of pregnancy

DEVIATIONS FROM THE NORMAL MATERNITY CYCLE IN THE NEWBORN
Neonatal respiratory distress

A. Asphyxia neonatorum occurs when respirations are not well established within 60 seconds after birth as a result of anoxia, cerebral damage, or narcosis

  1. Prevention—early prenatal care, prenatal education, early management of deviations from the normal pregnancy, adequate medical management during labor and delivery

  2. Signs and symptoms—asphyxia livida: persistent generalized cyanosis, good muscle tone; asphyxia pallida: marked pallor, poor muscle tone

  3. Treatment—after initial resuscitation keep baby under very close observation for first 24 hours, keep equipment for intubation and oxygen administration readily available

B. Atelectasis—an incomplete expansion of the lung or a partial or total collapse of the lung following initial expansion; common in prematurity, oversedation, damage to the respiratory center, or results from inhalation of mucus or amniotic fluid

  1. Signs and symptoms—cyanosis, rapid irregular respirations, flaring of the nostrils, intercostal or suprasternal retraction, grunting on expiration

  2. Treatment—maintain an open airway, administer oxygen with high humidity, stimulate respirations by frequently changing baby's position, administer antibiotics as ordered to prevent infection

C. Hyaline membrane disease—a condition in which a deficiency in surface-active (detergent-like) lipoproteins results in inadequate lung inflation and ventilation; common following cesarean section and in low birth weight infants

  1. Symptoms—cyanosis, dyspnea, and sternal retraction

  2. Treatment—keep airway patent, keep in Isolette with oxygen and high humidity, administer antibiotics as ordered

Birth injuries

A. Caput succedaneum—edema with extravasation of serum into scalp tissues caused by molding during the birth process; no treatment is necessary since it subsides in a few days

B. Cephalohematoma—edema of the scalp with effusion of blood between the bone and periosteum; reabsorption usually occurs in a few days

C. Intracranial hemorrhage—bleeding into cerebellum, pons, and medulla oblongata caused by a tearing of the tentorium cerebelli; occurs following prolonged labor, difficult forceps delivery, precipitate delivery, version or breech extraction

  1. Symptoms—abnormal respirations; cyanosis; sharp, shrill, or weak cry; flaccidity or spasticity;

restlessness; wakefulness; convulsions; poor sucking reflex

2. Treatment—keep in Isolette with oxygen, humidity, and minimal handling; place in high Fowler's position, administer vitamins C and K to control and prevent further hemorrhage; with impaired sucking reflex, gavage feeding is necessary; support of parents is vital because of guarded prognosis

D. Facial paralysis—asymmetry of face caused by damage to facial nerves from a difficult forceps delivery; temporary paralysis disappears in a few days

E. Erb-Duchenne paralysis (brachial palsy)—caused by a difficult forceps or breech extraction delivery; treatment depends on severity of paralysis; massage and exercise prevent contractures; when severe, splints and casts are applied

F. Dislocations and fractures are diagnosed by crepitation, immobility, and variations in range of motion; treatment depends on the site of fracture; therefore swaddling, positioning, splints, slings, or casts may be used; referral to a public health agency ensures continuity of care; if necessary, refer to community agencies

Infections

A. Thrush is a mouth infection caused by *Candida albicans;* it may be transmitted as the baby passes through the mother's vaginal canal, by unclean feeding utensils, or improper handwashing techniques by staff or mother
1. Symptoms are white patches on tongue, palate, and inner cheek surfaces that bleed on examination, and difficulty with sucking
2. Treatment—oral administration of nystatin (Mycostatin), application of 1% gentian violet, isolation of baby and equipment to prevent cross contamination

B. Impetigo is an infectious skin eruption characterized by vesicles or pustules caused by *Staphylococcus* or *Streptococcus* organisms; treatment consists of isolating infant, pHisoHex baths daily, breaking pustules with alcohol wipe, local application of gentian violet, neomycin, or bacitracin, and administration of antibiotics

C. Ophthalmia neonatorum is an eye infection caused by the *Neisseria gonorrhoeae* transmitted from the genital tract during delivery or by infected hands of personnel; prophylactic eye care is administered to all infants at birth; treatment for the eye infection consists of prompt antibiotic therapy to prevent eye damage; isolation of the infant, sterilization of all equipment, and strict handwashing are imperative

D. *Staphylococcus* infection—prevented by reduction of transient personnel in nurseries, adequate crib spacing, and medical asepsis

E. Epidemic diarrhea is caused by *Escherichia coli;* organism in stool characterized by forceful, watery, yellow-green stool; dry skin; rapid weight loss and acidosis; treatment—oral antibiotics, replacement of fluids parenterally, isolation to prevent cross contamination

F. Syphilis—a spirochetal infection characterized by maculopapular lesions of the palms of the hands and soles of the feet, restlessness, rhinitis, hoarse cry, enlargement of the spleen and palpable lymph nodes, enlarged ends of long bones on x-ray examination; penicillin is a specific treatment for syphilis with a 1- to 2-year follow-up
1. Prenatal syphilis is transmitted to fetus by the mother
2. Incidence of fetal infection varies with stage of the disease in the mother at the time of pregnancy
3. Fetus is seldom infected prior to fourth month of pregnancy; Langhan's cells in chorion are protective barrier
4. Pregnant women treated immediately with penicillin (prior to fourth month, fetus not infected; after fourth month of pregnancy the longer the infection goes untreated, the greater the damage to the fetus)

Congenital abnormalities

Defects present at birth are structural or metabolic (birth injuries are not included); they may be genetically determined or a result of environmental interference during intrauterine life (see Pediatrics for congenital abnormalities)

Hemolytic disease

Hemolytic disease—an ABO or Rh incompatibility in which there is a destruction of red cells and resulting anemia; caused by a transfer of incompatible blood from the fetal to the maternal circulation with antibody formation in mother; the antibodies are then transferred through the placental barrier to the fetus with a resulting agglutination and destruction of red cells

A. Symptoms are jaundice within the first 24 hours of birth, anemia, enlargement of the liver and spleen, lethargy, poor feeding pattern, vomiting, tremors and convulsions indicative of kernicterus (signs of kernicterus are absence of Moro reflex, severe lethargy, apnea, high-pitched cry, and assuming an opisthotonos position)

B. Treatment—during pregnancy amniotic fluid determinations are done by chemical and spectrophotometric analysis; elevated readings warrant either intrauterine transfusion or induction of labor depending on the weeks of gestation; following delivery exchange transfusion is done on the infant to decrease the antibody level and increase red blood cells and hemoglobin levels

C. Prevention—RhoGAM, a preparation of Rh_0 (D antigen) immune globulin is now given intramuscularly to the mother 72 hours after delivery or after abortion to prevent erythroblastosis fetalis in future pregnancies; mother must be negative for Rh antibodies to receive RhoGAM

Drug dependence

A. Definition—infant born with physiologic dependence on drugs as a result of maternal drug use and/or abuse

B. Source—many preparations including
  1. Alcohol
  2. Morphine derivatives
  3. Synthetic opiates
  4. Methadone

C. Perinatal mortality—6 to 8 times higher than in normal control group

D. Withdrawal symptoms—appear soon after birth, depending on the length of maternal addiction, amount of drug taken, and time taken prior to birth
  1. Jittery
  2. Hyperactive
  3. Shrill and persistent cry
  4. Frequent yawning and sneezing
  5. Tendon reflexes increased
  6. Moro reflex decreased
  7. If untreated, may develop fever, vomiting, diarrhea, dehydration, apnea, convulsions; death may result

E. Treatment—sedation and weaning from drugs

F. Nursing interventions
  1. Careful monitoring of infant
  2. Administering supportive care to prevent injury
  3. Promoting mother-infant attachment
  4. Assessing for long-term intervention

G. Fetal alcohol syndrome—may produce congenital defects and retardation

Low birth weight infant

A. Prevention
  1. Education of teenagers (prior to planning a family) in nutrition and general hygiene
  2. Education of teenagers to the hazards of drug use and smoking
  3. Adequate and early prenatal health supervision
  4. Provisions for adequate housing and financial aid to persons of lower socioeconomic means
  5. Adequate community agencies to facilitate available services to persons in need
  6. Higher prematurity rates and low birth weight babies are frequently associated with malnutrition and underweight in the mother

B. Definitions
  1. Classification of newborn infants is now made on the basis of gestational age as well as birth weight
  2. An infant born at term (37 weeks or over) is called full size; an infant born before term (36 weeks or less) is called premature
  3. A low birth weight infant is one who weighs 2500 g (5½ pounds) or less
  4. A full-term infant may be a low birth weight infant; a premature infant need not be a low birth weight infant

C. Management of mother in premature labor (before thirty-seventh week of pregnancy)
  1. Preanesthetic medications should be minimal to prevent depression of the fetus (barbiturates and opiates are especially contraindicated, since they depress respirations, depleting oxygen to the fetus)
  2. Regional anesthesias are safer than general anesthesias
  3. Added support to the mother, since she is concerned with the baby's welfare
  4. Adequate preparation for the infant at birth; a heated Isolette and equipment for aspiration and resuscitation should be available
  5. The pediatrician should be present at the time of delivery to care for the infant

D. Management of the low birth weight infant immediately following delivery
  1. Aspiration of mucus to maintain an open airway is vital
  2. Absence of respirations necessitates direct laryn-

goscopy, tracheal aspiration, intubation, and mouth-to-tube insufflation

3. Maintenance of body temperature is difficult because of heat loss by skin evaporation; heated Isolette is needed

4. Aspiration of stomach contents at birth facilitates respirations and is often indicated for the low birth weight infant

5. Infant should be moved to the nursery in the heated unit with oxygen and resuscitation equipment available

E. Differences in premature and full-size newborn

1. Premature infant has less subcutaneous fat, therefore the skin is wrinkled, blood vessels and bony structures are visible, lanugo present on face, eyebrows are absent, and ears are poorly supported by cartilage

2. The circumference of the head of the premature infant is quite large in comparison with the chest; the fontanels are small and bones are soft

3. Skin color changes when premature infant is moved; upper half of body pale and lower half red, known as harlequin color change

4. The premature infant's posture is one of complete relaxation with marked flexion and abduction of the thighs; random movements are common with slightest stimulus

5. Heat regulation poorly developed in the premature infant because of poor development of central nervous system; heat loss caused by large skin surface area; poorly developed respiratory center with diminished oxygen combustion causing asphyxia; weak heart action, therefore slower circulation and poor oxygenation; insufficient heat production caused by inadequate metabolism

6. Respirations are not efficient in the premature infant because of muscular weakness of lung and rib cage; retraction at xiphoid is evidence of air hunger; infant should be stimulated if apnea occurs

7. Greater tendency toward capillary fragility and intracranial hemorrhage in the premature infant; red and white blood cell counts are low with resulting anemia during first few months of life

8. Nutrition is difficult to maintain in the premature infant because of weak sucking and swallowing reflexes, small capacity of stomach, low gastric acidity, and slow emptying time of the stomach; the usual caloric intake of 110 to 130 calories per kilogram (50 to 60 calories per pound) of body weight may need to be increased to 200 to 220 calories per kilogram (100 calories per pound) for adequate growth and development

F. Nursing care of low birth weight and premature infants

1. Observe for changes in respirations, color, and vital signs

2. Check efficacy of Isolette—heat, humidity, and oxygen concentration

3. Maintain aseptic technique to prevent infection

4. Adhere to the techniques of gavage feeding for safety of infant

5. Determine blood gases frequently to prevent acidosis

6. Institute phototherapy should hyperbilirubinemia occur

7. Support parents by letting them verbalize and ask questions to relieve anxiety

8. Arrange follow-up before and after discharge by a visiting nurse

9. Provide flexible and liberal visiting hours for parents as soon as possible

10. Allow parents to do as much as possible for the infant after appropriate teaching

INFERTILITY AND STERILITY
Definitions

A. Sterility—the presence of an absolute factor that makes a person unable to produce offspring

B. Infertility—the inability on the part of a couple to reproduce after consistent attempts for a 1-year period

Male infertility and sterility

A. Coital difficulties—chordee or marked obesity

B. Spermatozoal abnormalities—small ejaculatory volume, low sperm count, increased viscosity, reduced mobility of spermatozoa and/or more than 30% abnormal sperm forms

C. Testicular abnormalities—agenesis or degenesis of testes, cryptorchidism, poor maturation of the spermatozoa, physical injury due to trauma, irradiation, or increased temperature for prolonged periods

D. Abnormalities of the penis or urethra—hypospadias or urethral stricture

E. Prostate and seminal vesicle abnormalities—chronic prostatitis or seminal vesiculitis

F. Abnormalities of the epididymis and vas deferens—inflammation or closure

G. Severe nutritional deficiencies

H. Emotional factors

Female infertility and sterility

A. Endocrine disorders—pituitary, thyroid, or adrenal

B. Vaginal disorders—absence or stenosis of vagina, imperforate hymen, vaginitis

C. Cervical abnormalities—cervicitis, obstruction by cervical polyps or tumors

D. Uterine abnormalities—hypoplasia, uterine neoplasms

E. Tubal disorders—obstruction (generally result of infection), perisalpingeal adhesions

F. Ovarian abnormalities—congenital abnormalities such as ovarian dysgenesis or agenesis, infections, tumors

G. Emotional problems—severe psychoneurosis or psychosis may cause anovulatory cycles

H. Coital factors—feminine hygiene preparation (including douches) that increase vaginal acidity may inactivate or destroy spermatozoa

I. Chronic disease states

J. Immunologic reactions to sperm

K. Nutritional factors such as a seriously faulty diet

Diagnostic measures

A. Male—history, physical examination, semen analysis

B. Female—history, physical examination, CBC, sedimentation rate, serologic tests, urinalysis, serum protein-bound iodine, x-ray films of the chest, basal metabolic rate determination, Sims or Huhner tests, endometrial biopsy, tubal insufflation, hysterosalpingography, culdoscopy

Treatment

Depends on causative factor

Nursing care

A. Apply principles of human relations and psychology

B. Listen to and discuss couple's particular problems, giving necessary support

C. Explain diagnostic procedure to alleviate anxiety and fear

D. Refer to visiting nurse service for continuity in care

Drugs that affect gonadal function and fertility

A. Androgens are used to replace deficient hormones in males after puberty and before the climacteric to improve development of secondary sex characteristics or as single-incident therapy controlling lactogenic activity in the nonnursing mother
   1. Drugs
      a. Fluoxymesterone (Halotestin, Ora-Testryl, Ultandren)
      b. Methyltestosterone (Metandren, Neo-Hombreol-M, Oreton-M)
      c. Testosterone (Androlan, Andronaq, Hormale Aqueous, Malogen, Neo-Hombreol-F, Oreton, Sterotate)
      d. Testosterone cypionate (Depo-Testosterone, Durandro, Malogen CYP, T-Ionate-P.A.)
      e. Testosterone enanthate (Delatestryl, Malogen LA, Repo-Test, Testate, Testostroval-P.A.)
      f. Testosterone propionate (Hormale Oil, Neo-Hombreol, Oreton Propionate, Testonate)
   2. Adverse effects—adolescent males may have premature epiphyseal closure (decreased skeletal development, height stops increasing)

B. Estrogens primarily used to replace deficient hormones to control hormonal balance in menopausal or postmenopausal women or to maintain menses and fertility in females during reproductive years
   1. Drugs
      a. Chlorotrianisene (Tace)
      b. Conjugated estrogens (Conestron, Conjutab, Equgen, Menotabs, Premarin, Theogen)
      c. Dienestrol (DV, Synestrol)
      d. Esterified estrogens (Amnestrogen, Estrifol, Evex, Femogen, Glyestrin, Menest, SK-Estrogens, Trocosone, Zeste)
      e. Estradiol (Aquadiol, Progynon)
      f. Estrone (Estrusol, Menformon [A], Theelin, Wynestron)
      g. Ethinyl estradiol (Estinyl, Feminone, Lynoral, Palonyl)
      h. Hexestrol
      i. Methallenestril (Vallestril)
      j. Promethestrol dipropionate (Meprane Dipropionate)
   2. Adverse effects—anorexia, nausea, vomiting, tissue fluid accumulation

C. Conception enhancers
   1. Menotropins (Pergonal) stimulates growth and maturation of ovarian follicles in women with deficient ovum production by creating an effect on ovarian follicles comparable to that of natural FSH and LH

2. Chorionic gonadotropin (A.P.L., Almetropin, Antuitrin-S, Chorex, Chorigon, Follutein, Glucotropin-Forte, Khorion, Libigen, Luton, Pregnyl, Riogon, Stemultrolin)

   a. Administered concurrently to support LH effect on ovulation when follicle maturation has occurred

   b. Adverse effects—20% of patients have multiple births

3. Clomiphene citrate (Clomid)

   a. Used during the fifth to the tenth day of the menstrual cycle to stimulate release of FSH and LH in anovulatory women

   b. Adverse effects—multiple births, visual changes, dizziness, light-headedness

FAMILY PLANNING
Goals

A. Maintain optimum emotional and physical health of the family

B. Involve both partners in planning family size

C. Inform parents of available methods of birth control and give them the freedom of choice

Contraceptive methods

A. Oral contraceptives—combined progestins and estrogens, which suppress ovulation, when taken as prescribed

1. Fixed combination program provides the estrogen component of the combination tablet to suppress secretion of FSH, and the progestogen inhibits midcycle release of LH from the pituitary when tablets are taken from the fifth to the twenty-fifth day and a placebo tablet is taken the remaining 7 days

   a. Ethinyl estradiol–ethynodiol diacetate (Demulen)

   b. Ethinyl estradiol–norethindrone acetate (Norlestrin)

   c. Ethinyl estradiol–norgestrel (Ovral)

   d. Mestranol–ethynodiol diacetate (Ovulen)

   e. Mestranol-norethindrone (Norinyl, Ortho-Novum)

   f. Mestranol-norethynodrel (Enovid)

2. Adverse effects—thrombophlebitis; during the first 4 months—headache, nausea, vomiting, breast fullness, depression, fatigue, brownish facial pigmentation, fluid retention, intermenstrual spotting, increased susceptibility to vaginal infection

B. Intrauterine devices (IUD)—mechanical devices inserted into isthmus of uterus; prevent pregnancy by increasing tubal motility so that ovum gets to uterus before lining is optimum for implantation; not as effective as oral contraceptives, since pregnancy may occur with device in place

C. Diaphragms—mechanical devices that fit over cervix and prevent sperm from entering cervical os

D. Condoms—rubber sheaths that cover penis and prevent semen from entering cervical os

E. Creams, jellies, foam tablets, and vaginal suppositories—spermicidal (generally low pH) preparations inserted into vaginal canal by applicator immediately prior to coitus (used in conjunction with the diaphragm and condom for added protection)

F. Coitus interruptus—the withdrawal of the penis during sexual intercourse prior to ejaculation; least effective method

G. Rhythm—the plotting of the basal body temperature to determine fertile period, with abstinence from coitus during that time

Sterilization

A. Male—accomplished by surgical severance and suturing of the vas deferens, preventing ejaculation of sperm (vasectomy); following vasectomy sperm are still produced; however, after 3 azoospermic specimens, sterility is achieved

B. Female—accomplished by abdominal laparotomy, laparoscopy, or culdoscopy; the fallopian tubes are severed and tied so there is no way the mature ovum can be impregnated by a mature sperm

Nursing implications

A. Method of contraception used should be acceptable to couple, since acceptability increases effectiveness

B. Ideal contraceptive is one that is completely safe, free of side effects, reversible, easily obtainable, and inexpensive

C. Periodic physical examination of all women using oral or mechanical devices should include pelvic examination and Pap smear

D. Discussion groups help couples expand their knowledge related to the anatomy and physiology of the reproductive systems

E. Assess couples individually and together prior to sterilization, since consideration of the physiologic and psychologic reactions to such procedures is vital

ABORTION
Methods of induced abortion

A. Vacuum aspiration—done under local paracervical, epidural, or general anesthesia in the first 12 weeks of pregnancy; the cervix is dilated and the products of conception are suctioned by a small hollow tube; the uterus is then curettaged to remove all fetal tissue
B. Dilation and curettage is performed during the first 12 to 14 weeks of pregnancy under local paracervical or general anesthesia; the cervix is dilated and uterus is curettaged
C. Saline injection—labor is induced when a pregnancy is 14 to 24 weeks in duration by injecting a sterile saline solution into the uterus by amniocentesis; labor usually begins within 20 to 36 hours after instillation of saline; produces a macerated fetus
D. Hysterotomy—performed after 16 weeks of pregnancy by surgically removing the fetus and placenta abdominally
E. Estrogen in high dosage after ovulation disrupts the estrogen-progesterone balance that usually maintains the dense endometrial nutrient bed for fertilized ova
F. Dinoprost tromethamine (Prostin F$_2$ Alpha)
  1. Action—used during second trimester to trigger vasoconstriction and uterine contractions that interfere with endocrine function of placenta
  2. Adverse effects—nausea, vomiting, diarrhea, pain at extrauterine sites, allergic reactions (not administered to patients with history of asthma)

Nursing considerations

A. Be aware of own feelings about abortion—essential if nurse is to therapeutically intervene with women having abortions
B. Nurse needs to encourage patient's expression of frustration, fear, and anger
C. Nurse needs to be objective and support the woman's decision about abortion
D. Complete history and physical examination, complete laboratory work-up, pelvic examination and Pap test, and a pregnancy test are essential for safe care prior to induced abortion
E. Postabortion counseling in contraceptive methods should be available
F. If prone to Rh sensitization, RhoGAM is given when patient's blood is negative for antibodies

Prerequisites for abortion facility (recommended by the College of Obstetricians and Gynecologists)

A. Verification of the diagnosis and duration of pregnancy
B. Preoperative instructions and counseling
C. Recorded preoperative history and physical examination
D. Laboratory procedures usually required for hospitalization, such as blood typing and Rh factor
E. Prevention of Rh sensitization
F. A receiving facility where client is prepared and may receive necessary preoperative medication and be observed prior to treatment
G. A recovery facility for care and observation following surgery, with a qualified anesthetist in attendance
H. Postoperative instructions and follow-up, including family planning
I. Adequate permanent records

GRIEF RESPONSES IN PREGNANCY
Causative factors

A. Spontaneous abortion
B. Elective abortion
C. Ectopic pregnancy
D. Antenatal fetal death
E. Removal of hydatidiform mole
F. Stillborn
G. Neonatal death

Emotional responses

A. Guilt
B. Loss of self-esteem
C. Denial
D. Anger

Nursing intervention

A. Assist parents in ventilating their feelings of guilt and/or self-shame
B. Assist parents in verbalizing their feelings about dead fetus or infant
C. Support parents if they want to see and/or hold dead infant
D. Assess support system and refer for assistance as required

MENOPAUSE

A period in a woman's life when there is gradual cessation of ovarian function and menstrual cycles

Physiologic changes

A. Ovary loses ability to respond to gonadotropic hormones
B. Dramatic decrease in levels of circulating estrogens and progesterone, since the ovary has run out of follicles
C. Increase in gonadotropin level in blood, since production is no longer inhibited (negative feedback) by ovaries; false positive pregnancy test may occur

Symptoms

A. Somatic—atrophic changes in reproductive organs resulting in dyspareunia, weight gain, facial hair growth, cardiac palpitations, hot flashes, profuse diaphoresis, constipation, pruritus, faintness
B. Psychic—headache, irritability, anxiety over loss of reproductive function, sexual feelings, and feelings of womanliness

Treatment

A. Support system to deal with stress
B. For dyspareunia—vaginal estrogen creams
C. Tranquilizers and phenobarbital if necessary
D. Hormonal therapy only if absolutely necessary and when no history of malignancy is present

Nursing care

A. Prepare women for the changes that may occur with menopause
B. Let women ventilate feelings
C. Refer for medical supervision

AGENCIES PROVIDING PARENT-CHILD HEALTH SERVICES
Government

A. World Health Organization—founded in 1948 by United Nations; 100 or more countries exchange knowledge and collaborate on elevating level of health throughout the world
B. Children's Bureau—founded in 1972 under Department of Health, Education and Welfare; its purpose is to improve services for maintenance of health in mothers and children through research, care, and teaching
C. Department of Family and Children's Services (HHS)—federal monies for food, shelter, and medical services for dependent children
D. Women's Bureau—under Department of Labor, provides supervision of places of employment for pregnant women
E. National Institutes of Health—monies provided for research on child health and human development

Private organizations

A. La Leche League—international, organized in 1956 by mothers interested in fostering breast-feeding
B. International Childbirth Education Association—federation of groups and individuals interested in fostering family-centered maternity and infant care, and to create an interest in education for childbirth
C. American Society for Psychoprophylaxis in Obstetrics (A.S.P.O.)—responsible for teaching Lamaze method in preparation for childbirth

MATERNITY NURSING REVIEW QUESTIONS

Situation: Mrs. Donira is a 29-year-old patient with a history of 3 spontaneous abortions. Questions 1 through 7 refer to this situation.

1 Mrs. Donira is being followed in the high-risk clinic and has expressed anxiety about remaining at home during this pregnancy. The nurse would question Mrs. Donira to determine her knowledge of the:
   1. Signs and symptoms of impending labor
   2. Causes of spontaneous abortion
   3. Mechanisms of early labor
   4. Interrelationship between rest, normal delivery, and diet

2 Mrs. Donira complains of heartburn. When counseling her, the nurse explains that during pregnancy:
   1. The pyloric sphincter relaxes and acid is regurgitated
   2. The cardiac sphincter relaxes and acid is regurgitated
   3. Gastric acidity and motility are increased
   4. There is increased gastric motility, which causes acid to be regurgitated

3 When involved in prenatal teaching, the nurse should also inform the patient that an increase in vaginal secretions during pregnancy is called leukorrhea and is caused by increased:
   1. Metabolic rate
   2. Functioning of the Bartholin glands

3. Production of estrogen
4. Supply of sodium chloride to the cells of the vagina

4 Mrs. Donira is trying to decide if she should breast-feed or bottle-feed her expected baby. She asks the nurse what advantage breast-feeding has over bottle-feeding. The nurse replies that one major group of substances in human milk that are of special importance to the newborn and cannot be reproduced in any bottle formula is:
1. Gamma globulins
2. Complex carbohydrates
3. Amino acids
4. Essential ions (electrolytes)

5 During labor Mrs. Donira receives continuous caudal anesthesia. When Mrs. Donira has a sudden episode of severe nausea and her skin becomes pale and clammy, the nurse's immediate reaction is to:
1. Notify the physician
2. Elevate the patient's legs
3. Monitor the fetal heart rate every 3 minutes
4. Check for vaginal bleeding

6 During delivery the physician performs an episiotomy. The nurse explains to Mrs. Donira that this is most commonly done to:
1. Prevent lacerations during birth
2. Limit postpartal discomfort
3. Stretch the perineum
4. Reduce trauma to the fetus

7 Mrs. Donira delivers a normal baby boy. When assessing the newborn's respiratory status, the nurse would expect respirations to be:
1. Shallow and thoracic
2. Deep and retracting
3. Abdominal and irregular
4. Stertorous and regular

---

8 The outermost membrane that helps form the placenta is the:
1. Amnion
2. Yolk sac
3. Chorion
4. Allantois

9 Progesterone is secreted in relatively large quantities by which of the following structures?
1. Corpus luteum
2. Adrenal cortex
3. Endometrium
4. Pituitary gland

10 The developing cells are called a fetus from the:
1. End of the second week to the onset of labor
2. Implantation of the fertilized ovum
3. Time the fetal heart is heard
4. Eighth week to the time of birth

11 The ischial spines are designated as an important land-mark in labor and delivery because the distance between the spines is:
1. A measurement of the floor of the pelvis
2. A measurement of the inlet of the birth canal
3. The widest measurement of the pelvis
4. The narrowest diameter of the pelvis

12 Which of the following is *not* characteristic of prodromal labor?
1. Intensification of uterine contractions with walking
2. Failure of presenting part to descend
3. Lack of cervical effacement or dilation
4. Cessation of uterine contractions with walking

13 During pregnancy the volume of tidal air increases because there is:
1. Increased expansion of the lower ribs
2. A relative increase in the height of the rib cage
3. Upward displacement of the diaphragm
4. An increase in total blood volume

Situation: Mrs. Greene, a 22-year-old primigravida, is attending prenatal clinic. She has missed 2 menstrual periods. She relates that the first day of her last menstrual period was July 22. Questions 14 through 19 refer to this situation.

14 Mrs. Greene's estimated date of confinement would be:
1. May 5
2. April 29
3. April 15
4. May 14

15 As the nurse prepares Mrs. Greene for the pelvic examination, she complains of feeling very tired and sick to her stomach, especially in the morning. The best response for the nurse to make is:
1. "This is common during the early part of pregnancy. There is no need to worry."
2. "This is a common occurrence during the early part of pregnancy because of all the changes going on in your body."
3. "These are common occurrences during pregnancy with all the body changes; can you tell me how you feel in the morning?"
4. "Perhaps you might ask the doctor when he arrives."

16 Mrs. Greene works as a secretary in a large office. Her job has implications for her plan of care during pregnancy. The nurse would most likely recommend that Mrs. Greene:
1. Ask for a break in the morning and afternoon so she can elevate her legs
2. Inform her employer that she cannot work beyond the second trimester
3. Ask for a break in the morning and afternoon for added nourishment
4. Try to walk about every few hours of her work day

17 The physician performs a pelvic examination and dis-

covers that Mrs. Greene has a normal female pelvis with
sacrum:
1. Well hollowed, coccyx movable, spines not prominent, pubic arch wide
2. Flat, coccyx movable, spines prominent, pubic arch
   wide
3. Deeply hollowed, coccyx immovable, pubic arch narrow, spines not prominent
4. Flat, coccyx movable, spines prominent, pubic arch
   narrow

18 Mrs. Greene is concerned because she has read that nutrition during pregnancy is important for proper
growth and development of the baby. She wants to know
something about the foods she should eat. The nurse
should:
1. Give her a list of foods so she can better plan her meals
2. Assess what she eats by taking a diet history
3. Emphasize the importance of limiting salt and
   highly seasoned foods
4. Instruct her to continue eating a normal diet

19 Mrs. Greene states, ''I'm worried about gaining too much
weight because I've heard it's bad for me.'' The nurse
should respond:
1. ''Yes, weight gain causes complications during pregnancy.''
2. ''Don't worry about gaining weight. We are more
   concerned if you don't gain enough weight to ensure
   proper growth of your baby.''
3. ''The pattern of your weight gain will be of more importance than the total amount.''
4. ''If you gain over 15 pounds, you'll have to follow a
   low-calorie diet.''

20 The uterus rises out of the pelvis and becomes an abdominal organ at about the:
1. Eighth week of pregnancy
2. Eighteenth week of pregnancy
3. Tenth week of pregnancy
4. Twelfth week of pregnancy

Situation: Mrs. Bey is pregnant and requests an abortion. Questions 21 through 24 refer to this situation.

21 During the salinization method of elective abortion, the
nurse should be alert for side effects such as:
1. Oliguria
2. Thirst
3. Bradycardia
4. Edema

22 After the salinization procedure, the patient should be
told that labor will probably begin within:
1. Two hours after the procedure
2. Several minutes following the procedure
3. Eight hours after the procedure
4. Twenty-four to 72 hours after the procedure

23 When Mrs. Bey returns to the clinic, she asks about an
intrauterine device for birth control. The nurse explains
that the copper intrauterine device provides contraception
by:
1. Blocking the cervical os
2. Increasing the mobility of the uterus
3. Setting up a nonspecific inflammatory cell reaction to
   the device
4. Preventing the sperm from reaching the fallopian tube

24 The nurse should also explain that the most common problem encountered by patients using an IUD is:
1. Development of vaginal infections
2. Discomfort associated with coitus
3. Spontaneous expulsion of the device
4. Perforation of the uterus

25 Most spontaneous abortions are caused by:
1. Physical trauma
2. Germ plasma defects
3. Unresolved stress
4. Congenital defects

26 In the dilation and suction evacuation method of elective
abortion, laminaria are used in the dilation stage of the
procedure because:
1. They are stronger in action than instruments
2. Dilation occurs within 2 hours
3. Less anesthesia is necessary with this method
4. They are hygroscopic and expand

Situation: Mrs. Johnson is in her first trimester and comes to the
prenatal clinic. She has a cold and appears farther into her pregnancy than the history indicates. Questions 27 through 32 refer
to this situation.

27 Mrs. Johnson asks if it is all right to take aspirin. The best
advice the nurse can give to a pregnant woman in her first
trimester is to:
1. Avoid all drugs, including aspirin, and refrain from
   smoking and ingesting alcohol
2. Take only prescription drugs, especially in the second
   and third trimesters
3. Cut down on drugs, alcohol, and cigarettes
4. Avoid smoking and all drugs except aspirin when
   needed, and limit alcohol to no more than 1 oz daily

28 Mrs. Johnson delivers twins during the seventh month,
and they are diagnosed as having hyaline membrane disease. The principle underlying the respiratory distress of
these infants is:
1. Surface tension
2. Pascal's principle
3. Second law of thermodynamics
4. Archimedes' principle

29 When caring for Mrs. Johnson's twins, the nurse should:
1. Keep them prone to prevent aspiration

2. Keep them in a high-humidity environment
3. Reduce oxygen concentration to prevent eye damage
4. Reduce caloric intake to decrease metabolic rate

30 While considering nursing measures to foster parent-child relationships, the nurse should be aware that the most important factor at this time is the:
1. Duration and difficulty of labor
2. Anesthesia during labor
3. Health status during pregnancy
4. Physical condition of the twins

31 Mrs. Johnson might experience postpartum hemorrhage for all the following reasons. The most common one is:
1. Retained secundines
2. Lacerations of the cervix
3. Atony of the uterus
4. Secondary infections

32 Overstretching of perineal supporting tissues as a result of childbirth can bring about a rectocele. The most common symptom is:
1. Protrusion of the bladder into the vagina
2. Crampy abdominal pain
3. Urinary stress incontinence
4. Recurrent urinary tract infections

Situation: Miss Daley, a 24-year-old secretary, is pregnant for the first time. She discussed the pregnancy with her boyfriend, who told her everything would work out fine. Two days later she received a letter from him with $500 and the news that he had left town. Miss Daley is very upset, feels at the end of her rope, and calls the crisis intervention center for help. Questions 33 through 37 refer to this situation.

33 Miss Daley is experiencing a crisis because:
1. She is under a great deal of stress
2. Her boyfriend left her when she was pregnant
3. She is going to have to raise her child alone
4. Her past methods of adapting are ineffective for this situation

34 Crisis intervention groups are successful because the:
1. Client is encouraged to talk about herself
2. Client is assisted to investigate alternative approaches to solving the identified problem
3. Crisis intervention worker is a psychologist and understands behavior patterns
4. Client is supplied with a workable solution to her problems

35 When talking with Miss Daley, the crisis intervention worker should:
1. Respect her and involve her in deciding what she will do and how she will do it
2. Restate the problem, putting it in the proper perspective
3. Explain to her that the center has helped many other people with the same problem

4. Explore her religious and cultural beliefs so that your instructions are within her value system

36 Miss Daley has decided to go through with the pregnancy and keep the baby. Now the crisis intervention worker's primary responsibility is to:
1. Support her for making a wise decision
2. Make an appointment for her to see a physician for prenatal care
3. Explore other problems she may be experiencing
4. Provide information about other health resources where she may receive additional assistance

37 Miss Daley is now excited and looking forward to caring for her baby. Her decision to attend prenatal child care classes is an example of:
1. Extrinsic motivation
2. Operant conditioning
3. Intrinsic motivation
4. Behavior modification

Situation: Miss Abigail Jones, age 17, is admitted to the obstetric unit in labor. Questions 38 through 40 refer to this situation.

38 The nurse asks about Abigail's marital status. Abigail refuses to answer and becomes very agitated, telling the nurse to leave. The nurse should:
1. Have restricted her questions to those relevant to the situation
2. Have this information to complete the patient's history
3. Question the family about the marital status of the patient
4. Refer the patient to Social Services for help

39 Following an 8-hour uneventful labor Miss Jones delivers a baby boy spontaneously under epidural block anesthesia. As the nurse places her baby in her arms immediately following delivery, she asks, "Is he normal?" Your most appropriate answer would be:
1. "Of course he is, your pregnancy and labor were so normal."
2. "Shall we unwrap him so you can look him over for yourself?"
3. "He must be all right, he has such a good strong cry."
4. "Most babies are normal; of course he is."

40 The major concern for a pregnant out-of-wedlock teenager is that she is:
1. Socially ostracized
2. Diabetogenic
3. Financially dependent
4. Prone to toxemia

Situation: Mrs. Unger delivers a baby spontaneously. Questions 41 through 46 refers to this situation.

41 Immediate critical observation for Apgar scoring includes:
1. Respiratory rate

2. Heart rate
3. Presence of meconium
4. Evaluation of Moro reflex

42 Within 3 minutes after birth the normal heart rate of the infant may range between:
1. 100 to 180
2. 130 to 160
3. 120 to 140
4. 100 to 130

43 Within this same period the normal respiratory rate may be as high as:
1. 100
2. 80
3. 60
4. 50

44 The nurse may best obtain a Moro reflex by:
1. Creating a loud noise suddenly
2. Changing infant's equilibrium
3. Stimulating the infant's feet
4. Grasping the infant's hand

45 The Moro reflex response is marked by:
1. Extension of arms
2. Extension of legs and fanning of toes
3. Adduction of arms
4. Abduction and then adduction of the arms

46 Asymmetric Moro reflexes are frequently associated with:
1. Cerebral or cerebellar injuries
2. Cranial nerve damage
3. Brachial plexus, clavicle, or humerus injuries
4. Down's syndrome

Situation: Mrs. Cohen, a 26-year-old primigravida, comes to the prenatal clinic during the first trimester. She states she weighed 105 lb before her pregnancy and currently weighs 109 lbs. Questions 47 through 51 refer to this situation.

47 Mrs. Cohen is concerned about regaining her figure after delivery and wishes to diet during pregnancy. The nurse should advise Mrs. Cohen that:
1. Dieting is recommended to make delivery easier
2. Inadequate food intake during pregnancy can cause some congenital anomalies
3. Dieting is recommended to lessen the incidence of stillbirth
4. Inadequate food intake during pregnancy can cause toxemia

48 The nurse should provide dietary teaching for Mrs. Cohen because:
1. Pregnant women must adhere to a specific pregnancy diet
2. Different sources of essential nutrients are favorite foods in different cultural groups
3. Most weight gain during pregnancy is fluid retention
4. Dietary allowances should not increase during pregnancy

49 During the seventh month of pregnancy Mrs. Cohen exhibits dependent edema. The nurse explains the treatment for fluid retention during pregnancy, which is:
1. Adequate fluid and a low-salt diet
2. Adequate fluid and elevation of the lower extremities
3. A low-salt diet and elevation of the lower extremities
4. Judicious use of diuretics and elevation of the lower extremities

50 Mrs. Cohen develops painless vaginal bleeding during the last trimester. The nurse realizes that this may be caused by:
1. Abruptio placentae
2. Frequent intercourse
3. Placenta previa
4. Excessive alcohol ingestion

51 Although the causative factors are not clear, 40% to 50% of all patients with abruptio placenta also have:
1. Polyhydramnios
2. Hypertension
3. Diabetes
4. Cardiac arrhythmias

52 The inner membrane that provides fluid medium for the embryo is the:
1. Amnion
2. Yolk sac
3. Chorion
4. Allantois

53 First fetal movements felt by the mother are known as:
1. Ballottement
2. Engagement
3. Lightening
4. Quickening

54 Growth is most rapid during which phase of prenatal development?
1. Implantation
2. First trimester
3. Second trimester
4. Third trimester

55 The chief function of progesterone is the:
1. Establishment of secondary male sex characteristics
2. Rupturing of follicles for ovulation to occur
3. Development of female reproductive organs
4. Preparation of the uterus to receive a fertilized ovum

Situation: Mrs. Elliot, 9 weeks pregnant, visits the obstetric clinic complaining of severe nausea and vomiting. Questions 56 through 62 refer to this situation.

56 Which of the following factors is unrelated to hyperemesis gravidarum?
1. High levels of chorionic gonadotropin
2. Decreased secretion of free hydrochloric acid
3. Preestablished stress-involved GI disturbances
4. Incidence of polyhydramnios

57 Mrs. Elliot asks the nurse if she can continue to have sexual relations. The nurse's response is based on the knowledge that coitus during pregnancy would only be contraindicated in the presence of:
1. Leukorrhea
2. Gestation of 30 weeks or more
3. Premature rupture of membranes
4. Increased fetal heart rate

58 On her expected date of delivery Mrs. Elliot has a bloody show but contractions have not began. The head is at station +1. An acceptable method to induce labor is:
1. IM injection of oxytocin
2. Artificial rupture of membranes
3. Administration of prostaglandins
4. A tap water enema

59 Mrs. Elliot has a persistent bloody show and crampy abdominal pain. The nursing intervention at this time is:
1. Typing and cross matching the patient's blood for a possible transfusion
2. Providing the patient with comfort measures used for women in labor
3. Teaching the patient how to avoid straining
4. Reviewing Lamaze breathing techniques with the patient

60 During the postpartum period it is important that Mrs. Elliot voids regularly. Retention of fluid in the bladder has no relation to the development of:
1. Atony of the bladder
2. Stasis of urine, causing infection
3. Diaphoresis following delivery
4. Postpartum bleeding

61 When Mrs. Elliot's male infant has been in the nursery for about 18 hours, the nurse caring for him notes that his breathing is below 35 per minute. No other changes are noted and, since the infant is apparently well, no record or report is made. Several hours later the infant experiences severe respiratory distress and emergency care is necessary. Legal responsibility in this instance would have to take into consideration that:
1. Any marked change in respirations is significant and should have been reported
2. Respirations in the newborn are irregular and a drop is rarley important
3. Most infants experience slow respirations during the first 24 hours
4. The respiratory tract is underdeveloped in newborns and respiratory rate is not significant

62 During the "taking hold" phase, the nurse would expect Mrs. Elliot to:
1. Be concerned with her own needs
2. Touch the baby with her fingertips
3. Call the baby by name
4. Talk about the baby

63 The practice of separating parents and child immediately after birth and limiting their time with the newborn in the first few days would appear to contraindicate studies based on:
1. Rooming in
2. Bonding
3. Taking-in behaviors
4. Taking-hold behaviors

64 Research indicates that the early mother-infant relationship is vital to future mental health. Which of the following statements is true?
1. Ambivalence and anxiety about mothering are common
2. A rejected pregnancy will result in a rejected infant
3. A good mother experiences neither ambivalence nor anxiety about mothering
4. Maternal love is fully developed within the first week after birth

Situation: Mrs. Portridge has been married for 6 years and has been unable to become pregnant. Mr. and Mrs. Portridge have decided to discuss this problem with a physician, who suggests that some studies be done. Questions 65 through 68 refer to this situation.

65 A test commonly used to determine the number, motility, and activity of sperm is the:
1. Rubin test
2. Huhner test
3. Papanicolaou test
4. Friedman test

66 In the female, evaluation of all the pelvic organs of reproduction is accomplished by:
1. Cystoscopy
2. Biopsy
3. Culdoscopy
4. Hysterosalpingogram

67 After ovulation has occurred, the ovum is believed to reman viable for:
1. 1 to 6 hours
2. 12 to 18 hours
3. 24 to 36 hours
4. 48 to 72 hours

68 A factor in sterility may be related to the pH of the vaginal canal. A frequent medication that is ordered to alter the pH is:
1. Sulfur insufflations
2. Sodium bicarbonate douches
3. Lactic acid douches
4. Estrogen therapy

Situation: Mrs. Winder, age 24, complains of menstrual irregularity and infertility. Questions 69 through 71 refer to this situation.

69 A drug the physician might prescribe to treat both of Mrs. Winder's complaints is:
1. Methallenestril (Vallestril)
2. Ergonovine (Ergotrate)
3. Norethynodrel with mestranol (Enovid)
4. Relaxin (Releasin)

70 Eventually Mrs. Winder becomes pregnant. She is hospitalized when her membranes rupture during the thirty-eighth week of pregnancy. If the obstetrician decides to induce labor, which of the following drugs will probably be used?
1. Ergonovine maleate
2. Progesterone
3. Oxytocin (Pitocin)
4. Lututrin (Lutrexin)

71 During the period of induction, Mrs. Winder should be observed carefully for signs of which of the following?
1. Uterine tetany
2. Severe pain
3. Prolapse of the umbilical cord
3. Hypoglycemia

Situation: Mrs. King is a primigravida at term and is admitted to the labor room. She has attended education for childbirth classes together with her husband. When Mrs. King is admitted, she is experiencing contractions every 5 to 8 minutes, which last approximately 30 seconds. She also has a slight bloody discharge. The physician's examination reveals that the cervix is about 3 cm dilated and almost fully effaced. The vertex is presenting at a +1 station, with the occiput toward the left side of the symphysis pubis. Mrs. King is quite cheerful and at ease. Questions 72 through 79 refer to this situation.

72 Mrs. King asks the nurse if it is all right for her to get up and walk around. Based on observations of Mrs. King's contractions and knowledge of the physiology and mechanism of labor, the best action for the nurse to take would be to tell Mrs. King:
1. "Please stay in bed; walking may interfere with proper uterine contractions."
2. "I can't make a decision on that, you will have to ask the doctor."
3. "You will have to stay in bed; otherwise your contractions cannot be timed and no one can listen to the fetal heart."
4. "It is quite all right for you to be up and about as long as you feel comfortable and your membranes are intact."

73 An enema is ordered for Mrs. King. Reasons for giving enemas to patients in labor include all the following reasons except:
1. Expulsion of feces during labor predisposes the patient to infection
2. A full rectum tends to hinder the progress of labor

3. It is a routine procedure carried out for every patient in labor
4. A full lower bowel predisposes to postpartum discomfort.

74 Mrs. King's contractions gradually increase in strength and become more frequent and last longer. Her membranes rupture. The first action for the nurse to take after putting Mrs. King to bed is to:
1. Listen to the fetal heart
2. Call the physician
3. Time the contractions
4. Check blood pressure and pulse

75 The nurse observes the amniotic fluid and decides that it appears normal, since it is:
1. Clear and dark amber colored
2. Milky, greenish yellow, containing shreds of mucus
3. Clear, almost colorless, containing little white specks
4. Cloudy, greenish yellow, containing little white specks

76 An examination reveals that Mrs. King is 7 to 8 cm dilated and that the vertex is low in the midpelvis. To alleviate discomfort during contractions, the nurse would instruct Mr. King to encourage his wife in:
1. Panting
2. Abdominal breathing
3. Pelvic rocking
4. Athletic chest breathing

77 Mrs. King becomes very tense with contractions and quite irritable. She frequently states "I cannot stand this a minute longer." This kind of behavior is indicative of the fact that she:
1. Is entering the transition phase of labor
2. Needs immediate administration of an analgesic or anesthetic
3. Is developing some abnormality in terms of uterine contractions
4. Has been very poorly prepared for labor in the parents' classes

78 Mr. King is becoming very tense at this time. He asks, "Do you think it is best for me to leave, since I don't seem to do my wife much good?" The most appropriate answer to this statement would be:
1. "If you feel that way, you'd best go out and sit in the father's waiting room for awhile because you may transmit your anxiety to your wife."
2. "I know this is hard for you. Why don't you go have a cup of coffee and relax and come back later if you feel like it?"
3. "This is the time your wife needs you. Don't run out on her now."
4. "This is hard for you. Let me try to help you coach her during this difficult phase."

79 The beginning of the second stage of labor can be recognized by the patient's desire to:
1. Relax during contractions

2. Push during contractions
3. Pant during contractions
4. Blow during contractions

Situation: Mrs. Kelly is a 27-year-old gravida I para 0 with a childhood history of rheumatic fever. She has been admitted to the hospital at 35 weeks' gestation because of shortness of breath. Questions 80 through 87 refer to this situation.

80 Normal hemodynamics of pregnancy that affect the pregnant cardiac patient include the:
1. Decrease in the number of red blood cells
2. Rise in cardiac output after the thirty-fourth week
3. Gradually increasing size of the uterus
4. Cardiac acceleration in the last half of pregnancy

81 Shortly after admission, Mrs. Kelly goes into labor. To prevent cardiac decompensation during labor the nurse should:
1. Position Mrs. Kelly on her side with shoulders elevated
2. Maintain an IV infusion of potassium chloride
3. Administer sodium IV infusion
4. Administer oxytocin to strengthen contractions

82 Nursing care of a patient in premature labor includes:
1. Reassuring patient that the situation is under control
2. Explaining why pain medication is kept at a minimum
3. Encouraging the patient not to bear down
4. Keeping the patient NPO to prevent abdominal distention

83 During the postpartum period the nurse is aware that the patient will have an increased cardiac output with tachycardia. She would observe the patient carefully for signs of:
1. Irregular pulse
2. Respiratory distress
3. Increased vaginal bleeding
4. Hypovolemic shock

84 Mrs. Kelly's infant weighs 4 lb, 9 oz. On admission to the nursery the nurse should routinely do all the following except:
1. Evaluate the newborn's status
2. Support body temperature
3. Administer oxygen
4. Record vital signs

85 The nurse must continuously monitor baby Kelly, since the most common complication in the preterm infant is:
1. Brain damage
2. Respiratory distress
3. Aspiration of mucus
4. Hemorrhage

86 The nurse must monitor baby Kelly's temperature and provide appropriate nursing care as the premature baby stabilizes body temperature at:
1. 36.4° to 37° C (97.5° to 98.6° F)

2. 36.1° to 37.2° C (97° to 99° F)
3. 35° to 36.1° C (95° to 97° F)
4. 34.4° to 35.6° C (94° to 96° F)

87 When meeting baby Kelly's hydration needs the nurse must consider the fact that urinary function of the premature baby:
1. Is the same as in a full-term newborn
2. Causes the loss of large amounts of urine
3. Maintains stability of acid-base and electrolyte balance
4. Tends to overconcentrate the urine

---

88 More than half the neonatal deaths in the United States are caused by:
1. Atelectasis
2. Prematurity
3. Respiratory distress syndrome
4. Congenital heart disease

89 The presence of multiple gestation should be detected as early as possible and the pregnancy managed with high risk in mind because:
1. Perinatal mortality is 2 to 3 times greater than in single births
2. Maternal mortality is much higher in multiple births
3. The mother needs time to adjust psychologically and physiologically
4. Postpartum hemorrhage is frequent

Situation: Mrs. Kim, a 22-year-old primigravida at term, is brought to the hospital by her husband. They have attended preparation for childbirth classes and plan to be together during labor. On admission Mrs. Kim is having 3- to 5-minute contractions, she has a bloody show, and her membranes are intact. On vaginal examination the cervix is fully effaced and 6 cm dilated, the vertex presenting at a +1 station. Vital signs are temperature 98.6°, pulse rate 76, respirations 20, fetal heart rate 140 L.L.Q., blood pressure 118/74. Mr. Kim is coaching and supporting his wife well, and Mrs. Kim appears to be quite relaxed. Questions 90 through 95 refer to this situation.

90 According to the above data, Mrs. Kim is in what phase of the first stage of labor?
1. Early phase
2. Midphase
3. Transition phase
4. Accelerated phase

91 Station +1 indicates that the presenting part is:
1. Slightly below the ischial spines
2. Slightly above the ischial spines
3. High in the false pelvis
4. On the perineum

92 Mrs. Kim is uncomfortable and asks for medication. Demerol, 50 mg, and Phenergan, 50 mg, are ordered to be administered intramuscularly. This medication would:
1. Induce sleep until the time of delivery
2. Increase her pain threshold, resulting in relaxation

3. Act as an amnesic drug

4. Act as a preliminary to anesthesia

93 A few hours later Mrs. Kim becomes very restless, her face is flushed, and she is irritable, perspiring profusely, and feels she is going to vomit. These symptoms are indicative of:

1. Second stage

2. Late stage

3. Transition phase

4. Third stage

94 When inspecting her newborn baby girl, Mrs. Kim notices a discharge from the nipples of both breasts. The nurse should explain that this is evidence of:

1. Monilia contracted during birth

2. Congenital hormonal imbalance

3. As infection contracted in utero

4. The influence of the mother's hormones

95 During the postpartum period the nurse examines Mrs. Kim and identifies the presence of lochia serosa and a fundus 4 finger breadths below the umbilicus. This indicates that the time elapsed is:

1. 1 to 3 days post partum

2. 4 to 5 days post partum

3. 6 to 7 days post partum

4. 8 to 9 days post partum

---

96 During the process of gametogenesis, the male and female sex cells divide and then contain:

1. A diploid number of chromosomes in the nuclei

2. A haploid number of chromosomes in their nuclei

3. Twenty-two pairs of autosomes in their nuclei

4. Forty-six pairs of chromosomes in their nuclei

97 The production of which of the following is not an endocrine function of the placenta?

1. Chorionic gonadotropin

2. Follicle stimulating hormone

3. Progesterone precursor substances

4. Somatotropin

98 During the first 2 months of pregnancy the chief source of estrogen and progesterone is the:

1. Anterior hypophysis

2. Placenta

3. Adrenal cortex

4. Corpus luteum

Situation: Mrs. Rowan is admitted to the high-risk obstetric unit with eclampsia. Questions 99 through 105 refer to this situation.

99 Mrs. Rowan is receiving magnesium sulfate. The nurse must be alert for the first sign of excessive blood levels, which is:

1. Development of cardiac arrhythmia

2. Disappearance of the knee-jerk reflex

3. Increase in respiratory rate

4. Disturbance of the bearing ability

100 In caring for Mrs. Rowan the nurse should:

1. Encourage her to drink clear fluids

2. Protect her against extraneous stimuli

3. Isolate her in a dark room

4. Maintain her in a supine position

101 The first sign of a convulsion in a patient with preeclampsia is frequently:

1. Rolling of the eyes to one side with a fixed stare

2. Spots or flashes of light before the eyes

3. Persistent headache and blurred vision

4. Epigastric pain, nausea, and vomiting

102 Mrs. Rowan has a convulsion. Following the convulsion she has an elevated temperature of 102° F (39° C). The nurse realizes that this may be caused by:

1. Development of a systemic infection

2. Dehydration caused by rapid fluid loss

3. Disturbance of the cerebral thermal center

4. Excessive muscular activity

103 Mrs. Rowan is afraid of having another convulsion and asks when the likelihood of convulsions will end. The nurse replies that the danger of a convulsion in a woman with preeclampsia ends:

1. After labor begins

2. After delivery occurs

3. 24 hours post partum

4. 48 hours post partum

104 Mrs. Rowan's labor is long and the baby is delivered in the breech position. Since Erb-Duchenne paralysis may be seen as the result of a difficult forceps or breech delivery, the nurse would look for which of the following symptoms?

1. A flaccid arm with the elbow extended

2. A negative Moro reflex on the unaffected side

3. Loss of grasp reflex on the affected side

4. Inability to turn the head to the affected side

105 If Erb-Duchenne paralysis occurred, nursing care of the infant would include:

1. Constant immobilization of the affected arm

2. Immediate active ROM exercises to the affected arm

3. Teaching the parents to manipulate the muscle

4. Daily measurement of girth and length of the affected arm

Situation: Mrs. Jackson, 2½ months pregnant, comes to the prenatal clinic for the first time. Questions 106 through 111 refer to this situation.

106 Mrs. Jackson asks the clinic nurse whether smoking will affect the baby. Her answer reflects the following knowledge:

1. Fetal and maternal circulation are separated by the placental barrier

2. The placenta is permeable to specific substances

3. Smoking relieves tension and the fetus responds accordingly

4. Vasoconstriction will affect both fetal and maternal blood vessels

107 Mrs. Jackson is concerned about the mask of pregnancy, her "dark nipples," and the "dark line" from her navel to her pubis. The nurse explains that these adaptations are caused by hyperactivity of the:
1. Adrenal gland
2. Thyroid gland
3. Ovaries
4. Pituitary gland

108 Mrs. Jackson complains of morning sickness. The nurse realizes that a predisposing factor which causes morning sickness during the first trimester of pregnancy is the adaptation to increased levels of:
1. Estrogen
2. Progesterone
3. Luteinizing hormone
4. Chorionic gonadotropin

109 The nurse can help Mrs. Jackson overcome morning sickness by suggesting she:
1. Eat nothing until the nausea subsides
2. Take an antacid before bedtime
3. Request her physician to prescribe an antiemetic
4. Eat dry toast before arising

110 Mrs. Jackson delivers a healthy baby boy. Two days post partum, after receiving a phone call from her babysitter informing her that her 2-year-old has been very upset since her admission to the hospital and is not eating, Mrs. Jackson elects to sign her baby and herself out of the hospital. Staff members have been unable to contact her physician. Mrs. Jackson arrives at the nursery ready to leave and asks that her infant be given to her to dress and take home. Appropriate nursing action would be:
1. Explain to Mrs. Jackson that her infant must remain in hospital until signed out by the physician and that she must leave the baby in the nursery
2. Allow Mrs. Jackson time with the baby to cuddle him before she leaves, but emphasize that the baby is a minor and legally must remain until orders are received
3. Tell Mrs. Jackson that under the circumstances hospital policy prevents you from releasing the infant into her care, but she will be informed when he is discharged
4. Give the baby to Mrs. Jackson to take home, making sure that she receives information regarding care and feeding of a 2-day-old infant and any potential problems which may develop

111 When Mrs. Jackson returns to the clinic for a postpartum examination, she is very depressed. The nurse realizes that the new mother who exhibits postpartum blues is probably adapting to:
1. A decrease in progesterone levels
2. Changes in body image
3. Psychologic letdown after labor
4. Rejection of her newborn

112 In which of the fetal blood vessels is the oxygen content highest?
1. Umbilical artery
2. Ductus arteriosus
3. Ductus venosus
4. Pulmonary artery

113 The blood vessels in the umbilical cord consist of:
1. Two arteries and 1 vein
2. Two arteries and 2 veins
3. One artery and 2 veins
4. One artery and 1 vein

114 When assessing the significance of estriol studies in an antenatal patient, the nurse should understand that:
1. Elevations in estriol levels indicate fetal postmaturity
2. Estriol is the hormone used in pregnancy tests
3. The fetus contributes precursors to the synthesis of estriol
4. Elevations in estriol levels indicate fetal demise

115 Physiologic anemia during pregnancy is a result of:
1. Increased blood volume of the mother
2. Decreased dietary intake of iron
3. Decreased erythropoiesis after first trimester
4. Increased detoxification demands on the mother's liver

116 The fetus is most likely to be damaged by the pregnant woman's ingestion of drugs during the:
1. First trimester
2. Second trimester
3. Third trimester
4. Entire pregnancy

Situation: Mr. and Mrs. Singer are Rh-incompatible partners. As the pregnancy progresses, the maternal serum antibody titer continues to rise. An amniocentesis is scheduled for the twenty-eighth week of pregnancy. Questions 117 through 120 refer to this situation.

117 A common method of locating the precise position of a fetus prior to an amniocentesis is:
1. X-ray examination
2. Holography
3. Fluoroscopy
4. Sonography

118 The results of the amniocentesis indicate that the fetus is only mildly affected but does, in fact, have Down's syndrome. Mr. and Mrs. Singer elect to have the pregnancy terminated. The nurse giving postoperative care to a patient who has had her pregnancy surgically terminated should be aware that:
1. The patient is emotionally unstable at this time
2. The patient needs to express her feelings of guilt, anger, and frustration
3. She should defer contraception counseling at this time
4. The risk of postoperative infection is high

119 Following the hysterotomy, Rh_oD was administered intramuscularly to:
1. Prevent antibody formation in the mother
2. Expand the antibody pool of the mother
3. Accelerate the mother's production of immune bodies
4. Suppress the activity of Rh-negative antibodies

120 It is important for the nurse to support the decisions made by the parents of a fetus with a birth defect, since:
1. The nurse's support will relieve the pressure associated with decision making
2. Supporting them will eliminate feelings of guilt
3. The parents are legally responsible for the decision
4. It is essential for maintenance of family equilibrium

---

121 The most common type of ectopic pregnancy is tubal. Within a few weeks after conception the tube may rupture suddenly, causing:
1. Sudden knifelike lower quadrant abdominal pain
2. Continuous dull lower quadrant abdominal pain
3. Painless vaginal bleeding
4. Intermittent abdominal contractions

122 Which symptom would the nurse be alert for when caring for a patient with a tentative diagnosis of hydatidiform mole?
1. Painless heavy vaginal bleeding
2. Usually rapid uterine enlargement
3. Hypertension
4. Decreased fetal heart rate

Situation: Mrs. Dowle delivers a 6-lb, 3-oz baby girl. Questions 123 through 125 refer to this situation.

123 While holding her baby, Mrs. Dowle calls the nurse and says, "My baby is sick; she sneezes a lot and look how she breathes. Her breathing is so rapid and shallow and not regular. My neighbor's baby had to return to the hospital after she was home a week because she had pneumonia. I hope this does not happen to my baby." The best action for the nurse to take is to:
1. Pick up the baby and tell the mother that she will watch her closely
2. Look the baby over and tell the mother that the baby is fine, there is nothing wrong with her
3. Look the baby over and explain to the mother that sneezing is normal and helps the baby to get rid of mucus and that a baby normally has rapid, shallow, irregular respirations
4. Look the baby over, take her to the nursery immediately, and return to the mother to tell her that the physician has been called, since the baby is obviously in respiratory distress

124 The nurse's response is based on the knowledge that a normal infant's respirations are:
1. Regular, initiated by the chest wall, 40 to 60 per minute, shallow

2. Irregular, abdominal, 40 to 50 per minute, shallow
3. Regular, abdominal, 40 to 50 per minute, deep
4. Irregular, initiated by chest wall, 30 to 60 per minute, deep

125 Mrs. Dowle, who has 3 children under 5 years of age at home, comments to the nursery nurse that she cannot hold the baby for feedings once she gets home. She has just too much to do, and anyhow it spoils the baby. The best response for the nurse to make is:
1. "That's entirely up to you, you have to do what works for you."
2. "Holding the baby when feeding is important for her development."
3. "It is most unsafe to prop a bottle. The baby could aspirate the fluid."
4. "You seem concerned about time. Let's talk about it."

Situation: Mrs. Ballen is admitted to the obstetric unit in labor with contractions about 15 minutes apart. Mrs. Ballen's cervix is moderately effaced and 4 cm dilated. Questions 126 through 131 refer to this situation.

126 During labor the nurse must be aware that fetal heart deceleration is evidenced by a fetal heart rate of:
1. 140 to 160 beats per minute
2. 120 to 140 beats per minute
3. 100 to 119 beats per minute
4. 80 to 100 beats per minute

127 Mrs. Ballen's labor progresses uneventfully and she enters the transitional stage. When Mrs. Ballen is positioned on the delivery table, both legs should be placed in the stirrups at the same time to prevent:
1. Excessive pull on the fascia
2. Pressure on the perineum
3. Trauma to the uterine ligaments
4. Venous stasis in the legs

128 During each contraction the fetal heart rate persistently drops from 140 to 110 per minute. The nurse should:
1. Continue to monitor the fetal heart rate during contractions
2. Notify the physician and prepare for immediate delivery
3. Decrease the drip rate of oxytocin to slow contractions
4. Change mother's position from back to side or side to side

129 Mrs. Ballen has decided to breast-feed her infant. When teaching breast-feeding the nurse should instruct Mrs. Ballen *not* to:
1. Try to empty the breast at each feeding
2. Use an alternate breast at each feeding
3. Wash breasts with soap and water before feeding
4. Wash breasts with water before each feeding

130 Mrs. Ballen complains of frequent leg cramps. The nurse should suspect:
1. Hypercalcemia and tell her to increase her activity

2. Hypokalemia and tell her to increase her intake of green, leafy vegetables
3. Hyperkalemia and tell her to see a physician immediately
4. Hypocalcemia and tell her to increase her intake of milk

131 Mrs. Ballen asks about the difference between cow's milk and the milk from her breasts. The nurse should respond that cow's milk differs from human milk in that it contains:
1. More protein, more calcium, and less carbohydrate
2. Less protein, less calcium, and more carbohydrate
3. Less protein, more calcium, and more carbohydrate
4. More protein, less calcium, and less carbohydrate

132 The pituitary hormone that stimulates the secretion of milk from the mammary glands is:
1. Prolactin
2. Oxytocin
3. Progesterone
4. Estrogen

133 Breast-feeding is *not* contraindicated in which of the following circumstances?
1. Pregnancy
2. Maternal tuberculosis
3. Inverted nipples
4. Mastitis

Situation: Baby Reisler is delivered at 29 weeks' gestation. He weighs 3 lb, 9 oz. Questions 134 through 137 refer to this situation.

134 Baby Reisler is considered to be in critical condition. According to his size and length of gestation, he would be classified as:
1. Premature
2. Immature
3. Nonviable
4. Low birth weight infant

135 Baby Reisler is being fed by gavage. This type of feeding is indicated in premature infants because:
1. The feeding can be given quickly, so handling is minimized
2. Vomiting is prevented
3. It conserves the baby's strength and does not depend on the swallowing reflex
4. The amount of food given can be more accurately regulated

136 Baby Reisler is placed in an incubator to maintain his body temperature at a constant level, since the heat regulation mechanism in premature infants is one of the least developed functions. Which of the following conditions is responsible for this?
1. The surface area of a premature baby is smaller than that of the normal newborn

2. A premature baby lacks subcutaneous fat, which would furnish some insulation
3. A premature baby perspires a great deal, thus losing heat almost constantly
4. A premature baby has a limited ability to produce antibodies against infections

137 In caring for a premature infant, which of the following precautions should be taken against retrolental fibroplasia?
1. Oxygen should be kept at less than 40% concentration and be discontinued as soon as feasible
2. Temperature and humidity should be controlled very carefully
3. A high concentration of oxygen (above 75%) should be maintained together with high humidity
4. Phototherapy should be used to prevent jaundice and retinopathy

138 Which of the following conditions is *unrelated* to postpartal hemorrhage?
1. Delivery of twins or hydramnios
2. Retained placenta
3. Toxemia of pregnancy
4. Overdistended bladder

139 Mrs. Pattern is admitted to the Emergency Room with vaginal bleeding. When taking a history, the nurse learns that the patient has had 5 missed periods. Later the nurse reads the chart, which states, "stillborn delivered at 8 P.M. . . ." The nurse understands this to mean that the products of conception:
1. Were completely expelled
2. Were previable
3. Weighed over 600 g
4. Measured 13.4 cm in length

140 A decision to withhold "extraordinary care" for a newborn with severe abnormalities is actually:
1. The same as pediatric euthanasia
2. A decision to let the newborn die
3. Presuming that the newborn has no rights
4. Unethical and illegal medical and nursing practice

141 The earliest clinical sign in idiopathic respiratory distress syndrome in the newborn is usually:
1. Sternal and subcostal retractions
2. Cyanosis
3. Rapid respiration
4. Grunting

Situation: Following a long and difficult delivery, Baby John is admitted to the newborn nursery. Questions 142 through 147 refer to this situation.

142 An Apgar score of 4 would most likely indicate which of the following?
1. Body pink, extremities blue
2. Heart rate over 100
3. Flaccid muscle tone
4. Respirations of 35

143 Baby John has muscle twitchings, convulsions, cyanosis, abnormal respirations, and a short shrill cry. The nurse should suspect that the infant has:
1. Tetany
2. Intracranial hemorrhage
3. Spina bifida
4. Hyperkalemia

144 When observing Baby John for signs of pathologic jaundice the nurse should be alert for:
1. Appearance of jaundice during the first 24 hours
2. Jaundice developing between 24 and 72 hours in a full-term infant
3. Neurologic signs during the first 24 hours
4. Muscular irritability at birth

145 The nurse observes Baby John lying in a supine position with his head turned to the side, his legs and arms extended on the same side and flexed on the opposite side. The nurse is aware that this is:
1. The Landau reflex
2. The tonic neck reflex
3. The Moro reflex
4. An abnormal reflex

146 Experience has shown that parents are better able to cope with the birth of an abnormal child if informed:
1. After the first 48 hours, when the mother's strength has returned
2. When bringing the baby to the mother for the first time
3. After the birth, while the mother is still in the delivery room
4. When the parents ask if something is wrong with their baby

147 Baby John's mother has decided not to nurse her baby. The medication used to suppress lactation would include the following hormone:
1. Testosterone
2. Cortisone
3. Oxytocin
4. Estrogen

Situation: Mr. and Mrs. Light want to practice the rhythm method of contraception but do not understand how it works. Questions 148 through 151 refer to this situation.

148 The nurse's explanation is based on ovulation occurring:
1. Seven days after the completion of the menstrual period
2. Fourteen days after the completion of the menstrual period
3. Seven days before the end of the menstrual cycle
4. Fourteen days prior to the onset of menstruation

149 The time of ovulation can be determined by taking the basal temperature. During ovulation the basal temperature:
1. Drops markedly

2. Drops slightly and then rises
3. Drops markedly and remains low
4. Rises suddenly and then falls

150 The nurse explains that the efficiency of rhythm is dependent on the basal body temperature. Which of the following factors will alter its effectiveness?
1. Frequency of intercourse
2. Age of those involved
3. Presence of stress
4. Length of abstinence

151 Mrs. Light has missed 2 periods. When she comes to the prenatal clinic, she complains of vaginal bleeding and left lower quadrant pain. The nurse suspects that Mrs. Light has:
1. An incomplete abortion
2. An ectopic pregnancy
3. Abruptio placentae
4. A rupture of the Graafian follicle

Situation: Mr. and Mrs. Quinn have been married almost 7 years when the physician confirms that Mrs. Quinn is 8 to 10 weeks pregnant. Mr. and Mrs. Quinn are overjoyed. About 10 days after her visit to the physician, at the time of her normal menstrual period, Mrs. Quinn starts to stain. The physician tells her to go to bed immediately and remain on complete bed rest for at least 72 hours. Since Mr. Quinn cannot stay at home and Mrs. Quinn has no one else to care for her, she is admitted to the hospital. Questions 152 through 155 refer to this situation.

152 Mrs. Quinn is admitted because of:
1. Threatened abortion
2. Inevitable abortion
3. Ectopic pregnancy
4. Missed abortion

153 After a few hours Mrs. Quinn begins to experience bearing-down sensations and suddenly expels the fetus in bed. To give safe nursing care the nurse should first:
1. Take her immediately to the delivery room
2. Check the fundus for firmness
3. Give her the sedation ordered
4. Immediately notify the physician

154 Following delivery the nurse should observe Mrs. Quinn for:
1. Dehydration and hemorrhage
2. Hemorrhage and infection
3. Subinvolution and dehydration
4. Signs of toxemia

155 When Mrs. Quinn returns to her room, both she and her husband are visibly upset. The nurse notices that Mr. Quinn has tears in his eyes and that Mrs. Quinn has her face turned to the wall and is sobbing quietly. The best approach for the nurse to take is to go over to Mrs. Quinn and say:
1. "I know how you feel, but you should not be so upset

now, it will make it more difficult for you to get well quickly.''
2. ''I can understand that you are upset, but be glad it happened early in your pregnancy and not after you carried the baby for the full time.''
3. ''I know that you are upset now, but hopefully you will become pregnant again very soon.''
4. ''I see that both of you are very upset. I brought you a cup of coffee and will be here if you want to talk.''

---

156 Abruptio placentae is most likely to occur in a woman with the following complication of pregnancy:
1. Toxemia
2. Cardiac disease
3. Hyperthyroidism
4. Cephalopelvic disproportion

157 A predisposing factor in determining whether a woman will have a postpartum hemorrhage is the knowledge that:
1. Her uterus is overdistended
2. She has had more than 5 pregnancies
3. Her duration of labor is very short
4. She is over 40 years of age

158 Which of the following fetal and neonatal hazards is *not* associated with breech delivery?
1. Intracranial hemorrhage
2. Cephalohematoma
3. Compression of cord
4. Separation of placenta prior to delivery of head

159 Which of the following is included in the care of a patient with placenta previa?
1. Limited ambulation until bleeding stops
2. Observation and recording of bleeding
3. Vital signs at least once per shift
4. A tap water enema before delivery

160 The nurse would suspect an ectopic pregnancy if the patient complained of:
1. Lower abdominal cramping present over a long period of time
2. Sharp lower right or left abdominal pain radiating to the shoulder
3. Leukorrhea and dysuria a few days after the first missed period
4. An adherent painful ovarian mass

161 The most effective position for a woman in labor when the nurse notes a prolapsed cord is:
1. Sims
2. Fowler
3. Trendelenburg
4. Lithotomy

Situation: Mr. and Mrs. James are attending the infertility clinic. Questions 162 through 167 refer to this situation.

162 In dealing with a couple who have an infertility problem, the nurse should know:

1. One partner has a problem that makes them unable to have children
2. The couple have been unable to have a child after trying for a year
3. Infertility is usually psychologic in origin
4. Infertility and sterility are essentially the same problem

163 A diagnostic test used to evaluate fertility is the postcoital test. It is best timed:
1. Immediately after menses
2. Within 1 to 2 days of presumed ovulation
3. One week after ovulation
4. Just prior to the next menstrual period

164 A tubal insufflation test is done to determine if there is a tubal obstruction. Infertility due to a defect in the tube is usually related to a:
1. Past infection
2. Fibroid tumor
3. Congenital anomaly
4. Previous injury to a tube

165 Mrs. James returns to the clinic because she has missed her menstrual period and thinks she is pregnant. The laboratory tests for pregnancy are based on the presence of:
1. Isoimmune bodies
2. Chorionic gonadotropin
3. Estrogen
4. Progesterone

166 In assessing Mrs. James' physical condition the nurse is aware of the fact that a normal adaptation of pregnancy is an increased blood supply to the pelvic region. The resulting bluish purple discoloration of the vaginal mucosa and cervix is known as:
1. Hegar's sign
2. Lodin's sign
3. Goodell's sign
4. Chadwick's sign

167 Mrs. James is concerned about gaining weight during pregnancy. The nurse explains that most of the weight gain during pregnancy is due to:
1. Metabolic alterations
2. Fluid retention
3. Increased blood volume
4. The fetus

Situation: Mrs. Page has been in labor for 18 hours and is exhausted. Questions 168 through 172 refer to this situation.

168 The most common indication for cesarean section is:
1. Cephalopelvic disproportion
2. Primary uterine inertia
3. Placenta previa
4. Vaginal atony

169 The anteroposterior diameter of the birth canal is one of the important measurements of the pelvis and is known as the:

1. Diagonal conjugate
2. Transverse conjugate
3. Conjugate vera
4. Transverse diameter

170 The most effective method of determining if there is cephalopelvic disproportion for the woman in labor is:
   1. Pelvimetry
   2. X-ray examination
   3. Amniocentesis
   4. Duration of labor

171 Mrs. Page eventually delivers her baby vaginally. The newborn has asymmetric gluteal folds, and the nurse suspects:
   1. A dislocated hip
   2. Peripheral nervous system damage
   3. An inguinal hernia
   4. Central nervous sytem damage

172 Mrs. Page asks the nurse why sugar is added to the baby's formula. The nurse's response would depend on the following understanding:
   1. Cow's milk contains fewer calories than breast milk
   2. Sugar in cow's milk is not assimilated well
   3. Diluted cow's milk provides less sugar than the baby needs
   4. Sugar in cow's milk is a disaccharide

---

173 The two most important predisposing causes of puerperal infection are:
   1. Hemorrhage and trauma during labor
   2. Toxemia and retention of placenta
   3. Malnutrition and anemia during pregnancy
   4. *Streptococcus* organism present in birth canal and trauma during labor

Situation: Mrs. Allen is 2 weeks past her expected date of delivery. The physician has decided to perform an oxytocin challenge test (OCT) in which IV oxytocin solution is administered and the fetal heart rate and uterine contractions are recorded. Questions 174 through 179 refer to this situation.

174 Which of the following would be an indication for the oxytocin challenge test?
   1. Previous obstetric problems
   2. Placenta previa
   3. Premature onset of labor
   4. Pregnancy of more than 40 weeks

175 Contraindications to an oxytocin challenge test would include:
   1. Prematurity
   2. Drug addiction
   3. Hypertension
   4. Uterine activity

176 Mrs. Allen responds well to the oxytocin challenge test and labor is induced. Several hours later Mrs. Allen is complaining of pain and asks for medication. A medi-cation given to a woman in labor that might cause respiratory depression of the newborn is:
   1. Meperidine (Demerol)
   2. Scopolamine
   3. Promazine (Sparine)
   4. Promethazine (Phenergan)

177 Mrs. Allen delivers a 9-lb, 6-oz baby. In assessing the newborn, the nurse observes an unequal Moro reflex on one side, the flaccid arm in adduction. The nurse suspects:
   1. Brachial palsy
   2. Supratentorial tear
   3. Fracture of the clavicle
   4. Crigler-Najjar syndrome

178 The evening following delivery, the nurse encourages Mrs. Allen to ambulate to:
   1. Increase the tone of the bladder
   2. Promote respiration
   3. Increase peripheral vasomotor activity
   4. Maintain tone of abdominal muscles

179 In caring for the family on a postpartum unit, the nurse must be aware that all the tasks, responsibilities, and attitudes which make up child care can be called mothering and that either parent can exhibit motherliness. A person is able to perform "mothering" due to:
   1. An inborn ability based on instinct
   2. Positive childhood roles and concepts
   3. A good education in growth and development
   4. A marriage with flexible roles

---

180 The most common symptom of congenital rubella syndrome that follows infection in the mother during the first trimester is:
   1. Hydrocephalus
   2. Phocomelia
   3. Cardiac anomaly
   4. Otosclerosis

181 Closure of the foramen ovale after birth is caused by:
   1. A decrease in the aortic blood flow
   2. An increase in the pulmonary blood flow
   3. A decrease in pressure in the left atrium
   4. An increase in the pressure in the right atrium

182 After birth, in a normal neonate the ductus arteriosus becomes the:
   1. Ligamentum teres
   2. Venous ligament
   3. Ligamentum arteriosum
   4. Superior vesical artery

183 An infant's intestines are sterile at birth, therefore lacking the bacteria necessary for the synthesis of:
   1. Prothrombin
   2. Bile salts
   3. Intrinsic factor
   4. Bilirubin

Situation: Mrs. Allen, a gravida III, para 2, has an uneventful labor and delivery. After a 7-hour labor she delivers an 8-lb, 2-oz baby girl spontaneously. Questions 184 through 189 refer to this situation.

184 In checking Mrs. Allen, the nurse finds the fundus firm, shifted to the right, and 2 fingers above the umbilicus. This would indicate:
1. A normal process
2. An abnormal process
3. A full bladder
4. Impending bleeding

185 After delivery, when checking Mrs. Allen's vital signs, the nurse should normally find:
1. An elevated basal temperature, a decrease in respirations
2. A decided bradycardia, no change in respirations
3. A slight lowering of basal temperature, increase in respirations
4. A decided tachycardia, a decrease in respirations

186 Eight hours following delivery the nurse notices that Mrs. Allen is voiding frequently in small amounts. Intake and output are important in the early postpartal period, since small amounts of output:
1. Are commonly voided and should cause no alarm
2. May be indicative of beginning glomerulonephritis
3. May indicate retention of urine with overflow
4. Are common because less fluid is excreted following delivery

187 In helping Mrs. Allen develop her parenting role the nurse would:
1. Do things for the baby in the mother's presence
2. Find out what she knows about babies and proceed from there
3. Demonstrate baby bathing and care before discharge
4. Provide enough time for her and the baby to be together

188 Mrs. Allen's infant develops a cephalohematoma. The nurse should be aware that:
1. This usually does not occur with natural delivery
2. It will resolve spontaneously in 3 to 6 weeks
3. The swelling may cross a suture line
4. The soft sac bulges when the infant cries

189 Nursing care of baby Allen is directed primarily toward:
1. Supporting the parents
2. Applying ice packs to the hematoma
3. Recording neurologic signs
4. Protecting the infant's head

190 Immunity transferred to the fetus from an immune mother through the placenta is:
1. Active natural immunity
2. Active artificial immunity
3. Passive natural immunity
4. Passive artificial immunity

191 Which of the following findings would probably necessitate placing the newborn in the intensive care nursery?
1. An initial Apgar score of 5
2. A birth weight of 3500 g
3. The aspiration of 20 ml of milky-colored fluid from newborn's stomach
4. An umbilical cord that contained only 2 vessels

192 The nurse encourages continued medical supervision for the pregnant woman with pyelitis because:
1. Antibiotic therapy is given until the urine is sterile
2. Toxemia frequently occurs following pyelitis
3. Pelvic inflammatory disease occurs with untreated pyelitis
4. A low-protein diet is given until pregnancy is terminated

193 A nurse tells a pregnant woman not to wear tight clothing around her abdomen because of possible damage to the fetus. The principle responsible for the potential damage is:
1. Pascal's
2. Archimedes'
3. Newton's
4. Einstein's

194 During pregnancy, the uterine musculature hypertrophies and is greatly stretched as the fetus grows. This stretching:
1. By itself inhibits uterine contraction until oxytocin stimulates the birth process
2. Is prevented from stimulating uterine contraction by high levels of estrogen during late pregnancy
3. Inhibits uterine contraction along with the combined inhibitory effects of estrogen and progesterone
4. Would ordinarily stimulate uterine contraction but is prevented by high levels of progesterone during pregnancy

195 During pregnancy a polypeptide similar to the adrenal steroids is responsible for:
1. Symptoms of morning sickness
2. Urinary frequency
3. Linea nigra and chloasma
4. Softening of the cervix

196 A normal woman who had a hemophilic father is mated to a man with normal blood clotting. What is the probable phenotype of the offspring?
1. All children are hemophiliacs
2. Half the male children are hemophiliacs
3. All male children are hemophiliacs
4. All children are normal

197 If anemia is present with a hemoglobin level of 8 g or lower, a mother with cardiac disease probably will go into:
1. Cardiac failure
2. Heart block
3. Atrial fibrillation
4. Cardiac compensation

Situation: Mrs. Evans, a diabetic, suspects that she is pregnant because she is experiencing breast changes, has missed 2 periods, and has some early morning nausea and excessive fatigue. Despite the nausea and fatigue, her urine tests are consistently negative for sugar. Mrs. Evans seeks the advice of an obstetrician who confirms the diagnosis of pregnancy. Mrs. Evans is taking 30 units of NPH insulin daily at this time. Questions 198 through 202 refer to this situation.

198 A diabetic mother's metabolism is significantly altered during pregnancy as a result of:
  1. The increased effect of insulin during pregnancy
  2. The effect of hormones produced in pregnancy on carbohydrate and lipoid metabolism
  3. An increase in the glucose tolerance level of the blood
  4. The lower renal threshold for glucose

199 Regulation of usual insulin coverage in a pregnant diabetic woman is difficult, since:
  1. Sugar can normally be found in the urine of a pregnant woman
  2. Sugar is metabolized more rapidly during pregnancy
  3. The basal metabolic rate is altered during pregnancy
  4. As a result of increased blood volume, insulin is absorbed more rapidly

200 Mrs. Evans is referred to the clinic nutritionist for nutrition assessment and counseling. The dietary program worked out for her would be:
  1. A low-carbohydrate, low-calorie diet to stay within her present insulin coverage and avoid hyperglycemia
  2. A diet high in protein of good biologic value and decreased calories
  3. Adequate balance of carbohydrate and fat to meet energy demands and prevent ketosis
  4. Insulin adjusted as needed to balance increased dietary needs

201 When Mrs. Evans' newborn is admitted to the newborn nursery, the nurse should be aware that babies of diabetic mothers show symptoms of tremors, apnea, cyanosis, and poor sucking reflex due to:
  1. Congenital depression of islets of Langerhans
  2. Hypoglycemia
  3. Central nervous system edema
  4. Hyperglycemia

202 Mrs. Evans' baby weighs 10 lb, 2 oz, and she is concerned about her size. The nurse should base her reply on the knowledge that babies of diabetic mothers are larger than other babies due to:
  1. Increased somatotropin and lowered glucose utilization
  2. Increased somatotropin and increased glucose utilization
  3. Decreased somatotropin and decreased glucose utilization
  4. Decreased somatotropin and increased glucose utilization

Situation: Mrs. Sawyer suspects she is pregnant when she attends the prenatal clinic for the first time. This is her first pregnancy and she is unsure whether the pregnancy should be terminated, since she and her husband depend on her salary. Questions 203 through 208 refer to this situation.

203 Pregnancy and birth are called crises because:
  1. They are periods of change and adjustment to change
  2. There are hormonal and physiologic changes in the mother
  3. There are mood changes during pregnancy
  4. Narcissism in the mother affects the husband-wife relationship

204 The nurse should intervene to alleviate crisis by:
  1. Involving the mother in preparation classes
  2. Helping the mother express her feelings
  3. Understanding the family interaction
  4. Involving the father in preparation classes

205 The nurse suggests a pregnancy test. This is possible because in early pregnancy the urine contains:
  1. Prolactin
  2. Chorionic gonadotropin
  3. Estrogen
  4. Luteinizing hormone

206 At the time of her second visit to the prenatal clinic Mrs. Sawyer requests information about abortion. She is 8 weeks pregnant at this time. The nurse tells her she feels abortion is immoral and that in her opinion many women had permanent guilt feelings following an abortion. The patient leaves the clinic in a very disturbed state. Legally the:
  1. Nurse had a right to state feelings as long as she identified them as her own
  2. Patient had a right to correct, unbiased information
  3. Physician should have been called in, since the nurse cannot talk about it
  4. Nurse's statements need not be based on scientific knowledge

207 Mrs. Sawyer returns to the clinic after deciding to continue with the pregnancy. She complains of nausea and urinary frequency. She states that she feels punished for her thoughts about abortion. The nurse explains that urinary frequency often occurs because the capacity of the bladder is diminished during pregnancy due to:
  1. Atony of the detrusor muscle
  2. Compression by the ascending uterus
  3. Constriction of the ureteral entrance at the trigone
  4. Compromise of the autonomic reflexes

208 The nurse also informs her that morning sickness is not punishment but is associated with pregnancy and usually ends by the end of the:
  1. Second month
  2. Third month
  3. Fifth month
  4. Fourth mouth

209 The most frequent side effect associated with the use of IUDs is:
1. Rupture of the uterus
2. Excessive menstrual flow
3. Expulsion of the IUD
4. Ectopic pregnancy

210 What is the menopausal implication for women taking oral contraceptives? They:
1. Prolong menses
2. Intensify menopausal symptoms
3. Cause menorrhagia
4. Have no effect on menopause

211 An abandoned infant has been brought to the hospital. Ophthalmia neonatorum is diagnosed. You know the infant's age is:
1. One day
2. Less than 24 hours
3. About 3 to 4 days
4. At least 2 days

Situation: Mrs. Pitis, a 28-year-old primipara, was admitted 8 hours ago, 2 cm dilated in active labor. She is now 3 or 4 cm dilated and the vertex is floating. Questions 212 through 219 refer to this situation.

212 One of the most common causes of hypotonic uterine dystocia is:
1. Toxemia
2. Maternal anemia
3. Pelvic contracture
4. Twin gestation

213 Nursing care would include a careful assessment for signs of maternal exhaustion such as:
1. Circumoral cyanosis
2. Lowered body temperature
3. Fruity odor to breath
4. Skeletal muscle irritability

214 When caring for Mrs. Pitis, who is having a prolonged labor, the nurse must be aware that the patient is very concerned when her labor deviates from what she sees as the norm. A response conveying acceptance of the patient's expressions of frustration and hostility would be:
1. ''Would you like to talk about what's bothering you?''
2. ''All women get weary and frustrated during labor.''
3. ''I'll rub your back; tell me if it helps.''
4. ''I'll leave so you can talk to your husband.''

215 Because Mrs. Pitis has developed secondary uterine inertia, the physician has ordered oxytocin to stimulate contractions. The most important aspect of nursing care at this time is:
1. Monitoring the fetal heart rate
2. Checking perineum for bulging
3. Timing and recording length of contractions
4. Preparing for an emergency cesarean section

216 After a trial labor with oxytocin and x-ray pelvimetry, the physician advises Mrs. Pitis that a cesarean section is necessary. In addition to the routine care given postpartum patients during the first 24 hours, the nurse should:
1. Check the fundus gently but firmly
2. Check vital signs for evidence of shock
3. Maintain IV infusion of oxytocin
4. Encourage early ambulation

217 Two-day-old Andrew Pitis, who weighs 6 lb, is fed Enfamil every 4 hours. Newborns need 2 to 3 oz of fluid per pound of body weight each day. Based on this information, the nurse knows at each feeding to give Andrew at least:
1. 2 to 3 oz
2. 1 to 2 oz
3. 3 to 4 oz
4. 4 to 5 oz

218 Andrew has begun to eat greedily and finishes the entire bottle of formula. Afterward he regurgitates and his mother is concerned. The nurse explains to the mother that this is normal and due to:
1. An undeveloped cardiac sphincter
2. A spasm at the pyloric valve
3. Intake of air while sucking
4. His position after feeding

219 Andrew has just been circumcised. The most essential nursing action the first day is to observe for:
1. Infection
2. Decreased urinary output
3. Shrill, piercing cry
4. Hemorrhage

Situation: Mrs. Coan, 9 months pregnant, is admitted to the hospital with bleeding due to possible placenta previa. The laboratory technician takes blood samples and IV fluids are begun. Questions 220 through 224 refer to this situation.

220 The nurse, following the physician's orders, begins administering oxygen by mask. The patient's apprehension is increasing and she asks the nurse what is happening. The nurse tells her not to worry, that she is going to be all right and everything is under control. The nurse's statements are:
1. Correct, since only the physician should explain why treatments are being done
2. Proper, since the patient's anxieties would be increased if she knew the dangers
3. Adequate, since all preparations are routine and need no explanation
4. Questionable, since the patient has the right to know what treatment is being given and why

221 Nursing care of Mrs. Coan includes:
1. Withholding food and fluids
2. Encouraging ambulation with supervision

3. Inspecting the bed for hemorrhage
4. Avoiding all extraneous stimuli

222 If a vaginal examination is to be performed on Mrs. Coan, the nurse must be prepared for an immediate:
1. Induction of labor
2. Cesarean section
3. Forceps delivery
4. X-ray examination

223 Which of the following should Baby Coan, weighing 6 lb, 4 oz, have daily?
1. Twenty-five ounces of fluid and 450 calories
2. Twenty ounces of fluid and 400 calories
3. Eighteen ounces of fluid and 375 calories
4. Thirty ounces of fluid and 500 calories

224 While working in the newborn nursery, the nurse observes a yellowish color in the skin of Baby Coan. The nurse should immediately:
1. Cover the baby's eyes with a blindfold and put the baby under the ultraviolet light

2. Notify the physician of the development
3. Take a heel blood sample and send it to the laboratory
4. Ascertain the age of the infant

225 If a woman with untreated gonorrhea is allowed to deliver, the infant is in danger of being born with:
1. Ophthalmia neonatorum
2. Congenital syphilis
3. Thrush
4. Pneumonia

226 In observing the newborn infant of a mother untreated for syphilis during the second trimester, the nurse would expect to find:
1. Normal size liver and spleen
2. A cleft palate and harelip
3. Maculopapular lesions of the soles
4. Hypotonicity of skeletal muscles

5 PEDIATRIC NURSING

Pediatric nursing encompasses the care of well and ill children, stressing preventive as well as restorative interventions. This section is divided into the descriptive age groups of childhood, that is, infancy, toddlerhood, preschool years, school-age years, and adolescence. Principles of growth and development, age-specific achievements, health maintenance objectives, and disease-related states are discussed for each age category. Such an organization attempts to present the nursing of children as one that incorporates their physical and psychologic needs toward optimum promotion of health.

BASIC CONCEPTS

A. Children are individuals, not little adults, who must be seen as part of a family
B. Family-centered care is the objective in the care of children to provide total health maintenance
C. Children are influenced by genetic factors, home and environment, and parental attitudes
D. Chronologic and developmental ages of children are the most important contributing factors influencing their care
E. Prevention of illness and maintenance of health are the main thrusts in health care of children
F. Play is a natural medium for expression, communication, and growth in children

THE FAMILY
Structure of family

A. The basic unit of a society
B. Composition varies although one member is usually recognized as head
C. Usually share common goals and beliefs
D. Roles change within the group and reflect both the individual's and the group's needs
E. Status of members determined by position in family in conjunction with views of society

Family functions

A. Reproduction—group developed to reproduce and rear members of a society
B. Maintenance to provide
   1. Clothing, housing, food, and medical care
   2. Social, psychologic, and emotional support for family members
   3. Protection, since immaturity of young children necessitates that care be given by adults
   4. Status—child is a member of a family that is also a part of the larger community
C. Socialization
   1. Child is ''humanized'' by introduction to social situations and instruction in appropriate social behaviors
   2. Self-identity develops through relationships with other family members

Disturbances in parent-child relationships

These can be viewed in terms of disturbed role theory
A. Parental child abuse
B. Maternal deprivation

HUMAN GROWTH AND DEVELOPMENT
Principles of growth

A. Traditional definition of growth is limited to physical maturation

B. Integrated definition includes functional maturation
C. Growth is complex with all aspects closely related
D. Growth is measured both quantitatively and qualitatively over a period of time
E. Although the rate is not even, growth is a continuous and orderly process
   1. Infancy—most rapid period of growth
   2. Preschool to puberty—slow and uniform rate of growth
   3. Puberty—growth spurt
   4. After puberty—decline in growth rate till death
F. There are regular patterns in the direction of growth and development, such as the cephalocaudal law and proximodistal law
G. Different parts of body grow at different rates; e.g.
   1. Prenatally—head grows the fastest
   2. During the first year—elongation of trunk dominates
H. Both rate and pattern of growth can be modified, most obviously by nutrition
I. There are critical periods in growth and development, such as brain growth during uterine life and infancy
J. Although there are specified sequences for achieving growth and development, each individual proceeds at own rate
K. Development is closely related to the maturation of the nervous system; as some primitive reflexes disappear they are replaced by a voluntary activity such as grasp

Characteristics of growth

A. Circulatory system
   1. Heart rate decreases with increasing age
      a. Infancy—130 beats per minute
      b. One year—100 to 110
      c. Childhood—70 to 80
      d. Adolescence to adulthood—60 to 70 (after maturity, women have slightly higher pulse rate than men)
   2. Blood pressure increases with age
      a. Ranges from 20 to 60 mm Hg diastolic to 60 to 90 mm Hg systolic
      b. These levels increase about 2 to 3 mm Hg per year
      c. Systolic pressure in adolescence—higher in males than in females
   3. Hemoglobin
      a. Highest at birth, 17 g, then decreases to 11.5 to 12 g per 100 ml of blood by 1 year

   b. Fetal hemoglobin (60% to 90%) gradually decreases during first year to less than 5% of total hemoglobin
   c. Gradual increase in hemoglobin level to 14.5 g between 1 and 12 years of age
   d. Hemoglobin level higher in males than in females
   e. Red blood cells in children contain less hemoglobin than in adults, but the hemoglobin has greater affinity for oxygen
B. Respiratory system
   1. Rate decreases with increase in age
      a. Infancy—30 to 40 per minute
      b. Childhood—20 to 24 per minute
      c. Adolescence and adulthood—16 to 20 per minute
   2. Vital capacity
      a. Gradual increase throughout childhood and adolescence with a decrease in later life
      b. Capacity in males exceeds that of females
   3. Basal metabolism
      a. Highest rate found in newborn
      b. Rate declines with increase in age, higher in males than females
C. Urinary system
   1. Premature and full-term neonates have some inability to concentrate urine
   2. Glomerular filtration rate greatly increased by 6 months of age
   3. Glomerular filtration rate decreases after 20 years of age
D. Digestive system
   1. Stomach size small at birth, rapidly increases during infancy and childhood
   2. Peristaltic activity decreases with advancing age
   3. Blood sugar levels gradually rise from 75 to 80 mg per 100 ml of blood in infancy to 95 to 100 mg during adolescence
   4. Premature infants have lower blood sugar levels than full-term infants
   5. Enzymes are present at birth to digest proteins and a moderate amount of fat, but only simple sugars (amylase is produced as starch is introduced)
   6. Secretion of hydrochloric acid and salivary enzymes increases with age until adolescence, then decreases with advancing age
E. Nervous system
   1. Brain reaches 90% of total size by 2 years of age

2. All brain cells are present by end of first year, although size and complexity will increase
3. Maturation of brain stem and spinal cord follows cephalocaudal and proximodistal laws

PLAY
Purposes

A. Educational
B. Recreational
C. Physical development
D. Social and emotional adjustment
   1. Learn moral values
   2. Develop idea of sharing
E. Therapeutic

Types

A. Active, physical
   1. Push-and-pull toys
   2. Riding toys
   3. Sports and gym equipment
B. Manipulative, constructive, creative, or scientific
   1. Blocks
   2. Construction toys such as erector sets
   3. Drawing sets
   4. Microscope and chemistry sets
   5. Books
C. Imitative, imaginative, and dramatic
   1. Dolls
   2. Dress-up costumes
   3. Puppets
D. Competitive and social
   1. Games
   2. Role playing

Criteria for judging suitability of toys

A. Safety
B. Compatibility
   1. Child's age
   2. Level of development
   3. Experience
C. Usefulness
   1. Challenge to development of child
   2. Enhancing social and personality development opment
   3. Increasing motor and sensory skills
   4. Developing creativity
   5. Expressing emotions

Criteria for judging nonsuitability of toys

A. Beyond child's level of growth and development
B. Unsafe
C. Overstimulating
D. Limited uses and transient value (see also Play for each age group)

The infant

GROWTH AND DEVELOPMENT
Developmental timetable

A. One month
   1. Physical
      a. Weight—gains about 150 to 210 g (5 to 7 oz) weekly during first 6 months of life
      b. Height—gains about 2.5 cm (1 inch) a month for first 6 months of life
   2. Motor
      a. Head sags, must be supported, may lift head temporarily
      b. Holds head parallel with body when placed prone
      c. Can turn head from side to side when prone or supine
      d. Asymmetric posture dominates, such as tonic neck reflex
      e. Primitive reflexes still present
   3. Sensory
      a. Follows light to midline
      b. Eye movements coordinated most of time
   4. Socialization and vocalization
      a. Smiles indiscriminately
      b. Utters small throaty sounds
B. Two to 3 months
   1. Physical—posterior fontanel closed
   2. Motor
      a. Holds head erect for short period of time and can raise chest supported on forearms
      b. Can carry hand or object to mouth at will
      c. Reaches for attractive object, but misjudges distances
      d. Grasp, tonic neck, and Moro reflexes are fading
      e. Can sit when back is supported; knees will be flexed and back rounded
      f. Step or dance reflex disappears
      g. Plays with fingers and hands

3. Sensory
   a. Follows light to periphery
   b. Has binocular coordination (vertical and horizontal vision)
   c. Listens to sounds
4. Socialization and vocalization
   a. Smiles in response to a person or object
   b. Laughs aloud and shows pleasure in making sounds
   c. Cries less

C. Four to 5 months
   1. Physical—drools because salivary glands are functioning and child has not learned to swallow saliva
   2. Motor
      a. No head lag; balances head well in sitting position
      b. Sits with little support; holds back straight when pulled to sitting position
      c. Symmetrical body position predominates
      d. Can sustain portion of own weight when held in a standing position
      e. Reaches and grasps object with whole hand
      f. Can roll over from back to side
      g. Lifts head and shoulders at a 90 degree angle when prone
      h. Primitive reflexes such as grasp, Moro, and tonic neck have disappeared
   3. Sensory
      a. Recognizes familiar objects and people
      b. Has coupled eye movements, accommodation is developing
      c. Visual acuity about 20/200
   4. Socialization and vocalization
      a. Coos and gurgles when talked to
      b. Definitely enjoys social interaction with people
      c. Vocalizes displeasure when an object is taken away

D. Six to 7 months
   1. Physical
      a. Weight—gains about 90 to 150 g (3 to 5 oz) weekly during second 6 months of life
      b. Height—gains about 1.25 cm (½ inch) a month
      c. Teething may begin with eruption of 2 lower central incisors, followed by upper incisors
   2. Motor
      a. Can turn over equally well from stomach or back

   b. Sits fairly well unsupported, especially if placed in a forward leaning position
   c. Hitches or moves backward when in a sitting position
   d. Can transfer a toy from one hand to the other
   e. Can approach a toy and grasp it with one hand
   f. Plays with feet and puts them in mouth
   g. When lying down, lifts head as if trying to sit up
   h. Transfers everything from hand to mouth
   3. Sensory
      a. Has taste preferences
      b. Will spit out disliked food
   4. Socialization and vocalization
      a. Begins to differentiate between strange and familiar faces and shows "stranger anxiety"
      b. Makes polysyllabic vowel sounds
      c. Vocalizes *m-m-m* when crying
      d. Cries easily on slightest provocation but laughs just as quickly

E. Eight to 9 months
   1. Motor
      a. Sits steadily alone
      b. Has good hand-to-mouth coordination
      c. Developing pincer grasp, with preference for use of one hand over the other
      d. Crawls, then creeps (creeping is more advanced because abdomen is supported off the floor)
      e. Can raise self to a sitting position but may require help to pull self to feet
   2. Sensory
      a. Depth perception is beginning to develop
      b. Displays interest in small objects
   3. Socialization and vocalization
      a. Shows anxiety with strangers by turning or pushing away and crying
      b. Definite social attachment is evident— stretches out arms to loved ones
      c. Is voluntarily separating self from mother by desire to act on own
      d. Reacts to adult anger—cries when scolded
      e. Has imitative and repetitive speech, using vowels and consonants such as *Dada*
      f. No true words as yet, but comprehends words such as *bye-bye*

F. Ten to 12 months
   1. Physical
      a. Has tripled birth weight

  b. Upper and lower lateral incisors usually have erupted, for total of 6 to 8 teeth
  c. Head and chest circumferences are equal
2. Motor
  a. Stands alone for short periods of time
  b. Walks with help—moves around by holding onto furniture
  c. Can sit down from standing position without help
  d. Can eat from a spoon and a cup but needs help, prefers using fingers
  e. Can play pat-a-cake and peek-a-boo
  f. Can hold crayon to make a mark on paper
  g. Helps in dressing, such as putting arm through sleeve
3. Sensory
  a. Visual acuity 20/100
  b. Amblyopia may develop with lack of binocularity
  c. Discriminates simple geometric forms
4. Socialization and vocalization
  a. Shows emotions such as jealousy, affection, anger
  b. Enjoys familiar surroundings and will explore away from mother
  c. Fearful in strange situation or with strangers; clings to mother
  d. May develop habit of ''security'' blanket
  e. Can say 2 words besides *Dada* or *Mama*
  f. Understands simple verbal requests, such as ''Give it to me.''
  g. Knows own name

PLAY DURING INFANCY (SOLITARY PLAY)

A. Mostly used for physical development
B. Toys need to be simple because of short attention span
C. Safety is chief determinant in choosing toys (aspirating small objects is one cause of accidental death)
D. Visual and audio stimulation is important
E. Suggested toys
  1. Rattles
  2. Soft stuffed toys
  3. Mobiles
  4. Push-pull toys
  5. Simple musical toys
  6. Strings of big beads and large snap toys

HEALTH PROMOTION DURING INFANCY
Developmental milestones associated with feeding

A. At birth full-term infant has sucking, rooting, and swallowing reflexes
B. Newborn feels hunger and indicates desire for food by crying
C. By 1 month of age is able to take food from a spoon
D. By 5 to 6 months of age can use fingers in eating zwieback or toast
E. By 6 to 7 months of age is developmentally ready to chew solids
F. By 8 to 9 months of age can hold a spoon and play with it during feeding
G. By 9 months of age can hold own bottle
H. By 12 months of age usually can drink from a cup, although fluid may spill and bottle may be preferred at times

Infant nutrition

A. Nutrition as it affects growth
  1. Birth weight usually doubled by 5 months of age and tripled by 1 year of age (small babies may gain more weight in a shorter period)
  2. Growth during first year should be charted to observe for comparable gain in length, weight, and head circumference
  3. Generally, growth charts demonstrate the percentile of the child's growth rate (below the third and above the ninety-seventh percentile are considered abnormal)
  4. Percentiles of growth curves must be seen in relation to
    a. Deviation from a steady rate of growth
    b. Hereditary factors of parents (size and body shape)
    c. Comparison of height and weight
  5. Satisfactory rate of growth judged by
    a. Weight and length (overweight and underweight constitute malnutrition)
    b. Muscular development
    c. Tissue tone and turgor
    d. General appearance and activity level of child
    e. Amount of crying and needed sleep
    f. Presence or absence of illness
    g. Mental status and behavior in relation to norms for age

B. Proper feeding essential to growth and development of child
   1. General good nutrition that promotes growth but prevents overweight
   2. Prevention of nutritional deficiencies
   3. Prevention of GI disturbances, such as vomiting or constipation
   4. Establishment of good eating habits later in life
   5. Consistency of feedings should progress from liquid to semisoft to soft to solids as dentition and jaw develop

Guidelines for infant feeding

A. Breast milk is most desirable complete diet for first 6 months but requires supplements of vitamin D, iron, and fluoride
B. Iron-fortified commercial formula is an acceptable alternative to breast-feeding; requires fluoride supplements in areas where fluoride content of drinking water is below 0.3 ppm (Table 5-1)
C. Breast milk or commercial formula is recommended for the first year, but after this age infants can be given homogenized vitamin D–fortified whole milk; the use of milk with reduced fat content (skimmed or low-fat) is not recommended because increased quantities of solids would be required to supply the caloric needs, leading to overfeeding
D. Solids can be introduced by about 6 months of age; the first food is usually commercially prepared iron-fortified infant cereals; rice is usually introduced first because of its low allergenic potential; infant cereals should be continued until 18 months of age

Table 5-1. Supplemental fluoride dosage schedule (mg/day*)†

	Concentration of fluoride in drinking water (ppm)		
Age	<0.3	0.3 to 0.7	>0.7
2 weeks to 2 years	0.25	0	0
2 to 3 years	0.50	0.25	0
3 to 16 years	1.00	0.50	0

*2.2 mg sodium fluoride contains 1 mg fluoride.
†From Committee on Nutrition, American Academy of Pediatrics: Fluoride supplementation: revised dosage schedule, Pediatrics **63:**150-152, 1979. Copyright American Academy of Pediatrics 1979.

E. With the exception of infant cereals, the order of introducing other foods is variable; recommended sequence is weekly introduction of other foods such as fruits, followed by vegetables, and then meats; breast-fed infants require more high-protein foods than those fed formula
F. First solid foods are strained, puréed, or finely mashed
G. Finger foods such as toast, zwieback, raw fruit, or crisp-cooked vegetables are introduced at 6 to 7 months
H. Chopped table food or commercially prepared junior foods can be started by 9 to 12 months
I. Fruit juices should be offered from a cup as early as possible to reduce the development of nursing bottle caries
J. Method
   1. Feed when baby is hungry, after a few sucks of breast milk or formula
   2. Introduce 1 food at a time, usually at intervals of 4 to 7 days to allow for identification of food allergies
   3. Begin spoon feeding by pushing food to back of tongue, because of infant's natural tendency to thrust tongue forward
   4. Use small spoon with straight handle; begin with 1 or 2 teaspoons of food; gradually increase to a couple of tablespoons per feeding
   5. As the amount of solid food increases, the quantity of milk needs to be decreased to approximately 900 ml (30 oz) daily to prevent overfeeding
   6. Never introduce foods by mixing them with the formula in the bottle
K. Weaning
   1. Giving up the bottle or breast for a cup is psychologically significant, since it requires the relinquishing of a major source of pleasure
   2. Usually, readiness develops during second half of first year because of
      a. Pleasure from receiving food by a spoon
      b. Increasing desire for more freedom
      c. Acquiring more control over body and environment
   3. Weaning should be gradual, replacing only 1 bottle at a time with a cup and finally ending with the nighttime bottle
   4. If breast-feeding needs to be terminated before 5 or 6 months of age, then a bottle should be used

to allow for the infant's continued sucking needs; after about 6 months wean directly to a cup

L. Diseases or conditions during infancy with possible diet modifications
1. Diarrhea—sterile feedings, decreased fat and carbohydrate
2. Constipation—increased fluids, added prune juice or strained fruit, change in type of carbohydrate
3. Celiac disease (malabsorption syndrome)—sometimes due to gluten sensitivity; diet is low in gluten, which is found in wheat, rye, and oat grains, so these grains are eliminated and rice and corn are substituted
4. Allergy—individual diet modification according to specific food sensitivity; e.g., if milk allergy exists, substitute forms of soybean or meat formula preparations are used
5. Lactose intolerance—found in non-Caucasian races; lactose-free diet used with Nutramigen as a milk substitute
6. Other examples of inborn errors of metabolism
   a. Galactosemia—missing enzyme to convert galactose to glucose, so galactose builds up in blood, leading to mental retardation, liver failure, cataracts; diet is galactose-free with Nutramigen as milk substitute
   b. Phenylketonuria (PKU)—missing enzyme to convert essential amino acid phenylalanine to another amino acid, tyrosine; increase of phenylalanine and abnormal metabolites in blood leads to mental retardation, central nervous system disturbances; diet is low in phenylalanine with milk substitute Lofenalac and calculated food selections from those foods low in phenylalanine

Immunizations (see Tables 5-2 and 5-3)

A. Specific characteristics of immunizations
1. Tetanus toxoid nearly 100% effective, induces prolonged immunity
2. Diphtheria toxoid about 80% effective; febrile reaction more commonly seen in older children, therefore adult type Td given
3. Pertussis vaccine (vaccine of whole organism) is least effective of DTP and has most side effects
   a. Started early since no passive immunity from mother, as with diphtheria and tetanus

Table 5-2. Recommended schedule for active immunization of normal infants and children*

2 mo	DTP[1]	TOPV[2a]
4 mo	DTP	TOPV
6 mo	DTP	[2b]
1 yr		Tuberculin test[3]
15 mo	Measles,[4] rubella[4]	Mumps[4]
1½ yr	DTP	TOPV
4 to 6 yr	DTP	TOPV
14 to 16 yr	Td[5]—repeat every 10 years	

*From American Academy of Pediatrics: Report of the Committee on Infectious Diseases, ed. 18, Evanston, Ill., 1977, The Academy.

[1]DTP—diphtheria and tetanus toxoids combined with pertussis vaccine.

[2a]TOPV—trivalent oral poliovirus vaccine. This recommendation is suitable for breast-fed as well as bottle-fed infants.

[2b]A third dose of TOPV is optional but may be given in areas of high endemicity of poliomyelitis.

[3]Frequency of repeated tuberculin tests depends on risk of exposure of the child and on the prevalence of tuberculosis in the population group. For the pediatrician's office or outpatient clinic, an annual or biennial tuberculin test, unless local circumstances clearly indicate otherwise, is appropriate. The initial test should be done at the time of, or preceding, the measles immunization.

[4]May be given at 15 months as measles-rubella or measles-mumps-rubella combined vaccines. (See further in Report, section 9, pp. 151 and 245.)

[5]Td—combined tetanus and diphtheria toxoids (adult type) for those more than 6 years of age, in contrast to diphtheria and tetanus (DT) toxoids which contain a larger amount of diphtheria antigen. *Tetanus toxoid at time of injury:* For clean, minor wounds, no booster dose is needed by a fully immunized child unless more than 10 years have elapsed since the last dose. For contaminated wounds, a booster dose should be given if more than 5 years have elapsed since the last dose.

Concentration and storage of vaccines

Because the concentration of antigen varies in different products, the manufacturer's package insert should be consulted regarding the volume of individual doses of immunizing agents.

Because biologics are of varying stability, the manufacturer's recommendations for optimal storage conditions (e.g., temperature, light) should be carefully followed. Failure to observe these precautions may significantly reduce the potency and effectiveness of the vaccines.

   b. Not given after child is 4 to 6 years old because of more severe reactions
4. Td, after 4 to 6 years of age, is given routinely every 10 years and at 5-year intervals in the event of a possibly contaminated wound
5. Measles vaccine (live attenuated vaccine) generally is not given before 15 months of age because of the presence of natural immunity from mother
   a. If given before 15 months of age, a second dose should be administered

Table 5-3. Primary immunization for children not immunized in early infancy*†

	Under 6 years of age	6 years of age and over
First visit	DTP, TOPV, tuberculin test	Td, TOPV, tuberculin test
Interval after first visit		
1 mo	Measles,‡ mumps, rubella	Measles, mumps, rubella
2 mo	DTP, TOPV	Td, TOPV
4 mo	DTP, TOPV§	
8 to 14 mo		Td, TOPV
10 to 16 mo or preschool	DTP, TOPV	
Age 14 to 16 yr	Td—repeat every 10 yr	Td—repeat every 10 yr

*From American Academy of Pediatrics: Report of the Committee on Infectious Diseases, ed. 18, Evanston, Ill., 1977, The Academy.
†Physicians may choose to alter the sequence of these schedules if specific infections are prevalent at the time. For example, measles vaccine might be given on the first visit if an epidemic is underway in the community.
‡Measles vaccine is not routinely given before 15 months of age.
§Optional.

    b. Tuberculin testing should be administered before the measles vaccine, since the vaccine can alter the findings
  6. Rubella given to children mainly to prevent occurrence of the disease in women during first trimester of pregnancy
    a. Not given if pregnancy is suspected in the mother because of potential infection of fetus
    b. Pregnancy must be prevented until 2 months after immunization of the child to eliminate danger to fetus
  7. Smallpox no longer routinely recommended in nonendemic areas, since occurrence of fatal and severe reactions to the vaccination outweigh the risk of contracting the disease
B. General contraindications for immunizations
  1. Presence of maternal antibodies
  2. Administration of blood transfusion or immune serum globulin within 6 weeks
  3. High fever, serious illness
  4. Diseases in which immunity is impaired
  5. Immunosuppressive therapy
  6. Generalized malignancy such as leukemia
  7. Allergy to egg protein
  8. Neurologic problems such as convulsions during administration of pertussis vaccine

Accident prevention

A. Accidents are one of the leading causes of death during infancy
  1. Mechanical suffocation causes most accidental deaths in children under 1 year of age
  2. Aspiration of small objects and ingestion of poisonous substances occurs most often during second half of first year and into early childhood
  3. Trauma from rolling off bed or falling down stairs can occur at any time
B. Teaching is an essential aspect—parents should never
  1. Leave plastic bags in crib
  2. Restrain infants with items that may choke them
  3. Leave infants alone on a high surface or near stairs without a proper gate to protect them from danger
  4. Give infant objects with sharp edges or detachable parts that can be swallowed
  5. Take infants in an automobile without restraining them in an infant seat or appropriate carrier
  6. Leave any poisons in a place that crawling infants can explore
  7. Leave burning cigarettes, candles, or incense within infants' reach
  8. Leave electric sockets uncovered or without plastic plugs
  9. Place crib near window where infant can fall or pull on blind cords

Nursing responsibilities for parental guidance during infant's first year

A. Birth
  1. Understand each parent's adjustment to newborn, especially mother's postpartal emotional needs
  2. Teach care of infant and assist parents to understand that infant expresses needs through crying

3. Encourage parents to establish flexible schedule to meet needs of child and themselves

B. First 6 months
1. Help parents understand infant's need for stimulation in environment
2. Support parents' pleasure in seeing child's growing friendliness and social response, especially smiling

C. Second 6 months
1. Prepare parents for child's "stranger anxiety"
2. Encourage parents to allow child to cling to mother or father and avoid long separation from either
3. Guide parents concerning discipline because of infant's increasing mobility
4. Teach accident prevention because of child's motor skills and curiosity
5. Encourage parents to leave child with suitable mother substitute to allow some free time

ACUTE AND CHRONIC HEALTH PROBLEMS
Hospitalization during infancy

A. Reactions to maternal separation (greatest from 6 months to 2 years of age)
1. Protest
   a. Prolonged loud crying, consoled by no one but mother or usual care giver
   b. Continually asks to go home
   c. Rejection of nurse or any other stranger
2. Despair
   a. Alteration in sleep pattern
   b. Decreased appetite and weight loss
   c. Diminished interest in environment and play
   d. Relative immobility and listlessness
   e. No facial expression or smile
   f. Unresponsive to stimuli
3. Detachment or denial
   a. Cheerful undiscriminating friendliness
   b. Lack of preference for parents

B. Prevention of separation anxiety
1. Encourage mother to stay with child in hospital or visit as frequently as possible
2. Provide consistent care giver
3. Provide individual attention, physical touch, sensory stimulation, and affection
4. Prepare mother for child's reaction to separation
5. Involve mother in child's care as much as possible
6. If mother is unable to visit, establish phone contact with her so that she is aware of child's progress and does not feel like a stranger

C. General problems in care of infant
1. Small size of infant
   a. Body warmth and temperature control
   b. Maintenance of fluids—prone to edema, dehydration, and electrolyte imbalance
      (1) Infants have a higher percentage of extracellular fluid than adults, which can be quickly excreted
      (2) Infants' kidneys are unable to concentrate urine
2. Immaturity of organ systems
   a. Primary defense mechanisms just developing—loss of antibodies from fetal life increases infant's susceptibility to infection
      (1) Antibody level lowest at 6 weeks to 2 months of age, then infant begins to develop own system
      (2) Problem subsides as child grows older
   b. Blood vessels are still developing; increased fragility causes hemorrhage
   c. Some essential enzymes such as glucuronyl transferase, which is necessary for conjugation of bilirubin, are still developing—more chance for jaundice and brain damage

Reaction of parents to a defective child

A. Parents exhibit a variety of responses, such as grief and mourning, chronic grief, and excessive use of defense mechanisms

B. Chronic grief
1. Shock and disbelief—parents tend to
   a. Learn about the deformity, but deny the facts
   b. Feel inadequate and guilty
   c. Feel insecure in their ability to care for the child
   d. "Doctor shop" in hope of finding solutions
2. Awareness of the handicap—parents tend to
   a. Feel guilty, angry, and depressed
   b. Envy well children—closely related to bitterness and anger
   c. Search for clues or reasons why this happened to them
   d. Reject and feel ambivalent toward child
3. Restitution or recovery phase—parents tend to
   a. See child's defect in proper perspective
   b. Function more effectively and realistically
   c. Socially and emotionally accept the child

d. Reintegrate family life without centering it around handicapped child

C. Implications for nursing
1. Helping parents gain awareness of child's defect
   a. Learning cannot take place until awareness of problem exists
   b. Help parents develop awareness through their own realization of problem rather than identifying problem for them
   c. Help parents see problem by drawing attention to certain manifestations of problem, such as failure to walk or talk
2. Help parents understand child's potential ability and assist them in setting realistic goals
   a. Help parents feel a sense of adequacy in parenting by emphasizing good care, identifying small steps in learning process of child, and acquainting them with parents of children with similar problems
   b. Teach parents how to work with their handicapped child in simple childhood tasks of walking, talking, toileting, feeding, and dressing
   c. Teach parents how to stimulate child's learning of new skills
3. Encourage parents to treat child as normally as possible
   a. Avoid overprotection and use consistent, simple discipline
   b. Help parents become aware of the effects of this child on siblings who may resent excessive attention given to this child
4. Provide family with an outlet for own emotional tensions and needs
   a. Acquaint them with organizations, especially parent groups, who have children with similar problems
   b. Be a listener, not a preacher
   c. Assist siblings who may fear the possibility of giving birth to children with similar defects

Congenital abnormalities

A. Chromosomal aberrations
1. Down's syndrome, or mongolism
   a. Chromosomal causes
      (1) Trisomy 21—associated with advanced maternal age (about a 2% risk over age of 40); can occur earlier
      (2) Translocation 15/21—translocated chromosome transmitted by mother who is a carrier; age is not a factor
      (3) Mosaicism—mixture of normal cells and cells trisomic for 21
   b. Resulting defects
      (1) Hypotonia
      (2) Congenital heart defects, particularly atrioventricular defects
      (3) Mental retardation—IQ frequently within trainable range
   c. Nursing considerations
      (1) Emotional support of parents
      (2) Genetic counseling appropriate for type of defect
      (3) Assist parents to set realistic expectations and goals for the child
      (4) Prevention of infection, especially respiratory
      (5) Activity consistent with defects
      (6) Physical supervision and habilitation
      (7) Careful testing of intellectual functioning for guidance
      (8) Same principles as in care of child with mental retardation and birth of a defective child
2. Trisomy 18
   a. Several physical anomalies of head, ears, mandible, hands, feet, heart, and kidneys
   b. Failure to thrive and short survival; if survive, severe mental retardation
   c. Nursing considerations
      (1) Genetic counseling
      (2) Because of short survival, preparation of parents for loss of their child
3. Turner's syndrome (gonadal dysgenesis)
   a. Chromosome monosomy (XO karyotype)
   b. Congenital malformations such as short stature, webbed neck, infantile genitalia, and developmental failure of secondary sexual characteristics at puberty
   c. Usually normal intelligence; problems in directional sense and space-form recognition
   d. Nursing considerations
      (1) Genetic counseling of parents
      (2) Preparation of child for lack of pubertal changes and need for hormonal replacement
      (3) Counseling with emphasis on adoption rather than person's inability to conceive

4. Klinefelter's syndrome
    a. Sex-chromosomal abnormality of XXY
    b. Physical characteristics—tall, skinny, long legs and arms, small firm testes, gynecomastia, and poorly developed secondary sex characteristics at puberty
    c. Behavioral disorders and mental defects are often present
    d. Nursing considerations
        (1) Counseling with emphasis on positive aspects such as adoption or donor insemination
        (2) May also be larger problem of psychopathology with need for counseling

B. Malformations (structural anomalies present at birth)
    1. Facial malformations
        a. Failure of union of embryonic structure of face
            (1) Fusion of maxillary and premaxillary processes between 5 and 8 weeks of fetal life
            (2) Palatal structures fuse between 9 and 12 weeks
        b. Cause unknown, evidence of hereditary influence
            (1) Incidence in general population is 1 in 800 births
            (2) If one child is born with cleft lip or palate but no history of anomaly in family, next child's chances are 1 in 150
            (3) If history of either anomaly in family and one child was born with it, next sibling has chance of 1 in 4
    2. Cleft lip
        a. Bilateral or unilateral; if unilateral, more common on left side
        b. More common in males
        c. Can be of several degrees; complete cleft is usually continuous with cleft palate
        d. Treatment is surgical repair, usually done soon after birth because of psychologic difficulties of parents associated with visual effects of defect and child's inability to meet sucking needs
        e. Nursing difficulties and interventions
            (1) Main difficulty is feeding
                (a) Child cannot form vacuum in mouth to suck
                (b) Should be fed with soft, large-holed nipple or rubber-tipped syringe

placed on top and side of tongue, toward back of mouth
                (c) Should be bubbled frequently because of swallowed air
            (2) Problem of swallowed air (mouth breather)
                (a) Distended abdomen, pressure against diaphragm
                (b) Mucous membranes of oropharynx become dried and cracked, leading to infection
                (c) Parent should be taught to give water after each feeding to cleanse mouth
            (3) Problem of infection from irritation of lip
                (a) Infant's hands may need restraining
                (b) May need pacifier to increase sucking pleasure
        f. Postoperative nursing care
            (1) Maintain patient airway
                (a) Problem because of edema of nose, tongue, and lips combined with child's habit of breathing through the mouth
                (b) Proper equipment such as laryngoscope, endotracheal tube, and suction at or near bedside
            (2) Cleanse suture line to prevent crust formation and eventual scarring
            (3) Prevent crying because of pressure on suture line (encourage parent to stay with infant)
            (4) Place child in supine position with arm or elbow restraints
                (a) Change position to side or sitting up to prevent hypostatic pneumonia
                (b) Remove restraints only when supervised
            (5) Feeding (same as before surgery)
            (6) Support parents by accepting and treating child as normal
    3. Cleft palate
        a. More common in girls
        b. May involve soft or hard palate and may extend into nose, forming oronasal passageway
        c. Age for repair is usually after child has grown, but before speech is well developed
        d. Nursing problems and interventions (only differences from cleft lip will be discussed)
            (1) Feeding

(a) Feed upright to prevent aspiration
(b) In severe cases, gavage feeding may be necessary
(c) Encourage early use of spoon and cup
(2) Infection, especially aspiration pneumonia
(3) Speech
    (a) Palate is needed to trap air in mouth
    (b) Tonsils usually not removed because they provide an additional mechanism to trap air
    (c) Child will need speech appliance to help prevent guttural sounds if repair is delayed beyond speech development
(4) Dental development
    (a) Excessive dental caries
    (b) Malocclusion from displacement of maxillary arch
    (c) Need for proper dental hygiene and regular dental supervision
(5) Hearing problems caused by recurrent otitis media (eustachian tube connects the nasopharynx and middle ear and easily transports foreign material to ear)
  e. Postoperative nursing care—same as for cleft lip except
(1) In maintaining patent airway, try to avoid use of suction that traumatizes operative site
(2) Place child in prone Trendelenburg position to prevent aspiration and promote postural drainage
(3) Avoid trauma to suture line by instructing child not to rub tongue on roof of mouth
(4) Feeding
    (a) Liquid diet; no milk because of curd formation on suture line
    (b) Avoid use of straw or spoon
(5) Need for emotional support of parents is greater, since recovery is longer and prognosis uncertain
4. Tracheoesophageal anomalies
  a. Absence of esophagus
  b. Atresia of the esophagus without a tracheal fistula
  c. Tracheoesophageal fistula
  d. The most common type of anomaly is proximal esophageal atresia combined with distal tracheoesophageal fistula

  e. Signs and symptoms
(1) Excessive drooling
(2) Excessive mucus in nasopharynx causing cyanosis, which is easily reversed by suctioning
(3) Choking, sneezing, and coughing during feeding, with regurgitation of formula through mouth and nose
(4) Inability to pass catheter into stomach
  f. Treatment—surgical correction
  g. Postoperative nursing care
(1) Frequent suctioning of mouth and pharynx
(2) Provision of high humidity to liquefy thick secretions
(3) Stimulation of crying and change of position to prevent pneumonia
(4) Proper care of chest tubes if used
(5) Maintenance of nutrition by oral, parenteral, or gastrostomy method
(6) Use of pacifier if oral feedings are contraindicated
(7) Need for comfort and physical contact because hospitalization is usually long
5. Intestinal anomalies
  a. Intestinal obstruction
(1) Signs alerting nurse to life-threatening obstruction
    (a) Abdominal distention
    (b) Absence of stools, especially meconium in newborn
    (c) Vomiting of bile-stained material that may be projectile
    (d) Cyanosis and weak grunting respirations from abdominal distention, causing diaphragm to compress lungs
    (e) Paroxysmal pain
    (f) Weak thready pulse
  b. Imperforate anus
(1) Most common intestinal anomaly
(2) Failure of membrane separating rectum from anus to absorb during eighth week of fetal life
(3) Fistulas within vagina, urinary tract, or scrotum are common
(4) Diagnosed by
    (a) Failure to pass meconium stool
    (b) Inability to insert thermometer or small finger into rectum
    (c) Abdominal distention

(5) Treatment—immediate surgical correction unless fistula is present
(6) Postoperative nursing care—dependent on type of surgery performed
    (a) Keep operative sites clean and dry, especially after passage of stool
    (b) If perineal sutures are present, position infant on side rather than abdomen to prevent pulling legs up under chest
    (c) Care of colostomy—prevent excoriation of skin by frequent cleansing and use of diaper held on by belly binder
    (d) Instruct parent about colostomy care (include avoidance of tight diapers and clothes around abdomen)

c. Diaphragmatic hernia
(1) Protrusion of abdominal viscera through opening into thoracic cavity
(2) Symptoms alerting nurse
    (a) Severe respiratory difficulty with cyanosis
    (b) Relatively large chest, especially on affected side
    (c) Failure of affected side of chest to expand during respiration and absence of breath sounds
    (d) Relatively small abdomen
(3) Treatment—immediate surgical repair
(4) Nursing care
    (a) Gastric suction is used to remove secretions and swallowed air from stomach and intestine before and after surgery
    (b) Preoperatively, to allow full expansion of unaffected side, position infant with head elevated on affected side
    (c) Postoperatively, to decrease chance of swallowing air, infant may be fed by gavage

6. Congenital laryngeal stridor (laryngomalacia)
  a. A crowing sound during inspiration caused by different factors, most often it is related flabbiness of the epiglottis
  b. May correct itself as infant grows, or may necessitate tracheostomy to sustain life
  c. Nursing problems and interventions

(1) Feeding
    (a) Infant must be fed slowly; stop frequently to allow breathing and then reoffer bottle or breast
    (b) Proper nipple hole size and position at breast important to regulate flow
    (c) Parent needs help to learn correct feeding method
(2) Breathing
    (a) Parents should be encouraged to listen to sound of stridor to detect a change
    (b) Needs to be protected from respiratory tract infection, which increases breathing difficulty

7. Choanal atresia
  a. Embryonic membrane obstructs posterior nares at junction with nasopharynx
  b. Bilateral obstruction causes mouth breathing and dyspnea that is relieved by crying and aggravated by sucking
  c. Nursing problems and interventions are the same as for laryngeal stridor

8. Congenital heart defects
  a. Normal circulatory changes that occur at or shortly after birth
    (1) Pulmonary circulation rapidly increases
    (2) Increased pressure from left side of heart results in closure of foramen ovale, ductus arteriosus, and ductus venosus
  b. General signs and symptoms of congenital heart defects in children
    (1) Dyspnea, especially on exertion
    (2) Feeding difficulty and failure to thrive often first signs discovered by mother
    (3) Stridor or choking spells
    (4) Heart rate over 200, respiratory rate about 60 in infant
    (5) Recurrent respiratory tract infections
    (6) In older child, poor physical development, delayed milestones, and decreased exercise tolerance
    (7) Cyanosis, squatting, and clubbing of fingers and toes
    (8) Heart murmurs
    (9) Excessive perspiration
  c. Classification of cardiac lesions
    (1) Acyanotic—shunt from left to right side of heart
      (a) No abnormal communication between pulmonary and systemic circulation

(b) If such a connection exists, pressure forces blood from arterial to venous side of heart, where it is reoxygenated

(2) Cyanotic—shunt from right to left side of heart

    (a) Abnormal connection between pulmonary and systemic circulation

    (b) Venous or unoxygenated blood enters systemic circulation

    (c) Polycythemia (increase in number of red blood cells) occurs as body tries to compensate for inadequate supply of oxygen

    (d) Squatting or knee-chest position is preferred because it decreases venous return by occluding the femoral veins, thus lessening the work load on the right side of the heart and increasing arterial oxygen saturation

    (e) Compensation and nature of defect cause clubbing of fingers and toes, retarded growth, increased viscosity of blood, and can lead to congestive heart failure

d. Types of acyanotic defects

  (1) Ventricular septal defect (VSD)

    (a) Abnormal opening between the 2 ventricles

    (b) Severity of defect depends on size of opening

    (c) High pressure in right ventricle causes hypertrophy, with development of pulmonary hypertension

    (d) Blowing type murmur heard throughout systole

    (e) Treatment procedure—close opening in septum

  (2) Atrial septal defect (ASD)—3 types

    (a) Ostium secondum defect, in which the foramen ovale fails to close

    (b) Ostium primum defect, in which there is inadequate development of the endocardial cushions

    (c) Sinus venosus defect, in which the superior portion of the atrial septum fails to form

    (d) Murmur heard high on chest, with fixed splitting of second heart sound

    (e) Treatment procedure—close opening in septum

(3) Patent ductus arteriosus (PDA)

    (a) Failure of closure of fetal connection between aorta and pulmonary artery

    (b) Blood shunted from aorta back to pulmonary artery; may progress to pulmonary hypertension and cardiomegaly

    (c) Machinery type murmur heard throughout heartbeat in left second or third interspace

    (d) Treatment procedure—close opening between aorta and pulmonary artery

(4) Coarctation of aorta

    (a) In utero, failure of aorta to develop completely; stricture usually occurs below level of aortic arch

    (b) Increased systemic circulation above stricture—bounding radial and carotid pulses, headache, dizziness, epistaxis

    (c) Decreased systemic circulation below stricture—absent femoral pulses, cool lower extremities

    (d) Increased pressure in aorta above defect causes left ventricular hypertrophy

    (e) Murmur may or may not be heard

    (f) Treatment procedure—resection of defect and anastomoses of the ends of the aorta

(5) Aortic stenosis

    (a) Narrowing of aortic valve

    (b) Causes increased work load on left ventricle, and lowered pressure base of aorta reduces coronary artery flow

    (c) Treatment procedures—divide the stenotic valves of the aorta or dilate the constricting ring

(6) Pulmonary stenosis

    (a) Narrowing of pulmonary valve

    (b) Causes decreased blood flow to lungs and increased pressure to right ventricle

    (c) Treatment procedures—valvulotomy or mechanical dilation

e. Types of cyanotic defects

  (1) Tetralogy of Fallot—4 associated defects

    (a) Pulmonary valve stenosis

    (b) Ventricular septal defect, usually high on septum

    (c) Overriding aorta, receiving blood

from both ventricles, or an aorta arising from right ventricle

(d) Right ventricular hypertrophy

(e) Treatment procedures—Waterston-Cooley procedure: aortic to pulmonary artery anastomosis; or Blalock-Taussig procedure: subclavian artery to pulmonary artery anastomosis

(2) Transposition of the great vessels

(a) Aorta arises from the right ventricle, and pulmonary artery arises from the left ventricle

(b) Incompatible with life unless there is a communication between the 2 sides of the heart, such as an atrial septal defect, ventricular septal defect, or a patent ductus arteriosus

(c) Treatment procedures—Rashkind procedure: nonsurgical creation of an atrial septal defect at the foramen ovale through the use of a cardiac catheterization balloon; Blalock-Hanlon procedure: surgical creation of an atrial septal defect; or Mustard procedure: complete surgical repair with creation of 2 new, functionally correct atrial chambers

(3) Tricuspid atresia

(a) Absence of tricuspid valve

(b) Incompatible with life unless there is a communication between 2 sides of heart, such as atrial septal defect, ventricular septal defect, or patent ductus arteriosus

(c) Palliative treatment procedures—Blalock, Potts, or Glen procedure: anastomosis of superior vena cava to right pulmonary artery

(d) Total correction—conversion of right atrium into outlet for pulmonary artery

(4) Truncus arteriosus

(a) Single great vessel arising from base of heart, serving as pulmonary artery and aorta

(b) Systolic murmur is heard, and single semilunar valve produces a loud second heart sound that is not split

(c) Palliative treatment—banding pulmo-nary arteries as they arise from truncus to decrease blood flow to lungs

(d) Rastelli's operation—corrective treatment involves excising pulmonary arteries from aorta and attaching them to right ventricle by means of a prosthetic valve conduit; septal defects also repaired

f. Treatment—besides surgical intervention, digitalization can be used to increase the efficiency of heart action

(1) Positive inotropic action is achieved by increasing permeability of muscle membranes to the calcium and sodium ions required for contraction of muscle fibrils

(a) Forceful contraction during systole improves peripheral tissue perfusion

(b) Chamber emptying allows additional venous blood to enter cardiac chambers during diastole

(2) Negative chronotropic effect is achieved by an action mediated by the vagus nerve that slows firing of the sinoatrial (SA) node and impulse transmission through the atrioventricular (AV) node (negative dromotropic action)

(3) Preparations have the same qualitative action on the heart but differ in potency, rate of absorption, amount of drug absorbed, onset of action, speed of elimination

(a) Digitalis—longer onset, peak action, and half-life

(b) Digoxin (Lanoxin)—rapid onset and peak action and short half-life; drug of choice in children, especially because risk of toxicity is lessened due to shorter half-life

(4) Digitalization

(a) Provides an initial loading dose for acute effect on the enlarged heart

(b) After desired effect is achieved, the dosage is lowered to maintainance level, replacing drug metabolized and excreted each day

(5) Adverse effects

(a) Most frequent—nausea, vomiting, headache, drowsiness, insomnia, vertigo, confusion are all attributable to drug action at central nervous system sites; oral forms also cause nausea and vomiting by irritation of gastric mucosa

(b) Bradycardia attributable to drug-induced slowing of SA node firing

(c) Arrhythmias are first evidence of toxicity in one third of patients; premature nodal or ventricular impulses; varying degrees of heart block caused by drug action that slows transmission of impulses through the AV node

(d) Xanthopsia (yellow vision) caused by drug effect on visual cones

(e) Gynecomastia (mammary enlargement) in males resulting from estrogen-like steroid portion of digitalis glycosides

(6) Considerations during therapy

(a) Premature contractions elevate the audible apical rate and mask the pacemaker conduction rate; apical pulse is taken before administration and drug is withheld when pulse rate drops to 110 to 90 in infants and below 70 in older children

(b) Immaturity of hepatic and renal systems in premature and newborn infants or depressed hepatic or renal function in children may result in cumulation

(c) Since potassium ions are required for interaction of digitalis glycosides with sodium-potassium dependent membranes, the lowering of serum levels of potassium ions may foster digitalis toxicity

(d) Since calcium ions act synergistically with digitalis on myocardial membranes, an elevation of serum calcium ion levels may increase sensitivity of cardiac muscle to digitalis action

(7) Drug interactions

(a) Phenobarbital, phenytoin, and phenylbutazone, by induction of hepatic microsomal enzymes, accelerate metabolism of digitalis glycosides, and serum levels are lower when the drugs are used concomitantly

(b) Diuretics that cause hypokalemia may contribute to the incidence of serious arrhythmias when administered concurrently with digitalis glycosides; supplemental potassium may be used for replacement of losses, or potassium-sparing diuretics may be prescribed to prevent potassium ion losses

g. Nursing responsibilities

(1) Correctly calculate dosage of digoxin; usually prescribed in micrograms; 1000 $\mu g = 1$ mg

(2) Take apical pulse prior to administering drug

(3) Observe for signs of digitalis toxicity

(4) Teach parents home administration of digoxin

h. Preoperative preparation

(1) Main assessment factor in preparation of child is the developmental and chronologic age, for example

(a) Explanation of heart differs according to age of child

(b) Children 4 to 6 years of age know heart is in chest, describe it as valentine shaped, and characterize its function by the sound of "tick-tock"

(c) Children 7 to 10 years of age, do not see heart as valentine shaped, know it has veins, have idea of function such as "It makes you live," but do not understand concept of pumping

(d) Children over 10 years of age have concept of veins, valves, circulation, and why death occurs when heart stops

(2) Based on principle that fear of unknown increases anxiety

(3) The same nurse should participate in preoperative and postoperative preparation as source of support for child

(4) Nurse must know what equipment is usual after open or closed heart surgery

(5) Let child play with equipment such as stethoscope, blood pressure machine, oxygen mask, suction, syringes

(6) For young child, especially preschooler, use dolls and puppets to describe procedures

(7) Preparation for cardiac catheterization prior to surgery is essential as well

(8) For young child, talk about size of bandage; for older child, discuss actual incision

(9) Familiarize child with postoperative environment such as recovery room and intensive care unit, stressing the strange noises such as the monitors

(10) Have child practice coughing, using blow bottles and breathing on intermittent positive pressure machine

(11) Explain to child why coughing and moving are necessary even though they will hurt

(12) Explain to child what tubes may be used and what they will look like

(13) For more specific discussion of the aforementioned, see specific age groups under Pediatric nursing

i. Preoperative assessment areas necessary for planning postoperative care

(1) Keep sleep record so care can be organized around child's usual rest pattern

(2) Constipation and straining after surgery must be avoided—this can be accomplished by

(a) Knowing child's elimination pattern

(b) Knowing words child uses

(c) Having child practice using bedpan

(3) Record level of activity and list favorite toys or games that require gradually increased exertion

(4) Determine child's fluid preferences for postoperative maintenance

(5) When recording vital signs, always indicate child's activity at the time of measurement

(6) Observe child's verbal and nonverbal responses to pain

(7) Specifics of postoperative care are similar to those for any major surgery

j. Adjustment of child and family to correction of cardiac defect

(1) Improved physical status is often difficult for the child who has become accustomed to the sick role and its secondary gains

(2) Improved physical status of the child is also difficult for the parents, since it reduces child's dependency

(3) Child may have difficulty learning to relate to peers and siblings on a competitive basis

(4) Child can no longer use disability as a crutch for educational and social shortcomings

(5) Parental expectations must be adjusted to accommodate child's new physical vigor and search for independence

9. Spina bifida

a. Malformation of the spine in which posterior portion of laminae of vertebrae fails to close; most common site is lumbosacral area

(1) Spina bifida occulta—defect only of vertebrae; spinal cord and meninges are intact

(2) Meningocele—meninges protrude through vertebral defect

(3) Meningomyelocele—meninges and spinal cord protrude through defect; most serious type

b. Associated defects include weakness or paralysis below defect, bowel and bladder dysfunction clubfeet, dislocated hip, and hydrocephalus

c. Arnold-Chiari syndrome—defect of occipitocervical region with swelling and displacement of medulla into the spinal cord

d. Nursing problems and intervention (meningomyelocele)

(1) Infection because breakdown of sac leaves spinal cord open to environment

(a) Area must be kept clean, especially from urine and feces

(b) Diaper is not used, but sterile gauze with antibiotic solution may be placed over sac

(2) Associated orthopedic defects

(a) Maintain function through proper position, which also decreases pressure on sac

(b) Clubfeet and dislocated hip—prone position, hips slightly flexed and abducted, feet hanging free of mattress, and slight Trendelenburg slope to reduce spinal fluid pressure

(3) Feeding because of restriction in position

(a) Must be fed prone; nurse should establish eye contact and encourage parents to visit and feed child

(b) If solids need to be introduced while infant still prone, may be mixed with formula in bottle with large-hole nipple

(4) Elimination, especially of neurogenic bladder

(a) Credé method or slight pressure against abdomen may be necessary to fully empty bladder

(b) While infant is prone, nurse can apply pressure to abdomen above symphysis pubis with sides of fingers and counterpressure with thumbs against buttocks

e. Postoperative nursing care

(1) Surgical repair of the sac may be done soon after birth to prevent infection and maintain neurologic function

(2) Care is same as for cardiac surgery, with emphasis on habilitation of child's abilities

(3) Head size should be measured to determine whether hydrocephalus is occurring

10. Hydrocephalus

a. Abnormal accumulation of cerebrospinal fluid within ventricular system

(1) Noncommunicating—obstruction within the ventricles such as congenital malformation, neoplasm, or hematoma

(2) Communicating—inadequate absorption of CSF resulting from infection or trauma

b. Clinical signs

(1) Increasing head size in infant because of open sutures and bulging fontanels

(2) Prominent scalp veins and taut shiny skin

(3) Sunset eyes (sclera visible above iris), bulging eyes, and papilledema of retina

(4) Head lag, especially important after 4 to 6 months

(5) Increased intracranial pressure—projectile vomiting not associated with feeding, irritability, anorexia, high shrill cry, convulsions

(6) Damage to brain because increased pressure decreases blood flow to cells, causing necrosis

c. Treatment

(1) Removal of obstruction

(2) Mechanical shunting of fluid to another area of body

(a) Ventriculoatrial shunt—catheter from lateral ventricle to internal jugular vein to right atrium of heart

(b) Ventriculoperitoneal shunt—catheter is passed subcutaneously to peritoneal cavity

d. General nursing problems and intervention

(1) Breakdown of scalp, infection, and damage to spinal cord

(a) Proper positioning—place in Fowler's position to facilitate draining of fluid, postoperatively positioned flat with no pressure on shunted side

(b) When held, neck and head must be supported

(c) Observe shunt site (abdominal site in peritoneal procedure) for infection

(2) Increasing intracranial pressure

(a) Careful observation, minimal use of sedatives or analgesics, which can mask signs

(b) Frequent checking of valve for patency

(c) Pumping valve per physician's orders to ensure proper functioning

(3) Nutrition

(a) Frequent vomiting, irritability, lethargy, and anorexia decrease intake of nutrients

(b) All care should be done before feeding to prevent vomiting; infant should be held if possible

(c) Observe for signs of dehydration

(4) Irritation of eyes if eyelid incompletely covers cornea

e. Specific postoperative nursing care—similar to that for cardiac surgery except

(1) Child is usually kept in bed after surgery with minimal handling to prevent damage to shunt

(2) Parents need much support

(a) Continued shunt revisions are usually necessary as growth occurs

(b) Usually very concerned about retardation

(3) Observe for brain damage by recording milestones during infancy

(4) Parental teaching must include

(a) Pumping of shunt

(b) Signs of increasing intracranial pressure

(c) Evidence of dehydration

11. Exstrophy of the bladder

a. Entire lower urinary tract from bladder to external urethral meatus is outside abdominal cavity

b. May be accompanied by defects such as epispadias, undescended testes, or short penis in boys and a cleft clitoris or absent vagina in girls

c. Treatment

(1) Plastic surgery

(2) Sigmoid implantation of ureters—may be complicated by

(a) Ascending infection (pyelonephritis from colon bacilli)

(b) Hydronephrosis from backup of urine into kidneys

(c) Electrolyte imbalance

d. Nursing problems and intervention

(1) Parental teaching is vital, but objectives can only be achieved after parents have accepted both the disorder and the long-term sequelae

(2) Infection and care of skin

(a) Scrupulous cleansing of area, application of sterile petroleum gauze, and care of skin around bladder

(b) Clothing should be light to avoid pressure over area

(c) Frequent change of clothing because of odor

(3) Control of urination in sigmoid implantation

(a) When old enough to control bowels, child can learn to tighten anal sphincter to prevent seepage of urine

(b) Parents need encouragement because accidents are common

12. Displacement of urethral opening

a. Hypospadias

(1) In boy, urethra opens on lower surface of penis from just behind the glans to the perineum

(2) In girl, urethra opens into the vagina

b. Epispadias

(1) Occurs only in boys

(2) Urethra opens on dorsal surface of penis, often associated with exstrophy of bladder

c. Nursing considerations

(1) Repair is usually of concern to parents, who need explicit explanation of child's future functioning

(2) Repair may be in several stages for boy, who needs preparation for surgery and help in coping with adjustment to voiding in a sitting position

(3) Defect can be sign of ambiguous genitalia

(4) Procreation may be interfered with in severe cases

13. Orthopedic deformities

a. Clubfoot

(1) Foot has been twisted out of position in utero

(2) Most common type—talipes equinovarus: foot is fixed in plantar flexion (downward) and deviates medially (inward)

(3) Treatment is most successful when started early, since delay causes muscles and bones of legs to develop abnormally, with shortening of tendons

(4) Treatment and nursing measures in infancy

(a) Denis Browne splint (appliance of a crossbar with shoes attached)

[1] Encourage activity since success of appliance depends on alternate kicking and extension of baby's legs

[2] Watch for circulatory impairment caused by swelling around ankles

[3] Pick up child frequently to prevent respiratory and other problems from immobility

(b) Gentle repeated manipulation of foot or forcible correction under anesthesia and application of a wedge cast
  [1] Observe toes for signs of circulatory impairment; make sure toes are visible at end of cast
  [2] Watch for signs of weakness and wear of cast, especially if child is allowed to walk on it
  [3] For other areas of cast care, see treatment of dislocated hip
  [4] Main nursing objective is teaching parents all of aforementioned, stressing need for follow-up care, which may be prolonged
(5) Follow-up care of patient
  (a) Extended medical supervision is required, since there is a tendency for this deformity to recur (considered cured when child able to wear normal shoes and walk properly)
  (b) Care emphasizes muscle reeducation (by manipulation) and proper walking
  (c) Heels and soles of braces or shoes prescribed following correction must be kept in repair
  (d) Corrective shoes may have sole and heel lifts on lateral border to maintain proper position

b. Dislocated hip
  (1) Trochanter (head of femur) does not lie deep enough inside the acetabulum and slips out on movement (may be caused by lack of embryonic development of joint)
  (2) Main clinical signs
    (a) Limitation in abduction of leg on affected side
    (b) Asymmetry of gluteal, popliteal, and thigh folds
    (c) Ortolani's sign—an audible click when abducting the leg on the affected side
    (d) Apparent shortening of the femur—Galeazzi's sign
    (e) Waddling gait and lordosis when child begins to walk

  (3) Treatment—directed toward enlarging and deepening the socket by placing the trochanter within the acetabulum and applying constant pressure
    (a) Proper positioning—legs slightly flexed and abducted
      [1] Frejka pillow—a pillow splint that maintains abduction of legs
      [2] Use of pillow or rolled diapers between legs
      [3] Bryant's traction
      [4] Spica cast—body cast from waist to below knee
    (b) Surgical intervention such as open reduction with casting
  (4) Specific nursing problems and intervention when spica cast is applied
    (a) Respiratory problems—hypostatic pneumonia
      [1] Need to change position from back to stomach frequently
      [2] Teach parents postural drainage and exercises such as blowing bubbles to increase lung expansion
      [3] Encourage parents to seek immediate medical care if child develops congestion or cough
    (b) Infection and excoriation of skin
      [1] Observe for circulation of toes, pedal pulses, and blanching
      [2] Do not let child put small toys or food inside cast
      [3] Gauze strips may be used inside cast as a scratcher
      [4] Alert parents to signs of infection such as odor
      [5] Protect cast edges with adhesive tape or waterproof material, especially around perineum
      [6] Minimize soiling of cast by feces and urine by using diapers and plastic lining
    (c) Constipation from immobility
      [1] Parents should observe for straining on defecation and constipation
      [2] Increase fluids and roughage to prevent constipation

(d) Nutrition
  [1] Provide small, frequent meals because of inflexibility of cast around waist
  [2] Adjust calorie intake, since less energy expenditure can lead to obesity
(e) Transportation and positioning
  [1] Use wagon or stroller with back flat
  [2] Protect child from falling when positioned
  [3] Child must not be picked up by bar between cast (use 2 people to provide adequate body support if necessary)
(f) Emotional needs
  [1] Since child cannot be picked up and cuddled, touch should be used as much as possible
  [2] Stimulate and provide for play activities appropriate to age
(g) Parents need help and support
  [1] Directions should be written
  [2] Home visits should be routine, with telephone counseling available
  [3] Treatment may be prolonged, so follow-up care must be stressed
  [4] Prepare parents for the possible use of an abduction brace after the cast is removed
c. Developmental anomalies of the extremities
  (1) Polydactyly—extra digits
  (2) Syndactyly—partial or complete fusion of 2 or more digits
  (3) Amelia—absence of a limb
  (4) Treatment—if possible, early correction and preparation for use of prosthesis
  (5) Nursing considerations
    (a) Recognize own reaction to deformity
    (b) Accept parents' reactions of guilt, anger, and hopelessness
    (c) Assist parents to set realistic goals for child
    (d) Prepare parents to answer child's questions about the deformity and what it will mean in the future
C. Inborn errors of metabolism

1. Phenylketonuria (PKU)
  a. Lack of enzyme phenylalanine hydroxylase, which changes phenylalanine (essential amino acid) into tyrosine
  b. Transmitted by autosomal recessive gene
  c. Clinical symptoms
    (1) Mental retardation, from damage to nervous system from build up of phenylalanine
      (a) Usually noticed by 4 months of age
      (b) IQ is usually below 50 and most frequently under 20
    (2) Strong musty odor in urine from phenylacetic acid
    (3) Absence of tyrosine reduces production of melanin and results in blond hair and blue eyes
    (4) Fair skin is susceptible to eczema
  d. Treatment
    (1) Prevention—test for PKU at birth
      (a) Guthrie blood test—effective in newborns, provided they have ingested a milk diet for 4 days
      (b) Ferric chloride urine test—only effective when infant is over 6 weeks of age
    (2) Dietary—low-phenylalanine diet: use Lofenalac as a milk substitute and foods restricted to those low in this amino acid (usually continued until child is 6 years of age)
  e. Nursing considerations
    (1) Parents need help in understanding the disease and the role of the diet
    (2) Genetic counseling
2. Galactosemia
  a. Missing enzyme that converts galactose to glucose
  b. Transmitted by autosomal recessive gene
  c. Treatment—dietary, reduction of lactose; use Nutramigen as a milk substitute and foods restricted to those low in lactose (usually continued until child is 3 years of age)
  d. Nursing considerations similar to those for phenylketonuria

Noncongenital conditions

A. Surgical problems
  1. Pyloric stenosis

a. Congenital hypertrophy of muscular tissue of pyloric sphincter, which usually is asymptomatic until 2 to 4 weeks after birth

b. Clinical signs
   (1) Vomiting, progressively projectile
   (2) Nonbile stained vomitus
   (3) Constipation
   (4) Dehydration and weight loss
   (5) Distention of epigastrium, visible peristalsis, and palpable olive-shaped mass in right upper quadrant

c. Treatment is usually surgical—the Fredet-Ramstedt procedure (longitudinal splitting of hypertrophied muscle)

d. Postoperative nursing care
   (1) Same as that for any abdominal surgery
   (2) Teach parents specific feeding method
      (a) Give small frequent feedings and feed slowly
      (b) Hold baby in high Fowler's position during feeding and place on right side after feeding with head of bed slightly elevated
      (c) Bubble frequently during feeding and avoid unnecessary handling afterward

2. Intussusception
   a. Telescoping of 1 portion of intestine into another; occurs most frequently at the ileocecal valve
   b. Clinical signs
      (1) Healthy, well-nourished infant who wakes up with severe paroxysmal abdominal pain, evidenced by kicking and drawing legs up to abdomen
      (2) One or 2 normal stools, then bloody mucous stool (''currant jelly'' stool)
      (3) Palpation of sausage-shaped mass
      (4) Other signs of intestinal obstruction are usually present
   c. Treatment
      (1) Medical—reduction by hydrostatic pressure (barium enema)
      (2) Surgical reduction and, if necessary, intestinal resection
   d. Nursing considerations
      (1) Same as that for any abdominal surgery
      (2) Since problem usually occurs when child is 6 to 8 months of age, separation anxiety is acute and provision must be made for parent's frequent visits

3. Megacolon (Hirschsprung's disease)
   a. Absence of parasympathetic ganglion cells in a portion of bowel, which causes enlargement of the bowel proximal to the defect
   b. Clinical signs may occur gradually
      (1) Constipation, or passage of ribbon or pelletlike stool
      (2) Intestinal obstruction
   c. Treatment
      (1) Medical
         (a) Use of laxatives, enemas
         (b) Dietary management—decrease bulk and residue
      (2) Surgical
         (a) Removal of aganglionic portion of bowel
         (b) Colostomy if necessary
   d. Nursing considerations
      (1) Teach parents correct procedure for enemas (point out danger of water intoxication)
      (2) General postoperative care

B. Medical problems
   1. Failure to thrive syndrome (often associated with maternal deprivation syndrome)
      a. Children are usually below third percentile in growth
      b. Lack of physical growth may be secondary to decreased emotional and sensory stimulation from parent or parent substitute
      c. Development delayed and demonstrates signs of parental understimulation
      d. Unpliable, stiff, uncomforted, and unyielding to cuddling
      e. Slow in smiling and responding to others
      f. History of difficult feeding, vomiting, sleep disturbance, and excessive irritability
      g. Characteristics of parent providing care
         (1) Difficulty perceiving assessing infant's needs
         (2) Frustrated and angered at infant's dissatisfied response
         (3) Frequently under stress and in crisis with emotional, social, and financial problems
         (4) Often have marital disturbances, such as absent spouse, or if present, one who gives little emotional support
         (5) Tend to lead lonely, solitary lives with few outside interests or friends

h. Nursing considerations
(1) Child needs consistent care giver, who can begin to satisfy child's routine needs
(2) Increased stimulation, appropriate to child's present developmental level
(3) Provide parent with opportunity to talk
(4) When necessary, relieve parent of child-bearing responsibilities until able and ready to emotionally support the child
(5) Demonstrate proper infant care by example, not lecturing (allow parent to proceed at own pace)
(6) Supply parent with emotional support without fostering dependency
(7) Promote parent's self-respect and confidence by praising achievements with child

2. Sudden infant death syndrome—SIDS (crib death)
a. A definite syndrome with cause unknown
b. Number one cause of death in infants between 2 weeks and 1 year of age with an incidence of 1 in every 350 live births
c. Peak age of occurrence—healthy infant 3 to 4 months of age
d. Nursing considerations to assist parents
(1) Know signs of sudden infant death to distinguish it from child neglect or abuse
(2) Reassure parents that they could not have prevented the death or predicted its occurrence
(3) An autopsy should be done on every child to confirm diagnosis
(4) Visit parents at home to discuss cause of death and help them with their guilt and grief
(5) Refer parents to National Sudden Infant Death Syndrome Parent Group

3. Diarrhea
a. Symptom of variety of conditions such as viral or bacterial infection or allergy
b. Metabolic acidosis from loss of water and electrolytes, which decreases available bicarbonate
c. Clinical manifestations
(1) Dehydration is severe when weight loss is greater than 10%
(2) Poor skin turgor and dry mucous membranes

(3) Depressed fontanels and sunken eyeballs
(4) Decreased urine output, increased specific gravity, and increased hematocrit
(5) Irritability, stupor, convulsions from loss of intracellular water and decreased plasma volume
d. Treatment and nursing considerations
(1) In severe diarrhea, medical treatment is necessary to correct fluid and electrolyte imbalance
(2) Isolate infant until stool culture results are reported
(3) Identify causative agent and institute proper therapy (antibiotics are used if bacterial agent is present)
(4) Explain to parents why antibiotics and an increase in food are ineffective in treating viral diarrhea
(5) Parents should be taught progressive increase in diet—alterations in diet may control mild diarrhea
(a) Clear fluids to decrease inflammation of mucosa
(b) If tolerated, half-strength skim milk may be given
(c) Regular diet of bland foods

4. Vomiting
a. A symptom of many conditions, such as poor feeding technique, chalasia (abnormal relaxation of cardiac sphincter), or infections
b. Results in metabolic alkalosis from loss of hydrogen ion
c. Clinical signs
(1) Dehydration
(2) Tetany and convulsions in severe alkalosis, resulting from hypokalemia and hypocalcemia
d. Nursing considerations
(1) Care directed toward correction of underlying problem
(2) Chalasia
(a) Thickened feeding
(b) Feed in upright position
(c) Maintain upright position 20 to 30 minutes after feeding

5. Colic
a. Paroxysmal intestinal cramps caused by accumulation of excessive gas
b. May be caused by excessive air swallowing,

feeding too fast or too much, excessive carbohydrate intake, or emotional tension

c. Treatment—directed toward correction of underlying cause

d. Nursing considerations
    (1) Nurse should observe parent feed infant before attempting to counsel
    (2) Teach parent to bubble the infant frequently and position on abdomen after feeding

6. Constipation
    a. Usually occurs as a result of diet although there may be a psychologic component
    b. Treatment should be dietary—enemas should be avoided
    c. If mineral oil is used, it should not be given with foods, since it decreases absorption of nutrients

7. Respiratory tract infections
    a. Frequent cause of morbidity
    b. Acute infection may be bacterial or viral (refer to Microbiology in Medical-surgical chapter)
        (1) Acute nasopharyngitis (common cold)
        (2) Pneumonia
        (3) Bronchitis
        (4) Tonsillitis
        (5) Epiglottitis
        (6) Croup
        (7) Acute laryngotracheobronchitis
    c. General nursing care for respiratory conditions
        (1) Increase fluid intake
            (a) Prevents dehydration from fever and perspiration
            (b) Loosens thickened secretions
        (2) Increase humidity and coolness
            (a) Liquefies secretions
            (b) Decreases febrile state and inflammation of the mucous membrane
            (c) Causes vasoconstriction and bronchiolar dilation
        (3) Promote nasal and pulmonary drainage
            (a) Clean nares with bulb syringes
            (b) Suction oronasal pharynx
            (c) Postural drainage, clapping, and vibrating
        (4) Provide rest by decreasing stimulation
        (5) Increase oxygen
        (6) Tracheotomy if necessary (see Medical-

surgical nursing for general nursing care of tracheotomy)

8. Otitis media
    a. Acute otitis media—infection of middle ear, causative organism usually *Haemophilus influenzae, Staphylococcus* organism, or *Streptococcus* organism
    b. Symptoms
        (1) Pain—infant frets and rubs ear or rolls head from side to side
        (2) Drum bulging, red, no light reflex, may rupture
    c. Serous otitis—accumulation of uninfected serous or mucoid matter in middle ear, cause unknown
    d. Symptoms
        (1) No pain or fever, but "fullness" in ear
        (2) Drum appears gray, bulging
        (3) May be loss of hearing from scarring of drum
    e. Nursing considerations
        (1) Proper instillation of eardrops
            (a) If child is under 3 years of age, auricle pulled down and back
            (b) Older child, auricle pulled up and back
        (2) Check for complications such as chronic hearing loss, mastoiditis, or possible meningitis

9. Meningitis
    a. Causative agent may be viral or bacterial, such as *Haemophilus influenzae, Neisseria meningitidis,* or *Diplococcus pneumoniae*
    b. Clinical manifestations (more severe in bacterial)
        (1) Opisthotonos—rigidity and hyperextension of neck
        (2) Headache
        (3) Irritability and high-pitched cry
        (4) Signs of increased intracranial pressure
        (5) Fever, nausea, and vomiting
    c. Nursing considerations
        (1) Provide for rest
        (2) Decrease stimuli from environment (control light and noise)
        (3) Position on side with head gently supported in extension
        (4) Respiratory isolation is used for bacterial meningitis

(5) Decrease fluids because of meningeal edema
    (a) Carefully record intake and output
    (b) Monitor IV fluid
(6) Provide emotional support for parents, since child usually becomes ill very suddenly
(7) Administer antibiotic therapy as prescribed

10. Eczema
  a. An atopic manifestation of a specific allergen that may have an emotional component
  b. Most common during first 2 years of life
  c. Clinical manifestations
    (1) Erythema and edema from dilation of capillaries
    (2) Papules, vesicles, and crusts
    (3) Itching that may precipitate infection from scratching
    (4) Periods of remission and exacerbation
    (5) Seen mostly on cheeks, scalp, neck, and flexor surfaces of arms and legs
  d. Nursing considerations
    (1) Support parents because this long-term problem is often discouraging, since the infant is difficult to comfort
    (2) Restrain hands to keep infant from scratching when unsupervised but provide supervised unrestrained play periods
    (3) Pick up frequently, since infant is irritable, fretful, and anorectic
    (4) Clothing or blankets of wool should be avoided
    (5) Provide parent with a list of foods permitted and omitted on elimination or allergenic diet
    (6) Instruct parent how to apply topical ointments prescribed

11. Febrile convulsions
  a. Caused by elevation of temperature
  b. Usually occur in children between 6 months and 3 years of age
  c. Nursing considerations
    (1) Reduce fever with antipyretic drugs and sponge baths
    (2) General seizure precautions
      (a) Protect child from injury, do not restrain, pad crib rails
      (b) Prevent tongue from blocking airway and protect it from injury
      (c) Record time of seizure, duration, and body parts involved
      (d) Suction nasopharynx, administer oxygen as required
      (e) Observe degree of consciousness and behavior after seizure
      (f) Provide rest after seizure
  d. For further discussion of convulsive disorders, see Medical-surgical nursing

The toddler

GROWTH AND DEVELOPMENT
Developmental timetable
A. Fifteen months
  1. Motor
    a. Walks well alone by 14 months, with wide-based gait
    b. Creeps upstairs
    c. Builds tower of 2 blocks
    d. Drinks from a cup and can use a spoon
    e. Enjoys throwing objects and picking them up
  2. Vocalization and socialization
    a. Ten to 15 single words
    b. Has learned "No," which may be said while doing requested demand
    c. Indicates when diaper is wet
B. Eighteen months
  1. Physical
    a. Growth has decreased and appetite lessened—"physiologic anorexia"
    b. Anterior fontanel is usually closed
    c. Abdomen protrudes, larger than chest circumference
  2. Motor
    a. Walks sideways and backward, runs well
    b. Climbs stairs or up on furniture
    c. Scribbles vigorously, attempting straight line
    d. Drinks well from a cup, still spills with a spoon
    e. May begin to control bowel movements
  3. Vocalization and socialization
    a. Uses phrases composed of adjectives and nouns
    b. Has new awareness of strangers

    c. Begins to have temper tantrums

    d. Very ritualistic, has favorite toy or blanket, thumb-sucking may be at peak

C. Two years

  1. Physical

    a. Weight—about 11 to 12 kg (26 to 28 pounds)

    b. Height—about 80 to 82 cm (32 to 33 inches)

    c. Teeth—16 temporary

  2. Motor

    a. Gross motor skills quite well refined

    b. Can walk up and down stairs, both feet on one step at a time, holding onto rail

    c. Builds tower of 5 cubes or will make cubes into a train

    d. Control of spoon well developed

    e. Toilet trained during daytime

  3. Sensory

    a. Accommodation well developed

    b. Visual acuity 20/40

  4. Vocalization and socialization

    a. Vocabulary of about 300 words

    b. Uses short 2- to 3-word phrases, using pronouns

    c. Obeys simple commands

    d. Still very ritualistic, especially at bedtime

    e. Can help undress self and pull on simple clothes

    f. Shows signs of increasing autonomy and individuality

    g. Does not share possessions, everything is "mine"

D. Thirty months

  1. Physical

    a. Full set of 20 temporary teeth

    b. Decreased need for naps

  2. Motor

    a. Walks on tiptoe

    b. Stands on 1 foot

    c. Builds tower of 8 blocks

    d. Copies horizontal or vertical line

  3. Vocalization and socialization

    a. Beginning to see self as separate individual from reflected appraisal of significant others

    b. Still sees other children as "objects"

    c. Increasingly independent, ritualistic, and negativistic

E. Toilet training—major task of toddler

  1. Physical maturation must be reached before training is possible

    a. Sphincter control adequate when child can walk

    b. Able to retain urine for at least 2 hours

    c. Usual age for bowel training—24 to 30 months

    d. Daytime bowel and bladder control—during second year

    e. Night control—by 3 or 4 years of age

  2. Psychologic readiness

    a. Aware of the act of elimination

    b. Able to inform parent of need to urinate or defecate

    c. Desire to please parent

  3. Process of training

    a. Usually begin with bowel, then bladder

    b. Accidents and regressions frequently occur

  4. Parental response

    a. Choose specific word for act

    b. Have specific time and place

    c. Do not punish for accidents

F. Discipline—need for independence without overprotection

  1. Should be consistent—set realistic limits

  2. Reinforce desired behavior

  3. Should be constructive, geared to teach self-control

  4. Punishment should be given immediately after wrongdoing

  5. Punishment should be appropriate

PLAY (PARALLEL PLAY)

A. Child plays alongside other children but not with them

B. Mostly free and spontaneous, no rules or regulations

C. Attention span is still very short, and change of toys occurs at frequent intervals

D. Safety is important

  1. Danger of breaking toy through exploration and ingesting small pieces

  2. Ingesting lead from lead-based paint on toys

  3. Danger of burns from potentially flammable toys

E. Imitation and make-believe play begins by end of second year

F. Suggested toys

  1. Play furniture, dishes, cooking utensils, dress-up clothes

  2. Telephone

  3. Puzzles with a few large pieces

  4. Pedal-propelled toys, such as tricycle

  5. Straddle toys and rocking horse

6. Clay, sandbox toys, crayons, finger paints
7. Pounding toys, blocks

HEALTH PROMOTION DURING CHILDHOOD
Childhood nutrition

A. Nutritional objectives
  1. Provide adequate nutrient intake to meet continuing growth and development needs
  2. Provide basis for support of psychosocial development in relation to food patterns, eating behavior, and attitudes
  3. Provide sufficient calories for increasing physical activities and energy needs
B. Diet—calorie and nutrient requirements increase with age
  1. Increased variety in types and textures of foods
  2. Increased involvement in feeding process, stimulation of curiosity about food environment, language learning
  3. Consideration for child's appetite, choices, motor skills
C. Possible nutritional problem areas
  1. Anemia—increase foods containing iron; e.g., enriched cereals, meat, egg, green vegetables
  2. Obesity or underweight—increase or decrease calories; maintain core foods
  3. Low intake of calcium, iron, vitamins A and C—usually caused by dietary fads
  4. Often omitting breakfast before school
  5. Influence of commercialism on selection of foods and emphasis on fast foods, "empty-calorie" snacks, and high-carbohydrate convenience foods

Accident prevention

A. Leading cause of death in children over 1 year of age
B. Children under 5 years of age account for over half of all accidental deaths during childhood
C. More than half of accidental child deaths are related to automobiles and fire
D. Accidents can be viewed in terms of child's growth and development, especially curiosity about the environment
  1. Motor vehicle
    a. Walking, running, especially after objects thrown into street
    b. Poor perception of speed, lack of experience to foresee danger
    c. Child often unseen because of small size, can be run over by car backing out of driveway, or when playing in leaves or snow
    d. Failure to restrain in car (sitting in person's lap, improper use of seat belts rather than appropriate car seat)
  2. Burns
    a. Investigating—pulls pots off stoves, plays with matches, inserts objects into wall sockets
    b. Climbing—reaches stove, oven, ironing board and iron, cigarettes on table
  3. Poisons
    a. Learning new tastes and textures, puts everything into mouth
    b. Developing fine motor skills—able to open bottles, cabinets, jars
    c. Climbing to previously unreachable shelves and cabinets
  4. Drowning
    a. Child and parents do not recognize the danger of water
    b. Child is unaware of inability to breathe under water
  5. Aspirating small objects and putting foreign bodies in ear or nose
    a. Puts everything in mouth
    b. Very interested in body and newly found openings
  6. Fractures
    a. Climbing, running, and jumping
    b. Still developing sense of balance
E. Prevention through parent education and child protection is goal

ACUTE AND CHRONIC HEALTH PROBLEMS
Hospitalization

A. Specific response of toddler is separation anxiety (see Hospitalization during infancy)
B. Toddler experiences basic fear of loss of love, fear of unknown, fear of punishment
C. Immobilization and isolation represent additional crises to toddler
D. Nursing considerations in preparing parents and child for hospitalization
  1. Primary consideration is maintaining parent-child relationship by preventing separation
  2. Through assessment, establish routines and rituals that child is accustomed to in the areas of
    a. Toilet training
    b. Feeding
    c. Bathing
    d. Sleep patterns
    e. Recreational activities

3. Prepare parent for regression of child to previous modes of behavior and loss of newly learned skills
4. Hospitalization is usually not a time for teaching child new skills
5. Allow child's release of tension, especially aggression, through play (banging a drum, knocking blocks over, or scribbling on paper)
6. Only minimal advance preparation of child for hospitalization is possible, since cognitive ability to grasp verbal explanation is limited

Burns

See Medical-surgical nursing
A. Principles of treatment
   1. Stop the burning process
      a. Remove from source of danger
      b. Remove smoldering clothes
      c. For superficial burns, immerse affected area in cool water
   2. Administer prompt first aid
      a. Maintain patent airway
      b. For first-degree burns, cleanse area, apply sterile dressing soaked in sterile saline if possible
      c. Do not apply creams, butter, or any household remedies
      d. For severe burns (more than 10% of body) oral fluids are not given
   3. Transport patient to proper care facility
      a. Children are hospitalized with burns of 5% to 12% of body surface or more
      b. Large body surface in proportion to weight results in greater potential for fluid loss
      c. Shock—primary cause of death in first 24 to 48 hours
      d. Infection—primary cause of death after initial period
B. Nursing problems and interventions
   1. Fluid and electrolyte loss
      a. Greatest in first 24 to 48 hours because of tissue damage
      b. Immediate replacement of both fluids and electrolytes is essential
      c. Accurate measurement of both intake and output is critical (daily weights, diaper count, and weight)
      d. Determination of hematocrit, hemoglobin, and chemistries should be done daily to provide a guide for replacement

2. Isolation
   a. Child has feelings of guilt and punishment
   b. Children under 5 years of age rarely understand reason for isolation
   c. Furthers separation between parents and child
   d. Encourage child to express feelings
   e. Allow child to play with gown, mask, and gloves so that they are less strange
3. Touch deprivation
   a. Touch, a child's main means of comfort and security, is now painful
   b. Pleasurable touch must be reestablished (apply lotion to unaffected areas and let child apply it to a doll)
   c. Prepare child for baths and whirlpool treatments, which can be frightening and painful
4. Nutrition
   a. High in protein, vitamins, and calories
   b. Child is frequently anorectic because of discomfort, isolation, emotional depression
   c. Provide child with food preferences when feasible; do not force eating or use it as a weapon; encourage parent participation
   d. Alter diet as needs change, especially when high-calorie foods are no longer needed and can cause obesity
5. Contractures
   a. Make moving a game; use play that utilizes affected part, such as throwing a ball for arm movement
   b. Provide for proper body alignment; place child so that attention is focused on an object that will keep body in specific position
   c. Do passive exercises during bath or whirlpool
6. Body image
   a. For younger child, more of a concern to parents whose reactions are communicated to child
   b. For older child, especially adolescent, body damage is of great concern
   c. Emphasize what can be done to improve looks (plastic surgery, wigs, appropriate clothing, makeup)
7. Pain
   a. Assessed by observing behavior of young child, rather than verbal complaints
   b. Distinguish pain from fear of dark, being left alone, or being in strange surroundings
C. Main nursing consideration—prevention
   1. Parent education especially in regard to child's

growth and development and specific dangers at each age level
2. Child education regarding fire safety
   a. Tell child to leave house as soon as smoke is smelled or flames seen, without stopping to retrieve a pet or toy
   b. Involve all members of the family in fire drills
   c. Demonstrate rolling rather than running if their clothes are on fire
3. Fire and burn prevention in the house
   a. Intelligent use of heaters, barbecue, and fireplace
   b. Children should be supervised at all times
   c. Maintain integrity of electric system
   d. Escape route must be maintained

Poisoning

A. Principles of treatment
   1. Identify poison
      a. Bring empty container to hospital
      b. Save any urine or vomitus and bring to hospital
      c. Call hospital before arrival
   2. Avoid excessive manipulation of child
   3. Prompt treatment
      a. Call Poison Control Center is specific ingredients of ingested substance are unknown or for specific antidote
      b. Administer specific or universal antidote
      c. Induce vomiting unless
         (1) Substance is corrosive (lye or drain cleaners) or petroleum distillate (turpentine or gasoline)
         (2) Child is comatose
      d. Vomiting can be induced by
         (1) Syrup of ipecac, 15 ml with 240 ml of water, may be repeated once within 20 to 30 minutes if necessary
         (2) Stimulate back of throat
         (3) Glass of milk or water with 1 tablespoon mustard
B. Common clinical symptoms
   1. Gastrointestinal—pain, vomiting, anorexia
   2. Respiratory and circulatory signs of shock
   3. Central nervous system—loss of consciousness, convulsions
C. Salicylate poisoning
   1. One of the most common drugs taken by children
   2. Toxic dose—3⅓ gr per kilogram of body weight or 6 adult aspirins for a 2-year-old

3. Clinical signs
   a. Hyperventilation—confusion, coma
   b. Metabolic acidosis—anorexia, sweating, increased temperature
   c. Bleeding, especially if chronic ingestion
4. Treatment
   a. Induce vomiting, gastric lavage
   b. IV fluids
   c. Vitamin K if bleeding
   d. Peritoneal dialysis in severe cases
5. Nursing considerations
   a. Parents need to explain to child that medicine is not candy
   b. All medication should be stored in locked cabinets
   c. Parents should have syrup of ipecac in house and know how to use it
D. Petroleum distillates—kerosene, gasoline, benzene
   1. Substance quickly absorbed
   2. Treatment—administer 1.5 ml of mineral oil per kilogram of body weight
   3. Vomiting is not induced—aspiration is a particular danger because of the nature of the substance
E. Corrosive chemicals—lye
   1. Symptoms—pain, dysphagia, prostration
   2. Treatment—neutralize substance with dilute vinegar or lemon juice
   3. Never induce vomiting, since regurgitation of the substance will cause further damage to the mucous membranes
F. Lead poisoning
   1. Most common between 18 months and 3 years of age because of ingestion of abnormal quantities of lead (usually from eating lead chips from peeling paint or sucking on objects painted with lead-based paint)
   2. Characteristics of child and parents
      a. About 50% of mothers had habit of pica (eating nonfood substances)
      b. High level of oral activity in child, such as use of pacifier, thumb-sucking
      c. Oral gratification used as method of relieving anxiety in child
      d. Maternal dependency, despair, passivity
         (1) Mother is absent from home
         (2) Mother present but unable to supervise child
   3. Clinical manifestations (chronic ingestion)
      a. Loss of weight, anorexia

b. Abdominal pain, vomiting
c. Constipation
d. Anemia, pallor, listlessness, fatigue
e. Lead line on teeth and density of long bone
f. Behavior changes such as impulsiveness, irritability, hyperactivity, or lethargy
g. Headache, insomnia, joint pains
h. Brain damage, convulsions, death
i. Increased blood lead level
  (1) Normal—below 40 μg per 100 ml of blood
  (2) Borderline—below 60 μg per 100 ml of blood
  (3) Treatment begun—usually 60 μg or higher
  (4) Convulsions and irreversible brain damage—about 80 μg

4. Treatment
a. Objective—reduce concentration of lead in blood and soft tissue by promoting its excretion and deposition in bones
  (1) Calcium disodium edetate (Calcium Disodium Versenate)
    (a) Urine lead content monitored; peak excretion in 24 to 48 hours
    (b) Adverse effects—acute tubule necrosis, malaise, fatigue, numbness of extremities, GI disturbances, fever, pain in muscles and joints
  (2) Dimercaprol (BAL)
    (a) Usually used in conjunction with calcium disodium edetate
    (b) Adverse effects—local pain at site of injection; may cause persistent fever in children receiving therapy; rise in blood pressure accompanied by tachycardia following injection
  (3) Use vitamin D, calcium, and phosphorus
b. Prevention of further ingestion

5. Nursing considerations
a. Prevention through education, proper housing, supervision of children
b. Screening for these children by recognizing signs, especially behavior changes
c. Careful planning for rotation of injection sites and preparation of child
d. Seizure precautions
e. Discharge planning and follow-up care of child
f. Teach parents to prevent further ingestion

Fractures

See Medical-surgical nursing
A. Greenstick fractures—an incomplete break and bending of a long bone occurring in young children because the bones are soft and not fully mineralized
B. Treatment of fractures—splint, traction, or cast
  1. Bryant's traction—for fractured femur
    a. Generally used for children under 2 years of age
    b. Legs are suspended vertically with buttocks slightly off bed and upper body maintaining contertraction
  2. Spica cast may be used for child any age
C. Nursing considerations
  1. Child must be kept flat on back
  2. A restraining jacket may be necessary to prevent moving
  3. Provide activity to keep child occupied and entertained

Aspiration of foreign objects

A. Symptoms
  1. Substernal retractions
  2. Cough and inability to speak
  3. Increased pulse and respiratory rate
  4. Cyanosis
B. Treatment
  1. Immediate first aid if object is in trachea
    a. Try to pull object out
    b. Turn small child upside down
    c. Heimlich maneuver—grasp victim from behind around upper abdomen and squeeze, forcing diaphragm up
    d. Do not slap victim on back because object may be forced lower in respiratory tract
  2. Medical removal by bronchoscopy
  3. Surgical relief by a tracheotomy below level of object
C. Prevention
  1. Keep small objects out of child's reach
  2. Inspect large toys for removable objects
  3. Teach child not to run or laugh with food or fluid in the mouth
  4. Avoid giving young children foods easily aspirated, such as nuts
  5. Teach child to chew food well before swallowing

Battered child syndrome

A. Refers to both physical abuse and emotional neglect
B. Majority of abused children are under 4 years of age

C. About 70% to 80% of abuse is by parents
D. One theory—role reversal: a reversal of dependency role in which parent turns to the child for nurturing and love
E. Characteristics of abusing parents
1. Their own childrearing included abuse
2. Have incorrect concept of what a small child is and can do
3. Plagued by deep sense of inferiority and lack of identify
4. Tend to be young, immature, and dependent
5. Frequently expect child to provide them with nurturing and love
6. Tend to be depressed, lonely people, yearning for love and understanding
7. Have no outside resources for emotional support or relief from responsibility, especially in time of crisis, thus they take out frustration on child
F. How to identify child neglect or abuse
1. Child has many unexplained injuries, scars, bruises
2. Parents offer inconsistent stories explaining child's injuries when questioned
3. Emotional response of parents is inconsistent with degree of child's injury
4. Parents may resist or fail to be present for questioning
5. Child exhibits physical signs of neglect—malnourished, dehydrated, unkempt
6. Child cringes when physically approached
7. Child responds in a manner that indicates avoiding punishment rather than gaining reward
G. Nursing considerations
1. Main objective—protect child from abusing environment (nurse must be aware of child abuse laws)
2. Be alert for clues that indicate child abuse
3. Focus on helping parents with their own dependency needs
a. Group therapy
b. Home visiting
c. Foster grandparents
4. Help parents learn to control frustration through other outlets
5. Educate parents about child's normal needs and development, new modes of discipline, and realistic expectations
6. Provide emotional support and therapy for the child, since abused children frequently grow up to be abusing parents

Mental retardation

A. Usually defined as low intelligence quotient of 70 or below, which represents about 3% of population
B. American Association on Mental Deficiency defines subaverage IQ as 83 or 84 associated with impairment in adaptive behavior, which represents about 16% of population
C. Retardation can be further classified by the use of the following intelligence test scores; it should be noted that the numbers are approximate and should not be used in a fixed manner for diagnosis
1. Normal—90 to 110 IQ
2. Slow—71 to 89 IQ
3. Mildly retarded—50 to 70 IQ
a. Educable, can achieve a mental age of 8 to 12 years
b. Can learn to read, write, do arithmetic, achieve a vocational skill and function in society
4. Moderately retarded—36 to 49 IQ
a. Trainable, can achieve a mental age of 3 to 7 years
b. Can learn activities of daily living, social skills, and can be trained to work in a sheltered workshop
5. Severely ratarded—below 35 IQ
a. Barely trainable—can achieve a mental age of 0 to 2 years
b. Totally dependent on others and in need of custodial care
D. Causes
1. Prenatal—heredity, PKU, Down's syndrome, severe malnutrition (relationship is under study), rubella
2. Natal—kernicterus (high bilirubin level), intracranial hemorrhage, anoxia
3. Postnatal—lead poisoning, meningitis, encephalitis, neoplasms, recurrent convulsions
E. Diagnosis
1. Delayed milestones
a. Infant fails to suck
b. Head lag after 4 to 6 months of age
c. Slow in learning self-help; slow to respond to new stimuli
d. Slow or absent speech development
2. Conditions that may lead to a false diagnosis of mental retardation
a. Emotional disturbance, such as autism or maternal deprivation

b. Sensory problems, such as deafness or blindness

c. Cerebral dysfunctions, such as cerebral palsy, learning disorders, hyperkinesia, epilepsy

F. Characteristics of mentally retarded children
   1. Mental abilities are concrete—abstract ability is limited
   2. Lack power of self-appraisal
   3. Do not learn from errors
   4. Cannot carry out complex instructions
   5. Do not relate with peers—more secure with adults
   6. Comforted by physical touch
   7. Learn rote responses and socially acceptable behavior
   8. May repeat words (echolalia)
   9. Short attention span, but usually attracted to music

G. Nursing considerations
   1. Always deal with child's developmental not chronologic age
      a. Educate parent regarding developmental age
      b. When child is nearing adolescence, sexual feelings accompany maturation and need to be explained according to child's mental capacity
   2. Set realistic goals, teach by simple steps for habit formation rather than for understanding or transference of learning
      a. When teaching a skill, break process down into simple steps that can be easily achieved
      b. Each step must be learned completely before teaching child next step
      c. Behavior modification is a very effective method of teaching these children
      d. Praise for accomplishment must be given to develop child's self-esteem
   3. Discipline must remain simple, geared toward learning acceptable behavior rather than developing judgment
   4. Routines are foundation of child's life style; hospitalization should be based on child's normal schedule
   5. See Parents' reaction to a defective child

Cerebral palsy

A. Neuromuscular disability or difficulty in controlling voluntary muscles (caused by damage to some portion of brain, with associated sensory, intellectual, emotional, or convulsive disorders)

B. Characteristics of cerebral palsy
   1. Affects young children, usually becoming evident before 3 years of age
   2. Nonprogressive, but persists throughout life
   3. Some motor dysfunction is always present
   4. Mental deficiency may or may not be present

C. Major causes
   1. Anoxia of brain caused by a variety of insults at or near the time of birth
   2. Infection of central nervous system

D. Types—classified according to predominant clinical manifestation
   1. Spasticity (65%)—hyperactivity of muscle stretch reflex, which becomes worse with rapid passive motion
   2. Athetosis—slow, wormlike, involuntary purposeless movement
   3. Rigidity—persistent stiffness of muscles on movement, which becomes less severe with rapid passive motion
   4. Ataxia—disturbance in sense of balance
   5. Tremor—rhythmic purposeless movement, which becomes worse with excitement or intentional movement
   6. Flaccidity—decreased muscle tension

E. Clinical manifestations
   1. Difficulty in feeding, especially sucking and swallowing
   2. Asymmetry in motion or contour
   3. Delayed motor development and speech
   4. Excessive or feeble cry
   5. Any of the muscular abnormalities listed under types

F. Nursing problems and interventions
   1. Feeding
      a. Drooling results from difficulty in swallowing
      b. Use spoon and blunt fork, with plate attached to table for easier self-feeding
      c. Require increased calories because of excessive energy expenditure, increased protein for muscle activity, and increased vitamins (especially B_6) for amino acid metabolism
   2. Relaxation
      a. Provide rest periods in area with few stimuli
      b. Set limits and control activity level
   3. Safety
      a. Protect from accidents resulting from poor balance and lack of muscle control

b. Provide helmet for protection against head injuries

c. Always restrain in chair, bed, etc.

d. Institute seizure precautions

4. Play
   a. Keep safety as main objective
   b. Must not be overstimulating, should have educational value, appropriate to child's developmental level and ability

5. Elimination
   a. Difficulty in toilet training because of poor muscle control
   b. May need special bowel and bladder training

6. Speech
   a. Poor coordination of lips, tongue, cheeks, larynx, and poor control of diaphragm make formation of words difficult
   b. May need speech therapy

7. Breathing
   a. Poor control of intercostal muscles and diaphragm causes child to be prone to respiratory tract infection
   b. Need to protect child from exposure to infection as much as possible; be alert for symptoms of aspiration pneumonia

8. Dental problems
   a. Problems in muscular control affect development and alignment of teeth
   b. Frequent dental caries occur, and there is a great need for dental supervision and care
   c. Parent may have to be taught to brush child's teeth because of muscular dysfunction

9. Vision
   a. Common ocular problems such as strabismus and refractive errors may be related to poor muscular control
   b. Must look for such disorders to prevent further problems such as amblyopia

10. Hearing problems may be present depending on the basic cause of the brain damage

Hearing disorders

A. Types
   1. Conductive—loss from damage to middle ear
      a. Accounts for about 80% of reduced hearing
      b. Conductive loss of 30 dB or more may require a hearing aid
   2. Sensorineural—damage to inner ear structures or auditory nerve
      a. Distortion in clarity of words
      b. Problem in discrimination of sounds
   3. Mixed conductive—sensorineural
   4. Central auditory
      a. Not explained by other 3 causes
      b. Child hears but does not understand

B. Causes
   1. Maternal factors—rubella, syphilis
   2. Perinatal—anoxia, kernicterus, prematurity, excessive noise
   3. Postnatal—mumps, otitis media, head trauma, drugs such as streptomycin

C. Developmental and behavioral manifestations of hearing loss
   1. Lack of Moro reflex in response to sharp clap
   2. Failure to respond to loud noise
   3. Failure to localize a source of sound at 2 to 3 feet (61 to 95 cm) after 6 months of age
   4. Absence of babble by 7 months of age
   5. Inability to understand words or phrases by 12 months of age
   6. Use of gestures rather than verbalization to establish wants
   7. History of frequent respiratory tract infections and otitis media

D. Nursing considerations
   1. Detection—can and should be identified within the first year of life
   2. Specific guidelines for working with a deaf child
      a. Face child to facilitate lipreading
      b. Do not walk back and forth while talking
      c. Have good light on speaker's face
      d. Be level with child's face and speak toward good ear
      e. Always enunciate and articulate carefully
      f. Do not talk too loudly, especially if the loss is sensorineural
      g. Use facial expressions, since verbal intonations are not communicated
      h. Encourage active play to build self-confidence

Visual disorders

A. Strabismus—imbalance of extraocular muscles causing a physiologic incoordination of the eyes
   1. A cause of blindness—amblyopia develops in the weak eye from disuse
   2. Must be corrected before 4 years of age to prevent blindness
   3. Treatment

a. To force weak eye to fixate—patch good eye and exercise weak eye

b. Surgery to lengthen or shorten extraocular structures

B. Functional definition of blindness—visual loss of acuity to read print, must use braille, may have light perception

C. Causes other than strabismus
1. Maternal—albinism, congenital cataracts, rubella, galactosemia
2. Perinatal—retrolental fibroplasia
3. Postnatal—trauma, diabetes, syphilis, tumor

D. Developmental and behavioral manifestations indicating a reduction in vision
1. Retarded motor development
2. Rocking for sensory stimulation
3. Squinting, rubbing eyes
4. Sitting close to television, holding book close to face
5. Clumsiness, bumping into objects

E. Nursing considerations
1. Early detection of loss
2. Specific nursing intervention when working with a blind child
   a. Always talk so child can hear clearly
   b. Use noise so child can locate your position
   c. Help child learn through other senses, especially touch through play activities
   d. Facilitate eating by
      (1) Arranging food on plate at clock hours and teaching child location
      (2) Providing finger foods when possible
      (3) Providing light spoon and deep bowl so child can feel weight of food on spoon

Pinworms

Most common intestinal parasites

A. Children reinfect themselves by fingers to anus to mouth route

B. Can also be infected by breathing air-borne ova

C. Symptoms
1. Severe pruritus of anal area
2. Vaginitis
3. Irritability and insomnia
4. Poor appetite and weight loss
5. Eosinophilia

D. Diagnosis—cellophane tape test to isolate eggs from anal area (must be done in morning before first bowel movement)

E. Treatment—anthelmintics
1. Hexylresorcinol (Caprokol, Crystoids)
   a. Paralyzes worms (hookworms, roundworms, pinworms, whipworms, threadworms, tapeworms, intestinal flukes), and worms are inactive when excreted
   b. Adverse effects—burning sensation of skin, oral and anal mucous membrane
2. Methylrosaniline chloride—paralyzes pinworms, threadworms, and liver flukes
3. Piperazine citrate (Antepar Citrate, Multifuge, Ta-Verm, Vermidol)
   a. Paralyzes musculature of pinworms and roundworms by curare-like action
   b. Within 3 days pinworms are passed active and alive; roundworms paralyzed and alive
4. Pyrantel pamoate (Antiminth)
   a. Blocks neuromuscular transmission in roundworms, hookworms, pinworms
   b. Adverse effects—anorexia, nausea, vomiting, diarrhea, abdominal cramps, headache, dizziness, drowsiness, rash
5. Pyrvinium pamoate (Povan)
   a. Inhibits respiratory enzymes and anaerobic metabolism to inactivate pinworms, threadworms
   b. Adverse effects—nausea, vomiting, abdominal cramps, cyanine dye origin of drug colors stool, emesis, and most materials bright red

F. Nursing considerations
1. Prevent reinfestation
   a. Child should not be allowed to scratch anus; may need to wear mittens
   b. Fingernails should be kept short
   c. Should wear a tight diaper or underpants
   d. Wash anal area thoroughly at least once a day
   e. Change clothes daily; wash in hot water
   f. Air out bedroom, dust and vacuum house thoroughly
2. Teach parent administration of medication
   a. Overdose will not produce a quicker recovery
   b. Stools may turn bright red from medication

Anemia

A. Most prevalent nutritional disorder among children in the United States, caused by lack of adequate sources of dietary iron
1. Infant usually has iron reserve for 6 months

2. Premature infant lacks reserve
3. Children receiving only milk have no source of iron
B. Insidious onset, usually diagnosed because of an infection
C. Clinical manifestations
   1. Pallor, weakness
   2. Slow motor development
   3. Poor muscle tone
   4. Hemoglobin level below 10 g
D. Treatment
   1. Food sources rich in iron
   2. Iron replacement
      a. Oral iron sources
         (1) Drugs
            (a) Ferrocholinate (Chel-Iron, Ferrolip)
            (b) Ferrous fumarate (Ircon, Toleron)
            (c) Ferrous gluconate
            (d) Ferrous lactate (Ferro Drops)
            (e) Ferrous sulfate
         (2) Adverse effects—nausea, vomiting, fatalities in children ingesting enteric coated tablets, thinking they are candy
         (3) Drug interactions—ferrous sulfate binds tetracycline and decreases absorption; magnesium trisilicate decreases absorption of iron preparations
      b. Parenteral iron sources
         (1) Drugs
            (a) Iron-Dextran injection (Imferon)
            (b) Iron sorbitex (Jectofer)
         (2) Adverse effects—tissue staining (use Z tract for injection), fever, lymphadenopathy, nausea, vomiting, arthralgia, urticaria, severe peripheral vascular failure, anaphylaxis, secondary hematochromatosis
E. Nursing considerations
   1. Prevention
      a. Teach pregnant women importance of their iron intake
      b. Encourage feeding of fortified cereal
      c. Introduce foods high in iron
   2. Good nutrition and proper administration of supplemental iron
      a. Vitamin C aids absorption
      b. Hydrochloric acid aids absorption
      c. Oxalates, phosphate, and phytates decrease absorption

d. Use a straw, since some liquid preparations stain teeth
e. Discolors stools; may cause gastric irritation or constipation

Celiac disease

A. Chronic intestinal malabsorption and inability to digest gluten, a protein found mostly in wheat and rye
B. Usually begins in infancy or toddler stage, but later in breast-fed infants
C. Clinical manifestations
   1. Progressive malnutrition—secondary deficiencies: anemia, rickets
      a. Stunted growth
      b. Wasting of extremities
      c. Distended abdomen
   2. Steatorrhea—fatty, foul, frothy, bulky stools
   3. Celiac crisis—severe episode of dehydration and acidosis from diarrhea
D. Treatment—dietary
   1. Low in glutens, eliminate wheat, rye, oats, and barley
   2. High in calories and protein
   3. Low fat
   4. Smooth, soft foods with low roughage and residue
   5. Small, frequent feedings; adequate fluids
   6. Vitamin supplements, all in water-miscible form
   7. Supplemental iron
E. Nursing considerations—parental education
   1. Protect child from infection
   2. Strict adherence to dietary regimen
   3. Need for frequent follow-up supervision, home visits

Cystic fibrosis of the pancreas

A. Autosomal recessive disorder affecting mucus-secreting glands
B. Pathology—defect in overproduction of mucus or an absence of normal mucus-removing mechanism
   1. Pancreas—becomes fibrotic with a decreased production of pancreatic enzymes
      a. Lipase—causes steatorrhea
      b. Trypsin—causes increased nitrogen in stool
      c. Amylase—inability to break down polysaccharides
   2. Intestines—increased mucus production preventing enzymes from reaching duodenum and resulting in an inability to absorb fat

3. Sweat glands—high electrolyte content of sodium and chloride (3 to 5 times higher than normal)
4. Respiratory system—increased viscous mucus in trachea, bronchi, and bronchioles resulting in
   a. Obstruction interfering with expiration (emphysema)
   b. Infection
5. Liver—possible cirrhosis from biliary obstruction, malnutrition, or infection
C. Clinical manifestations
   1. Based on above pathophysiology
   2. Similar to celiac disease
   3. Some early manifestations during infancy
      a. Meconium ileus at birth (about 15%)
      b. Failure to regain normal 10% weight loss at birth
      c. Presence of cough or wheezing during first 6 months of age
   4. Because of respiratory involvement, there may be clubbing of fingers, barrel-shaped chest, cyanosis, distended neck veins
   5. Cardiac enlargement, particularly right ventricular hypertrophy (cor pulmonale)
D. Nursing problems and interventions
   1. Prevention of respiratory tract infection
      a. Postural drainage, percussion, vibrating
      b. Croupette at home with high humidity, additional oxygen as needed
      c. Use of expectorants and antibiotics
   2. Nutrition
      a. Replacement of pancreatic enzymes, given with cold food
      b. Replacement of fat-soluble vitamins in water-miscible form
      c. High-protein diet of easily digested food, normal fat, high calories
      d. Small frequent feedings
   3. Mobility and activity
      a. May have little tolerance for exertion
      b. Help child regulate own tolerance
      c. Provide frequent rest periods
   4. Body image
      a. Barrel-shaped chest, poor weight gain, thin extremities, bluish coloring, smell of stools, poor posture
      b. Encourage good hygiene and select clothes that compensate for protuberant abdomen and emaciated extremities

5. Counseling
   a. Long-term problem causing financial and emotional stresses
   b. Illness can become a major controlling factor in family
      (1) Child begins to recognize that wheezing brings attention and uses this knowledge
      (2) Helps parents deal with such behavior by recognizing false attacks and using consistent discipline
   c. Encourage family to join the Cystic Fibrosis Foundation

Sickle cell anemia

A. Autosomal recessive disorder affecting hemoglobin
B. Defective hemoglobin causes red blood cells to become sickle shaped and clump together under reduced oxygen tension
C. Clinical manifestations of a sickle cell crisis
   1. Severe pain in abdomen, legs, and flank area
   2. Fever
   3. Anemia, pallor, weakness
   4. Vomiting, anorexia
   5. Convulsion, stiff neck, coma
   6. Jaundice
   7. Enlarged spleen, liver, heart
D. Nursing problems and interventions
   1. Prevention of crisis
      a. Avoid infection, dehydration, and other conditions causing strain on body, which precipitates crisis
      b. Avoid hypoxia
         (1) Avoid drugs that depress respiratory center
         (2) Treat respiratory tract infections immediately
         (3) Administer additional oxygen with high humidity
      c. Avoid dehydration
         (1) May cause a rapid thrombus formation
         (2) Daily fluid intake should be calculated according to body weight (130 to 200 ml per kilogram [2 to 3 oz per pound])
         (3) During crisis, fluid needs to be increased, especially if patient is febrile
   2. Care during crisis—provisions should be made for
      a. Adequate hydration (may need IV therapy)
      b. Proper positioning, careful handling

    c. Exercise as tolerated (immobility promotes thrombus formation and respiratory problems)

    d. Adequate ventilation

    e. Control of pain (avoid narcotics or barbiturates)

    f. Blood transfusions for severe anemia

  3. Genetic counseling

    a. Disorder mostly of black race

    b. Parents need to know risk of having other children with trait or disease

    c. Screen young children for disorder, since clinical manifestations usually do not appear until after 1 year of age

The preschool-age child

GROWTH AND DEVELOPMENT
Developmental timetable

A. Three years

  1. Motor

    a. Walks backward

    b. Rides a tricycle, using pedals

    c. Walks upstairs, alternating feet

    d. Begins to use scissors

    e. Constructs a 3-block bridge

    f. Can unbutton front or side button

    g. Usually toilet trained at night

  2. Sensory—visual acuity 20/30

  3. Vocalization and socialization

    a. Vocabulary of about 900 words, uses 8- to 9-word sentences

    b. May have normal hesitation in speech pattern

    c. Uses plurals

    d. Begins to understand ideas of sharing and taking turns

  4. Mental abilities

    a. Little understanding of past, present, future, or aspect of time

    b. Stage of magical thinking

B. Four years

  1. Motor

    a. Climbs and jumps well

    b. Walks up and down stairs like an adult

    c. Can button buttons and lace shoes

    d. Throws ball overhand

  2. Vocalization and socialization

    a. Vocabulary of 1500 words or more

    b. May have imaginary companion

    c. Tends to be selfish and impatient, but takes pride in accomplishments

    d. Exaggerates, boasts, and tattles on others

  3. Mental abilities

    a. Reading readiness is present

    b. Can repeat 4 numbers and is learning number concept

    c. Knows which is longer of 2 lines

    d. Has poor space perception

C. Five years

  1. Motor

    a. Gross motor abilities well developed

    b. Can balance on 1 foot for about 10 seconds

    c. Can jump rope, skip, and roller skate

    d. Can draw a picture of a person

    e. Prints first name and other words as learned

    f. Dresses and washes self

    g. May be able to tie shoelaces

  2. Sensory

    a. Minimal potential for amblyopia to develop

    b. Color recognition is well established

  3. Vocalization and socialization

    a. Vocabulary of about 2100 words

    b. Talks constantly

    c. Asks meaning of new words

    d. Generally cooperative and sympathetic toward others

    e. Basic personality structure is well established

  4. Mental abilities (Piaget's phase of intuitive thought)

    a. Beginning understanding of time in terms of days as part of a week

    b. Can determine difference in weights

    c. Has not mastered concept that parts equal a whole regardless of their appearance

PLAY (COOPERATIVE PLAY)

A. Loosely organized group play where membership changes readily and rules are absent

B. Through play, child deals with reality, learns control of feelings, and expresses emotions more through words than actions

C. Play is still physically oriented but is also imitative and imaginary

D. There is increasing sharing and cooperation among preschool children, especially 5-year-olds

E. Suggested toys (same principles as discussed before)

  1. Puppets

  2. Additional dress-up clothes, dolls, house, furniture, small trucks, animals, etc.

3. Painting sets, color books, paste, and cut-out sets
4. Illustrated books
5. Puzzles with large pieces and more shapes
6. Tricycle, swing, slide, and other playground equipment

ACUTE AND CHRONIC HEALTH PROBLEMS
Hospitalization

A. Reaction of child
  1. Fears about body image are now greater than fear of separation
  2. The fears include
     a. Intrusive experiences—needles, thermometer, otoscope
     b. Punishment and rejection
     c. Pain
     d. Castration and mutilation
B. Preparation
  1. Can prepare child beforehand, since increased cognitive and verbal ability makes explanations possible
  2. General considerations for nursing intervention
     a. Should begin a few days before, but not too soon because of poor concept of time
     b. Clarify cause and effect because of child's phenomenalistic thinking (in child's mind proximity of 2 events relates them to each other)
     c. Explain routines of hospital admission but not all procedures at one time, since this would be overwhelming
     d. Play is an excellent medium for preparation (use dolls, puppets, make-believe equipment, dress-up doctor and nurse clothes)
     e. Provide time for play as an outlet for fear, anger, and hostility, as well as a temporary escape from reality
     f. Verbal explanation should be as simple as possible and always honest
     g. Add details about procedures, drugs, surgery, and the like as child's cognitive level and personal experiences increase

Cancer

A. Second leading cause of death in children
B. Leukemia—principal type of cancer
  1. Peak incidence—3 to 4 years of age
  2. Malignant neoplasm of blood-forming organs
  3. In children, overproduction of immature leukocytes—blast-cell or stem-cell leukemia

  a. Lymphocytic—about 85% of cases, better prognosis than for myelogenous
  b. Myelogenous—about 10%, extremely poor prognosis
4. Symptoms—caused by overproduction of immature nonfunctional cells
   a. Anemia—pallor, weakness, irritability
   b. Infection—fever
   c. Tendency toward bleeding—petechiae and bleeding into joints
   d. Pain in joints caused by seepage of serous fluid
   e. Tendency toward easy fracture of bones
   f. Enlargement of spleen, liver, lymph glands
   g. Abdominal pain and anorexia resulting in weight loss
   h. Necrosis and bleeding of gums and other mucous membranes
   i. Later symptoms—central nervous system involvement and frank hemorrhage
5. Treatment objectives
   a. Induce remission by chemotherapy
      (1) Prednisone—steroid
      (2) Vincristine
      (3) Methotrexate—folic acid antagonist
      (4) 6-Mercaptopurine—purine antagonist
      (5) Cyclophosphamide—alkylating agent
      (6) Daunorubicin—cytotoxic antibiotic
   b. Prevent CNS involvement by use of irradiation and intrathecal methotrexate because leukemic cells invade brain, but most antileukemic drugs do not pass blood-brain barrier
   c. Transfusions to replace and provide blood factors such as platelets, white cells, and clotting factors
   d. See Antineoplastic drugs in Medical-surgical nursing
6. Nursing considerations
   a. Prognosis—improving
      (1) Adjustment of parents may be difficult because of potential long-term status
      (2) Must deal with child's idea of death—discussion should be appropriate to level of understanding
         (a) Preschooler—concept that death is reversible; greatest fear is separation
         (b) Child 6 to 9 years of age—concept that death is personified; person actually comes and removes child

(c) Child over 9 years of age—adult concept of death as irreversible and inevitable
b. Treatment
   (1) Be alert for and attempt to support the child experiencing side effects of drugs, for example
      (a) Cytoxan—severe nausea and vomiting
      (b) Vincristine—constipation, alopecia, neurotoxicity
   (2) Prevent infection with use of reverse isolation
   (3) Handle child carefully because of pain and hemorrhage
   (4) Provide gentle oral hygiene, soft, bland foods, and increased liquids
   (5) Provide for frequent rest periods, quiet play
c. See Behavioral sciences for further details on behavioral changes that result from physical illness

Nephrosis or nephrotic syndrome

A. Pathology—abnormal, increased permeability of glomerular basement membrane to plasma albumin
B. Cause unknown—theories include
   1. Hypersensitivity
   2. Antigen-antibody response (rationale for use of glucocorticoids and other immunosuppressive drugs)
C. Peak incidence—2 to 5 years of age
D. Clinical manifestations
   1. Generalized edema, especially genital, periorbital, and ascites
   2. Proteinuria
   3. Hypoproteinemia—poor general health, loss of appetite
   4. Hyperlipemia
   5. May also see symptoms usually associated with nephritis
      a. Hematuria
      b. Hypertension
E. Nursing problems and interventions
   1. Infection—both disease state and drug therapy increase susceptibility
      a. Should be protected from others who are ill
      b. Teach parents signs of impending infection and encourage them to seek medical care

2. Malnutrition caused by loss of protein and poor appetite
   a. Regular diet is usually allowed; added salt and salty foods discouraged
   b. Protein is usually not adjusted; encourage child to select foods likes from high-protein choices
   c. Fluids may be restricted, but this generally causes more discomfort than benefit
3. Respiratory difficulty caused by ascites
   a. Proper positioning—place in Fowler's position to decrease pressure against diaphragm
   b. Frequent change of position is vital because of dependent edema
4. Discomfort caused by edema, pressure areas
   a. Positioning and skin care provide some relief
   b. Support genitalia if edematous
5. Change in body image caused by edema and steroids
   a. Of greater concern as child grows older
   b. Emphasize clothes, hairdo, etc. that make child attractive
   c. Stress that "diets" will not help weight loss
6. Behavioral changes such as irritability and depression
   a. Parents need to understand that mood swings are influenced by physical condition
   b. Encourage child to participate in own care
   c. Encourage diversionary activities that provide satisfaction

Urinary tract infection

A. Very common in females because of anatomy of lower urinary tract—urethra is short and meatus is close to anus
B. Nursing considerations—teach prevention
   1. Proper cleansing of genitalia
   2. Voiding when necessary as opposed to holding urine in bladder
   3. Increased fluids, particularly those which acidify urine
   4. Identification of asymptomatic infections

Allergy

A. Altered tissue response to a substance, either inhaled, ingested, or contacted on skin
B. Most common types in children
   1. Eczema
   2. Allergic rhinitis
   3. Asthma

C. General nursing considerations
1. Family history can be a significant factor
2. A comprehensive study of child and environment is essential
   a. Prepare child for skin tests
   b. Study environment in terms of emotional stresses as well as physical allergens
3. Teach parents to eliminate allergenic substances and to administer drugs properly
D. Asthma
1. Pathology
   a. Bronchiolar spasm
   b. Bronchiolar constriction
   c. Increased secretions
   d. Respiratory acidosis from buildup of carbon dioxide
2. Clinical manifestations
   a. Wheezing, especially on expiration
   b. Labored breathing, cough, increased secretion
   c. Flaring nares, distended neck veins
E. Treatment for respiratory allergies
1. Bronchodilators
   a. Theophyllines
      (1) Drugs
          (a) Aminophylline
          (b) Dyphylline (Dilor, Neothylline)
          (c) Oxtriphylline (Choledyl)
          (d) Theophylline (Aqualin, Elixophyllin)
      (2) Actions
          (a) Act directly on bronchial smooth muscle to decrease spasm and relax smooth muscle of the vasculature
          (b) Direct stimulatory effect on myocardium increases cardiac output, which improves blood flow to kidneys
          (c) Direct action on renal tubules provides diuretic effect by increasing excretion of sodium and chloride ions
      (3) Adverse effects—oral forms cause gastric irritation
      (4) Considerations during therapy—cumulation of drug can occur unless dosage is regulated; parenteral drug must be administered slowly over a 4- to 5-minute period to avoid peripheral vasodilation (hypotension, facial flushing), cerebral vascular constriction (headache, dizziness), cardiac palpitation, and precordial pain

b. Epinephrine hydrochloride—the drug of choice in respiratory emergency, such as status asthmaticus
   (1) Actions
       (a) Acts at beta-adrenergic receptors in bronchus to relax smooth muscle and increase respiratory volume
       (b) Inhalants have a local action causing vasoconstriction that reduces congestion or edema
   (2) Adverse effects—cardiac palpitation; overuse of inhalants may cause ''congestive rebound''
c. Isoproterenol hydrochloride (Isuprel Hydrochloride, Proternol)
   (1) Action—similar to that of theophyllines
   (2) Adverse effects—action at cardiovascular beta receptors causes tachycardia, peripheral blood vessel dilation (hypotension)
d. Metaproterenol (Alupent, Metaprel)
e. Terbutaline (Bricanyl) has little effect on cardiac tissue
f. Oral drugs that relax bronchi and decrease glandular and tissue fluid in bronchi
   (1) Drugs
       (a) Methoxyphenamine hydrochloride (Orthoxine)
       (b) Phenylpropanolamine hydrochloride (Propadrine)
       (c) Pseudoephedrine hydrochloride (Sudafed)
   (2) Adverse effects—transient elevation in pulse and systolic blood pressure, dry oral tissues
g. Cromolyn sodium (Aarane, Intal) acts primarily by preventing release of mediators of type I allergic reactions (histamine, slow-reacting substance of anaphylaxis) from sensitized mast cells; prophylactic use by inhaling capsule contents lessens bronchoconstriction
h. Adverse effects common to bronchodilator group—anxiety, nervousness, tremors, nausea, vomiting, headache, dizziness
2. Expectorants—increase production of thinner, less viscid secretions that protect bronchial tissues
   a. Hydriodic acid—administered diluted, sipped through straw to avoid damage to teeth
   b. Elixir of terpin hydrate—42.5% alcohol con-

tent of compounds provides expectorant action
3. Mucolytics
   a. Drugs
      (1) Calcium iodide
      (2) Glyceryl guaiacolate (Robitussin)
      (3) Iodinated glycerol (Organidin)
      (4) Potassium iodide (Enkide)
   b. Act to raise the osmolality of bronchial glandular secretions causing fluids to move to dilute the secretions
   c. Adverse effects—nausea, skin eruptions; long-term use of iodides may cause iodism (inflammation of respiratory tract tissues, skin eruptions, accumulation of fluid in nasal passages, lungs, eyelids)
4. Corticosteroids
   a. Anti-inflammatory effect diminishes inflammatory component of asthma and reduces airway obstruction
   b. Used in status asthmaticus; less often used for long-term control because of side effects
F. Nursing considerations
   1. Treatment—use of antispasmodic drugs and bronchodilators; parents must know how to give medication and why it must be given even if child does not have an attack
   2. Good respiratory hygiene; teach parents postural drainage, need for increased fluids, and the use of a cool mist humidifier to provide high humidity in home
   3. Proper environment
      a. Free of as many allergens as possible
      b. Avoid exertion, exposure to cold air, and people with infections
      c. Avoid as much as possible emotional factors that precipitate attacks

Tonsillectomy and adenoidectomy

Not done routinely, since lymphoid tissue helps prevent invasion of organisms
A. Indications for surgical removal
   1. Recurrent tonsillitis or otitis media
   2. Enlargement that interferes with breathing or swallowing
B. Contraindications for removal
   1. Occasional infections that clear up rapidly
   2. Cleft palate, hemophilia, or debilitating disease such as leukemia

C. Complications after surgery
   1. Hemorrhage—first 24 hours
      a. Frequent swallowing, bright red blood in vomitus
      b. Restlessness
      c. Increased pulse, pallor
   2. Hemorrhage from sloughing of tissue—5 to 10 days postoperatively
D. Nursing considerations
   1. Keep child on abdomen or side with head turned to side
   2. After surgery, child should have cool liquids, not red in color and not thick or mucus-producing
   3. Ask child to talk; provide assurance that it is possible
   4. Ice collar to decrease edema
   5. Attempt to limit crying

The school-age child

GROWTH AND DEVELOPMENT
Developmental timetable

A. Physical growth
   1. Permanent dentition, beginning with 6-year molars and central incisors at 7 or 8 years of age
   2. Growth has decreased, about 1 inch (2.5 cm) in height a year
   3. Tends to look lanky because bone development precedes muscular development
B. Motor
   1. Refinement of coordination, balance, and control is occurring
   2. Motor development necessary for competitive activity becomes important
C. Sensory—visual acuity of 20/20
D. Mental abilities
   1. Readiness for learning, especially in perceptual organization—names months of year, knows right from left, can tell time, can follow several directions at once
   2. Acquires use of reason and understanding of rules
   3. Trial and error problem solving becomes more conceptual rather than action oriented
   4. Reasoning ability allows greater understanding and use of language
   5. Quantity conservation (Piaget)—child knows that quantity remains the same even though appearance differs

PLAY
Play activities vary with age

A. Number of play activities decreases while amount of time spent in one particular activity increases
B. Likes games with rules because of increased mental abilities
C. Likes games of athletic competition because of increased motor ability
D. Child should learn how to work as well as play, with a beginning appreciation for economics and finances
E. In beginning of school years, boys and girls play together but gradually separate into sex-oriented type of activities
F. Suggested play for 6- to 9-year-olds
   1. More housekeeping toys that work, doll accessories, paper doll sets, simple sewing machine, and needlework
   2. Simple work and number games, games calling for increased skills
   3. Physically active games such as hopscotch, jump rope, climbing trees
   4. Stamp collecting and the like and building simple models
   5. Bicycle riding
G. Suggested play for 9- to 12-year-olds
   1. Handicrafts of all kinds
   2. Model kits, collections, hobbies
   3. Archery, dart games, chess, jigsaw puzzles
   4. Sculpturing materials such as pottery clay
   5. Science toys, magic sets

ACUTE AND CHRONIC HEALTH PROBLEMS
Diabetes mellitus

A. Symptoms—juvenile diabetes may be more severe and variable than diabetes in adults
   1. Onset—rapid, obvious
   2. Child usually thin, underweight; obesity does not appear to be a factor
   3. Increased thirst, fluid intake, appetite, and urinary output
   4. Hypoglycemia and ketoacidosis common
B. Differences between childhood and adult diabetes
   1. Onset
      a. Rapid in child
      b. Insidious in adult
   2. Obesity
      a. Does not appear to be a factor in child
      b. Predisposing factor in adult
   3. Dietary treatment

      a. Rarely adequate for child
      b. Possible in one third of adults
   4. Oral hypoglycemics
      a. Contraindicated for child
      b. Helpful in one third of adults
   5. Insulin
      a. Almost universally necessary in children
      b. Necessary for only one third of adults
   6. Hypoglycemia and ketoacidosis
      a. Quite frequent in children
      b. More uncommon in adults
   7. Degenerative vascular changes
      a. Develop after adolescence in child
      b. May be present at time of diagnosis in adult
C. Hypoglycemia—insulin shock
   1. Causes
      a. Overdose of insulin
      b. Decreased food intake
      c. Excessive physical exercise—increases muscle activity and movement of glucose into muscle cells
   2. Signs
      a. Sweating, flushing, pallor
      b. Numbness, trembling, chilliness
      c. Unsteadiness, nervousness, irritability
      d. Hunger
      e. Hallucinations
      f. Late signs—convulsions, coma, death
   3. Emergency treatment—immediate supply of readily available glucose
D. Hyperglycemia—ketoacidosis or diabetic coma
   1. Causes
      a. Decreased insulin
      b. Emotional stress
      c. Fever
      d. Infection
      e. Increased food intake
   2. Signs
      a. Weakness, drowsiness
      b. Lack of appetite, thirst
      c. Abdominal and/or generalized pain
      d. Acetone breath
      e. Late signs—Kussmaul breathing (deep, rapid respirations), cherry red lips, loss of consciousness, death
   3. Treatment—hospitalization with administration of insulin
E. Hereditary influence
   1. Inherited as a recessive characteristic

2. "Anticipation"—manifestation of disease occurs earlier in succeeding generations
F. Peak ages of incidence in the school-age group
  1. Six years of age
  2. Twelve years of age
G. Treatment
  1. Control calorie, carbohydrate, fat, and protein intake
  2. Insulin (see Endocrine section in Medical-surgical nursing)
H. Nursing problems and interventions—main objective is control of diabetes and education of child and family
  1. Explain differences between childhood and adult diabetes to parents who may think child is faking because their own illness does not cause serious problems
  2. Teach factors that affect insulin requirements and signs of insulin overdose and diabetic coma
    a. Give family written list explaining symptoms
    b. Emphasize that sugar can be given if insulin shock is suspected, but insulin should not be increased if diabetic coma is developing
    c. Emphasize need for close medical supervision
  3. Infection—teach need for
    a. Good skin care, frequent baths
    b. Properly fitting shoes
    c. Prompt treatment of any small cut
    d. Protection from undue exposure to illness
  4. Diet—should be well balanced, with fairly equal quantities of food eaten frequently and regularly, usually unrestricted within reason
  5. Urine testing—child should learn how to do this to increase independence
  6. Administration of insulin
    a. Child should be taught as early as motor and mental ability allows, usually by 7 or 9 years of age
    b. Explanation should be simple; diagrams for rotating sites should be used
    c. Periodic observation by an adult should be routine to discover faulty or careless technique

Hemophilia

A. Defects in clotting mechanism of blood—3 most common deficiencies
  1. Factor VIII, classic hemophilia
  2. Factor IX, Christmas disease
  3. Factor XI

B. Hereditary influence—sex-linked recessive gene, classically occurring in males
C. Clinical manifestations
  1. Prolonged bleeding from any wound
  2. Bleeding into the joints (hemarthrosis), resulting in pain, deformity, and retarded growth
  3. Anemia
  4. Intracranial hemorrhage
D. Treatment
  1. Control of bleeding
  2. Prevention of bleeding with use of factor replacement
    a. Drugs that replace deficient coagulation factors
      (1) Antihemophilic factor (Hemofil)
        (a) Obtained from human sources
        (b) Provides concentrated factor VIII
      (2) Antihemophilic plasma
      (3) Factor IX complex (Konỹne) contains factors II, VII, IX, X (concentrated)
    b. Clotting factor replacement
      (1) Epsilon-aminocaproic acid (Amicar) inhibits the enzyme that destroys formed fibrin and increases fibrinogen activity in clot formation
      (2) Fibrinogen (Parenogen) maintains plasma fibrinogen levels required for clotting materials
      (3) Thrombin supplies physiologic levels of natural material at superficial bleeding sites to control bleeding
E. Nursing problems and interventions
  1. Bleeding
    a. Instruct child and parents on treatment of bleeding, especially of joints
      (1) Immobilization of area
      (2) Compression of area
      (3) Elevation of body part
      (4) Application of cool compresses
    b. Appropriate activity that lessens chance of trauma, which is often difficult since boys are so physically active
  2. Pain
    a. Avoid use of aspirin or phenylbutazone
    b. Control joint pain so child uses extremity to prevent muscle atrophy
  3. Repeated hospitalizations—objective now is to strive for home care, with self-administration of coagulation factors such as cryoprecipitate

4. Guilt of parents
   a. Provide counseling, since disease is genetic and parents need assistance
   b. Encourage parents to treat child as normally as possible, avoiding overprotection or over-permissiveness

Rheumatic fever

A. Collagen disease—characterized by damage to connective tissue and usually blood vessels
B. Cause unknown—frequently follows infection with group *A beta hemolytic streptococci*
C. One of chief causes of death in school-age children, peak incidence between 6 and 8 years of age, with familial incidence
D. Predisposing factors—crowded living conditions, general lack of hygiene, temperate climate, poor nutrition
E. Clinical manifestations
   1. Carditis—possible damage to mitral valve
      a. Increased pulse, especially at night, poor pulse quality
      b. Low-grade fever in afternoon
      c. Anemia, pallor, weakness
      d. Anorexia, weight loss
      e. Increased respirations
   2. Arthritis
      a. Enlarged joints, with migratory pain
      b. Joint is red, hot, swollen, and tender, but deformity does not result
   3. Sydenham's chorea (St. Vitus's dance)
      a. Gradual onset
      b. Involuntary, purposeless movements
      c. Facial grimaces
      d. Restlessness and inability to maintain same position
      e. Emotional instability
   4. Subcutaneous nodules on extensor tendons of hands, feet, elbows, scapulae, patellae, vertebrae
      a. Nonpainful
      b. Skin moves freely over nodules
F. Laboratory findings
   1. Increased erythrocyte sedimentation rate
   2. Antistreptolysin-O titer
   3. Presence of C-reactive protein
   4. Aschoff bodies—in heart, arteries, nodules
   5. Leukocytosis
G. Treatment—antibiotics to eradicate organism and prevent recurrence

1. Penicillin preparations—drugs of choice
   a. Disrupt bacterial cell wall synthesis when new cells are forming by interfering with the synthesis and cross-linkage of mucopeptides in the final stage of cell wall synthesis
   b. Adverse effects—allergic reactions (highest incidence with parenteral administration)
      (1) Penicillinase (Neutrapen) used to inactivate circulating penicillin by its enzymatic action that converts the drug to penicilloic acid
      (2) Superinfection; e.g., *Candida* and *Pseudomonas* organisms in vagina, respiratory and intestinal tracts
   c. Drug interactions—salicylates and sulfonamides compete with penicillin for nephron tubule transport sites for secretion from the blood; blocking may cause high blood levels of penicillin; probenecid (Benemid) is a sulfonamide used therapeutically with penicillin to slow tubule secretion and allow lower dosage of penicillin
2. Erythromycins and similar drugs
   a. Compete for receptor sites on the ribosome unit to inhibit mRNA synthesis of protein required for reproduction
   b. Excretion route is in the bile through the intestine (90%), which allows use with compromised renal function
   c. Adverse effects—GI disturbances (nausea, vomiting, pyrosis, diarrhea, abdominal pain, stomatitis, black tongue)
   d. Drug interactions—decrease tolerance to alcohol ingestion
3. Sulfonamides—sulfadiazine
   a. Actions
      (1) Act by substitution of a false metabolite for para-aminobenzoic acid required for bacterial synthesis of folic acid
      (2) Plasma protein-binding maintains tissue levels by liberating drug when tissue levels are low
      (3) Tenacious plasma protein-binding may hold drug until it reaches renal sites, producing high levels in tubule urine
      (4) Many forms require alkalinization of urine and high fluid intake to maintain urine volume and decrease incidence of nephron crystals

(5) Recycling of drug in nephron delays excretion and maintains blood levels of drug
  (a) Tubule cells excrete drug into tubule urine after removal from plasma protein–binding sites
  (b) Tubule cells also reabsorb drug from tubule urine and it returns to tissue and liver sites to be metabolized
  (c) Alkalinization of urine slows recycling and increases excretion rate

b. Adverse effects—anorexia, nausea, vomiting (caused by gastric irritation and action at vomiting centers in medulla), malaise, blood dyscrasias (leukopenia, thrombocytopenia, erythrocytopenia) and hypoprothrombinemia, allergic reactions (generalized skin eruptions, high fever, severe headache, stomatitis, conjunctivitis, rhinitis, destructive skin lesions, death can result), hepatotoxicity, kernicterus in fetus (replaces protein-bound bilirubin)

c. Drug interactions—enhances action of oral anticoagulants and methotrexate

H. Nursing problems and interventions
  1. Bed rest—to reduce workload of heart
    a. Often difficult to maintain when child is feeling better
    b. Encourage child to do schoolwork and keep up with class
    c. Stimulate the development of quiet hobbies and collections
    d. Gradually increase activities over a period of weeks to months
  2. Pain
    a. Handle painful joints carefully
    b. Maintain proper body alignment to prevent deformities
    c. Monitor need for pain medication and administer when necessary
  3. Nutrition
    a. Increase fluids
    b. Provide small, frequent, nutritious meals
  4. Emotional support
    a. Prevent invalidism by emphasizing abilities rather than limitations
    b. Maintain child's status in home and school by keeping channels of communication open during illness

c. Help parents with home problems that may have served as predisposing factors
5. Public health prevention
  a. Proper and prompt treatment of streptococcal infections with antibiotics
  b. School screening and health promotion programs
  c. Improvement of poor housing conditions
  d. Teach proper standards of hygiene

Juvenile rheumatoid arthritis

A. Collagen disease, cause unknown, may occur in response to stress
B. Clinical manifestations
  1. Joint enlargement
    a. Stiffness, pain, and limited motion, especially in morning on awakening
    b. Spindle-fingers—thick proximal joint with slender tip
  2. Low-grade fever
  3. Erythematous rash on trunk and extremities
  4. Weight loss, fatigue, weakness
  5. Tachycardia
  6. Enlargement of spleen, liver, and lymph nodes
C. Treatment
  1. Salicylates—used in large doses for anti-inflammatory properties
    a. Drugs
      (1) Acetylsalicylic acid (A.S.A., Aspirin, Asteric, Ecotrin)
      (2) Carbaspirin calcium (Calurin)
      (3) Choline salicylate (Arthropan)
      (4) Salicylamide (Amid-Sal, Liquiprin, Raspberin, Salamide, Salicim, Salrin)
      (5) Sodium salicylate
    b. Adverse effects—gastric irritation, salicylism with long-term use (visual disturbances, tinnitus, dizziness, mental confusion, diaphoresis, nausea, vomiting, intense thirst)
    c. Drug interactions
      (1) Salicylates have an intrinsic hypoglycemic effect and require a decrease in the dosage of oral hypoglycemics for diabetics (they displace sulfonylurea hypoglycemics from protein-binding sites, which causes a greater hypoglycemic effect)
      (2) Salicylates decrease absorption of

indomethacin from the intestinal tract and lower its effective circulating level

    (3) Salicylates antagonize the effect of sulfinpyrazone and probenecid in reducing serum uric acid levels by inhibiting tubular secretion of uric acid

    (4) Salicylates have a hypoprothrombinemic action and potentiate effect of oral anticoagulants primarily by inhibiting platelet aggregation

  2. Steroids

  3. Physical therapy

D. Nursing problems and interventions

  1. Joint deformity and pain

    a. Emphasize that aspirin must be taken regularly, even in period of remission, to decrease inflammation and pain

    b. Promote proper body alignment and provide passive range of motion

    c. Encourage warm bath in morning to decrease stiffness and increase mobility

    d. Encourage exercises such as swimming

  2. Acceptance of disease by family and child

    a. Encourage parents to accept the child's illness but to limit the use of the disease to foster dependency or control relationships

    b. Teach family why aspirin is given in large dosages and why other medications are not used

  3. Aspirin toxicity—demonstrated by tinnitus, vertigo, nausea, vomiting, sweating, and other signs of salicylate poisoning

Skin infections

A. Pediculosis—lice

  1. May infest head, body, pubic area

  2. Eggs (greenish, translucent oval bodies) attach to hair

  3. Severe itching may lead to secondary infection

  4. Treatment—special shampoo, use of fine-toothed comb to remove nits, or eggs

  5. Prevention

    a. Cleanliness

      (1) Teach proper hair care

      (2) Encourage frequent bathing and change of clothes

    b. Screening in schools to identify source of infection

B. Scabies—produced by itch mite

  1. Female burrows under skin to lay eggs (usually in folds of skin)

  2. Intensely pruritic—scratching can lead to secondary infection with the development of papules and vesicles

  3. Treatment—all members of the family must be treated, since it is highly contagious

    a. Must wear clean clothes

    b. Must wash with sulfur or other special soap

C. Ringworm—fungus disease

  1. Scalp (tinea capitis)

    a. Reddened, oval or round areas of alopecia

    b. Treated topically or orally with an antifungal drug such as griseofulvin

    c. Head should be covered to prevent spread of infection

  2. Feet (athlete's foot)

    a. Scaly fissures between toes, vesicles on sides of feet, pruritus

    b. Particularly common in summer; contacted in swimming areas and gymnasium locker rooms

    c. Prevention—do not walk barefooted, dry feet carefully, wear lightweight shoes to decrease heat, disinfect shoes and socks

    d. Treatment—griseofulvin, micronized (Fulvicin-U/F, Grifulvin V, Grisactin)

      (1) Acts as an analog of purine and is incorporated into new epithelial cells during synthesis of nucleic acids

      (2) Adverse effects—peripheral neuritis, vertigo, fever, dryness of mouth, arthralgia, mild transient urticaria, nausea, diarrhea, headache (may disappear as therapy continues), drowsiness, fatigue

D. Intertrigo—excoriation of any adjacent body surfaces caused by moisture and chafing (diaper rash)

  1. Keep area clean and dry, rinse wastes from skin

  2. Expose area to light and air

  3. Apply bland ointment at night

  4. Avoid strong alkalis such as bleach in clothes washing

E. Impetigo

  1. Bacterial infection of skin by streptococci or staphylococci

  2. Sequelae of streptococcal infection—rheumatic fever, glomerulonephritis

3. Highly contagious, other areas of body frequently become infected
4. Treatment—antibiotics systemically and locally, isolate child, keep from scratching other areas of the body

Minimal brain dysfunction (MBD)

A. A disturbance of central nervous system functioning in which specific motor, sensory, or intellectual impairment exists
B. Characteristics of children with minimal brain dysfunction
   1. Difficulty in attention span
   2. May be hyperkinetic or underactive but are awkward and clumsy
   3. Impulsive acting out
   4. Problems with remembering, language, conceptualization, and perception
   5. Normal intellectual functioning
C. Nursing considerations—teach parents to
   1. Avoid overstimulation, provide frequent rest periods throughout day
   2. Structure situations to provide less frustration (play with only one other child rather than group)
   3. Provide firm and consistent discipline; ignore temper tantrums
   4. Learning is best done through play and use of concrete examples, such as 2 halves of an orange to teach fractions
   5. Provide exercises in perceptual-motor coordination and balance
   6. Structure learning experience to utilize child's ability
   7. Provide opportunities so that child can experience success and satisfaction
   8. Administration of drugs such as amphetamines to reduce hyperactivity

The adolescent

GROWTH AND DEVELOPMENT
Developmental timetable

A. Physical growth—includes the physical changes associated with puberty such as secondary sexual characteristics
B. Mental abilities
   1. Abstract thinking

   a. New level of social communication and understanding
      (1) Can comprehend satire and double meanings
      (2) Can say one thing and mean another
   b. Can conceptualize thought, more interested in exploring ideas than facts
   c. Can appreciate scientific thinking, problem solve, and theoretically explore alternatives
   2. Perception
   a. Can appreciate nonrepresentational art
   b. Can understand that the whole is more than the sum of its parts
   3. Learning
   a. Much longer span of attention
   b. Learns through process of inference, intuition, and surmise, rather than repetition and imitation
   c. Enjoys regressing in terms of language development by using jargon to suit changing moods
C. Social patterns
   1. Peer group identity
   a. One of strongest motivating forces of behavior
   b. Extremely important to be part of the group and like everyone else in every way
   c. Clique formation; usually based on common denominators such as race, social class, ethnic group, or special interests
   2. Interpersonal relationships
   a. Major goal is learning to form close intimate relationship with opposite sex
   b. Adolescents may develop many crushes and worship many idols
   c. Time of sexual exploration and questioning of one's sexual role
   3. Independence
   a. By 15 or 16 years of age, adolescents feel they should be treated as adults
   b. Ambivalence—adolescent wants freedom but is not happy about corresponding responsibilities and frequently yearns for more carefree days of childhood
   c. Parental ambivalence and discipline problems are common as parents try to allow for increasing independence but continue to offer constructive guidance and enforce discipline

HEALTH PROMOTION
Adolescent nutrition

A. Nutritional objectives
  1. Provide optimum nutritional support for demands of rapid growth and high energy expenditure
  2. Support development of good eating habits through variety of foods, regular pattern, good quality snacks (high in protein, low in refined carbohydrate, primarily sugar)
B. Nutrient needs increased in all respects, so adequate intakes of all nutrients should form basis of diet
C. Possible nutritional problems
  1. Low intakes of calcium, vitamin A and C, iron in girls
  2. Anemia—increase foods containing iron
  3. Obesity or underweight—decrease or increase calories as needed
  4. Skin problems—use well-balanced diet high in protein, vitamins, minerals
  5. Nutritional deficiencies related to
    a. Psychologic factors—food aversions, emotional problems
    b. Fear of overweight or crash diets—mainly in girls; cultural pressure
    c. Fad diets—caused by misinformation; need for sound counseling
    d. Poor choice of snack foods—usually high in sugar; use more fruit and protein forms
    e. Irregular eating pattern

6. Additional stress of pregnancy—need high protein and calorie intake
D. Nutrition education may be made through association with teenagers' concerns about physical appearance, figure control, complexion, physical fitness, athletic ability

Accident prevention

A. Appropriate education regarding sexual maturity, reproduction, and sexual behavior
B. Driver education
C. Education regarding use and abuse of drugs, especially alcohol
D. Education on health hazards associated with smoking

Problems of adolescence

A. Accidents—still number one cause of death, with motor vehicle accidents causing most fatalities
B. Suicide—one of chief causes of death among this age group
C. Drug abuse
D. Delinquency
E. Alcoholism
F. Many problems of adolescence similar to those of adults; see specific areas in Psychiatric and Medical-surgical nursing for further discussion

PEDIATRIC NURSING REVIEW QUESTIONS

Situation: Mr. Crew, a nursing student, is doing therapeutic play with the children in the playroom of the well-baby clinic. To understand how to plan for children of various ages, he needs to have knowledge of their developmental norms. Questions 1 through 4 refer to this situation.

1 Mr. Crew observes that 2-year-old Mark:
  1. Builds houses with blocks
  2. Is very possessive of toys
  3. Attempts to stay within the lines when coloring
  4. Amuses himself with a picture book for 15 minutes
2 Four-year-old Colin is having difficulty playing with the other children. Mr. Crew observes Colin's behavior and understands that it is normal for Colin to:
  1. Exaggerate and boast to impress others
  2. Have fierce temper tantrums and negativism

  3. Engage in parallel or solitary play
  4. Be almost totally dependent on parents
3 Fifteen-month-old Nadia is playing in the playpen. Mr. Crew observes her activities and realizes that her physical tasks are within the norms when she is able to:
  1. Build a tower of 6 blocks
  2. Stand in the playpen holding onto the sides
  3. Throw all the toys out of the playpen
  4. Walk across the playpen with ease
4 Mr. Crew would encourage two 6-year-old boys in the playroom to play with:
  1. A board game
  2. An erector set
  3. Checkers
  4. Clay

5 Play during infancy is:
1. Initiated by the child
2. A way of teaching how to share
3. More important than in later years
4. Mostly used for physical development

6 The primary developmental task to be accomplished between 12 and 15 months of age is to learn to:
1. Use a spoon
2. Give up the bottle
3. Walk
4. Say simple words

7 Preschool children role play. This is an important part of socialization, since it:
1. Encourages expression
2. Helps children think about careers
3. Teaches children about stereotypes
4. Provides guidelines for adult behavior

8 Learning processes associated with a particular stage of development often are referred to as "developmental tasks." What is characteristic about these tasks?
1. There is no uniform time for learning a task
2. Tasks are learned at the same age in children
3. Tasks occur with predictable rhythm
4. Most developmental tasks are learned by school age

Situation: Mr. and Mrs. B were emotionally upset when their baby girl Sue was born with a cleft palate and double cleft lip. Questions 9 through 13 refer to this situation.

9 How could the nurse give the most support to the parents?
1. Discourage them from talking about the baby
2. Encourage them to express their worries and fears
3. Tell them not to worry because the defect could be repaired
4. Show them postoperative photographs of babies who had similar defects

10 What is the most critical factor in the immediate care of Sue after repair of the lip?
1. Maintenance of a patent airway
2. Administration of drugs to reduce oral secretions
3. Administration of parenteral fluids
4. Prevention of vomiting

11 Additional nursing care for the infant with a surgical lip repair includes:
1. Placing the infant in a semisitting position
2. Keeping the infant from crying
3. Spoon-feeding for the first 2 days after surgery
4. Keeping baby NPO

12 At 2 years of age Sue returned for palate surgery. What was the most important factor in preparing her for this experience?
1. Her previous hospital visits
2. Gratification of all her wishes

3. Never leaving her with strangers
4. Assurance of affection and security

13 A toothbrush was not used on Sue immediately after palate surgery because:
1. The suture line might be injured
2. She was not accustomed to a brush at home
3. She had no teeth
4. It might be frightening to her

Situation: David, age 1 year, weighs 28 pounds (12.6 kg) but is pale and lethargic. His hemoglobin level is 5 g and he has an enlarged heart. When taking a nursing history from his mother, the nurse learns that he refuses food, so she gives him a quart of milk per day from a bottle. Questions 14 through 20 refer to this situation.

14 The nurse suggests that his mother:
1. Put a large hole in the nipple and put baby food in with his milk
2. Take him to the metabolic clinic for a check-up
3. Immediately begin the weaning process
4. Give him finger foods such as raisins and chopped meat

15 David should have been started on solid foods by at least 4 or 5 months of age because:
1. His fetal reserve of iron was depleted
2. It would have taught him how to chew
3. His bone marrow activity had slacked off at this time
4. It would have helped control his weight

16 The most prevalent nutritional disorder among children in the United States is iron deficiency anemia. A major reason for this in young children is:
1. Overfeeding of milk
2. Lack of adequate iron reserves from mother
3. Blood disorders
4. Introduction of solid foods too early for proper absorption

17 Anemia, a nutritional problem encountered in children and adults, involves several different nutrients. The nutrients include proteins, iron, vitamin B_{12}, and:
1. Carbohydrates
2. Thiamin
3. Calcium
4. Folic acid

18 Which of the following foods would you emphasize to David's mother as a source of iron to be included in his diet daily?
1. Orange juice
2. Lamb
3. Egg yolk
4. Milk

19 David's mother also states that he has 8 teeth and asks when she should take him to the dentist. For dental prophylaxis, the nurse encourages her to take him:

1. The next time another family member goes to the dentist
2. Before starting school
3. Between 2 and 3 years of age
4. When he begins to lose deciduous teeth

20 Your background knowledge of the basic nutrients that act as partners in building red blood cells will form the basis for a teaching plan. These nutrient partners are iron:
   1. Calcium and vitamins
   2. Carbohydrates and thiamine
   3. Proteins and ascorbic acid
   4. Vitamin D and riboflavin

21 Parents can predispose their children to problems with nutrition by using food in early childhood as a means of:
   1. Socializing
   2. Reward and punishment
   3. Aculturization
   4. Maintaining control

22 The major influence on eating habits of the *early* school-age child is the:
   1. Example of parents at mealtime
   2. Food preferences of the peer group
   3. Availability of food selections
   4. Smell and appearance of food

Situation: Four-year-old Ann weighs 40 pounds (18 kg) and is in a private pediatric room on "hand and linen precaution." She was admitted for weight loss, anorexia, vaginitis, and insomnia. A diagnosis of pinworm infestation was made. Questions 23 through 27 refer to this situation.

23 The most effective time for the nurse to do a cellophane tape test for pinworms is:
   1. At bedtime before bathing
   2. Just following a bowel movement
   3. Immediately after meals
   4. Early morning before arising

24 Pinworms cause a number of symptoms besides anal itching. A rare sequela of pinworm infestation that the nurse would observe for is:
   1. Pneumonitis
   2. Stomatitis
   3. Hepatitis
   4. Appendicitis

25 Pyrvinium pamoate (Povan) is an effective single-dose drug to eliminate pinworms. How many milligrams will you give Ann if 5 mg per kilogram of body weight are ordered?
   1. 90 mg
   2. 18 mg
   3. 40 mg
   4. 200 mg

26 After administering pyrvinium pamoate (Povan) to Ann, it is important to alert the staff that a normal side effect of this drug is that it colors the stool or vomitus:
   1. Dark brown
   2. Light green
   3. Bright red
   4. Gentian blue

27 The nurse's decision to alert the staff is based on her knowledge that:
   1. Irritation by pinworms in the rectum may cause ulceration and bleeding
   2. The cyanine dye origin of the drug colors the stool
   3. The stool contains hemoglobin-like metabolic products of disintegrating pinworms
   4. The drug is irritating to the intestinal mucosa and may cause transient bleeding

Situation: Seven-year-old Johnny has been admitted for a tonsillectomy. Questions 28 through 30 refer to this situation.

28 An essential nursing action preoperatively is to:
   1. Encourage parent to stay until Johnny goes to the operating room
   2. Provide him with his favorite toy
   3. Observe his ASO titer
   4. Check for loose teeth and report to physician

29 The nurse suspects hemorrhage postoperatively when Johnny:
   1. Snores noisily
   2. Becomes pale
   3. Complains of thirst
   4. Swallows frequently

30 Johnny is complaining of pain in his throat. Which of the following medications for pain would be best for him at this time?
   1. Aspirin, 300 mg
   2. Tylenol, 300 mg
   3. Phenobarbital, 15 mg
   4. Demerol, 50 mg

Situation: Two-day-old Edward has a myelomeningocele. He is scheduled for surgery. Questions 31 through 33 refer to this situaton.

31 Prior to the surgical correction, a primary nursing goal is to:
   1. Observe for hydrocephalus
   2. Prevent infection
   3. Prevent skin breakdown
   4. Observe for increasing paralysis

32 Following the closure of Edward's myelomeningocele, it is essential that his nursing care include:
   1. Decrease of environmental stimuli
   2. Strict limitation of leg movement
   3. Measurement of head circumference daily
   4. Observation of serous drainage from the nares

33 To meet a major developmental need of Edward's, the nurse should:
1. Provide a soft cuddly toy
2. Provide him with a pacifier
3. Warm his formula before feeding
4. Put a mobile over his crib

Situation: Eight-year-old John Kee is being discharged following treatment for sickle cell crisis. He is allowed to return to school and resume normal activities. Questions 34 through 38 refer to this situation.

34 The nurse explains to Mrs. Kee that a very important aspect of care for John at home should include:
1. At least 14 hours sleep per day
2. Avoidance of all strenuous play and activities
3. Ingestion of large quantities of liquids
4. Protection from emotional upsets

35 Infants with sickle cell anemia may not be diagnosed as having this disorder because of:
1. The presence of fetal hemoglobin during the first year of life
2. Compensation of increased hematocrit and hemoglobin if well fed
3. Absence of respiratory disorders
4. General good health and an excellent growth curve

36 The sickling process of the red blood cell occurs in conditions of:
1. Hypovlemia
2. Hypoxia
3. Anemia
4. Hypocalcemia

37 To prevent thrombus formation in capillaries, as well as other problems from stasis and clotting of blood in the sickling process, the main nursing intervention is:
1. Administration of oxygen
2. Increasing fluids by mouth and a humidifier
3. Complete bed rest
4. Use of heparin or other anticoagulants

38 Common nursing care that helps prevent both sickle cell crisis and celiac crisis is:
1. Limitation of activity
2. Protection from infection
3. High-iron, low-fat, high-protein diet
4. Careful observation of all vital signs

Situation: Roy Brown, an 18-month-old boy, is admitted to the hospital with an upper respiratory tract infection. This is his first hospitalization and prolonged separation from his mother. Questions 39 through 44 refer to this situation.

39 Based on this information, the nurse may expect to see which type of behavior during the initial admission?
1. Generally crying when people enter the room, but does respond with a smile after a few minutes

2. Crying relentlessly, consoled by no one except his mother or father
3. Withdrawn, sitting quietly, not interested in playing
4. Initially unhappy and crying, but contented after meeting his roommates

40 After a prolonged period of hospitalization, Roy becomes depressed, withdrawn, and apathetic toward his mother. Eventually, he begins playing with toys and relating to others, even strangers. The nurse should realize that he has:
1. Accepted his hospitalization well and has matured because of this experience
2. Grown out of the stage of separation and realizes that he has to depend on others
3. Probably become somewhat detached because of this traumatic separation
4. Finally recognized that the staff is not out to hurt him

41 Studies of young children institutionalized for some time indicate that they show signs of retarded development. Not all aspects of development are equally affected. The least affected is:
1. Neuromuscular development
2. Hearing
3. Ability to understand
4. Ability to express himself

42 The major depriving factor in long-term hospitalization is usually the:
1. Absence of interaction with a mother figure
2. Lack of multisensory inputs
3. Care provided only by a mother substitute
4. Lack of play objects

43 Studies of histories of children who have suffered prolonged maternal deprivation early in life indicate that these children:
1. Are unable to love
2. Establish warm relationships with a mother substitute
3. Recall past experiences vividly
4. Are particularly conscious of time

44 When Roy's mother is getting ready to take him home, she asks the nurse what kind of behavior she should expect Roy to display. The nurse informs her that Roy will probably be:
1. Hostile toward her
2. Make excessive demands of both parents
3. Cheerful but have a shallow attachment to all adults
4. Apathetic and withdrawn from all emotional ties to her

45 Selection of drugs of choice for the treatment of pneumonia depends primarily on:
1. Selectivity of the organism
2. Tolerance of the patient
3. Preference of the physician
4. Sensitivity of the organism

46 Mrs. Legere and her son Johnny are seen at the clinic.

They both have severe upper respiratory tract infections, and the physician plans to prescribe tetracycline (Achromycin). The nurse reminds him that Johnny is 6 years old and that Mrs. Legere is in her eighteenth week of pregnancy. The data are important because the drug may cause:

1. Persistent vomiting when given to small children and pregnant women
2. Tooth enamel defects in children under 8 years of age and in the maturing fetus
3. Lower red blood cell production at times in their development when anemia is a common problem
4. Changes in the bone structure of young children and pregnant women

Situation: Baby boy Charles Brown, 7 days old, is admitted to the Pediatric Unit from the nursery with a diagnosis of Down's syndrome. Questions 47 through 53 refer to this situation.

47 Which of the following problems can be expected in caring for Baby Brown?
1. Slowed development as child reaches 1 or 2 years of age
2. High incidence of circulatory problems
3. Proneness to respiratory tract infections
4. Difficulty in hearing

48 The symptom of Down's syndrome most evident to the nursery nurse during the initial newborn assessment would be:
1. Asymmetric gluteal folds
2. Hypertonicity of skeletal muscles
3. A rounded occiput
4. Simian creases on the palms and soles

49 Special nursing care for Baby Brown should include:
1. Frequent handling and rocking to keep him from crying
2. Helping parents to learn about their child
3. Teaching infant to nipple-feed
4. Preventing aspiration of formula by frequent bubbling

50 When observing a newborn with Down's syndrome, the nurse should be aware that a common defect associated with the condition is:
1. Deafness
2. Congenital heart defects
3. Hydrocephaly
4. Muscular hypertonicity

51 Which of the following factors would probably be most significant for the nurse working with the Brown family? Mr. and Mrs. Brown's:
1. Response to family's and friends' reactions to their infant
2. Ability to give physical care to their infant
3. Ability to talk about changing plans they had made for their infant

4. Understanding of the factors causing Down's syndrome

52 As Charles grows, his development lags and it is found that he is moderately retarded. Which of the following suggestions would be most helpful to his parents? They should:
1. Offer challenging, competitive situations
2. Offer simple, repetitive tasks
3. Concentrate on teaching detailed tasks
4. Offer complete directions at the beginning of the task to be accomplished

53 The handicapped child has the same needs as the normal child, although his means of satisfying these needs are limited. This limitation frequently causes:
1. Emotional disability
2. Overcompensation
3. Frustration
4. Rejection

---

54 A viral infection characterized by red blotchy rash and Koplik's spots in the mouth is:
1. Rubeola
2. Rubella
3. Chickenpox
4. Mumps

55 Under certain circumstances the virus that causes chickenpox can also cause:
1. Athlete's foot
2. Infectious hepatitis
3. Herpes zoster
4. German measles

56 Using live virus vaccines against measles is contraindicated in children receiving corticosteroids or antineoplastic or irradiation therapy because these children may:
1. Have had the disease or have been immunized previously
2. Be unlikely to need this protection during their shortened life span
3. Be allergic to rabbit serum, which is used as a base for these vaccines
4. Be susceptible to infection due to their depressed immune response

57 An injection consisting of bacterial cells that have been modified is:
1. A vaccine
2. An antitoxin
3. A toxoid
4. A toxin

Situation: Johnny Smith, 12 months of age, is brought to the Preventive Health Clinic for a regular physical assessment. Questions 58 through 61 refer to this situation.

58 In reviewing his immunizations for the past 10 months the nurse would expect him to have been immunized against:
1. Measles, rubella, polio, TB, and pertussis
2. Polio, pertussis, tetanus, and diphtheria
3. Measles, mumps, rubella, and TB
4. Pertussis, tetanus, polio, and measles

59 Mrs. Smith asks the nurse how the DPT injection works. The nurse, in formulating a response, recalls that in active immunity:
1. Blood antigens are aided by phagocytes in defending the body against pathogens
2. Protein antigens are formed in the blood to fight invading antibodies
3. Protein substances are formed by the body to destroy or neutralize antigens
4. Lipid agents are formed by the body against antigens

60 The measles immunization is usually routinely given after 15 months of age because of the:
1. Increased hazard of side effects in infants
2. Presence of maternal antibodies during the first year
3. Interference it causes with effectiveness of pertussis, diphtheria, and tetanus immunizations
4. Rare incidence of measles infection prior to 12 months of age

61 In terms of preventive teaching for a 1-year-old, the nurse would speak to Mrs. Smith about:
1. Adequate nutrition
2. Accidents
3. Sexual development
4. Toilet training

---

62 A child comes to the hospital after exposure to diphtheria and is given antitoxin. This is what type of immunity?
1. Active natural immunity
2. Active artificial immunity
3. Passive natural immunity
4. Passive artificial immunity

63 Immunity by antibody formation during the course of a disease is:
1. Active natural immunity
2. Active artificial immunity
3. Passive natural immunity
4. Passive artificial immunity

64 A viral disease with grave complications producing respiratory tract inflammation and skin rash is:
1. Rubeola
2. Rubella
3. Yellow fever
4. Chickenpox

65 Mary has had her primary immunizations and so her mother asks the nurse which ones she should receive prior to starting kindergarten. The nurse suggests the following booster doses:
1. DPT, TOPV
2. Measles, DPT
3. TOPV, rubella
4. DPT, tuberculin test

66 Occasionally infants are born without an immune system. These infants can live normally with no apparent problems during their first months after birth because:
1. Limited antibodies are produced by the fetal thymus during the eighth and ninth months of gestation
2. Antibodies are passively received from the mother through the placenta and milk
3. Limited antibodies are produced by the infant's colonic bacteria
4. Exposure to pathogens during this time can be limited

Situation: Nancy Hand, a 5-year-old only child, is admitted to the hospital with rheumatic fever. She requires bed rest, a soft diet, liberal fluid intake, and ampicillin, 250 mg, po qid. Nancy is restless and fretful and tells you that her legs hurt. Questions 67 through 74 refer to this situation.

67 Nancy may be more comfortable if her:
1. Position is changed frequently
2. Bed is elevated at the head
3. Legs are supported on a pillow
4. Body alignment is maintained

68 The immediate priority in Nancy's nursing care is:
1. Nutrition
2. Rest
3. Exercise
4. Elimination

69 Nursing care likely to be most effective in alleviating Nancy's fretfulness is:
1. Giving her a jigsaw puzzle
2. Putting her in a room by herself
3. Letting her play with a doll
4. Reading a story to her

70 The best choice of between-meal nourishment for Nancy is:
1. Fresh fruit
2. Hard candy
3. Fruit gelatin
4. Creamed soup

71 The most serious complication that may threaten Nancy is:
1. Endocarditis
2. Pneumonitis
3. Tenosynovitis
4. Rheumatoid arthritis

72 When you bring Nancy her dinner tray she says, ''I'm too sick to feed myself.'' You should tell her to:
1. Try to eat as much as she can
2. Be a big girl and not to act like a baby
3. Let it go until she feels better
4. Wait 5 minutes and you will help her

73 Nancy's statement is most likely indicative of:
1. Immaturity

2. Lonesomeness
3. Regression
4. Temper tantrum

74 Nancy is apathetic about eating. Nursing care directed toward supporting her nutrition ought to include:
1. Providing diversional activity at mealtime
2. Eliminating all between-meal nourishment
3. Asking her parents to visit at mealtime
4. Giving her only the foods she likes best

Situation: Eighteen-month-old Molly Brown is admitted with croup. She is clinging to her mother crying and responds negatively to all suggestions. Questions 75 through 81 refer to this situation.

75 The nurse, in assessing Molly, would expect to find:
1. Bronchospasm, whooping cough
2. Expiratory stridor, rales
3. Laryngospasm, barking cough
4. Productive cough, inspiratory stridor

76 Mr. and Mrs. Brown ask the nurse what they should do if Molly has another attack of croup at home. The nurse suggests that Molly's parents interrupt the croup attack by administering:
1. Cheracol syrup
2. Syrup of ipecac
3. Hydrocortisone succinate (Solu-Cortef)
4. Epinephrine

77 The nurse's teaching is based on the action of this drug, which results in:
1. Dilation of the bronchi
2. Reduction of the inflammation
3. Interruption of the spasm
4. Depression of the cough center

78 When Mrs. Brown returns with Molly to the physician's office for medical follow-up, she tells the nurse that Molly has been ''driving her crazy'' by saying no to everything she suggests. She asks the nurse for help in handling her. The nurse explains to Mrs. Brown that Molly's negativism is normal for her age and that it is helping her meet her need for:
1. Discipline
2. Independence
3. Attention
4. Trust

79 Mrs. Brown states, ''This morning I gave Molly her juice and she said 'no.' She says 'no' and I get angry, but she needs her fluids. What shall I do?'' The nurse suggests that she:
1. Be firm and hand her the glass
2. Distract her with some food
3. Let her see that she is making her mother angry
4. Offer her a choice of 2 things to drink

80 The nurse plans to talk to Mrs. Brown about toilet train-

ing Molly, knowing that the most important factor in the process of toilet training is the:
1. Child's desire to be dry
2. Approach and attitude of the parent
3. Ability of the child to sit still
4. Parent's willingness to work at it

81 Before Mrs. Brown leaves the clinic, the nurse tells her that she can best help her daughter learn to control her own behavior by:
1. Rewarding her for good behavior
2. Allowing her to learn by her mistakes
3. Punishing her when she deserves it
4. Setting limits and being consistent

Situation: Mrs. Bronson is informed that her infant daughter has phenylketonuria (PKU). Questions 82 through 86 refer to this situation.

82 Which of the following statements is true concerning PKU?
1. PKU is transmitted by an autosomal dominant gene
2. The infant is tested for PKU immediately after delivery
3. If untreated, mental retardation occurs
4. Treatment for PKU includes life-long diet therapy

83 A test that was done on Baby Bronson in the nursery to detect PKU is:
1. Guthrie blood test
2. Ferric chloride urine test
3. Phenistix test
4. Clinitest serum phosphopyruvic acid

84 Primary treatment of an infant who has an inherited inborn error of metabolism consists mostly of:
1. Hormonal therapy
2. Dietary control
3. Enzyme replacement
4. Vitamin supplement

85 When teaching Mr. and Mrs. Bronson about their daughter's disorder, the nurse should state that:
1. Phenylalanine is not necessary for growth
2. Other amino acids can be increased to substitute for phenylalanine
3. A low-phenylalanine diet is required
4. Phenylalanine can be administered to correct the deficiency

86 In terms of dietary counseling, the parents need much help and support in adhering to specific regimens. A frequent question asked by parents is, ''How long will my child have to be on this diet?'' An appropriate response by the nurse is:
1. ''Unfortunately, this is a life-long problem and dietary management must always be maintained.''
2. ''Usually, if the child does well for 1 year, she then can gradually begin eating regular foods.''
3. ''As of now, research shows that a child needs to be on

this diet until she is about 6 to 8 years of age. Then she can gradually begin to eat other foods.''
4. ''No one knows, but why don't you discuss it with your doctor.''

Situation: Mrs. Simmons brings 3-year-old Sam to the emergency room, indicating he has had a fever for several days, has held his neck rigid, and is now vomiting. While being examined he has a convulsion and is admitted to the Pediatric Unit. Questions 87 through 91 refer to this situation.

87 While instituting nursing measures to reduce Sam's fever, the nurse recognizes that an important consideration is to:
   1. Monitor vital signs every 10 minutes
   2. Force oral fluids
   3. Measure output every hour
   4. Limit exposure to prevent shivering
88 Febrile convulsions are not uncommon and:
   1. Rarely occur during the first year of life
   2. The cause is usually readily identified
   3. May occur in minor illnesses
   4. Occur more frequently in females than males
89 The physician orders A.S.A., 150 mg, po q 4 h prn for fever above 101° F (38° C). You have on hand A.S.A. labeled ''1 tablet equals 1¼ gr.'' How many tablets should be administered?
   1. ½ tablet
   2. 1 tablet
   3. 1½ tablets
   4. 2 tablets
90 Sam is diagnosed as having meningococcal meningitis. The nurse observes Sam for the:
   1. Identifying purpuric skin rash
   2. Continual tremors of the extremities
   3. Low-grade nature of the fever
   4. Palatal paralysis and glossitis
91 The most serious complication of meningitis in young children is:
   1. Hydrocephalus
   2. Blindness
   3. Peripheral circulatory collapse
   4. Epilepsy

---

92 James, a 2-year-old child, is admitted to the hospital with a diagnosis of pneumonia. He is given antibiotics, forced fluids, and oxygen. James' temperature continued to rise until it reached 39.4° C (103° F). The nurse calls the physician at the mother's request, but the physician sees no cause for alarm or change in treatment, even though James has a history of convulsions during previous periods of high fever. Even though the nurse is concerned, she takes no further action. Later James has a convulsion that results in neurologic impairment of the left arm and leg. Legally:
   1. The nurse's actions did not derive from observations, patient's history, or scientific fact

2. The physician's decision takes precedence over the nurse's concern
3. High temperatures are common in children, and this situation presented little cause for undue concern
4. The physician is totally responsible for the patient's health history and treatment regimen
93 Four-year-old Bobby has a seizure disorder and has been taking phenytoin (Dilantin) for 3 years. An important nursing measure for Bobby would be to:
   1. Offer the urinal frequently
   2. Administer scrupulous oral hygiene
   3. Check for pupillary reaction
   4. Observe for flushing of the face
94 When teaching parents at the PTA about communicable diseases, the nurse reminds them that these diseases are serious, and that encephalitis can be a complication of:
   1. Chickenpox
   2. Pertussis
   3. Poliomyelitis
   4. Scarlet fever
95 A viral disease caused by one of the smallest human viruses that infects the motor cells of the anterior horn of the nerve cord is:
   1. Rubeola
   2. Rubella
   3. Poliomyelitis
   4. Chickenpox

Situation: Three-month-old Matt Quincy is admitted to the hospital with bile-stained vomitus and abdominal distention. Questions 96 through 99 refer to this situation.

96 The nurse should also observe for:
   1. Constant severe pain and absence of stools
   2. Bounding pulse and hypotonicity
   3. Paroxysmal pain and grunting respirations
   4. High-pitched cry and weak thready pulse
97 Prior to surgery for the intestinal obstruction, Matt is kept NPO and has a Levin tube in place. To calm Matt and also to best meet his developmental needs, the nurse should:
   1. Allow him to suck on a pacifier
   2. Hang a brightly colored mobile in his crib
   3. Place him on his abdomen and permit him to crawl
   4. Allow him to hold his favorite toy
98 Matt develops diarrhea postoperatively and is given IV fluids. The rate of flow must be observed often by the nurse to:
   1. Avoid IV infiltration
   2. Prevent increased output
   3. Prevent cardiac embarrassment
   4. Replace all fluids lost
99 When Mrs. Quincy returns to the surgical clinic for follow-up care, the nurse includes the following preventive suggestion in her teaching:
   1. Remove all tiny objects from the floor

2. Keep crib rails up to the highest position
3. Cover electric outlets with safety plugs
4. Remove poisonous substances from low areas

Situation: After an uneventful labor and delivery Mrs. Handler delivers a 7-pound (3.15 kg) boy with a bilateral cleft lip and palate. She does not see the baby in the delivery room. Mr. Handler has been told of the defect and has seen the baby. He is very upset, but his major concern is for his wife and her reaction. Questions 100 through 104 refer to this situation.

100 While looking at the baby, Mr. Handler says to the nursery nurse, "Oh, what am I going to do, how could this happen to us, what is my wife going to do? It would have been better if she had never become pregnant." The most appropriate response for the nurse to make is:
   1. "How can you say that? You have a lovely healthy baby; the cleft lip can be fixed and then the baby will be fine."
   2. "I know how hard this must be for you. But believe me, you will love the baby so much, you won't even notice that he is disfigured."
   3. "This must be very hard on you. Would it help if I went with you when the doctor talks to your wife?"
   4. "I know that this is very difficult for you. But you can't think of yourself now. Your wife needs you. You must be strong."

101 After the physician talks to Mrs. Handler, she seems quite composed and asks to see the baby. To assess Mrs. Handler's reaction, the nurse would:
   1. Bring the baby to her immediately
   2. Tell her exactly what the baby looks like before bringing him to her
   3. Encourage her to express and explore her feelings; bring the baby to her and stay with her during this time
   4. Show her some pictures and give her some literature on harelip and cleft palate and discuss the treatment with her before bringing the baby to her

102 When Mrs. Handler sees the baby, she becomes very disturbed, pushes him away, and says, "Oh, take him away, I never want to see him again." This reaction would indicate that Mrs. Handler is:
   1. Unable to cope with the situation and that arrangements will have to be made to place the baby into a foster home, at least for the first few months
   2. Responding as most normal new mothers do, who find it difficult to accept that their baby is less than perfect
   3. Severely emotionally disturbed and is in immediate need of psychiatric help
   4. Rejecting the baby and he will have to be placed for adoption

103 Mr. and Mrs. Handler decide to take the baby home as soon as feasible. The nurse has many concerns relating to the baby's welfare and the ability of the mother to care for him. The most important of these is:

1. Mother-infant relationship
2. Feeding of the infant
3. General physical care for the infant
4. Long-range plans for repair of the defects

104 Afterward Mrs. Handler asks how she is going to feed the baby if his mouth is deformed and he cannot suck properly. The nurse teaches her carefully and gently how feedings are to be given and states:
   1. "Try using a soft nipple with an enlarged opening so that he can get the milk through a chewing motion"
   2. "Since he tries easily, it is best to have him lying in bed while he is being fed"
   3. "He should be held in a horizontal position and fed slowly to avoid aspiration"
   4. "Give him brief rest periods and frequent burpings during feedings to expel swallowed air"

Situation: Five-year-old Sam has been hospitalized with acute glomerulonephritis. Questions 105 through 108 refer to this situation.

105 The nurse observes Sam primarily for:
   1. Polyuria, high fever
   2. Dehydration, hematuria
   3. Hypertension, circumocular edema
   4. Oliguria, hypotension

106 When planning nursing care for Sam, the nurse realizes that he needs help in understanding his restrictions, one of which is:
   1. Bed rest for at least 4 weeks
   2. A bland diet high in protein
   3. Daily doses of IM penicillin
   4. Isolation from other children with infections

107 The average 5-year-old is incapable of:
   1. Making decisions
   2. Tying his shoelaces
   3. Abstract thought
   4. Hand-eye coordination

108 Sam loves to ride his bike, and his parents are very concerned about his activity when he returns home. You base your answer to them on the fact that after the urinary findings are nearly normal:
   1. He must remain in bed for 2 weeks
   2. Activity does not affect the course of the disease
   3. He must not play active games
   4. Activity must be limited for 1 month

---

109 A *Streptococcus* infection characterized by swollen joints, fever, and the possibility of endocarditis and death is:
   1. Whooping cough
   2. Measles
   3. Tetanus
   4. Rheumatic fever

110 A skin infection that can be a sequela of rheumatic fever or glomerulonephritis is:
1. Herpes simplex
2. Scabies
3. Intertrigo
4. Impetigo

111 A small toddler is admitted to the hospital because of sudden hoarseness and an insistence on continuous and somewhat unintelligible speech. In talking with the mother, the nurse will be particularly concerned about:
1. Acute respiratory tract infection
2. Undetected laryngeal abnormality
3. Respiratory tract obstruction due to a foreign body
4. Retropharyngeal abscess

Situation: Eight-year-old John has rheumatic fever. He has a low-grade fever in the afternoon, is anemic, and his shoulder, elbow, and knee joints are painful, hot, and enlarged. His therapy includes bed rest, and he is receiving large amounts of A.S.A. daily. Questions 112 through 114 refer to this situation.

112 During the acute phase, to help relieve the pain in John's joints, the nurse should maintain body alignment, support the joints with pillows, and:
1. Apply heat to the joints
2. Give passive range of motion exercises once a day only
3. Elevate the extremities
4. Move him as little as possible

113 While John is in bed convalescing, he becomes very bored and irritable. The nurse plans activities that a school-age child would like and suggests he:
1. Play chess
2. Start a collection
3. Watch game shows on TV
4. Do arithmetic puzzles

114 John *must* remain in bed until his pulse rate and hemoglobin level are normal and the:
1. C-reactive protein is negative
2. Fever is decreased to 100° F (37.8° C)
3. Pain is totally gone from the joints
4. Rash has disappeared

Situation: Sue Green, a 2-year-old girl, is admitted to the Pediatric Unit with respiratory wheezing, dyspnea, and cyanosis. One of the tentative diagnoses is cystic fibrosis. Questions 115 through 121 refer to this situation.

115 Cystic fibrosis can predispose Sue to bronchitis mainly because:
1. Tenacious secretions obstruct the bronchioles and respiratory tract and provide a favorable medium for growth of bacteria
2. Increased salt content in saliva can irritate and necrose mucous membranes in nasopharynx
3. Neuromuscular irritability causes spasm and constriction of the bronchi

4. The associated heart defects of cystic fibrosis cause congestive heart failure and respiratory depression

116 The problem of cystic fibrosis is sometimes first noted by the nurse in the newborn nursery because of:
1. Increased heart rate
2. Abdominal distention
3. Excessive crying
4. Sternal retractions

117 Sue is small and underdeveloped for her age primarily because she:
1. Ingested little food for several months because of poor appetite
2. Failed to absorb nutrients because of a lack of pancreatic enzymes
3. Secreted less than normal amounts of pituitary growth hormone
4. Developed muscular and bony atrophy from lack of motor activity

118 When caring for the child with cystic fibrosis the nurse should:
1. Promote postural drainage
2. Help the child conserve energy
3. Prevent coughing
4. Provide small frequent feedings

119 The foul-smelling, frothy characteristic of the stool in cystic fibrosis results from the presence of large amounts of:
1. Sodium and chloride
2. Semidigested carbohydrates
3. Undigested fat
4. Lipase, trypsin, and amylase

120 Medications that will probably be used for Sue in her therapeutic regimen include:
1. A steroid and an antimetabolite
2. Antibiotics, a multivitamin preparation, and cough drops
3. Pancreatic enzymes and antibiotics
4. Aerosol mists, decongestants, and fat-soluble vitamins

121 In cystic fibrosis, frequent stools and tenacious mucus often produce:
1. Intussusception
2. Anal fissures
3. Meconium ileus
4. Rectal prolapse

Situation: Two-year-old Mike Cox is admitted to the hospital for the second surgical repair of his clubfoot. Mrs. Cox cannot stay overnight with her son, since visiting hours are restricted. On the morning after admission, Mike is standing in his crib crying. He refuses to be comforted and calls for his mother. Questions 122 through 125 refer to this situation.

122 The nurse approaches Mike to bathe him and he screams louder. She recognizes this behavior as the stage of protest and:

1. Picks him up and walks with him around the room
2. Sits by his crib and bathes him later when his anxiety decreases
3. Decides he really does not need a bath when he is this upset
4. Fills the basin with water and proceeds to bathe him

123 On the third postoperative day Mike begins to regress and lies quietly in his crib with his blanket. The nurse recognizes that Mike is in a stage of:
1. Denial
2. Mistrust
3. Rejection
4. Despair

124 During his second week of hospitalization, Mike smiles easily, goes to all the nurses happily, and no longer cries when his mother goes home. After leaving Mike's room, Mrs. Cox tells the nurse she is pleased that Mike is adjusting well. Before responding to Mrs. Cox, the nurse understands Mike's behavior and realizes that he:
1. Is repressing his feelings for his mother
2. Has established a routine and feels safe
3. Feels better physically so his behavior has improved
4. Has given up fighting and accepts the separation

125 The nurse explains the meaning of Mike's behavior to Mrs. Cox and tells her that after he goes home she should expect that:
1. Mike will miss the nurses and hospital routine
2. It will be easier for Mike to adjust to his home situation
3. Mike will continue his happy, normal behavior
4. It will take some time before the mother-child relationship is reestablished

---

126 Sara, 12 years old, was diagnosed at the orthopedic clinic as having idiopathic scoliosis. Proper exercising and avoidance of fatigue are essential components of Sara's care. Early in Sara's treatment the nurse can suggest which of the following sports as therapeutic?
1. Bowling
2. Swimming
3. Badminton
4. Golf

127 To assist her curvature correction, Sara is fitted with a Milwaukee brace. The nurse explains to Sara and her parents that the length of time the brace must be worn varies, but it is usually worn until:
1. Cessation of bone growth at the time of physical maturity
2. The curvature of the spine is completely straightened
3. Pain on prolonged standing diminishes
4. The iliac crests are at equal levels

128 One of the earliest signs of sexual maturity in the young female is:

1. Interest in the opposite sex
2. Attention to grooming
3. An increase in the size of the external genitalia
4. The appearance of axillary and pubic hair

129 An infection caused by the yeast *Candida albicans* often occurring in infants and debilitated individuals is:
1. Typhoid fever
2. Thrush
3. Malta fever
4. Dysentery

130 A mother talks to the nurse about her sick infant and she is disturbed because she did not realize the baby was ill. Which of the following is frequently the only sign of illness that her infant may have?
1. Longer periods of sleep
2. Grunting and rapid respirations
3. Perspiring profusely
4. Desire for increased fluids during the feedings

131 Among the last signs of heart failure in the infant and child is:
1. Rapid respiratory rate in the supine position
2. Orthopnea
3. Tachypnea
4. Peripheral edema

132 A newborn of a few hours appears to be less cyanotic when he cries. The nurse should observe for:
1. Twitching of the body for neural damage
2. Equality of chest expansion for an atelectasis problem
3. Heart rate for an atrioventricular septal defect
4. Sternal retractions of respiratory distress syndrome

133 A mother brings her week-old newborn to the clinic because he continually regurgitates. Chalasia is suspected. The nurse instructs the mother to:
1. Keep the infant prone following feedings
2. Not permit the infant to cry for prolonged periods
3. Keep the infant in a semisitting position, particularly after feedings
4. Administer a minimum of 8 oz of formula at each feeding

Situation: At 2 weeks of age Baby Williams begins to vomit after his feedings and is admitted to the hospital for observation with a tentative diagnosis of pyloric stenosis. Questions 134 through 138 refer to this situation.

134 The nurse was careful to note:
1. Signs of dehydration
2. Coughing and gagging after feeding
3. Quality of cry
4. Quality of stool

135 When vomiting is uncontrolled in an infant, the nurse should observe for signs of:
1. Tetany
2. Alkalosis

3. Acidosis
4. Hyperactivity
136 The maintenance of fluid and electrolyte balance is more critical in children than in adults because:
1. Renal function is immature in children
2. Cellular metabolism is less stable than in adults
3. The proportion of water in the body is less than in adults
4. The daily fluid requirement per unit of body weight is greater than in adults
137 What is the most critical factor confronting the nurse in the administration of IV fluids to a small, dehydrated infant?
1. Maintenance of the prescribed rate of flow
2. Maintenance of the fluid at body temperature
3. Calculation of the total intake
4. Maintenance of sterility
138 Surgery is performed and Baby Williams' condition is good. The nurse caring for him notices that his postoperative orders are similar to those for other infants having such surgery and include:
1. Withholding of all feedings for the first 24 hours
2. Additional glucose feedings after the first 24 hours
3. Thickened formula 24 hours after surgery
4. Diluted formula feeding 24 hours after surgery

---

139 In many states, failure by the nurse to report a suspected case of child abuse is punishable by law. Child abuse is one of the major causes of death in young children. When a child is admitted to the hospital with traumatic injuries, a common clue that the child was battered is that he:
1. Cries for longer periods of time and has large hematomas
2. Ignores offers of toys and favors and cries when picked up
3. Shows no expectation of being comforted
4. Does not cry during painful procedures
140 There are many common reactions of parents who batter their children. One reaction the nurse should be aware of is that the parent:
1. Seldom touches or looks at the child
2. Show signs of guilt about the child's injury
3. Is quick to inquire about the discharge date
4. Is very concerned about his own physical health
141 Another behavior that is most typical of the parents of the battered child is that they:
1. Present many details related to how the trauma occurred
2. Blame the child for the accident
3. Become irritable about having the history taken
4. Give contradictory explanations about what happened
142 The best legal definition of assault is:
1. The application of force to another person without lawful justification

2. Threats to do bodily harm to the person of another person
3. A legal wrong committed by one person against the property of another
4. A legal wrong committed against the public and punishable by law through the state and courts
143 In legal terminology, the term battery means:
1. Doing something that a reasonable person with the same education or preparation would not do
2. A legal wrong committed by one person against the property of another
3. The application of force to the person of another person without lawful justification
4. Maligning the character of an individual while threatening to do bodily harm

Situation: Karen Vale, a 5-year-old girl, is admitted to the hospital 1 week before surgery for tetralogy of Fallot. Questions 144 through 148 refer to this situation.

144 The defects associated with this heart anomaly include:
1. Right ventricular hypertrophy, atrial and ventricular defects, and mitral valve stenosis
2. Right ventricular hypertrophy, ventricular septal defect, stenosis of pulmonary artery, and overriding aorta
3. Origin of the aorta from the right ventricle and of the pulmonary artery from the left ventricle
4. Abnormal connection between the pulmonary artery and the aorta, right ventricular hypertrophy, and atrial septal defects
145 A common finding in most children with cardiac anomalies is:
1. Mental retardation
2. Cyanosis and clubbing of fingertips
3. A family history of cardiac anomalies
4. Delayed physical growth
146 Karen is to receive digoxin (Lanoxin) elixir, 0.010 mg, po. Based on developmental norms for a 5-year-old, the nurse would withhold the medication and notify the physician if the apical rate is below:
1. 60 beats per minute
2. 80 beats per minute
3. 90 beats per minute
4. 100 beats per minute
147 Karen's laboratory analysis indicates a high red blood cell count. This polycythemia can best be understood as a compensatory mechanism for:
1. Cardiomegaly
2. Low iron level
3. Low blood pressure
4. Tissue oxygen need
148 Karen has heart surgery to repair the anomaly. Postoperatively it is essential that the nurse prevent which of the following?

1. Constipation
2. Unnecessary movement
3. Crying
4. Coughing

149 Meg, 2 years old, has a cyanotic congenital heart disease. The nurse would expect to observe:
1. Edema in extremities
2. An elevated hematocrit
3. Absence of pedal pulses
4. Orthopnea

150 Baby boy Vics has been found to have a patent ductus arteriosus, which is:
1. A narrowing of the pulmonary artery
2. An abnormal opening between the right and left ventricles
3. A connection between the pulmonary artery and the aorta
4. An enlarged aorta and pulmonary artery

151 The nurse is caring for a child with an acyanotic heart disease. A major *common* symptom of acyanotic heart disease is:
1. Polycythemia
2. Clubbing of fingers and toes
3. Severe retarded growth
4. The presence of an audible heart murmur

152 Alma has coarctation of the aorta. When taking her vital signs, the nurse is expecting to observe:
1. Weak, thready radial pulses
2. Higher blood pressure in upper extremities
3. Bounding femoral pulses
4. Notching of the clavicle

Situation: Johnny, a 10-year-old, is taken to the emergency room of the local hospital because he stepped on a nail. Questions 153 and 154 refer to this situation.

153 The puncture wound is cleansed by the nurse and a sterile dressing applied. She asks the mother if Johnny has been immunized against tetanus. The reply is affirmative. Penicillin is administered and the child sent home with instructions to return if there is any change in the wound area. A few days later, Johnny is admitted to the hospital with a diagnosis of tetanus. Legally:
1. The possibility of tetanus could not have been foreseen, since he had been immunized
2. The nurse's judgment was adequate in view of the patient's symptoms
3. Assessment by the nurse was incomplete and the treatment was inadequate
4. Hospital protocol should govern treatment in emergency room care

154 After Johnny's admission, one of the most important aspects of nursing care should be directed toward:
1. Maintaining body alignment

2. Encouraging high intake of fluid
3. Carefully monitoring urinary output
4. Decreasing external stimuli

Situation: Three-day-old Patty is diagnosed as having congenital hip dysplasia. Questions 155 through 157 refer to this situation.

155 An early sign able to be observed by the nurse in the newborn nursery is:
1. Limitation in adduction of leg
2. Shortening of leg on unaffected side
3. Depressed dance reflex
4. Asymmetry of gluteal folds

156 At 3 months of age Patty has a spica cast applied from below the axilla to below the knee. To prevent a serious complication that often occurs in infants in a spica cast, the nurse teaches Patty's parents to:
1. Seek immediate medical care if Patty develops a cough
2. Limit movement to prevent cast damage
3. Change Patty's diapers frequently
4. Place Patty on a low-calorie diet

157 When elevating Patty's head, the nurse is aware that it is important to:
1. Limit this position to 1 hour at a maximum
2. Raise the entire mattress and spring at the head of the bed
3. Use at least 2 pillows under her shoulders
4. Place folded diapers at the edge of the cast

158 Dietary treatment of PKU consists of a:
1. Low-phenylalanine diet
2. Phenylalanine-free diet
3. Dietary supplement for phenylalanine
4. Protein-free diet

159 Alan has been diagnosed as having cretinism. Even if care is instituted early, Alan will probably:
1. Have myxedema
2. Be somewhat mentally retarded
3. Have abnormal deep tendon reflexes
4. Have thyrotoxicosis

160 Three-month-old Lisa is diagnosed as having cretinism. She is to receive thyroxine sodium, 0.35 mg, od po. The medication is available in elixir form, 0.25 mg/ml. How many minims would the nurse give?
1. 16 minims
2. 21 minims
3. 18 minims
4. 20 minims

161 Three-year-old Karen Allen may have celiac disease. One symptom common in children with celiac disease is stools that are:
1. Large, frothy, dark green
2. Small, pale, mucoid

3. Large, pale, foul smelling
4. Moderate, green, foul smelling

162 Mrs. Joyce asks the nurse how to tell the difference between measles (rubeola) and German measles (rubella). The nurse tells Mrs. Joyce that with rubeola the child has:
1. A high fever and Koplik spots
2. Symptoms similar to a cold, followed by a rash
3. Nausea, vomiting, and abdominal cramps
4. A rash on the trunk with pruritus

163 Six-month-old Bart has roseola and is febrile. The physician orders a tap water enema. The nurse considers that giving Bart an enema could:
1. Cause a fluid and electrolyte imbalance
2. Increase his fear of intrusive procedures
3. Result in shock from a sudden drop in temperature
4. Result in loss of necessary nutrients

164 Chickenpox can sometimes be fatal to children who are receiving which of the following medications?
1. Antibiotics
2. Steroids
3. Anticonvulsants
4. Insulin

165 The nurse explains to the parent group that the most important complication of mumps in postpubertal males and females is:
1. Decrease in libido
2. Hypopituitarism
3. Sterility
4. A decrease in androgens

Situation: John, 17 years old, is admitted to the hospital because of minor injuries suffered in an automobile accident. During the examination the physician notices a rash on the skin and finds that John has suffered from a sore throat for several days. Based on the clinical examination the physician makes a tentative diagnosis of secondary syphilis, pending a report on the serologic test. Questions 166 through 168 refer to this situation.

166 Secondary syphilis is classified as which of the following?
1. Primary syphilis
2. Latent syphilis
3. Infectious syphilis
4. Late syphilis

167 The report of the serologic test is reactive. In view of the clinical examination and history of exposure, the physician confirms the diagnosis of secondary syphilis. The nursing care of the patient should include the following:
1. Thorough hand-washing after patient care
2. Isolation for 7 days
3. Autoclaving linens
4. Boiling dishes

168 John was exposed to syphilis through sexual contact with an infected person. It is important to locate the source of his infection and also persons whom he may have infected. Therefore all sexual contacts from how long ago should be located and examined?

1. Past 3 months
2. Past 6 months
3. Past 30 days
4. Past 3 weeks

Situation: Ten-year-old Jim Smith is admitted to the emergency room after a car accident. However, normal measures to stop his bleeding are unsuccessful, and, on further study, Jim is found to have a mild case of classic hemophilia. Mr. and Mrs. Smith are very concerned about this and wonder how it happened. Questions 169 through 171 refer to this situation.

169 The nurse should explain that:
1. Hemohilia is a sex-linked recessive disorder in which the mother is usually the carrier of the illness but is not affected by it
2. Hemophilia is a sex-linked dominant disorder in which the woman carries the trait
3. Hemophilia follows regular laws of mendelian inherited disorders such as sickle cell anemia
4. This disorder can be carried by either male or female but occurs in the sex opposite that of the carrier

170 Jim's parents are very worried about their other children, 2 girls and another boy, and want to know what the chances are concerning their having the disorder or being a carrier. An appropriate answer to this question would be that:
1. All the girls will be normal and the other son a carrier
2. Each son has a 50% chance of being a victim and each daughter a 50% chance of being a carrier
3. All the girls will be carriers and one half the boys will be victims
4. Each son has a 50% chance of being either a victim or carrier, and the girls will all be carriers

171 The most common site of internal bleeding in hemophiliacs is:
1. Cerebrum
2. Ends of long bones
3. Intestines
4. Joints

Situation: Cara has rheumatic fever. Drug therapy includes the administration of sodium salicylate, 10 gr, 4 times daily. Questions 172 through 174 refer to this situation.

172 During the salicylate therapy the nurse should observe Cara for which of the following groups of symptoms?
1. Nausea, dizziness, edema, headache
2. Gastric distress, nausea, vomiting, tinnitus
3. Constipation, deafness, nausea, headache
4. Diarrhea, gastric distress, edema of the face

173 Sodium salicylate is classified as an:
1. Antibiotic and antipyretic
2. Analgesic and antipyretic
3. Analgesic and sedative
4. Antipyretic and hypnotic

174 In working with parents in the preventive aspects of rheumatic fever, the nurse would stress:
  1. Prevention of exposure to childhood diseases
  2. Early treatment of upper respiratory tract infections
  3. Isolating the child with rheumatic fever from siblings
  4. Early immunization

Situation: Nellie, a newborn, is admitted to the Pediatric Unit with the diagnosis of choanal atresia. Questions 175 through 177 refer to this situation.

175 Choanal atresia is an anomaly located in the:
  1. Nasopharynx
  2. Intestinal tract
  3. Pharynx and larynx
  4. Anal area

176 While feeding Nellie, the nurse notices that she:
  1. Lacks a swallow reflex
  2. Chokes on her feeding
  3. Does not appear to be hungry
  4. Takes very little feeding

177 When reviewing the data recorded on Nellie's chart, what information might indicate to the nurse that the baby requires special attention?
  1. Birth weight of 3500 g
  2. 20 ml of milky-colored fluid was aspirated from her stomach
  3. The infant has a positive Babinski reflex
  4. The Apgar score at birth was 3

Situation: Three-year-old Roger is admitted to the Pediatric Unit with a diagnosis of nephrosis. Questions 178 through 181 refer to this situation.

178 The most important nursing intervention for Roger is:
  1. Encouraging fluids
  2. Regulating his diet
  3. Maintaining bed rest
  4. Preventing infection

179 As Roger gets older and has repeated attacks of nephrosis, it is most important for the nurse to help him develop:
  1. Fine muscle coordination
  2. Acceptance of possible sterility
  3. A positive body image
  4. The ability to test his own urine

180 During his nap, Roger wets the bed. The best approach by the nurse would be to:
  1. Change his clothes and make no issue of it
  2. Explain that big boys should try to call the nurse
  3. Tell him to help you remake the bed
  4. Change his bed, putting a rubber sheet on it

181 When providing nursing care to a preschool-age child, the nurse should remember that his greatest fear is of:
  1. Isolation
  2. Intrusive procedures

  3. Death
  4. Pain

Situation: Mary is hospitalized with a severe asthma attack. Questions 182 through 185 refer to this situation.

182 The acid-base imbalance complicating this condition is:
  1. Respiratory alkalosis caused by the accelerated respirations and loss of CO_2
  2. Respiratory acidosis caused by the impaired respirations and increased formation of H_2CO_3
  3. Metabolic acidosis caused by excessive production of acid metabolites
  4. Metabolic acidosis caused by the kidney's inability to help compensate for the increased H_2CO_3 formed

183 Mary is in a Croupette and is given prednisone, 15 mg, po bid. The nurse should:
  1. Check her eosinophil count daily
  2. Prevent exposure to infection
  3. Keep Mary NPO
  4. Have her rest as much as possible

184 Mary has IV therapy of 5% dextrose in ½ normal saline started. Aminophylline is to run in via piggyback for 20 minutes every 8 hours. Before administering the drug, the nurse should:
  1. Check her temperature
  2. Monitor blood pressure
  3. Administer oxygen
  4. Take her pulse

185 When Mary's parents take her home, they should be taught to increase her fluid intake and to have her:
  1. Avoid exertion and exposure to cold
  2. Stay in the house for at least 2 weeks
  3. Increase her calorie intake
  4. Avoid foods high in fat

Situation: Two-month-old Paul Carr is brought to the clinic, and a diagnosis of colic is made. Mrs. Carr appears exhausted. Questions 186 through 189 refer to this situation.

186 The nurse realizes that Mrs. Carr needs help coping with Paul and suggests that she:
  1. Provide Paul with warm sweetened tea when he begins to cry
  2. Arrange for some time away from Paul each day to rest
  3. Sit comfortably in a quiet darkened room to hold Paul when he cries
  4. Give Paul a warm bath to calm him down

187 The behavior of an infant with colic is usually suggestive of:
  1. Inadequate peristalsis resulting in constipation
  2. A protective mechanism designed to rid the GI tract of foreign proteins
  3. Paroxysmal abdominal pain due to excessive gas
  4. An allergic response to certain proteins in milk

188 Paul returns with his mother for his 6-month check-up. When teaching Mrs. Carr how to prevent accidents when caring for her 6-month-old, the nurse should emphasize that this age child can usually:
1. Sit up
2. Stand while holding onto furniture
3. Roll over
4. Crawl lengthy distances

189 When Mrs. Carr returns with Paul for his 9-month check-up, she expresses concern about his development. The baby no longer has the same strong grasp that he had shortly after birth, nor does he have a similar response to startle that he had at an early age. The nurse should discuss with Mrs. Carr that:
1. Neurologic examination is desirable
2. Failure of these responses may be related to mental retardation
3. These responses are usually replaced by voluntary activity at 5 to 6 months of age
4. The infant needs additional sensory stimulation to aid in the return of these responses

---

Situation: Loren, age 14, is admitted to the hospital and is scheduled to have orthopedic surgery the following day. Questions 190 through 193 refer to this situation.

190 At the conclusion of visiting hours, Loren's mother hands the nurse a bottle of capsules and says, "These are for Loren's allergy. Will you be sure she takes one about 9 o'clock?" The nurse might best respond with which of the following statements?
1. "One capsule at 9 P.M.? Of course, I will give it to her."
2. "Did you ask the doctor if she should have this to-night?"
3. "I am certain the doctor knows about Loren's allergy."
4. "We will ask Loren's doctor to write an order so we can give this medication to her."

191 In relation to obtaining an informed consent, the nurse should remember that the adolescent:
1. Does not have the legal capacity to give consent
2. Is not able to make an acceptable or intelligent choice
3. Is able to give voluntary consent when parents are not available
4. Will most likely be unable to choose between alternatives when asked to consent

192 Postoperatively, Loren complains of pain and is given 15 mg of codeine sulfate as ordered q 3 to 4 h prn. Two hours after she is given this medication she complains of severe pain. The nurse should:
1. Administer another dose of codeine within 30 minutes, since it is a relatively safe drug
2. Tell Loren she cannot have any additional medication for 1 more hour

3. Report that Loren has an apparent idiosyncrasy to co-deine
4. Request that the physician evaluate Loren's need for additional medication

193 About 8 hours later, Loren complains of itching. A drug that can be ordered to relieve this symptom is:
1. Chlorpheniramine (Chlor-Trimeton)
2. Nitrofurazone (Furacin)
3. Salicylanilide (Salinidol)
4. Hyaluronidase (Alidase)

---

194 Paula, a 3-year-old with eczema of the face and arms, has not heeded her nurse's warnings to "stop scratching—or else!" The nurse finds Paula scratching so intensely that her arms are bleeding. With great flurry, the nurse ties Paula's arms to the crib sides saying, "I'm going to teach you one way or another." In this situation, the nurse:
1. Had to protect Paula's skin and acted as any reasonably prudent nurse would do
2. Tried to explain to Paula and rightly expected her to understand and cooperate
3. Has used actions that can be interpreted as assault and battery
4. Has merely done her job with considerable account-ability

195 Nancy, age 8, is receiving tetracycline (Achromycin). Her fever is down and secretions have lessened, but she is eating pooly, is withdrawn, lethargic, and irritable, and sobs readily. The nurse should promptly discuss the problem with the physician because:
1. She needs a higher food intake to fight the infection
2. Anemia is a frequent occurrence after infection and treatment with antibiotics
3. Concurrent bladder infection may be present as an extension of her gram-negative infection
4. Generalized physical symptoms and behavior problems may procede drug-induced liver damage

---

Situation: Two-year-old Sue McMichael, fractures her femur and is placed in Bryant's traction. Questions 196 through 199 refer to this situation.

196 While caring for Sue, the nurse should know that Bryant's traction:
1. Helps by allowing child to turn side to side
2. Is skin traction with weights hanging from the end of the bed
3. Is skin traction and elevates the hips slightly from the bed
4. Is attached to a pin placed in the affected femur

197 Sue becomes constipated and the physician orders an iso-tonic enema. The nurse is aware that the maximum amount of fluid to be given a small child without a physician's specific order is:
1. 100 to 150 ml
2. 150 to 250 ml

3. 250 to 350 ml
4. 350 to 500 ml

198 One evening Sue screams and cries frequently, particularly after her mother's visit. Her loud crying disturbs others on the unit, and the nurse finds it impossible to quiet her. She is in a 4-bed room, adjacent to which is a storeroom large enough to hold a crib. When her crying is particularly loud and prolonged, the nurse puts her crib in the storeroom and closes the door. She is left there until her crying ceases, a matter of 30 or 45 minutes. Legally:
1. The other children had to be considered, so Sue needed to be removed
2. Sue needed to have limits set to control her crying
3. Sue had a right to remain in the room with the other children
4. Keeping the child by herself for more than 30 minutes was too long

199 Several days later, Mrs. McMichael asks the nurse what to do when Sue has her temper tantrums. The nurse suggests that Mrs. McMichael allow Sue another way of expressing her anger, such as the use of:
1. A ball and bat
2. A pounding board
3. Clay or play dough
4. A punching bag

200 Fourteen-year-old Evelyn is severely hurt while on a skateboard and develops muscle contractures in all her limbs. She refuses to move, so the nurse could encourage her by:
1. Explaining that some pain is inevitable
2. Allowing friends to visit every day
3. Permitting her to make decisions regarding her care
4. Setting strict limits to increase her security

201 Nine-year-old Harold has a fractured femur and has just had a full leg cast applied. One of the following observations made by the nurse that should be reported to the physician immediately is:
1. Pedal pulse of 90
2. Cast still damp and warm after 4 hours
3. Inability to move toes
4. Increased urinary output

Situation: Karina, 7 years old, is to have an exploratory laparotomy and possible appendectomy. Questions 202 through 205 refer to this situation.

202 The physician orders atropine, 1/300 gr, IM preoperatively. The vial reads "atropine 0.4 mg/ml." How much should the nurse administer?
1. 0.5 ml
2. 1 ml
3. 0.25 ml
4. 0.75 ml

203 Postoperatively, to help relieve Karina's anxiety, the nurse should:

1. Tell her a story about a girl with similar surgery
2. Allow her time to talk about her feelings
3. Provide her with bandage, tape, scissors, and a doll
4. Asks her mother to room with her for a few days

204 Karina begins thumb-sucking after her surgery. Although this was not Karina's behavior preoperatively, the nurse should:
1. Report this behavior to the physician
2. Distract her by playing checkers
3. Accept the thumb-sucking
4. Tell her thumb-sucking causes buck teeth

205 Karina develops a urinary tract infection. The physician orders a sulfonamide preparation. A major nursing responsibility when administering this drug is to:
1. Weigh the child daily
2. Administer the drug at the prescribed times
3. Give milk with the medication
4. Monitor the temperature frequently

Situation: Mr. Gioni, the father of 3 young children, is diagnosed as having tuberculosis. Questions 206 through 208 refer to this situation.

206 Members of the family who have a positive reaction to the tuberculin test are candidates for treatment with:
1. Old tuberculin
2. BCG vaccine
3. INH and PAS
4. Purified protein derivative of tuberculin

207 If a person has been exposed to tuberculosis but shows no signs or symptoms except a positive tuberculin test, prophylactic drug therapy is usually continued after the last exposure for a period of:
1. 3 weeks
2. 6 months
3. 1 year
4. 5 years

208 Children in the family who have been exposed to but show no evidence of tuberculosis:
1. Can be considered to be immune
2. Should be treated with INH and PAS
3. Are usually given massive doses of penicillin
4. Are given x-ray examinations every 6 months and observed for evidence of tuberculosis

209 Two-year-old Jimmy swallowed kerosene from a soda bottle stored in the garage. Immediate treatment for ingestion of petroleum distillates is to have the child swallow:
1. Milk of magnesia
2. Strong tea
3. Weak salt solution
4. Mineral oil

210 A toddler has swallowed a liquid drain cleaner containing lye. The immediate intervention is to administer:
1. Syrup of ipecac

2. Two ounces of milk
3. Dilute vinegar solution
4. Sodium bicarbonate and water

211 Susan is found by her mother playing with an open bottle of diuretic tablets. The physician tells Susan's mother to give syrup of ipecac to Susan. The effect of the drug will be enhanced by:
1. Resting until vomiting occurs
2. Drinking 2 to 3 glasses of water
3. Actively playing until vomiting occurs
4. Stimulating the gag reflex

Situation: The nurse in the outpatient Pediatric Clinic is talking to a group of parents whose children have been diagnosed as having minimal brain dysfunction. Questions 212 and 213 refer to this situation.

212 One of the major behavioral characteristics of children with minimal brain dysfunction is their:
1. Inability to use abstract thought
2. Overreaction to stimuli
3. Continued use of rituals
4. Retarded speech development

213 In helping the parents to cope with their children's behavior, the nurse suggests that one of their best approaches would be to:
1. Write a list of expectations to avoid confusion
2. Be consistent and firm about established rules
3. Avoid asking specific questions
4. Allow the child to set up his own routines

214 The primary reason for using prednisone in the treatment of acute leukemia in children is that it is able to:
1. Suppress mitosis in lymphocytes
2. Reduce irradiation edema
3. Decrease inflammation
4. Increase appetite and sense of well-being

215 A combination of drugs, which includes vincristine (Oncovin) and prednisone, is prescribed. The toxic symptom(s) that the nurse should expect are:
1. Neurologic
2. Irreversible alopecia
3. Anemia and fever
4. Gastrointestinal

216 Which of the following responses is unusual in infants exposed to prolonged hospitalization?
1. Lack or slowness of weight gain
2. Looking at ceiling lights rather than persons caring for them
3. Limited emotional response to stimuli
4. Excessive crying and clinging when approached

217 A characteristic of infants and young children who have experienced maternal deprivation is:
1. Extreme activity
2. Proneness to illness

3. Responsiveness to stimuli
4. Tendency toward overeating

218 Naomi, 9 years old, is about to have surgery. The physician orders meperidine (Demerol), 20 mg, IM preoperatively. The container reads "50 mg/ml." How many minims would the nurse administer?
1. 4 minims
2. 6 minims
3. 8 minims
4. 10 minims

219 An infant scheduled for surgery is diagnosed as having a diaphragmatic hernia. A measure that a nurse would expect to be employed at this time includes:
1. Positive pressure oxygen by mask
2. Positive pressure oxygen by intratracheal tube
3. Increased oxygen concentration by any method
4. Humidity of 40%

220 It is expected that, after some surgical intervention for atelectasis, lung expansion will recur within:
1. An hour
2. 48 to 72 hours
3. 4 hours
4. 12 to 48 hours

221 Dina, 18 months old, is to receive 5% dextrose and Ringer's lactate, 1000 ml IV, in 24 hours. The drop factor of the minidropper is 60 gtt/ml. The nurse should regulate the IV to run at:
1. 34 gtts per minute
2. 38 gtts per minute
3. 42 gtts per minute
4. 21 gtts per minute

222 When picked up by either the mother or the nurse, an 8-month-old infant screams. The scream seems to be that of pain. At his clinic visit the nurse will note and talk particularly to the mother about:
1. The infant's food and specific vitamins given to him, including vitamins C and D
2. Accidents and injuries and the importance of their prevention
3. Any other behavior of the infant that may have been noticed by the mother
4. Limiting the play time and activities that this infant has with other children in the family

223 Eleven-year-old Harry has gained weight. His mother is concerned that Harry, who loves sports, may become obese. The nurse:
1. Urges a decreased caloric intake
2. Explains this is normal for a preadolescent
3. Advises an increase in activity
4. Discusses the relationship of genetics and weight gain

224 Hepatitis occurs in sporadic cases and isolated outbreaks. Exposure to virus B homologous serum hepatitis (SH) may be expected to occur in hospitals because of which of the following?

1. Increased use of blood and blood products
2. Careless handling of excreta
3. Asymptomatic carriers
4. Increasing use of ventilating systems

225 Elouise, 8 months old, has a gastrostomy tube and is given 240 ml of tube feeding q 4 h. One of the primary nursing responsibilities at the time of the feeding is to:
1. Elevate the tube 12 inches (30 cm) above the mattress
2. Give 10 ml of normal saline before and after feeding
3. Position on right side following feeding
4. Open the tube 1 hour before feeding

226 Prior to administering a tube feeding to an infant, the nurse should:
1. Slowly instill 5 ml of water
2. Aspirate the tube

3. Provide the baby with a pacifier
4. Place in semi-Fowler's position

227 Sal has been admitted to the hospital for surgery to correct his congenital megacolon. Enemas are ordered preoperatively to cleanse the bowel. The nurse should use:
1. Soapsuds
2. Hypertonic phosphate
3. Isotonic saline
4. Tap water

228 If monocular strabismus is not corrected early enough:
1. Vision in both eyes will be diminished
2. Peripheral vision will disappear
3. Dyslexia will develop
4. Amblyopia develops in the weak eye

6 HISTORICAL AND LEGAL ASPECTS OF NURSING IN THE UNITED STATES AND CANADA

Nursing as it is known today has had a relatively short history—only slightly over 100 years. Modern nursing is usually said to have begun with the work of Florence Nightingale. However, nursing has its roots in ancient days, and many would claim that nursing really antedates all other kinds of health and medical care. Nursing has a history, the knowledge of which should serve to make the modern nurse proud of nursing's heritage and determined to make contemporary nursing meet modern challenges.

Knowledge of nursing development and progress should help in viewing the current problems of nursing in perspective. As each generation enters the nursing field, failure to recognize what has gone before will cause that generation to repeat the mistakes of the past. As knowledge advances, as societies change, as economic situations differ, so will nursing if it is to meet society's needs. The history of nursing then reflects how the leaders in nursing have attempted to meet new demands in new ways without losing sight of the original and fundamental goals of nursing. Modern nursing is fortunate in having as its founder a woman of the stature and wisdom of Florence Nightingale. Continued study of her writings brings new insights and appreciations of her work and its influence.

In the material that follows, emphasis is placed on the modern world, particularly the twentieth century. The various movements that have occurred are treated chronologically because in this way changes and trends can be viewed more easily. Nursing cannot be seen in isolation. Since nursing acts on society and is acted on by society, it must be viewed within the context of that society.

The system of laws is a part of the fabric of a society and will affect the practice of nursing. In the United States, the system of laws has a long history and is still evolving. The influence of other legal systems, notably that of Great Britain, is obvious. All citizens are affected by the laws of the nation and the state, but some laws affect certain segments of society more than others because they specifically apply to that group. Some laws, such as those of licensure, are specific for nurses, whereas others are applied to nurses, if appropriate, such as when nurses are sued for negligence.

NURSING IN THE UNITED STATES
The twentieth century

Studies affecting nursing and nursing education

A. *Nursing and Nursing Education in the United States*—1923

1. Study resulted from a conference sponsored by the Rockefeller Foundation for the purpose of discussing the status of public health nursing
2. Committee for the Study of Public Health Nursing Education was formed with C. E. A. Winslow as chairman

3. Josephine Goldmark was chosen as director of the study and the report is popularly called *The Goldmark Report*
4. Original intent was to study only public health nursing but later expanded to include all nursing
5. Report included recommendations relative to
   a. The desirability of establishing university schools of nursing that would be adequately financed, administered by a qualified dean, and include liberal arts in the curriculum
   b. The inadequacy of many schools and disadvantages of the apprenticeship system
   c. The need for 2 types of workers in nursing
   d. Admission requirements in hospital schools and curriculum and teaching needs
   e. The kind of training needed by nurses in public health
   f. Postgraduate courses
B. *Nursing Schools Today and Tomorrow*—1934
   1. Committee on the Grading of Nursing Schools was initiated by the National League of Nursing Education but supported by the American Nurses' Association, National Organization of Public Health Nurses, and American Medical Association; this report is popularly called *The Grading Committee Report*
   2. Dr. May Aynes Burgess directed the study
   3. Two ''gradings'' of schools were done in 1929 and in 1932
   4. Two thirds of all schools participated
   5. Recommendations included
      a. Employment of graduate nurses to replace students
      b. The closing of inadequate schools
      c. Collegiate level education with enriched curriculum
      d. Better prepared students
      e. Better prepared faculty
C. *Nursing for the Future*—1948
   1. Sponsored by the National Nursing Council, the successor to the National Nursing Council for War Service
   2. Directed by Dr. Esther Lucile Brown and popularly called *The Brown Report*
   3. Included nursing service and nursing education in terms of what was best for the public, not for the profession
   4. Recommendations included
      a. Term *professional* to be used only by those

graduated from professional schools or by achievement in some system of examination
      b. Both academic and professional training and basic alterations in the curriculum
      c. Requirements relative to administrative structure, facilities, faculty, and financing of nursing education
      d. Mandatory free accreditation of schools of nursing
      e. Improved training for practical nurses
   5. As a result of this study, Margaret Bridgman was employed by the National League for Nursing as a consultant to university nursing schools; this service was financed by the Russell Sage Foundation and a report was published as *Collegiate Education for Nursing* in 1953
D. *A Program for the Nursing Profession*—1949
   1. A Committee on the Function of Nursing was formed under the aegis of the Division of Nursing Education, Teachers College, Columbia University
   2. Eli Ginsberg, economist, was chosen as chairman; the report is popularly called *The Ginsberg Report*
   3. Recommendations in many ways paralleled those of *Nursing for the Future,* which was going on concurrently
E. *Liberal Education and Nursing*—1959
   1. A study done under the aegis of the Institute of Higher Education, Teachers College, Columbia University as part of a series covering those professions that admit students directly from high school
   2. Findings included
      a. More lip service than reality to inclusion of liberal arts
      b. Some confusion as to what constitutes liberal arts
F. *Community College Education for Nursing*—1959
   1. The Cooperative Research Project in Junior and Community College Education for Nursing, sponsored by the Division of Nursing Education, Teachers College, Columbia University, studied the possibility of 2-year, associate degree programs, to prepare for the technical practice of nursing
   2. Dr. Mildred L. Montag, whose dissertation, *The Education of Nursing Technicians,* laid the foun-

dations for the associate degree program, was named project director

3. Financed by an anonymous donor
4. Cooperated with 7 community colleges and 1 hospital school
5. Findings included
   a. Graduates passed licensing examinations
   b. Evaluated by employers as satisfactory in practice
   c. Colleges could support these programs financially

G. *Abstract for Action*—1970
1. National Commission for the Study of Nursing and Nursing Education established by the American Nurses' Association and National League for Nursing as a result of the recommendation of the Surgeon General's Consultant Group in Nursing
2. Distributed questionnaires to many schools and nurse educators relative to role, function, goals, and future of nursing
3. Compiled data that had been secured through many studies, large and small
4. Recommendations included
   a. Desirability of regional planning
   b. Necessity of research
   c. Single licensure for all in nursing occupation
   d. Academies to recognize excellence in the several specialized areas
   e. Preparation for episodic and distributive nursing
5. Following the report the Commission assumed the responsibility for implementation of its recommendations

H. *The Study of Credentialing in Nursing*—1979
1. Inaugurated by the American Nurses' Association and carried on by an independent study committee
2. Purpose to assess adequacy of current credentialing in nursing and to recommend future directions
3. Process included literature review, use of secondary data, and survey of certified nurses
4. Identified issues relative to credentialing
5. Recommendations included
   a. Licensing only one group of nurses—professional
   b. Registration of qualified individuals in nursing other than professional
   c. A national credentialing center
6. No decision at present as to implementation of

any or all recommendations; they are significant recommendations and would require many changes in current practice

Changes in nursing organizations

A. The American Nurses' Association
1. 1911—name changed from Nurses' Associated Alumnae of United States and Canada
2. 1952—restatement of functions following a study of various nursing organizations; all concerns of individual professional nurses retained by American Nurses' Association
3. 1962—the House of Delegates of the American Nurses' Association amended the purposes of the organization
4. 1964—Study Committee appointed to recommend organizational structure to carry out functions
5. 1966—new structure adapted
   a. Three commissions formed
      (1) Economic and General Welfare
      (2) Nursing Education
      (3) Nursing Service
6. 1970—a Commission on Research added
7. Individual members may choose to belong to a division of practice
   a. Medical-surgical nursing
   b. Maternal and child health nursing
   c. Psychiatric and mental health nursing
   d. Geriatric nursing
   e. Community health nursing
8. Academy for Nursing Practice, established 1970—its members, known as Fellows, are certified as qualified
9. Academy of Nursing established in 1973
   a. Purpose is to explore broad issues and problems concerning nursing and health care
   b. Charter members named in January, 1974
10. Congress of Nursing Practice established in 1968
11. Structure of American Nurses' Association
    a. President
    b. Three Vice-Presidents
    c. Secretary
    d. Treasurer
    e. Ten Directors
    f. House of Delegates
    g. Ten standing committees
    h. Four commissions
    i. Five divisions of practice
    j. Ten occupational forums

12. Membership available to all registered professional nurses
13. State associations are divided into districts and are constituent associations of the American Nurses' Association
14. American Nurses' Foundation—founded in 1955 by American Nurses' Association
    a. Supported by public funds as well as contributions by nurses
    b. Sponsors and conducts research, disseminates research, and gives consultation
15. *American Journal of Nursing,* published by American Journal of Nursing Company, official journal
16. American Nurses' Association headquarters in Kansas City, Missouri
17. Conventions held biennially

B. National League for Nursing Education
1. Name changed from American Society of Superintendents of Training Schools for Nurses in 1912
2. Membership limited to those involved in nursing education until 1943, when lay members were admitted
3. Served as the education committee of the American Nurses' Association
4. Sponsored curriculum studies and reports
    a. 1917—Standard Curriculum for Nursing Schools
    b. 1927—Curriculum for Schools of Nursing
    c. 1937—Curriculum Guide for Schools of Nursing
5. 1952—became part of the new organization, National League for Nursing

C. National Association for Colored Graduate Nurses
1. Organized in 1908
2. In some states black graduates were not eligible for membership in district, state, and national associations
3. Dissolved in 1951 after American Nurses' Association (1950) absorbed its functions and responsibilities

D. National Organization of Public Health Nursing
1. Organized in 1912
2. Promotion of public health nursing—coordination and standardization of public health nursing was major interest
3. Nurse and lay membership even though it was primarily a nursing organization

4. The official publication was *Public Health Nursing*
5. 1952—became part of the new National League for Nursing

E. Association of Collegiate Schools of Nursing
1. Organized in 1932
2. Membership open only to those accredited programs offering college degrees
3. Purpose was to
    a. Develop nursing on professional and collegiate level
    b. Strengthen relationships between schools of nursing and institutions of higher education
    c. Stimulate research and experimentation
4. Had total of 37 members
5. Dissolved in 1952, becoming a part of the new National League for Nursing

F. American Association of Industrial Nurses
1. Organized in 1942
2. Growth of industry, especially in war time, prompted greater attention to welfare of workers and their families
3. American Nurses' Association had industrial nurse section from 1946 to 1952
4. Was 1 of 6 national organizations that participated in reorganization study but withdrew in 1952 maintaining its own organization

G. National League for Nursing
1. Organized in 1952 as a result of structure study combining the functions and activities of
    a. National League of Nursing Education
    b. National Organization of Public Health Nursing
    c. Association of Collegiate Schools of Nursing
2. Membership included
    a. Individual members—anyone interested in nursing (registered nurses, practical nurses, nurses' aides, and lay people)
    b. Agency members—hospitals, nursing homes, public health agencies, educational programs, and public schools
3. Functions included
    a. Identifying needs of society and fostering programs designed to meet these needs
    b. Developing and supporting services to improve nursing care and nursing service
    c. Working with American Nurses' Association for advancement of nursing
    d. Working with governmental agencies toward achievement of comprehensive health care

4. Structure made provision for
   a. Officers
      (1) One President and President-Elect
      (2) Two Vice-Presidents
      (3) Treasurer
      (4) Board of Directors
   b. Two divisions
      (1) Division of Individual Members—forms Council on Community Planning for Nursing
      (2) Division of Agency Members with the following councils
         (a) Associate Degree Programs
         (b) Baccalaureate and Higher Degree Programs
         (c) Diploma Programs
         (d) Practical Nursing Programs
         (e) Hospital and Institutional Nursing Services
         (f) Public Health Nursing Services
5. Services provided
   a. Shares responsibility for recruitment with American Nurses' Association
   b. Accreditation of nursing programs
   c. Test construction
   d. Biennial convention
   e. Headquarters at 10 Columbus Circle, New York 10019

H. National Student Nurses' Association
  1. Organized in 1953
  2. Individual membership preferred
  3. Purpose is chiefly that of preparing for membership in the American Nurses' Association on graduation
  4. Annual conventions
  5. Headquarters at 10 Columbus Circle, New York 10019

I. National Association for Practical Nurse Education and Service, Inc.
  1. Organized in 1940
  2. Active in stimulating interest in practical nursing, accrediting programs, and seeking financial support for practical nursing

J. National Federation of Licensed Practical Nurses, Inc.
  1. Founded in 1949
  2. Membership limited to licensed practical nurses
  3. Recognized by American Nurses' Association as official organization for practical nurses

Special interest organizations
A. Association of Operating Room Nurses
  1. Founded in 1957
  2. Membership includes nurses engaged in operating room work at all levels
  3. Interested in new practices and developments in operating room nursing
  4. Holds annual congress
B. American Association of Nurse Anesthetists
  1. Founded in 1931
  2. Membership open to registered nurses who have taken a 12-month course and passed a qualifying examination
  3. Purpose is to further art of anesthesiology and develop educational standards
  4. Accredits schools of nurse anesthetists
C. American Association of Colleges of Nursing
  1. Founded in 1969
  2. Purpose is to promote university nursing programs and to take positions on issues relevant to higher education in nursing
D. Other specialty associations form as specializations increase

International organizations
A. International Council of Nurses
  1. Founded in 1899 in Boston
  2. A federation of National Nursing Organizations of which American Nurses Association is a member
  3. Membership automatic for individual nurses belonging to national organizations
  4. Congress meets every 4 years—1973 in Mexico City; 1977 in Tokyo; 1981 in Los Angeles
  5. Purposes are to raise worldwide standards of nursing education and promote general welfare of nurses
  6. Oldest continually functioning international council
  7. Headquarters at Geneva, Switzerland
B. International Red Cross
  1. Founded by Henri Dunant, a Swiss, in 1863
  2. Geneva Convention of 1864 confirmed Dunant's original principles
  3. International Red Cross Committee coordinates national committees
  4. The Florence Nightingale medal was authorized to be given to nurses of special distinction in 1912
  5. American Red Cross—a component part of the International Red Cross

a. Any graduate nurse may be a member of the Red Cross Nursing Service
b. The services include
   (1) Teaching home nursing
   (2) Blood collection
   (3) Disaster nursing
   (4) Providing educational materials
C. World Health Organization
1. Organized in 1946 as an agency of the United Nations
2. Nursing recognized as integral part
3. Influential in showing nursing as an essential part of medical and health teams
4. Expert Committees on Nursing organized in 1950 and still serving
5. Reports of Expert Committees, guides for nursing surveys, reports of regional conferences, and seminars help to disseminate knowledge and recommendations about nursing

Advances in education
A. Early developments in collegiate education
1. First nursing program in the world that was an integral part of a university was developed by the University of Minnesota in 1909
2. By 1931, there were 67 schools of nursing with some connection to a college or university
3. Collegiate programs for graduates of diploma programs were also developed
4. Curriculum influenced by publication of 3 works on curriculum—1917, 1927, 1937—plus additional works relative to faculty and other essentials required for a good school of nursing
5. Accreditation of schools of nursing began in 1939 by the National League of Nursing Education in cooperation with the North Central Association of Colleges and Secondary Schools; first list of accredited schools was issued in 1941 and contained 70 schools
6. Nursing schools responded in 2 war crises
   a. World War I
      (1) Vassar Training Camp during the summer of 1918 prepared 400 college graduates to transfer to nursing schools in the fall
      (2) Army School of Nursing developed
   b. World War II
      (1) Authorization by Congress of the Cadet Nurse Corps (Bolton Act) in 1943 (discontinued in 1948)
      (2) Accelerated program mandated, all essen-

tial theory and practice within 2½-year period with 6 months' experience in military, federal, civilian hospitals, or public health agencies
B. Developments in the second half of the century
1. Development of the associate degree nursing program
   a. The Cooperative Research Program in Junior and Community College Education for Nurses resulted from a proposal in M. Montag's *The Education of Nursing Technicians* (1952-1957)
      (1) Purpose was to develop and test a new program preparing for those functions commonly associated with the registered nurse
      (3) Seven colleges and 1 hospital program cooperated
      (3) Results of the 5-year project published in *Community College Education for Nursing* and stated
         (a) Graduates capable of passing licensing examinations
         (b) Graduates rated by employers as good or better than other graduates of similar experience
   b. The program developed differed greatly from existing programs and had the following characteristics
      (1) Controlled and financed by community college
      (2) Faculty employed by the college
      (3) Curriculum developed by the faculty with at least one third of total credits in general education, with remainder in nursing
      (4) Broad grouping of subject matter in contrast to many small courses
      (5) Students met admission and graduation requirements of the college
      (6) Faculty met college requirements for appointment and enjoyed all faculty privileges and responsibilities
      (7) Students eligible for associate degree
      (8) Graduates eligible to take state licensing examinations
      (9) Students provided own housing
   c. These programs had very rapid growth, on the average of 50 per year
   d. In 1978 the number of programs was 677

e. Almost half the students admitted to nursing programs are in associate degree programs

2. Developments in baccalaureate degree nursing programs
   a. Designation of the baccalaureate degree as the minimal preparation for the practice of professional nursing resulted from a recommendation in *Nursing for the Future*
   b. All specialized programs leading to a baccalaureate degree were discontinued in 1957
   c. Graduates of diploma programs seeking a baccalaureate degree are admitted to the generic program with advanced standing (usually verified by examination)
   d. Curriculum changed to include
      (1) More emphasis on liberal arts
      (2) Reorganization of the nursing major
      (3) More selective clinical laboratory experiences
      (4) More independent study
   e. Better qualified faculties
   f. The control of the programs is now fully by the universities
   g. Federal funding of construction, special projects, grants to programs, and scholarships and loans to students have helped these programs appreciably
   h. Accreditation of programs has tended to improve quality
   i. The number of programs has increased and in 1978 was 353; about 31,000 students admitted annually

3. Growth of higher degree nursing programs
   a. Master's degree nursing programs
      (1) Although graduate programs existed before 1959, they have received increased attention since that date
      (2) Programs include those which
         (a) Provide functional preparation for teaching or administration in addition to clinical study
         (b) Provide only a clinical nursing specialty
      (3) Federal funding of students through traineeships has assisted in preparing nurses for careers in teaching, administration, or a clinical specialty
      (4) Programs numbered 179 in 1978 and enrolled 6561 full-time students

   b. Doctoral degree nursing programs
      (1) Increased recognition that doctoral preparation is necessary if nursing is to develop true professional status
      (2) University faculty positions often require doctoral preparation
      (3) Research essential to a profession requires doctoral preparation
      (4) Number of nurses holding earned doctorates has increased greatly since 1950; however, the exact number holding doctorates can only be estimated because many nurses receive doctorates in areas other than nursing

4. Diploma nursing programs
   a. The number has declined since 1955
   b. In 1978 the number of programs was 344; admissions are declining
   c. Changes in curriculum have occurred as a result of the influence of college-based programs, especially the associate degree program
   d. Length has been shortened from 36 months to 27 or 24 months, often following the academic year pattern
   e. Tuition is usually charged
   f. Required living in nurses' dormitories declining, with students usually choosing own place of residence
   g. More flexible admission requirements are common
   h. The term *generalist* for these graduates voted by National League for Nursing Council of Diploma Programs because of emphasis on the term professional for the baccalaureate degree graduate

5. Practical nurse programs
   a. Functions stated by American Nurses' Association and National Federation of Licensed Practical Nurses, Inc.
      (1) Personal and environmental hygiene, comfort and safety, spiritual needs, observing and recording signs and symptoms not requiring professional judgment
      (2) Contribution to the understanding of the employing institution and staff relationships
      (3) Personal growth
   b. Most programs are now 12 months in length

   c. Integrated programs of study and clinical experience the pattern by the middle 1960s

   d. The number of programs has increased considerably caused, in large measure, by federal and state financial assistance

     (1) 1951—W. K. Kellogg Foundation gave funds for 5 years to 5 states to expand practical nursing programs (number of programs increased from 5 to 41)

     (2) 1956—the Health Amendments Act provided $5,000,000 for improvement and expansion of practical nursing programs in public vocational schools

     (3) 1962—Manpower Development and Training Act provided funds for retraining the unemployed and by 1963, 129 practical nurse projects were in operation

   e. In 1974 the programs numbered 1329, admitting almost 40,000 students annually

  6. American Nurses' Association Position Paper on Nursing Education—1965

   a. All nursing programs to be within the organized educational system of the United States

   b. Recognized 2 types of practice

     (1) Technical—preparation in the associate degree program

     (2) Professional—preparation in the baccalaureate degree program

   c. Aides to be prepared in vocational schools or adult programs instead of on-the-job training

  7. American Nurses' Association's statement on diploma programs in 1973 really nullified its earlier stand on education, although some attempts were made to change the wording after criticism

Advances in nursing service

A. Early developments

  1. Employing graduate nurses as part of nursing staff and thus relieving students from total responsibility for patient care began in 1930s partly as a result of

   a. Closing of small and poor schools resulting from *Grading Committee Study*

   b. Decrease in private duty nurses as a result of the depression

  2. Study of nursing service administration sponsored by W. K. Kellogg Foundation in 1951; 14 universities developed master's degree programs preparing for nursing service administration

  3. Introduction of team nursing

   a. Result of a combination of recommendations in *Nursing for the Future* and *A Program for the Nursing Profession*

   b. Nursing team organized to meet the needs of the patient rather than relying on acuteness of illness or techniques needed

     (1) Professional nurse—team leader—plans, directs, participates in implementation and evaluates care

     (2) Other nursing personnel—practical nurses and aides—contribute to planning and give such care as delegated

     (3) Daily team conference held to plan, delegate, and evaluate care

   c. The term is still used, but the concept has been so misunderstood and misused that it has lost its original purpose; where properly interpreted, it can be a useful way of organizing nursing care

  4. Proliferation of workers in nursing

   a. Increased use of auxiliary workers during war years

   b. Increased development of practical nursing programs

   c. Redefinition of practical nursing makes it seem virtually like that of registered nursing

B. Later developments

  1. Introduction of clinical specialists

   a. Engaged in giving nursing care

   b. Assisting as consultants

  2. Changing baccalaureate curricula produced nurses better prepared for professional practice

  3. Increased numbers of nurses with baccalaureate degrees

  4. Introduction of associate degree graduate pointed out the obvious need for orientation of new staff and in-service education

  5. Emphasis on economic security and welfare by American Nurses' Association

   a. Increased salaries and benefits

   b. Introduced collective bargaining

   c. Produced possibility of strikes

  6. Primary nursing—one way of organizing nursing service to permit the nurse to give total care to the patient and to be held accountable for it

Legislation related to nurses and nursing

A. Licensure to practice nursing

  1. Purpose of licensure is to protect the public

  2. American Nurses' Association, from the time of

its inception, saw need for legislation to set standards for nursing

3. First states to have nurse licensing laws were
   a. North Carolina—1903
   b. New York—1903
   c. New Jersey—1903
4. 1952—all states and territories had nurse practice acts
5. Early laws were permissive, with New York the first state to pass a mandatory licensing law in 1938 that, because of the war, did not become effective until 1948
6. All but a few states now have mandatory laws
7. The laws are administered by a state board of nursing either as a department of state government or as an autonomous agency
8. The definition of the practice of nursing is included in the law

B. National Council of State Boards, Inc. (NCSBN)—a separate, autonomous, nonprofit body established in 1978
   1. Membership open to any board of nursing
   2. Delegate assembly composed of one member of each board
   3. State Board Test Pool Examinations under control of this body
   4. Executive director with office in Chicago

C. The State Board Test Pool Examination was begun in 1944 and is now used by all jurisdictions
   1. Each state board agrees to adopt the Test Pool Examination as its licensing examination
   2. Blueprint Committee develops the plan for the tests
      a. Uses item writers nominated by state boards to write the questions
      b. Reviews the final drafts of examinations
   3. Each state board reviews and accepts each examination
   4. Examination administered by each state board of nursing 2 times a year
   5. In 1982 a comprehensive examination will be given replacing the current 5-part examination
   6. Passing score determined by each state board of nursing
   7. The National League for Nursing Test Construction Unit works with the Blueprint Committee in the test construction
   8. Facilitates the licensing of nurses as they move from state to state

   a. Renewal of licenses usually required every 2 or 3 years
   b. Different licensing laws and examinations are required for practical nursing
   c. Licenses can be revoked for cause by the state board of nursing

D. Federal legislation
   1. Works Progress Administration (1935)—depression resulted in many nurses being unemployed and this Act made employment possible
   2. Federal Security Agency Appropriations Act—1941
      a. Administered by United States Public Health Service
      b. $1,200,000 appropriated to assist in training nurses for national defense
      c. Appropriation increased to $3,500,000 in 1942
   3. Nurse Training Act (The Bolton Act) (1943) established the Cadet Nurse Corps
   4. Health Amendments Act (1956) provided traineeships for those preparing for teaching, supervision and administration, and public health nursing
   5. Nurse Training Acts
      a. 1964—first comprehensive federal legislation to provide for increase in supply of nurses and to assist in modernizing nursing education
      b. 1968—Title II of the Health Manpower Act provided aid to students and to schools of nursing
      c. 1971—Nurse Training Act expanded and extended federal aid until 1974; extensions continue
      d. 1965 to 1971—over $334,000,000 awarded for
         (1) Scholarships and loans
         (2) Traineeships
         (3) Construction
         (4) Support for nursing schools
         (5) Projects to improve nursing education and recruitment

E. Legislation affecting nurses and nursing
   1. Social Security Act—1935
      a. Nurses became eligible for benefits—1951
      b. Amendments in 1965 provided for hospital and medical care for persons 65 years of age and older (Medicare)

c. Some funds concerned with maternal-child care, blind and crippled children, and the training and employment of nurses in this care
2. Hill-Burton Act (1947) provided financial aid for construction of hospitals, nursing homes, and other health facilities

Accreditation of nursing programs

A. State Board of Nursing approval of schools is a form of accreditation but it is mandatory rather than voluntary; no school of nursing can function without state approval under nurse practice acts
B. National League for Nursing has had responsibility for the accrediting of schools of nursing since 1952
1. Forerunners in the voluntary accreditation of schools were
a. National Organization of Public Health Nursing
b. National League of Nursing Education
c. National Nursing Accrediting Service
2. Purpose was to improve standards and to make available to the public the names of schools meeting approved criteria
3. Criteria are set for each type of program
4. Period of accreditation—6 to 8 years, with re-evaluation required if school is to continue on accredited list
5. National League for Nursing recognized as approved agency for accrediting by the National Commission on Accreditation
6. The Nurse Training Act of 1964 recognized the National League for Nursing as the accrediting agency for those programs desiring federal funds
7. List of accredited schools published annually in *Nursing Outlook*

Current developments

A. Changes in the legal definition of nursing
1. 1972—New York state law for the registered professional nurse was changed to include
a. Diagnosing and treating human response to actual or potential health problems through
(1) Case finding
(2) Health teaching
(3) Health counseling
b. Providing care supportive to or restorative of life and well-being
c. Executing the medical regimen prescribed by a licensed physician or dentist

2. Several other states are broadening their laws in similar fashion; e.g., Nevada, California, Colorado, Pennsylvania, New Jersey
B. Mandatory continuing education for relicensure being advocated in many states to ensure current competency; bills have been introduced in several state legislatures to mandate this requirement
C. American Nurses' Association's move to organize for collective action
1. Emphasis to be on achieving quality care
2. Assure the public of accountability of nurses
3. Increase accessibility of health services
4. Interest in economic welfare not abandoned but emphasis decreased
D. Commission on Education of the American Nurses' Association after a period of relative inactivity becoming more aggressive
E. Increasing numbers of professional nurses are going into private practice as individual practitioners or in groups under partnership arrangements
1. Conduct screening
2. Give nursing care
3. Teach preventive health measures
F. Nurses Coalition for Action in Politics (N-CAP) organized in 1974
1. Purpose is to promote health care of people by encouraging nurses to take a more active and effective part in government
2. Voluntary, nonprofit organization
3. Membership available through contributions
G. Nursing education
1. The career ladder
a. Advocates of this concept desire a curriculum that begins at either practical nurse or associate degree level and articulates with each succeeding level up to master's degree level
b. Opponents of this concept contend that this would virtually destroy the integrity of each program and further confuse the use of the products of each program
c. Several programs have been designed to carry out the idea; the success of these programs remains to be proved
2. The external degree program
a. A nontraditional program that does not require enrollment in or attendance at any nursing program
b. Competency validated by both written and performance examinations

    c. Examinations include those in general education and nursing

    d. Performance examinations given in a hospital setting with actual patients

    e. Program attractiveness can be judged by the number of applicants enrolled

    f. Currently offered only in New York State

  3. Curriculum change in baccalaureate programs

    a. Focus of organization changing from the traditional ''Big 5'' to emphasis on nursing process and nursing functions

    b. Changes necessary to implement the role of nurses as described in the new definitions of nursing

    c. Enlarging to include the expanded role of the nurse in

      (1) Health maintenance

      (2) Primary care

      (3) Screening

      (4) Community health

    d. Increasing use of independent study

  4. Increasing number of practitioner programs

    a. Nurse practitioner—one skilled in assessment and management of psychosocial and developmental problems and able to function independently

    b. Specialty nurse practitioner; e.g., family nurse practitioner, pediatric nurse practitioner

  5. Increasing number of programs leading to doctorates in nursing

H. Nursing service

  1. Primary nursing

    a. A plan of organization by which a nurse is responsible for total care of the patient or a group of patients using the nursing process

    b. Primary nurse—plans and carries out plan of care

    c. Requires greater attention to nurse's comments regarding patient, and integrating nurses' notes with notes of other health professionals

  2. Problem-Oriented Medical Records (POMR)

    a. Increasing use of this method of categorizing patient's problems rather than using diagnostic classification

    b. Method is criticized by some physicians and nurses

      (1) No panacea for poorly written notes by physicians or nurses

      (2) Too well-defined and categorized problems

      (3) Repetitive

  3. Peer review

    a. Nurses actively engaged in nursing appraise the quality of individual nursing care according to established standards of practice

    b. Essential if nurses are to be held accountable for care given

    c. Useful in helping individual nurses improve their own practice

    d. Useful in recommending nurses for advancement or merit increases

  4. Clinical specialist

    a. High degree of knowledge, skill, and competence in a specialized area

    b. Use is increasing as more nurses are prepared in master's degree programs

I. Institutional licensure

  1. Proposal that health care facilities would have the authority to determine proper utilization of personnel according to specific job descriptions

  2. Individual licensing laws for nurses and other health workers except physicians and dentists would be eliminated

  3. Proponents argue this would increase flexibility, permit better utilization of personnel, and improve health care

  4. Opponents contend that, although new ways are needed in institutions, this proposal would not improve the situation

    a. Knowledge and judgment needed because the tasks rather than the mechanics of the tasks should be the controlling factor

    b. Job descriptions already present

    c. Educators cannot prepare workers unless they know what is needed

    d. Competency is an individual responsibility, not exclusively the responsibility of the employer

J. Developments related to and influencing nursing

  1. Moves toward national health insurance

    a. For several years bills have been introduced but none has become law

    b. Believed inevitable within a few years

  2. Social and economic factors

    a. Increased cost of medical care

    b. Increase in persons over 65 years of age in population

c. Declining birth rate

d. Family planning

e. Need for consideration of minority groups in education and employment

f. Housing needs

g. Hunger and malnutrition

3. Increase in number and types of health professionals; e.g., respiratory therapists, operating room technicians, emergency technicians

4. Changes in medical practice include

a. Increased specialization

b. Increased skill in organ transplants

c. Improved anesthetic agents increasing safety of surgical intervention

d. Drug research and screening—more scrutiny of drugs reaching the market

e. Introduction of physician's assistants

5. Increase in hospital beds with concurrent emphasis on ambulatory care

6. Proliferation of nursing homes and extended care centers

7. Shortage of nurses—a controversial subject

a. Largest number of registered nurses employed in history—800,000

b. Maldistribution a factor in supply and demand

c. Economic situation in the nation influences employment

d. The existence of an oversupply and overuse of practical nurses is a debatable subject

8. The Patient's Bill of Rights—American Hospital Association—a bill of particulars designed to protect patients by establishing standards governing the hospital's and professional staff's responsibility to patients and their families

NURSING IN CANADA
The twentieth century

Studies affecting nursing and nursing education

A. *Special Committee on Nurse Education*—1916

1. Report presented to the Canadian National Association of Trained Nurses

2. Recommendations included

a. Nurse training schools or colleges should be established within the educational system of each province

b. Nurse training schools should be separated in organization from hospitals that were still to be used for practical training

B. *Survey of Nursing Education in Canada (the Weir Report)*—1932

1. A study of nursing education in Canada jointly sponsored by the Canadian Nurses' Association and The Canadian Medical Association under the chairmanship of Dr. Stewart Cameron

2. Purpose was to investigate growing criticism about nursing and its training system across the 5 main sections of Canada

3. Report contained recommendations on

a. Delivery of health care; e.g., the need for a comprehensive system of supervision and control of nursing personnel

b. Nursing as a profession; e.g., Provincial Registration Acts required amendments in areas related to nursing education

c. Private duty nursing; e.g., only registered graduates should be allowed to use the title *nurse*

d. Institutional nursing; e.g., training schools should be established within educational institutions

e. Student nurses; e.g., a period of internship as part of regular nurses' training may be desirable

f. Teachers of nursing; e.g., the number of full-time qualified teachers should be increased

g. Examination system; e.g., only graduates of approved training schools should be permitted to write the examination

C. *Proposed Curriculum for Schools of Nursing*—Canadian Nurses' Association

The 1939 curriculum proposal and a 1940 supplement, *Improvement of Nursing Education in the Clinical Field,* arose from recommendations in the Weir Report

D. *Evaluation of the Metropolitan School of Nursing (The Lord Report)*—1952

1. A study to examine all aspects of this demonstration program (less than 3 years in length) jointly sponsored by the Canadian Nurses' Association and the Canadian Red Cross under the direction of Nettie Fidler

2. Concluded that

a. The average graduate of this program compared with the average graduate of the control school in both bedside skills and achievement on the Registered Nurse Examination

b. Schools with complete control of students can

prepare nurses in 2 years as well as those prepared in 3 years

E. *Report on the Experiment in Nursing Education at the Atkinson School of Nursing of the Toronto Western Hospital*—1955
   1. Before the project at the Metropolitan School was completed, a project under the direction of W. Stewart Wallace was begun at the Toronto Hospital
   2. Program was to follow the same curriculum as Metropolitan School, but an "intern" third year under the control of Nursing Service was added
   3. Study showed problems developed because of the 2 plus 1 nonintegrated pattern of the program and the division of authority between the school and hospital

F. *Study of Nursing Education in New Brunswick*—1956
   1. Sponsored by the New Brunswick Department of Health and Social Service and reported by Kathleen Russell
   2. Recommendations included
      a. Hospital schools should reorganize to become independent by 1957
      b. Students should be ensured more direct patient care during clinical experience
      c. Interprovincial reciprocal registration should be established
      d. The establishment of a School of Nursing at the University of New Brunswick
      e. The inclusion of a 3-month psychiatric affiliation in all nursing programs
      f. The Provincial Association should hold 3-month institutes for the preparation of clinical instructors until postgraduate courses can be established
      g. Policies for the organization and preparation of nursing assistant groups should be written

G. *Report of the Pilot Project for the Evaluation of Schools of Nursing in Canada (Spotlight on Nursing Education)*—1960
   1. Sponsored by the nursing profession through the Canadian Nurses' Association under the direction of Helen K. Mussallem to study readiness for voluntary national accreditation
   2. Recommendations included
      a. A reexamination of nursing education in Canada be undertaken

b. An improvement program to upgrade programs be started
c. The evaluation of the quality of nursing service in clinical agencies be established
d. An accreditation program for schools be established by the Canadian Nurses' Association

H. *Royal Commission on Health Services Briefs*—1961
   Projected evolvement of 2 levels of nurses—those required for leadership roles and those technically skilled for bedside nursing

I. *Report of Royal Commission on Health Services*
   1. Suggested expansion of university schools of nursing especially at masters and doctoral levels
   2. Recommended that baccalaureate programs in nursing develop integrated curriculum
   3. Recommended establishment of a comprehensive, compulsory, universal health service program for all Canadians
   4. Specifically recommended that
      a. Schools of nursing have budgets separate from nursing service
      b. Diploma nurses be registered and graduated from 2-year nursing programs
      c. Salaries comparable with education and responsibility in other fields be paid nurses
   5. Recommendations that were implemented as a result included new patterns of nursing curricula, home care programs, health councils, and group practices

J. *Report of the Nursing Education Survey Committee for the Province of Alberta (Scarlett Report)*—1961-1963
   1. Sponsored by the Department of Health in Alberta
   2. Recommendations included that
      a. A Provincial Council of Nursing be established for licensing of all nursing personnel; licensure be mandatory for those who nurse for hire in Alberta
      b. Nursing education remain under the aegis of the University of Alberta and the program be shortened to 4 years
      c. The 2-year program as demonstrated by the Nightingale School in Toronto not be instituted in Alberta because of the costs of such a program

K. *Report on the Canadian Nurses' Association School*

Improvement Program (Glenna S. Rowsell)—1961-1964

1. Report emerged from recommendation of *The Report of the Pilot Project for the Evaluation of Schools of Nursing in Canada* in 1960; examined 168 diploma schools (98% of all such schools in Canada)
2. Reaffirmed impracticality of an accreditation program of schools of nursing at this time; based on task force recommendations
3. Task force also made following recommendations relative to the School Improvement Program
    a. The Canadian Nurses' Association create a Department of Nursing Education to act in consultant capacity to new programs and in nursing research
    b. The Canadian Nurses' Association clarify beliefs about nursing education and nurses' roles in society
4. Indicated need for continued study in areas of philosophy and school objectives, organization and administration, curriculum, facilities, and residence living

L. *A Study of the Development of a Diploma Program in Nursing at the Ryerson Institute of Technology, Toronto*—1963

1. Submissions were made to the Royal Commission on Health Services by nursing leaders that a nursing program be conducted at a level after high school under the jurisdiction of an educational institution; program approved in 1963 by College of Nurses of Ontario and conducted at Ryerson Institute of Technology
2. The 5-year experimental program had its own governing body and budget, a well-qualified teaching staff, 1 full-time teacher per 10 students, and control of student time and experience over a maximum 30-hour week
3. In 1973, the success of the program was made evident, since provision was made for its continuance following an evaluation by Moyra Allen

M. *Plan for the Development of Nursing Education Programs Within the General Educational System of Canada*—1964

1. Sponsored by the Canadian Nurses' Association under the direction of Helen K. Mussallem and popularly called *A Path to Quality*

2. Basic elements advocated by the project and rebuffed by the Canadian Hospital Association were that
    a. Nursing programs be developed within educational systems
    b. Two categories of nursing personnel be prepared
        (1) The professional nurse to be prepared in a 4-year university program
        (2) The technical nurse to be prepared in a 2-year program under educational auspices
    c. Two categories to be prepared in a ratio of 1 professional to 3 technical nurses

N. *Royal Commission on Health Services Nursing Education in Canada* (Dr. Helen K. Mussallem)—1964

1. Purpose was to examine and analyze all types of formal educational programs for personnel providing nursing care with emphasis primarily on those preparing nurses for registration in the provinces
2. Recommended that
    a. Deplorable lack of qualified teachers be remedied as soon as possible
    b. Diploma schools of nursing be part of the provinces' systems after high school
    c. Educational programs be revised to prepare 2 levels of nurses—the university and diploma nurses, with the former providing leadership in nursing practice and the latter assisting the professional nurse
    d. More graduate programs be designed to prepare nurses in research, consultation, and nursing specialties

O. *A Plan for the Education of Nurses in the Province of New Brunswick (Portrait of Nursing)*—1965

1. Sponsored by the New Brunswick Association of Registered Nurses and directed by Katherine MacLaggan
2. Purposes of the undertaking were
    a. To project a plan for educating 2 categories of nurses
    b. To present a plan for nurse education
        (1) To those in the general educational system of the province
        (2) To those responsible for nursing education and its development
3. The Canadian Hospital Association wanted hos-

pitals to continue operation of nursing schools even though 84 junior college programs had been initiated in the United States by this time
4. Recommendations included that
   a. Federal, provincial, and local governments finance nurse education at Institutes of Health Sciences
   b. Four health service groups be formed with clearly written levels of function (nurses Grades I and II, secretaries, wardkeepers)
5. That Provincial Councils on Education for Health Services be formed and be responsible to the Ministry of Education
6. Local management boards be responsible for
   a. Setting and receiving tuition
   b. Approving personnel appointments
   c. Approving all programs of education prior to submission to the Provincial Council for consideration
   d. Contracting for clinical experience

P. *Committee on the Healing Arts*
1. Established by Province of Ontario, July, 1966
2. Study invesitgated role and function of nursing personnel, nature of nursing activities, supply and demand, curriculum, teaching staff requirements
3. Recommendations included
   a. That the provincial association merge with the Ontario Association of Registered Nursing Assistants
   b. That studies be done to improve nurse resource utilization
   c. That activities representing the practice of nursing be defined
   d. That Labor Relations Act be amended according to the British Columbia model
   e. That Canadian Nurses' Association continue to develop uniform standards of registration

Q. *Report on the Project for the Evaluation of the Quality of Nursing Service* (sponsored by Canadian Nurses' Association)—1966
1. First attempt to evaluate the quality of nursing service, administration, and nursing care being provided within the concept of total patient care
2. Recommendations were that
   a. Nursing service departments evaluate care given
   b. Roles, functions, and relationships of physi-

cians, nurses, and administrators within patient care area be defined
   c. Standards for nursing service and hospital accreditation programs be set
   d. Nursing personnel be used more economically
   e. Individual nursing care plans be implemented
   f. More challenging clinical experiences be structured for students using problem-solving approaches

R. *Ad Hoc Committee on Nursing Education, Department of Public Health, Province of Saskatchewan—1966*
1. Formed after the recommendation of the Royal Commission on Health Services that Nursing Education Planning Committees be established provincially
2. Submitted basic guidelines for a system of educating nurses in Saskatchewan based on the belief that authority and responsibility for nurse education belonged to an agency whose primary concern was education
3. Recommendations included
   a. That Department of Education be responsible for education of nurses including the diploma level
   b. That Provincial Nurses' Association determine minimum admission standards and standards for registration
   c. That 2 central schools be established by Department of Education and hospital schools be phased into these
   d. That present 5-year university program be altered to 4-year integrated baccalaureate program and enrollment be increased by 50%
   e. That university certificate courses be eventually phased out

S. *Community Colleges and Nursing Education in Ontario* (R. G. Quittendon)—1968
1. Study initiated to provide data for optimum development of nurse training in relation to community needs
2. Findings were that
   a. Nonuniversity, postsecondary school enrollments increased 400% between 1955 and 1966 in Canada
   b. Ontario University enrollments increased 250% between 1955 and 1965
   c. Diploma nursing enrollment in Ontario in-

creased 35% between 1955 and 1965, whereas nursing assistant enrollment increased 100%

   d. Health science divisions needed to be developed in community colleges for training health team members

T. *Ontario Council of Health Report*—1969

   1. Ontario Council of Health received legislative approval in 1968, becoming Senior Advisory body to Minister of Health

   2. Guidelines for study were inherent in The Royal Commission on Health Services and included health care delivery, health manpower, education of health disciplines, and regional organization of health services

U. *Report of the Ontario Health Council on Health Care Delivery Systems*—1970

   1. Prepared by a subcommittee on community health and presented to the Ontario Council of Health

   2. Recommendations included

      a. Urgent need to make primary care more accessible from existing health workers

      b. Development of ambulatory care facilities

      c. Involvement of health science centers and professional faculties in primary health care delivery

      d. Examination of the role of the community health nurse in health services

      e. Establishment of health resource centers

V. *Task Force Reports on Cost of Health Services in Canada-Public Health Services*—1970

   1. Suggested that public health practice was not as effective or economically sound as it might be

   2. Recommendations included that

      a. Health services be regionalized

      b. Levels of community care be available to the public

      c. Home care programs be expanded

      d. University programs in public health be strengthened

      e. Community health centers be constructed

      f. Governments subsidize group practice by physicians

      g. Studies be done in use of physician-associates

W. *Task Force Reports on Cost of Health Service in Canada*—1970

   1. Established by Conference of Ministers of Health of Canada in 1968 to inquire into ways of restraining escalating health services expenditures

   2. Areas of inquiry related to hospital services

   3. Recommendations included that

      a. Nursing units not be staffed for maximum nursing care loads, adding personnel as required

      b. A uniform classification of care functions be established for Canada

      c. Specialized service units be encouraged

      d. Ambulatory care facilities be developed, along with community health centers

      e. Home care programs be expanded

      f. Standards for nursing care be formulated and measured

      g. Accreditation be mandatory for all hospitals of a national, nongovernmental nature

      h. Community mental health clinics be developed

      i. Further studies related to use of physician-associates be done

Changes in nursing organizations

A. Canadian Nurses' Association

   1. In 1951, *Structure Study of the Canadian Nurses' Association* was undertaken by Dr. Pauline Jewett and the structure was changed in 1954

   2. Structure was changed in 1962, and in 1966 standing committees were reduced

   3. The Canadian Nurses' Association is now a federation of 11 member associations (10 provinces and 1 territory); as of 1979 it represented 121,000 professional nurses

   4. Affairs of the Canadian Nurses' Association are managed by a 23-member board of directors, which serves a 2-year term and is composed of 9 directors elected at a general meeting, 11 directors from association members, and 3 public-appointed representatives

   5. The Canadian Nurses' Association offers the following services and functions

      a. Research and advisory aid

      b. Library

      c. Information services

      d. Labor relations

      e. Testing service

      f. International role through International Council of Nurses

   6. Objectives of the Canadian Nurses' Association as stated in the Constitution are to

      a. Promote the best interests of the members of the nursing profession and the general public

      b. Formulate policies in the fields of nursing ser-

vice, nursing education, and employment relations, for the purpose of advising provincial associations with regard to the maintenance and improvement of the ethical and professional standards of nursing education and nursing service, and the economic standards of nursing employment
   c. Provide effective media for the exchange of information within the National Association and with other organizations
7. Canadian Nurses' Association celebrated its fiftieth anniversary in 1958, the year in which the first French-Canadian, Alice M. Girard, was elected President
8. Activities included
   a. 1961—Canadian Nurses' Association and Kellogg Foundation established bilingual Nursing Unit Administration Extension Program
   b. 1962—established Canadian Nurses' Foundation
   c. 1965—carried out first national inventory of registered nurses
   d. 1967—undertook development of Canadian Nurses' Association Testing Service (CNATS) to be used by provincial associations for registration and for licensing purposes instead of the National League for Nursing Examinations
   e. Comprehensive Examination for Registered Nurses for registration/licensing purposes implemented August, 1980
      (1) Offered in both French and English
      (2) Blueprint relates to a nursing model rather than the previously used medical model
B. Student Nurses' Association—first organized system of student government in Canadian schools of nursing was established in 1917 at the Toronto General Hospital
C. Canadian University Nursing Student Association
D. Canadian Association of University Schools of Nursing (C.A.U.S.N.)
   1. Originally formed as Canadian Conference of University Schools of Nursing
   2. In 1971, name was changed from Canadian Conference of University Schools of Nursing to allow for French translation—''Association Canadienne des Écoles Univérsitaires de Nursing''
   3. As of 1980, 23 university schools are represented

4. Objectives are to
   a. Develop criteria for university education in nursing
   b. Promote research in nursing
   c. Promote interchange of nursing knowledge
   d. Foster the idea that university education in nursing contributes to development of Canada's health services
5. C.A.U.S.N. is official accrediting agency for university nursing programs in Canada
6. Assisted in Kellogg-sponsored conference on doctoral preparation for nurses in Canada

Advances in education

A. Early developments in university education
   1. Several trends strengthened need for more advanced education for nurses
      a. Rapid, widening scope of medical practice
      b. General public concern regarding health and social welfare
      c. Increasingly critical evaluation of professional education
   2. University of British Columbia offered the first baccalaureate degree course in nursing in the British Empire in 1919; patterned on the 2+2+1 pattern already established at the University of Minnesota
   3. 1920—6 universities began certificate or diploma courses of 1-year duration in public health nursing and teaching and administration with grants from the Canadian Red Cross
      a. First course in public health nursing at Dalhousie University in Halifax
      b. First course in teaching and administration established at McGill University, Montreal
   4. 1924—Grey Nuns organized first French language course in nursing education and ward administration for graduate nurses at University of Montreal
   5. 1925—first French language public health nursing course in Canada established at University of Montreal
   6. 1933—University of Toronto received Rockefeller Grant utilized in establishment of 4-year, integrated basic baccalaureate degree program that prepared graduates for varied types of nursing service (first program of this nature in Canada)
   7. 1941—first joint conference of the Canadian Nurses' Association Executive Committee and directors of Canadian University Schools of Nursing

8. Problems in establishing university programing for nurses continued even in the 1940s because of
   a. Ambivalent approach of many nurses
   b. Lack of qualified staff
   c. Unwillingness of hospitals to accept loss of student time and service
   d. Increased costs involved in higher education programs
9. No parallel development in graduate nursing education was occurring, with the result that Canadian nurses went to the United States for postgraduate studies, a move that further delayed postgraduate programing in Canada

B. Developments in the second half of the century
   1. Esther Lucile Brown's study, *Nursing for the Future* (published in the United States in 1948) had implications for nursing education in Canada
   2. Only 2 significant national studies in nursing education had been done by the Canadian Nurses' Association
   3. Hospitals owned and operated 90% of schools of nursing
   4. Major development in the late 1950s was the establishment of a prepaid hospital insurance program that included the cost of operating nursing schools in hospitals despite the opposition of the nursing profession
   5. Various types of nursing programs leading to the diploma rather than the baccalaureate degree exist in Canada today
      a. The traditional course in a hospital school of nursing in Alberta, British Columbia, Manitoba, New Brunswick (phased out in 1976), Nova Scotia, and Newfoundland
      b. The community college system in Quebec (Colleges d'Enseignement Général et Professional; the CEGEP Programs), Ontario, Alberta, Saskatchewan (Institutes of Applied Arts and Sciences), Newfoundland (started in 1975), British Columbia, and Manitoba
      c. The system of Regional and Independent Schools of Nursing in Prince Edward Island and New Brunswick
      d. The Programs for Psychiatric Nurses in British Columbia and Manitoba
   6. Nightingale School of Nursing—Toronto
      a. Began in 1960
      b. A regional school that controlled the educational program and utilized resources within a given geographic area
      c. Supported by the Board of Governors of New Mount Sinai Hospital, Toronto
      d. Operating costs borne by the government of Ontario with monies derived from the health insurance program
      e. Nightingale School was an alternative to the centralized school system in Alberta and the community college system in Quebec and British Columbia
   7. Quo Vadis Nursing Program
      a. Founded in Toronto in 1964 somewhat as a result of a recommendation made by Dr. Mussallem in *Nursing Education in Canada* (1962)
      b. A nursing education for women between 30 and 50 years of age with privileges of living at home, and working a regular workday for 5 days per week
      c. First students graduated in 1966
      d. Program transferred into the community college system in 1973
   8. Development of diploma programs in Ontario after 1965
      a. Minister of Health challenged pattern of diploma programs in Ontario by announcing that
         (1) Annual number of graduates would be doubled
         (2) Length of program would be reduced to 2 years within regional schools
         (3) A third internship year in a hospital nursing service would be required from 1965 to 1975
         (4) Schools would have own budgets with monies supplied by the Department of Health
      b. In 1969 the Provincial Association supported the abolition of the internship year as well as urging the financing of nurse education in the same way as other postsecondary programs
      c. In 1971 the internship program was phased out, leaving nursing with a 2-year program pattern
      d. By 1973 all nursing education programs at the diploma level had been transferred to the system of Colleges of Applied Arts and Technology

e. In 1980 The Ministry of Colleges and Universities decreed a change in minimum hours for diploma nursing programs from 1200 to 1625 hours of clinical practice and 750 hours of theory

9. Accelerated nursing program at Grey Nun's Hospital School of Nursing—1966
   a. An experimental 2-year nursing program in the general educational system
   b. System for which students paid tuition
   c. Students were not used for hospital service
   d. Structured liberal education component was included
   e. Students wrote registration examinations at end of 2 years

10. 1966—Saskatchewan became first province in Canada to transfer authority for hospital schools of nursing from Department of Public Health to Department of Education

11. The Colleges d'Enseignement Général et Professional (CEGEP) Schools
    a. *Report of the Royal Commission of Inquiry on Education* (Parent Report) in Quebec suggested that nursing education move into the general educational system, a transfer approved by the Association of Nurses for the Province of Quebec (A.N.P.Q.)
    b. Provincial legislature adopted the *Criteria for College Education* from the Parent Report in 1964; among these were
       (1) All college teachers to have appropriate academic preparation
       (2) System of accreditation be established
       (3) Definite student-teacher ratio to be used
    c. 1966—Concept of nursing education in Colleges d'Enseignement Général et Professional (CEGEP) introduced with 3 colleges starting nursing options in 1967
    d. In 1972, last of schools of nursing based within hospitals closed their doors, ending three fourths of a century of history

12. Diploma nursing programs in community college settings (including CEGEP programs)
    a. 1970—119 community colleges across Canada had 100,701 students enrolled in nursing programs—32,426 in university *stream* courses, 68,275 in vocational courses
    b. 1973—of 142 diploma programs, 101 were in educational institutions; 12,882 enrolled

in initial programs, and 89% of these entered at diploma level; graduations from initial programs decreased to 9514
    c. A 2-year, unique educational program distinct from both secondary and higher levels of education is offered by 35 Quebec CEGEP schools
    d. In 1974 a brief presented to the Superior Council of Education on the advantages and perpetual deficiencies of the Nursing Option in the CEGEP system; recommendations include
       (1) Information sessions on different levels of nurse training be offered by Department of Education and Order of Nurses of Quebec for vocational counselors
       (2) Professional improvement programs and incentives be established to allow employed teachers to take needed courses; in 1973 57.6% of teachers were still without a bachelor's degree
       (3) Programs of study be established to facilitate articulation between college and university programs with a minimum of upgrading
       (4) Clinical training periods be revised to inprove intensity and continuity; clinical ratio be maintained at 1:6
       (5) Hospital centers devise procedures to facilitate integration of graduates into labor market and include adequate budgets for orientation, in-service, and continuing education programs

13. Development of baccalaureate degree programs
    a. 1961—in a brief presented to the *Royal Commission on Health Services in Canada,* The Canadian Association of University Schools of Nursing stated that a baccalaureate degree provided generalized preparation, whereas masters and doctoral programs would prepare nursing consultants, experts in the clinical fields, and researchers
    b. 1961—beginning of Extension Course in Nursing Unit Administration in Toronto, sponsored by the Canadian Nurses' Association with the financial support of the Kellogg Foundation, to assist head nurses in upgrading their skills in administration
    c. 1962—University of Montreal became first

university in Canada to establish a faculty of nursing with Alice M. Girard as Dean

d. First basic integrated degree program taught in French in the world instituted at Institut Marguerite d'Youville, Montreal, in 1962

e. 1967—Institut Marguerite d'Youville amalgamated with the University of Montreal, becoming the first university in the world to offer both undergraduate and graduate degrees in nursing taught in French

f. Following *Royal Commission on Health Services in Canada,* nursing education began a new era with the major development being the general increase in the numbers of basic integrated baccalaureate programs

   (1) 1963—16 programs, 8 integrated and 8 nonintegrated

   (2) 1964-1973—graduations from baccalaureate degree programs increased from 2% to 6% of total graduations

   (3) 1973—ratio of basic degree graduates to diploma graduates was 1:15

   (4) 1973—22 programs were integrated, basic baccalaureate programs having 14% of 28,028 enrollment to initial programs

   (5) 1974—nonintegrated programs phased out of universities

g. 1973—University of British Columbia Program permits students to become registered nurses on completion of first 2 years of baccalaureate program

14. Higher degree programs

a. Nurses wanting to pursue graduate study in nursing beyond baccalaureate degree until 1959 were required to do so in the United States

b. Masters programs in Canada could not evolve until sufficient numbers of baccalaureate programs and graduates had been produced

c. 1959—University of Western Ontario established the first Canadian masters degree program in nursing, followed by McGill University

d. 1962—Canadian Nurses' Foundation was incorporated to provide monies for study at masters and doctoral levels and for research in nursing service

e. 1974—McGill University School of Nursing revised the masters program to offer 2 options: nurse clinician and nurse researcher programs

f. No doctoral programs are yet available in Canada, but plans are being drawn up to provide for these in the near future

15. University programs offered through schools of nursing as of 1980 according to *The Canadian Nurse Journal* (January, 1980)

a. Baccalaureate degree courses

   (1) Integrated, 4-year courses for studies following high school offered by 20 universities

   (2) Baccalaureate degree courses for registered nurses offered by 18 universities; also 5 French language universities

b. Masters degree programs

   (1) Two-year offered by 7 universities

   (2) One-year offered by 1 university

c. Certificate courses offered by 5 universities

d. Family practice nurse program offered by 1 university

e. Outpost nursing program offered by 1 university

f. Doctoral programs not offered in any Canadian university

g. Health science centers are integrated with nursing programs at 2 universities

h. 1978—only 50 of 190,000 nurses have doctoral degrees

16. Nonuniversity programs for preparation of nursing personnel as per Canadian Hospital Directory 1974

a. Hospital schools offering a diploma in nursing—26

b. Diploma nursing programs in provincial educational systems—76

c. Diploma nursing programs in regional and independent schools—5

d. Psychiatric nurse preparation programs in British Columbia, Alberta, Saskatchewan, and Manitoba—7

e. Postdiploma programs for registered nursing assistants available in

   (1) Operating room technician at Humber College, Toronto, Ontario

   (2) Operating room nursing and techniques

at the Wascana Institute of Applied Arts and Sciences, Regina, Saskatchewan
  f. Program for registered nursing assistants certificate of achievement in the practice and supervision of care in long-term facilities at Centennial College, Scarborough, Ontario
17. Licensed practical nurse programs
  a. Uncommon in Canada
  b. Graduates eligible for licensure as practical nurses (LPN) are those from nursing orderly program and the Nursing Assistant Program
18. *Canadian Nurses' Association Position Paper on Nursing Education* (1960s)—supported the following
  a. All nursing education programs should be under the jurisdiction of institutes whose primary aim is education
  b. Two types of nurses be prepared—university and nonuniversity
  c. Graduates of diploma programs to possess high degree of technical skill and to be prepared to assist in assessment of nursing needs and problems
  d. A merging of the roles of the diploma program registered nurse and registered nursing assistant be considered
19. Canadian Testing Service Examinations
  a. Established in 1970 by the Canadian Nurses' Association Testing Service (CNATS); now used in all jurisdictions
  b. Operation of testing service is directed by Test Service Board
  c. Master blueprint committee constructs overall plan for examinations
  d. Blueprint subcommittees have representatives from Canada's main regions—Atlantic, Ontario, Quebec, West, and French language representatives
  e. In 1976 all jurisdictions accepted 350 as a passing score
  f. In 1977 Blueprint for a Comprehensive Examination for Nurse Registration/Licensure developed by CNATS
  g. The Comprehensive Nurse Registration Examination using the nursing model was implemented in August, 1980

Advances in nursing service
A. The crisis after World War II
  1. World War II left nursing in an even greater state of chaos than World War I because the demands for nursing service were rapidly increased (as a result of newer treatment methods and social changes), whereas number of students entering nursing programs declined
  2. Nurses with leadership preparation were lacking as a direct result of the economic depression following the war and the absence of educational programs above the basic level
B. In 1961 the Canadian Nurses' Association in cooperation with the Canadian Hospital Association sponsored an extension course in Nursing Unit Administration in Toronto; financial support for the project was provided by the W. K. Kellogg Foundation
C. Development of programs for nursing assistants
  1. A large group of young women needed to be absorbed from women's military forces into civilian life, and government funds were used to organize schools for the preparation of nursing assistants from the group of ex-service women
  2. Approval and support of the nursing profession was given to the proposal to initiate courses of 9- to 12-month duration in educational settings
  3. Title for new worker suggested by the Canadian Nurses' Association was "nursing assistant" and with it came the thrust of the nursing assistant program across Canada
  4. In 1960, 43 nursing assistant programs were operating with certification or registration of the graduate on completion of the program and writing of examination administered through the Provincial Department of Health, the Provincial Registered Nurses' Associations, and the Boards of Registration of Nursing Assistants
D. Problems with proliferation developed
  1. The categories of workers in nursing proliferated in the 1960s and included
    a. Registered nurses (university and diploma programs)
    b. Nursing assistants
    c. Psychiatric nurses
    d. Orderlies and attendants
    e. Operating room technicians
  2. Problems with proliferation included
    a. A great deal of direct nursing care being given by nursing assistants
    b. A blurring of roles between the registered nurse and the registered nursing assistant
    c. Increasing need for nurses to spend time in teaching and supervisory functions

d. Increasing desire of nursing assistants for advancement

3. In 1968 at the general meeting of the Canadian Nurses' Association, the recommendation to gradually phase out programs from which practitioners on graduation were not eligible for licensure as registered nurses was approved

E. In its *Statement of Delivery of Nursing Care* the Nurses' Association recommended that
1. Standards of determining the levels of nursing care be formulated from within the nursing profession
2. A clear distinction be made between nursing and nonnursing activities
3. Objectives of the health agency as well as the means for achieving stated goals be defined by the nursing service

F. Team nursing
1. See background material under American section
2. In 1968 Registered Nurses' Association of Ontario offered practical experience in team nursing in a demonstration center supported by Ontario Hospital Services Commission, Ontario Department of Health, and Ontario Public Health Association
3. Team nursing development project served to teach nurses how to coordinate care of patients in hospitals, but more important how to coordinate care by involving hospitals, voluntary agencies, and public health teams to promote continuity of patient care

G. Accreditation of health care facilities
1. In 1970 Canadian Council on Hospital Accreditation expanded its program to include accreditation of the 3000 extended care facilities across Canada
2. In 1974 the Canadian Nurses' Association withdrew its official support for mandatory accreditation of all health agencies and joined with the Canadian Hospital Association in supporting voluntary accreditation

Legislation related to nurses and nursing

A. Economic security and nurse welfare
1. Labor relations and collective bargaining
   a. 1944—Canadian Nurses' Association recognized collective bargaining as a useful process in bettering socioeconomic status of nurses
   b. 1946—British Columbia became first province to introduce collective bargaining

   c. 1970s—nurses in British Columbia, Alberta, Manitoba, Ontario, Quebec, New Brunswick, and Nova Scotia had become organized and certified under provincial labor legislation
   d. "Strike right"—some Canadian nurses have right to strike according to provincial legislation in Quebec, Ontario (except for hospitals), Nova Scotia, British Columbia
   e. Provincial Nurses' Association in Quebec does not bargain for nurses, as a collective bargaining unit; Quebec nurses are members of professional syndicates—English Chapter formed the United Nurses of Montreal in 1966 and La Fédération des Syndicats Professionels d'Infirmières du Quebec, which includes nurses, physiotherapists, etc.
   f. Labor Relations Department of Canadian Nurses' Association to provide services related to collection and analysis of data, information distribution, educational programs, and research activities

B. National Health Insurance
1. 1966—following a recommendation from the *Royal Commission on Health Services* (1961), the Medical Care Act received royal assent
2. 1971—all provinces were participants in National Health Insurance except Northwest and Yukon territories, which implemented programs by 1972
3. 1973—Hospital Insurance and Diagnostic Services and Medical Care Directorates amalgamated to administer the 2 national health insurance schemes—Hospital Insurance and Medicare
4. National Health Insurance increased the demand for medical and nursing services in agencies other than hospitals and institutions; e.g., health clinics

C. The Health Disciplines Act—Ontario
1. Received royal assent in 1974 but was not proclaimed law until July, 1975
2. Incorporated recommendations from Committee on the Healing Arts and *Royal Commission Inquiry into Civil Rights*
3. Allowed for lay representation in the professional governing council
4. Created health disciplines board to conduct hearings related to complaints and applications for licensing
5. Gave Council of the College of Nurses of Ontario authority to
   a. Initially register new members and renew registration of standing members

b. Require nursing personnel to be currently registered with College of Nurses
c. Discipline any person granted initial registration
d. Protect titles—Registered Nurse and Registered Nursing Assistant
e. Establish, maintain, and develop standards of knowledge, skill, and professional ethics

D. Nurse practice acts
1. Nursing is recognized by provincial statutes (Nurses' Acts)
2. Purpose of registration
   a. Registration allows for protection of the general public by distinguishing the trained nurse from the untrained nurse
   b. Protects title of registered nurse for persons who have successfully passed registration examinations
3. Enactment
   a. Was first enacted in Nova Scotia (1910), followed by Manitoba (1913), New Brunswick and Alberta (1916), Ontario (1922)
   b. Is administered by provincial associations except in Ontario where College of Nurses registers nurses and in Quebec where Order of Nurses of Province of Quebec licenses nurses for nursing practice
4. Control
   a. In Ontario, with the Nurses' Act of 1961 amended, the College of Nurses of Ontario was established as the governing body of nursing with provision also for governing of nursing assistants (now titled Registered Nursing Assistant)
   b. As of February, 1974, only 1 nurses' association had right of appeal to a legal definition of nursing written into law—the Order of Nurses of Quebec
   c. Three provinces (Quebec, Prince Edward Island, and Newfoundland) protect the title nurse as well as the registered nurse
   d. Remaining provinces and territory have permissive registration/licensure based on approval of nursing programs and successful passing of CNATS
   e. The trend in remaining provinces/territory is toward mandatory licensure
   f. The Order of Nurses of Quebec
      (1) Professional Code of the Province of Quebec proclaimed in February, 1974, the changing of the title of Association of the Nurses of the Province of Quebec (A.N.P.Q.) to the Order of Nurses of Quebec (O.N.Q.) whose chief purpose is protection of the public
      (2) Passage of the Professional Code created professional groups of which 11 have exclusive rights to practice and 10 regulate only title of the health worker
      (3) Quebec Nurses' Act now defines profession of nursing as identification of persons' health needs, assisting with diagnosis, employing nursing interventions, and communication of health problems to clients
   g. Northwest Territories Registered Nurses' Association (N.W.T.R.N.A.)
      (1) January, 1975, the Ordinance Respecting the Nursing Profession in the Northwest Territories was approved by Territorial Council
      (2) Gave Northwest Territories Registered Nurses' Association the authority to
         (a) Join with the Canadian Nurses' Association
         (b) Grant and/or revoke certificates of registration to nurses practicing in the Northwest Territories
         (c) Discipline members of the nursing profession
         (d) Lay claim to being the first professional group north of the sixtieth parallel to acquire registration control over its members
5. Purposes of Nurses' Acts
   a. In most provinces Acts do not define legal boundaries in terms of nursing functions, although there is concerted effort by provincial associations to define nursing practice
   b. Provide for interprovincial registration if credentials are equivalent
   c. In some provinces, provide for the licensing of nursing assistants

Accreditation of nursing programs
A. Approval of programs
1. Nursing programs are provincially controlled within the general health category

2. Provincial associations establish minimum standards and approve nursing programs on satisfactory inspection
3. Some provinces utilize other approval channels
   a. In Manitoba an accrediting committee of nurses and nonnurses establishes minimum standards that are approved by the Board of the Provincial Association
   b. In Ontario the Council of Regents establishes minimum standards for diploma nursing in the CAAT system. College of Nurses continues to inspect
4. Approved nursing programs listed in the *Canadian Hospital Directory* and Canadian Nurses' Association publications
5. Association of Community Colleges in Canada is implementing a process by which National Standards for Health Science Programs will be promoted
6. Nursing programs cannot function without approval as specified under individual provincial Nurses' Acts
B. Accreditation
   1. 1967—Executive Director of Canadian Nurses' Association consulted with the National League for Nursing on the accreditation process
   2. 1972—publication of *Canadian Nurses' Association Position on Accreditation*
   3. 1973—self-evaluation tools formulated on which criteria for accreditation would be based
   4. 1974—optimum standards for nursing education developed by Canadian Nurses' Association
   5. Canadian nursing education programs have no national accreditation process
   6. C.A.U.S.N. has developed and tested in at least 3 universities an accreditation program for University Schools of Nursing
   7. A.C.C.C. involved in accreditation of programs other than nursing
   8. 1978—Resolution passed at Canadian Nurses' Association convention that Canadian Nurses' Association together with C.A.U.S.N. and A.C.C.C. develop a national accreditation program for nursing education programs; initial plan developed has been tested at 3 universities
   9. First meeting of Steering Committee for Development of National Standards of Nursing Practice held in 1978; National Standards of Nursing Practice available in 1980

Current developments

A. Need for a clear legal definition of nursing
   1. Canadian Health Manpower statistics in 1974 showed 14 professional classifications engaged in health care with a fragmentation of care and a clouding of roles
   2. New definition of nursing must
      a. Establish a well-defined role
      b. Provide for accountability
B. Mandatory versus voluntary continuing education for nurses
   1. Debate continues as to whether continuing education should be a mandatory or voluntary requirement for nurse registration and licensure
   2. The pressure for continuing education as a prerequisite for renewal of the license to practice nursing is becoming more urgent
C. The Canadian Nurses' Association—continuing leadership for the present and the future
   1. With a 1979 membership of 122,000 nurses, the Canadian Nurses' Association continues to
      a. Promote highest possible standards of nursing care
      b. Strive for structure that will ensure nurse accountability
      c. Encourage preparation of guidelines for standards of nurse preparation, continuing competence in practice, and legal protection especially in areas of expanded nurse roles
      d. Explore ways of raising the level of nurse awareness to life-styles that foster optimum health
      e. Explore development of standards for ongoing education as a requirement for registration/licensure
      f. Stimulate and develop interest in ongoing research in nursing
   2. The established priorities
      a. Evaluation of nursing care
      b. Evaluation of educational programs for nurses
      c. Evaluation of nurse competence
      d. Advancement of nursing research
      e. Advancement of the health and rights of the the individual
   3. Code of Ethics, uniquely Canadian, will be developed by the Association utilizing as a base
      a. The International Council of Nurses' Code of Ethics (1973)

b. The Canadian Nurses' Association Statement Related to Ethics of Nursing Research (1972)

c. Provincial legislation and policies

4. Economic welfare for members of the nursing profession remains a major concern of the Association

D. Research in nursing—Canadian Council of Nurse Researchers

1. 1974—Third National Conference on Research in Nursing, projecting that numbers of nurse researchers would increase at all levels, appointed a task force to explore development of a Canadian Council of Nurse Researchers

2. 1974—research unit set up by McGill University in nursing and health care to develop, study, and evaluate the nurse's expanded function, especially in primary care

3. 1975—Fourth National Conference on Nursing Research focused on developing indicators for nursing research

4. Canadian Nurses' Association publishes research in Index of Canadian Nursing Studies

5. In 1977 Canadian Nurses' Association, Canadian Nurses' Foundation, and C.A.U.S.N. developed joint approach to nursing research

E. Nursing education

1. Career ladder concept

a. Supports curriculum that allows articulation with succeeding levels so that one may proceed from nursing assistant level to diploma level, etc.; a program is available in Saskatchewan where practical nurses can become diploma graduates

b. Report of a Royal Commission headed by Dr. Leonard Miller strongly supports the career ladder in Newfoundland

c. Humber College of Applied Arts and Technology in Toronto has developed an experimental curriculum that

(1) Offers core courses for nurses and allied health workers

(2) Allows students to elect to continue toward a nursing diploma or a registered nursing assistant certificate after the common initial semester

d. Success of the career ladder approach still remains unproved

2. Changes in curriculum

a. Revision of baccalaureate degree programs to include increased content on community health

b. Graduation of larger numbers of 2-year diploma (community college) and baccalaureate students

c. Specialization at masters level has resulted in the introduction of clinical specialists into health care agencies

d. 1972—Canadian Nurses' Association issued *Statement of the Expanded Role of the Nurse* urging modification of educational programs to allow nurses to enter a variety of health care settings

3. Nurse practitioner programs

a. 1971—The National Conference on Assistance to the Physician recommended that Canada not develop programs to produce "physician's assistants" but rather to augment nursing programs to develop nurse practitioners

b. *Report of the Committee on Nurse Practitioners* (Boudreau Report) (1972)—special Committee established by Minister of National Health and Welfare to study role of the nurse practitioner; offered description of nurse practitioners' role and recommended

(1) The delegation of specific, defined tasks by physicians to appropriately prepared nurses

(2) That nurse practitioner preparation be eventually incorporated within baccalaureate programs

(3) That development of nurse practitioner programs become a priority

(4) That basic preparations of nurses at diploma and university levels reflect broadened concept of nursing

(5) That nurse practitioners receive courses in educational institutions affiliated with university health science centers; by 1972, 1 pilot project in nurse practitioner programs was operating; several universities were conducting ad hoc classes for family practice nurses; 6 universities were providing outpost nursing courses; Quebec nurses were exploring the *community nurse* concept

c. 1973—Canadian Nurses' Association issued *Statement on Specialization in Nursing* supporting degrees or levels of specialization in nursing after a basic diploma or baccalaureate program

F. Nursing service
  1. Expanded role
     a. Four patterns of expanding role of nurse in primary care are emerging
        (1) Physician's associate
        (2) Community health nurse
        (3) Northern Health Service nurse
        (4) Primary health care worker
     b. Definitions of nurse practitioner are drafted in 7 provinces, and 4 provinces (Alberta, Saskatchewan, Ontario, Manitoba) are amending their Nurse Practice Acts to provide for the nurse's expanded role
  2. Problem-oriented medical records
     a. Approach to health records that requires a patient-centered focus to define presenting problems
     b. 1974—Science Council of Canada submitted a report, *Science for Health Services,* recommending that health care be organized into an integrated system using computer-based health information systems and standardized health records
     c. Canadian Nurses' Association recognized value of application of science technology to the health care system (problem-oriented medical records) but deferred endorsement of a single approach as the solution to problems in the health care system
  3. Peer review
     a. Quality of nursing care given to clients is evaluated in terms of formulated standards of nursing practice
     b. A useful evaluation tool for assisting individual nurses to improve their care and for assessing nurses for advancement
     c. Essential for nurse accountability for care provided
  4. Clinical specialists
     a. Definition—nurses prepared at the masters level who possess advanced knowledge, skill, and clinical competence in specialized areas
     b. Use—it is predicted that use will increase as more nurses are prepared
G. Developments related to and influencing nursing
  1. *Community Health Center Project* (The Hasting Report) (1972)

  a. Initiated by Minister of National Health and Welfare to describe community health centers and to determine problems in health center development
  b. Recommendations included that
     (1) Provinces develop community health centers
     (2) Patient-centered, problem-solving approaches be used by all health personnel
     (3) A comprehensive system for evaluation of community health centers be instituted
     (4) Public health functions continue as a vital part of the health services system
  2. *A New Perspective on the Health of Canadians* (1974)—published by the Minister of National Health and Welfare
     a. A document that presents policies to be developed in the health care system within the next 10 to 15 years
     b. Report presented a study of the major causes of death and illness and from these identified the major health problems of the Canadian population
     c. Major focus is on the *health field concept* composed of 4 principal parts—human biology, environment, life-style, and health care organization
     d. Recommendations included that
        (1) The value system of health care organizations be revised
        (2) Programs be initiated to create safer environments and life-styles that foster good health
        (3) Programs geared to the reduction of self-imposed health risks be implemented through government involvement in public education programs
        (4) Programs directed at "neglected" areas of Canadian population be initiated; i.e., programs for the aged, mentally ill, economically deprived, chronically ill, troubled parents and children, etc.
     e. Key proposition for nursing related to
        (1) Reduction of environmental hazards and self-imposed health risks in the population
        (2) Family counseling
        (3) Care of the mentally and chronically ill
        (4) Care of the aged population
        (5) Provision of home care

3. Proliferation of personnel in health care field
4. Changes in medical practice patterns
5. Other social and economic factors that will influence the delivery of health care include
   a. Spiraling costs of health care
   b. Increasing number of aged
   c. Malnutrition
   d. Cost of housing
   e. Unemployment

NURSING PRACTICE AND THE LAW— UNITED STATES AND CANADA
Typology of laws

A. Legal systems of modern nations influenced by both Roman civil law and English common law
B. Law arises from
   1. Statutory law (legislation)
      a. Body of law enacted by federal, provincial, state, or local government
      b. That which commands or prohibits
      c. Licensing laws belong in this category
   2. Common law (custom and precedent)
      a. Unwritten; based on customs
      b. Precedent plays large part in judge's decisions, thus giving uniformity to decisions in like situations
      c. Nurses practice under common as well as statutory law
C. British North America Act (1867) has served as basic law of Canada; gives provincial governments power in health care activities
D. The Constitution of the United States gives states the power to police the health and welfare of its citizens
E. Military law
   1. Applies to nurses only when members of one of the military nurse corps
   2. Applies to all citizens when martial law declared
F. Private law
   1. Property law—wills, patents, copyrights, trademarks
   2. Contract law—agency, conditional sales, mortgages, bail
   3. Tort law—intentional aggression, negligence, strict liability, defamation, invasion of privacy
G. Public law
   1. Constitutional law—government structures, federal division of powers, fundamental rights
   2. Administrative law—consumer protection, social welfare

3. Criminal law—serious offenses against the individual and society
   a. Felonies—more serious; e.g., grand larceny, homicide
   b. Misdemeanors—less serious; e.g., burglary
H. Civil law—acts contrary to a criminal statute; may result in a civil suit, since the act has violated civil law

Torts and crimes especially important to nurses

A. Torts
   1. Violates civil law
   2. Failure to use care or failure to prevent injury
   3. Malpractice and negligence fall into this category and are unintentional torts
      a. No precise statute describes malpractice
      b. Terms often used interchangeably, but some legal experts make a distinction between them
         (1) Malpractice—professional misconduct; negligence performed in professional practice; any unreasonable lack of skill in professional duties or illegal or immoral conduct that results in injury or death to the client, patient, consumer
         (2) Negligence—practice without a license; measurement of negligence is "reasonableness"; involves exposure of person or property of another to unreasonable risk of injury by acts of commission or omission
   4. Usual standard of conduct is that which a prudent nurse would or would not do
   5. Tort different from crime, but serious tort can be tried as both civil and criminal action
   6. Necessary to prove negligence—if proven, this means act was performed incorrectly or not at all and nurse is responsible for injury
   7. Elements essential to prove negligence
      a. Lack of conformity to standards
      b. Breach of duty
      c. Proved cause-effect relationship between act and injury
      d. Not dependent on a contract
   8. Nurse responsible for own acts; if employed, employer may also be held responsible under the doctrine of *respondeat superior;* when responsibility shared, nursing actions must lie within the scope of employment

9. Reasonableness and prudence in actions are usually determining factors in a judgment; increasing attention is being paid to the law governing the practice of nursing

10. Examples of malpractice/negligence include leaving sponges inside a patient; causing burns from hot water bottles, heating pads, hot solutions, and electric, steam, or vapor sources; medication errors; failure to prevent falls by neglecting to raise bed or crib rails; incompetent assessment of patient situations, such as ignoring complaints of chest pain leading to subsequent inappropriate actions; improper identification of patients for operative or diagnostic procedures; and carelessness in caring for a patient's property, such as dentures, clothing, valuables

11. Intentional torts occur when a person does damage to another person in a willful, intentional way and without just cause and/or excuse; includes fraud and deceit, assault and battery, false imprisonment, exposure of person or body after death, eavesdropping, libel and slander (defamatory torts)
    a. Assault
       (1) Knowingly threatening or attempting to do violence to another
       (2) Forcing a medication or treatment on a person who does not want it constitutes assault
    b. Battery
       (1) Actually wounding or touching a person in an offensive manner
       (2) Hitting or striking a patient would constitute battery
    c. Fraud
       (1) False presentation of facts purposefully to create deception
       (2) Presenting false credentials for purposes of entering a nursing program or gaining registration, licensure, or employment
    d. Invasion of privacy
       (1) Encroachment or trespass on another's body and/or personality includes
          (a) False imprisonment—the intentional confinement without authorization by a person who physically constricts another using force, the threat of force, or who uses confining structures and/or clothing. Even without force or malicious intent, to detain another without consent in a specified area constitutes grounds for a charge of false imprisonment; the charge is not false imprisonment if it is necessary to protect an emotionally disturbed person from harming self or others or if it is necessary to confine to defend self, others, or property or to effect a lawful arrest
          (b) Exposure of a person—any unnecessary exposure or discussion of the patient's case is actionable unless authorized by the patient; after death, the patient's right to be unobserved, excluded from unwarranted operations, and unauthorized touching of the body persists
          (c) Defamation—concerns privileged communications and privacy; law grants right of privacy to everyone; divulgence of privileged communication whether from charts, conversation, interview, or observation in a way that exposes the person to hatred, contempt, aversion, or a lowering of opinion; includes slander (oral) and libel (written, pictured, telecast), both of which are dependent on communication to a third party

B. Crimes
   1. Criminal act—an act contrary to a criminal statute; in Canada, one contrary to the Criminal Code of Canada; violates societal law; includes felonies and misdemeanors
   2. Criminal Code of Canada is determined by the Parliament of Canada, is applicable to all provinces and territories, and may be amended by Parliament to reflect society's changing values; e.g., suicide is no longer a crime
   3. Crimes are wrongs punishable by the state, committed against the state, usually demonstrate that intent was present, and are reported by the state as the complainant
   4. Commission of crime requires 2 fundamental factors
      a. Committing a deed contrary to criminal law

b. Omitting an act when there is a legal obligation to perform such an act; e.g., refraining from assistance with the birth of a child if such refusal results in injury to the newborn
5. Criminal conspiracy occurs when 2 or more persons agree to commit a crime
6. Giving aid to another in the commission of a crime makes the person equally guilty of the offense if awareness is present that a crime is being committed
7. Ignorance of the law is usually not an adequate defense when a crime or civil wrong is committed
8. Assault may be justified in instances of self-defense if only as much force as is absolutely necessary for self-protection is used
9. Search warrants are required before property can be searched
10. Administration of narcotics by nurse is legal only when authorized by a physician who is legally registered under the Controlled Substances Act
    a. If a nurse knowingly administers a drug that causes a major disability or death, a crime may be charged
    b. Illegal possession or sale of a controlled substance makes nurse liable, as is any citizen
11. Those involved in decisions to discontinue life-support systems may be liable to charge of murder; there is a strong movement against dramatic life-saving measures in cases of terminally ill patients; these questions are as much moral as legal; nurse should know decision must be made on knowledge; nurse is accountable; "living will" aims at giving the individual the authority to say whether life-support systems should be used at all or discontinued if in use; legality of "living will" and effectiveness of legislation permitting it are under dispute

Malpractice insurance

A. Liability can be defined as a person's legal responsibility to be accountable for wrongful acts by making financial restitution to the party wronged
B. Malpractice insurance can be purchased from nurses' associations, bargaining organizations, and private insurance companies
C. Amount of malpractice/liability insurance is dictated by factors such as

1. Type of nursing practiced, such as private practitioner, nursing instructor, acute care nursing
2. Increasing inclination to sue professionals, including nurses
3. Any limits of liability established in area where nursing is practiced; e.g., in Ontario, Canada, $200,000 per incident and $500,000 per calendar year are limits
D. An employer's insurance protects the nurse while on duty in the course of employment (concept of vicarious liability, *respondeat superior*); a nurse can, however, be personally sued and held liable for negligent or malpractice actions
E. Malpractice insurance provides monetary settlement if a suit by a client is decided in favor of the client; most policies pay legal fees and costs, as well as bond for the nurse in an appeal

Informed consent

A. Purposes of informed consent
   1. Makes possible a contract between 2 individuals with each sharing equally
   2. Makes competent decision possible for patient who has the final decision
B. Consent essential for any treatment, except in an emergency where failure to institute treatment may constitute negligence
C. Major question is what constitutes informed consent
   1. Elements of consent
      a. Explanation of treatment to be done
      b. Advantages and disadvantages
      c. Possible alternatives
      d. Time for decision making
      e. No undue pressure
   2. Problems arise in determining
      a. What constitutes adequate information
      b. Who should give explanation
      c. Whether to give alternatives where one treatment is clearly preferable
   3. Patient has right to know, right to agree, or right to refuse
D. Nurse's responsibility is to respect rights of individual patient, thus avoiding legal action

Registration/licensure

A. Used interchangeably but are not synonymous
B. Registration—entrance of name in a registry
   1. Maintained by individual states in United States

2. Maintained by individual provincial professional nurses' associations in Canada
3. Authorizes practice as a registered nurse
4. Protects the title of registered nurse
5. Follows automatically after licensure

C. Licensure—granting of a license following successful completion of State Board Test Pool Examination in the United States and the Canadian Nurses' Association Testing Service Registration Examination in Canada
1. Protects the public and nursing practice; issued by individual states or provinces
2. Mandatory licensure—all who practice nursing must be licensed; employees of federal government are not bound by state or provincial mandatory licensure laws
3. Permissive licensure—protects the titles Reg N or RN, but does not protect the practice of nursing; the practice of nursing is not prohibited as long as the unlicensed person does not represent himself as a registered nurse; thus anyone, licensed or not, may practice nursing so long as the title Reg N or RN is not used
4. May be obtained by examination, waiver, or endorsement (reciprocity)

The nurse in the courts

A. Nurse may be in court either as a witness if involved personally in a case or as an expert witness because of knowledge and expertise
B. Expert witness
1. Not an advocate
2. If called into court, the nurse must be
   a. Informed as to standards of care that prudent, reasonable nurse would give relative to incident in question
   b. Knowledgeable in the field specific to the incident
   c. Without opinion unless specifically asked
3. Although a professional may join in a "conspiracy of silence" when asked to testify against another professional, the basic question is ethical and concerns the willingness of the professional to deal adequately with the incompetence of another professional
4. Patient's charts, to which nurses contribute, may be used in court, therefore placing nurses in court vicariously; notes should be accurate, complete, factual, and give evidence of knowledge and judgment

The nurse's legal status

A. Employee
1. Nurse acts and performs service for another and is known as agent; this does not eliminate the independence of the nurse in practice
2. Contract made with the employer that sets forth the nature of the services expected, the conditions of employment, and compensation
3. Elements of a written contract
   a. Services to be rendered
   b. Environment in which services are to be rendered
   c. Duration of contract
   d. Termination conditions
B. Collective bargaining increasingly involved in arranging contracts between employees and the employing agency
1. Contracts binding on both parties even though individual nurse not directly involved with the deliberations; if majority of employees agree, all are bound
2. Damages may be sought in court if contract broken
C. Independent contractor
1. Independent contractor is one who renders direct services to clients and is in control of that service, including setting fee for service
2. A small number of nurses setting up independent practices
3. Joint practice is an adaptation of the independent contractor
   a. Nurse and physician practice independently and collaboratively, each rendering service to the same group of patients
   b. The client's needs determine which professional gives the service
4. Private duty nurse is an independent contractor

Patients' complaints

A. Clients/patients have the right to lodge complaints about a nurse and the care received when complaints are related to
1. Incompetence
2. Professional misconduct
3. Physical or mental incapacity
B. Nursing's licensing body disciplines members of the profession of nursing according to the mechanisms described in Nurse Practice Acts
C. Self-regulation practices are criteria of a profession, along with autonomy and expertise

COMPREHENSIVE TEST 1

TO SIMULATE THE COMPREHENSIVE STATE BOARD EXAMINATION YOU SHOULD COMPLETE THIS TEST WITHIN TWO HOURS.

Situation: Mrs. Penny, a gravida II para 1, is admitted to the labor unit by ambulance, and delivery is imminent. She keeps bearing down, and after 2 contractions the baby's head is crowning. Questions 1 through 15 refer to this situation.

1 The nurse should:
1. Tell her to breathe through her mouth and pant during contractions
2. Tell her to breathe through her mouth and not to bear down
3. Transfer her immediately by stretcher to the delivery room
4. Tell her to pant while supporting the perineum with her hand to prevent tearing

2 With the next contraction Mrs. Penny delivers a large baby boy spontaneously. The nurse's initial action should be to:
1. Ascertain the condition of the fundus
2. Establish an airway for the baby
3. Quickly tie and cut the umbilical cord
4. Move mother and baby to delivery room

3 The physician arrives and cares for the baby and delivers the placenta. Pitocin, an oxytocic, is administered intramuscularly. Since Mrs. Penny has had a precipitous delivery, it is important to observe for:
1. Bleeding and infection
2. Sudden chilling
3. Elevation in blood pressure
4. Respiratory insufficiency in the baby

4 If involution is progressing normally, immediately after birth the nurse would expect the fundus to be located:
1. Three centimeters above the umbilicus
2. At the level of the umbilicus
3. Two centimeters below the umbilicus
4. Two centimeters above the symphysis pubis

5 Mrs. Penny's newborn infant is taken from the delivery room to the nursery, where it is the policy for the nurse to appraise the infant. In the examination the nurse notes that the temperature, pulse, and respiration are in normal range. Other physical characteristics are also normal. The nurse notes all observations on the baby's record. Which of the following statements is correct?
1. The nurse was making a medical diagnosis
2. Only the physician should determine the infant's physical status
3. According to the Nurse Practice Act the nurse performed correctly
4. Assessment by the nurse is not equivalent to the physician's assessment

6 Mr. and Mrs. Penny name their baby Andrew. At 10 hours of life he has a large amount of mucus and becomes slightly cyanotic. The nurse should:
1. Give the infant oxygen
2. Insert a Levin tube
3. Note the incident on the chart
4. Suction the mucus as needed

7 Baby Andrew must be observed carefully for the first 24 hours, particularly for:

1. Respiratory distress
2. Change in body temperature
3. Frequency in voiding
4. Duration of cry

8 When Andrew's mother removes his blanket and starts to examine her infant, she becomes concerned because he assumes a fencing position as she turns his head; the mother suspects neurologic damage. The nurse would discuss with the mother that:
1. This is a normal response
2. The physician had been notified of this suspicious response
3. This reflex disappears around 2 months of age
4. Tonic neck reflex may indicate neurologic damage in the newborn

9 Supportive nursing care in the beginning mother-infant relationship should include:
1. Encouraging Mrs. Penny to decide between breast-feeding and bottle-feeding
2. Allowing Mrs. Penny ample time to inspect the baby
3. Requiring Mrs. Penny to assist with simple aspects of infant's care
4. Unobtrusive observation to pick up disturbed mother-infant relationship

10 Mrs. Penny has decided to breast-feed this baby. However, she has some doubts as to whether she will be successful, since her breasts are small. She is also concerned about putting on weight, since she is proud of her petite figure. Concerning Mrs. Penny's statement about the size of her breasts, the nurse's best response should be:
1. "The size of your breasts has nothing to do with the production of milk."
2. "The amount of fat and glandular tissue in the breasts determines the amount of milk produced."
3. "You seem to have some concern about breast-feeding."
4. "Everybody can be successful at breast-feeding."

11 It is now 2 days post partum and Mrs. Penny asks the nurse about cleansing the nipples. The nurse's best response would be:
1. "Thoroughly scrub the nipples with soap and water before each feeding."
2. "Cleanse the nipples with sterile water before each feeding."
3. "Cleanse the nipples with an alcohol sponge before and after each feeding."

4. "Wash the breasts and nipples daily with water."

12 On the third day following delivery Mrs. Penny states that she has a great deal of pain in her breasts and that she is afraid that the baby will hurt her when he tries to grasp the nipple. The most appropriate action for the nurse to take is to explain the reasons for the patient's discomfort and to:
1. Call the physician to obtain advice
2. Administer a medication for pain
3. Express some of the milk manually before putting the baby to breast
4. Suggest that the patient limit fluids and not try to nurse the baby for the next 2 days

13 Mrs. Penny is concerned because she heard that her neighbor's breasts suddenly dried up when she got home and she had to discontinue nursing. An appropriate comment for the nurse to make is:
1. "This commonly happens with the excitement of going home. Putting the baby to breast more frequently will reestablish lactation."
2. "This commonly happens; however, we will give you a formula to take home so the baby won't go hungry until your milk supply returns."
3. "This is not true; once lactation is established, this rarely happens."
4. "You have little to worry about, since you already have a good milk supply."

14 Mrs. Penny has heard of demand feeding and wonders how anyone ever finds time to do anything but feed the baby. The nurse's best response would be:
1. "Most mothers find babies on breast do better on demand feeding, since the amount of milk ingested varies at each feeding."
2. "Perhaps a schedule might be better, since the baby is already accustomed to hospital routine."
3. "Although the baby is on demand feedings, he will eventually set his own schedule, so there will be time for your household chores."
4. "Most mothers find that feeding the baby whenever he cries works out fine."

15 Mrs. Penny wants to know whether it is true that she will not have to use contraceptives while nursing. The nurse's most appropriate response should be:
1. "Since lactation suppresses ovulation, you probably don't have to worry about becoming pregnant."

2. As long as you have no menstrual period you won't have to worry about using contraceptives.''
3. ''It is best to use contraceptive measures, since ovulation may occur without a menstrual period.''
4. ''It is best to delay any sexual relations until you have your first menstrual period.''

Situation: Andrew Penny is now 1 month old. He has been vomiting for 1 week. Mrs. Penny explains that the vomiting has been progressively more forceful and contains undigested formula. Presently Andrew is dehydrated and has abdominal distention. A tentative diagnosis of pyloric stenosis has been made. Questions 16 through 22 refer to this situation.

16 Vomiting caused by pyloric stenosis is usually non-bile stained because:
1. The obstruction is above the opening of the common bile duct
2. The bile duct is also obstructed
3. The obstruction of the cardiac sphincter prevents bile from entering the esophagus
4. The sphincter of the bile duct is connected to the hypertrophied pyloric muscle

17 While doing the physical assessment of Andrew the nurse should particularly observe for visible peristaltic waves and:
1. An olive-shaped mass in the right upper quadrant
2. Decreased bowel sounds
3. Severe cramping movements in the lower intestine
4. A boardlike abdomen

18 The physician orders a gavage tube for Andrew. How should the nurse determine the distance needed to advance the gavage tube?
1. Advance the tube until resistance is met
2. Measure the distance from the nose to the earlobe to the epigastric area of the abdomen
3. Measure from the mouth to the umbilicus and add half the distance
4. Advance the tube as far as necessary to aspirate gastric contents

19 During insertion of the tube, which sign or reaction would be considered abnormal by the nurse if demonstrated by Andrew?
1. Choking
2. Cyanosis
3. Flushing
4. Gagging

20 A Fredet-Ramstedt procedure is performed and, postoperatively, the nurse instructs Mrs. Penny regarding proper feeding techniques, such as:
1. Feed child in semi-Fowler's position and afterward place child in prone position
2. Rock the child after feedings to reduce crying and ingestion of air
3. Feed child in supine position to reduce pressure on sutures
4. Feed child in an upright position and afterward place on right side with head slightly elevated

21 One month after his discharge, Mrs. Penny brings Andrew into the Pediatric Clinic and asks about the introduction of new foods. The nurse suggests:
1. ''Mix the pureed food with the formula and give through the bottle to help him learn new tastes.''
2. ''Offer a new food every day until he likes one.''
3. ''Offer a new food after he has had some milk when he is still hungry.''
4. ''Offer a new food after he has had his regular feeding.''

22 Mrs. Penny also asks about what foods she should begin to introduce. A likely choice would be to start with:
1. Rice cereal and fruit, then add egg yolk
2. Cereal, and add a soft-boiled egg for breakfast
3. Fruit first, then add meat and vegetables
4. Sweets, such as fruits and puddings

Situation: Mrs. Mager, age 20, is 37 weeks pregnant. She is admitted to the hospital with preeclampsia and sudden abdominal pain. Questions 23 through 35 refer to this situation.

23 On Mrs. Mager's admission to the unit the nurse should observe for:
1. Decrease in size of uterus, cessation of contractions, visible or concealed hemorrhage
2. Firm and tender uterus, concealed or external hemorrhage, shock
3. Increase in size of uterus, visible bleeding, no associated pain
4. Shock, decrease in size of uterus, absence of external bleeding

24 The nurse realizes that the abdominal pain associated with abruptio placentae is caused by:
1. Hemorrhagic shock
2. Inflammatory reactions
3. Blood in the uterine muscle
4. Concealed hemorrhage

25 Mrs. Mager is given a unit of blood. The nurse realizes that this is necessary, since the bleeding following severe abruptio placentae is usually caused by:
1. Hypofibrinogenemia
2. Hyperglobulinemia
3. Thrombocytopenia
4. Polycythemia

26 Mrs. Mager delivers a stillborn baby girl. To foster a healthy grieving response to the birth of a stillborn child, the nurse's best response to an expression of anger from Mrs. Mager would be:
1. "It's God's will; we have to have faith that it was for the best."
2. "You are young; you'll have other children."
3. "This often happens when something is wrong with the baby."
4. "You may be wondering if something you did caused this."

27 Mrs. Mager has difficulty resolving her grief and, in 6 months, appears to be increasingly anxious over her inability to conceive again. She visits her physician and after examination is admitted to the hospital with a tentative diagnosis of hyperthyroidism. The nurse would expect Mrs. Mager to exhibit:
1. Nervousness, weight loss, increased appetite
2. Protruding eyeballs, slow pulse, sluggishness
3. Increased appetitie, slow pulse, dry skin
4. Loss of weight, GI disturbances, listlessness

28 When teaching Mrs. Mager about the diagnostic tests to be done, the nurse should include:
1. Radioactive iodine uptake and T_3
2. Protein-bound iodine and SMA 12
3. T_4 and x-ray films
4. Basal metabolism rate and P_{0_2}

29 The major nursing problem in caring for Mrs. Mager would be:
1. Providing an adequate diet
2. Keeping the bed linen neat
3. Providing sufficient rest
4. Modifying hospital routines

30 The purpose of propylthiouracil, which was ordered for Mrs. Mager, is to:
1. Interfere with the synthesis of thyroid hormone
2. Produce atrophy of the thyroid gland
3. Increase the uptake of iodine
4. Decrease the secretion of thyroid-stimulating hormone

31 The physician decides that Mrs. Mager should have a subtotal thyroidectomy. In preparation for surgery, Lugol's Iodine Solution is ordered. This medication is given to:
1. Maintain the function of the parathyroid glands
2. Decrease the total basal metabolic rate
3. Block the formation of thyroxin by the thyroid gland
4. Decrease the size and vascularity of the thyroid gland

32 Mrs. Mager is concerned that the thyroidectomy will interfere with her ability to become pregnant. The nurse bases her response on the following information:
1. As long as medication is taken as ordered, ovulation will occur
2. Pregnancy is not advisable for the patient with a thyroidectomy
3. Hyperthyroidism can cause abortions or fetal anomalies
4. Pregnancy will affect metabolism and will require greatly increased thyroid hormone

33 When Mrs. Mager returns to her room after surgery, the nurse should:
1. Instruct her not to speak
2. Inspect the incision
3. Keep her flat in bed for 24 hours
4. Place a tracheostomy set at the bedside

34 Postoperatively the nurse should carefully observe Mrs. Mager for signs of thyroid storm. These include:
1. Loss of consciousness
2. Elevated serum calcium
3. Rapid heart action and tremors
4. Sudden drop in pulse rate

35 Thyroid storm is caused by:
1. Removal of the parathyroid gland
2. Increased amount of thyroid hormone in the blood
3. Increased iodine in the blood
4. A rebound increase in metabolism following anesthesia

Situation: Mrs. Kraft, a 45-year-old woman, is a severe diabetic who is admitted to the hospital for a midthigh amputation of her right leg because of a gangrenous leg ulcer. She also has a history of closed-angle chronic glaucoma and has been using pilocarpine 2 % eyedrops 4 times a day for the past year. Questions 36 through 45 refer to this situation.

36 The chief aim of medical treatment in chronic glaucoma is:
1. Controlling intraocular pressure
2. Dilating the pupil to allow for an increase in visual field
3. Resting the eye to reduce pressure
4. Preventing secondary infections that can add to the visual problem

37 Mrs. Kraft seems able to accept the amputation but appears to have difficulty dealing with the glaucoma. The nurse arranges to spend more time with her, since she realizes the patient with glaucoma needs assistance in learning to accept the disease because:
1. There is usually restriction in the use of both eyes
2. Lost vision cannot be restored
3. Total blindness is inevitable
4. Surgery will only temporarily help the problem

38 Which of the following ocular symptoms should the nurse expect Mrs. Kraft to exhibit?
1. A complete loss of forward vision
2. Attacks of acute pain
3. Impairment of peripheral vision
4. Constant blurred vision

39 Before the amputation, the anesthesiologist prescribes meperidine (Demerol), 50 mg, and atropine, 0.4 mg, for Mrs. Kraft. The nurse should:
1. Withhold the atropine, since it is contraindicated
2. Give the medication as ordered
3. Administer the pilocarpine before the atropine
4. Ask the anesthesiologist to verify the order

40 Postoperatively, to prevent contractures of the hip, the nurse should:
1. Place pillows under the stump
2. Encourage Mrs. Kraft to lie in the prone position several times daily
3. Remove pillows from under the stump and elevate the head of the bed
4. Encourage Mrs. Kraft to sit in a chair as much as possible

41 To promote early and efficient ambulation when Mrs. Kraft is allowed out of bed, the nurse should encourage her to:
1. Keep hip in extension and abduction
2. Keep hip in extension and adduction
3. Keep hip in flexion and adduction
4. Keep right shoulder raised when swinging stump

42 Stump shrinkage is an important step in the healing process. There are 2 factors that contribute to stump shrinkage: one is atrophy of the muscles, and the other is:
1. Postoperative edema
2. Development of skin turgor
3. Reduction of subcutaneous fat
4. Loss of tissue and bone during operation

43 In helping Mrs. Kraft prepare her stump for a prosthesis, the nurse should encourage her to:
1. Abduct the stump when ambulating
2. Hang the stump off the bed frequently
3. Soak the stump in warm water twice a day
4. Periodically press the end of the stump against a pillow

44 When preparing Mrs. Kraft for dinner, it is the nurse's responsibility to:
1. Remove the pillow under the stump and raise the head of the bed
2. Check Mrs. Kraft's urine for sugar and acetone
3. Get Mrs. Kraft out of bed and into a chair
4. Make sure that Mrs. Kraft uses sugar substitutes

45 In planning with Mrs. Kraft for discharge the nurse discusses stump care; considering her glaucoma, she encourages Mrs. Kraft to:
1. Use mydriatrics regularly
2. Restrict fluid intake
3. Avoid bright lights or darkness
4. Exercise in moderation

Situation: Two-year-old Tommy is brought to the Pediatric Clinic. His mother states he has been irritable and that she noticed swollen glands on the left side of his neck. After examination a diagnosis of otitis media is made and antibiotic eardrops ordered. Questions 46 through 51 refer to this situation.

46 To teach the correct way to administer eardrops to a small child, the nurse should instruct the parent to position the child on the right side and instill the drops while pulling the auricle:
1. Straight back
2. Up and back
3. Forward
4. Down and back

47 Physiologically the middle ear (containing the 3 ossicles) serves primarily to:
1. Communicate with the throat via the eustachian tube
2. Amplify the energy of sound waves entering the ear

3. Translate sound waves into nerve impulses
4. Maintain balance

48 Tommy's condition does not improve, and he is admitted for a myringotomy. Postoperatively the nurse would expect Tommy to have:
1. Symptoms of central nervous system irritation
2. Difficulty voiding and slight hematuria
3. Irrigations to the lacrimal glands
4. Purulent drainage into the external auditory canal

49 When Tommy is ill and has temporary dietary restrictions, the best way for the nurse to avoid future feeding problems is to have the restrictions:
1. Limited to foods that are not essential
2. Be administered by someone other than parents
3. Explained to the child by the dietitian
4. Handled in a matter-of-fact way

50 Before discharge, while his mother is talking to the nurse about his care at home, Tommy joins the other children in the playroom. You would expect him to engage in:
1. Parallel play
2. Competitive play
3. Solitary play
4. Tumbling-type play

51 While successfully learning autonomy and independence, Tommy would be learning:
1. Trust and security
2. Roles within society
3. Superego control
4. To accept external limits

Situation: May Ann Lewis, age 18, is admitted to the Mental Health Unit of the general hospital. She has always been a shy, inroverted person, but within the past few days she has retreated into a world of fantasy. She makes up her own vocabulary and talks to an imaginary person. She has taken to wearing several sets of clothing at the same time and has made up her face like a clown. The day of admission she retreats to her room, telling the family that she is wired to the television, which informed her that the family was out to kill her. Questions 52 through 59 refer to this situation.

52 Which initial action by the admitting nurse would be most therapeutic for May Ann?
1. Taking her to the day room and introducing her to the other patients
2. Telling her that the door is locked and no one can harm her here
3. Reassuring her that she will not be frightened here, away from her family

4. Introducing her to the primary nurse who will be working with her

53 When May Ann says ''My lacket hss kelong mon,'' the nurse should respond by:
1. Trying to learn the language of the patient
2. Telling the patient she is not understood
3. Communicating in simple terms directed toward the patient
4. Recognizing that the patient needs a nurse who can understand her fantasies

54 May Ann, unprovoked, attacks another patient. A short-term goal for her would be to:
1. Protect others from her impulsive acts by secluding her
2. Keep her actively participating and in contact with reality
3. Have a staff member whom she trusts stay with her
4. Get May Ann to apologize for her behavior

55 May Ann tells you the voices have told her she is no good. She asks if you have also heard the voices. Which response is most appropriate?
1. ''No, I do not hear your voices, but I believe you can hear them.''
2. ''The voices are coming from within you and only you can hear them.''
3. ''This is a voice of your conscience, which only you can control.''
4. ''Oh, the voices are a symptom of your illness; don't pay attention to them.''

56 May Ann holds herself aloof; she ridicules and is sarcastic to other patients. She identifies with the staff. The nursing care goal at this time should be to:
1. Assign activities with the staff only
2. Accept the negative emotions; praise the positive ones
3. Explain that she should be more accepting of others
4. Encourage group participation with withdrawn patients

57 The physician has ordered chlorpromazine (Thorazine), 300 mg po tid. Which of the following nursing actions can alleviate the side effect May Ann might experience the first week she takes the drug?
1. Have her increase her fluid intake
2. Take her blood pressure before giving the drug
3. Give her coffee with the medication and meals
4. Give her benztropine (Cogentin) with the medication

58 The major reason for treating psychoses with tranquilizers is to:
1. Make the patient more amenable to psychotherapy
2. Prevent destructivness by the patient
3. Reduce the neurotic symptoms
4. Prevent secondary complications

59 May Ann is much improved and, with a group of other patients, is preparing for a social evening in town. They are to go with a staff member. The purpose of visits into the community under the supervision of a professional is to:
1. Assist patients in adjusting to anxieties in the community
2. Observe a patient's ability to cope with a more complex society
3. Help the patient return to reality under controlled conditions
4. Broaden the patients' experiences by providing exposure to cultural activities

Situation: As a result of an industrial accident, Mr. Jones has suffered second- and third-degree burns on his left leg, left arm, and face. Questions 60 through 66 refer to this situation.

60 Burns classified as third degree involve destruction of the:
1. Epidermis layer
2. Subcutaneous tissue
3. Dermis
4. Fatty layer

61 What percent of Mr. Jones' total skin surface has been burned?
1. 18%
2. 27%
3. 36%
4. 45%

62 The major objective during the early postburn phase is to:
1. Prevent infection
2. Replace blood loss
3. Restore fluid volume
4. Relieve pain

63 One difficult problem for the nurse to deal with concerning a recently admitted burned patient is:
1. Severe pain
2. Alteration in body image
3. Frequent dressing changes
4. Maintenance of sterility

64 In assessing Mr. Jones for respiratory involvement during the first 2 days, the nurse should interpret which of the following observations as indicative of this complication? Sputum that is:
1. Frothy
2. Sooty
3. Yellow
4. Tenacious

65 The nurse should assess the patient for symptoms of hypovolemic shock, which is often associated with burns because of:
1. Sodium retention as a result of the aldosterone mechanism
2. Decreased rate of glomerular filtration
3. A shift of proteins and water out of intravascular compartment
4. Excessive blood loss through the burned tissues

66 An individual with serious burns requires frequent checks of potassium levels because:
1. Damaged cells absorb potassium, causing hyperkalemia
2. Burned individuals excrete excessive potassium, resulting in hypokalemia
3. Damaged cells release potassium, causing hyperkalemia
4. Potassium loss from damaged skin may cause hypokalemia

Situation: Mr. Smith, 55, has had difficulty sleeping and eating. He has lost a great deal of time from work because he "wasn't feeing well." Lately he has just sat in his room staring at the floor with a sad look on his face. His one wish is that he would die. Questions 67 through 74 refer to this situation.

67 Mr. Smith is brought to the general hospital after taking an overdose of phenobarbital. After a gavage, Mr. Smith states, "Let me die, I'm no good." The nurse's most appropriate response would be:
1. "Of course you're good, we'll take care of you."
2. "You must have been upset to try to take your life."
3. "Do you feel like telling me why you did this?"
4. "You have been through a rough time; let me take care of you."

68 Mr. Smith has been placed on suicide precautions. A therapeutic community would provide these precautions by:
1. Removing all "cutting" objects
2. Not allowing him to leave his room
3. Giving him an opportunity to ventilate his feelings

4. Assigning a staff member to be with him at all times

69 Mr. Smith is to receive a series of electroconvulsive therapy (ECT). The nurse, in explaining this procedure to the patient, should emphasize that:
1. He will have amnesia afterward
2. The treatments will make him better
3. Someone will be with him all the time
4. He should not be afraid; it will not hurt

70 One of the side effects of ECT that Mr. Smith may experience is:
1. Loss of appetite
2. Postural hypotension
3. Confusion for a time after treatment
4. Complete loss of memory for a time

71 Mr. Smith is given a muscle relaxant just before the ECT. The major disadvantage of this drug is that it inhibits which muscles?
1. Intercostal and diaphragmatic
2. Biceps and triceps
3. Facial and thoracic
4. Sternocleidomastoid and abdominal

72 Which of the following aspects of ECT can result in the most serious complication?
1. Thiopental sodium (Pentothal) to induce sleep
2. Succinylcholine to relax muscles
3. Positive pressure to inflate alveoli
4. Electric voltage to induce convulsions

73 A treatment program is planned for Mr. Smith. The staff set specific goals directed toward helping the patient:
1. Develop trust in others
2. Express his hostile feelings
3. Set realistic life goals
4. Get involved in activities

74 Which of the following activities would be least helpful to a severely depressed patient such as Mr. Smith:
1. Allowing the patient to plan own projects
2. Specific simple instructions to be followed
3. Simple, easily completed short-term projects
4. Monotonous, repetitive projects and activities

Situation: Mr. Sill, age 45, who has smoked 3 to 4 packs of cigarettes per day for the last 25 years, was treated with irradiation of his larynx 3 months ago for squamous cell carcinoma. For the past 2 weeks he has noted recurrent hoarseness that has progressively worsened. He now enters the hospital for evaluation and further therapy. He plays the harmonica professionally. Except for findings of hoarseness and a small mass in the left vocal cord, the remainder of his physical examination is unremarkable. Total laryngectomy with block dissection of the cervical lymph nodes is performed after appropriate diagnostic studies and preparation for surgery have been carried out. Mr. Sill is discharged 14 days after surgery. Questions 75 through 81 refer to this situation.

75 An important aspect of preoperative nursing care includes:
1. Adequate explanation of the nature of the surgery to be performed
2. Instruction in breathing exercises and/or equipment used postoperatively to prevent complications
3. Basing instruction on those areas which Mr. Sill questions
4. Having a speech therapist visit Mr. Sill

76 Among neoplasms of the head and neck, cancer of the larynx is a major concern. Which factor would *not* predispose an individual to this disorder?
1. Heavy alcohol ingestion
2. Poor dental hygiene
3. Air pollution
4. Chronic respiratory infections

77 Immediate postoperative management for Mr. Sill would *not* include:
1. Placing the patient in a high semi-Fowler's position
2. Removing the outer tracheostomy tube prn
3. Application of suction to the tracheostomy tube at least every 10 or 15 minutes
4. Instructing the patient not to talk

78 Mr. Sill asks how long he will have to be fed through a tube. The nurse should explain that nasogastric feedings will be required:
1. For the rest of Mr. Sill's life
2. Until healing has occurred
3. Until Mr. Sill develops the ability to belch
4. Until Mr. Sill can tolerate oral feedings

79 Mr. Sill's initial feedings are by nasogastric tube. Soon afterward he begins to develop diarrhea. A possible solution to this problem would be to:
1. Increase the carbohydrate content of the formula to give it more energy value
2. Decrease the protein content to make it easier to digest
3. Dilute the formula with water to give it more volume
4. Decrease the carbohydrate content of the formula and give it more slowly

80 On the day Mr. Sill is being discharged he exhibits concern about the possibility of his laryngectomy tube becoming dislodged. The nurse should teach him to:
1. Notify the physician at once
2. Keep calm, since there is no immediate emergency
3. Recognize that prompt closure of the tracheal opening may occur
4. Reinsert another tube immediately

81 Since Mr. Sill's tracheostomy is permanent, which of the following factors should be included in the teaching plan?
1. The sterile technique necessary for care of his tracheostomy tube
2. The establishment of a regular pattern for suctioning the tube
3. The importance of cleanliness around the site
4. The importance of covering the tube opening while bathing and swimming

---

Situation: Ten-year-old Marc has rheumatoid arthritis. His joints are enlarged, and he has a low-grade fever with an erythematous rash on his trunk. Questions 82 through 85 refer to this situation.

82 When planning nursing care for Marc, the nurse should know that he will most often have pain and limited movement of his joints:
1. When the latex fixation test is positive
2. When the room is cool
3. In the morning on awakening
4. After assistive exercise

83 A major difference between juvenile rheumatoid arthritis and the polyarthritis of rheumatic fever is that with rheumatoid arthritis there may be:
1. Some permanent cardiac damage
2. An exacerbation during the winter months
3. Some residual joint deformity
4. A link with the *Streptococcus* organism

84 In a patient receiving prolonged aspirin therapy, the nurse should be alert for symptoms of:
1. Urinary calculi
2. Prolonged clotting time
3. Atrophy of the liver
4. Premature erythrocyte destruction

85 When 10-year-old Marc is able to move to a two-bed room, the best suited roommate would be:
1. An 11-year-old boy with an appendectomy
2. A 10-year-old girl with a fractured femur
3. A 9-year-old boy with asthma
4. A 12-year-old girl with colitis

Situation: Mr. Leonard is an alcoholic and has cirrhosis of the liver. Questions 86 through 92 refer to this situation.

86 Mr. Leonard is brought to the emergency room in the midst of protracted clonic convulsions. He is given diazepam (Valium), which decreases central neuronal activity and:
1. Dilates the tracheobronchial structures
2. Relaxes peripheral muscles
3. Slows cardiac contraction
4. Provides amnesia for the convulsive episode

87 Mr. Leonard's serum albumin level is low, and the physician prescribes 50 ml of salt-poor albumin IV. Albumin replacement is expected to:
1. Decrease tissue fluid accumulation and decrease the hematocrit level
2. Decrease ascites and the blood ammonia level
3. Increase capillary perfusion and decrease the blood pressure level
4. Decrease venous stasis and the blood urea nitrogen level

88 While Mr. Leonard is receiving the albumin, the planned therapeutic effect will be greater if the infusion is regulated to run:
1. Slowly, and fluid intake is restricted
2. Rapidly, and fluids are encouraged
3. Slowly, and fluids are encouraged liberally
4. Rapidly, and fluid intake is withheld

89 Mr. Leonard is having delirium tremens and is given paraldehyde (Paral) IM. Elimination of the drug can be assessed by monitoring:
1. Urination
2. Salivation
3. Diaphoresis
4. Breathing

90 Mr. Leonard is receiving neomycin sulfate (Mycifradin) orally. The purpose for administration of the drug is to:
1. Protect against infection while immune mechanisms are deficient
2. Suppress ammonia-forming bacteria in the intestinal tract
3. Increase urea digestive activity of enteric bacteria
4. Protect regenerative nodules in the liver from invading bacteria

91 Immediately before an abdominal paracentesis, the nurse should ask the patient to void because:

1. A urine specimen must be obtained at this time to check level of nonprotein nitrogen
2. A full bladder increases the danger of puncture of the bladder
3. An empty bladder will decrease the intra-abdominal pressure
4. A full bladder decreases the amount of fluid in the abdominal cavity

92 Mr. Leonard, participating in an alcohol abstinence program, has a cold when he comes to the clinic. He tells the nurse he plans to use elixir of terpin hydrate for his cough. The nurse would advise him not to take it while he is taking disulfiram (Antabuse) because it will cause:
1. Abdominal cramps and muscle twitching
2. Epigastric pain and headache
3. Jitteriness and nausea
4. Dizziness and violent vomiting

Situation: Jane Bond, a 15-year-old girl, is brought into the emergency room after being found unconscious in the locker room at school. There is a strong odor of acetone to her breath and her face is flushed. Questions 93 through 99 refer to this situation.

93 After developing a relationship with the nurse, Jane tells her that she has not been adhering to her diabetic regimen. As a first step in attempting to help Jane develop some understanding of the importance of a diabetic regimen, the nurse should:
1. Give her printed material about diabetes in teenagers
2. Impress on the parents that it is their responsibility to help and understand Jane
3. Allow Jane to express her feelings about diabetes
4. Assume that Jane has not been properly taught previously

94 When teaching Jane about diabetes and giving herself insulin, the first step for the nurse should be to:
1. Begin the teaching program at Jane's present level
2. Find out what Jane knows about her health problem
3. Set specific and realistic short- and long-term goals
4. Collect all the equipment needed to demonstrate giving an injection

95 Jane exhibits a need for cognitive learning when she asks:

1. "What is diabetes?"
2. "How do I give myself an injection?"
3. "When do I test my urine for S and A?"
4. "Can I still be a cheerleader?"

96 After initial treatment to correct the acidosis, Jane is moved to the medical ward. Her height and weight are average (5 feet 3 inches, 114 pounds), and the diet ordered for her is 2200 calories, 75 g protein, 250 g carbohydrate, and 100 g fat. She is receiving NPH insulin mixed with regular insulin, according to need. In planning a menu for a juvenile diabetic such as Jane, the nurse considers a meal pattern that:
1. Limits calories to encourage weight loss
2. Allows for normal growth and developmental needs
3. Avoids using potatoes, bread, and cereal
4. Discourages substitutions on the menu pattern

97 The nurse instructs Jane and her parents to:
1. Weigh all her food on a gram scale
2. Eat all her meals at home
3. Prepare her food separately from that of the rest of the family
4. Always carry some form of sugar with her

98 The nurse plans an evening snack including milk, crackers, and cheese to provide:
1. High-carbohydrate nourishment for immediate use
2. Nourishment with latent effects to counteract late insulin activity
3. Encouragment for her to stay on her diet
4. Added calories to help her gain weight

99 A week after the nurse speaks with Jane, Mrs. Bond, whose sister died of diabetes, asks the nurse for information about the disease. The nurse should recognize that Mrs. Bond is:
1. Too upset to learn new information
2. Transferring attitudes about her sister to her daughter
3. Exhibiting readiness for learning
4. Expressing her attitudes through her behavior

Situation: Mr. Ray is admitted to the surgical unit with a diagnosis of cancer of the colon. His physician plans to do a colon resection with a permanent colostomy. During the 3 days prior to surgery, Mr. Ray is very cooperative in all preoperative procedures, responds pleasantly when approached by the nurses, and does not question staff about what is being done to him. Questions 100 through 106 refer to this situation.

100 From his behavior, the nurse recognizes that Mr. Ray most likely:
1. Is totally denying his illness
2. Has been fully informed by his physician about what to expect
3. Is not verbalizing his feelings about what will happen to him
4. Feels reassured by his frequent contacts with the nurses

101 The night before Mr. Ray's surgery the nurse notices that each time she makes rounds he is awake, despite adequate sedation. He has no requests but invites her to have a cigarette with him. Based on her understanding of Mr. Ray's behavior, the nurse's response should be to:
1. Send in a nurse's aide to keep him company while he smokes
2. Point out to him that nurses cannot smoke in patients' rooms
3. Light his cigarette and tell him to call her again if he still can't sleep
4. Light his cigarette and indicate she has noticed his inability to sleep

102 During the rehabilitation period, when discussing with Mr. Ray the regaining of some measure of bowel control, the nurse should emphasize:
1. Having a set time each day for his colostomy irrigation
2. The importance of a soft low-residue diet
3. The importance of managing his fluid intake
4. The necessity for a high-protein diet

103 After surgery the most effective way of helping Mr. Ray accept his colostomy would be to:
1. Give him literature containing factual data about colostomies
2. Point out to him the number of important people who have had colostomies
3. Begin to teach him self-care of his colostomy immediately
4. Contact a member of Colostomies, Inc. to speak with him

104 During a colostomy irrigation, if Mr. Ray complains of abdominal cramps, the nurse should:
1. Raise the irrigating can so that the irrigation can be completed quickly
2. Reassure Mr. Ray and continue the irrigation
3. Pinch the tubing so that less fluid enters the colon
4. Clamp the tubing and allow Mr. Ray to rest

105 Mr. Ray's colostomy is located on the left side of the abdomen. What type of stools would the nurse expect Mr. Ray to expel?
1. Moist, formed
2. Pencil shaped
3. Liquid
4. Mucus coated

106 Mr. Ray's postoperative diet order reads "diet as tolerated." Principles that should guide food choices include:
1. A low-residue diet should be followed indefinitely to avoid overstimulating the intestine
2. A return to a regular diet as soon as possible gives psychologic support and more rapid physical rehabilitation
3. Many foods will cause all individuals with colostomies the same discomfort
4. More rigid dietary rules limiting food choices are needed to provide security

Situation: Mr. Gold, a 42-year-old insurance broker, is admitted to the hospital with a diagnosis of coronary occlusion and is experiencing pain and distress. Questions 107 through 114 refer to this situation.

107 The nurse realizes that the pain associated with coronary occlusion is caused primarily by:
1. Arterial spasm
2. Irritation of nerve endings in the cardiac plexus
3. Ischemia of the heart muscle
4. Blocking of the coronary veins

108 On Mr. Gold's admission the nurse immediately gives him oxygen to:
1. Prevent dyspnea
2. Prevent cyanosis
3. Increase oxygen concentration to heart cells
4. Increase oxygen tension in the circulating blood

109 During the acute period of Mr. Gold's illness the nurse should make the bed by:
1. Changing the top linen and only the necessary bottom linen
2. Changing the linen from top to bottom without lowering the head of the bed
3. Sliding him onto a stretcher, remaking the bed, then sliding him back to the bed
4. Lifting rather than rolling him from side to side while changing the linen

110 Mr. Gold's orders include strict bed rest and a clear liquid diet. The nurse should explain to the patient that the primary reason for this diet is to reduce:

1. Gastric acidity
2. The metabolic work load associated with digestion
3. His weight
4. The amount of fecal elimination

111 Two days after admission Mr. Gold develops a temperature of 38.3° C (101° F). The nurse should realize that this elevation indicates:
1. Possible infection
2. Tissue necrosis
3. Pulmonary infarction
4. Pneumonia

112 In creating a therapeutic environment for Mr. Gold the nurse should provide for:
1. Daily papers in the morning
2. Telephone communication
3. Short family visits
4. Television for short periods

113 The monitor shows a PQRST wave for each beat and indicates a rate of 120. The rhythm is regular. The nurse should note that the patient is experiencing:
1. Atrial fibrillation
2. Ventricular fibrillation
3. Sinus tachycardia
4. First-degree heart block

114 Mr. Gold complains of severe nausea, and his heartbeat is irregular and slow. The nurse should recognize these symptoms as toxic effects of:
1. Lanoxin
2. Lidocaine
3. Morphine sulfate
4. Meperidine hydrochloride

Situation: Johnny has been attending a day care center for autistic children. Questions 115 through 120 refer to this situation.

115 Autism can usually be diagnosed when the child is about:
1. 6 months of age
2. 1 to 3 months of age
3. 2 years of age
4. 6 years of age

116 In planning activities for Johnny the nurse must remember that autistic children respond best to:
1. Loud cheerful music
2. Own self-stimulating acts
3. Individuals in small groups
4. Large group activity

117 Since autistic children withdraw into their own world, relationships are difficult to establish. The nurse may be able to reach Johnny by:
1. Body contact, such as cuddling
2. Encouraging his participation in group activities
3. Imitating and participating in his activities
4. Providing a quiet, safe place for rocking

118 The nurse would expect Johnny to demonstrate:
1. Sad, blank facial expressions
2. Flapping of hands and rocking
3. Inappropriate smiling with flat emotions
4. Lack of response to any stimulus

119 When using play as therapy with Johnny the nurse should:
1. Play music and dance with Johnny
2. Provide mechanical and inanimate objects for him to play with
3. Talk with Johnny while touching his hands
4. Provide brightly colored toys and blocks that he can handle

120 Given a choice, the autistic child would usually enjoy playing with a:
1. Cuddly toy
2. Large red block
3. Small yellow block
4. Playground merry-go-round

COMPREHENSIVE TEST 2

TO SIMULATE THE COMPREHENSIVE STATE BOARD EXAMINATION YOU SHOULD COMPLETE THIS TEST WITHIN TWO HOURS.

Situation: Mrs. Wyer, 21 years old, is 6 months pregnant with her second child and is being visited at home by a community health nurse as part of her prenatal care. Her first child is 15 months old. While in the kitchen with Mrs. Wyer, the nurse notes that her lunch includes salami, cheese, and a cola drink. During assessment the nurse notes increased edema in Mrs. Wyer's ankles. Questions 1 through 13 refer to this situation.

1 Besides advising rest with legs elevated, the nurse discusses the foods Mrs. Wyer has been eating and gives instructions concerning her diet. In this instance:
   1. Dietary preferences must influence the food that is eaten
   2. The food selected should have a low salt content
   3. The nutritionist should be brought in to plan a diet
   4. The patient should be advised to attend the prenatal clinic to see the physician

2 Mrs. Wyer complains of constipation. The nurse should explain that constipation frequently occurs during pregnancy due to:
   1. Pressure of the growing uterus on the anus
   2. Increased intake of milk as recommended during pregnancy
   3. The slowing of peristalsis in the gastrointestinal tract
   4. Changes in the metabolic rate

3 Mrs. Wyer begins labor close to her expected date of delivery and is admitted to the hospital. The nurse notices a gush of fluid from the vagina of the patient. After checking the fetal heart rate the nurse should:
   1. Notify the physician immediately about the gush of fluid from the vagina
   2. Place the patient in modified lithotomy position and inspect the perineum
   3. Keep the patient flat in bed and elevate the legs
   4. Place the patient on her side and take the blood pressure

4 After several hours of labor the physician orders oxytocin (Pitocin). When a patient in labor is being infused with oxytocin, it is the nurse's responsibility to:
   1. Obtain a physician's order to slow the IV in the presence of hypertonic contractions
   2. Flush the IV tubing if the flow slows
   3. Shut off the IV in the presence of hypertonic contractions
   4. Monitor fetal heart tones every 2 hours

5 The nurse knows that Mrs. Wyer has begun the transitional phase of labor when she:
   1. Complains of pains in the back
   2. States the pain has lessened
   3. Perspires and her face flushes
   4. Assumes the lithotomy position

6 Shortly following delivery Mrs. Wyer says she feels as if she is bleeding. On checking the fundus the nurse finds a steady trickling of blood from the vagina. The first action should be to:
   1. Call the physician immediately
   2. Hold the fundus firmly and gently massage it

3. Check Mrs. Wyer's blood pressure and pulse
4. Take no action, since this is a common occurrence

7 The nurse, while checking Mrs. Wyer's fundus 2 days postpartum, observes that it is at the umbilicus and displaced to the right, the nurse recognizes that the patient probably has:
1. A full, overdistended bladder
2. Overstretched uterine ligaments
3. A slow rate of involution
4. Retained placental fragments

8 Mrs. Wyer is discharged 5 days after delivery and is referred for home care follow-up. The initial visit to Mrs. Wyer will be more productive if scheduled when:
1. The nurse has more time to expend
2. She is feeding the children
3. Her husband is at work
4. It is convenient for the family

9 The role most likely to foster sound interpersonal relationships during the first visit to the Wyer home is that of:
1. Stranger
2. Teacher
3. Counselor
4. Surrogate

10 When the nurse first talks with Mrs. Wyer, the type of interview that is likely to be most productive is:
1. Information-giving
2. Problem-solving
3. Exploratory
4. Directive

11 On arrival for the first visit at 10 A.M., the nurse finds Mr. Wyer at home. He is temporarily collecting unemployment benefits, and the family is on welfare. Mrs. Wyer is worried and ill at ease in the situation. The infant is due for bottle-feeding and the toddler is playing on the floor. At this time the nurse's best action would be to ask Mr. Wyer if he would mind:
1. Giving the baby a bottle
2. Taking the toddler for a walk
3. Leaving you and Mrs. Wyer alone
4. Participating in the discussion

12 The 15-month-old child has had no inoculations. Mr. Wyer says he does not believe in them. The nurse's best choice of response to this statement would be:
1. "Scientific evidence proves you wrong."

2. "Have you discussed this with a doctor?"
3. "How can you risk the life of your child?"
4. "You feel they may be harmful?"

13 Following discussion with the nurse, Mr. and Mrs. Wyer agree to have their 15-month-old immunized. The initial immunizations on the first visit to the health clinic are:
1. Diphtheria and tetanus toxoids (DTP) and trivalent oral poliovirus vaccine (TOPV)
2. Measles, rubella, and mumps combined vaccines
3. Diphtheria and tetanus toxoids (DTP), trivalent oral poliovirus vaccine, and tuberculin test
4. Combined tetanus and diphtheria toxoid (Td), trivalent oral poliovirus vaccine, and tuberculin test

---

Situation: Julie Syms, a 12-month-old girl, is admitted to the hospital with a diagnosis of failure to thrive. Her weight is below the third percentile, her development is retarded, and she shows signs of neglect. Questions 14 through 18 refer to this situation.

14 Based on this assessment, what behaviors might also support the possibility of parental deprivation?
1. Infant is cuddly, responsive to touch, and wants to be held
2. Infant is stiff, unpliable, and uncomforted by touch
3. Infant is a poor eater, sleeps soundly, and is easily satisfied
4. Infant is responsive to adults, rarely cries but shows no interest in her environment

15 A plan of care that would best meet the needs of this child should include:
1. A vigorous schedule of stimulation geared to the infant's present level of development
2. A plan to have all staff members pick her up and play with her whenever they can
3. A schedule of care that allows the infant stimulation and physical contact by several staff members
4. As consistent a caregiver as possible, with stimulation that is moderate and purposeful

16 During the nurse's assessment of Julie, she observes that the child has good head control, can roll over, but cannot sit up without support or transfer an object from one hand to the other. Based on these facts, the nurse concludes that Julie is developmentally at age:
1. 2 to 3 months

2. 3 to 4 months
3. 4 to 6 months
4. 6 to 8 months

17 Which toys would be unsuited for Julie based on her present developmental age?
1. Brightly colored mobiles
2. Soft stuffed animals that she can hold
3. Small rattle that she can hold
4. Snap toys, large snap beads

18 The nurse who has been caring for Julie decides on a plan of care for the mother as well. The main objective is to:
1. Set up a schedule for teaching the mother how to care for her baby
2. Discuss the matter with her in a nonthreatening manner
3. Show by example how to care for the infant and satisfy her needs
4. Supply emotional support to the mother and encourage her dependency

Situation: John Gray, a 21-year-old physical education major in college, sustained a crushing fracture of the third and fourth lumbar vertebrae with severance of the cord while practicing on the trampoline. Three days after the injury the physician explained to him that he was a paraplegic and what this diagnosis entailed. Questions 19 through 30 refer to this situation.

19 The nurse understands that paraplegia involves:
1. Paresis of both lower extremities
2. Paralysis of one side of the body
3. Paralysis of upper and lower extremities
4. Paralysis of both lower extremities

20 When caring for John, the initial responsibility of the nurse is to:
1. Prevent contractures and atrophy
2. Protect the patient from flexion or hyperextension of the spine
3. Prevent urinary tract infections
4. Prepare the patient for vocational rehabilitation

21 Considering the diagnosis, the nurse knows that John must be encouraged to drink a lot of fluids to prevent:
1. Urinary tract infections
2. Fluid and electrolyte imbalance
3. Dehydration
4. Constipation

22 John was placed on a Circ-O-letric bed primarily to:
1. Promote mobility

2. Prevent loss of calcium from long bones
3. Prevent pressure sores
4. Promote orthostatic hypotension

23 Two weeks after the accident John begins vomiting thick coffee-ground material and appears restless and apprehensive. The nurse should:
1. Change the patient's diet to bland
2. Prepare for insertion of a nasogastric tube
3. Check laboratory reports for hemoglobin level
4. Collect stool specimen and check for occult blood

24 While caring for John the nurse would immediately report which of the following observations?
1. Tachycardia, diaphoresis, and cold extremities
2. Complaints of thirst and warm flushed skin
3. Nausea, weakness, and headache
4. Dyspepsia, distention, and diarrhea

25 Perforation has occurred, so a gastrectomy is performed. In the immediate postoperative period John's nasogastric tube is draining a bright red liquid. The nurse should expect this drainage for:
1. 1 to 2 hours
2. 3 to 4 hours
3. 10 to 12 hours
4. 24 to 48 hours

26 John is returned to his room on the second postoperative day. An IV of 1000 ml of 5% glucose in water containing 40 mEq potassium chloride is running. Parenteral preparations of potassium are administered slowly and cautiously to prevent which of the following complications?
1. Acidosis
2. Cardiac arrest
3. Edema of the extremities
4. Psychotic-like reactions

27 John's IV stopped and was restarted by the IV team in his other arm. The nurse coming on duty checked the IV bottle, noting that it was practically full and seemed to be dripping adequately. She did not count the drip rate or check the site of infusion. Later in the morning it was noted that a large infiltrated area had developed, and the needle had to be removed. The area of infiltration became reddened, and ultimately sloughing of tissue occurred. In situations such as this:
1. The staff nurse is not responsible for IVs when the hospital has an IV team
2. The rate of flow should have been regulated and maintained at a slow rate

3. Sloughing of tissue is a frequent complication of IV therapy
4. The rate of flow is unrelated to the problem of infiltration

28 After the nasogastric tube is removed, John is placed on a gradually increasing diet, which he tolerates fairly well. As the diet is increased, John develops the dumping syndrome. Dumping syndrome refers to:
1. Buildup of stool and gas within the large intestine
2. Rapid passage of osmotic fluid into the jejunum
3. Reflux of intestinal contents into the esophagus
4. Nausea due to a full stomach

29 Management of the dumping syndrome is best accomplished by maintaining the patient on:
1. Low-protein, high-carbohydrate diet
2. Low-residue, bland diet
3. Fluid intake below 500 ml
4. Small frequent feedings

30 Three weeks after his injury, John explains to the nurse that he must get out of the hospital soon to practice for the upcoming intercollegiate gymnastic tournament. In light of what the patient is saying, the nurse should realize that John is:
1. No longer able to adapt
2. Extremely motivated to get well
3. Verbalizing a fantasy
4. Exhibiting denial

Situation: Baby Ginger Little is admitted to the newborn nursery. The nurse weighs her and performs a newborn evaluation. Questions 31 through 41 refer to this situation.

31 The most important weak or absent reflex for the nurse to report in her initial evaluation of the newborn is:
1. Moro
2. Tonic neck
3. Gag
4. Babinski

32 Baby Ginger has small whitish, pinpoint spots over her nose, which the nurse knows are caused by retained sebaceous secretions. When charting this observation, the nurse identifies it as:
1. Lanugo
2. Milia
3. Whiteheads
4. Mongolian spots

33 When changing Baby Ginger, the nurse notices a brick red stain on the diaper. The nurse should realize that this is:
1. Common during the first week
2. A symptom of low iron stores
3. Due to medication given to the mother
4. Expected in female babies

34 Three days after birth, Ginger is slightly jaundiced. The nurse knows that this is due primarily to her:
1. Immature liver function
2. Mother's high hemoglobin level
3. High hemoglobin and low hematocrit levels
4. Inability to synthesize bile

35 The physician orders phototherapy. During the therapy the nurse should apply eye patches to Ginger's eyes to:
1. Be sure the eyes are closed
2. Prevent injury to conjunctiva and retina
3. Reduce overstimulation from bright lights
4. Limit excessive rapid eye movements and anxiety

36 At 3 months Ginger is admitted to the hospital because of increasing head size and a possible diagnosis of hydrocephalus. In performing a developmental appraisal, what clue would be most important to the nurse in light of the diagnosis?
1. Absence of Moro, tonic neck, and grasp reflexes
2. Presence of Babinski reflex
3. Head lag
4. Inability to sit unsupported

37 Because of the diagnosis, the nurse is especially alert to signs of increasing intracranial pressure, such as:
1. Bulging fontanel, ''sunset'' eyes, projectile vomiting not associated with feeding
2. Depressed fontanel, bulging eyes, irritability
3. Dilated scalp veins, depressed and sunken eyeballs, decreased blood pressure
4. High shrill cry, decreased skin turgor, elevated fontanels

38 Proper positioning of Ginger is essential to prevent breakdown of the scalp. A suitable position would be:
1. Prone, with legs elevated about 30 degrees
2. Prone or supine, with head elevated about 45 degrees
3. Positioned on either side and flat
4. Supine and Trendelenburg

39 Hydrocephalus, if untreated, can cause mental retardation because:
1. Hypertonic CSF disturbs normal plasma concentration, depriving nerve cells of vital nutrients
2. CSF dilutes blood supply, causing cells to atrophy
3. Increasing head size necessitates more oxygen and nutrients than normal blood flow can supply
4. Gradually increasing size of ventricles presses the brain against the bony cranium; anoxia and decreased blood supply result

40 After several tests have been performed, the diagnosis of noncommunicating hydrocephalus is confirmed and a ventriculoperitoneal shunt is performed. Postoperative care of Ginger includes all the following except:
1. Positioning her flat for about 48 hours
2. Administering sedatives and analgesics to keep her quiet
3. Encouraging the parents not to pick up Ginger even to prevent crying
4. Checking the valve frequently and pumping it as ordered

41 Mr. and Mrs. Little have been very anxious during their child's admission and especially concerned about the prognosis. The nurse should explain that:
1. The prognosis is excellent and the valve is permanent
2. The shunt may need to be revised as the child grows older
3. If any brain damage has occurred, it is reversible during the first year of life
4. Hydrocephalus usually is self-limiting by 2 years of age and then the shunt is removed

---

Situation: Mrs. Hanson is an obese 59-year-old secretary with a long history of asthma dating back to her childhood. She has varicose veins and has been admitted to the hospital for surgery. Questions 42 through 56 refer to this situation.

42 Varicose veins are usually the result of:
1. Atherosclerotic plaques along the veins
2. External compression of the muscles of the legs
3. Defective valves within the veins
4. The formation of thrombophlebitis

43 The nurse should expect Mrs. Hanson to complain of:
1. Continued edema of the affected extremity
2. A positive Homans' sign

3. Coolness and pallor of the affected extremity
4. Cramping sensations in the calf muscle

44 A simple test for varicose veins is the:
1. Trendelenburg test
2. Babinski reflex
3. Romberg's sign
4. Arteriography

45 Mrs. Hanson is going to have a vein ligation and stripping. Prior to performing this surgery, the physician must be certain that:
1. Mrs. Hanson understands the need to lose weight
2. The deep veins of the leg are not occluded
3. The saphenous vein has no sign of aneurysms
4. Mrs. Hanson is aware of the need for several weeks of bed rest

46 The nurse should base her preoperative teaching on the fact that Mrs. Hanson:
1. Can control and limit her asthmatic attacks if she wants
2. Should try to limit coughing, since this causes distention of the chest
3. Can control her anxiety and decrease the severity of postoperative asthma attacks
4. Will be quite prone to other respiratory tract infections

47 When Mrs. Hanson returns from the recovery room, the nurse should position her:
1. Supine with legs elevated 30 degrees
2. Flat with knee gatch engaged
3. In a semi-Fowler's position with knees slightly flexed
4. Head elevated, feet tight against footboard

48 The evening of surgery, after Mrs. Hanson is fully reacted, the nurse should:
1. Apply a binder for support
2. Assist her out of bed to a chair
3. Perform passive range of motion exercises to legs
4. Ambulate her in the room

49 Five days postoperatively Mrs. Hanson develops an acute episode of bronchial asthma. Mrs. Hanson is experiencing difficulty in breathing due to:
1. Spasms of the bronchi, which trap the air
2. A too rapid expulsion of air
3. An increase in the vital capacity of the lungs
4. Hyperventilation due to an anxiety reaction

50 Nursing management of Mrs. Hanson is now directed toward:

1. Raising mucus secretions from the chest
2. Limiting pulmonary secretions by decreasing fluid intake
3. Curing the condition permanently
4. Convincing the patient that her condition is emotionally based

51 The nurse administers aminophylline via suppository to Mrs. Hanson as ordered. The effect of this therapy is:
1. Rest and relaxation
2. Evacuation of lower bowel
3. Relaxation of bronchial muscles
4. Reduction of intestinal bacteria

52 Mrs. Hanson has an IV infusion to keep the vein open for emergency medications. What should the nurse initially do when the IV infusion infiltrates?
1. Attempt to flush the tube
2. Elevate the IV site
3. Discontinue the infusion
4. Apply warm, moist soaks

53 The physician orders daily sputum specimens to be collected from Mrs. Hanson. When is the most appropriate time for the nurse to collect this specimen?
1. On awakening
2. Before meals
3. Before an IPPB treatment
4. After activity

54 The nurse understands that Mrs. Hanson's asthmatic wheeze is thought to be:
1. An impairment of cardiovascular function
2. An unexpressed rejection of independence
3. A dilation of the bronchii
4. An expression of hypochondriasis

55 Mrs. Hanson is found to be allergic to dust. The teaching plan for her should include the fact that:
1. She will probably be unable to do her own housework in the future
2. It is imperative that her entire house be redecorated, since she must live in a dust-free environment
3. Damp-dusting her house will help limit dust particles in the air
4. She may as well accept her condition, since dust cannot be avoided

56 Before discharge Mrs. Hanson is instructed on the use of elastic stockings. Which of the following instructions would be most appropriate concerning the stockings? They should be:

1. Left in place until the physician advises otherwise
2. Worn only at night when she is less active
3. Put on before getting out of bed in the morning
4. Alternately kept on 2 hours and off 2 hours

Situation: Maria Lory, a 12-year-old girl, is admitted to the hospital with the diagnosis of acute lymphocytic leukemia. Questions 57 through 64 refer to this situation.

57 Which signs and symptoms would the nurse consider unusual with this diagnosis?
1. Multiple bruises, petechiae
2. Marked fatigue, pallor
3. Enlarged lymph nodes, spleen, and liver
4. Marked jaundice and generalized edema

58 A pathophysiologic change underlying the production of symptoms in leukemia is:
1. Progressive replacement of bone marrow with fibrous tissue
2. Destruction of red blood cells and platelets by overproduction of white blood cells
3. Proliferation and release of immature white blood cells into the circulating blood
4. Excessive destruction of blood cells in the liver and spleen

59 To induce a remission, Maria is placed on a drug regimen that includes prednisone, vincristine, and L-asparaginase. Which of the following side effects of these drugs requires the greatest preparation of this patient?
1. Constipation
2. Generalized, short-term paralysis
3. Retarded growth in height
4. Alopecia

60 A major objective of nursing care related to Maria's disease and drug regimen is to:
1. Maintain reverse isolation
2. Reduce unnecessary stimuli
3. Check her vital signs every 2 hours
4. Prevent all physical activity

61 Understanding the side effects of vincristine, the nurse prepares a diet for Maria that is:
1. Low in residue with increased fluids
2. High in iron with decreased fluids
3. High in both roughage and fluids
4. Low in fat, and regular fluids

62 Because Maria's platelet count is very low, the nurse plans to observe her urine for the presence of:
1. Erythrocytes

2. Leukocytes
3. Casts
4. Lymphocytes

63 Maria's physician also plans a program of irradiation of the spine and skull. This treatment is used mainly because:
1. Leukemia cells invade the nervous system more slowly, but the usual drugs are ineffective in the brain
2. Radiation will retard growth of cells in bone marrow of the cranium
3. Neoplastic drug therapy without radiation is effective in most cases, but this is a precautionary treatment
4. Radiation will decrease cerebral edema and prevent increased intracranial pressure

64 One day Mr. Lory asks the nurse whether he should tell his son, who is 7 years old, the truth about Maria. The nurse should reply:
1. "A child of his age cannot comprehend the real meaning of death, so don't tell him until the last moment."
2. "Your son probably fears separation most and wants to know that you will care for him, rather than what will happen to his sister."
3. "Your son probably doesn't understand death as we do but fears it just the same. He should be told the truth to let him prepare for his sister's possible death."
4. "Why don't you talk this over with your doctor, who probably knows best what is happening in terms of Maria's prognosis?"

Situation: David King is a 34-year-old sales manager. He frequently experiences weakness and difficulty in moving his right hand. A thorough medical examination reveals no physical pathologic condition. The physician now believes the symptoms are a conversion reaction. Questions 65 through 71 refer to this situation.

65 A conversion reaction is:
1. A psychosomatic reaction to stress
2. An unconscious means to control conflict
3. A psychologic defense against stress
4. A conscious defense against anxiety

66 A person who habitually converts anxiety into physical symptoms is displaying which of the following patterns of behavior?
1. Psychoneurotic
2. Psychosomatic

3. Regressive
4. Projective

67 *Hysterical conversion* is the term used to describe the phenomenon whereby anxiety associated with stress or conflict has been repressed and converted into specific physical manifestations. One of the characteristics of the patient's reaction to the physical symptom is:
1. Agitation
2. Indifference
3. Anger
4. Anxiety

68 The basic difference between psychosomatic illness and hypochondria is that in psychosomatic illness there is:
1. An emotional cause
2. A feeling of illness
3. An actual tissue change
4. A restriction of activities

69 David is scheduled for an occupational therapy group. While listening to instructions for the group project, he experiences the feeling of weakness and is unable to move his right arm. After a check of pulse and respirations, the nurse's best response should be:
1. "Exactly when did the weakness begin?"
2. "Is this similar to what you usually experience?"
3. "What emotion were you feeling before you felt the weakness?"
4. "Would you like to leave the group for a while?"

70 The occurrence of this pattern of behavior can be reduced if the nurse:
1. Decreases anxiety by limiting discussion of problems with the patient
2. Provides patient teaching regarding medical care
3. Teaches the family how to decrease stress at home
4. Assists the patient in developing altered life patterns

71 During group therapy other members accuse David of intellectualizing and avoiding his feelings. He asks the nurse if she agrees with the others. The nurse's best answer would be:
1. "It seems that way to me, too."
2. "I'd rather not give my personal opinion."
3. "What is your perception of my behavior?"
4. "You seem to need my opinion."

Situation: Mr. Dime, age 39, a single, executive producer for one of the major television networks was in a serious auto accident. He is admitted with multiple fractures and deep lacerations with hemorrhage. When admitted he is in severe shock and is rushed to the operating room. He is given a blood transfusion that proves incompatible with his blood type. Questions 72 through 83 refer to this situation.

72 The initial sign of such a transfusion reaction, which the nurse should observe for, is:
1. Dyspnea
2. Backache
3. Cyanosis
4. Shock

73 As a result of this transfusion reaction, Mr. Dime suffers kidney damage. In determining kidney damage, the most significant clinical response that the nurse should assess is:
1. Acute pain over kidney area
2. Decreased urinary output
3. Hematuria
4. Polyuria

74 Although Mr. Dime does not request an analgesic, the nurse should be alert for a sign of an involuntary reaction to pain, which is:
1. Perspiration
2. Crying
3. Pulling knees up to abdomen
4. Grimacing

75 Mr. Dime's kidney function has not returned and is currently about 10% of normal. Peritoneal dialysis is ordered when his BUN begins to rise. Peritoneal dialysis once instituted:
1. Is largely a nursing responsibility
2. May be maintained from 12 to 48 hours
3. Requires checking of vital signs every 15 minutes
4. Should be discontinued if patient complains of abdominal pain

76 The purpose of peritoneal dialysis is to:
1. Reestablish kidney function
2. Clean the peritoneal membrane
3. Remove toxins and metabolic wastes
4. Provide fluid for intracellular spaces

77 Mr. Dime complains of nausea, pain in the abdomen, diarrhea, and muscular weakness. The nurse notes an irregularity in pulse and signs of pulmonary edema. These are probably manifestations of:
1. Calcium deficiency

2. Calcium excess
3. Sodium deficiency
4. Potassium excess

78 Between dialysis treatments, Mr. Dime is maintained on a modified Giordano-Giovannetti diet. Which of the following statements is not true of this dietary regimen?
1. Protein is low, which causes the body to use excess urea nitrogen to synthesize necessary amino acids for tissue protein synthesis
2. Potassium is high to replace losses
3. Sodium is allowed according to need
4. Calories are allowed as needed within designated food lists

79 In caring for Mr. Dime when he is being dialyzed, the nurse should:
1. Maintain the patient in a flat, supine position during the entire procedure
2. Notify the physician if there is a deficit of 200 ml in the drainage fluid
3. Apply firm manual pressure on the lower abdomen if fluid is not draining properly
4. Remove the cannula at the end of the procedure and apply a dry, sterile dressing

80 If Mr. Dime is observed to have severe respiratory difficulty, the most immediate nursing action would be to:
1. Change the patient's position
2. Drain fluid from the peritoneal cavity
3. Notify the physician
4. Discontinue the treatment

81 Mr. Dime has been immobilized in traction for 3 weeks. The nurse realizes that he may develop renal calculi as a complication because:
1. He has more difficulty urinating in a supine position
2. His dietary patterns have changed
3. Lack of muscle action and normal tension cause calcium withdrawal from the bone
4. Fracture healing requires more calcium and thus increases total calcium metabolism

82 Mr. Dime's leg is set in a long leg cast. The nurse should observe for which of the following signs that indicates compromised circulation in a patient with a long leg cast?
1. Foul odor
2. Swelling of toes
3. Increased temperature
4. Drainage on cast

83 Mr. Dime is waiting for a renal transplant. In teaching Mr. Dime, the nurse informs him that:
1. He will require immunosuppressive drugs daily for the rest of his life
2. He will be unable to follow a full program of work and recreation, including sports
3. Symptoms of rejection include fever, proteinuria, hypotension, and edema
4. Urine production will be delayed after surgery

Situation: Mrs. Loft, 42 years of age, is admitted to the hospital with a tentative diagnosis of chronic adrenal insufficiency. Questions 84 through 91 refer to this situation.

84 A room assignment contraindicated for Mrs. Loft would be one:
1. With an elderly CVA patient
2. With a middle-aged woman with pneumonia
3. That is private and away from the nurses' station
4. Next to a 17-year-old girl with a fractured leg

85 Mrs. Loft complains of weakness and dizziness on arising from bed in the morning. The nurse realizes that this is most probably caused by:
1. Postural hypertension
2. A hypoglycemic reaction
3. A lack of potassium
4. Increased extracellular fluid volume

86 After a Thorn test shows an increased eosinophil count, Mrs. Loft is advised that she has Addison's disease. It is most important that the nurse discuss with her the need for:
1. Frequent visits to the physician
2. Restriction of physical activity
3. A special low-salt diet
4. Hormone replacement therapy

87 In teaching Mrs. Loft about her diet, the nurse should tell her to:
1. Add a little extra salt to her food
2. Limit intake to 1200 calories
3. Omit protein foods at each meal
4. Restrict her daily intake of fluids

88 In the event Mrs. Loft neglects to continue the hormone therapy, an adrenal crisis may occur. Usually the predominant symptom is:
1. Hypertension
2. A high body temperature
3. Muscle spasms
4. Diarrhea

89 Patients on prolonged cortisone therapy may ex-
hibit adaptations caused by its glucocorticoid and mineralocorticoid actions. The nurse should teach Mrs. Loft and her family to observe for:
1. Hypoglycemia and anuria
2. Weight gain and moon face
3. Anorexia and hyperkalemia
4. Hypotension and fluid loss

90 When Mrs. Loft shows concern about the fact that she is developing signs of masculinity, the nurse should tell her:
1. It is a further sign of the illness
2. That this is due to the therapy
3. Not to worry, since it will disappear with therapy
4. That this is not important, so long as she gets better

91 In observing Mrs. Loft for cortisone overdose, the nurse should be particularly alert for:
1. Behavioral changes
2. Severe anorexia
3. Hypoglycemia
4. Anaphylactic shock

Situation: Gail, 17, has a history of being a loner. She made excellent grades in school, but often her thinking was highly symbolic. During her senior year in high school she refused to get out of bed, there was a loss of appetite, and she displayed disorganized speech. She was hospitalized at one of the community hospitals. Questions 92 through 99 refer to this situation.

92 One of the primary goals in providing a therapeutic environment for Gail is to:
1. Get her involved in a group with her peers
2. Remove her from the home
3. Foster a trusting relationship
4. Give her medication on time

93 While in the hospital Gail still refuses to get out of bed and becomes very hostile with the staff when approached. The most immediate therapeutic nursing approach would be:
1. Require that Gail get out of bed at once
2. Stay with her until she calms down
3. Give her the prn tranquilizer that is ordered
4. Allow her to stay in bed for now but leave her alone

94 Gail sits huddled in a chair and seldom leaves it. She occasionally lets out a scream and runs to the end of the hallway and crouches in a corner. The nurse realizes that this type of behavior is classified as:

1. Reactive
2. Regressive
3. Involutional
4. Paranoid

95 To begin to establish a therapeutic relationship with Gail, the nurse must:
1. Obtain a complete history from her family
2. Ascertain what topics are of interest to her
3. Protect her from herself
4. Plan to keep her anxiety at a minimum

96 The priority goal is for Gail to develop:
1. A sense of identity
2. Ego strengths
3. Trust
4. An ability to socialize

97 Gail is taking chlorpromazine (Thorazine), 2000 mg, every day. She comes to the nurse complaining that her fingers are twitching.
The best reply would be:
1. ''This is a temporary situation until your body adjusts to the medication.''
2. ''I will get the doctor to order a medication that will help overcome this. It is a side effect of the drug you are taking.''
3. ''You need the medication that we are giving you. You will soon get used to the side effects.''
4. ''Let's wait a few days and see whether the side effects of the drug you are taking go away.''

98 Which of the following symptoms would cause the nurse to stop giving chlorpromazine to Gail until further laboratory work was done?
1. Photosensitivity
2. Shuffling gait
3. Yellow sclera
4. Grimacing

99 On being discharged Gail should be encouraged to:
1. Go back to her regular activities
2. Continue in the after-care clinic
3. Call the unit whenever upset
4. Find a group that has similar problems

Situation: Mrs. Sims is returned to her room after a radical neck dissection for a malignant tumor. Questions 100 through 106 refer to this situation.

100 Mrs. Sims has an endotracheal tube still in place. The nurse should:
1. Change the dressing to observe for covert bleeding
2. Irrigate the tube to maintain patency

3. Reposition the endotracheal tube when the gag reflex returns
4. Have a tracheostomy set at the bedside

101 When Mrs. Sims' color improves and she is able to breathe on her own, the anesthesiologist removes the endotracheal tube. That evening the nurse decides Mrs. Sims is showing signs of respiratory embarrassment and notifies the physician immediately. Which of the following signs might the nurse have observed?
1. Decreased pulse and respirations
2. Restlessness and confusion
3. Cyanosis and clubbing of the fingers
4. Anxiety and dilated pupils

102 A tracheostomy is performed and Mrs. Sims is placed on a mechanical ventilator. For a patient on a ventilator, the nurse must be sure to check the cuff of the tracheostomy tube, which:
1. Must be inflated during suctioning
2. Must remain deflated for 10 minutes every hour
3. Should allow only a slight air leak at the height of inspiration
4. Should create a tight seal between the trachea and the tube

103 When doing deep tracheal suction for a patient after a tracheostomy, the nurse should:
1. Be sure the cuff of the tracheostomy is inflated during suctioning
2. Instill acetylcysteine (Mucomyst) into the tracheostomy prior to suctioning to loosen secretions
3. Apply negative pressure as the catheter is being inserted
4. Suction the patient with the head turned to either side

104 When doing tracheostomy care for Mrs. Sims the nurse must:
1. Take pulse and respirations before and after procedure
2. Use gloves during procedure
3. Use Betadine to clean inner cannula when removed
4. Place Mrs. Sims in semi-Fowler's position

105 As a result of the tracheostomy the nurse is aware that which one of the following drugs would be contraindicated for Mrs. Sims?
1. Pyrvinium pamoate (Povan)
2. Atropine
3. Chloral hydrate
4. Nalorphine (Nalline)

106 Mrs. Sims' tracheostomy tube has an inner cannula. In providing tracheostomy care the nurse should remove the inner cannula:
1. And use sterile applicators to cleanse the outer cannula
2. Only after the cuff is deflated
3. And cleanse it with peroxide
4. Only when the obturator is in place

Situation: Mrs. Simon, a 72-year-old with congestive heart failure, is having difficulty breathing as a result of pulmonary edema. She is being treated with digitalis and diuretic therapy and also with a 1-gram sodium diet. Questions 107 through 113 refer to this situation.

107 At 9 P.M. Mrs. Simon asks for a glass of juice. The nurse knows that the only kinds on the ward are pear nectar, apple, and tomato; she should:
1. Explain to Mrs. Simon that she should not have juice between meals, but she will give her a glass of water
2. Ask her which she prefers, the apple juice or the pear nectar
3. Explain to her that the only kind she can have is tomato juice
4. Tell her that she cannot have any kind of juice because she is on a low-sodium diet

108 Mrs. Simon is to receive 0.2 mg of digoxin IM. The ampule is labeled 0.5 mg = 2 ml. How many milliliters should be administered?
1. 8 ml
2. 0.8 ml
3. 1 ml
4. 1.2 ml

109 Mrs. Simon's ankles are swollen on admission. The nurse should:
1. Restrict fluids
2. Elevate the legs
3. Applying elastic bandages
4. Do ROM exercises

110 Assuming all the food involved is cooked without salt, which of the following meal plans would the nurse not order for Mrs. Simon, who is on a 1-gram sodium diet?
1. Baked chicken, boiled potatoes, broccoli, coffee
2. Mixed fruit salad bowl with cottage cheese; crackers, relish dish (celery, carrot, olives, sweet pickles), tea
3. Soft cooked egg, salt free toast, jelly, skim milk
4. Fillet of sole, baked potato, lettuce and tomato salad, fresh fruit cup, milk

111 To help monitor Mrs. Simon's physical status, a central venous catheter is inserted. The nurse can take a correct central venous pressure reading when the water level in the manometer:
1. Drops and then rises
2. Synchronizes with the blood pressure
3. Rises and stops at a specific plateau
4. Fluctuates with respirations

112 Mrs. Simon is receiving hydrochlorothiazide (Diuril) and furosemide (Lasix) to relieve edema. The nurse should observe for evidence of:
1. Excessive loss of potassium ions
2. Elevation of the urine specific gravity
3. Negative nitrogen balance
4. Excessive retention of sodium ions

113 Mrs. Simon will be taking digitalis at home. She asks the nurse why this is necessary. The nurse bases the answer on the fact that digitalis:
1. Slows and strengthens cardiac contraction
2. Lengthens the refractory phase of the cardiac cycle
3. Reduces edema in extracellular spaces
4. Increases ventricular contraction

Situation: Mr. Norman, a husky 6-foot man, 30 years of age, is hospitalized with a diagnosis of manic-depressive psychosis. He is active and sometimes combative. Since his admission he has been alone in a room. A 45-year-old man was admitted and placed in the room with Mr. Norman. Mr. Norman seemed to accept the man in his room. The nurse paid little attention to them for the rest of the afternoon. Questions 114 through 120 refer to this situation.

114 Suddenly a commotion is heard and Mr. Norman is found beating the other patient. Legally:
1. The admitting office should not have put the patient in with Mr. Norman
2. Knowing that Mr. Norman was frequently combative, close observation was indicated
3. Patients who are combative should never be left unsupervised
4. A combative patient like Mr. Norman should have been sedated with tranquilizers

115 Mr. Norman is receiving lithium carbonate. While the patient is on this medication, it is important that the nurse:
1. Restrict the patient's sodium intake
2. Test the patient's urine weekly
3. Withhold other medications for the first week
4. Monitor the patient's blood level regularly

116 While the nurse is talking with Mr. Norman in his room, the patient's conversation becomes embarrassingly vulgar. The nurse should respond to his behavior by:
1. Restricting Mr. Norman's contact with staff until this symptom passes
2. Tactfully teasing him about the use of such vulgarity
3. Asking him to limit his vulgarity and continuing the conversation with him
4. Discreetly refusing to talk to him when he is speaking in this manner

117 Activities that would be most therapeutic for Mr. Norman and that the nurse should encourage include:
1. Carving figures out of wood
2. Sanding and varnishing wooden bookends
3. Stenciling designs on copper sheeting
4. Lacing tooled leather wallets

118 Mr. Norman is noisy, loud, and disruptive. The nurse informs him that, unless he is more quiet, he will be isolated and put in restraints, if necessary. Legally:
1. Restraint of Mr. Norman is justified for his own protection
2. Information given to Mr. Norman is actually a threat
3. Patients like Mr. Norman cannot be expected to give consent
4. Mr. Norman's behavior is to be expected and should be ignored

119 During a period of hyperactivity, Mr. Norman demands to be allowed to go downtown to do his shopping. He has no privileges at the present time. Which of the following responses would be the best response?
1. "I'm sorry, Mr. Norman, you can't go. Let's look through this new catalog."
2. "You cannot leave the ward, Mr. Norman."
3. "You'll have to ask your doctor, Mr. Norman."
4. "Not right now, Mr. Norman. I don't have a staff member to go with you."

120 One day while the nurse is staying with Mr. Norman, who is shaving, he states, "I have hidden a razor blade and tonight I am going to kill myself." The nurse's best reply is:
1. "You're going to kill yourself?"
2. "You'd better finish shaving, since it's time for lunch."
3. "I'm sure you don't really mean that."
4. "Things can't really be that bad."

COMPREHENSIVE TEST 3

TO SIMULATE THE COMPREHENSIVE STATE BOARD EXAMINATIONS YOU SHOULD COMPLETE THIS TEST WITHIN TWO HOURS.

Situation: Mrs. Winet, a 32-year-old gravida III, para 2, spontaneously delivers a 9 pound baby boy en route to the hospital after a brief labor. Questions 1 through 13 refer to this situation.

1 The nurse should be aware that the chief hazard to a child in precipitate delivery is:
   1. Brachial palsy
   2. Intracranial hemorrhage
   3. Dislocated hip
   4. Fractured clavicle

2 Perineal laceration is a common complication of precipitate delivery. In addition to regular perineal care, Mrs. Winet's nursing care would include:
   1. Encouraging early and frequent ambulation
   2. Encouraging perineal exercises to strengthen muscles
   3. Telling the patient to expect slower healing
   4. Providing a high-protein, high-roughage diet

3 Baby Winet has sustained and intracranial hemorrhage because of a tear in the tentorial membrane. The nurse would expect the baby to display which one of the following symptoms?
   1. Extreme lethargy
   2. Weak, timorous cry
   3. Abnormal respirations
   4. Generalized purpura

4 The nurse checks Baby Winet's Babinski reflex and finds it to be positive. The nurse understands that this is due to:
   1. Immaturity of the central nervous system
   2. Hypoxia during labor and delivery
   3. Hyperreflexia of the muscular system
   4. Neurologic impairment

5 Nursing care of Baby Winet would include:
   1. Stimulating frequently to monitor level of consciousness
   2. Elevating his head higher than his hips
   3. Checking reflexes every 15 minutes
   4. Weighing him daily before feeding

6 A diagnosis of cerebral palsy is suggested in the nursery and confirmed when Baby Jimmy Winet visits the health clinic at 6 weeks. Mrs. Winet cries, "What did we do to deserve this?" The nurse responds:
   1. "Why do you feel you are being punished?"
   2. "You didn't do anything; let me tell you about this disorder."
   3. "Let's sit down and have a cup of coffee."
   4. "I know you must be upset, but it's too early to tell."

7 As Jimmy Winet develops, his vision, hearing, and speech are fine but he does have a slight general sensory loss in position, pain, and temperature in both legs. He uses braces and self-help appliances to provide self-care. He is admitted to the hospital when he is 7 years old for a tendon lengthening. While in bed after surgery, Jimmy must wear his braces and shoes for at least 8 hours a day. This is to:
   1. Continue his acceptance of physical restraints
   2. Maintain hip and knee alignment and prevent footdrop

3. Stretch his ligaments and strengthen muscle tone
4. Encourage ambulation as soon as possible

8 The orthopedic surgeon is anxious to get Jimmy onto crutches. In preparing Jimmy for crutch walking the nurse must determine:
1. The weight-bearing ability of Jimmy's upper and lower extremities
2. Whether Jimmy has the power in his trunk to drag his legs forward when erect
3. When Jimmy's circulation can tolerate an erect position
4. The ability of Jimmy's shoulder girdle to support his body weight when it leaves the floor

9 It is decided that Jimmy be taught the 4-point alternate crutch gait. This gait was probably chosen because:
1. There are always 2 points of support on the floor
2. Jimmy has more power in the upper extremities than in the lower extremities
3. It provides for equal but partial weight-bearing on each limb
4. Jimmy has no power or step ability in the lower extremities

10 In light of his slight sensory loss in the legs, Jimmy and his parents should be taught to:
1. Keep braces in good repair and pad them well
2. Check alignment of braces (brace joints should coincide with body joints)
3. Select shoes which have heels that are wide and low
4. Examine skin for evidence of pressure points

11 When teaching Jimmy to ambulate with crutches, the nurse should remember that:
1. Learning progresses on a line forward and upward
2. Because of his age, Jimmy's experiential background is limited
3. Learning is a result of adequate teaching
4. Jimmy must first understand normal walking patterns

12 Because of Jimmy's diminished sensation in the legs, he should be taught the following safety precautions:
1. Test temperature of water in any water-related activity
2. Set the clock 2 times during the night to awaken and change position
3. Tighten straps and buckles more than usual on braces when ambulating

4. Look down at lower extremities when crutch walking to determine proper positioning of legs

13 When planning long-term care for Jimmy, it is important for the nurse to recognize that:
1. Cerebral palsy is unstable and unpredictable
2. Jimmy should have genetic counseling before planning a family
3. His illness is not progressively degenerative
4. Jimmy probably has some degree of mental retardation

Situation: Mrs. White, a 73-year-old widow, lives with her daughter. While picketing for senior citizens' rights at the state legislature, she fell and fractured her right hip. Mrs. White is admitted to the hospital for reduction of the fracture and insertion of a pin. On admission her blood pressure is 180/102 with some dependent edema. Questions 14 through 24 refer to this situation.

14 During the day the nurse puts Mrs. White's side rails up specifically:
1. As a safety measure because of the patient's age
2. Because all patients over 65 years of age should use side rails
3. Because elderly people are often disoriented for several days after anesthesia
4. To be used as hand holds and to facilitate the patient's mobility

15 Mrs. White is apprehensive about being hospitalized. The nurse realizes that one of the stresses of hospitalization is the strangeness of the environment and activity. A nurse can best limit extension of this stress by:
1. Listening to what Mrs. White has to say
2. Calling the patient by her first name
3. Visiting Mrs. White frequently
4. Explaining to Mrs. White what is expected of her

16 Mrs. White is placed on a 1-gram sodium diet and is to receive furosemide (Lasix) IM. Mrs. White does not like her diet and tells the nurse her sister is bringing in some "good old home-cooked food." The initial, most effective nursing action should be to:
1. Call in the dietitian for patient teaching
2. Tell Mrs. White that she cannot have salt, since it will raise her blood pressure
3. Wait for Mrs. White's sister and discuss the diet with both of them
4. Catch Mrs. White's sister before she goes into the room and tell her about the diet

17 Since sodium is the major cation controlling fluid outside the cells, diet therapy in congestive heart failure with subsequent cardiac edema is aimed at reducing the sodium intake. In teaching Mrs. White about her diet, the nurse should encourage her to exclude which group of foods?
1. Fruits
2. Vegetables
3. Grains
4. Processed foods

18 The nurse should explain to Mrs. White that sodium restriction is an effective therapeutic tool in the treatment of congestive heart failure because its restriction:
1. Helps to prevent the potassium accumulation that occurs when sodium intake is higher
2. Helps to control food intake and thus weight
3. Causes excess tissue fluid to be withdrawn and excreted
4. Aids the weakened heart muscle to contract and improves cardiac output

19 While Mrs. White has gluteal edema in the unaffected hip, the nurse will use the deltoid muscle for administration of drugs IM, mainly because at edematous sites:
1. Deposition of an injected drug causes pain
2. Blood supply is insufficient for drug absorption
3. Fluid leaks from the site for long periods after injection
4. Tissue fluid dilutes the drug before it enters the circulation

20 An independent nursing action that could be used to prevent thrombus formation in the unaffected leg would be:
1. Gentle massage
2. Passive range of motion exercises
3. Encouraging fluids
4. Elastic stockings

21 While assisting Mrs. White to transfer from the bed to a wheelchair, the nurse should remember that:
1. When performing a weight-bearing transfer, the patient's knees should be slightly bent
2. Transfers to and from the wheelchair will be easier if the bed is higher than the wheelchair
3. The transfer can be accomplished by pivoting while bearing weight on both upper extremities and not on the legs
4. To maintain appropriate proximity and visual relationship of wheelchair to bed

22 To prepare Mrs. White for crutch walking, the nurse should encourage the patient to:
1. Sit up straight in a chair to develop back muscles
2. Keep the affected limb in extension and abduction
3. Do exercises in bed to strengthen her upper extremities
4. Use the trapeze to strengthen the biceps muscles

23 When assisting Mrs. White to ambulate, the nurse should be standing:
1. In front of the patient
2. Behind the patient
3. On the left side of the patient
4. On the right side of the patient

24 Mrs. White is being discharged from the hospital; however, she needs assistance with several activities of daily living and needs to learn how to use a cane, since her daughter works full time and cannot care for her. The most appropriate place for Mrs. White to go to convalesce would be:
1. Her own home with visits from the public health nurse
2. A nursing home
3. An adult facility
4. An extended care facility

Situation: Mrs. Malone, 48 years old, has discovered a lump in her breast on self-examination. It is fixed, and the physician can aspirate no fluid. She is admitted for a possible right radical mastectomy. Questions 25 through 35 refer to this situation.

25 A priority of nursing intervention for Mrs. Malone in the preoperative period would be to:
1. Teach isometric arm exercises
2. Ascertain how patient will adjust to radical mastectomy
3. Cleanse operative site with Betadine several times
4. Have a representative from Reach to Recovery visit her

26 During her morning care Mrs. Malone tells the nurse that she is worried about what she will look like after the surgery. The nurse's most appropriate *initial* response is:
1. "Try not to think about the surgery now."
2. "Why don't you discuss this with your husband."
3. "I can understand that you'd be concerned."
4. "Everyone having this surgery feels the same way."

27 Following the surgery the nurse would position Mrs. Malone's right arm:
1. In abduction surrounded by sandbags
2. Lower than the level of the right atrium on pillows
3. In adduction supported by sandbags
4. With the hand higher than the arm on pillows

28 When teaching Mrs. Malone postmastectomy arm exercises, it is important for the nurse to:
1. Simultaneously exercise both arms
2. Exercise the right arm only
3. Have Mrs. Malone wear a sling in-between exercises
4. Alternately exercise right then left arm

29 Mrs. Malone's physician plans chemotherapy 2 weeks after the surgery. The delay in instituting the plan for drug therapy is because the drugs:
1. Interfere with cell growth and delay wound healing
2. Cause vomiting that endangers the integrity of the large incisional area
3. Decrease red blood cell production, and the resultant anemia would add to postoperative fatigue
4. Increase edema in areas distal to the incision by blocking lymph channels with destroyed lymphocytes

30 Mrs. Malone is symptom free for 3 years. At her next 6-month visit she complains of headaches and difficulty with her embroidery. Her blood pressure is elevated and her pupils react sluggishly. She is admitted to the hospital for further evaluation. Which of the following findings should the nurse recheck in doing an assessment of Mrs. Malone for increased intracranial pressure?
1. Jacksonian seizures
2. Rapid pulse
3. Psychotic behavior
4. Nausea and vomiting

31 Which of the following orders written by Mrs. Malone's physician should the nurse question?
1. Administer osmotic diuretic as ordered
2. Place the patient in reverse Trendelenburg position
3. Administer steroids as ordered
4. Apply rotating tourniquets

32 The nurse assists the physician in performing a lumbar puncture. When pressure is placed on the jugular vein during a lumbar puncture, there is normally a rise in the spinal fluid pressure. This is referred to as:
1. Chvostek's sign
2. Romberg's sign
3. Queckenstedt's sign
4. Homans' sign

33 Mrs. Malone has a tumor of the cerebellum. In view of the functions of this organ, what symptom should the nurse expect to observe?
1. Absence of the knee-jerk and other reflexes
2. Inability to execute smooth, precise movements
3. Inability to execute voluntary movements
4. Unconsciousness

34 Before preparing Mrs. Malone for cranial surgery, the nurse should:
1. Wash the patient's hair with pHisoHex
2. Help the patient chose a wig
3. Obtain consent for shaving the head
4. Wait to shave the head until the patient is anesthetized

35 In caring for Mrs. Malone postoperatively, the nurse should:
1. Take only axillary temperatures
2. Encourage deep breathing but discourage coughing
3. Report yellow drainage on dressing to the physician immediately
4. Administer narcotics and sedatives at the first sign of irritability

---

Situation: Mrs. Janeway is 36 weeks pregnant and is attending a class in preparation for childbirth with her husband. Questions 36 through 48 refer to this situation.

36 Mrs. Janeway verbalizes, "I am sick and tired of wearing these same old clothes; how I wish all this would be done and over with." The nurse's best response would be:
1. "Is there something bothering you? You sound discouraged."
2. "Most women feel the same way you do at this time."
3. "I understand how you feel; what do you know about labor?"
4. "Yes, this is the most uncomfortable time during pregnancy."

37 In the preparation for childbirth class the nurse would teach that labor:
1. Should be painless and uneventful
2. May be uncomfortable, but medication is available when needed

3. Will be painful, but patients will be taught how to tolerate it
4. Will be uncomfortable; however, medication will not be needed

38 Mrs. Janeway is admitted to the labor and delivery unit in extreme discomfort with contractions occurring 3 minutes apart. The nurse realizes that the perception of pain for a woman in labor is influenced most by the:
1. Difficulty of the labor
2. Length of the labor
3. Tension of the patient
4. Parity of the patient

39 The nurse takes the fetal heart rate during a contraction and finds it is 115 per minute. The nurse should:
1. Notify the physician immediately
2. Take a second reading during decrement
3. Take a second reading during the acme of the next contraction
4. Administer oxygen immediately

40 The nurse knows that Mrs. Janeway has begun the the advanced stage of labor when:
1. She feels she has to move her bowels
2. She complains of sudden intense back pain
3. The cervix is dilated to 6 cm
4. Restlessness and thrashing increase

41 One hour following delivery the nurse finds that Mrs. Janeway's uterus has become boggy. The nurse's initial response should be to:
1. Notify the physician
2. Check the blood pressure
3. Massage it until firm
4. Observe the amount of bleeding

42 Mrs. Janeway's baby girl has a unilateral cleft lip and palate. The lip defect extends through the floor of the nostril and communicates with the defect in the palate. The physician recommends that the lip be repaired as soon as possible after birth because the baby is otherwise in good physical condition. Cleft lip is usually repaired early because of:
1. The emotional impact on the parents
2. Feeding difficulty
3. Infection
4. Obstruction of breathing

43 Mr. and Mrs. Janeway are very concerned about the defect and ask the nurse, "What caused our baby to be born deformed?" The nurse should reply:
1. "I don't know, but you don't need to worry because surgery can correct it."

2. "I am glad that you are able to ask these kinds of questions."
3. "Are you feeling guilty?"
4. "It sounds as if you are wondering what you might have done to cause this situation."

44 In informing the parents about the significance and etiology of cleft lip and palate, the nurse should:
1. Assess the family history for presence of the defect in other siblings or relatives
2. Emphasize that the 2 defects follow laws of mendelian genetics
3. Prepare the parents for the likelihood of mental and psychologic problems in the child
4. Stress that the defect is rare and will probably never happen twice in the same family

45 Before Baby Sarah was born, Mrs. Janeway had wanted to breast-feed. Now feeding will probably be:
1. With a rubber-tipped syringe or medicine dropper
2. Too difficult because of breathing problems
3. With a soft, large-holed nipple
4. IV fluids

46 Sarah's cleft lip predisposes her to infection primarily because:
1. Of poor nutrition from disturbed feeding
2. Of poor circulation to the defective area
3. Mouth breathing dries the mucous membranes of the oropharynx
4. Of the accumulation of waste products along the defect

47 Mrs. Janeway has walked to the nursery numerous times to see Sarah each day. Three days post partum she complains of pain in her right leg. The nurse's initial response should be to:
1. Encourage ambulation and exercise
2. Massage the affected area
3. Apply hot soaks
4. Maintain bed rest and notify the physician

48 Baby Sarah's lip is repaired 4 days after birth. In caring for her postoperatively the nurse should do all the following *except:*
1. Observe for swelling of the tongue, lips, and mucous membranes
2. Place her on her abdomen to prevent aspiration
3. Keep the suture line clean and free of crusting
4. Encourage the parents to visit as much as possible to prevent the infant from crying

Situation: Mrs. Jones, a 35-year-old mother of 4 children, has been diagnosed as having Cushing's syndrome. Questions 49 through 60 refer to this situation.

49 In planning her care the nurse should take into consideration the fact that Mrs. Jones would:
1. Be bothered by frequent urination
2. Probably have hypotension
3. Have muscle weakness due to protein depletion
4. Probably have hyperkalemia

50 Mrs. Jones would probably demonstrate which of the following symptoms?
1. Lability of mood
2. Decrease in the growth of hair
3. Ectomorphism with a gaunt expression
4. Increased resistance to bruising

51 Prior to Mrs. Jones undergoing an adrenalectomy the nurse should:
1. Withhold all medications for 48 hours
2. Administer steroids prior to surgery
3. Provide a high-protein diet
4. Collect a 24-hour urine specimen the day before surgery

52 Postoperatively, prior to maintenance steroid therapy, the nurse would expect to see signs of:
1. Hyperglycemia
2. Sodium retention
3. Potassium excretion
4. Hypotension

53 In teaching Mrs. Jones about her medications, the nurse should emphasize the fact that:
1. Once she is regulated, her dosage will remain the same for life
2. Taking her medications late in the evening may cause sleeplessness
3. While she is taking medications, her salt intake might have to be restricted
4. Steroid therapy will be given in conjunction with insulin

54 The nurse finds Mrs. Jones very upset after visiting hours. She tearfully tells the nurse that her 2-year-old son Alex is being admitted to the hospital in the morning for a circumcision due to phimosis. After quieting Mrs. Jones, the nurse notifies the physician, since Mrs. Jones:
1. Will probably require mild sedation to ensure her rest
2. Should have her steroid medication dosage reduced

3. Has a decreased ability to handle stress despite steroid therapy
4. Will have feelings of exhaustion and lethargy as a result of stress

55 Alex is admitted in the morning for the circumcision and is now ready to go to the OR in 1 hour. As the nurse enters his room with a preoperative injection, he begins to scream and flail about the bed. His father is sitting at his bedside and gets up to leave. The nurse's best response to this situation is to:
1. Leave the room and ask another nurse to come in to hold Alex during the injection
2. Allow Alex to say goodbye to his father before giving the injection
3. Tell Mr. Jones he can return to comfort Alex after the injection is given
4. Ask Mr. Jones to stay to comfort and hold Alex while the injection is given

56 Attendance of parents during painful procedures on their children should be:
1. Based on the type of procedure to be performed
2. Encouraged and permitted if child desires their presence
3. Based on individual assessment of the parents
4. Discouraged for the benefit of the parents and child

57 The gluteal muscle is generally not used when giving IM injections to infants and young children because they:
1. Fear intrusive procedures
2. Are able to wiggle and change their position when placed on abdomen
3. Have an undeveloped muscle mass in this area
4. Associate this area with punishment

58 A major nursing responsibility in caring for Alex postoperatively is to:
1. Limit oral fluids
2. Monitor IV fluids carefully
3. Apply ice packs to the penis
4. Observe for bleeding at operative site

59 Mrs. Jones and Alex are being discharged together. Alex is eating a regular diet. Mrs. Jones' therapy includes a low-sodium, high-potassium diet because:
1. Excessive secretions of aldosterone and cortisone cause renal retention of sodium and loss of potassium
2. Her use of salt had probably contributed to her disease

3. She is losing excess salt in her urine and requires less renal stimulation

4. She will gain excessive weight if sodium is not limited

60 After discharge Mrs. Jones begins to develop signs of diabetes mellitus. The nurse recognizes that diabetes mellitus may develop because:
1. The cortical hormones had created a too rapid weight loss
2. The excessive glucocorticoids secreted by the adrenal gland caused excess tissue catabolism and consequent gluconeogenesis
3. A negative nitrogen balance resulted from the tissue catabolism
4. The excessive ACTH had damaged pancreatic tissue

Situation: Mr. Burn, 55, is admitted to the hospital with benign prostatic hypertrophy. Surgery is scheduled for the next day. Questions 61 through 67 refer to this situation.

61 The night nurse reports that Mr. Burn is complaining of inability to void. On making the morning rounds it is noted that his bladder is distended. Nursing intervention should be to:
1. Force fluids to induce voiding
2. Encourage use of a urinal
3. Apply pressure over the pubic area
4. Assist him into a warm tub bath

62 Mr. Burn has a suprapubic prostatectomy. After the surgery, in addition to the placement of a Foley catheter, the nurse should expect the patient to have:
1. A rectal incision and a ureteral catheter
2. A ureterostomy with gravity drainage
3. A nephrostomy tube with tidal drainage
4. An abdominal incision and a cystostomy tube

63 The most significant complication immediately following this surgery is:
1. Hemorrhage
2. Impotence
3. Urinary incontinence
4. Spasms

64 Mr. Burn has just returned from the recovery room following the suprapubic prostatectomy. He accidently pulls out the urethral catheter. The nurse should:
1. Check for bleeding by irrigating the suprapubic tube

2. Have the male nurse reinsert a new catheter
3. Notify the physician immediately
4. Take no immediate action if the suprapubic tube is draining

65 In implementing postoperative care for Mr. Burn an important action to prevent secondary bladder infection is to:
1. Observe for signs of uremia
2. Attach the catheter to suction
3. Clamp off the connecting tubing
4. Change the dressings frequently

66 Mr. Burn complains of pain in the operative area. The initial response of the nurse should be to:
1. Administer the prescribed analgesic
2. Take vital signs before administration of analgesic
3. Inspect drainage tubing for occlusion
4. Encourage intake of fluids to dilute urine

67 Following prostatectomy the nurse should:
1. Have the patient stand to void
2. Aspirate catheter with a bulb syringe
3. Discourage straining for a bowel movement
4. Notify the physician if the patient does not void in 12 hours

Situation: Mr. Jay is admitted to the Psychiatric Service by his parents, who can no longer deal with him. He is a handsome, smooth-talking, bright young man who has been married 3 times and has a child by each wife. He states he has never loved any of his wives, does not intend to support his children, and has no reason to be sorry for anything he has ever done. Questions 68 through 74 refer to this situation.

68 The nurse would expect Mr. Jay's behavior to demonstrate a defect in:
1. Id development
2. Ego development
3. Superego development
4. Sexual development

69 In working with Mr. Jay the nurse should adopt which of the following attitudes?
1. Sincere, cautious, and consistent
2. Strict, punishing, and restrictive
3. Accepting, supportive, and friendly
4. Sympathetic, motherly, and encouraging

70 Mrs. Jones, one of the nurses, is taking a new patient on an orientation tour of the unit when Mr. Jay rushes down the hallway and asks her to sit and talk to him. Which would be the most appropriate action by the nurse?

1. Excuse herself from the new patient and speak with Mr. Jay
2. Suggest to Mr. Jay that he talk with another staff member
3. Introduce Mr. Jay and suggest that he join them on the tour
4. Tell Mr. Jay that she will speak with him later

71 Mr. Jay responds by smiling broadly and saying ''Mrs. Jones, you sure do look messy today.'' Which would be the most appropriate response by the nurse?
   1. ''That's not a nice thing to say, Mr. Jay.''
   2. ''Don't you feel well today, Mr. Jay?''
   3. ''I didn't get a chance to set my hair last night.''
   4. ''You're angry with me, Mr. Jay.''

72 Mr. Jay takes Mrs. Jones by the shoulder, suddenly kisses her, and shouts ''I like you.'' Which would be the most appropriate response for the nurse to make?
   1. ''I like you too, but please don't do that again.''
   2. ''I wish you wouldn't do that.''
   3. ''Don't ever touch me like that again.''
   4. ''Thank you, I like you too.''

73 Mr. Jay has just been given his first day pass from the hospital. He is due to return at 6 P.M. At 5 P.M. Mr. Jay telephones the nurse in charge of the ward and says ''Six o'clock is too early. I feel like coming back at 7:30.'' Which approach by the nurse would be most therapeutic at this time? Tell him to:
   1. Return immediately, to demonstrate control
   2. Return on time or he will be restricted
   3. Come back by 6:45, as a compromise to set limits
   4. Come back as soon as he can or you'll have to send police

74 Mrs. Jones is leaving in 2 weeks and tells Mr. Jay. Which response would indicate that he is progressing in his ability to maintain more mature relationships? He:
   1. Tells her that he must get well enough by then so that he may also leave
   2. Wishes her good luck and thanks her for helping him
   3. Tells her that her leaving is just another loss he must adjust to
   4. Informs her that, since she is leaving, this should be their last meeting

Situation: Mr. Brown, a 48-year-old man with a long history of chronic obstructive lung disease, is admitted to the hospital for a segmental resection of the right lower lobe. Questions 75 through 82 refer to this situation.

75 Intermittent positive pressure breathing is given preoperatively to:
   1. Encourage respiration at a faster rate than that established by respiratory center control
   2. Provide more adequate lung expansion than could be achieved by unassisted breathing
   3. Force air through the infected secretions that accumulated in the lung bases
   4. Remove air and fluid from the pleural cavity

76 Because of Mr. Brown's history of COPD, the nurse should be aware of complications involving:
   1. Kidney function
   2. Peripheral neuropathy
   3. Cardiac function
   4. Joint inflammation

77 When scheduling intermittent positive pressure breathing treatments, the nurse should realize that the least appropriate time of day to receive an IPPB treatment is:
   1. On awakening
   2. Before a meal
   3. At bedtime
   4. After a meal

78 Immediately following Mr. Brown's arrival in the recovery room, the nurse should undertake which of the following measures concerning the closed chest drainage apparatus?
   1. Secure the chest catheter to the wound dressing with a sterile safety pin
   2. Mark the time and the fluid level on the side of the drainage bottle
   3. Raise the drainage bottle to bed level to check patency of the system
   4. Add 3 to 5 ml of sterile saline to the water seal

79 The purpose of the water in the closed chest drainage bottle is to:
   1. Facilitate emptying bloody drainage from the chest
   2. Foster removal of chest secretions by capillarity
   3. Prevent entrance of air into the pleural cavity
   4. Decrease the danger of sudden change in pressure in the tube

80 Mr. Brown has a large amount of respiratory secretions. Independent nursing care should include:
1. Turning and positioning
2. Cupping
3. Clapping
4. Postural drainage

81 Mr. Brown requires oxygen. Which of the following factors is of major concern in determining the method of oxygen administration to be used for a specific patient? The patient's:
1. Facial anatomy
2. Pathologic condition
3. Age and mental capacity
4. Level of activity

82 A preventive measure to be taken by the nurse regarding the untoward effects of oxygen therapy is:
1. Padding elastic bands of face masks
2. Humidifying the gas
3. Taking apical pulse before starting therapy
4. Placing patient in orthopneic position

Situation: Mr. Paley, a 56-year-old plumber, is hospitalized with a recent myocardial infarction. Questions 83 through 90 refer to this situation.

83 The nurse goes to Mr. Paley's bedside to administer his 10 A.M. dose of digitoxin. He has a lidocaine hydrochloride (Xylocaine) IV drip running at 3 mg/minute for control of premature ventricular contractions. The cardiac monitor shows 20 PVCs per minute, and his heart rate is 78. The nurse's first actions should be to:
1. Increase the lidocaine hydrochloride flow rate and check for sources of excess neural stimuli
2. Check the availability of the defibrillator and run an ECG rhythm strip
3. Administer the digitoxin and increase the lidocaine hydrochloride flow rate
4. Run an ECG rhythm strip and administer the digitoxin

84 The nurse should recognize that the greatest danger of premature ventricular contractions is that they can lead to ventricular fibrillation if they strike on the:
1. P wave
2. PR interval
3. R wave
4. T wave

85 Three days after admission Mr. Paley has a cardiac arrest and is successfully defibrillated. The nurse is aware that the use of electric currents to defibrillate the heart during cardiac arrest depends on the body fluids:
1. Containing electrolytes
2. Containing base elements
3. Being a colloidally dispersed medium
4. Resembling pure water

86 After the arrest Mr. Paley is receiving levarterenol bitartrate (Levophed) intravenously for regulation of blood pressure. The planned effect of the drug is based on the fact that it:
1. Stimulates adrenergic receptors at arterial sites
2. Stimulates adrenergic receptors in the heart
3. Depresses cholinergic receptors in the arteries
4. Increases adrenal output of epinephrine

87 The nurse should place a second clamp on the IV tubing because:
1. The drug must be infused slowly, since it is irritating to the vein
2. Administration of the drug above the established rate may cause generalized arterial constriction
3. Extravasation of the drug into subcutaneous tissues causes sloughing
4. Headache and cerebral hemorrhage occur when the infusion runs rapidly

88 Mr. Paley is receiving digitoxin IM at 10 A.M. daily. At 9 A.M. he states that he has been nauseated since awaking. He has a prn order for trimethobenzamide (Tigan) and receives Amphojel every 2 hours. The nurse should:
1. Give the Amphojel now and give the digitoxin at 10 A.M.
2. Give the trimethobenzamide now, the Amphojel at 10 A.M., and withhold the digitoxin
3. Hold the digitoxin for 1 hour and give the Amphojel now
4. Give the Amphojel and trimethobenzamide now and give the digitoxin at 10 A.M.

89 Mr. Paley questions the nurse about the length of time it takes the heart to heal. The nurse replies that myocardial tissue usually heals within:
1. 3 to 4 weeks
2. 6 to 8 weeks
3. 10 to 14 weeks
4. 20 to 24 weeks

90 Mr. Paley is being discharged from the hospital. He has a prescription for procainamide hydrochloride (Pronestyl) that he is to take for control of ventricular irritability. He should be taught that:

1. His heart rate will be slower and he may experience fatigue
2. The drug must be taken at exact time intervals prescribed to maintain the therapeutic effect
3. He should plan a schedule for taking the drug during highest periods of activity
4. The total daily dosage of drug must be maintained, but he may modify the schedule to allow taking the drug with meals

---

Situation: Mrs. Grite, who is 35 weeks pregnant and a diabetic, is admitted to the hospital to await delivery. Questions 91 through 95 refer to this situation.

91 The nurse can answer Mrs. Grite's questions about why she is being hospitalized if the nurse understands that in diabetic pregnant women:
1. Complete rest prior to the work of delivery is essential
2. Fetal death usually occurs after the thirty-sixth week of gestation
3. Fetal development is completed and should be monitored
4. Insulin needs to be administered intravenously before labor begins

92 The nurse should be aware that diabetic pregnant women such as Mrs. Grite require:
1. Increased dosage of insulin
2. Administration of estrogenic hormones
3. Decreased caloric intake
4. Administration of pancreatic enzymes

93 Mrs. Grite asks why she cannot take the oral hypoglycemic pills she used to take for her diabetes. The nurse should base her response on the fact that oral hypoglycemics are not used during pregnancy because:
1. The fetal pancreas compensates for the mother's inability to secrete adequate insulin
2. The effect of exogenous insulin on the fetus is uncertain
3. They may produce deformities in the fetus
4. During the later part of pregnancy, diabetes can usually be controlled by diet alone

94 Mrs. Grite's delivery is induced and she delivers a baby girl. A sign of hypoglycemia in Baby Grite, which the nurse should be alert for, is:
1. Excessive birth weight
2. Excessive body movement
3. Pallor of the skin and mucosa
4. Poor sucking reflex

95 In caring for Baby Grite the nurse should provide:
1. A decreased glucose intake
2. Routine newborn care
3. For administration of insulin
4. Special high-risk care

Situation: Mr. Osgood is admitted to the hospital for surgery for an incarcerated hernia. Questions 96 through 100 refer to this situation.

96 The nurse recognizes that a diagnosis of incarcerated hernia means that:
1. The blood supply to the intestine has been cut off
2. The hernia contents cannot be reduced
3. There is an erosion of the involved intestinal tissue
4. The bowel has twisted on itself

97 Prior to Mr. Osgood's hernia repair the nurse should:
1. Place the patient in the supine position
2. Periodically check the patient's vital signs
3. Observe the patient's bowel movements
4. Monitor the patient's serum enzyme levels

98 The physician returns the incarcerated tissue to the abdominal cavity and uses a stainless steel mesh to reinforce the muscle wall, thereby preventing a future recurrence. This procedure is referred to as a:
1. Herniorrhaphy
2. Herniotomy
3. Herniectomy
4. Hernioplasty

99 After Mr. Osgood's surgery, to help limit a common complication of this surgery, the nurse should:
1. Place a rolled towel under the scrotum
2. Encourage a high-carbohydrate diet
3. Cough and deep breathe Mr. Osgood frequently
4. Apply a Scultetus binder

100 An important part of discharge planning is educating Mr. Osgood about body mechanics. Which of the following statements is an important concept in body mechanics?
1. Bending at the waist reduces tension on the inguinal muscles
2. Keeping the body straight when lifting reduces pressure on the abdomen
3. Placing the feet apart will increase the stability of the body
4. Relaxing the abdominal muscles and using the extremities prevent strain

Situation: Mr. Walter is admitted to the Psychiatric Unit with a diagnosis of paranoid schizophrenia. Questions 101 through 108 refer to this situation.

101 During the admission procedure Mr. Walter appears to be responding to voices. He cries out at intervals, "No, no, I didn't kill him," and states, "You know the truth, tell that policeman. Please help me!" The nurse should:
  1. Respond by saying, "Mr. Walter, I want to help you and I realize you must be very frightened."
  2. Sit there quietly and not respond at all to his statements
  3. Respond by saying, "Who are they saying you killed, Mr. Walter?"
  4. Respond by saying, "Mr. Walter, do not become so upset. No one is talking to you; we are alone. This is part of your illness."

102 Mr. Walter has delusions that his food is poisoned and he refuses to eat. The nurse tells him that it is foolish for him to believe that, since his food comes from the same kitchen as for all other patients. The nurse states "Unless you eat, you will have to be fed by other means." This response indicated that:
  1. Mr. Walter needed nourishment and therefore had to eat
  2. Mr. Walter's misinterpretations had to be corrected
  3. Mr. Walter had to be reminded about needing to eat
  4. The nurse really did not know how to handle the situation

103 One evening the nurse finds Mr. Walter trying to leave the unit. He says, "Please let me go. I trust you. The Mafia are going to kill me tonight." The nurse should respond:
  1. "Nobody here wants to harm you, you know that. I'll come with you to your room."
  2. "Mr. Walter, you are frightened. Come with me to your room and we can talk about it."
  3. "Thank you for trusting me, Mr. Walter. Maybe you can trust me when I tell you no one can kill you while you're here."
  4. "Come with me to your room. I'll lock the door and no one will get to you to hurt you."

104 In caring for Mr. Walter, whose behavior is characterized by pathologic suspicion, one of the goals of nursing care should be to:

  1. Help him realize these suspicions are unrealistic
  2. Remove as much environmental stress as possible
  3. Help him feel accepted
  4. Ask him to explain the reasons for his feelings

105 The nurse has been observing Mr. Walter for some time. He is quite delusional, talking about people who are out to get him. Staff notices he is pacing more than usual. One afternoon the nurse decides that Mr. Walter is beginning to lose control of himself. The best nursing intervention would be to:
  1. Allow him to use a punching bag
  2. Move him to a quiet place on the unit
  3. Allow him to continue pacing
  4. Suggest that he sit down for a while

106 Mr. Walter is receiving large doses of chlorpromazine (Thorazine) and the nurse is concerned, since the phenothiazine derivatives produce a wide variety of untoward side effects. The presence of which side effect should signal the nurse to withhold the drug?
  1. Masklike facies
  2. Blurred vision
  3. Edema
  4. Jaundice

107 Mr. Walter tells the nurse that he used to believe that he was God, but now he knows that this is not true. The nurse's best response would be:
  1. "You really believed that?"
  2. "You must be getting well."
  3. "What caused you to think you were God?"
  4. "Many people have this delusion."

108 Mr. Walter is to be discharged with orders for chlorpromazine therapy. In developing a teaching plan for discharge the nurse should include cautioning Mr. Walter against:
  1. Taking medications containing aspirin
  2. Staying in the sun
  3. Driving at night
  4. Ingesting wines and cheeses

Situation: Mrs. Garvin, age 38, has cancer of the cervix. She is hospitalized for internal radiation therapy with radium. Questions 109 through 113 refer to this situation.

109 When Mrs. Garvin returns to her room, after the insertion of radium, the nurse should:
  1. Immediately place Mrs. Garvin in high Fowler's position to prevent dislodging of the radium

2. Check Mrs. Garvin's voiding and catheterize if necessary, since a distended bladder can interrupt the path of radiation
3. Check that Mrs. Garvin is on a low-residue diet to prevent bowel movements and the possibility of dislodging the radium
4. Stay with the patient for half an hour to watch for symptoms of radiation sickness

110 Six months later Mrs. Garvin is readmitted for an abdominal hysterectomy. During her preoperative care Mrs. Garvin asks how the surgery will affect her periods. The nurse should respond:
1. "Initially your periods will increase."
2. "You will no longer menstruate."
3. "Your monthly periods will be more regular."
4. "Your monthly periods will be lighter."

111 Mrs. Garvin is admitted to the Recovery Room following surgery. Which of the following observations should be reported to the physician immediately?
1. Increase in drainage from Levin tube
2. Serosanguinous drainage on perineal pad
3. Decrease in urinary output
4. Apical pulse of 90

112 Mrs. Garvin develops abdominal distention. Which of the following measures would most likely provide immediate relief?
1. Restriction of oral intake and frequent change of position
2. Ambulation and bicarbonated drink
3. Insertion of a rectal tube and application of heat to the abdomen
4. Nasogastric intubation and administration of cholinergic agents

113 Mrs. Garvin's physician has ordered that she wear a girdle while out of bed. The nurse should explain that this is to:
1. Prevent pooling of blood in the pelvic area
2. Increase wound healing
3. Prevent feelings of nausea
4. Support abdominal muscles

Situation: Mrs. Gold is a 50-year-old woman with a diagnosis of involutional depressive psychosis. She is agitated, paces in her room almost continuously, and has difficulty sleeping at night. Questions 114 through 120 refer to this situation.

114 Mrs. Gold frequently states that she will die. The nurse tells her this is not true and she should not dwell on the subject. The nurse urges Mrs. Gold to go to the day room to talk with the other patients. Mrs. Gold becomes more agitated and ultimately has to be sedated. In instances such as this:
1. The nurse must be accepting and should not try to talk a patient out of a delusion
2. The sleeplessness and agitation should have been treated as a symptom
3. Mrs. Gold had to be encouraged to relate to the other patients
4. Mrs. Gold should have been given a tranquilizer before this incident developed

115 The treatment plan for Mrs. Gold would probably include:
1. High doses of mood elevators
2. Psychoanalysis
3. Electroconvulsive therapy
4. Nondirective psychotherapy

116 In caring for Mrs. Gold the nurse should keep in mind that:
1. Patients with simple depressions rarely attempt suicide
2. Once the severe depression begins to lift, the danger of suicide is no longer a problem
3. Depressed patients are potentially suicidal during the entire course of their illness
4. Opportunities to attempt suicide are practically absent on a closed psychiatric ward

117 Mrs. Gold appears preoccupied. She remains seated when it is time for the patients to go to eat. The nurse's best approach would be to:
1. Overlook her not eating and leave snacks in the room
2. Tell her she must eat now, since no food will be served later
3. Ask her whether she would like to eat in her room instead of the dining room
4. Take her by the hand and accompany her to the dining room

118 Mrs. Gold is eating very little at this time. A part of the nursing care plan should be to assist her with her meals. Besides encouraging nourishment, this action also:
1. Shows her she is a worthwhile individual
2. Gets her out of the dining room with the rest of the patients
3. Proves to her that she can tolerate food
4. Provides her with some special attention

119 Mrs. Gold is taking isocarboxazid (Marplan). The nurse should observe for evidence of drug effect on body tissues, which can result in:
  1. Hypotension and edema
  2. Increased psychomotor activity and appetite
  3. Diarrhea and anorexia
  4. Flushing of face and neck and increased salivation

120 Mrs. Gold is much improved and is permitted passes to leave the hospital. She tells the nurse that she is going to a cocktail party later in the day. The nurse should advise her to:
  1. Drink only wines or diluted drinks
  2. Have a snack with milk before going to the party
  3. Avoid participation in heavy discussions
  4. Avoid drinking wines or eating cheeses

COMPREHENSIVE TEST 4

TO SIMULATE THE COMPREHENSIVE STATE BOARD EXAMINATIONS YOU SHOULD COMPLETE THIS
TEST WITHIN TWO HOURS.

Situation: Mr. Wilson, a 57-year-old man with a history of myocardial infarction, is admitted to the hospital to have a hemorrhoidectomy. Questions 1 through 9 refer to this situation.

1 The nurse should expect Mr. Wilson's preoperative diet to be:
   1. High protein
   2. Low residue
   3. Bland
   4. Clear liquid

2 Mr. Wilson is in pain on the second postoperative day. A method ordered to relieve pain, which the nurse uses, is:
   1. Medicated suppository
   2. Application of water-soluble jelly
   3. Sitz baths
   4. Ice packs

3 Mr. Wilson is having his first postoperative bowel movement. When cleansing the rectum, Mr. Wilson should be instructed to use:
   1. Moist cotton swabs
   2. Betadine pads
   3. Sterile 4 × 4-inch gauze pads
   4. Soft facial tissue

4 The nurse turns from preparing Mr. Wilson's sitz bath and discovers he is lying on the floor. After ascertaining that the patient is unconscious, the nurse should:
   1. Help the patient back to bed
   2. Check the blood pressure
   3. Check the carotid pulse
   4. Call for assistance

5 The nurse sends the nurse's aide for help and begins CPR. When there is only one person to perform cardiopulmonary resuscitation, the rate of ventilation to cardiac compression is:
   1. 1:5
   2. 1:10
   3. 2:15
   4. 4:15

6 In performing external cardiac compression on Mr. Wilson the nurse should exert downward vertical pressure on the lower sternum by placing:
   1. The heels of each hand side by side, extending the fingers over the chest
   2. The heel of one hand on the sternum and the heel of the other on top of it, interlocking the fingers
   3. The fingers of one hand on the sternum and the fingers of the other hand on top of them
   4. The fleshy part of the clenched fist on the lower sternum

7 The cardiac arrest team arrives and places Mr. Wilson on a monitor. To prepare the skin area for placement of the electrodes for cardiac monitoring, the nurse:
   1. Uses a scrubbing motion while cleansing the skin
   2. Scrubs the area with tincture of benzoin
   3. Makes certain the area is moistened with normal saline before applying the electrodes

547

4. Applies electrode paste only if the skin becomes excoriated

8 The cardiac monitor shows ventricular fibrillation. The nurse from the Coronary Care Unit should prepare for:
1. An IM injection of digoxin (Lanoxin)
2. An IV line for emergency medications
3. Immediate defibrillation
4. Elective cardioversion

9 As the cells are deprived of oxygen in the patient with cardiac arrest, metabolic acidosis develops. The nurse should be prepared to administer:
1. Potassium chloride
2. Calcium gluconate
3. Sodium bicarbonate
4. Regular insulin

Situation: Mr. and Mrs. June are a young married couple. John is 24 and has a history of colitis; Mary is 21. John is the first of his family to attend college. Mary is supporting the family by working as a keypunch operator at a large insurance company. They had decided to postpone having a family until John finishes his education in 2 years. Mary has therefore taken oral contraceptives since shortly before the marriage. Mary has always had a regular menstrual cycle. She therefore became concerned when she missed her regular menstrual period. After 3 weeks passed she decided to go to a physician for a check-up. She told the nurse interviewing her that she suspected she may be pregnant because she had missed taking her contraceptive pills for more than a week when she had the flu. Questions 10 through 24 refer to this situation.

10 Concerning the patient's statement about her possible pregnancy, the best response for the nurse to make is:
1. "Contraceptive pills are very unpredictable anyhow. You probably would have become pregnant even if you had taken them regularly as prescribed."
2. "You may well be correct; one of the reasons for prescribing an exact schedule is that the effect of contraceptive drugs depends on the regularity with which they are taken."
3. "Don't think about that now. It's too late to worry anyhow. First find out whether you really are pregnant. If you are, you may want to consider having an abortion."
4. "That's the trouble with using contraceptive pills. People become too careless and don't use proper restraint. If you had used the rhythm method, this probably would not have happened."

11 While Mrs. June is being prepared for the examination, she complains of feeling very tired and being sick to her stomach, particularly in the morning. The best response for the nurse to make is:
1. "This is a common occurrence during the early part of pregnancy and you need not worry."
2. "This is a common occurrence due to all the change going on in your body."
3. "These are common occurrences; you say your sick feelings bother you most often in the morning?"
4. "Perhaps you might discuss this with the doctor when he arrives."

12 Mrs. June asks, "Is it true the doctor will do an internal examination today?" The nurse should answer:
1. "Yes, an internal is done on all mothers on the first visit."
2. "Yes, an internal is done on all mothers, but it is only slightly uncomfortable."
3. "Are you fearful of having an internal examination done?"
4. "Yes, he will; have you ever had an internal examination done before?"

13 Mrs. June asks when she may expect her baby. She states that her last menstrual period was April 14, 1980. Her expected date of delivery most likely is:
1. December 21, 1980
2. January 7, 1981
3. January 21, 1981
4. February 1, 1981

14 Mrs. June is concerned, since she has read that nutrition during pregnancy is important for proper growth and development of the baby. She wants to know something about the foods she should be eating. The nurse should proceed by:
1. Giving her a list of foods to refer to in planning meals
2. Asking her what she usually eats at each meal
3. Emphasizing the importance of limiting salt and highly seasoned foods
4. Instructing her to continue eating a normal diet

15 Mrs. June's work as a keypunch operator would necessarily have implications for her plan of care during pregnancy. The nurse should recommend that Mrs. June:
1. Ask for time in the morning and afternoon to elevate her legs

2. Tell her employer she cannot work beyond the second trimester
3. Ask for time in the morning and afternoon to obtain nourishment
4. Try to walk about every few hours during the workday

16 Since Mrs. June is a primigravida, she should be told to come to the hospital when:
1. Contractions are 2 to 3 minutes apart and she cannot walk about
2. Contractions are 10 to 15 minutes apart
3. She has a bloody show and back pressure
4. Membranes rupture or contractions are 5 to 8 minutes apart

17 During the examination the nurse asks Mrs. June if she would like to listen to her baby's heartbeat. She is delighted and after listening comments on how rapid it is. She appears frightened and asks if this is normal. The nurse should respond:
1. "The baby's heart rate is usually twice the mother's pulse rate."
2. "The baby's heartbeat is rapid to accommodate the nutritional needs."
3. "The baby's heart rate is normally rapid, so you needn't worry."
4. "It is far better that the heart rate is rapid; when it is slow, there is need to worry."

18 Mrs. June spontaneously delivers a 6-pound, 8-ounce baby daughter. Although Mr. June expresses delight, he appears anxious and tends to avoid physical contact with the baby. One evening he says to the nurse, "My wife seems so wrapped up with the baby, I hope she has time for me when she gets home." The nurse should respond by saying:
1. "Do you think your parents will be able to help out, Mr. June?"
2. "I can understand your concern about the changes you'll have to make."
3. "You seem to feel you'll have to fend for yourself."
4. "You'll both be so busy you won't even miss her attention."

19 When the baby is 2 months old, Mr. June, pale, thin, and dehydrated, is admitted to the hospital with an exacerbation of colitis. He is placed on a residue-free, bland, high-protein diet, and vitamins B, C, and K parenterally. An IV solution containing electrolytes is also started. The type of person who most frequently develops ulcerative colitis is:

1. Hard driving and immature
2. Sensitive and dependent
3. Quick tempered and hostile
4. Unassuming and secure

20 The nurse administers vitamins parenterally because:
1. More rapid action results
2. They are ineffective orally
3. They decrease colon irritability
4. Intestinal absorption may be inadequate

21 Mr. June is to receive 2000 ml of IV fluid in 12 hours. The drop factor is 10 gtt/1 ml. The nurse should regulate the flow so the number of drops per minute is approximately:
1. 27 to 29
2. 30 to 32
3. 40 to 42
4. 48 to 50

22 Which of these food combinations should be included on his residue-free diet?
1. Lean roast beef, buttered white rice with egg slices, white bread with butter and jelly, tea with sugar
2. Creamed soup and crackers, omlet, mashed potatoes, roll, orange juice, coffee
3. Stewed chicken, baked potato with butter, strained peas, white bread, plain cake, milk
4. Baked fish, macaroni with cheese, strained carrots, fruit gelatin, milk

23 Mr. June's diet is designed to reduce:
1. Gastric acidity
2. Colonic irritation
3. Electrolyte depletion
4. Intestinal absorption

24 In addition, the nurse encourages a high-protein diet to:
1. Correct anemia
2. Slow peristalsis
3. Improve muscle tone
4. Repair tissues

Situation: Mrs. O'Hanlon, a childless widow, was born in Ireland. She has been an outpatient in the medical clinic for 6 months, under treatment for diabetes and hypertension. Her regimen includes tolbutamide (Orinase), a low-sodium, diabetic diet, and reserpine (Serpasil) bid. On the occasion of a regular visit her urine sample shows sugar 3+ and a trace of acetone. She is employed as a cook in the sandwich shop of the local department store. Questions 25 through 37 refer to this situation.

25 The nurse interviewing Mrs. O'Hanlon would first be most concerned to find out about any changes in her:
   1. Eating habits
   2. Blood pressure
   3. Weight range
   4. Serum glucose

26 In discussing the patient's present metabolic state, the nurse should mention that people taking oral antidiabetic agents:
   1. Should not work where food is readily accessible
   2. Consciously or unconsciously may tend to relax dietary rules
   3. Are not as threatened by their disease as those on insulin
   4. Need not be concerned about serious complications

27 Mrs. O'Hanlon tells the nurse she can't eat big meals and prefers to snack throughout the day. The nurse should carefully explain that:
   1. Small, frequent meals are better for digestion
   2. Large meals can contribute to a weight problem
   3. Salt and sugar restriction is her main concern
   4. Regulated food intake is basic to her control

28 When promoting affective learning (developing attitudes), the nurse must remember the influence of the:
   1. Patient's personal resources
   2. Type of onset of the disease
   3. Physical and emotional stress of the situation
   4. Patient's past experiences

29 Mrs. O'Hanlon complains that she finds the low-salt foods very tasteless. The nurse's best response is:
   1. "Salt can be very harmful to your health."
   2. "I know how difficult it is for you."
   3. "You miss your ham and cabbage?"
   4. "Ask the doctor if you can splurge occasionally."

30 Mrs. O'Hanlon is scheduled to have a serum glucose test the following morning. To ensure accuracy in the result, the nurse should instruct her to:
   1. Take her regular dose of tolbutamide
   2. Abstain from food and fluid
   3. Have clear fluids for breakfast
   4. Eat her usual diet

31 Mrs. O'Hanlon has a cough. She tells the nurse that she takes Robitussin cough syrup about every 2 hours when she has a cold. The nurse should tell her that she:
   1. May take the cough syrup if her urine test remains negative
   2. Must calculate the sugar in her daily carbohydrate allowance
   3. Can substitute an elixir for the syrup
   4. Can increase her fluid intake and humidify her bedroom to control the cough

32 Mrs. O'Hanlon complains of difficulty seeing at night. The nurse knows this frequently occurs in diabetes due to:
   1. Poor glucose supply to rods and cones
   2. Lack of glucose in the retina
   3. The effect of ketones on retinal metabolism
   4. Atherosclerotic changes in blood vessels within the eyes

33 One week after admission Mrs. O'Hanlon has a cerebral vascular accident. Three weeks later she still has left-sided paresis but is able to ambulate fairly well with a cane. She is very frustrated and angry because of her expressive aphasia. The nurse anticipates she will have difficulty with:
   1. Following specific instructions
   2. Recognizing words for familiar objects
   3. Speaking and/or writing
   4. Understanding speech and/or writing

34 Mrs. O'Hanlon gets frustrated and upset when she tries to communicate with the nurse. To help alleviate this frustration the nurse should:
   1. Face the patient and raise her voice so that Mrs. O'Hanlon can see and hear her better
   2. Limit Mrs. O'Hanlon's contact with other patients to limit the frustration
   3. Anticipate Mrs. O'Hanlon's needs so that she does not have to ask for help
   4. Give Mrs. O'Hanlon plenty of time to speak and respond so she does not have to formulate a response under pressure

35 Although Mrs. O'Hanlon has regained control of her bowel movements, she is still incontinent of urine. To help her reestablish bladder function, the nurse should encourage her to:
   1. Assume her normal position for voiding
   2. Void every 3 hours and attempt to hold urine between set times
   3. Drink a minimum of 4000 ml of fluid equally divided among the hours she is awake
   4. Attempt to void more frequently in the afternoon than in the morning

36 Mrs. O'Hanlon is using a cane specifically to:
1. Prevent further injury to weakened muscles
2. Maintain balance and improve stability
3. Relieve pressure on weight-bearing joints
4. Aid in controlling involuntary muscle movements

37 When teaching Mrs. O'Hanlon to ambulate with a cane, the nurse should instruct her to:
1. Hold it in the hand on the same side as the affected lower extremity
2. Lean the body toward the cane when ambulating
3. Advance the cane and the affected extremity simultaneously
4. Shorten the stride of the unaffected extremity

Situation: Mrs. Lobinski, a 52-year-old Polish woman, is admitted for diagnostic evaluation for arteriosclerotic heart disease. In the year since her husband's death she has lived with her son and daughter-in-law. Currently she is not physically distressed but is apprehensive and alienated. Questions 38 through 48 refer to this situation.

38 Nursing care that may help Mrs. Lobinski to feel more at ease includes:
1. Telling her that everything is all right
2. Giving her a copy of hospital regulations
3. Reassuring her that staff will be available if she becomes upset
4. Orienting her to the environment and unit personnel

39 In understanding Mrs. Lobinski's diagnosis, the nurse knows that atherosclerosis is:
1. A loss of elasticity in and thickening and hardening of the arteries
2. Development of atheromas within the myocardium
3. A mobilization of free fatty acid from adipose tissue
4. Development of fatty deposits within the intima of the arteries

40 The nurse's initial approach to creating a therapeutic environment for Mrs. Lobinski should give priority to:
1. Accepting her individuality
2. Promoting her independence
3. Providing for her safety
4. Explaining everything that is being done for her

41 On one occasion after her family has been visiting, the patient is angry and says to the nurse, "My daughter-in-law says they can't take me home until the doctor lets me go. She doesn't understand; she isn't Polish." The nurse should best:
1. Ignore the statement
2. Point out that the physician makes decisions about discharge
3. Reflect on her feelings about her daughter-in-law
4. State, "You feel she doesn't want you home."

42 Mrs. Lobinski is placed on nitroglycerine therapy for angina. In administering nitroglycerine the nurse should:
1. Make certain the medication is stored in a dark container
2. Discontinue the medication if the patient complains of a headache
3. Limit the number of tablets to 4 daily
4. Replace the tablets if patient complains of sublingual tingling sensation on the tongue

43 Mrs. Lobinski demonstrates an increasing lability of mood and forgetfulness. She becomes disoriented to both time and place. A diagnosis of Alzheimer's disease is made. The nurse knows that Alzheimer's disease is characterized by:
1. Slowly progressive deficits in intellect, which may not be noted for a long time
2. Transient ischemic attacks
3. Remissions and exacerbations
4. Rapid deterioration of mental functioning due to arteriosclerosis

44 Mrs. Lobinski frequently switches from being pleasant and happy to being hostile and sad without apparent external cause. The nurse can best care for Mrs. Lobinski by:
1. Avoiding her when she is angry and sad
2. Attempting to give nursing care when she is in a pleasant mood
3. Encouraging her to talk about her feelings
4. Trying to point out reality to her

45 The nurse should provide Mrs. Lobinski with an environment that is:
1. Challenging
2. Nonstimulating
3. Variable
4. Familiar

46 It is important for a team working with patients having chronic organic brain disorders to adapt a common approach of care because the patients need to:
1. Learn that the staff cannot be manipulated

2. Relate in a consistent manner to staff
3. Accept external controls that are fairly applied
4. Have sameness and consistency in their environment

47 Patients with chronic brain syndromes need assistance in maintaining contact with society for as long as possible. Which one of the following groups might help Mrs. Lobinski achieve this goal?
1. Psychodrama
2. Recreation therapy
3. Remotivation therapy
4. Occupational therapy

48 The objective of remotivational therapy in psychiatry is to stimulate:
1. Face-to-face contact with other patients
2. Diminished psychologic faculties
3. Interaction with environment
4. Participation in educational activities

Situation: Melanie, a 21-year-old heroin addict, delivers a 5-pound baby boy. On the third day after delivery she leaves the hospital because the person caring for her 3-year-old, Mary, can no longer do this. She assures the staff she can care for both Mary and Baby Jesse. Questions 49 through 57 refer to this situation.

49 The nurse administers vitamin K, IM to Jesse immediately after birth to:
1. Prevent increased levels of serum bilirubin
2. Promote the synthesis of prothrombin
3. Substitute for normal bacterial flora
4. Decrease calciferol until renal clearance can take over

50 Typical signs of drug dependence in babies are due to withdrawal and usually begin within 24 hours after birth. The nurse should observe for:
1. Prolonged periods of sleep
2. Hyperactivity
3. Dehydration and constipation
4. Hypotonicity of muscles

51 Nursing care of Jesse should include:
1. Increasing environmental stimuli
2. Reducing elevated body temperature
3. Offering small frequent feedings
4. Administering methadone

52 When preparing Melanie prior to her discharge the nurse should:
1. Keep Melanie and the baby separated until Melanie is drug free
2. Refer Melanie to a drug rehabilitation program

3. Support Melanie's positive maternal responses
4. Help Melanie understand that Jesse's problems are due to her drug intake

53 Two weeks after Melanie and Baby Jesse are discharged, 3-year-old Mary is admitted with second- and third-degree burns over 30% of her body. She is placed in a warm isolation room with a humidifier, and strict sterile technique is instituted. The physician orders a Foley catheter to be inserted and IV therapy to begin immediately. One nurse is assigned to care for Mary each shift for the first 48 hours. Nursing observations in the first 48 hours of hospitalization are directed primarily toward preventing:
1. Pneumonia
2. Contractures
3. Dehydration
4. Shock

54 Despite Mary's physical distress and discomfort, her weight must be accurately taken because it provides a:
1. Baseline for future growth
2. Measure of the burned surface area
3. Basis for fluid replacement and medications
4. Guideline for dietary and fluid management

55 On the second day of hospitalization the nurse observes that Mary has decreased urinary output with edema. She recognizes this as one sign of possible complications that commonly occur in the first 2 days. The nurse observes Mary for other signs of complications, which are:
1. Vomiting, bradycardia
2. Subnormal temperature, slow pulse
3. High fever, disorientation
4. Rapid pulse, low blood pressure

56 The nurse must accurately measure Mary's urinary output each hour to evaluate kidney function. The minimum safe output of urine per hour is:
1. 10 to 20 ml
2. 25 to 50 ml
3. 40 to 60 ml
4. 75 to 100 ml

57 As Mary's burns begin to heal, the nurse attempts to involve her in therapeutic play to give her the opportunity to:
1. Learn to accept the hospital situation
2. Know the other children on the unit
3. Forget the reality of the situation for a while
4. Work out ways of coping with her fears

Situation: Mrs. Felton is admitted after an argument with her daughter, during which she incurred a sucking stab wound of the left thorax. Questions 58 through 72 refer to this situation.

58 In the emergency room the nurse should position Mrs. Felton:
1. On her back with her feet elevated
2. On her left side with head elevated
3. In high Fowler's position with left side supported
4. On her right side flat in bed

59 When assessing Mrs. Felton the nurse should be concerned primarily with the:
1. Quality and depth of respirations
2. Blood pressure and pupillary response
3. Amount of serosanguineous drainage
4. Degree and level of pain

60 Mrs. Felton has a large pressure dressing over the stab wound. The nurse recognizes that the purpose of this dressing is to:
1. Seal off major vessels
2. Prevent additional contamination
3. Protect the pleura
4. Maintain negative intrathoracic pressure

61 Postoperatively Mrs. Felton is given 24-hour IV feedings. The current fluid orders read: Bottle 1: 1000 ml 5% D/W; bottle 2: 1000 ml 5% D/0.9% NaCl; bottle 3: 1000 ml 5% D/0.33% NaCl. What is the approximate flow rate in drops per minute (IV tubing = 20 gtt/ml)?
1. 22
2. 27
3. 36
4. 42

62 The nurse should encourage Mrs. Felton to perform deep breathing exercises. The nurse recognizes that deep breathing exercises help to:
1. Counteract respiratory acidosis
2. Expand the alveoli
3. Increase blood volume
4. Decrease the partial pressure of oxygen

63 Mrs. Felton has chest tubes attached to a Pleurevac suction. When caring for Mrs. Felton, the nurse should:
1. Change the dressing daily using aseptic techniques
2. Palpate the surrounding area for crepitus
3. Empty the drainage bottles at the end of the shift
4. Clamp the chest tubes when ambulating the patient

64 Mrs. Felton complains of severe pain 2 days postoperatively. Initially the nurse should:
1. Have the patient rest
2. Take vital signs
3. Administer prn analgesic
4. Check time of patient's last medication

65 Arlene Felton, the 23-year-old daughter of Mrs. Felton, is arrested and is admitted to the psychiatric service for observation. On admission she has delusions of persecution and auditory hallucinations. The nurse greets Ms. Felton by saying "Good evening, Arlene. How are you?" Ms. Felton answers, "Arlene is bad." This is an example of:
1. Dissociation
2. Reaction formation
3. Displacement
4. Transference

66 Which of the following factors is most important in caring for a confused or delusional patient such as Arlene?
1. Maintain quiet, dim surroundings to minimize stimuli
2. Encourage realistic activity considering the patient's ability
3. Recognize she is completely unable to differentiate fantasy from reality
4. Provide physical hygiene and comfort to demonstrate she's worthy of receiving care

67 That evening Arlene appears quite upset. As the nurse approaches Arlene states, "I am hearing voices that are saying bad things about me." The nurse should:
1. Tell her she does not hear the voices
2. Encourage her not to listen to what the voices are saying
3. Suggest she join other patients playing cards
4. Let her know the staff understands she is frightened and stay with her

68 One day the nurse and Arlene sit together and draw. Arlene draws a face with horns on top of the head and says, "This is Arlene. She is a devil." The nurse should respond:
1. "Arlene, you are not a devil. Don't talk about yourself like that."
2. "Let's go to the mirror, Arlene, and see what you look like."
3. "Arlene, when I look at you, I see a young woman not a devil."
4. "I don't see a devil. Why do you see a devil?"

69 Arlene is receiving a major tranquilizer bid. Two thirds of the daily dose is given in the evening, one third in the morning. This is done to:
1. Help her sleep at night
2. Reduce sedation during the daytime
3. Maintain diurnal rhythms
4. Reduce increased assaultiveness in the evening

70 After 2 weeks of drug therapy the nurse notices that Arlene has become jaundiced, but she continues to give the tranquilizers until the psychiatrist can be consulted. In situations such as this:
1. Jaundice is sufficient reason to discontinue the tranquilizers
2. The psychiatrist's order for tranquilizers should be reduced by the nurse
3. Jaundice is a benign side effect and has little significance
4. The blood level of tranquilizers must be maintained once established

71 Arlene describes her delusions to the nurse. The nurse should:
1. Change the topic as soon as she begins to discuss her delusions
2. Encourage Arlene to discuss her delusions
3. Get Arlene involved in a repetitive project
4. Accept this as Arlene's reality without argument

72 After a couple of weeks in the hospital the nurse notices Arlene's hair is dirty and asks if she would like to wash it. Arlene answers, ''Yes, and I'd like to set it, too.'' The nurse uses this information to assess that Arlene:
1. Has some feelings of self-worth
2. Has a need for social reassurance and approval
3. Is quite open to suggestions
4. May be entering a hyperactive phase

Situation: Eight-year-old Kim is admitted to the hospital for the first time with a diagnosis of diabetes. Questions 73 through 77 refer to this situation.

73 Juvenile diabetes:
1. Has a more rapid onset than adult diabetes
2. Occurs more often in obese children
3. Does not always require insulin
4. Involves early vascular changes

74 The nurse plans to include the entire family in Kim's care and is especially concerned that:
1. The parents receive immediate instruction about urine testing

2. Kim is taught to give injections before being discharged
3. The parents and child be helped to understand their feelings about diabetes
4. Kim's activity be limited and the parents understand the need for this

75 The physician orders 12 units of NPH insulin daily for Kim. The vial reads 1 ml = 40 units of NPH. The nurse does not have an insulin syringe so, using a regular syringe, gives:
1. 6 minims
2. 4.5 minims
3. 4 minims
4. 3.5 minims

76 A night feeding planned for a juvenile diabetic includes milk, crackers, and cheese. This will provide:
1. High-carbohydrate nourishment for immediate utilization
2. Nourishment with latent effect to counteract late insulin activity
3. Encouragement for the child to stay on a diet
4. Added calories to help the child gain weight

77 Before Kim goes home, the nurse reviews with the family the importance of their knowing that Kim's insulin needs will be decreased when:
1. There is an emotional upset
2. An infectious process is present
3. She reaches puberty
4. She participates in active exercise

Situation: Mr. Boise, a 45-year-old tunnel guard, is diagnosed as having emphysema and is waiting for the examining physician. He has cyanosis of his lips and fingernails and is short of breath. Questions 78 through 85 refer to this situation.

78 In which position should the nurse place Mr. Boise?
1. Moderate Fowler's supported with pillows
2. Semirecumbent with one pillow
3. Sitting on the edge of the bed
4. Supine with his head slightly elevated

79 Mr. Boise's difficulty in breathing is caused by:
1. Spasm of the bronchi that traps the air
2. A too rapid expulsion of the air from the alveoli
3. An increase in the vital capacity of the lungs
4. Difficulty in expelling the air trapped in the alveoli

80 The nurse administers epinephrine hydrochloride (Adrenalin) immediately. The therapeutic effect of the drug is an outcome of action at:

1. Beta-adrenergic receptors in the bronchus and heart
2. Alpha-adrenergic receptors in the arteries and veins
3. Beta-adrenergic receptors in the arteries and veins
4. Alpha-adrenergic receptors in the bronchus and heart

81 The physician orders O_2 given in low concentration and intermittently, rather than in high concentration and continuously, to prevent:
1. Depression of the respiratory center
2. Decrease in red blood cell formation
3. Rupture of emphysematous bullae
4. Excessive drying of respiratory mucosa

82 Mr. Boise has been advised to use an isoproterenol hydrochloride (Isuprel) inhaler for intermittent periods of bronchial constriction. The nurse should tell him he might have:
1. Slow pulse, headache, muscle tension
2. Facial flushing, tingling in his fingers, dizziness
3. Rapid pulse, dizziness, pounding of his heart
4. Coldness of fingers and toes, muscle cramps, headache

83 When teaching the method of inhalation to Mr. Boise, the nurse explains that he should:
1. Inhale the vapors until all the drug has been nebulized
2. Stop inhaling the vapors as soon as he obtains relief
3. Never inhale more than 0.3 ml during any 20-minute period
4. Not repeat the dose more frequently than every 4 hours

84 The nurse also tells Mr. Boise that problems occurring with use of the inhaler will be lessened by:
1. Limiting use of the drug to the time required for relief of dyspnea
2. Using rapid, shallow (panting) respirations while using the inhaler
3. Interrupting the spray of inhalent while continuing normal breathing patterns
4. Gradually decreasing pressure on the spray control after initial relief is obtained

85 At home Mr. Boise had been taking aminophylline for control of his asthma. The planned effect of the drug is to:
1. Increase the ventilation-perfusion ratio of the bronchioles

2. Stimulate chemoreceptor control of bronchial dilation
3. Dilate the bronchial and coronary arteries
4. Dilate the smooth muscles of the bronchi

Situation: Mrs. Ryan, 82 years of age, is hard of hearing and has severe painful rheumatoid arthritis. She was admitted to a nursing home when she became incontinent and her family could no longer care for her. Questions 86 through 91 refer to this situation.

86 Mrs. Ryan's condition indicates that a primary consideration in her care would be her need for:
1. Immobilization of joints
2. Bladder control reeducation
3. Control of pain
4. Motivation and teaching

87 The nurse should be aware that the drug of choice in rheumatoid arthritis is:
1. Methocarbamol (Robaxin)
2. Aspirin
3. Cortisone
4. Gold salts

88 As to bed position, the nurse should encourage Mrs. Ryan to:
1. Assume the position in which she is most comfortable
2. Place pillows beneath her knees
3. Assume the Fowler's position
4. Maintain the limbs in extension

89 Since Mrs. Ryan's admission to the nursing home she has not been incontinent. While discussing her past and present elimination patterns the patient told the nurse of her anger at being bedridden and inability to go anywhere or see anyone. The nurse deducted that the patient's incontinence at home was:
1. An unconscious expression of hostility
2. A method to determine her family's love for her
3. A physiologic response expected with elderly bedridden patients
4. A way of maintaining control

90 When caring for Mrs. Ryan the nurse should:
1. Frequently ask if she needs the bedpan to void
2. Create an environment that prevents sensory monotony
3. Limit her fluid intake in the evening
4. Provide television or radio when the patient is alone

91 Mrs. Ryan uses an air-conduction hearing aid. This

hearing aid increases hearing sensitivity in instances of:
1. Diminished sensitivity of the cochlea
2. Perforation of the tympanic membrane
3. Immobilization of the auditory ossicles
4. Destruction of the auditory nerve

Situation: Mrs. Cole brought her son Johnny to the emergency room with severe gastrointestinal distress symptoms. Johnny is a normal infant who weighed 16 lb (7.2 kg) on his 6-month check-up last week. Questions 92 through 98 refer to this situation.

92 The nurse immediately prepares for:
1. Type and cross match
2. Intestinal intubation with continuous suction
3. Placement in an Isolette
4. Insertion of an IV line

93 Johnny is admitted to the hospital. The most important clinical manifestation of the degree of dehydration would be:
1. Sunken fontanel
2. Weight loss
3. Decreased urine output
4. Dry skin

94 When observing Johnny's laboratory reports, the nurse should be especially concerned about a decrease in sodium and:
1. Potassium
2. Chlorides
3. Calcium
4. Phosphates

95 Johnny is receiving parenteral therapy. His IV orders are 400 ml of 5% D/W and 0.45 NaCl to run in 8 hours. How many drops per minute should the IV run? (A minidropper is not available, so the nurse selects an IV set with a drop factor of 20 gtt per milliliter)
1. 10 to 11 gtt
2. 14 to 15 gtt
3. 16 to 17 gtt
4. 18 to 19 gtt

96 Johnny may be given liquids in small amounts. Which of the following liquids would be most beneficial for the nurse to give?
1. Cranberry juice
2. Liquefied gelatin
3. Ginger ale
4. Skim milk

97 An essential nursing action when caring for the small child with severe diarrhea is to:
1. Force fluids orally
2. Take daily weights
3. Replace lost calories
4. Keep body temperature below 100° F (37.7° C)

98 Johnny improves, and prior to discharge the nurse discusses Johnny's diet with Mrs. Cole. Mrs. Cole asks when Johnny should be able to drink from a cup. The nurse responds:
1. Five months
2. Seven months
3. Twelve months
4. Eighteen months

Situation: Mrs. Palecek, a 33-year-old housewife, is admitted to the hospital with a diagnosis of acute cholecystitis, biliary colic, and possible obstructive jaundice. She has a history of manic-depressive psychosis, which is currently under control. Questions 99 through 110 refer to this situation.

99 In addition to pain in the right upper quadrant, what other manifestations should the nurse expect Mrs. Palecek to have?
1. Intolerance of foods high in lipids
2. Vomiting of coffee-ground emesis
3. Gnawing pain when the stomach is empty
4. Melena and diarrhea

100 A cholecystectomy is scheduled. Vitamin K is administered to Mrs. Palecek prior to surgery, since vitamin K is used in the formation of:
1. Bilirubin
2. Prothrombin
3. Thromboplastin
4. Cholecystokinin

101 After surgery Mrs. Palecek is transferred to the Recovery Room with a nasogastric tube in place. She vomits 30 ml of bile-colored fluid. The nurse should:
1. Administer an antiemetic
2. Check the patency of the tube
3. Elevate the head of the bed
4. Encourage the patient to breathe deeply

102 Once Mrs. Palecek is returned to her unit, the nurse continues to make frequent checks of the wound area to note any tendencies toward excess bleeding or hemorrhage. These observations are made because:
1. Mrs. Palecek is exceedingly anxious about her incision

2. Mrs. Palecek's temperature is slightly elevated
3. Blood clotting may be hindered by lack of vitamin K absorption
4. Mrs. Palecek is complaining of much pain

103 Mrs. Palecek is prone to upper respiratory tract complications because of the:
1. Proximity of the incision to the diaphragm
2. Length of time required for surgery
3. Lowering of resistance caused by bile in the blood
4. Invasion of the bloodstream by infection from the biliary tract

104 Three days after the cholecystectomy Mrs. Palecek begins a full fluid diet. When the breakfast tray arrives, it has whole milk and cream for cereal. The luncheon tray includes whole milk and ice cream. When the surgeon visits at lunchtime he notes the tray's contents, is disturbed that the diet is not low in fat, and takes the tray away. In situations such as this the:
1. Dietitian should check the diet the patient receives
2. Physician orders the diet, and the order should be carried out as written
3. Nurse shares responsibility, since the physician's order was not questioned
4. Patient should have followed the physician's directions

105 When Mrs. Palecek is ready to be discharged, the dietitian instructs her to remain on her prescribed diet for several more weeks. Afterward she asks her nurse, "Will I have to stay away from fat for the rest of my life?" Which of the following responses would be most appropriate?
1. "You'll have to remain on a fat-free diet from now on to avoid problems."
2. "It's too early to say. Later, when we see whether your operation is successful, we'll know the answer."
3. "Only the doctor can answer that. Why don't you ask him about it before you are discharged from the hospital?"
4. "After you have fully recovered from surgery, you'll probably be able to eat a normal diet, avoiding excessive fat."

106 Six months later Mrs. Palecek is readmitted to the hospital. She has been eating and sleeping very little and has charged hundreds of dollars worth of purchases to her husband. The symptoms that the nurse should expect Mrs. Palecek to exhibit in the hospital would include:
1. Decreased psychomotor activity
2. Increased interest in the environment
3. Depressed mood and crying
4. Increased insight into her behavior

107 In view of Mrs. Palecek's elated state, the nurse should arrange for her to be in a room:
1. That will provide a great deal of stimuli
2. With as little furniture as possible
3. With a patient scheduled for a cholecystectomy
4. With another patient who is very quiet

108 Mrs. Palecek becomes loud and insulting and says to a staff member, "Get lost you old buzzard!" The nurse should say:
1. "Now, Mrs. Palecek, he isn't an old buzzard."
2. "Don't be so rude, Mrs. Palecek, it isn't necessary."
3. "Here is something I feel you might be interested in, Mrs. Palecek."
4. "Could you tell me why you are angry, Mrs. Palecek?"

109 Mrs. Palecek leaves group therapy in the middle of the session. She is obviously upset and crying when she meets the nurse. She tells the nurse that the group's discussion is too much for her. The most therapeutic nursing action would be to:
1. Suggest kindly but firmly that she return to the group to work out the conflict
2. Suggest that she accompany you to her room so that the 2 of you can talk about it
3. Respect her right to decline therapy at this time and simply report the incident to the rest of the health team
4. Ask the group leader what happened in the group and base your intervention on this additional information

110 Mrs. Palecek is to receive lithium carbonate. Which of the following studies should the nurse ensure is done prior to drug administration?
1. Neurologic studies
2. Fluid and electrolyte studies
3. Enzyme studies
4. Renal studies

Situation: Mrs. Wallace is a 22-year-old primigravida who is 6½ months pregnant. Questions 111 through 116 refer to this situation.

111 When she is seen by the physician Mrs. Wallace's blood pressure is 135/85 and she has gained 5 lb in the last 2 weeks. The nurse should:
1. Give Mrs. Wallace an appointment for 2 weeks hence
2. Prepare Mrs. Wallace for a vaginal examination
3. Take Mrs. Wallace's temperature and pulse
4. Prepare the equipment for testing Mrs. Wallace's urine

112 Preeclampsia is first suspected in a pregnant woman when there is:
1. An excessive weight gain
2. Fluctuation of the blood pressure
3. Progressive ankle edema
4. Presence of albuminuria

113 Mrs. Wallace has been diagnosed as having preeclampsia. When counseling Mrs. Wallace the nurse instructs her to follow a diet that includes:
1. Normal sodium with ample calories and protein
2. High sodium and calories and low protein
3. Moderate sodium, low calories, and ample protein
4. Low sodium and calories and high protein

114 Mrs. Wallace is receiving magnesium sulfate, 10 mg IM, every 4 hours. The nurse should check which of the following before giving the drug?
1. Respirations and patellar reflex
2. Blood pressure and apical pulse
3. Urinary output equal to fluid intake
4. Temperature and pulse rate

115 When giving $MgSO_4$ IM the nurse should:
1. Add 1% normal saline to maximize the dispersion of the drug
2. Add 1% procaine to minimize the pain caused by the drug
3. Use a large-gauge needle to expedite the dispersion of the drug
4. Give the injection in the outer aspect of the thigh

116 In severe preeclampsia, changes in blood values include an elevation of the hematocrit. This results from:
1. Hemodilution of pregnancy caused by increases in blood volume
2. Vasodilation due to an alteration in circulating fluid
3. Agglutination of red cells due to membrane fragility
4. Hemoconcentration due to a decrease in plasma volume

Situation: Mrs. Ivy is a 35-year-old woman who compulsively washes her hands. Her ritual includes 4 separate scrubs, which are carried out methodically. Questions 117 through 120 refer to this situation.

117 Although the nurse becomes tense as the ritual is carried out, it should be recognized that a compulsive act is one which:
1. A person performs willingly
2. Is performed after long urging
3. Is purposeful but useless
4. Seems absurd but is necessary to the person

118 Mrs. Ivy's basic personality is probably characterized by:
1. Marked emotional maturity
2. Elaborate delusional system
3. Doubts, fears, and indecisiveness
4. Rapid, frequent mood swings

119 In caring for Mrs. Ivy it is most important that the nurse:
1. Promote reality by showing that the ritual serves little purpose
2. Try to ascertain the meaning of the ritual by discussing it with the patient
3. Interrupt the ritual to demonstrate that the ritual does not control what happens
4. Allow the patient sufficient time to carry out the ritual

120 If interrupted in the performance of the ritual, Mrs. Ivy would most likely react with:
1. Aggression
2. Anxiety
3. Withdrawal
4. Hostility

ANSWERS AND RATIONALES

REVIEW QUESTIONS: Medical-surgical nursing
                         Psychiatric nursing
                         Maternity nursing
                         Pediatric nursing
COMPREHENSIVE TEST 1
COMPREHENSIVE TEST 2
COMPREHENSIVE TEST 3
COMPREHENSIVE TEST 4

REVIEW QUESTIONS
Medical-surgical nursing

1. (2) The hypothesis is the identification of the nursing problem after patient assessment. (c)
2. (4) The primary nurse provides or oversees all aspects of care, including assessment, implementation, and evaluation of that care. (b)
3. (2) Immunization programs prevent the occurrence of disease and are considered a primary intervention. (b)
4. (4) Specimens can be analyzed for specific information, which is objective. (c)
5. (4) When a plan does not adequately effect the desired outcome, the plan should be changed. (b)
6. (3) Nursing process is more than identifying a nursing problem; it is a step-by-step process that scientifically provides for patient-nursing needs. (b)
7. (3) The initial step in any process using problem solving is the collection of data. (a)
8. (3) Feedback permits the patient to ask questions and express feelings and allows the nurse to verify patient understanding. (b)
9. (1) The first action should be to remove the victim from a source of further injury. (b)

10. (2) The victim should be moved with great care to avoid additional spinal cord damage, which may be caused by such movement and can be irreversible. (b)
11. (4) Trendelenburg position is useful in treating shock, since it promotes gravity-induced venous return; warmth and fluids are also supportive to the patient. (a)
12. (3) People in panic could initiate the panic reaction in those who appear to be in control. (c)
13. (2) This group would succumb quickly to severe blood loss if dressings as indicated were not applied. (c)
14. (2) This organism is the specific causative agent for gas gangrene. (a)
15. (2) Tetanus antitoxin provides antibodies, which confer immediate passive immunity. (c)
16. (1) In active immunity, plasma cells provide antibodies in response to a specific antigen. (c)
17. (3) Painless enlargement of the cervical lymph nodes is often the first sign of Hodgkin's disease, a malignant lymphoma of unknown etiology. (c)
18. (2) For reasons unknown, Hodgkin's disease occurs most frequently between 15 and 30 years of age. (b)

559

19. (2) Radiation exposure may lead to depression of the bone marrow with subsequent insufficient WBCs to combat infection. (b)

20. (1) Depression of the bone marrow interferes with hemopoiesis and results in anemia. (a)

21. (3) Radiation in controlled doses is therapeutic. When uncontrolled or in excess amounts it is carcinogenic. (a)

22. (4) Paradoxical response to a drug is directly opposite to the desired therapeutic response. (c)

23. (2) Many antihypertensive agents such as methyldopa (Aldomet), which lower peripheral vascular resistance, may cause orthostatic hypotension, especially when the patient first gets up. Therefore blood pressure should be monitored in both a supine and an upright position. (c)

24. (4) Hypokalemia causes a flattening of the T wave in the ECG because of its effect on muscle function. (c)

25. (2) Potassium follows insulin into the cells of the body, thereby raising the cellular potassium and preventing fatal arrhythmias. (c)

26. (4) Methyldopa decreases tissue concentration of norepinephrine and interferes with its release in response to sympathetic stimulation. Therefore the vasoconstriction caused by norepinephrine is inhibited. (c)

27. (4) Sitting on the edge of the bed before getting up is recommended because it gives the body a chance to adjust to the effects of gravity on circulation in the upright position. (b)

28. (4) Unexpressed rage or anger affects the sympathetic nervous system, precipitating the release of epinephrine and norepinephrine, constricting the blood vessels, and thus raising arterial blood pressure. (b)

29. (2) If there is a decreased output with increased conservation of body fluid, the blood pressure will be increased and vice versa. (c)

30. (1) Because propranolol (Inderal) competes with catecholamines at the beta-adrenergic receptor sites, the normal increase in heart rate and contractility in response to exercise does not occur. This, combined with the drug's hypotensive effect, may lead to dizziness. (c)

31. (2) Streptococcal infections occurring in childhood may result in damage to the heart valves; an autoimmune reaction occurs between antibodies (made against the bacteria) and the heart valves, particularly the mitral. (b)

32. (2) Pulse should be assessed, since a cutdown may interfere with venous flow distal to the site. There is also a danger of phlebitis in the area. (a)

33. (2) The nurse should foster open lines of communication with the patient. (a)

34. (1) Due to pooling of blood in the extremities, there is an increased hazard of peripheral emboli in patients who have had mitral replacement. (c)

35. (3) Temperatures over 102.2° F (38.9° C) result in increased metabolism and cardiac work load. (a)

36. (4) Fluid will accumulate in the intrapleural space following thoracic surgery because of trauma and the inflammatory response. During the first 24 hours 500 ml of fluid is not uncommon. Gradually this amount will decrease. When less than 150 ml of fluid is aspirated in 24 hours and there is no air leak, the chest tube may be removed. The other responses are excessive and may indicate complications. (c)

37. (1) Chills, headache, nausea, and vomiting are all signs of a transfusion reaction. (a)

38. (3) Shivering should be prevented because peripheral vasoconstriction results in increases in temperature, circulatory rate, and oxygen consumption. (b)

39. (1) Adams-Stokes syndrome is a result of complete atrioventricular block. The ventricles take over the pacemaker function in the heart, but at a much slower rate than that of the SA node. As a result there is decreased cerebral circulation, causing syncope. (a)

40. (4) Ventricular fibrillation and ventricular standstill are both death-producing arrhythmias because the heart is not functioning as a pump. Immediate action is required or death will occur as a result of anoxia to brain and other vital organs. (a)

41. (4) Pulse pressure is obtained by subtracting the diastolic from the systolic readings after taking a blood pressure. (b)

42. (4) A culture and testing of the antibiotic sensitivity of secretions or drainage identify the causative organism (culture) and those antibiotics to which the organism is particularly sensitive or resistant. (a)

43. (4) This is the causative organism of tuberculosis and is acid fast. (a)

44. (2) The respiratory membrane, comprising the alveolar and capillary walls, is extremely thin, facilitating exchange of respiratory gases. (a)

45. (1) Tidal air is defined as the amount of air exhaled normally after a normal inspiration. The volume of air exhaled forcibly after a normal expiration is the expiratory reserve volume. The volume of air that can be forcibly inspired over and above a normal inspiration is the inspiratory reserve volume. The air trapped in the alveoli that cannot be exhaled is the residual volume. (b)

46. (2) The dosage of streptomycin sulfate is carefully regulated according to the combination of drugs prescribed and the severity of the illness because of potential eighth cranial nerve and vestibular damage (ototoxicity). (b)

47. (3) INH often leads to pyridoxine (vitamin B_6) deficiency because they compete for the same enzyme. This is most often manifested by peripheral neuritis, which can be controlled by regular administration of vitamin B_6. (b)

48. (3) Streptomycin is ototoxic and may cause damage to the auditory and vestibular portions of the eighth cranial nerves. (c)

49. (1) The etiology of a spontaneous pneumothorax is com-

monly the rupture of blebs on the lung surface. Blebs are similar to blisters. A spontaneous pneumothorax may also occur secondary to a variety of pulmonary diseases such as COPD and TB. (b)

50. (2) A patient with a spontaneous pneumothorax will generally experience sudden chest pain on the affected side, which may also involve the arm and shoulder. (b)

51. (3) As a person with a tear in his lung (such as a ruptured bleb) inhales, air moves through that opening into the pleural space. This creates a positive pressure and causes partial or complete collapse of the lung. (c)

52. (4) Pressure within the pleural cavity causes a shift of the heart and great vessels to the unaffected side. This not only decreases the capacity of the unaffected lung, but also impedes the filling of the right side of the heart. This in turn leads to a decreased cardiac output. (c)

53. (3) A pneumothorax results in decreased surface area for gaseous exchange. If the unaffected pleural regions cannot compensate, CO_2 builds up in the blood (hypercapnia). The patient becomes drowsy and may lose consciousness. The body attempts to compensate by increasing the respiratory and pulse rate and by the renal retention of bicarbonate. (c)

54. (4) Oxygen is supplied to prevent anoxia but cannot be given in higher concentrations because, in an individual with emphysema, a low P_{O_2} (not high P_{CO_2}) is the only respiratory stimulus. (b)

55. (4) Fluctuations occur with normal inspiration and expiration until the lung is fully expanded. If these fluctuations do not occur, the chest tube may be clogged. The nurse should milk the chest tube q 1 to 2 h and avoid kinking the tube. (a)

56. (4) Chest x-ray films or radiographs reveal the degree to which the lung fills the pleural cavity and also the presence of any mediastinal shift. (c)

57. (1) Carbon monoxide binds with hemoglobin more avidly than does oxygen; the progressive results are dyspnea, asphyxia, and death. CO does not block CO_2 transport, it does not inhibit vasodilation, and it does not form bubbles in plasma. (b)

58. (4) With an oxygen debt a muscle would show primarily low levels of oxygen and low levels of ATP due to the low levels of aerobic respiration and high levels of lactic acid. Such conditions bring about weakness and pain. Glycogen and calcium levels might be low, high, or moderate, depending on the recent dietary history of the individual, but such conditions do not have direct bearing on the concept of oxygen debt. (c)

59. (3) Accumulated CO_2 will powerfully stimulate the breathing center of the brain stem, forcing resumption of respiration even if the person has fainted first. (b)

60. (1) Vomiting may result in aspiration of vomitus, since it cannot be expelled, causing pneumonia or asphyxia. (b)

61. (1) $C° = {}^5/_9 (F° - 32)$
$= {}^5/_9 (99.8 - 32)$
$= {}^5/_9 (67.8)$
$= 37.7$ (b)

62. (3) The pulse increases to meet increased tissue demands for O_2 in the febrile state. (a)

63. (3) Vincent's angina (trenchmouth) is an infection of the mouth resulting in bleeding gums, pain on swallowing and talking, and fever. (c)

64. (1) Pain and swelling should subside prior to 1 week postoperatively. Continued pain may indicate infection. (b)

65. (3) Following an SMR, hemorrhage from the nares is frequently detected by vomiting of blood that has been swallowed. (b)

66. (3) Personality and psychologic stresses cause changes that influence the development of ulcerative colitis. (b)

67. (1) Potassium, the major intracellular cation, functions with sodium and calcium to regulate neuromuscular activity and contraction of muscle fibers, particularly heart muscle. In hypokalemia these symptoms develop. (b)

68. (4) All diagnostic tests should be explained to a patient to allay anxiety and promote cooperation. (b)

69. (1) To take advantage of the anatomic position of the sigmoid colon and the effect of gravity, the patient should be placed in a left Sim's position for the enema. (b)

70. (3) If the height of the enema can increases, the force and rate of flow also increase. If the can is raised excessively, damage to the mucosa may result and it will make it much more difficult for the patient to tolerate the procedure. (b)

71. (3) Administration of additional fluid when a patient complains of abdominal cramps adds to discomfort because of additional pressure. By clamping the tubing a few minutes the cramps generally subside, and the enema can be continued. (b)

72. (1) Since the soft tissues of the GI tract lack sufficient quantities of x ray–absorbing atoms (as are naturally present in the dense calcium salts of bone) an x ray–absorbing coating of barium is used for radiologic studies. (c)

73. (2) Milk and the caffeine in cola are chemically irritating to the intestinal mucosa; they also promote secretion of gastric juice. (b)

74. (3) Close proximity to the nurses' station is vital so that the patient may be frequently observed, since behavior is unpredictable. (a)

75. (4) Paraldehyde is a sedative that is ordered to reduce psychomotor stimuli. (b)

76. (2) Protein helps to correct severe malnutrition; moderate fat limits the need for bile; high calorie and high vitamin diet prevents the need for tissue breakdown. (b)

77. (2) The liver detoxifies alcohol and is the organ most often damaged in chronic alcoholism; the high-caloric

diet prevents tissue breakdown, which produces additional amino acids and nitrogen. (a)

78. (2) Thiamine and nicotinic acid help convert glucose for energy and therefore nerve activity. (a)

79. (3) The parasympathetic nervous system (a branch of the autonomic nervous system) causes increased GI motility and secretions. The adrenal cortex releases glucocorticoids which also stimulate the GI tract, increasing the acidity of the secretions. (b)

80. (2) A nurse must actively try to understand her own feelings and prejudices, since these will affect her ability to assess the patient's behavior objectively. (b)

81. (3) Ulcerative colitis is linked to psychoemotional stress and generally is exacerbated when conflicts exist. (c)

82. (1) Due to influence of glucocorticoids and acetylcholine, peristalsis is increased, causing cramping and diarrhea with subsequent weight loss. As ulceration occurs, loss of blood leads to anemia. (b)

83. (2) Occult blood in the stool could indicate active bleeding; the stool should also be examined for microorganisms to detect early infections that could easily become systemic by spread through the damaged intestinal mucosa. (b)

84. (2) As a result of chronic irritation, the colon becomes thin and may perforate. (b)

85. (4) Fruits and vegetables contain cellulose, which is not absorbed and provides bulk to encourage defecation. Low-residue diets are necessary in the acute phase of ulcerative colitis to prevent irritation of the colon. (c)

86. (2) Milk and milk products are not tolerated well because they contain lactose, a sugar that is converted to galactose by lactase. (c)

87. (3) Sleeping on pillows raises the upper torso and prevents reflux of the gastric contents through the hernia. (a)

88. (2) Oral hypoglycemics may be helpful when some functioning of the beta cells exists, as in adult onset diabetes. (a)

89. (2) Many people are ashamed or have a distorted body image when they know they have a long-term disorder. (a)

90. (2) Ketones are given off when fat is broken down for energy. (a)

91. (1) Infection increases the body's metabolic rate, and insulin is not available for increased demands. (b)

92. (3) During treatment for acidosis the patient may develop hypoglycemia, and this complication should be observed for carefully by the nurse, even without an order. (b)

93. (2) Hypokalemia promotes mental confusion and apathy and poor muscular contractions and weakness; these effects are related to the diminished magnitude of the neuronal and muscular cell resting potentials. Abdominal distention is due to flaccidity of the abdominal musculature. (b)

94. (2) Each patient should have an individually devised diet

selecting commonly used foods from the American Diabetic Association exchange diet; family members should be included in the diet teaching. (b)

95. (3) The concept of nursing care and rehabilitative care are synonymous. All nursing intervention aims to assist an individual in maximizing capabilities and coping with modifications in life-style. (b)

96. (2) Orange juice has a higher proportion of simple sugars, which are readily available for conversion to energy. (c)

97. (4) The ketones produced in excess in the diabetic are acetoacetic acid, beta hydroxybutyric acid, and acetone. The major ketone, acetoacetic acid, is an alpha ketoacid that lowers the blood pH (acidosis). (c)

98. (4) The urinary catheter and drainage bag should always remain a closed sterile system; fractional urine should only be drawn from the catheter, not the collection bag. (b)

99. (4) ADH from the posterior pituitary promotes water uptake by the kidney tubules; the result is decreased urinary output—an antidiuretic effect. An antidiuretic effect also occurs due to aldosterone secreted by the adrenal cortex, but this is a secondary, osmotic effect to sodium reabsorption and not a direct antidiuretic effect. (c)

100. (3) Resorption of sodium and water in the tubule decreases urinary output and retains body fluids. (c)

101. (3) Antidiuretic hormone aids the body in retaining fluid by causing the nephrons to reabsorb water. (b)

102. (1) The respiratory and urinary systems interact with the bicarbonate buffer system to preserve the normal body pH of 7.4 (7.35 to 7.45). Consider the following equation: $CO_2 + H_2O \rightleftarrows H_2CO_3 \rightleftarrows H^+ + HCO_3^-$. Increased respiration blows off CO_2 and pulls the equation to the left; this decreases H^+ and the pH rises (less acidity). Decreased respiration results in CO_2 buildup, which pushes the equation to the right; this increases H^+ and the pH falls (more acidity). Similarly, the kidneys either conserve or excrete bicarbonate, which respectively shifts the equation to the left or the right, thereby helping to adjust the pH. (a)

103. (3) Mineralocorticoids, such as aldosterone, cause the kidneys to retain Na^+ ions. With Na^+, water is also retained, serving to elevate blood pressure. Absence of this hormone thus causes hypotension. (b)

104. (2) Patients with Addison's disease have decreased ability to adapt to exposure to infectious agents because of deficit of glucocorticoids. (b)

105. (1) Glucocorticoids help maintain blood sugar and liver and muscle glycogen content. A deficiency of glucocorticoids causes hypoglycemia, resulting in breakdown of protein and fats as energy sources. (c)

106. (4) Exertion, either physical or emotional, places additional stress on the adrenal glands, which may precipitate Addisonian crisis. (b)

107. (1) Lack of mineralocorticoids causes hyponatremia, hypovolemia, and hyperkalemia. Dietary modification,

as well as administration of cortical hormones, is aimed at correcting these electrolyte imbalances. (a)

108. (1) Lack of mineralocorticoids (aldosterone) leads to loss of Na$^+$ ions in urine and subsequent hyponatremia. (a)

109. (1) Hydrocortisone is a glucocorticoid that has antiinflammatory action and aids in metabolism of carbohydrate, fat, and protein, causing elevation of blood sugar. Thus it enables the body to adapt to stress. (b)

110. (3) Fludrocortisone acetate has a strong effect on sodium retention by the kidneys, which leads to fluid retention (weight gain and edema.) (a)

111. (3) Hydrocortisone succinate (Solu-Cortef) is a glucocorticoid. A patient undergoing a bilateral adrenalectomy must be given adrenocortical hormones to enable adjustment to the sudden lack of these hormones, which occurs with this surgery. (c)

112. (3) Glucocorticoids (e.g., cortisone) and mineralocorticoids (e.g., aldosterone) are secreted by the adrenals. The pancreas secretes insulin and glucagon. The anterior hypophysis (pituitary gland) secretes STH, FSH, LH, LTH, TSH, and ACTH. The gonads secrete testosterone (primarily in males) and estrogen and progesterone (primarily in females.) (a)

113. (3) Hyperplasia of the adrenal cortex leads to increased secretion of cortical hormones, which causes signs of Cushing's syndrome. (c)

114. (1) Cushing's syndrome results from excess adrenocortical activity. Signs include slow wound healing, buffalo hump, hirsutism, weight gain, hypertension, acne, moon face, thin arms and legs, and behavioral changes. (c)

115. (4) Adrenal insufficiency results after an adrenalectomy, causing hypotension due to fluid and electrolyte alterations. (b)

116. (3) The adrenal gland, stimulated by the sympathetic nervous system, secretes epinephrine during stressful situations. The ensuing alarm reaction involves rapid adjustment of the body to meet the emergency situation. There may be modifications in the secretion of hormones from the pituitary, thyroid, and pancreas due to varying physiologic situations, but such modification is not directly related to meeting emergency situations. (a)

117. (1) Adrenal steroids help an individual adjust to stress. Unless received from external sources, there would be no hormone available to cope with surgical stresses following adrenalectomy. (c)

118. (2) Fowler's position facilitates localization of the infection by pooling pelvic drainage. (b)

119. (3) The period of time between ovulation and the next menstruation is relatively constant at about 14 days; variations in the total cycle time are due to variations in the preovulatory phase. Within a 30-day cycle the first 15 days are preovulatory, ovulation occurs on day 16, and the next 14 days are postovulatory. Ovulation therefore occurs on January 17. (b)

120. (4) Although the usual incubation period of syphilis is about 3 weeks, clinical symptoms may appear as early as 9 days or as long as 3 months after exposure. (b)

121. (4) The FTA test utilizes fluorescent treponemal antibody to conclusively confirm a diagnosis of syphilis; the Wasserman, Kahn, and VDRL tests use nonspecific antigen and, although convenient for screening, may give false positives (e.g., glandular fever, systemic lupus erythematosus) and false negatives with late syphilis. (c)

122. (2) The tertiary stage is noncontagious; tertiary lesions contain only small numbers of treponemes; fatal cases involve the aorta, CNS, or the eye. (c)

123. (1) Condylomata acuminata are variably sized cauliflower-like warts occurring principally on the genitals or rectum (anogenital skin or mucosa) of both females and males; they are generally associated with poor hygiene. (c)

124. (3) The gonococcus *Neisseria gonorrhoeae* possesses fastidious growth requirements that are met by the columnar epithelium of the urethra, prostate, seminal vesicles, and epididymis in males and the urethra, endocervix, fallopian tubes, and Skene and Bartholin glands in the female. (b)

125. (2) Gonorrhea frequently is an ascending infection and affects the fallopian tubes. (b)

126. (1) The *Candida* genus consists of several species of fungi commonly found in the mouth, sputum, vagina, and stools of otherwise normal people. Candidiasis (*Candida* infection) arises in certain individuals when local resistance is decreased through prolonged antibiotic therapy or with certain diseases (e.g., diabetes) and special debilitating conditions (e.g., drug addiction). (a)

127. (1) *Neisseria gonorrhoeae* is a gram-negative diplococcus commonly infecting the urogenital tract of both males and females. (b)

128. (2) Laparoscopy involves direct visualization of the uterus via fiberoptics. The procedure is carried out through a stab wound below the umbilicus. (a)

129. (1) Increased intracranial pressure places tension on vital brain centers, causing signs such as increased systolic blood pressure, slow bounding pulse, elevated temperature, and changes in the respiratory pattern. (b)

130. (2) An unconscious individual loses control of voluntary sphincters surrounding the urethra and anus. (b)

131. (3) It is important to help the patient with expressive aphasia regain maximum communicative abilities early during the hospital stay. This action provides hope but it avoids the patient. (b)

132. (2) Atony permits the bladder to fill without being able to empty. As pressure builds within the bladder the urge to void occurs, and just enough urine is voided to relieve the pressure and the urge to void. The cycle is repeated as pressure again builds up. Thus small amounts are voided without emptying the bladder. (c)

133. (4) A strange environment, as well as the anxiety associated with private body functions such as elimination, interferes with the patient's ability to relax the urinary sphincter to void. (a)

134. (4) This is considered a routine procedure to meet basic physiologic needs and is covered by a consent signed on admission. (c)

135. (4) After a CVA the patient should be repositioned frequently, and passive ROM exercises should be instituted to prevent deformity. (b)

136. (1) Footboards provide a broad flat surface that helps to keep the foot in a position of dorsiflexion. (a)

137. (1) Although patients who have suffered a CVA are expected to be emotionally labile, the major factors determining the reaction to illness are past experiences and coping mechanisms. (a)

138. (2) Change of position every 2 hours helps prevent the respiratory, urinary, and cutaneous complications of immobility. (a)

139. (2) The nurse should focus on the positive aspects of the patient's progress to aid in motivation. (c)

140. (1) As part of the rehabilitative process after a CVA a patient must be encouraged to participate in his own care to the extent to which he is able and extend the abilities by establishing short-term goals. (b)

141. (3) The brain's blood supply through vessels branching from the circle of Willis provides excellent collateral circulation; partial blockage of one vessel is compensated for by flow from other vessels. (b)

142. (2) After removal of arterial obstruction by endarterectomy, adequate circulation may be monitored by observation of skin color, pulses, and skin temperature. (b)

143. (4) Polycythemia vera results in pathologically high concentrations of erythrocytes in the blood; the consequent increase in viscosity increases the tendency toward thrombosis. (b)

144. (4) Vitamin C is an intercellular cement substance. (c)

145. (3) According to the Nurse Practice Act, a nurse may independently treat human responses to actual or potential health problems. (c)

146. (1) Viscosity, a measure of a fluid's internal resistance to flow, is increased as the number of red cells suspended in plasma increases. (a)

147. (1) Anxiety causes an increase in body secretions, which stimulates tissue changes. (c)

148. (3) This test allows the physician to perform a biopsy of gastric mucosa. (c)

149. (3) The nurse was negligent in using a stretcher with worn straps because her actions did not reflect those of a reasonably prudent nurse. (b)

150. (4) Barium salts used in GI series and barium enemas coat the inner lining of the GI tract and then absorb x rays passing through, thereby giving an outline of the surface features of the tract on a photographic plate. The GI tract, without barium salts, would be virtually transparent to x rays, and a photographic plate would not show any contrast. The barium salts do not give off any visible light, do not fluoresce, and are not dyes in the sense that gentian violet is a dye and absorbs specific wavelengths of visible light. (a)

151. (3) Anxiety or stress causes a hypersecretion of hydrochloric acid, which results in actual physiologic changes in the tissue itself. (a)

152. (2) Hemorrhage following erosion of blood vessel walls is often the first symptom that leads patients to seek medical assistance. (b)

153. (2) Applesauce, cream of wheat, and milk are bland foods that do not irritate the gastric mucosa. (c)

154. (2) Some weight-bearing on the uninvolved leg helps to maintain its muscle tone. (c)

155. (1) This position causes no strain by supporting the fracture site. The involved leg must be maintained in alignment, avoiding adduction. (a)

156. (3) The palms should take all the weight to prevent nerve damage in the axillary area. (a)

157. (3) Following a fracture, if blood supply is cut off or impaired, necrosis to the bond may occur due to lack of oxygen and nutrient perfusion. (c)

158. (3) This type of contracture frequently occurs when the patient lies in bed with knees bent and thighs not abducted. (b)

159. (1) Intramedullary nails are used to maintain bone alignment and provide support along the femur's length. (c)

160. (1) Paralysis of sympathetic vasomotor nerves after administration of spinal anesthesia results in dilation of blood vessels, which causes a subsequent drop in blood pressure. (c)

161. (1) Turning the patient to the side promotes drainage of secretions and prevents aspiration, especially when the gag reflex is not intact. This position also brings the tongue forward, preventing occlusion of the airway by the relaxed tongue. (a)

162. (3) Since pain is an all-encompassing and often demoralizing experience, the patient should be kept as pain free as possible. (b)

163. (1) A latex test can determine autoimmune rheumatoid factor in the blood. (a)

164. (3) Heat causes muscles to relax, and therefore injury during exercise can be minimized. (c)

165. (1) The nurse's positive attitude encourages and motivates the patient. (a)

166. (1) A long-range goal should be to involve the patient in many activities of daily living; such a program can help to reestablish the patient in her former life-style. (b)

167. (2) Braces would restrict movement of the joint, causing increased deformity. (a)

168. (1) Laminar air flow decreases the risk of bone infection, since potentially contaminated air continuously flows

away from the sterile field, decreasing the concentration of air-borne pathogens. (c)

169. (4) Warm compresses at or slightly above body temperature increase blood flow to the area and decrease edema. (c)

170. (1) The temperature range for tepid applications is slightly below body temperature. (c)

171. (4) Conduction is the conveyance of energy such as heat, cold, or sound by direct contact. (a)

172. (4) Cold reduces the sensitivity of receptors for pain in the skin. In addition, local blood vessels constrict, limiting the amount of interstitial fluid and its related pressure and discomfort. (b)

173. (3) In transfer, the suspected back-injured patient should be positioned to keep the vertebral column in perfect alignment (back straight) to prevent further spinal cord damage by vertebral (bone) movements. (a)

174. (4) Both legs and generally the lower part of the body are paralyzed in paraplegia (quadriplegia involves paralysis of all four limbs). (a)

175. (2) The anterior root of a spinal nerve consists of axons of motor neurons located in the ventral horns of the gray matter; the axons carry (motor) impulses to skeletal muscles. (c)

176. (4) Lack of or reduced body movement predisposes paraplegic or quadriplegic patients to urinary infection and stone formation. (a)

177. (4) Care should be aimed at encouraging independence. (a)

178. (1) The bones respond to the stress of walking (running, etc.) by laying down bone substance along lines of stress; inactivity leads to reduced bone deposition and actual bone decalcification. (b)

179. (1) Bowel or bladder distention results in autonomic nerve impulses ascending the cord to the point of injury; here the reflex is completed and autonomic outflow causes piloerection (goosebumps), sweating, and splanchnic vasoconstriction; the latter causes hypertension and a pounding headache. (c)

180. (4) The woman is unconscious, and although her husband can consent, he has no legal power to refuse a treatment for her unless he was previously given power of attorney; the court can make a decision for her. (b)

181. (2) The confused or delerious patient protects herself by assimilating small amounts of information at a time, since the mental status prevents total awareness of reality. (b)

182. (2) The pain may prevent the patient from ingesting anything by mouth. (b)

183. (2) Tic douloureux, also referred to as trigeminal neuralgia, is an inflammation of the fifth cranial nerve, which innervates the midline of the face and head. (c)

184. (1) The patient was in severe constant pain prior to admission, and the emotional stress, muscle tensing, and diminished nutritional intake led to exhaustion and fatigue. (c)

185. (1) The nurse should avoid swiftly walking past the patient, since drafts or even slight air current can initiate pain. (c)

186. (1) Carbamazepine (Tegretol) is an analgesic, anticonvulsive drug used for the treatment of epilepsy and trigeminal neuralgia. (c)

187. (2) Recurrence of pain would be unusual, since the nerve is severed. (a)

188. (2) Since neurectomy eliminates sensations, the patient must be counseled to get regular dental check-ups to prevent local infection from becoming systemic. (c)

189. (4) Electrodes are attached to sensory nerves or over the dorsal column; a transmitter is worn externally and, by electric stimulation, may be used to interfere with the transmission of painful stimuli, as needed. (c)

190. (3) A rhizotomy is the resection of posterior nerve roots to eliminate nerve impulses associated with severe pain from the thoracic area (as in lung cancer). (c)

191. (2) Due to cellular destruction, Na^+ is lost in the interstitial fluid, whereas K^+ is liberated from the injured cells, causing hyperkalemia. (c)

192. (4) As a result of fluid loss and sodium retention, urine output is diminished. Output of less than 30 ml per hour, however, is considered a sign of shock. (c)

193. (3) Since a great deal of intravascular fluid is lost during the first 48 hours in evaporation, exudate, and edema, urinary output is not expected to equal the intake but increases from that of the first day. An output of less than 30 ml per hour is an indication of shock. (c)

194. (3) Vitamin C is essential for wound healing, since it provides a component of intercellular ground substance that develops into collagen and is necessary to build supportive tissue. (a)

195. (1) The skin is the first line of defense against infection. When much of the skin is destroyed, the individual is left vulnerable to infection. (a)

196. (1) Curling's ulcer, an ulcer of the GI tract, is related to the excess secretion of stress-related hormones that increase hydrochloric acid. (a)

197. (2) The fluid in a bottle hung over a person lying down possesses potential energy. When that fluid is allowed to run into a person intravenously, the fluid's potential energy is then converted to kinetic energy (energy of motion). (c)

198. (4) Blood albumin, a protein, establishes the plasma colloid osmotic pressure because of its high molecular weight and size. Red cell formation occurs in red marrow and can be related to albumin only indirectly; albumin is the blood transport protein for thyroxin, which stimulates metabolism in all cells, including those in red bone marrow. White cells may be activated by antigens and substances released from damaged or diseased cells. Blood

clotting involves blood protein fractions other than albumin; for example, prothrombin and fibrinogen are within the alpha and beta globulin fractions. (b)

199. (2) Plasma proteins do not easily pass through the capillary endothelium; O_2, CO_2, glucose, ions, amino acids, and water pass through more easily. However, the slight leakage of plasma proteins through the capillary endothelium is important and results in edema if not corrected (one of the lymphatic system's functions is to return "leaked" plasma proteins to the blood). (a)

200. (3) Osmosis is the diffusion of water through a selectively permeable membrane. Such membranes include cellular membranes and capillary walls, and osmosis occurs in the kidney tubules and in all capillary beds. Dialysis is the diffusion of small molecules down their concentration gradients through a selectively permeable membrane; even though water is a small molecule, its diffusion through a selectively permeable membrane is defined as osmosis. Active transport is the movement of molecules against a concentration gradient and requires energy input; osmosis, dialysis, and diffusion are passive processes. (a)

201. (1) Malaria is caused by the protozoan parasite *Plasmodium*. Plasmodia appear in the bloodstream during chills and fever. (b)

202. (1) Parasites invade the erythrocytes, subsequently dividing and causing the cell to burst. The spleen enlarges due to sloughing of red blood cells. (c)

203. (3) Although it is not possible to prevent infection once an individual is bitten by an infected mosquito, early treatment with quinine sulfate, a selective parasiticide, can arrest disease and prevent recurrence. (b)

204. (4) *Plasmodium falciparum,* in persons who have been treated with quinine, causes hemoglobinuria, intravascular hemolysis, and renal failure as a result of destruction of red blood cells. (c)

205. (3) Fluid and electrolyte disturbances occur due to fever, excess diaphoresis, vomiting, and diarrhea. (c)

206. (3) Maintaining adequate nutritional and fluid balance is essential to life and must be accomplished during periods when intestinal motility is not excessive so that absorption can occur. (b)

207. (2) Since 650 mg of quinine are present in 1000 ml of solution, administration of more than 77 ml of solution per minute would exceed the recommended rate of 50 mg per minute. (c)

208. (2) Signs of cinchonism, such as tinnitus, headache, dizziness, and nausea, indicate that the maximum therapeutic level of quinine has been attained. (c)

209. (2) Quinine, when administered orally, can cause gastric irritation resulting in nausea and vomiting. By administering such a medication after meals, the irritating effect is minimized. (c)

210. (1) Quinine sulfate is used in malaria when the plasmodia are resistant to the less toxic chloroquine. However, a new strain of *Plasmodium*, resistant to quinine, must be treated with a combination of quinine (quick acting) and pyrimethamine and sulfonamide (slow acting). (b)

211. (2) The patient still had the right to make decisions regarding hours of sleep and time of medication. The concept of invasion of rights or intrusion applies. (b)

212. (1) A definitive diagnosis of the cellular changes associated with benign prostatic hypertrophy is made by biopsy with subsequent microscopic evaluation. (c)

213. (1) The phenolsulfonphthalein test (PSP) and the urea clearance evaluate the kidney's ability to excrete a particular substance from the blood; the urine concentration of specific gravity is an indicator of the kidney's ability to concentrate urine. (b)

214. (2) Inability to empty the bladder, as a result of pressure exerted by the enlarging prostate on the urethra, causes a backup of urine into the ureters and finally the kidneys (hydronephrosis). (b)

215. (3) The total amount of irrigation solution instilled into the bladder is eliminated with urine and therefore must be subtracted from the total output to determine the volume of urine excreted. (b)

216. (3) The excreted ammonia combines with H^+ in glomerular filtrate to form an ammonium ion (NH_4^+), which is excreted from the body. This mechanism helps to rid the body of excess H^+, maintaining acid-base balance. (b)

217. (3) The prostate gland is a tubuloalveolar gland shaped like a ring, with the urethra passing through its center. (a)

218. (2) Protein breakdown liberates cellular potassium, leading to hyperkalemia, which can cause cardiac arrhythmia and standstill. The failure of the kidneys to maintain a balance of K^+ is the main indication for dialysis. (b)

219. (4) Hemodialysis exposes the blood to a solution that contains normal concentrations of nutrients and low concentrations of waste products; the blood and dialyzing solution are separated by a selectively permeable membrane. The diffusion of small molecules (wastes) from the blood to the dialyzing solution is an example of dialysis. (c)

220. (4) Serum hepatitis is transmitted by blood or blood products. The hemodialysis and routine transfusions needed for a patient in renal failure constitute a great risk of exposure. (b)

221. (2) Insertion of an arteriovenous shunt represents a break in the first line of defense against infection, the skin. An infection of an arteriovenous shunt can be avoided by strict aseptic technique. (a)

222. (3) Homologous serum hepatitis is caused by the B virus and is transmitted by contact with the blood of carriers of the disease. (c)

223. (2) Urine is strained to determine if any calculi or calcium gravel has been passed. (a)

224. (4) Dietary intake of calcium, as well as parathormone excretion, will increase calcium blood levels. (c)

225. (4) Roast beef and a baked potato have only moderate amounts of calcium compared with the other choices. (b)

226. (2) Cystolithiasis denotes the presence of stones in the bladder, whereas cystolithectomy refers to the removal of the bladder stones. (c)

227. (4) Calcium and phosphorus are components of these stones and should therefore be avoided while an acid environment is not favorable to their development. (a)

228. (1) Calcium oxalate renal stones can be prevented by adhering to a diet low in ash, calcium, and oxalate. (b)

229. (1) Patient should have sufficient intake to produce a liter of fluid per day while taking this drug to prevent crystal fomation. (b)

230. (3) Because furosemide and aspirin compete for the same renal excretory sites, salicylate toxicity may occur even with lower dosages. (c)

231. (1) Congestive heart failure is the failure of the heart to pump adequately to met the needs of the body, resulting in a backward buildup of pressure in the venous system. Adaptations include edema, ascites, hepatomegaly, tachycardia, dyspnea, and fatigue. (a)

232. (2) Right-sided heart failure causes increased pressure in the systemic venous system, which leads to a fluid shift into the interstitial spaces. Because of gravity, the lower extremities are first affected in an ambulatory patient. (b)

233. (4) In right-sided heart failure blood backs up in the systemic capillary beds; the increase in plasma hydrostatic pressure causes edema. (c)

234. (3) Measuring an area is an objective assessment and is not subject to individual interpretations. (b)

235. (1) Failure of the right ventricle causes an increase in pressure in the systemic circulation. To equalize this pressure, fluid moves into tissues, causing edema, and into the abdominal cavity, causing ascites. (c)

236. (3) The CVP measures the pressure within the right atrium. For an accurate reading the zero point must be level with the right atrium. This is approximately the midaxillary line. (a)

237. (2) Oxygen perfusion is impaired during prolonged edema, leading to tissue ischemia. (b)

238. (1) The presence of excess solute (Na$^+$) in the nephric tubules effectively decreases the water concentration of the glomerular filtrate and urine; water passively diffuses (osmosis) from the kidney tubule cells into the urine to equalize the water concentration. (b)

239. (2) Chlorothiazide (Diuril) affects electrolyte absorption in the nephron, causing an increased excretion of sodium and chloride. (b)

240. (1) Shock may have different etiologies (i.e. hypovolemic, cardiogenic, septic, anaphylactic) but always involves a drop in blood pressure and failure of the peripheral circulation because of the involvement of the sympathetic nervous system. (b)

241. (4) Burger's disease (thromboangiitis obliterans) is characterized by vascular inflammation, usually in the lower extremities, leading to thrombus formation. As a result of impaired circulation, there is burning pain and intermittent claudication. (a)

242. (2) Constriction of the peripheral blood vessels and the resulting increase in blood pressure impair circulation and limit the amount of oxygen being delivered to body cells, particularly the extremities. (a)

243. (4) Injured tissue cannot heal properly because of cellular deprivation of oxygen and nutrients; ulceration and gangrene may result; diminished sensation decreases awareness of injury. (b)

244. (1) Myocardial infarction may cause an increased irritability of tissue or interruption of normal transmission of impulses. Arrhythmias occur in about 90% of patients after an MI. (b)

245. (2) LDH, CPK, and SGOT are enzymes released into the blood from cardiac muscle cells when the myocardium is damaged. (a)

246. (2) Lidocaine (Xylocaine) decreases the irritability of the ventricles and is used in the treatment of ectopic beats originated by a ventricular focus. (b)

247. (2) Asystole refers to the absence of atrial and ventricular contractions, which can cause death within several minutes. (b)

248. (1) Irreversible brain damage will occur if a patient is anoxic for more than 4 minutes. (a)

249. (1) Resuscitative efforts are futile unless an airway is patent so that oxygen expired by the resuscitator can reach the alveoli. (a)

250. (1) When 2 people implement CPR, one inflates the lungs and the other performs cardiac compression. A ratio of 1 breath per 5 compressions with a rate of 60 compressions per minute is considered most effective. (a)

251. (4) The sternum must be depressed at least 1½ to 2 inches (3.7 to 5 cm) to compress the heart adequately between the sternum and vertebrae to simulate cardiac pumping action. (c)

252. (1) Blood samples from the right atrium, right ventricle, and pulmonary artery would all be about the same with regard to oxygen concentration. Such blood has slightly more CO_2 than does pulmonary vein blood, which already has had some of its CO_2 expelled into the alveoli. Such blood also contains slightly less oxygen than does systemic arterial blood and pulmonary vein blood that has been charged with oxygen in the alveoli of the lungs. (b)

253. (2) A coenzyme is the nonprotein part of an enzyme and serves as a catalyst in chemical changes. (a)

254. (4) Lipoproteins are simple proteins combined with lipid to facilitate circulation of fat in blood. (b)

255. (4) Fruits contain less natural sodium than do other foods. (b)

256. (3) Saturated fats found in animal tissue are more dense than unsaturated fats, which are found in vegetable oils; the denseness has nothing to do with digestibility. (c)

257. (4) Animal fats are high in dense saturated fats. (a)

258. (4) Since triglycerides are constructed from fatty acids bonded (esterfied) to glycerol, their breakdown releases fatty acids as well as glycerol. (a)

259. (3) Cholesterol is an absolutely essential structural and functional component of most cellular membranes. That it is associated with atherosclerotic plaques does not detract from its essential functions in membrane structure and steroid hormone metabolism. (b)

260. (2) Cholesterol is a sterol found in tissue and is attributed in part to diets high in saturated fats. (a)

261. (1) Epidemiologic studies have linked inhalation of asbestos, ferrous ore, and chromate to increased incidence of lung cancer. Incidence also increases with age. (b)

262. (4) A spirometer measures lung volumes such as tidal volume, inspiratory reserve volume, and expiratory reserve volume. From these measurements capacities such as the vital capacity can be calculated. (b)

263. (2) The tidal volume is the amount of air inhaled and exhaled while breathing normally. (b)

264. (4) After administration of local anesthetic during a bronchoscopy, fluids and food should be withheld until the gag reflex returns. Since a biopsy will have been performed, coughing should not be encouraged because it may initiate bleeding. (a)

265. (3) The phrenic nerve stimulates the diaphragm. After destruction of the nerve on the operative side, the diaphragm will move upward, decreasing the size of the empty space. This will help prevent mediastinal shift. (c)

266. (3) Because Mrs. Smith has just had major surgery and has an ET tube in place, secretions could be loosened by administering humidified air and by frequent turning and coughing. (b)

267. (1) After a pneumonectomy the patient should be positioned on the operative side or back to maintain normal expansion of the remaining lung. (c)

268. (2) After a pneumonectomy the mediastinum may shift toward the remaining lung, or the remaining lung could shift toward the empty space, depending on the pressure within the empty space. Either of these shifts would cause the trachea to move from its normal midline position. (The trachea is palpated above the suprasternal notch.) (c)

269. (2) The phrenic nerves conduct motor nerve impulses to the diaphragm; cutting one phrenic nerve will paralyze the portion of the diaphragm innervated by that nerve. (c)

270. (3) The orthopneic position is a sitting position that enables maximum lung expansion for gaseous exchange, since the abdominal organs do not provide pressure against the diaphragm and gravity facilitates the descent of the diaphragms. (c)

271. (4) Isoproterenol stimulates the beta receptors of the sympathetic nervous system, causing bronchodilation and increased rate and strength of cardiac contractions. (b)

272. (2) Isoproterenol is a synthetic catecholamine that causes increased heart contraction (positive inotropic effect) and increased heart rate (positive chronotropic effect). If toxic levels are reached, side effects occur and the drug should be withheld and the physician notified. (c)

273. (2) As a result of the narrowed airways, exhalation is difficult, leaving air trapped in the lung. Distention of alveolar walls to accommodate this volume leads to emphysema. (b)

274. (4) Destruction of the alveolar walls leads to diminished surface area for gaseous exchange and an increased CO_2 level in the blood. (b)

275. (2) Loss of elasticity causes difficult exhalation with subsequent air trapping. Patients with emphysema are taught to use accessory abdominal muscles and to breathe out through pursed lips to help keep the air passages open until exhalation is complete. (b)

276. (1) Retention of CO_2 after exhausting the available bicarbonate ions as buffers will cause a lower pH (respiratory acidosis). (b)

277. (3) Thoracic pressure is reduced because thoracic volume is increased as the diaphragm descends. Rising pressure in the alveoli and the intrapleural space or relaxation of the diaphragm would expel air from the alveoli. (c)

278. (4) An Ambu bag is a piece of equipment that can be compressed at regular intervals by hand to temporarily ventilate the patient in respiratory arrest. (a)

279. (1) During suctioning of a patient, negative pressure (suction) should not be applied until the catheter is ready to be drawn out because, in addition to the removal of secretions, oxygen is being depleted. (b)

280. (2) Hypersensitivity to a foreign substance can cause an anaphylactic reaction. Histamine is released, causing bronchial constriction, increased capillary permeability, and dilation of arterioles. This decreased peripheral resistance is associated with hypotension and inadequate circulation to major organs. (c)

281. (3) Hypersensitivity results from the production of antibodies in response to exposure to certain foreign substances (allergens). Prior exposure is necessary for the development of these antibodies. (c)

282. (4) Diphenhydramine hydrochloride (Benadryl), like other antihistamines, competes with histamine at receptor sites. This alleviates the effects of histamine, which include increased dilation and permeability of capillaries (the cause of urticaria). (c)

283. (3) Penicillinase alters the structure of the penicillin molecule so that it loses its antibiotic and allergenic capabilities. (c)

284. (3) Soap and water reduce surface tension, facilitating the removal of microorganisms by friction; without friction the other 3 factors would have little, if any, value. (b)

285. (4) Vitamin K, synthesized by the bacterial flora of the intestine, promotes the liver's synthesis of prothrombin, an important blood clotting factor. (c)

286. (2) Prevention of serum hepatitis from blood transfusions can be accomplished through screening donors. (b)

287. (1) This is an enzyme that is released early in the course of liver damage. (c)

288. (3) Gamma globulin, an immune globulin, contains most of the antibodies circulating in the blood. When injected into an individual, it prevents a specific antigen from entering a host cell. (b)

289. (4) Phenobarbital depresses the CNS, particularly the motor cortex, producing side effects such as lethargy, loss of appetite, depression, and vertigo. (b)

290. (3) The virus is present in the stool of patients with infectious hepatitis, so special handling is required. The virus may also be present in the urine and in the nasotracheal secretions of such patients. (b)

291. (1) Various aspects of hospitalization and diagnosis could cause the patient anxiety. The nurse should determine what factor(s) disturbs the patient. (b)

292. (2) The facial nerve may be damaged during surgery, and drooping of the area results due to loss of muscle tone. (b)

293. (2) This position minimizes discomfort and decreases facial edema. (b)

294. (2) If the dressing is too tight, impaired cerebral circulation may result. (b)

295. (4) Pitressin is a vasoconstrictor that is used with great success in controlling GI bleeding. (c)

296. (2) Removal of the fundus of the stomach destroys those parietal cells which secrete intrinsic factor needed to complex vitamin B_{12} as a preliminary to its absorption in the ileum. (c)

297. (3) The antrum is responsible for gastrin production, which stimulates HCl secretion; its removal reduces HCl secretion and thus reduces irritation of the gastric mucosa. (c)

298. (4) The act of eating allows the hydrochloric acid in the stomach to work on and be neutralized by food rather than to irritate the gastric mucosa. (b)

299. (1) Peptic ulcers may occur when there is a conflict between a strong drive for independence in an individual who has an unconscious need to be dependent. (c)

300. (4) The patient should be encouraged to rest mind and body, and sedatives may be indicated to achieve this goal. (b)

301. (2) Irritation of the mucosa may cause increased bleeding or perforation and therefore should be avoided. (b)

302. (3) Iron is needed in the formation of hemoglobin. (b)

303. (3) The heart may be strained by prolonged anemia because the blood's decreased viscosity eases its return to the heart from the periphery. In accordance with Starling's law, the greater volume of blood returning to the heart will stretch it and result in greater cardiac output. The increased blood viscosity occurring in polycythemia forces the heart to strain to maintain adequate peripheral blood flow; the heart must exert greater force to propel the more viscous blood through the circulatory system. (a)

304. (3) Ileostomy drainage is liquefied and continuous, so irrigations are not generally indicated. Emotional stress of any kind can stimulate peristalsis and thereby increase the volume of drainage. (b)

305. (1) Vitamin B_{12} (extrinsic factor) combines with intrinsic factor, a substance secreted by the parietal cells of the gastric mucosa; forming hemopoietic factor. Hemopoietic factor is only absorbed in the ileum, from which it travels to bone marrow and stimulates erythropoiesis. (c)

306. (4) Trauma to the abdominal wall and to the stoma should be avoided, so contact sports are contraindicated. (a)

307. (2) A rectal catheter should be inserted approximately 4 inches (10 cm), since this will be far enough to pass the rectal sphincter. This depth is less likely to cause damage to the mucosa than deeper insertions. (b)

308. (2) A rectal tube promotes maximum benefits in 30 minutes. This allows adequate time for gas escape. (b)

309. (2) Intussusception is a telescoping or prolapse of a segment of the bowel within the lumen of an immediately connecting part. (a)

310. (3) A flat plate film of the abdomen visualizes abdominal organs as they are. (b)

311. (1) Semi-Fowler's position aids in drainage and prevents spread of infection throughout the abdominal cavity. (b)

312. (2) Paralytic ileus occurs when neurologic impulses are diminished, as from anesthesia, infection, or surgery. (a)

313. (4) Thrombophlebitis is an inflammation of the vein that occurs with the formation of a clot. Signs include pain (especially on dorsiflexion of the foot), redness, warmth, tenderness, and edema. (a)

314. (1) Coumarin derivatives are ordered day by day, based on the prothrombin time of the patient; this test gives a good index of the individual's clotting ability. (b)

315. (3) Dicumarol depresses prothrombin activity and inhibits the formation of several of the clotting factors by the liver. Its antagonist is vitamin K, which is involved in prothrombin formation. (c)

316. (4) In the absence of insulin, which facilitates the transport of glucose into the cell, the body breaks down proteins and fats to supply energy ketones, a byproduct of fat metabolism. These accumulate, causing metabolic acidosis (pH < 7.35). (b)

317. (3) In the absence of insulin glucose cannot enter the cell or be converted to glycogen, so it remains in the blood. Breakdown of fats as an energy source causes an accumulation of ketones, which results in acidosis. The lungs, in an attempt to compensate for lowered pH, will blow off CO_2 (Kussmaul respirations). (c)

318. (2) Regular insulin is rapid acting and is used to meet a patient's current insulin needs, as in diabetic coma or in coverage for fractional urine test results. (b)

319. (1) Once treatment with insulin for diabetic ketoacidosis is begun, potassium ions reenter the cell, causing hypokalemia; therefore potassium, as well as replacement fluids, is generally supplied. (b)

320. (1) Ice milk is a dairy product, whereas bread is not. Exchanges must be from the same food group, supplying approximately equal amounts of nutrients. (b)

321. (2) Glucagon is an insulin antagonist produced by the alpha cells in the islets of Langerhans. It causes breakdown of glycogen and protein to glucose. (b)

322. (2) The Nurse Practice Act states that the nurse will do health teaching and administer nursing care supportive to life and well-being. (a)

323. (2) A triglyceride comprises 3 fatty acids and a glycerol molecule. When energy is required, the fatty acids are mobilized from adipose tissue for fuel. (b)

324. (2) Insulin stimulates cellular uptake of glucose and also stimulates the membrane-bound pump for Na^+ and K^+, resulting in K^+ influx into insulin's target cells. The resulting hypokalemia is offset by parenteral K^+ administration. (c)

325. (3) Since oral hyperglycemics stimulate the islets of Langerhans to produce insulin, a regular interval between doses should be maintained. (a)

326. (3) Blood has a narrow pH range of 7.35 to 7.45. Venous blood (pH 7.35) is more acidic and closer to 7.35 than is arterial blood, which is normally closer to a pH of 7.45. (a)

327. (1) Somatotropin promotes growth by accelerating amino acid transport into cells. Oversecretion after full growth and epiphase close results in acromegaly, with enlargement of bones and overlying soft tissue in feet, hands, jaw, and cheeks. Growth hormone also increases blood glucose levels. (b)

328. (4) The hypophysis does not directly regulate insulin release. This is controlled by blood glucose levels. Since somatotropin release will cease following the hypophysectomy, any elevation of blood glucose due to somatotropin will also cease. (a)

329. (1) ACTH is released in response to decreased blood levels of cortisol. The ACTH then stimulates release of more adrenocortical hormone. (c)

330. (3) Because of the location of the pituitary gland, there is swelling in the brain after the gland's removal. This edema may result in increased intracranial pressure. (c)

331. (2) Endocrine gland secretions (hormones) are inactivated by the liver and other tissues fairly rapidly; continuous hormonal secretion by endocrine glands is regulated by immediate feedback controls, and the body's metabolism is always close to being suitable to the body's immediate needs. (b)

332. (1) Metrorrhagia refers to uterine bleeding at any time other than during the menstrual period. (a)

333. (2) Since hysterectomy indicates removal of the uterus but no other female organs, menstruation will cease, but the hypophyseal and ovarian hormone cycles will continue. (a)

334. (4) Thrombophlebitis is an inflammation of the vein, which is associated with the formation of a clot (thrombus). The signs of inflammation include pain, redness, swelling, and heat. (a)

335. (1) Menstruation is the shedding of the endometrial lining of the uterus. A patient who has had a hysterectomy has had her uterus removed and will no longer menstruate. (b)

336. (2) Flushing of the head and neck with accompanying diaphoresis is known as hot flashes and is a symptom of estrogen deprivation. (c)

337. (1) Uninformed consent constitutes an artificial consent. Sufficient information was not given. (b)

338. (1) The ovaries are responsible for producing the female sex hormones estrogen and progesterone. A bilateral oophorectomy causes an abrupt cessation in the production of most of these hormones (the adrenal cortex produces small quantities of female sex hormones) and results in surgical menopause. (b)

339. (4) Depletion of ovarian hormones causes vasomotor instability. Periodic systemic vasodilation is then triggered by the sympathetic nervous system, causing the feeling of warmth. (c)

340. (3) The lack of utilization of gonadotropin by the ovaries causes an elevation of gonadotropin in the blood. Ovarian function is diminished; there is little or no follicular activity. (c)

341. (1) Ovulation occurs when the blood levels of FSH and LH are both relatively high, but it is the surge of LH secretion in midcycle that is responsible for ovulation. (a)

342. (2) High levels of plasma estrogen inhibit pituitary secretion of FSH; this effect appears to be mediated by the hypothalamus and its releasing factors. (c)

343. (3) Rectal temperature is the most accurate. Oral temperature is contraindicated, since dysphagia may cause excessive salivation. (a)

344. (1) Dysphagia is difficulty in swallowing. (a)

345. (3) Dysphasic patients have difficulty in communicating verbally, and alternate means may be indicated. (b)

346. (3) The paralyzed side has decreased muscle tone, which affects blood pressure readings. (b)

347. (4) The maximum amount of fluid to be administered at the first tube feeding is 250 ml to prevent distention and/or aspiration. (c)

348. (2) Although tube feedings are often administered at room temperature, formula at body temperature is tolerated best. (b)

349. (2) Since the cardiac sphincter of the stomach is slightly opened because of the nasogastric tube, rapid feeding could result in regurgitation. (b)

350. (3) The optic chiasm is the point of crossover of some

optic nerve fibers in the cranial cavity at the base of the brain. The optic tracts conduct nerve impulses from the optic chiasm to other brain regions. (b)

351. (4) The thalamus associates sensory impulses with feelings of pleasantness and unpleasantness; therefore it is partly responsible for emotions. The cortical limbic system is also involved in expression of emotions. (c)

352. (3) The arteries communicating (anastomosing) at the base of the brain are referred to as the circle of Willis. The blood vessel anastomosis in the palm is the volar arch. The brachiocephalic sinus is a single large branch of the aorta, and the brachial plexus is a nerve communication network in the region of the neck and axilla. (b)

353. (1) Dendrites of the cochlear nerve terminate on the hair cells of the organ of Corti in the cochlea. (a)

354. (3) The ear bones that transmit and amplify air pressure waves from the tympanic membrane to the oval window of the cochlea are located in the inner ear. The tympanic membrane separates the outer from the middle ear. The cochlea and semicircular canals mainly compose the inner ear. The eustachian tube links the middle ear and nasopharynx. (b)

355. (1) Since the organ of hearing is the organ of Corti, located in the cochlea, nerve deafness would most likely accompany damage to the cochlear nerve. Since the vestibular and cochlear nerves fuse to form cranial nerve VIII, infection in the vestibular might also affect the cochlear nerve, but this is less likely to cause nerve deafness than direct injury and infection to the cochlear nerve itself. The trigeminal and vagus nerves are not concerned with hearing. (b)

356. (4) The medulla has centers for control of breathing, heartbeat, and blood vessel diameter. Sexual development is initiated by changes in hypothalamic and pituitary metabolism at puberty. Body temperature control and water balance are also hypothalamic functions. Voluntary movements are mediated through the somatomotor area of the frontal cerebral lobe. The opercular-insular area of the parietal cerebral lobe is concerned with taste sensations. (a)

357. (1) One of the centers for reflex control of respiration is in the medulla. Another important reflex respiratory center is in the pons. The other brain regions—cerebral cortex, hypothalamus, and cerebellum—may influence respiration, but not so directly as the centers in the medulla and pons. (a)

358. (2) The labyrinth is the inner ear and consists of the vestibule, cochlea, semicircular canals, utricle, saccule, cochlear duct, and the membranous semicircular canals. A labyrinthectomy is performed to alleviate the symptom of vertigo but results in deafness, since the organ of Corti and cochlear nerve are located in the inner ear. (b)

359. (4) In otosclerosis there is an overgrowth of bone in the middle ear, fusing the 3 ossicles. The ossicles can no longer vibrate, and conduction is impaired; therefore hearing aids are generally of no use. Removal of the stapes eliminates this obstruction. (b)

360. (1) Decadron is a corticosteroid that acts on the cell membrane to prevent the normal inflammatory responses as well as stabilize the blood-brain barrier. (c)

361. (2) Decadron increases glucogenesis, which may case hyperglycemia. (c)

362. (2) Decadron increases the production of hydrochloric acid, which may cause GI ulcers. Patients should also be instructed to take Decadron with meals. (c)

363. (4) Peristalsis and gastric motility should not be increased, to help prevent ulcer formation in the gastric mucosa. (c)

364. (3) Prolonged use of sodium bicarbonate may cause systemic alkalosis as well as retention of sodium and water. (b)

365. (2) Any hormone normally produced by the body must be withdrawn slowly to allow the appropriate organ to adjust and resume production. (b)

366. (2) In myasthenia gravis the effectiveness of acetylecholine is reduced, interfering in muscle contraction. Inadequate contraction of the ocular muscles results in double vision (diplopia). (c)

367. (2) Tensilon is an anticholinesterase compound that drastically increases muscle strength when administered to an individual with myasthenia gravis. (c)

368. (2) Myasthenia gravis is a chronic degenerative disorder with exacerbations precipitated by emotional stress, ingestion of alcohol, and physical stress such as infection. (a)

369. (3) It is a degenerative disease that occurs equally in both sexes during adulthood. (b)

370. (1) Neostigmine is an anticholinergic that increases the peristaltic activity of the intestines, resulting in hyperactive bowel sounds. (b)

371. (4) The response should be kept as optimistic as possible while still being realistic. (b)

372. (2) Swimming would help to keep muscle tone supple, without requiring fine motor activity. (b)

373. (1) The aerobic oxidation of glucose occurring in the mitochondrion produces 38 moles of ATP for every mole of glucose oxidized. (b)

374. (4) Prostigmin, an anticholinesterase drug, causes temporary relief of symptoms of myasthenia gravis in patients who have the disease and is therefore an effective diagnostic aid. (b)

375. (2) Prolonged use of steroids may cause leukopenia due to bone marrow depression. (c)

376. (4) Open-ended questions provide a milieu in which people can verbalize their problems rather than be placed in a situation of forced response. (a)

377. (4) Rheumatoid arthritis is a chronic systemic disease of

inflammatory and degenerative changes in the body's connective tissue. (c)

378. (2) Gold salts, bound to plasma proteins, are distributed irregularly throughout the body, but the highest concentration occurs in the kidneys. The slow excretion of gold salts cannot keep up with their intake, and they accumulate in the kidneys, causing damage. (b)

379. (2) Allopurinol interferes with the final steps in uric acid formation by inhibiting xanthine oxidase. (a)

380. (2) Colchicine decreases the formation of lactic acid, which may promote the deposition of uric acid in the joints. It also decreases the inflammatory responses. (b)

381. (1) The connective tissue degeneration of SLE results in the involvement of the basal cell layer, producing a butterfly rash over the bridge of the nose and the malar region. (b)

382. (3) Scleroderma is an immunologic disorder characterized by inflammatory, fibrotic, and degenerative changes. (c)

383. (3) Not only the skin but also major organs are affected, including the heart, lungs, liver, kidney, and intestine. Death usually occurs due to cardiac arrest, renal failure, or cachexia. (c)

384. (2) Open-angle glaucoma has an insidious onset with increased intraocular pressure, causing pressure on the retina and blood vessels in the eye. Peripheral vision is decreased as the visual field progressively diminishes. (b)

385. (1) In glaucoma, intraocular pressure is elevated and must be returned to normal. (b)

386. (4) The contraction permits the lens to return to its normal bulge, decreasing focal length and allowing focus on near objects. (c)

387. (1) Sedatives have no effect on intraocular pressure. (b)

388. (3) Since continued use of eyedrops is indicated, an extra supply should always be available. (b)

389. (1) Eye medications are applied directly to the eye. (a)

390. (1) Acetazolamide (Diamox) is a carbonic anhydrase inhibitor that decreases the inflow of aqueous humor and controls intraocular pressure. (c)

391. (4) Cortisone, a steroid, stabilizes lysosomal membranes, inhibiting the release of proteolytic enzymes during inflammation. This anti-inflammatory drug also maximizes vasoconstrictor effects. (b)

392. (4) A second-degree burn over 30% of the body is considered critical. Shock, infection, electrolyte imbalance, and respiratory distress are life-threatening complications that can occur. (a)

393. (3) Extravasation of fluid into the interstitial spaces results in hemoconcentration and decreased volume. Pain is present in both first- and second-degree burns, and inhalation of hot air can cause tracheal edema. (b)

394. (3) Potassium replacement is generally not indicated in the management of burns because hyperkalemia results from liberation of potassium from injured cells. (c)

395. (3) Tetanus immune globulin provides the individual with antibodies against tetanus. This is used if the patient has never received tetanus toxoid or antitoxin, which confer active immunity (the body makes its own antibodies in response to the antigen). (c)

396. (4) Sulfisoxazole (Gantrisin) is a short-acting sulfonamide. These drugs have an antibacterial effect by acting as antimetabolites and interfering with the microorganism's ability to manufacture folic acid. (a)

397. (1) Bethanechol (Urecholine) improves the muscle tone of an atonic bladder, facilitating micturition. (c)

398. (3) Application of a solution of sodium bicarbonate (a mild alkali) after thoroughly flushing with water is the best way to treat acid-splashed skin, since the alkali will neutralize residual acid on the skin. Although sodium hydroxide is also an alkali and would neutralize acid, it is too strong and can also cause burns. Sodium chloride or sulfate are neutral salts whose application to burned skin would serve no immediate (first aid) benefit. (b)

399. (1) A good first aid treatment for an alkali burn is to wash it with water and then to wash it with a weak acid, which will chemically neutralize residual alkali still on the skin. This procedure will not reverse the chemical damage already done by the alkali (burns) but will minimize additional chemical change. (a)

400. (2) The average adult human body is about 60% water. A newborn infant is about 80% water and reaches the 60% figure about a year after birth. (a)

401. (1) The osmoreceptors are located in the hypothalamus. Under conditions of dehydration they stimulate the neurohypophysis to release the hormone ADH into the blood. The kidney tubules are the target organ for ADH; they reabsorb more water from glomerular filtrate. (b)

402. (2) The kidneys regulate fluid balance by adjusting the amount of fluid reabsorbed from glomerular filtrate. (b)

403. (1) Interstitial fluid constitutes about 16% of body weight, which is 10 to 12 L in an adult male of 150 lb. (b)

404. (3) The concentration of potassium is greater inside the cell and is extremely important in establishing a membrane potential, which is an important factor in a cell's ability to function. (b)

405. (1) Approximately 25 of the 40 L of the body's fluid are in the cells. (c)

406. (1) Blood plasma and interstitial fluid are both part of the extracellular fluid and are of the same ionic composition. (b)

407. (4) Since the plasma colloid osmotic pressure (COP) opposes glomerular filtration, a decrease in blood proteins will increase the GFR. (b)

408. (2) A balloon tube is inserted into the renal pelvis to drain urine, necessitating an incision into the kidney (nephrostomy). (c)

409. (4) The ureters are implanted in a segment of the ileum, and urine drains continually because there is no sphincter. (b)

410. (3) Dressings retain an undetermined amount of drainage, which would result in an inaccurate reading. (c)

411. (4) Because of the anatomic position of the incision, drainage would flow by gravity and accumulate under the patient lying in the supine position. (b)

412. (2) Maintenance of a patent airway is always the priority, since airway obstruction impedes breathing and may result in death. (c)

413. (3) A drop in blood pressure, a rapid pulse, cold clammy skin, and oliguria are all signs of shock, which, if not treated promptly, can lead to death. (a)

414. (4) When mixing two compatible drugs, if one is a narcotic, it should be drawn up first. This prevents contaminating the second vial with a narcotic. (c)

415. (1) Cystitis is an inflammation of the bladder that causes frequency, urgency, pain on mitricurition, and hematuria. (a)

416. (2) The length of the urethra is shorter in a female than in a male; therefore microorganisms have a shorter distance to travel to reach the bladder. The proximity of the meatus to the rectum in females also increases this incidence. (b)

417. (1) Ammonium chloride causes metabolic acidosis. As a result, the kidneys secrete the excess hydrogen ions, increasing the acidity of the urine. An acid urine is essential for methenamine mandelate's (Mandelamine) antibacterial action. (c)

418. (2) Since the female urethra is shorter than that in the male, the bacteria can more easily invade the bladder. (a)

419. (2) Bundle branch block interferes with the conduction of impulses from the AV node to the ventricle supplied by the affected bundle. The conduction through the ventricles is delayed, which is evidenced by a widened QRS complex. (c)

420. (3) The PM electrode is inserted via the venous system into the right ventricle where PM-generated impulses can directly stimulate the ventricles. (c)

421. (4) The SA node is the heart's natural pacemaker. An electronic pacemaker is used in some individuals to supply an impulse that stimulates the heart to bring about more efficient heart action. (a)

422. (3) Atropine blocks vagal stimulation of the SA node, resulting in an increased heart rate. (c)

423. (3) A demand pacemaker only functions when the heart rate falls below the set rate of the pacemaker. The patient can detect pacemaker malfunctions by monitoring his pulse rate and noting a drop below the set rate. (b)

424. (2) Ventricular fibrillation will cause irreversible brain damage and then death within a few minutes because the heart is not pumping blood. Defibrillation or CPR (until defibrillation is possible) must be initiated immediately. (a)

425. (4) Bradycardia refers to a heart rate of less than 60 per minute. It may be a physiologic adaptation to a long-term exercise, cardiac disease, or digitalis toxicity. (a)

426. (2) Six to 8 L provide enough oxygen without altering the patient's blood gases, which would cause increased respiratory distress. (b)

427. (4) Open flames or spark production from static electricity (e.g., leather-soled shoes, wool, silk, nylon and Dacron blankets, ungrounded electric appliances) can initiate explosions and fire in the presence of higher than normal O_2 levels. (a)

428. (3) Irritability and restlessness increase metabolic rate (including increased heart rate) and pressure, which complicates congestive heart failure. (a)

429. (2) O_2 via cannula is the most comfortable and the least intrusive, since the cannula extends minimally into the nose. It is also the least oppressive, since it does not cause the feeling of suffocation often associated with the use of masks, tents, or catheters. (a)

430. (3) The patient is made to feel that the nurse cares about him personally and will have time for his special emotional needs; such an approach allays anxiety and reduces emotional stress, which is beneficial in cases of cardiovascular disease. (a)

431. (2) Since digoxin slows the heart, the apical pulse should be counted for 1 minute prior to administration. If the apical rate is below 60 (bradycardia), digoxin should be withheld, since its administration could further depress the heart rate. (b)

432. (3) Potassium is lost with the urine during diuresis. Hypokalemia, in turn, predisposes the patient to developing digitalis toxicity. (a)

433. (2) The Swan-Ganz catheter is placed in the pulmonary artery; information regarding left ventricular functions is obtained when the catheter balloon is inflated. (c)

434. (1) Mitral stenosis impairs blood flow from the left atrium to the left ventricle; this backs up blood into the pulmonary veins and lungs. The result may be pulmonary edema. (c)

435. (3) Since cortisol and other glucocorticoids promote involution of lymphatic tissue, lymphocyte and antibody production decreases, and the body's inflammatory response is reduced. (a)

436. (4) Since many chemotherapeutic agents function by interfering with DNA replication associated with normal cellular reproduction (mitosis), those tissues with high mitosis rates are most affected. The normal rapid mitoses of the stratified epithelium of the mouth and anus result in their being powerfully affected by the drugs, with resultant soreness and possible ulceration. (b)

437. (3) Unwashed hands are considered contaminated and are used to turn on sink faucets. Foot pedals or the use of a paper towel barrier prevents recontamination of washed hands. (c)

438. (3) Bargaining is one of the stages of dying in which the patient promises some type of desirable behavior in exchange for temporary postponement of death. (a)

439. (2) Once a patient reaches the point where he can intellectually and psychologically accept death, anxiety is reduced and the individual becomes detached from his environment. (c)

440. (2) Since 1 oz approximately equals 30 ml and the patient drank a total of 21.5 oz, 21.5 × 30 yields the answer in milliliters. (a)

441. (4) Denial, bargaining, and detachment are coping mechanisms often needed by the patient, especially when facing a devastating illness, and should be accepted by the nurse. (a)

442. (1) Seeking other opinions to disprove the inevitable is a form of denial employed by individuals having illnesses with a poor prognosis. (b)

443. (4) In the stage of acceptance the patient frequently detaches himself from the environment and may become indifferent to family members. In addition, the family may take longer to accept the death than does the patient. (c)

444. (2) The nurse's presence communicates concern and provides an opportunity for the patient to initiate communication if needed. Silence is an effective interpersonal technique that permits the patient to direct the content and extent of his verbalizations without the nurse imposing on his privacy. (b)

445. (1) Methotrexate is a folic acid antagonist that can cause depression of bone marrow. This serious toxic effect is sometimes prevented by administration of folic acid. (c)

446. (4) Prolonged chemotherapy may slow down leukocyte production in bone marrow and lymph nodes, thus suppressing the activity of the immune system. Antibiotics may be required to help counter infections the body can no longer handle easily. (b)

447. (4) Aspirin can cause a lowered prothrombin blood level, increasing the risk of undesired bleeding that may occur with administration of anticoagulants. (a)

448. (4) The patient who is immobilized must do exercises such as dorsiflexion of the feet to prevent venous stasis and thrombus formation. (a)

449. (2) The high vascularity of the nose, combined with its susceptibility to trauma (e.g., sneezing, nose-blowing), makes it a frequent region for hemorrhage. (a)

450. (4) Hemoptysis is expectoration of blood-stained sputum derived from the lungs, bronchi, or trachea. (a)

451. (3) Orthopneic position refers to sitting up and leaning slightly forward. This drops the diaphragm, allowing the lungs more room for expansion. (a)

452. (4) An appendectomy is a relatively simple operation; the patient is generally out of bed the same day. With an ambulatory patient there is less risk of venous stasis, a condition that predisposes the individual to thrombus formation and emboli. (a)

453. (1) Since an elevated plasma bilirubin level could indicate an increased rate of red cell destruction (bilirubin is a product of free hemoglobin metabolism), the individual may have a hemolytic anemia (such as sickle cell anemia or glucose-6-phosphate dehydrogenase deficiency in erythrocytes). (b)

454. (3) The salts in bile act as detergents to physically break large fat droplets into smaller ones (emulsification), providing a larger surface area for the enzymatic action of fat-splitting enzymes (lipases). (a)

455. (3) When bile is not mixing with foods in the intestine, emulsification of fats cannot occur and fat digestion is retarded; stomach motility is also reduced, since increased stomach peristalsis is dependent on fat digestion in the small intestine. (b)

456. (2) Vitamin K, a fat-soluble vitamin, is not absorbed from the GI tract in the absence of bile. Bile enters the duodenum via the common bile duct. (a)

457. (3) Cholescystography is an x-ray examination of the gallbladder after ingestion or IV injection of a radiopaque drug that is concentrated by the normally functioning gallbladder. (b)

458. (1) Cholecystokinin is a widely distributed hormone whose functions include stimulation of gallbladder contraction and the release of pancreatic enzymes; it also functions as a neurotransmitter in the CNS. (b)

459. (2) A drain is inserted to remove fluid that could cause pressure on the operative site and delay healing. The nurse should anticipate drainage and must reinforce the surgical dressings as needed. (a)

460. (4) Localized sensory changes may indicate nerve damage, which may occur during surgery. (a)

461. (2) Low-fat diets are indicated, since fat requires bile to be absorbed; spasms in the biliary system result in pain. (a)

462. (1) When protein intake is inadequate, the liver is unable to manufacture albumin, the major plasma protein. There is a drop in intravascular colloidal osmotic pressure, resulting in a fluid shift to the interstitial spaces. (c)

463. (3) Observation for glycosuria is of the utmost importance in hyperalimentation, since too rapid infusion of a hypertonic solution can cause cellular dehydration as well as specific metabolic derangements. (c)

464. (1) Hyperalimentation should be infused at a slow constant rate to prevent cellular dehydration due to too rapid infusion of hypertonic solutions or to prevent water intoxication from fluid overload. (b)

465. (3) Gastrostomy is an opening directly through the abdomen into the stomach. When tube feedings are given via this route, they bypass the upper GI tract and reduce the risk of tracheal aspiration. (b)

466. (4) Rise of feeding fluid in the tube indicates a full stomach. (a)

467. (2) Water is administered after the tube feeding to prevent the thicker feeding solution from obstructing the lumen of the tube. (b)

468. (2) A temperature of 70° to 75° F will not cause gastric spasm or irritation. (b)

469. (1) Since mastication of food is a psychologically satisfying activity, patients are advised to chew their food before putting it in the blender. (c)

470. (1) Carcinoma can only be ruled out by tissue biopsy, which is obtained during surgery. (c)

471. (2) Patients should turn every 2 hours to promote drainage of different lung regions; deep breathing inflates alveoli and promotes fluid drainage. (b)

472. (2) Pernicious anemia occurs due to the lack of vitamin B_{12}, which is produced by the parietal cells of the gastric mucosa and is required for erythropoiesis. B_{12} absorption requires intrinsic factor, which binds B_{12}, and the ileum, which absorbs B_{12}-intrinsic factor combination (hemopoietic factor). (b)

473. (1) Patency of the tube should be maintained to ensure continued suction; physiologic saline is used to prevent fluid and electrolyte disturbances during irrigation. (a)

474. (3) Overbathing and use of soap can cause increased dryness and skin breakdown; emollients help to relieve dryness. (b)

475. (2) The patient with a history of diverticulitis should eat foods that are nonirritating, bland, and seed free. (a)

476. (4) A colostomy is a surgical opening proximal to the tumor between the colon and the skin surface. (a)

477. (3) Neomycin sulfate is poorly absorbed from the GI tract and is often used for sterilization of the intestines prior to bowel surgery. (a)

478. (3) Preparations such as aluminum paste can be used on the skin around the stoma to prevent excoriation of the skin due to ostomy drainage. (a)

479. (3) Surgery on the bowel has no direct anatomic or physiologic effect on sexual performance; however, psychologic factors could hamper this function, and the nurse should encourage verbalization. (b)

480. (1) Ample time in the bathroom must be ensured for the actual irrigation process and the fecal returns, which may not be immediate. (c)

481. (3) Rapid rate of enema or ostomy irrigation administration often causes cramping, with additional fluid leading to more discomfort. Cramping will generally subside if the enema tubing is clamped for a few minutes; the procedure can then be continued. (b)

482. (2) This is far enough to direct the flow of solution into the bowel; further insertion may cause trauma to the mucosa. (c)

483. (1) A colostomy irrigation is much like a tap water enema. The solution must be held high enough to allow it to flow into the bowel, but not so high that it flows rapidly, or it can cause cramping or mucosal injury. (b)

484. (3) Fat freely circulates as a lipoprotien, the combination of a simple protein and a lipid that is easily and quickly utilized in various metabolic processes. (c)

485. (1) The liver stores carbohydrates as glycogen, which is a polymer of glucose. (a)

486. (3) Fatty acids are insoluble and must combine with bile to form water-soluble substances. (a)

487. (1) The symptoms indicate hepatic coma. Protein is reduced according to tolerance, and calories are increased to prevent tissue catabolism. (a)

488. (4) The liver manufactures albumin, the major plasma protein. A deficit of this protein will lower the osmotic pressure in the intravascular space, leading to a fluid shift. (c)

489. (3) With obstruction of the portal vein there is an increase in pressure in abdominal veins, which empty into the portal system. These veins develop collaterals to circumvent the obstruction. The collaterals are usually in the paraumbilical, hemorrhoidal, and esophageal areas. (a)

490. (2) The elevated pressure within the portal circulatory system causes elevated pressure in areas of portal systemic collateral circulation (most important, in the distal esophagus and proximal stomach). Hemorrhage is a possible complication. (a)

491. (1) Since lipoproteins, a combination of a fat and simple protein, have not been formed due to poor protein intake, fat accumulation in the liver occurs. (c)

492. (2) IV fluids do not provide proteins required for tissue growth, repair, and maintenance. (b)

493. (2) The pH of blood is maintained within the narrow range of 7.35 to 7.45. When there is an increase in H^+ ions, acidosis results, and this is reflected in the lower pH. (a)

494. (3) Sodium bicarbonate is a base and one of the major buffers in the body. (b)

495. (4) The sodium bicarbonate–carbonic acid buffer system helps maintain the pH of the body fluids. In metabolic acidosis there is a decrease in bicarbonate due to retention of metabolic acids. Since there is a decrease in bicarbonate, the carbonic acid will increase to maintain the balance between these 2 buffers. (c)

496. (4) Regular insulin is rapid acting and should be used when immediate action is desired. (b)

497. (1) There are 100 units of insulin in 1 ml or in 16 minims; 6 minims must be administered to provide the patient with 40 units of insulin. (b)

498. (2) Glucagon, an insulin antagonist produced by the alpha cells in the islets of Langerhans, leads to the conversion of glycogen to glucose in the liver. (b)

499. (1) Different types of insulin are compatible and are administered in the same syringe; the regular insulin is generally drawn up first. (c)

500. (3) Glucose catabolism is the main pathway for cellular energy production. Cell membrane, protein, and nucleic acid (genetic material) synthesis require energy but do not directly utilize glucose. (b)

501. (3) Ingested glucose not immediately used for energy

needs is stored in the liver as glycogen and broken down when the blood glucose level falls. (a)

502. (2) IV fluids are given to combat dehydration in acidosis and to keep an IV line open for administration of medications. Once electrolyte levels are evaluated, potassium may be added if needed. (b)

503. (2) All patients should have adequate understanding of their disease to increase compliance with treatment. (b)

504. (1) Glucagon, produced by the alpha cells in the islets of Langerhans, is an insulin antagonist. It mobilizes glycogen storage in the liver, leading to an increased blood glucose level. (c)

505. (4) Insulin functions by facilitating the transport of glucose through the cell membrane and by increasing the deposits of muscle glycogen. Both the cellular glucose and muscle glycogen can be utilized for energy. (a)

506. (3) Refrigeration retards the growth of bacteria and may preserve the specimen for several hours. (b)

507. (2) The method of preservation can affect the test results. Depending on the purpose of the 24-hour study, the urine may be iced, kept with preservatives, or stored in a routine collection bag. (b)

508. (2) Most chemotherapeutic agents used in the treatment of breast cancer are cytotoxic and they cause bone marrow depression. (a)

509. (3) Doxorubicin hydrochloride (Adriamycin) is a chemotherapeutic agent classified as an antibiotic. It achieves its therapeutic effect by inhibiting the synthesis of RNA. This effect blocks protein synthesis and cell division. (c)

510. (1) Doxorubicin, an antitumor antibiotic, causes nausea, diarrhea, and cardiac toxicity because it interferes with cell division. (c)

511. (3) A sarcoma is defined as a malignant tumor whose cells resemble those of the supportive (connective) tissues of the body. (c)

512. (3) Gliomas account for about 45% of all brain tumors. (c)

513. (2) A teratoma is defined as a neoplasm originating in the embryo composed of bizarre and chaotically arranged tissues that are embryologically and histologically foreign to the region containing the tumor. (c)

514. (1) Some spermatozoa will remain viable in the vas deferens for a variable period of time after vasectomy. (c)

515. (4) Cerebral damage on one side of the cortex causes alterations on the opposite side, since three fourths of the fibers originating in the cortex decussate (cross over) in the medulla before extending down the spinal cord. When there is cranial nerve damage, the same side of the body is affected, since the cranial nerves do not decussate but rather leave the cranial cavity by way of the small foramina in the skull. (c)

516. (2) The nurse should provide the patient with an environment that permits exploration of feelings without judgment, punishment, or rejection. As soon as a patient gives a clue that she is ready to talk about her feelings, the nurse should proceed with the conversation using communication techniques to encourage further ventilation. (a)

517. (4) Bowel training is a program for the development of a conditioned reflex that controls regular emptying of the bowel. The key to success in a conditioning program is adherence to a strict time for evacuation based on the patient's individual schedule. (c)

518. (3) Success is a basic motivation for learning. Individuals receive satisfaction when a goal is reached. The more frequent the success, the greater the satisfaction, which in turn motivates the individual to continue striving toward realistic goals. (b)

519. (3) Reasonably prudent behavior in dealing with an immobile patient is to change the patient's position at least every 2 hours to relieve pressure on tissues and promote circulation. The nurse is negligent in not doing this. (b)

520. (4) The enzymatic action of Debrisan helps to clean decubitus ulcers and promotes healing. (c)

521. (3) Due to the presence of feces in the colon, a patient with a fecal impaction has the urge but is unable to defecate. (a)

522. (3) When the bowel is impacted with hardened feces, there is often seepage of liquid feces around this obstruction and thus uncontrolled diarrhea. (a)

523. (3) Sensory impulses from temperature, touch, and pain travel via the spinothalamic pathway to the thalamus and then to the postcentral gyrus of the parietal lobe, the somatosensory area. (a)

524. (4) The thalamus receives impulses from the spinothalamic tract and relays these sensory impulses to the cerebral cortex. (c)

525. (3) The autonomic nervous system functions to regulate visceral effectors to maintain internal equilibrium. (b)

526. (3) Vagal stimulation slows the heart. As the principal nerve of the parasympathetic portion of the autonomic nervous system, the axon terminals of the vagus nerve release acetylcholine; the response of the viscera to this substance varies, but in general the organism is in a relaxed state. (c)

527. (2) As a result of the muscle contracting and pulling on the 2 portions of bone, there is a characteristic shortening of the femur and external rotation of the extremity. (c)

528. (3) A fracture in the neck of the femur will cause shortening of the femur and external rotation. To correct this malalignment, the patient's leg should be extended and maintained in slight internal rotation. (c)

529. (1) Buck's traction is frequently used in the treatment of a fractured hip to align the bones (reduction of fracture). If such traction was not employed, the muscles would go into spasm, causing pain and shifting of the bone fragments. (b)

530. (3) Assessment of any peripheral pulse should include

characteristics of pulse, such as amplitude, rhythm, and rate. Symmetry, correspondence of homologous parts on opposite sides of the body, provides a way to assess data that should be identical. (b)

531. (4) The 3-point gait, which requires considerable arm strength, is used when a limb cannot bear weight. The affected leg and crutches are advanced together, and the strong leg swings through. (c)

532. (3) In the 4-point gait the patient brings the left crutch forward first, followed by the right foot; then the right crutch is brought forward followed by the left foot. Thus both legs must be able to bear some weight. (c)

533. (1) Because of its high blood supply and general fragility, the spleen, when ruptured, must be removed to prevent possible total hemorrhage. (b)

534. (1) Due to the vascularity of the spleen, hemorrhage may occur and result in abdominal distention. (c)

535. (1) Head injuries can cause trauma to the brain, and the patient should be observed for signs of increased intracranial pressure such as headache, dizziness, and visual disturbances. (b)

536. (4) Release of the adrenocortical steroids (cortisol) by the stress of surgery causes renal retention of Na^+ and K^+ excretion. Potassium can also be depleted by nasogastric suction. (b)

537. (2) On inspiration excursion of the fractured ribs is limited, pressing on the pleura and causing pain. (b)

538. (3) Changes in amount of blood in the urine may indicate progressive increases in kidney damage. (b)

539. (1) Hematuria occurs when there is kidney damage due to leakage of erythrocytes through the glomerular filtration membrane. (b)

540. (3) The gamma globulin fraction in the plasma is the fraction including the antibodies. (a)

541. (2) Platelets (thrombocytes) adhere to the intima of damaged vessels within seconds after injury, releasing substances that promote hemostasis. (b)

542. (1) Isotonic solutions are those which cause no change in the cellular volume or pressure, since their concentration is equivalent to that of body fluid. (a)

543. (2) REM (rapid eye movement) sleep is necessary for psychologic coping. The nurse should be aware that some medications affect this sleep stage and thereby alter emotional health. (b)

544. (2) Fiber absorbs water, swells, and consequently stretches the bowel wall promoting peristalsis, mass movements, and defecation. Smooth muscle tends to contract when stretched due to the reflex activity of stretch receptors. (c)

545. (1) Adrenalin is used to treat shock because the induced vasoconstriction reduces the blood pooling (vessels cannot hold as much blood) and increases venous return and cardiac output. (c)

546. (2) An autograft is one taken from an uninjured area of the same person's body. (b)

547. (3) A heterograft or xenograft involves the grafting of tissues from 2 different species. (b)

548. (3) Increased hematocrit level is indicative of hemoconcentration secondary to fluid loss. (b)

549. (1) As the amount of tissue involved increases, there is greater extravasation of fluid into the tissues; thus the relationship of fluid loss to body surface is directly proportionate. Several formulas, such as the Evans Formula, Baxter Formula, and Brooke Army Hospital Formula, are used to estimate fluid loss based on percent of body surface burned. (b)

550. (3) *Clostridium tetani* can develop in wounds in which there is dead tissue. (b)

551. (3) Mafenide (Sulfamylon) interferes with the kidneys' role in hydrogen ion excretion, resulting in metabolic acidosis. (b)

552. (4) Negative pressure such as suction should never be exerted on the bladder, since this might injure the sensitive tissue. Solution should be allowed to drain by the force of gravity alone. (b)

553. (1) Although other solutions may be ordered, irrigations of the bladder usually employ normal saline (0.9% NaCl), which is a solution of approximately the normal tonicity of body fluids. (b)

554. (2) The bladder is a sterile body cavity, and any time a solution or catheter is introduced into the urinary meatus, strict surgical asepsis is required to prevent infection. (b)

555. (4) Patients, when adapting to illness, frequently feel afraid and helpless and strike out at health team members as a way of maintaining control or denying their fear. (b)

556. (1) Chlordiazepoxide (Librium) is a sedative that depresses the central nervous system and therefore promotes rest. (b)

557. (4) Drowsiness is a side effect of Librium and is indicative of excessive depression of the central nervous system. (b)

558. (3) Reserpine is an antihypertensive because it reduces norepinephrine levels in peripheral nerve endings. (a)

559. (4) An improper reading of the level of mercury will be obtained if the reader is not perpendicular to the column. (a)

560. (2) An honest nurse-patient relationship should be maintained so that trust can develop. (a)

561. (3) At this time the patient is using this behavior as a defense. Silence can be an effective interpersonal technique, since it is nonjudgmental. (c)

562. (2) Orthopneic position allows maximum lung expansion because gravity reduces the pressure of the abdominal viscera on the diaphragm and lungs. Breathing is also difficult in the recumbent position probably because of a shift of blood to the lung vessels, which exacerbates edema, increasing the respiratory effort. (b)

563. (3) Application of rotating tourniquets keeps blood in the extremities, decreasing venous return, which reduces pulmonary artery pressure and relieves congestion. (b)

564. (4) Diuretic therapy generally involves use of drugs that directly or indirectly increase urinary sodium excretion. Increased urinary excretion of sodium also promotes potassium loss. (a)

565. (1) CVP is to be recorded when the patient is horizontal and the zero point of the manometer is at the midaxillary line (level of the right atrium). (a)

566. (2) With air conditioning, blood vessels in the skin remain partially constricted, preventing extensive blood flow through the skin. Such extensive skin blood flow would ordinarily occur in hot weather to promote radiation of heat from the body; however, the heart must then work to pump the blood through many extra miles of blood vessels in the skin. (a)

567. (2) Since Mr. Roger's condition is described as terminal, nursing priority should be directed toward providing comfort. (b)

568. (4) Small meals are not as psychologically overwhelming and do not upset the stomach as easily. They are therefore better tolerated. (a)

569. (1) Anorexia refers to loss of appetite. (a)

570. (2) IPPB treatments loosen bronchial secretions and dilate the air passages, but coughing is needed to raise the secretions for expectoration. (a)

571. (3) Meperidine is the generic name for Demerol. (a)

572. (4) Patients with COPD respond only to the chemical stimulus of low oxygen levels. Administration of high concentrations of oxygen will eliminate the stimulus to breathe, leading to decreased respirations and lethargy. (c)

573. (3) Since family members are old enough to understand his needs, they should be encouraged to participate in his care. (c)

574. (4) Gastroscopy permits visualization of the stomach and biopsy of the tissue. (a)

575. (4) An American relative can serve as interpreter and provide emotional support and security. (b)

576. (4) $\dfrac{\text{Amount to be infused} \times \text{Gtt factor}}{\text{Time of infusion in minutes}}$ (a)

577. (4) After 24 hours there is increased risk of contamination of the solution. (b)

578. (2) In sprue there is malabsorption of nutrients and macrocytic anemia. Folic acid is an important growth factor for a large number of cells and participates in the synthesis of amino acids and DNA. (c)

579. (1) Gluten is found in rye, wheat, and oat products. (a)

580. (2) These foods are low in gluten. (c)

581. (3) Since the patient with cancer of the esophagus is frequently anorexic, any nutrients he will take should be encouraged. (b)

582. (2) The respiratory center in the medulla responds primarily to increased CO_2 concentration in the blood. (a)

583. (2) The lower the Po_2 and the higher the Pco_2, the more rapidly the oxygen dissociates from the oxyhemoglobin molecule. (c)

584. (2) This is the organism that causes botulism. (a)

585. (3) *Entamoeba histolytica,* the organism that causes amebic dysentery, is transmitted through excreta. (a)

586. (1) In starvation there are inadequate carbohydrates available for immediate energy, and stored fats are used in excessive amounts. (a)

587. (3) Fluid and electrolytes are lost through intestinal decompression; on a daily basis about one fifth the total body water is secreted into and almost completely reabsorbed by the GI tract. (a)

588. (1) Dehydration is a danger because of fluid loss in GI suction. (b)

589. (2) Isotonic saline will not pull out extra fluids and electrolytes and cause an imbalance. (a)

590. (1) Open communication lines are always important in relieving anxiety and reducing stress, which might interfere with postoperative recovery. (b)

591. (2) The patient must be ready to accept changes in body image and function; this acceptance will facilitate mastery of techniques of colostomy care, special dieting, and optimistic utilization of community resources. (b)

592. (2) A transverse colostomy is an opening in the transverse colon. The rectal tube should be pointed to the proximal intestine to evacuate the bowles. (b)

593. (3) Hemostasis and thrombus formation in the deep veins of the calves may result in pulmonary embolism, since the pulmonary capillary beds are the first small vessels (capillary beds) the embolus encounters once it is released from the calf veins. (b)

594. (3) The absorption of fluids by gauze is due to the adhesion of water to the gauze threads. The surface tension of water causes contraction of the water fiber pulling fluid up the threads. (c)

595. (4) Alcohol stimulates pancreatic enzyme secretion and an increase in pressure in the pancreatic duct. The backflow of enzymes into the pancreatic interstitial spaces results in partial digestion and inflammation of pancreatic tissue. (b)

596. (2) A pseudocyst of the pancreas contains blood, necrotic tissue, and enzymes and is surrounded by connective tissue. (c)

597. (4) That is the unique function of pancreozymin, which is secreted by the duodenum. (a)

598. (2) Lipase is a pancreatic enzyme that aids the digestion of fat. (c)

599. (1) The duodenum secretes several digestion-related hormones, including secretin, which elicits sodium bicarbonate secretion from the pancreas, and pancreozymin, which elicits enzyme secretion from the pancreas. It also brings about gallbladder contraction and secretion of bile; in this function it is known as cholecystokinin. (b)

600. (4) The nurse should show the patient that she recognizes her concerns and is available to listen. (c)

601. (2) Certain diagnostic tests such as CBC, urinalysis, and chest x-ray examination are done preoperatively to rule out the existence of other health problems that could increase the risks involved with surgery. (c)

602. (4) Anxiety experienced by a preoperative patient can be a disruptive force affecting the patient's ability to adapt psychologically and physiologically. It must be alleviated for other nursing measures to be effective. (b)

603. (3) Interpretation of pain sensations by each patient is highly individual and is based on the patient's past experiences, which include cultural values. (b)

604. (1) When a patient has been confined to bed for a time or has been receiving certain antihypertensives, the patient's neurocirculatory reflexes may have some difficulty adjusting to the force of gravity in an upright position. Postural or orthostatic hypotension occur, and there is a temporary decreased blood supply to the brain. (a)

605. (4) Used for its analgesic effects, morphine is a central nervous system depressant. The major adverse effect of morphine is respiratory depression, but it could also cause lethargy, capillary constriction, and depressed reflexes, and it could lead to coma and death. (b)

606. (3) Pain in the calf may be a sign of thrombophlebitis, a possible postoperative complication. If the thrombus becomes dislodged, it may lead to pulmonary embolism. Any patient with this complaint should immediately be confined to bed, and the physician should be notified. (a)

607. (1) Almost all peptic ulcers in the stomach develop along the lesser curvature of the antral (pyloric) region. About 85% of all peptic ulcers, in general, occur within the first 2 cm of the duodenum. These regions are most exposed to acid conditions. (b)

608. (4) Propantheline (Pro-Banthine) reduces the motility of the GI tract and thereby facilitates healing. (c)

609. (1) Physiologic normal saline is used in gastric irrigation to prevent electrolyte imbalance. Because of the fresh gastric sutures, slow and gentle irrigation should be performed. However, most surgeons prefer gastric instillations. (a)

610. (4) The vagus nerve stimulates the stomach to secrete hydrochloric acid. By severing the vagus nerve this neural pathway is interrupted, and there will be a decrease in stomach secretions. (b)

611. (4) To calculate rate of fluid infusion:

$$\frac{\text{Amount of fluid to be infused} \times \text{Drop factor}}{\text{Amount of time in minutes}} \quad \text{(b)}$$

612. (2) Since IV solutions enter the body's internal environment, all solutions and medications utilizing this route must be sterile to prevent the introduction of microbes. (b)

613. (1) Symptoms of dumping syndrome occur to some degree in about 50% of all individuals having gastrectomy or vagotomy and include weakness, faintness, heart palpitations, and diaphoresis. It is therefore important to explain to Mr. Smith that such symptoms may be minimized by resting after meals in semi-Fowler's position and eating small meals omitting concentrated, highly refined carbohydrates. (b)

614. (3) An individual treated for a thyroid problem by intake of radioactive ^{131}I becomes mildly radioactive, particularly in the region of the thyroid gland, which preferentially absorbs the iodine; such individuals should be treated with standard precautions. (b)

615. (1) Because of the individual's increased metabolic rate, a high-calorie diet is needed to meet the energy demands of the body and prevent weight loss. (b)

616. (3) Lugol's Solution adds iodine to the body fluids, exerting negative feedback on thyroid tissue and decreasing its metabolism and vascularity. (a)

617. (3) During surgery, if the laryngeal nerves are injured bilaterally, the vocal cords will tighten interfering with speech. If one cord is affected, hoarseness develops. This can be evaluated simply by having the patient speak every hour. (b)

618. (3) These signs may indicate tetany due to calcium depletion. If this occurs following a thyroidectomy, one might suspect inadvertent removal of the parathyroids. (c)

619. (1) Parathyroid removal eliminates the body's source of parathyroid hormone, which functions to increase blood calcium. Consequently, normal decreases in blood calcium cannot be balanced by additions to the blood from calcium reservoirs in bone, increased calcium reabsorption from kidney tubules, or increased intestinal calcium absorption. Low body fluid calcium tetanizes muscles including the diaphragm, resulting in dyspnea, asphyxia, and death. (a)

620. (1) Parathyroid hormone increases osteoclast activity, resulting in bone substance breakdown and release of calcium into the blood. Blood calcium and phosphate levels rise. The hormone calcitonin, released from the thyroid gland, increases calcium incorporation into bone. (b)

621. (4) Parathormone increases the blood concentration of calcium by accelerating calcium absorption from the intestine, bones, and kidneys. Vitamin D is essential for calcium to be absorbed from the intestines. (b)

622. (2) Calcitonin, a thyroid gland hormone, prevents bone reabsorption of calcium. It also inhibits the release of calcium from the bone. The net result is lowered serum calcium levels. (a)

623. (1) Myxedema is the severest form of hypothyroidism. Decreased thyroid gland activity causes a reduced production of its hormones. (b)

624. (2) The thyroid gland produces thyroxine, which directly helps to regulate oxidation in all body cells. The pituitary is also involved in regulating cellular oxidation rate through its secretion of TSH, which helps to regulate

thyroid functioning through TSH secretion. However, this function is considered a secondary regulation of cellular oxidation rate. (b)

625. (1) Any abnormal signs of vaginal bleeding may be indicative of cervical cancer and must be checked by a physician. (c)

626. (4) During radiation therapy with radium implants the patient is placed in isolation to decrease exposure to radiation by family and staff. (a)

627. (2) Radium atoms are unstable and spontaneously disintegrate into other atomic species. This atomic disintegration produces potentially harmful radiation, which is absorbed by lead. (a)

628. (3) Time, distance, and shielding are the important factors in determining the amount of radiation the individual receives. Restriction of each visitor to a 10-minute stay minimizes the risk of exposure. Many institutions will not allow visitors while an implant is in place. (c)

629. (3) Prior to discharge it is important for the nurse to instruct the patient to follow through with medical care at specified intervals. (b)

630. (2) A sharp rise in the luteinizing hormone triggers the rupture of the follicle and ovulation. (c)

631. (1) The function of progesterone is to relax the uterus and maintain a succulent endometrium to foster implantation of the fertilized ovum. (c)

632. (2) Estrogen is found in the follicular fluid of the ovaries and aids in the growth of the endometrium. (b)

633. (2) Persistent pain of any kind is usually a symptom, and the patient should seek medical attention. (b)

634. (1) Mild hypocalcemia sometimes occurs during menstruation. An increase in dietary calcium just before and during menstruation may eliminate or relieve the occasional abdominal cramps resulting from the temporary hypocalcemia. (c)

635. (2) Although sympathetic impulses usually control most visceral effectors in times of stress, parasympathetic fibers also stimulate and can result in increased gastric contractions and increased peristalsis. Sympathetic fibers also inhibit organs such as the bladder and cause relaxation of this organ. (c)

636. (2) The sympathetic nervous system constricts smooth muscle of blood vessels in the skin when a person is under stress. (a)

637. (2) Parasympathetic nerves increase peristalsis of the digestive tract and secretion by the gastric hydrochloric acid glands. (b)

638. (2) Only axon terminals secrete acetylcholine, so nerve impulse propagation only occurs in one direction: from axon terminal to dendrite or cell body of the next neuron or from axon terminal to effector organ (muscle or gland). The action of cholinesterase to inactivate acetylcholine only has physiologic meaning at the synapse where acetylcholine is active; its presence all along the axon would not affect the direction of the nerve impulse. (b)

639. (1) Axon terminals release acetylcholine at the myoneural junction; as acetylcholine contacts the sarcolemma, it stimulates the muscle fiber to contract. (a)

640. (3) Phenytoin (Dilantin) is an anticonvulsant, most effective in controlling grand mal seizures. Data collection before planning nursing care for a patient with epilepsy should always include a history of seizure incidence (type and frequency). (c)

641. (4) Therapeutic blood levels of phenytoin must be maintained to achieve its anticonvulsant effect. If the patient is not able to take the prescribed oral preparation, the physician should be questioned about alternate routes of administration. (b)

642. (2) When an oral medication is available in a suspension form, the nurse should use it for patients with dysphagia. (c)

643. (1) Gingival hyperplasia is a frequently occurring adverse effect of long-term phenytoin therapy. The incidence can be decreased by meticulous oral hygiene. (c)

644. (4) Phenytoin inhibits folic acid absorption and potentiates the effects of folic acid antagonists. Folic acid therapy is often helpful in correcting certain anemias that can result from administration of phenytoin. (c)

645. (4) Lesions affecting the facial nerve (seventh cranial) cause paralysis of the eyelids. (c)

646. (2) The third cranial, or oculomotor, nerve contains autonomic fibers that control size of pupil. (c)

647. (2) The facial nerve has motor and sensory functions. The motor function is concerned with facial movement, including smiling and pursing the lips. Nonconduction of either right or left will cause drooping on the opposite side. (c)

648. (1) Anterior horn neurons are also known as lower motoneurons. Their cell bodies are located in the anterior gray columns and are part of the reflex arc. (c)

649. (1) Extrapyramidal tracts of motor pathways assist in maintaining muscle tonus. (c)

650. (3) This is where spinal fluid is located. (b)

651. (1) Pain and temperature sensations enter the posterior horn of the spinal cord, cross to the contralateral side, and travel upward via the spinothalamic tract to the thalamus, where they synapse with another sensory neuron for transmission to the cortex. (c)

652. (2) Parkinson's disease involves destruction of neurons of the substantia nigra, caudate nucleus, and globus pallidus of the basal ganglia. The cause of this destruction is unknown. (b)

653. (3) The destruction of the neurons of the basal ganglia results in decreased muscle tone. Therefore patients with Parkinson's disease may have a masklike appearance and monotonous speech patterns that can be interpreted as flat affect. (b)

654. (2) L-Dopa acts as a replacement drug but after prolonged use frequently is associated with side effects of nausea, vomiting, orthostatic hypotension, and mental confusion. (b)

655. (1) L-Dopa is the precursor of dopamine. It is converted to dopamine in the brain cells where it is stored until needed by axon terminals where it functions as a neurotransmitter. (b)

656. (3) The cerebellum coordinates muscular activity and promotes balance. The other brain regions govern motor, sensory, and high integrative functions. (a)

657. (3) Rehabilitating exercises carried out under water minimize strain on the partially atrophied and painful joints because the buoyant force of the water makes the limbs easier to move. (b)

658. (2) Ankylosing spondylitis (Marie-Strümpell disease) is a chronic, progressive polyarthritis. Ossification of cartilage, particularly of the spine, causes fixation of the involved joints. (a)

659. (1) ROM exercises must be instituted to maintain mobility of joints, but overuse may prevent resolution of the inflammation. (a)

660. (3) As a result of the normal stresses on the body, the incidence of chronic illness increases in the elderly population. (a)

661. (3) A balanced diet consisting of the basic 4 food groups is essential in maintaining good nutrition. (b)

662. (2) Osteoarthritis affects the hips and knees first because they are the weight-bearing joints and undergo the most stress and strain. (b)

663. (1) Psoriasis is characterized by dry scaly lesions that occur most frequently on the elbows, knees, scalp, and torso. (a)

664. (3) Steroids are applied locally and usually covered with plastic or Saran Wrap at night to reverse the inflammatory process. (b)

665. (1) Scabies is caused by the itch mite (*Acarus scabiei*), the female of which burrows under the skin to deposit eggs. It is intensely pruritic and is transmitted by direct contact or in a limited way by soiled sheets or undergarments. (b)

666. (4) Pemphigus is a serious skin disease characterized by large vesicles called bullae. Although potentially fatal, pemphigus has been relatively controlled by steroid therapy. (b)

667. (1) The Stryker wedge frame provides for horizontal changes of position to prone or supine while maintaining proper body alignment. (a)

668. (3) The main nursing principles in turning a patient on the Stryker frame are the maintenance of alignment and safety. Securing all bolts and straps ensures that the patient is snug, yet comfortably wedged between the frames. (b)

669. (2) Progressive patient care is based on the precept that different levels of patient needs require different kinds of services and facilities. The care provided is specialized and individualized to meet the patients' needs in an appropriate, continuous, and dynamic pattern. (b)

670. (4) During prolonged inactivity bone reabsorption proceeds faster than bone formation, and lack of therapeutic weight-bearing on bone results in disuse atrophy. A tilt table provides gradual progressive weight-bearing, which counters these effects. (c)

671. (1) Patients with quadriplegia do not and never will have the muscle innervation necessary for the strength or balance needed for ambulation. (b)

672. (1) The serum acid phosphatase is elevated when the cancer extends beyond the prostate, whereas the serum alkaline phosphatase is elevated in bony metastasis. (b)

673. (4) Dysuria, nocturia, and urgency are all signs of an irritable bladder following radiation therapy. Bleeding would not necessarily indicate this. (b)

674. (3) An enlarged prostate constricts the urethra, interfering with urine flow and causing retention. When the bladder fills and approaches capacity, small amounts can be voided. (b)

675. (1) Catheter patency ensures drainage and prevents bladder distention and other complications; therefore patency of a catheter should be established prior to notifying the physician. (a)

676. (2) Cleansing the urinary meatus and adjacent skin removes accumulated bacteria, limiting the possible introduction of microbes into the urinary tract. (c)

677. (4) The Foley catheter is always positioned so that the level of the bladder with catheter inserted is higher than the level of the drainage container; gravity causes urine flow. (a)

678. (1) An indwelling catheter dilates the urinary sphincters, keeps the bladder empty, and short-circuits the normal reflex mechanism based on bladder distention. Once the catheter is removed, the body has to adapt to functioning once again. (b)

679. (1) When the testes are twisted, there is a decrease in blood supply to the testicles, which can result in gangrene. (c)

680. (3) The tourniquets must be rotated in a clockwise direction at 15-minute intervals so that venous outflow in any one extremity is not occluded for more than 45 minutes at a time. (b)

681. (3) Application of rotating tourniquets keeps blood in the extremities, decreasing venous return to reduce pulmonary artery pressure and relieve pulmonary congestion. (b)

682. (4) The exact mode of action of morphine sulfate is unknown; however, it has a rapid onset, producing euphoria and an elevated pain threshold. (c)

683. (2) Ethacrynic acid interferes with the concentrating and diluting mechanism of the decending and ascending

limbs of the loop of Henle and the concentrating process in the collecting duct. It inhibits the active transport of chloride back into the blood. Copious amounts of dilute urine high in chloride and sodium are excreted. (c)

684. (3) Aminophylline, a theophylline derivative, relaxes smooth muscle, stimulates cardiac muscle and the central nervous system, and promotes diuresis. It is also irritating to the gastric mucosa and can cause GI irritation, nausea, anxiety, restlessness, and hypotension. (b)

685. (2) The fluid level in the manometer fluctuates with respiration because the changes in thoracic pressure affect the pressure in the right atrium. The positive pressure of a ventilator would alter the CVP readings, so the ventilator must be removed when the CVP is taken. (b)

686. (3) Deslanoside (Cedilanid-D) can be administered slowly by IV route. The other medications should never be administered intravenously. (c)

687. (3) Cardioversion involves administration of precordial shock, which is synchronized with the R wave to interrupt the heart rate. It is used for atrial fibrillation, proximal atrial tachycardia (PAT), and ventricular tachycardia when pharmaceutical preparations fail. The heart is stopped by the electric stimulation, and it is hoped that the SA node will take over as pacemaker. (c)

688. (2) Ventricular fibrillation is a death-producing arrhythmia and, once identified, must be terminated immediately by precordial shock (defibrillation). This is usually a standing physician's order in a cardiac care unit. (c)

689. (2) The precordial shock during cardioversion must not be delivered on the T wave, or ventricular fibrillation may ensue; by placing the synchronizer in the "on" position, the machine will be preset and will not deliver the shock on the T wave. (b)

690. (2) The height of the ventricular complexes must be sufficient to be picked up by the voltmeter, which will set an alarm if the heart rate is outside the parameters set by the high- and low-rate alarms. (c)

691. (1) Atrial fibrillation is rapid discharge of impulses from a focus other than the SA node. Since not all these impulses are transmitted through the AV node, the ventricular response varies. Quinidine inhibits discharge of electric impulses from such ectopic foci, whereas digoxin delays the conduction of impulses from the AV node, slowing down the rate of ventricular response to impulses from the atria. (b)

692. (3) The apex of the heart is between the third and fourth ribs at the midclavicular line. (b)

693. (1) Adverse effects of digoxin include many types of arrhythmias. An apical pulse rate less than 60 or above 120 contraindicates administration of the drug. Since the patient will be taking the medication at home, he must be taught to take his own pulse and to contact the physician if his pulse falls outside the parameters mentioned. (b)

694. (4) The Nurse Practice Act states that nurses diagnose human responses to actual or potential health problems. The nurse used her knowledge. (b)

695. (2) The 2 coronary arteries are the first branches of the aorta and carry high–oxygen content blood to the myocardium. (c)

696. (1) Angina pectoris is the pain referred to the chest wall due to hypoxia of the cardiac muscle. (b)

697. (2) Anginal pain, which can be anticipated to occur during certain activities, may be prevented by dilating the coronary arteries immediately before engaging in the activity. (b)

698. (1) Nitroglycerin tablets are affected by light, heat, and moisture. A loss of potency can be detected by absence of a tingling sensation when the tablet is placed under the tongue or by its ineffectiveness in relieving pain. A new supply should be obtained immediately. (c)

699. (4) In addition to GI disturbances, digitalis toxicity may be evidenced by visual disturbances such as blurred vision. Heart rates over 120 may also indicate toxicity. (b)

700. (3) Toxic levels of digitalis overstimulate the vagus nerve, leading to depressed conduction through the AV node (AV block of any degree) as well as SA node depression (sinus bradycardia). In addition, ectopic pacemakers are accelerated, leading to multiple premature beats. Such pathologic effects are enhanced by low serum potassium levels due to diuretics, vomiting, and nasogastric drainage, as well as chronic arterial hypoxemia and impaired renal function. (b)

701. (1) Whole milk is high in fat. (a)

702. (4) Vegetable oils, like most lipids from plants, are high in unsaturated fats, whereas meats and most animal-derived products such as butter, milk, and eggs are high in saturated fats. (b)

703. (3) Thromboplastin is one of the substances released by platelets that accelerate coagulation. Other factors such as serotonin constrict blood vessels. (b)

704. (2) Fibrinogen is a soluble plasma protein that becomes the insoluble clot, fibrin, during the clotting process. (c)

705. (2) Calcium acts as a catalyst to convert prothrombin to thrombin. Thrombin accelerates formation of insoluble fibrin from the soluble fibrinogen. (c)

706. (4) In the process of rocking the Trendelenburg position facilitates venous return from the lower extremities, whereas reverse Trendelenburg decreases the pressure of the abdominal organs on the diaphragm, allowing maximum lung expansion. (c)

707. (2) The residual volume is the amount of air remaining in the lungs after maximum exhalation. (b)

708. (3) Sodium polystyrene sulfonate, a cation exchange resin used in the treatment of hyperkalemia, will release sodium ions in the intestines in exchange for potassium ions. Sorbitol has a hyperosmotic effect in the intestinal tract concomitantly maintaining the liquid content of the

feces and counteracting the constipating effect of the resin. (b)

709. (4) The nurse needs to ascertain how the patient tolerates the turning. Orthostatic hypotension can occur, and the physician should be alerted if the vital signs do not stabilize in 5 to 10 minutes. (b)

710. (4) The Circ-O-lectric bed turns patients from a horizontal supine position vertically to a horizontal prone position. The bed can also remain stationary in a vertical position. The change of position alters the body pressures periodically while the patient is confined to bed. (c)

711. (2) Asepsis around the site of insertion must be maintained, since it is a break in the first line of defense. (b)

712. (2) The Schwann cells that compose the neurilemma of peripheral nerve fibers (dendrites and axons) are capable of supporting nerve fiber regeneration. The oligodendrocytes that cover the central nervous system nerve fibers are not capable of supporting fiber regeneration. The myelin sheath, produced peripherally by Schwann cells and centrally by oligodendrocytes, is not involved directly with the regenerative process. (b)

713. (4) Since the phrenic nerves innervate the diaphragm, a crushing spinal cord injury above the level of the phrenic origins would stop diaphragmatic contractions and result in respiratory paralysis. Choice 3 could be correct, but the question mentioned the ''phrenic nerve origins,'' which implicates respiratory paralysis as the best choice. Activities regulated by the vagus nerve would be unaffected because the vagi originate in the medulla, which is superior to the cervical region (the phrenic nerves originate from the cervical plexuses). (b)

714. (3) In hepatic coma there is an accumulation of nitrogenous wastes, which affect the nervous system. In the second stage of this disease this effect is evidenced by flapping tremors and generalized twitching. (b)

715. (4) Bile deposits will cause a yellowish tinge (jaundice or icterus) to the skin, often first observed in the sclera. (c)

716. (3) In liver cirrhosis, fibrous scarring within the liver parenchyma due most often to alcohol toxicity compresses portal veins and causes a backup of blood and increased pressure within the portal system. Ascites fluid (interstitial fluid) forms in excess and seeps into the abdominal cavity mainly from the surface of the liver. (b)

717. (2) The increased plasma hydrostatic pressure in the extremities due to heart failure or liver cirrhosis, possibly combined with a genetic weakness in the vein walls, may lead to varicose veins. (c)

718. (4) Increased ammonia levels indicate the inability of the liver to detoxify protein by-products. Neomycin cuts down on the ammonia-forming bacteria in the intestines. (c)

719. (2) The hepatic portal vein carries blood from the capillary beds of the viscera (small and large intestinal walls, stomach, spleen, pancreas, and gallbladder) to the sinu-

soids of the liver. The hepatic veins drain the liver sinusoids into the inferior vena cava. (b)

720. (1) Prothrombin, which is normally present in the plasma, is synthesized in the liver in the presence of vitamin K from the amino acid glutamine. Vitamin K initiates the vital process of coagulation. (b)

721. (4) Vitamin K is a fat-soluble vitamin and needs bile salts for absorption from the upper segment of the small intestine. It is a catalyst in the carboxylation of glutamine to prothrombin. (c)

722. (2) This is negligence. The patient should have been informed. Also, the nurse was responsible for collecting the specimen. (b)

723. (4) Vitamin K is synthesized by intestinal bacteria but is also found in liver, egg yolks, and cheese. (b)

724. (2) Liver cirrhosis results in development of extensive scar tissue within the liver structure; such scar tissue contracts around hepatic blood vessels, impeding blood flow and raising the pressure in the hepatic portal system. The physiologic response to slowly developing portal circulatory obstruction is the growth of collateral vessels linking portal veins with esophageal veins; as destruction progresses, the collaterals become so large that they bulge into the esophageal lumen and are called esophageal varices. (b)

725. (4) Iced saline is instilled via a nasogastric tube to control hemorrhage; cold promotes blood vessel constriction. (a)

726. (2) Neomycin destroys intestinal flora, which breaks down protein and in the process gives off ammonia. Ammonia at this time is poorly detoxified by the liver and can build up to toxic levels. (b)

727. (1) This tube has an esophageal balloon that, on inflation, exerts pressure, which retards hemorrhage. (b)

728. (2) The patient's breath has a sweet odor due to failure of the liver to metabolize the amino acid methionine. (b)

729. (1) Since protein breakdown gives off ammonia that cannot be detoxified by the liver, protein should be eliminated from the diet. (b)

730. (2) Low sodium controls fluid retention, blood pressure, and consequently edema; low protein controls ammonia formation in proportion to the liver's ability to detoxify ammonia in forming urea; moderate fat and high calories and vitamins help repair long-standing nutritional deficit. (b)

731. (1) Protein intake should be further restricted when coma is inevitable due to the liver's inability to detoxify ammonia to urea. (b)

732. (3) Patients with aphasia must be encouraged to speak so that communication ability is regained. However, needs should be anticipated so that frustration is avoided. (b)

733. (2) A patient who is comatose loses voluntary control but may still exhibit spontaneous movement and respond to pain. (a)

734. (1) Absence of a gag reflex is common after a CVA. To

prevent aspiration, the patient is positioned on the side or semiprone to allow gravity to drain mucus in the nasopharyngeal area away from the trachea. (b)

735. (2) Passive ROM exercises prevent development of deformities and yet do not require any energy expenditure by the patient who is confined to bed. Instituting ROM exercises is an independent nursing function. (b)

736. (3) Changes in self-image and family role can initiate a grieving process with a variety of emotional responses. (a)

737. (4) Family members should be involved in planning and implementing care to foster communication and cooperation. (a)

738. (2) The brachial plexus is a maze of nerves extending from the axilla to the neck in the shoulder area. Trauma to the arm may also injure the brachial plexus. (a)

739. (1) The medulla contains the vital respiratory, cardiac, and vasomotor centers. (a)

740. (1) The hypothalamus in the brain connects with the autonomic area for vasoconstriction, vasodilation, and perspiration and with the somatic centers for shivering; therefore the hypothalamus is an important area for regulating body temperature. (a)

741. (2) The eighth cranial nerve has 2 parts—the vestibular nerve and the cochlear nerve. Sensations of hearing are conducted by the cochlear nerve. (a)

742. (2) The primary site of action is the motor cortex, where seizure activity is limited by maintaining the sodium gradient of neurons. (b)

743. (4) The respiratory tract can be obstructed during a seizure, and therefore a plastic airway should be available at all times for patients with convulsive disorders. (b)

744. (3) Seizure disorders are usually associated with marked changes in the electric activity of the cerebral cortex, requiring prolonged or life-long therapy. (b)

745. (3) There are no dietary restrictions, but iron and vitamins should be encouraged to normalize any underlying nutritional deficiencies. (b)

746. (2) Aspirin, because of its anti-inflammatory effect, is useful in treating arthritis symptoms. (a)

747. (3) Exercise of involved joints is important to maintain optimal mobility and to prevent build-up of calcium deposits. (c)

748. (2) Steroids have an anti-inflammatory effect, which can reduce arthritic pannus formation. (c)

749. (4) Marie-Strümpell disease is synonymous with ankylosing spondylitis, which involves fixation of joints (usually vertebral). (c)

750. (2) Synovial fluid minimizes friction at joints by providing lubrication for the moving parts. (b)

751. (3) The patient had a right to know what medication she was receiving (informed consent). This also constituted an invasion of the patient's rights. (b)

752. (2) Synovial joints, like the knee, shoulder, or joints

between the middle ear bones, are lined with synovial membrane. (a)

753. (3) The nurse should obtain the drug from the pharmacy to meet the patient's need for relief from pain immediately. Other medications must not be substituted nor another patient's supply depleted. (a)

754. (2) Decubiti easily develop when one position is maintained because the body weight, directed continuously in one region, restricts circulation and results in tissue necrosis. (a)

755. (4) The paraplegic patient is unable to actively exercise. (c)

756. (3) Calcium leaves long bones during periods of prolonged bed rest; the tilt table places the patient in an upright position. (b)

757. (4) Calcium that has left the bones as a response to prolonged inactivity enters the blood and may precipitate in the kidneys, forming calculi. (b)

758. (1) All rehabilitation should begin on admission to the hospital to promote optimism and facilitate optimum functioning. (a)

759. (4) Bladder function may be impaired with lower spinal cord injuries due to the location of the micturition reflex center in the sacral region of the spinal cord. (b)

760. (1) Correct positioning prevents the patient from assuming incorrect positions, which could result in contracture formation. (a)

761. (3) The precentral gyrus is the most posterior convolution of the frontal lobe and the primary motor area. Other gyri also contain motor neurons. (c)

762. (3) Sneezing, as well as lifting and straining, causes an increase in intraspinal pressure, resulting in pain. (c)

763. (4) Compresses are not required after a spinal puncture. Responses 1 through 3 must be employed to monitor and limit the body's response to the trauma of a myelogram. (c)

764. (3) Ambulation is commenced after several days of bed rest, not immediately. (b)

765. (3) A laminectomy, which involves the removal of portions of several vertebrae, is generally done in conjunction with removal of a herniated disc. Inflammation from the trauma of surgery could lead to compression of the spinal cord with consequent motor or sensory dysfunction. (b)

766. (2) Sore throat and oral secretions are additional problems of the patient after cervical laminectomy. (c)

767. (2) Radium, a radioactive isotope, is used to destroy or delay the growth of malignant cells. Special care is taken to maintain normal tissue and not allow it to come closer to the radioactive substance than is necessary. Distance, along with time and shielding, is a way of limiting exposure. (b)

768. (4) While the patient is receiving therapy, alpha, beta, and gamma rays will be emitted. Therefore the nurse should employ the principles of time, distance, and

shielding when providing care. Extent of exposure to the patient must be monitored and kept within safe limits depending on the type and amount of rays emitted. (a)

769. (2) Nausea, vomiting, restlessness, irritability, and vaginal discharge are to some degree all expected side effects of internal radiotherapy. Pain and elevated temperature may indicate toxic effects; excessive sloughing of tissue can cause hemorrhage or infection. (b)

770. (4) Radium, a radioactive substance, should be handled with forceps, since distance helps to limit exposure to the source of radiation. Foil-lined rubber gloves do not provide adequate shielding. (b)

771. (2) Bicarbonate buffering is limited, hydrogen ions accumulate, and acidosis results. (c)

772. (1) Although ADH and aldosterone have a direct effect on the function of the nephron, the kidneys are ultimately responsible for maintaining fluid and electrolyte balance by excretion or retention based on the body's needs. (b)

773. (4) The Giordano-Giovannetti diet includes very low protein (20 g) and controlled potassium (1500 mg) daily. (b)

774. (3) In renal failure, as the glomerular filtration rate decreases, phosphorus is retained. As hyperphosphatemia occurs, calcium is excreted. Calcium depletion (hypocalcemia) causes tetany. (b)

775. (1) An elevated BUN indicates uremia, which is toxic to the central nervous system and causes mental cloudiness, confusion, and loss of consciousness. (a)

776. (4) Since an external shunt provides circulatory access to a major artery and vein, special safety precautions must be taken to prevent disconnection of the cannulas. Disconnection can cause unimpeded excessive blood loss and death. Clamps should be carried at all times by the patient in case this emergency should arise. (c)

777. (4) The kidneys help control blood pH; therefore the pH of the urine will vary with the needs of the blood and the number of hydrogen ions excreted by the kidney tubules. (c)

778. (2) Since the plasma COP is the major force drawing fluid from the interstitial spaces back into the capillaries, a drop in COP due to albuminuria results in edema. (c)

779. (4) Intact skin is the first line of defense against entry of microorganisms. A surgical incision is a portal of entry. (c)

780. (1) These symptoms result from failure of bile to enter the intestines and subsequent backup into the biliary system and diffusion into the blood. The bilirubin is carried to all body regions including the skin (itching) and kidneys (excretion with coloring of urine). The absence of bilirubin in the intestine results in clay-colored stools. (c)

781. (1) Vitamin C (ascorbic acid) plays a major role in wound healing because it is necessary for the maintenance and formation of strong collagen, the major protein of most connective tissues. (b)

782. (3) Location of the incision results in pain on inspiration or coughing. The subsequent reluctance to cough and

deep breathe facilitates respiratory complications due to retained secretions. (b)

783. (4) Bile, a natural antioxidant, helps to stabilize the vitamin and prevents destruction by oxygen. In addition, bile serves as a transport vehicle for fat through the intestinal wall. (c)

784. (3) Vitamin A is a fat-soluble vitamin that accumulates in the body and is not significantly excreted even if extremely large amounts are ingested. After prolonged ingestion of extremely large doses, toxic effects can occur. (c)

785. (3) Pancreatic enzymes and bile enter the small intestine at the sphincter of Oddi. (c)

786. (4)

Intake		Output	
IV fluid	350 ml	Voiding	150 ml
Gastric tube	600 ml		220 ml
formula			235 ml
Water	150 ml	Aspirated stom-	25 ml
Vitamin	30 ml	ach contents	
TOTAL	1130 ml	TOTAL	630 ml

(b)

787. (2) Excessive loss of gastric juice results in excessive loss of HCl and can lead to alkalosis; the HCl is not available to neutralize the sodium bicarbonate secreted into the duodenum by the pancreas. The intestinal tract absorbs excess HCO_3^- and alkalosis results. (a)

788. (1) The high Fowler's position promotes optimal entry into the esophagus due to gravity. (c)

789. (2) As the uterus drops, the vaginal wall relaxes. When the bladder herniates into the vagina (cystocele) and the rectal wall herniates into the vagina (rectocele), the individual feels pressure or pain in the lower back and/or pelvis. When there is an increase in intra-abdominal pressure in the presence of a cystocele, incontinence results. (b)

790. (1) Relaxation of the pelvic musculature causes the uterus to drop with a subsequent relaxation of the vaginal walls. A rectocele is the protrusion of the rectal wall into the vagina, whereas a cystocele is the protrusion of the bladder into the vaginal wall. (b)

791. (4) Since Mrs. Gorham is past the child-bearing age, a plastic surgical repair designed to tighten the vaginal wall will probably be performed. A hysterectomy is only performed if there is uterine disease, and a pessary is a device employed for a prolapsed uterus. (b)

792. (2) A Foley catheter serves to keep the bladder empty and has nothing to do with preventing bleeding. (a)

793. (1) A generous supply of blood is carried to the uterine arteries and branches of the internal iliac arteries. The vaginal and ovarian arteries also supply the uterus with blood by anastomosing with the uterine vessels. (b)

794. (4) Gonadotropins, follicle-stimulating hormone (FSH),

and luteinizing hormone (LH) are concerned with ovarian changes that produce ovulation. Estrogen levels are high between the end of menses and ovulation because of secretion from the developing follicle. Progesterone levels are high between ovulation and the onset of menses because of secretion from the corpus luteum. The hormones work in concert to stimulate the menstrual cycle. (a)

795. (4) This position maximally exposes the rectal area and facilitates the entry of the sigmoidoscope. (b)

796. (3) The bowel must be cleansed with a nonirritating enema prior to the examination to permit adequate visualization of the mucosa during the sigmoidoscopy. (a)

797. (4) The nurse should pick up all clues to patient anxiety and allow for verbalization. (a)

798. (4) Because neomycin is poorly absorbed from the GI tract, most remains in the intestines and exerts its antibiotic effect on the intestinal mucosa. In preparation for GI surgery the level of microbial organisms will be reduced. (a)

799. (2) Drainage from the colostomy can quickly cause a breakdown of the skin around the stoma if the area is not kept both clean and dry. This, in combination with a warm, moist surface, also predisposes the individual to infection. (a)

800. (3) The stoma of a colostomy must be dilated with a lubricated, gloved finger to prevent strictures and subsequent obstruction of the stoma. (b)

801. (1) Although foods that produce gas are generally avoided, the diet of an individual with a colostomy should be as close to normal as possible for optimum physiologic and psychologic adaptation. (b)

802. (1) The acetabulum is the socket in the pelvis with which the head of the femur articulates. (b)

803. (2) Nails, pins, plates, and screws maintain bone alignment while bone replacement (healing) occurs. (a)

804. (3) Turning and periodic deep breathing promote drainage of and circulation in lung alveoli, which helps to prevent circulatory and pulmonary complications; patients should not be turned onto the affected side to prevent strain and possible misalignment or pressure at fracture site. (b)

805. (2) When lying on the unaffected side there is an increased risk of adduction of the affected thigh, which can result in displacement of the prosthesis. (c)

806. (3) Prune juice and warm water can be administered prophylactically by the nurse to promote defecation; prune juice irritates the bowel mucosa, stimulating peristalsis. Increased fiber in the diet may also improve intestinal motility. (b)

807. (2) Bones become more fragile with advancing age due to osteoporosis, often associated with lower circulating levels of estrogens or testosterone. (a)

808. (2) Gonorrhea is caused by a gram-negative diplococcus called *Neisseria gonorrhoeae*. (a)

809. (2) In the male, the inflammatory process associated with the infection may lead to the destruction of the epididymis. In the female, the gonorrheal infection causes destruction of the tubal mucosa and eventually tubo-ovarian abscesses. (a)

810. (3) Gonorrhea is a highly contagious disease transmitted through sexual intercourse. The incubation period varies, but symptoms usually occur 2 to 10 days after contact. Early effective treatment prevents complications. (a)

811. (1) Penicillin inhibits the synthesis of bacterial cell walls. It is effective against *Neisseria gonorrhoeae*, a gram-negative diplococcus. (b)

812. (1) Penicillin is specific for *Neisseria gonorrhoeae* and eradicates the microorganism. (a)

813. (3) Flexion contractures of the hip can occur when the patient is kept supine with the leg raised on a pillow; therefore the patient should be prone periodically to extend the hip. (b)

814. (1) This position offsets the development of hip deformities due to contractures; it also maintains correct center of gravity when the patient is upright. (b)

815. (2) Preparing muscles that will do the work in crutch walking is imperative. (b)

816. (2) Four-point gait provides for weight-bearing on all 4 extremities and maximum support during ambulation. (b)

817. (2) Practicing ambulation without proper preparation of ambulation techniques and strengthening involved muscle groups would not be helpful in the rehabilitation process. (a)

818. (1) Rehabilitation should begin on admission; this includes preoperative discussion of the nature of the operation and rehabilitation techniques. (b)

819. (1) Bleeding between periods is abnormal. The occurrence of bleeding other than during the menstrual period is known as metrorrhagia. (b)

820. (4) A hysterectomy only involves the removal of the uterus. The ovaries, which secrete estrogen and progesterone, are not removed. Therefore menopause will not be precipitated but will occur naturally. (b)

821. (3) The prescribing of medications is the legal responsibility of physicians. In addition, the use of hormones is controversial and depends on the physician's beliefs and the patient's needs. (b)

822. (1) This response reflects back and verbalizes the patient's feelings in a nonjudgmental way. (a)

823. (4) Oral contraceptives contain hormones that help to regulate the menstrual cycle. (b)

824. (4) Compact bone is stronger than cancellous bone because of its greater density. Compact bone forms from cancellous bone by addition of concentric rings of bone substance to the marrow spaces of cancellous bone; the large marrow spaces are reduced to haversian canals. (a)

825. (2) The ache in muscles that have been vigorously worked without adequate oxygen supply is caused in part by the buildup of lactic acid. During rest the lactic acid is oxidized completely to CO_2 and H_2O, providing ATP for further muscular contraction. (a)

826. (3) A cataract is a clouding of the crystalline lens or its capsule. (b)

827. (2) Activities such as bending, coughing, and rigorous hair and teeth brushing cause increased intraocular pressure and may result in hemorrhage in the anterior chamber. (b)

828. (2) Retinal detachment is a separation between the sensory retina and the retinal pigment epithelium. These layers are not attached by any special structures and can separate as a result of various pathologic processes. (c)

829. (1) Scar formation seals the hole and promotes attachment of the 2 retinal surfaces. (c)

830. (1) Vitamin A is used in the formation of retinene, a component of the light-sensitive rhodopsin molecule. (a)

831. (2) Deep green and yellow vegetables contain large quantities of the pigments, α-, β-, and γ-carotene; β-carotene is the major chemical precursor of vitamin A in human nutrition. (a)

832. (4) Malignant melanoma of the eye is an intraocular tumor that metastasizes rapidly; therefore enucleation—removal of the eye—is the treatment of choice. (c)

833. (4) Alterations in pH of the vaginal tract cause cellular alteration and destruction. (c)

834. (3) Douches with acidic solutions such as vinegar and water bring back the normal acidity of the vaginal tract. (b)

835. (3) The dorsal position takes advantage of the anatomic position of the vaginal tract and prevents undue retention or too rapid a return of the douche. (a)

836. (3) This is the anatomic direction of the vaginal tract in the back-lying position. (b)

837. (2) Erosion of the cervix frequently occurs at the squamo-columnar junction, the most common site for carcinoma of the cervix. (a)

838. (3) Any product containing aluminum, magnesium, or calcium ions should not be taken the hour before or after an oral dose, since it decreases absorption by as much as 25% to 50%. (c)

839. (2) Since pressure is force developed per unit of area over which the force is applied, as the area decreases the pressure increases. The tip of a needle or the point of a knife has an extremely small area, and consequently a very high pressure can be developed for a given force. (c)

840. (2) Amino acids are absorbed into blood in intestinal capillaries with the aid of vitamin B_6 via the energy-dependent system—active transport. (b)

841. (2) Complete proteins contain sufficient amounts of all essential amino acids and are of animal origin. (b)

842. (1) These amino acids are needed to maintain life and are not produced by the body. (a)

843. (2) Phospho-Soda is a saline cathartic, increasing the osmotic pressure within the intestines so that body fluids are drawn into the bowel, stimulating bowel stretching, peristalsis, and defecation. (c)

844. (4) Antibodies produced against group A beta-hemolytic streptococci sometimes interact with antigens in the heart's valves, causing damage and symptoms of rheumatic heart disease. (b)

845. (2) Streptococci are present on the skin at all times. They cause many infections common in humans. (b)

846. (1) In gangrene the release of iron from hemoglobin as erythrocytes disintegrate in necrotic tissue results in ferrous sulfide formation, causing darkening of the tissues. (c)

847. (3) A one normal solution is defined as containing 1 gram equivalent weight of solute per liter of solution. In human body fluids the milliequivalent (1/1000 of the gram equivalent) is a more convenient term for expressing concentration, since the gram equivalent is rather large. Isotonic solutions have equal osmotic pressure. A one molar solution contains 1 gram-molecular weight of a solute per liter of solution. Molarity is not as informative as normality because the latter is based on the actual chemical-combining properties of the substance involved. (c)

848. (1) Unless Mr. Manor has been certified as incompetent, he retains the right of informed consent. (c)

849. (3) An individual is held legally responsible for actions committed against another individual or his property. (c)

850. (2) False imprisonment and battery are wrongs committed by one person against another. The individual is legally responsible for the acts. (c)

851. (1) The reporting of possible child abuse is required by law, and the nurse can remain anonymous. (b)

852. (1) Each state or province is charged with the responsibility of protecting the health and welfare of its populace, which it does by regulating nursing practice. (b)

853. (4) Coumarin anticoagulants are administered orally and take 2 to 3 days to achieve the desired decrease in prothrombin level, whereas heparin, which must be administered parenterally, has immediate effects. (c)

854. (3) Warfarin (Coumadin) has been shown to inhibit the metabolism of phenytoin (Dilantin), which results in an accumulation of this drug in the body. (b)

855. (2) Coumarin derivatives cause an increased prothrombin time, leading to increased risk of bleeding. Any abnormal or excessive bleeding must be reported, since it may indicate toxic levels of the drug. (b)

856. (4) Compliance with the prescribed regimen, which includes taking the drug and having prothrombin times performed by the laboratory, is necessary for safe and effective warfarin (Coumadin) therapy. The dosage of warfarin is adjusted according to the prothrombin time, and if

the patient fails to take the drug as prescribed, the tests are not reliable in monitoring the response to therapy. (a)

857. (2) Secobarbital sodium (as well as other barbiturates) decreases the body's response to warfarin (Coumadin), and as a result there is less suppression of prothrombin. (c)

858. (4) a subjective symptom such as ringing in the ear can be felt only by a patient. (b)

859. (3) Massive doses of penicillin may limit CNS damage if treatment is started before neural deterioration occurs due to syphilis. (c)

860. (1) Since stomach distention (after eating) results in contractions of the colon (gastrocolic reflex) promoting defecation, establishing some regularity of meals that include adequate bulk or fiber will help to establish routine patterns of defecation. (b)

861. (4) *Trichomonas vaginalis* is a protozoan that favors an alkaline environment. (c)

862. (2) Since *Trichomonas vaginalis* favors an alkaline environment, vinegar, an acid, is utilized to decrease the pH of the vagina. (c)

863. (3) Metronidazole is a potent amebicide. It is extremely effective in eradicating the protozoan *Trichomonas vaginalis*. (c)

864. (3) Primitive sex cells, called spermatogonia, are present in newborn males. At puberty these cells mature and form spermatozoa. (b)

865. (3) Sperm cells are very fragile and can be destroyed by heat, resulting in sterility. (b)

866. (2) This recognizes that the patient is upset and by indirect questioning helps facilitate communication. (b)

867. (4) This recognizes the patient's feeling of anxiety as valid; informing her honestly of a fact may help to decrease the anxiety. (b)

868. (1) Polyps are usually benign but should undergo biopsy, since epidermoid cancer occasionally arises from cervical polyps. (a)

869. (1) When the cancerous cells are completely confined within the epithelium of the cervix without stromal invasion, it is stage 0 and called carcinoma in situ. (c)

870. (3) The endocervical surface is frequently altered by metaplasia or covered by a variant of squamous epithelium. It is thus called the transitional zone. This area is often distorted by eversion and laceration, especially in pregnancy. Therefore it is a frequent site for carcinoma. (c)

871. (3) Conization (conical excision of the lesion), cryosurgery, and hysterectomy can be used in treatment of squamous cell carcinoma in situ. If treatment is initiated during the preinvasive stage, it is 100% curable. (b)

Psychiatric nursing

1. (4) The unconscious stores past experiences and the emotional feelings associated with them. These emotional feelings influence one's perceptions, attitudes, and behavior. (c)

2. (1) Mild anxiety motivates one to action, such as learning or emotional changes; higher levels of anxiety tend to blur the individual's perceptions and interfere with functioning. (b)

3. (2) The individual using sublimation attempts to fulfill desires by selecting a socially acceptable activity rather than those which are socially unacceptable (e.g., pursuing a career in nursing as a means of giving and receiving love). (b)

4. (3) When acting out against the primary source of anxiety creates even further anxiety or danger, the individual may use displacement to express feelings on a safer object. (a)

5. (2) The parameters set by birth, the psychologic experiences, and the environment make each individual unique; although other factors may impinge to a slight degree, these factors form the personality. (b)

6. (3) When the individual experiences a threat to self-esteem, anxiety increases and the normal defense mechanisms are used to protect the ego. (a)

7. (4) Incorporation of parental and societal values into the superego leads to the development of a sense of right and wrong; guilt and shame are experienced when these values are broken. Thus the superego is the conscience. (b)

8. (1) The child views his own worth by the response received from the parents. This sense of worth sets the basic ego strengths and is vital to the formation of the personality. (a)

9. (4) The sympathetic or autonomic nervous system reacts to stress by releasing epinephrine, which prepares the body to fight or flee by increasing the heart rate, constricting peripheral vessels, and increasing oxygen supply to the muscles. (b)

10. (3) Conscience and a sense of right and wrong are expressed in the superego, which acts to counterbalance the id's desire for immediate gratification. (b)

11. (4) Learning from others occurs in a group setting and is reinforced by group acceptance of the norms; group pressure is peer pressure, which is more easily accepted if the individual wants to stay in the group. (a)

12. (2) Socialization, values, and role definition are learned within the family and help develop a sense of self; once established in the family, the child can more easily move into society. (a)

13. (3) Socialization occurs through communication with others; without some form of communication there can be no socialization. (a)

14. (3) Before this age the infant has not developed enough ego strength to have an identity or personality. (c)

15. (2) The toddler learns to say ''no'' and to express independence, yet because of human nature the toddler is both physically and emotionally dependent on the parents. (c)

16. (1) The child is learning to identify own needs but is also still involved in attempting to please parents; the conflict that arises when trying to toilet train before the child is ready can be severe and overwhelming. (b)

17. (2) Testing the self both physically and psychologically occurs during the toddler stage after trust has been achieved. (c)

18. (1) The infant and toddler are dependent on significant others and react strongly to separation and loss, which they view as rejection and abandonment; these needs are strongest during the ''taking in'' or oral phase of development. (c)

19. (3) A sense of one's self and a feeling of belonging form the basis for mental health, since it provides comfort with self and group. (c)

20. (1) Rivalry between siblings is normal and arises because one child resents the care and attention given another child; one child unconsciously wishes the other would disappear and frequently acts out negatively against him. (a)

21. (2) The individual who cannot communicate cannot test reality; without this connection to others or reality severe emotional problems will develop. (b)

22. (1) Feelings of resentment toward children by parents is a normal response, and it is vital to help parents realize this to relieve feelings of guilt and shame. (a)

23. (3) During the oedipal stage (between 2½ and 6 years of age) the child has many fears about his body; any invasive techniques done at this time can create severe emotional problems. (c)

24. (1) The mature personality does not respond to the immediate gratification demands of the id or the oppressive control of the superego because the ego is strong enough to maintain a balance between them. (a)

25. (3) Values and beliefs from parents and society are expressed through the child's play world; these values become part of the child's system through the process of internalization (introjection). (c)

26. (4) Freud's theory is that a child develops a sexualized love for the parent of the opposite sex and becomes jealous of the parent of the same sex; these thoughts result in feelings of guilt, anxiety, fear, and hate toward the parent of the same sex, which are repressed. (a)

27. (2) Child resolves oedipal conflicts by learning to identify with the parent of the same sex and accomplishes this by mimicking the role of this parent. (b)

28. (1) When props are needed to blur reality, the individual is not able to rely on self to test out situations, and dependence on others therefore increases. (c)

29. (4) During a crisis one may regress to a stage provoking less anxiety in an attempt to cope with an unacceptable situation. (b)

30. (4) The defense mechanism is called conversion because the individual actually reduces emotional anxiety by converting it to a physical disability. (b)

31. (2) By developing skills in one area the individual compensates or makes up for a real or imagined deficiency, thereby maintaining a positive self-image. (a)

32. (3) An illusion is a misperception or misinterpretation of actual external stimuli. (b)

33. (3) Mediating frustration within the real world is an ego function and requires ego strength. (b)

34. (1) The ego develops during childhood as a result of positive experiences; when the situation in childhood is such that severe anxiety is unresolved, the ego seems to be permanently traumatized and is unable to totally recover. (b)

35. (3) The child realizes that the parent of the same sex cannot be bested in a struggle for the affection of the parent of the opposite sex; the role and behavior of the same sex parent are therefore assumed by the child to attract the parent of the opposite sex. (b)

36. (1) Any behavioral therapy or learning new methods of dealing with situations requires modifications of approach and attitudes; hence personality change. (b)

37. (2) The superego incorporates all experiences and learning from external environments (society, family, etc.) into the internal environment. (b)

38. (2) Slips of the tongue, also called ''Freudian slips,'' are material from the unconscious that slips out in unguarded moments. (a)

39. (4) Poor interpersonal relationships, inappropriate behavior, and learning disabilities prevent these children from emotionally adapting or responding to the environment despite possible high level of intelligence. (b)

40. (1) From infancy the child is nonresponsive. Not wanting to eat demonstrates a further withdrawal. (c)

41. (3) The drug of choice in this diagnosis. It appears to act by stimulating release of norepinephrine from nerve endings in the brain stem. (b)

42. (3) When the individual consciously pretends an illness with no physical basis it is called malingering. (c)

43. (1) Her stated feelings of distrust of others and her inability to mix socially can best be defined in these terms. (a)

44. (4) Demonstrating that the staff can be trusted is a vital initial step in the therapy program. (b)

45. (1) Patients cannot be argued out of delusions, so the best approach is a simple statement of reality. (c)

46. (2) It is important to help the patient focus on her feelings, and this is the only response that does so. (c)

47. (4) If patients feel a need to be punished, it is best to permit them to engage in controlled activities that expiate guilt feelings. (b)

48. (1) Bringing another patient into a set situation would be the most therapeutic, least threatening approach. (b)

49. (1) Since patient has feelings that people are trying to harm her, assignment to a 4-bed room would be very threatening. (b)

50. (2) Patient is too anxious to sleep in 4-bed room and should simply be told she is being moved to a private room. (c)

51. (3) Sitting quietly gives the patient the message that the nurse accepts her feelings and cares. (a)

52. (4) Needing to be dependent while wanting to be independent creates a struggle that makes all movement psychologically difficult. Symptoms develop and remove psychologic choice, making movement physically impossible. (b)

53. (3) This type of defense (conversion reaction) tends to be a learned behavioral response that the individual will use when put under stress. (b)

54. (1) Patient is caught between two equally compelling needs and movement is impossible; paralysis justifies inability to move to the patient. (b)

55. (2) From the history you can determine that the patient's contacts were limited, her schedule fixed, and her demands on self quite rigid. (b)

56. (2) Her suicidal impulses take priority, and she must be stopped from acting on them while her treatment is in progress. (b)

57. (1) These patients can usually be fairly easily distracted by getting them involved in repetitious, simple tasks. (b)

58. (4) Points out reality while accepting the fact that the patient believes they are real. (b)

59. (2) Nurse's response again urges patient to reflect on feelings and encourages communication of feeling tones. (c)

60. (3) Patients frequently report suicidal feelings so that staff will have the chance to stop them; they really ask, "Do you care enough to stop me?" (c)

61. (4) The patient is using this compulsive behavior to control anxiety and needs to continue with it until anxiety is reduced and more acceptable methods are developed to handle it. (b)

62. (2) By carrying out the compulsive ritual, the patient unconsciously tries to control the situation so that unacceptable impulses and feelings will not be acted on. (b)

63. (2) Helping patients understand that the behavior is being used to control impulses usually makes them more amenable to psychotherapy. (b)

64. (3) The patient with senile psychosis rarely expresses any concern about personal appearance, and the staff must meet most of the needs in this area. (a)

65. (1) When an elderly person's brain atrophies, some unusual deposits of iron are scattered on nerve cells. Throughout the brain, areas of deeply staining amyloid, called senile plaques, can be found; these plaques are end stages in the destruction of brain tissue. (c)

66. (1) Patients with senile psychosis need a simple environment and are unable to make choices due to brain cell destruction. (b)

67. (3) The senile patient attempts to utilize those defense mechanisms which have worked in the past but uses them in an exaggerated manner; because of brain cell destruction they are unable to focus on one defense mechanism or to develop new ones. (b)

68. (2) Damaged brain cells do not regenerate, so care is directed toward preventing further damage; patient will always need protective and supportive care in the future. (b)

69. (1) The patient with senile psychosis will be most comfortable with the familiar, repetitive daily routine, since it creates less anxiety. (b)

70. (3) Simply states facts without getting involved in role conflict. (b)

71. (2) The patient has the right to decide how he will be introduced, and the staff should accept his wishes. (b)

72. (2) A patient out of control needs controls set for him. Staff must understand that patient is not deliberately setting out to disrupt the unit. (c)

73. (4) The hyperactive patient is usually rather easily distracted, so the excess energy can be redirected into constructive channels. (a)

74. (1) A firm, warm consistent approach will help reduce the patient's anxiety, thereby reducing hyperactivity. (b)

75. (4) Hyperactive patients frequently will not take the time to sit down to eat because they are overinvolved in everything that is going on. (b)

76. (3) The hyperactive patient will frequently eat hand foods that do not require sitting down to eat. (b)

77. (1) Anxiety is communicated and is contagious, since it is an interpersonal experience. (b)

78. (3) These actions make the environment as emotionally unthreatening as is realistically possible. (b)

79. (2) Response demonstrates acceptance of the patient but does set limits on the patient's behavior. (c)

80. (3) Helps the patient focus on situations that precipitate feelings. (b)

81. (2) Sitting with her indicates acceptance and demonstrates that the nurse feels she is worthy of spending time with. (b)

82. (4) Everyone has the right to personal sexual preference, but limits must be set on acting out behavior within the hospital. (c)

83. (3) Adult homosexuality is a regression to an earlier, oral and anal stage rather than acceptance of the more mature genital heterosexual level. (b)

84. (1) Hyperactive behavior in individuals such as this is

typical of the hypermanic flight into reality associated with affective disorders. (a)

85. (3) Recognizing it as part of the illness makes it easier to tolerate, but limits must be set for staff and other patients' benefit. Setting limits also demonstrates to the patient that you care enough to stop her. (b)

86. (2) Hyperactive patients burn up large quantities of calories, which must be replenished; since these patients will not take the time to sit down to eat, providing them with food they can carry with them sometimes helps. (b)

87. (1) Physical activity will help utilize some of the excess energy without requiring her to make decisions or forcing other patients to deal with her. (c)

88. (4) Experience can be used to keep patient in contact with reality. (b)

89. (3) Behavior demonstrates increased anxiety; since it was directed toward the new staff, it was probably precipitated by their arrival. (b)

90. (4) When individuals use these defense mechanisms to blur the pains of reality, they are unable to test out their feelings or differentiate the real world from their personal intrapsychic perceptions. (b)

91. (3) A delusion of persecution is a firm, fixed belief or feeling of being harassed, in danger, or at the mercy of others. (a)

92. (2) Nursing care must be a steady attempt to draw the patient into some response. This can best be accomplished by focusing on nonthreatening subjects that do not demand a specific response. (b)

93. (3) Keeping the withdrawn patient oriented to reality prevents him from withdrawing even further into his private world. (a)

94. (1) By observing the patient's behavior, the nurse is able to better understand the feelings, since behavior usually serves a purpose and is directed toward satisfaction of needs. (b)

95. (3) A one-to-one trusting relationship is essential to help the patient become more involved and interested in interpersonal relationships. (a)

96. (1) Depression is a disturbance in the mood or affect (classified as an affective disorder) that usually develops when the ego suffers a real or imagined loss. (c)

97. (3) No organic pathology has as yet been identified in schizophrenia. The process of behavioral response seems to be learned in childhood, causing the individual to distort events and relationships and lose the ability to relate to the world. (a)

98. (2) Disinterest in or fear of personal involvement creates distancing behavior and lack of response to the environment. (b)

99. (1) Mental illness is characterized by the use of abnormal defense mechanisms or the abnormal use of normal defense mechanisms; these defenses build a wall and interrupt interpersonal relationships. (a)

100. (4) Shows acceptance for the patient yet sets firm limits on the behavior. This response also points out reality to the patient. (b)

101. (2) Family interaction patterns and role identification and definition lay the foundations for the child's future emotional response. (b)

102. (3) Inner psychic stress and environmental difficulties can interfere with the function of organically sound organs resulting in a loss of ability to communicate. (a)

103. (2) The nurse's response really was a threat by attempting to put pressure on the patient to speak or be left alone. (b)

104. (3) Patients who are out of control are seeking control and frequently respond to simple directions stated in a firm voice. (b)

105. (4) The nurse's response provides an example to the patient that feelings can be expressed by words rather than by action. This response also demonstrates that the nurse cares enough to set limits on behavior. (b)

106. (3) The nurse has to base nursing intervention on a patient's problems. Since retarded depression is due to the patient's feelings of self-rejection, it is important for the nurse to have the patient identify these feelings before a plan of action can be taken. (b)

107. (4) This attitude conveys to others that Mr. Long feels he is not really significant enough for anyone to listen to. (b)

108. (2) The best approach is the direct approach at the first interview, since this sets the focus and concern and lets you know what the patient is feeling now. (b)

109. (4) This is the most therapeutic approach. The staff member also provides the patient with special attention to meet his dependency needs and reduce his self-defeating attitude. (c)

110. (1) Routines should be kept simple and no demands should be made that the patient cannot meet. The patient is depressed, and all his reactions will be slow. Putting pressure on the patient will only increase anxiety and feelings of worthlessness. (c)

111. (2) Patient is expressing his hostility symbolically by not being cooperative. He has a right to feel this way. If the staff criticizes him, it will only increase his feelings of guilt. (c)

112. (3) Patient is very dependent, and these individuals can never get enough attention to fill this dependence. This unfulfilled need causes anger, which he has problems expressing for fear of losing the person he is dependent on. (c)

113. (1) Patients fear this therapy because of the expected pain. If they are reassured that they will be asleep and have no pain, there will be less anxiety and more cooperation. (b)

114. (3) The development of glaucoma is one of the side effects of imipramine (Tofranil), and the patient should be alerted to these symptoms. (c)

115. (2) This response demonstrates understanding that the

newly discharged patient needs to have the support of the therapeutic unit when he goes home. He needs to feel that in a crisis he can turn to them for this support. (b)

116. (2) Acting out anxiety with antisocial behavior is most commonly found in individuals with personality disorders rather than psychoneurotic disorders. (c)

117. (4) In phobias the individual transfers anxiety to a rather safe inanimate object. Therefore the anxiety and resulting feelings will only be precipitated when in direct contact with the object. (b)

118. (2) The longer the child stays out, the more difficult it is to get him to return to school, since more fantasies and fears develop. (c)

119. (3) Having poor superego control, these individuals cannot set limits for themselves and require an environment in which appropriate limits for behavior are set for them. (a)

120. (3) Accepting the patient and the symptomatic behavior sets the foundation for the nurse-patient relationship; setting limits provides external controls and helps to lower anxiety. (c)

121. (1) If the patient is prevented from using the ritualistic behavior to control anxiety, he has been deprived of his defense and has no way of relieving tension. (a)

122. (4) The problem is psychologic, and therefore the initial approach by the nurse should be directed toward establishing trust. (a)

123. (3) If seizures were physiologically based, the patient would not be able to continue to chew gum. This "attack" should be reported as a behavioral response, with the precipitating factors noted. (c)

124. (3) Accepts patient as a person of worth rather than being cold or implying rejection; however, the nurse maintains a professional rather than a social role. (a)

125. (1) Individuals with this personality disorder tend to be self-centered and impulsive; they lack judgment and superego controls and do not profit from their mistakes. (c)

126. (4) The lack of superego control allows the ego and the id to control the behavior. Self-motivation and self-satisfaction are of paramount concern. (c)

127. (4) Patient is in the hospital for treatment and evaluation not judgment of behavior. Since he feels people will judge him, it is important to point out that at this time he is the only one filling this role. (c)

128. (4) Lets patient know you realize he is having difficulty without asking direct questions or focusing on specific behavior. (a)

129. (3) By staying physically close the nurse provides the patient with the message that somebody cares enough to be there and that she is a person worth caring for. (c)

130. (2) When tension is reduced, anxiety diminishes and the person feels more comfortable, safe, and secure. (b)

131. (2) Anxiety is a normal human response, causing both physical and emotional changes that everyone experiences when faced with stressful situations. (b)

132. (1) Providing support, understanding, and acceptance of feelings the patient is experiencing is essential for reducing stress. (b)

133. (1) The "fight or flight" responses of the autonomic nervous system would be stimulated and result in these findings. (b)

134. (4) Learning a variety of coping mechanisms helps reduce anxiety in stressful situations. (a)

135. (3) The patient with conversion hysteria literally converts the anxiety to the symptom. Once the symptom develops, it acts as a defense against the anxiety and the patient is almost diagnostically anxiety free. (b)

136. (2) The physical symptoms are not the patient's major problem and therefore should not be the focus for care. This is a psychologic problem, and the focus should be on this level. (b)

137. (2) The patient's anxiety results from being unable to psychologically choose between 2 conflicting actions; the conversion to a physical disability removes the choice and therefore reduces the anxiety. (c)

138. (3) The symptoms are problematic to the patient and thus have caused emotional pain that is beyond conscious control. (a)

139. (3) Recognizes the importance of feelings and provides an opening so that patient may talk about her feelings. (b)

140. (2) Puts focus on the feelings, not on a statement of what did or did not happen. (b)

141. (2) Ambivalance about life and death plus the introspection commonly found in patients with emotional problems would result in increased anxiety and fear in the group members. (b)

142. (2) The first step in a nursing care plan should be the establishment of a meaningful relationship because it is through this relationship that the patient can be helped. (b)

143. (2) Assisting patients with grooming keeps them in contact with reality and allows them to see that the staff cares enough to help and places value on appearance. (a)

144. (4) Sets limits on behavior as well as showing the patient that staff care enough to protect her; accepts patient but rejects behavior. (c)

145. (3) Echolalia is the repetition of another person's remarks, words, or statements. It occurs when individuals are fearful of saying their own words and therefore just echo the words of others. (b)

146. (3) Patient is not voiding on the floor to express hostility, but is confused; taking her to the toilet frequently limits the voiding in inappropriate places. (b)

147. (1) Patient needs limits set; response by the nurse sets limits, rejects the behavior, but accepts the patient. (b)

148. (3) Lets patient know you are available if she needs you and demonstrates an acceptance of her. (b)

149. (4) A delusion is a fixed, false personal belief that is not founded in reality. (a)
150. (2) Nurse's response reflects on patient's feelings rather than focusing on verbalization. (b)
151. (3) Succinylcholine causes paralysis of the diaphragm and the intercostal muscles as well as other muscles; this paralysis causes a cessation of respiration. (a)
152. (2) Patients are confused when they awaken after electro-convulsive therapy and have a loss of recent memory, so it is important to orient them to time, place, and situation. (b)
153. (2) The anniversary frequently reemphasizes the feeling of loss and abandonment and serves to heighten the current feelings of depression and hopelessness. (c)
154. (3) Gives the patient the nonverbal message that someone cares and that she is worthy of attention and concern. (b)
155. (2) Telling the patient you will spend time with her communicates that you find her worthy of your time and you care. (c)
156. (3) Depression is usually on both emotional and physical levels, so a simple daily routine is the least stressful and least anxiety-producing. (b)
157. (4) The liquid concentrate is a highly irritating substance on contact with skin and eyes and can cause uncomfortable dermatologic conditions. (c)
158. (3) Acute dystonic reactions, parkinsonian syndrome, and akathisia are observable side effects of chlorpromazine hydrochloride therapy. (b)
159. (1) Checks liver functioning, since liver damage may occur from use of the drug. Cholestatic hepatitis with obstructive jaundice is the most frequent form of liver disturbance and can be identified by jaundiced sclera and clay-colored stools. (c)
160. (1) The physician is responsible for medication orders but depends on the nurse's observations in making decisions. (b)
161. (3) Occurs as a late and persistent extrapyramidal complication of long-term chlorpromazine therapy. Can take many forms such as torsion spasm, opisthotonos, oculogyric crisis, drooping of the head, protrusion of the tongue, and other facial disturbances. (c)
162. (4) Lithium carbonate does not impair intellectual activity, consciousness, or range or quality of emotional life, yet it is able to control the manic behavior in manic-depressive psychosis. (b)
163. (2) Unintentional tremors are one of the extrapyramidal side effects of the major tranquilizers and are considered common and manageable. (a)
164. (3) The monoamine oxidase inhibitors can cause a hypertensive crisis if food or beverages that are rich in amines or amino acids are ingested. (b)
165. (1) Patient taking chlorpromazine should be told to stay out of the sun to avoid severe sunburn, since photosensitivity makes skin susceptible to burning. (b)

166. (4) The major tranquilizers modify the behavior of the psychotic patient so that the patient can more effectively cope with the environment and benefit from therapy. (a)
167. (1) These drugs are used to control the extrapyramidal symptoms (parkinsonism-like symptoms) that often develop as a side effect of major tranquilizer therapy. (b)
168. (3) These drugs control the extrapyramidal parkinsonism symptoms associated with the major tranquilizers and are classified as antiparkinsonian drugs. (b)
169. (2) Naloxone hydrochloride (Narcan) is a narcotic antagonist that counteracts and reverses respiratory depressive action of narcotics without causing sedation or analgesia. Nalorphine (Nalline) could also be used but can precipitate a severe withdrawal reaction. (b)
170. (3) Narcan is used when narcotic-induced apnea occurs, since the drug competes for central nervous system receptor sites, thus acting as a narcotic antagonist. (c)
171. (3) When Narcan is metabolized and its effects are diminished, the respiratory distress due to the original drug overdose returns. (b)
172. (4) The strength of this drug is controlled and remains constant from dose to dose, which is uncertain in illicit drugs. (c)
173. (3) Drug is not taken for medical reasons but for the favorable, pleasant, unusual, or desired effects it produces. It is often taken in doses that would be fatal if the individual had not established a tolerance to it. (b)
174. (3) The addict tries to avoid stress and reality, and the drug produces a blurring of these feelings to the point that the addict becomes dependent on it. (a)
175. (3) The symptoms of withdrawal begin within 8 hours, become more severe 24 hours later, and reach a peak on the third day. (c)
176. (1) The addictive personality is marked by low self-esteem, fear of stress, and dependence with poor self-boundaries and a need for immediate gratification. (b)
177. (1) When methadone is reduced, a craving for narcotics may occur; without narcotics anxiety will increase, agitation will occur, and the patient may try to leave the hospital to secure drugs. (b)
178. (4) Alcoholics have a low self-image and overwhelming guilt feelings; they drink to relieve these feelings, but the drinking only adds to them. (b)
179. (3) Addresses the emotional impact of this delusion; the nurse's presence can reduce anxiety and provide comfort. (c)
180. (2) The individual is unaware of gaps in memory, so the use of stories is an unconscious attempt to deny or cover up the gaps. (a)
181. (4) The patient is using denial as a defense against feelings of guilt. (a)
182. (3) Focuses on patient's feelings rather than the organization itself; organization is effective only when the patient is able to openly discuss feelings. (a)

183. (2) Sharing problems with others who are also open and concerned because of similar problems can reduce guilt and shame and begin to increase ego strengths. (a)

184. (3) The nurse's failure to observe what was brought in for the patient constituted negligence. Her knowledge of the alcoholic would warrant checking to see what the patient was consuming. (b)

185. (4) Thiamine is a coenzyme in producing energy from glucose. If thiamine is not present in adequate amounts, nerve activity is diminished and damage or degeneration of myelin sheaths occurs. (b)

186. (1) Polydrug users abuse a variety of drugs in their search for the ultimate ''high.'' They usually will include alcohol in their search and frequently combine their abuses. (b)

187. (4) Members find sympathy, patience, and understanding in the group. They are able to have their dependence needs met while helping others who are even more dependent than themselves. (a)

188. (4) Self-help groups are successful because they support a basic human need for acceptance. A feeling of comfort and safety and a sense of belonging may be achieved in a nonjudgmental, supportive, sharing experience with others. (b)

189. (1) Self-help groups deal with behavior and changes in behavior rather than the underlying causes of behavior. Small steps are encouraged and when attained are reinforced by the group. (c)

190. (4) according to the philosophy of Alcoholics Anonymous, the alcoholic must identify his own need to seek help and is thus the primary rehabilitator. (a)

191. (1) Intrinsic motivation, stimulated from within the learner, is essential if rehabilitation is to be successful. Often the patient is most emotionally ready for help when he has ''hit bottom.'' Only then is he motivationally ready to face reality and put forth the necessary energy and effort to change his behavior. (a)

192. (4) Past level of success demonstrates ego strengths that can be built on. (b)

193. (3) Helps patient to realize the staff cares about him and that he is worthy of care. (b)

194. (3) Encourages the patient to talk about feelings without really setting the focus for the discussion. (b)

195. (4) The nurse failed to use her knowledge regarding suicidal patients and did not protect the patient from this ever-present danger. Her failure could be legally defined as negligence. (b)

196. (1) The nurse's major tool in psychiatric nursing is the therapeutic use of self. Psychiatric nurses must learn to be aware of their own feelings and how they affect the situation. (c)

197. (2) The therapeutic milieu is directed toward helping the patient develop effective ways of dealing with interpersonal situations. (b)

198. (2) Permits the patient to see that his feelings are not unique but are shared by others. (a)

199. (1) By sensing, supporting, and verbalizing the emotional feelings of others the individual emerges as the leader. (a)

200. (3) Sharing problems with others who have similar problems, thoughts, and feelings helps the individual learn new ways of coping. (b)

201. (1) The group setting provides the individual with the opportunity to learn that others share the same problems and needs; the group also provides an arena where new methods of relating to others can be tried. (c)

202. (2) Group therapy should focus on the present and how current problems and feelings are affecting current behavior. In the group setting the individual members have the opportunity to receive feedback on their behavior. (b)

203. (3) A person able to cope with life situations usually has developed fairly strong ego defenses. In a crisis situation these individuals frequently just need support to regroup their strengths and reestablish their ability to cope. (b)

204. (2) The current trend in psychiatry is to treat the patient and maintain him in the community. This trend includes the family and community in the plan and has reduced the number of patients in psychiatric hospitals. (a)

205. (1) The day hospital provides the patient with a therapeutic setting for a few hours daily during the transitional stage between hospital and total discharge. (b)

Maternity nursing

1. (1) If the patient is to remain at home, she must be aware of when to notify her physician of her symptoms. (b)

2. (2) Tension may be the precipitating cause of gastroesophageal regurgitation early in pregnancy. Displacement of the stomach and delayed emptying of stomach contents due to the enlarged uterus may be the cause of heartburn later in pregnancy. (c)

3. (3) The increase in estrogen during pregnancy causes hyperplasia of the vaginal mucosa, which results in increased production of mucus by endocervical glands that contains many exfoliated epithelial cells. (b)

4. (1) The antibodies in human milk provide the newborn infant with immunity against all or most of the pathogens that the mother has encountered. (b)

5. (2) Maternal hypotension is a common complication of conduction anesthesia for labor. Nausea is one of the first clues that this has occurred. Elevating the extremities restores blood to central circulation. (c)

6. (1) A neat surgical incision is easier to repair and quicker to heal than an irregular laceration. (a)

7. (3) Respirations are normally abdominal, diaphragmatic, irregular, and 30 to 50 per minute. (b)

8. (3) The chorion is the outermost membrane that helps to

form the placenta. The chorion develops villi and, through its interaction with the endometrium, becomes part of the placenta. (c)

9. (1) Progesterone is secreted mainly by the corpus luteum; it helps to prepare the endometrium for possible implantation of a fertilized ovum. The adrenal cortex secretes only small amounts of progesterone. (b)

10. (4) Gestation is divided into 3 stages—the blastocyst, the embryo, and the fetus. (b)

11. (4) A determination of the station (descent) of the fetus is based on the relationship of the presenting part and the spine. If too small, delivery cannot occur. (c)

12. (1) The true regular contractions of labor increase in intensity and regularity with activity. (c)

13. (1) To allow for the larger intake of air, the normal adaptation is to increase the size of the thoracic cavity. (c)

14. (2) Naegle's Rule is an indirect noninvasive method for estimating the date of delivery:

$$EDC = LMP + 7 \text{ days} - 3 \text{ months} + 1 \text{ year} \quad (b)$$

15. (3) Response encourages further elaboration of what Mrs. Greene means by feeling very tired and sick to her stomach. It is always best to let the client explain her symptoms rather than the nurse drawing conclusions immediately. (b)

16. (4) A frequent change from one sitting position is important for good circulation. Walking is an excellent form of exercise to promote circulation. (b)

17. (1) Although pure types are unusual, the normal female pelvis is the one most favorable for normal delivery. Characteristics include well-rounded inlet, straight sidewalls, well-formed sacrosciatic notches, good sacral curvature and inclination, movable coccyx, moderately sized ischial spines, and well-rounded suprapubic arches. (b)

18. (2) By taking a diet history the nurse can assess the woman's level of nutrition knowledge and gain clues for appropriate methods of counseling. (a)

19. (3) A sudden sharp increase near the twentieth week of pregnancy may indicate water retention and the beginning of preeclampsia. (b)

20. (4) By this time the fetus and placenta have grown, expanding the size of the uterus, and the extended uterus expands into the abdominal cavity. (b)

21. (2) The saline may have gotten into the vascular system rather than into the amniotic sac. (c)

22. (4) The saline causes puffing of placenta, fetal death, placental separation, release of fibrin, then labor and paradoxical hemorrhaging. This takes at least 24 hours in most cases. (c)

23. (3) The uterine lining, due to the irritation, is not receptive to the implantation of the fertilized egg. (c)

24. (3) The IUD may cause irritability of the myometrium, inducing contraction of the uterus and expulsion of the device. (c)

25. (2) About 75% of all spontaneous abortions take place between 8 and 12 weeks of gestation and show embryonic defects. (b)

26. (4) This is a seaweed that expands in a moist environment. It is a natural, safe method of dilating the cervix. (c)

27. (1) The first trimester is the period at which all major organs are being laid down, and drugs, alcohol, and tobacco may cause major defects. (a)

28. (1) The physical principle underlying the respiratory distress of infants with hyaline membrane disease is surface tension. Since the lung tissue of the infants lacks the group of detergents known as surfactant, water molecules strongly interact with each other (by hydrogen bonding) and the alveolar sacs and respiratory passages do not easily expand, resulting in extremely labored, if not impossible, breathing. (b)

29. (2) Humidity may liquefy the tenacious secretions, making gas exchange possible. (b)

30. (4) Bonding between parent and baby is most successful when interaction is possible right after birth. If the child is ill, contact is limited. (c)

31. (3) The overdistended uterus does not contract readily. (b)

32. (3) The posterior vaginal wall is pushed forward by the herniation of the rectum, thus increasing intravesical pressure, which causes the incontinence. (c)

33. (4) A crisis is defined as a situation whereby the clients' previous methods of adaptation are inadequate to meet present needs. (b)

34. (2) A crisis intervention group helps clients reestablish psychologic equilibrium by assisting them to explore new alternatives to coping. Realistic situations are considered using rational and flexible problem-solving methods. (a)

35. (1) Behavior that reflects the recognition of the intrinsic worth of each individual is essential in all supportive relationships. Problem-solving potential is increased when clients are involved in exploring alternatives that will affect the direction of their own lives. (a)

36. (4) The crisis center's main responsibility is to assist the client in utilizing the problem-solving process in exploring alternative solutions to a situation and to provide information regarding other agencies, facilities, and services. (b)

37. (3) Intrinsic motivation is stimulated from within the learner. It is most effective because the learner recognizes the need to know, is self-directed, and is ready to learn. (b)

38. (1) Any other action would be an invasion of privacy. The marital status has little bearing on the needs of the patient at this time. (b)

39. (2) Mothers need to explore their infants visually and tactually to assure themselves that the infant is normal in all respects. (a)

40. (4) The pregnant teenager is more prone to toxemia because of age, poor diet, and often poor prenatal care. (c)

41. (2) Respiratory effort rather than rate is included in Apgar score because the rate is very erratic. Heart rate is vital. (c)

42. (3) Rate varies with activity; crying will increase rate, whereas deep sleep will lower it. Rate below 120 beats per minute is considered bradycardia, and rate above 160 beats per minute is considered tachycardia. (b)

43. (3) Rate is associated with activity and can be as rapid as 60 breaths per minute. Over 60 breaths per minute is considered tachypnea in the infant. (b)

44. (2) Changes in equilibrium stimulate this neurologic reflex in an infant under the age of 6 months. The movements should be bilateral and symmetric. Reflex causes the same reaction to a loud noise (startle reflex), but using the noise as a stimulus really tests hearing. (c)

45. (4) Moro reflex is the sudden extension and abduction of arms at the shoulders and spreading of fingers, with the index finger and thumb forming the letter ''C,'' followed by flexion and adduction; legs might weakly flex and the infant may cry vigorously. (b)

46. (3) Injury to the brachial plexus, clavicle, or humerus prevents the abductive and adductive movements of the upper extremities. (b)

47. (2) The Committee on Maternal Nutrition of the National Research Council recommends a weight gain of *at least* 25 lb during pregnancy. Inadequate nutrition results in underweight babies. Specifically, excess vitamin A can cause bone malformation and skeletal pain; folate deficiency is associated with fetal malformation. (a)

48. (2) The nurse should become informed about cultural eating patterns of her patients to ensure that foods containing the essential nutrients are part of these dietary patterns and will be included in the diet. (c)

49. (3) The National Research Council reports routine use of *salt-free* diets and diuretics is potentially dangerous. Salty foods can be eliminated to decrease intake. Ankle edema is common during the second and third trimesters and is cause for concern when accompanied by hypertension or proteinuria. Elevation of the extremities several times daily is recommended to decrease the edema. (b)

50. (3) During the painless contractions of pregnancy, the lower edge of the placenta separates from the walls of the uterus, opening placental sinuses and allowing blood to escape. (b)

51. (2) The vascular changes associated with hypertension may cause a reduction in the blood supply to the uterus, resulting in placental infarcts and separation of the placenta from the decidua. (b)

52. (1) The amnion encloses the embryo and the shock-protective amniotic fluid in which the embryo floats. (a)

53. (4) The word originates from the Old English word ''quick,'' which means life. (c)

54. (4) This is the period in which the fetus stores deposits of fat. (b)

55. (4) The chief function of progesterone is to prepare the uterus to receive a fertilized ovum by stimulating differentiation of the endometrium into a secretory type of tissue. (b)

56. (4) Polyhydramnios (excessive fluid) is associated with multiple gestation. Dehydration is generally associated with hyperemesis gravidarum. (b)

57. (3) Intact membranes act as a barrier against organisms that may cause an intrauterine infection. (b)

58. (2) An amniotomy is a painless procedure with labor usually following in 6 to 8 hours. (c)

59. (2) The patient is experiencing the expected discomforts of labor, and the nurse should initiate those nursing measures which promote relaxation. (b)

60. (3) Diaphoresis is a normal adaptation of the postpartum period and does not relate to bladder distention. It is caused by the reduction of the antidiuretic hormone leading to profuse perspiration. (b)

61. (1) A respiratory rate below 40 in the newborn is not within the normal range. The normal is 40 to 60 breaths per minute. (b)

62. (3) Mother has completed the taking in phase and has moved into taking hold phase, when she calls the baby by name. (c)

63. (3) There is a sensitive period in the first minutes or hours after birth during which it is necessary that the mother and father have close contact with their neonate for later development to be normal. (b)

64. (1) Almost all mothers, including multiparas, report some ambivalence and anxiety about their ability to be good mothers, since mothering is not an inborn instinct. (a)

65. (2) The Rubin test is for tubal patency, the Papanicolaou test is for cancer, and the Friedman test is for pregnancy. (b)

66. (4) This test visualizes the uterus and fallopian tubes, the pelvic organs for reproduction. (a)

67. (3) The ovum is capable of being fertilized for only 24 to 36 hours after ovulation. After this time the ovum travels a variable distance between the fallopian tube and uterus, disintegrates, and is phagocytized by leukocytes. (b)

68. (2) Sperm mobility is increased at pH values that are near neutral or slightly alkaline. Sodium bicarbonate douche will reduce the acidity of fluids in the vagina and help to optimize the pH. (c)

69. (3) The action of Enovid is to inhibit ovulation and establish regular menstrual cycles. This is one of the first steps in treating infertility problems. (b)

70. (3) Oxytocin is a small polypeptide hormone normally synthesized in the hypothalamus and secreted from the neurohypophysis during parturition or suckling. The hormone promotes powerful uterine (smooth muscle) contractions and thus is used to induce labor. (c)

71. (1) Since oxytocin promotes powerful uterine contractions, exogenous administration of this hormone may produce uterine tetany, which does not optimize progression of labor and may restrict fetal blood flow. (b)

72. (4) Contractions are stronger and more regular when the woman is standing. Also, during walking the diameter of the pelvic inlet increases and allows for easier entrance of the head into the pelvis. (b)

73. (3) Each patient in labor is an individual with individual needs. The enema is never a routine procedure. (b)

74. (1) When membranes rupture, there is always the possibility of a prolapsed cord leading to fetal distress, which would manifest itself in a slowed heartbeat. (b)

75. (3) By 36 weeks' gestation normal amniotic fluid is colorless, with small particles of vernix caseosa present. (a)

76. (2) This slow deep breathing expands spaces between the ribs and raises the abdominal muscles, allowing room for the uterus to expand and preventing painful pressure of the uterus against the abdominal wall. (a)

77. (1) The contractions become stronger, last longer, and are erratic during this stage. The intervals during the contractions are shorter than the contractions themselves. Much concentration and effort are needed by the mother to pace herself with each contraction. (b)

78. (4) Both the father and mother need additional support during the transitional stage of labor. (b)

79. (2) The contractions in this phase of labor are expulsive in nature and cause the patient to push or bear down. (a)

80. (4) The heart rate increases by about 10 beats per minute in the last half of pregnancy. This increase plus the increase in total blood volume can strain a damaged heart beyond the point at which it can efficiently compensate. (c)

81. (1) The side lying position takes the weight off large blood vessels, and blood flow to the heart is increased. Elevating the shoulders relieves pressure on the diaphragm. (c)

82. (2) Any medication that might further depress a premature infant is given with extreme caution. (b)

83. (2) An early symptom of congestive heart failure is respiratory distress. (c)

84. (3) Oxygen, as a drug, has the potential for complications such as retrolental fibroplasia when used injudiciously. The physician orders the prescribed oxygen concentration based on chemical findings and laboratory blood gas analyses. (b)

85. (2) Immaturity of the respiratory tract in preterm infants can be evidenced by a lack of functional alveoli, a smaller lumen with increased possibility of collapse of the respiratory passages, weakness of respiratory musculature, and insufficient calcification of bony thorax leading to respiratory distress. (a)

86. (3) The premature infant has difficulty with heat conservation because of high metabolic rate and large surface area compared to body weight. Use of an incubator is often required to maintain skin temperature as high as 36.7° C (98° F) (c)

87. (2) The premature infant has a reduced glomerular filtration rate and reduced ability to concentrate urine or conserve water. (c)

88. (2) About two thirds of neonatal deaths are caused by prematurity. There appears to be a correlation with teenage pregnancy, lack of prenatal care, nonwhite mothers, and chronic health problems. (c)

89. (1) Perinatal morbidity and mortality are greatly increased in multiple pregnancy because the high metabolic demands increase the potential for medical and obstetric complications. (b)

90. (2) Characteristics of the midphase of labor for the primiparous patient include regular contractions 30 to 45 seconds long and 3 to 5 minutes apart, station of presenting part at +1 to 2 cm, and pink to bloody show in a moderate amount. (c)

91. (1) In reporting progress in the descent of the presenting part the level of the tip of the ischial spines is considered to be zero and the position of the bony prominence of the fetal head is described in centimeters—minus (above the spines) or plus (below the spines.) (b)

92. (2) Meperidine (Demerol) is classified as a narcotic analgesic drug and is effective for the relief or pain. Promethazine (Phenergan) can be classified as an analgesic-potentiating drug that permits the effective use of analgesics in lower dosages. (a)

93. (3) The physiologic intensification of labor occurring during transition is caused by a greater energy expenditure and increased pressure on the stomach; this results in feelings of fatigue, discouragement, and nausea. (b)

94. (4) The oxytocin secreted by the maternal posterior pituitary promotes parturition but also induces contractions of many smooth muscles, including those of the breasts. Some maternal oxytocin crosses the placenta and induces secretion of fluids that have accumulated in the fetal breasts (such secretions are sometimes called witch's milk). (a)

95. (2) The fundus descends one finger breadth per day from the day after delivery; lochia serosa begins to flow on the fifth day. (b)

96. (2) This is the result of the reduction of the chromosome number from 46 to 23, readying the sex cells for fertilization. (c)

97. (2) Follicular-stimulating hormone is secreted from the anterior portion of the pituitary gland. (c)

98. (4) The corpus luteum supplies the estrogen and progesterone needed to sustain the pregnancy until the placenta is ready to take over after the eighth week. (b)

99. (2) Magnesium sulfate has a CNS depressant effect; therefore toxic levels will be reflected in decreased respiration and the absence of the knee-jerk reflex. (c)

100. (2) Absolute bed rest, a quiet room, and minimal stimu-

lation are essential components to reduce the risk of precipitating a convulsion. (b)

101. (1) This is a sign of CNS involvement that the nurse can observe without obtaining subjective data from the patient. The other choices are all subjective symptoms. (c)

102. (3) Increased electric charges in the brain during a convulsion may disturb the cerebral thermoregulation center. (b)

103. (4) The danger of convulsion in a woman with preeclampsia ends when postpartum diuresis has occurred, usually 48 hours after delivery. (c)

104. (1) In Erb-Duchenne paralysis there is damage to the spinal nerve C_5 and C_6, which causes paralysis of the arm. (c)

105. (3) Range of motion exercises must be done to prevent contractures. (c)

106. (4) Heavy cigarette smoking or continued exposure to a smoke-filled environment causes both maternal and fetal vasoconstriction, resulting in fetal growth retardation and increased fetal and infant mortality. (a)

107. (4) This pigmentation is caused by the anterior pituitary hormone melanotropin, which increases during pregnancy. (c)

108. (4) Altered hormone levels and metabolic changes may be precipitating factors to nausea and vomiting in early pregnancy. (b)

109. (4) Nausea and vomiting of pregnancy can be relieved with small snacks of dry crackers or toast before rising, since the ingestion of carbohydrates helps to settle the stomach. (a)

110. (4) Once the patient signs herself and baby out of the hospital, she is legally responsible for her infant and must be given the baby. (c)

111. (1) Hormone decrease causes an emotional letdown. (a)

112. (3) The umbilical vein carries high oxygen from the placenta and empties into the vena cava by way of the ductus venosus. (a)

113. (1) Two umbilical arteries arise from the fetus and go to the placenta, where waste products are exchanged for oxygen and nutrients and then returned via one umbilical vein to the baby. (a)

114. (3) If the fetus is in a compromised state, it does not contribute to the synthesis of estriol and estriol levels fall, indicating a need for intervention. (c)

115. (1) There is a 30% to 50% increase in maternal blood volume at the end of the first trimester, leading to a decrease in the concentration of hemoglobin and erythrocytes. (b)

116. (1) The greatest danger of drug-induced malformation is during the first trimester of pregnancy, since this is the period of organogenesis. (b)

117. (4) Sonography, based on sound wave reflection and detection, locates the position of the fetus prior to insertion of the needle in amniocentesis; this minimizes fetal damage during the procedure. (b)

118. (2) The patient must feel comfortable enough to verbalize her feelings of guilt if she is to be able to complete the grieving process. (b)

119. (1) Rh_oD globulin attacks fetal red cells that have gained access to the maternal bloodstream at the time of delivery and prevents antibody formation. (b)

120. (4) Although support will help minimize guilt, it will not eliminate it. Neither will the support affect the legal responsibility of the parents. However, support will sustain family cohesion and unity. (a)

121. (1) A symptom of sudden rupture of the fallopian tubes is pain on the affected side, usually sudden, excruciating, and spreading over the lower abdomen. Sometimes the pain is associated with nausea, vomiting, and diarrhea. (a)

122. (2) The proliferation of trophoblastic tissue filled with fluid causes the uterus to enlarge more quickly than it does with a normally growing fetus. (b)

123. (3) Sneezing is the way in which the newborn clears mucus from the nose. The newborn's breathing is normally rapid and irregular. (a)

124. (2) Normally the newborn's breathing is diaphragmatic and irregular in depth and rhythm. The rate ranges from 40 to 50 breaths per minute. (b)

125. (4) Opens up an area of communication to get at what really is troubling the mother about feeding the baby. (a)

126. (3) A rate of 100 to 119 per minute indicates moderate bradycardia, and 100 or below indicates marked bradycardia. (a)

127. (3) As the uterus rises into the abdominal cavity, the uterine ligaments become elongated and hypertrophied. Raising both legs at the same time limits the tension placed on these ligaments. (b)

128. (2) Persistent deceleration during contractions indicates fetal hypoxia because of deficient placental perfusion; bradycardia is not a requirement. (b)

129. (3) Soap irritates, cracks, and dries breasts and nipples, making it difficult for the baby to suck. (b)

130. (4) The most likely cause is a disturbance in the ratio of calcium to phosphorus, with the amount of serum calcium reduced and the amount of phosphorus increased; milk is an excellent source of calcium. (a)

131. (1) Cow's milk is diluted with water and has sugar added to make it resemble human milk. (c)

132. (1) Prolactin is the hormone from the anterior pituitary that stimulates mammary gland milk secretion. Oxytocin is a posterior pituitary hormone that assists in milk ejection from the breasts as well as uterine contractions at birth. Progesterone and estrogen are ovarian hormones that influence breast development and other female sexual characteristics. (a)

133. (3) Breast-feeding is not contraindicated with inverted nipples, since a breast shield can provide mild suction to help pull out a nipple. (b)

134. (1) The term "premature" describes a neonate delivered at 37 weeks' gestation or less, regardless of weight. (a)

135. (3) Gavage feeding is preferred for immature and weak infants, those with respiratory distress or poor sucking-swallowing coordination, and those who are easily fatigued. (b)

136. (2) Much of a full-term infant's birth weight is gained during the last month of pregnancy (almost a third), and most of this final spurt is subcutaneous fat, which serves as insulation; the premature baby has not had the time to grow in the uterus and has a paucity of this insulating layer. (a)

137. (1) Prolonged O_2 administration at relatively high concentrations in a premature infant whose retina is incompletely differentiated and/or vascularized may result in retrolental fibroplasia; when O_2 therapy is discontinued, capillary overgrowth in the retina and vitreous body may result and include capillary hemorrhage, fibrosis, and retinal detachment. (b)

138. (3) Toxemia does not interfere with uterine involution, return of uterine tone, or constriction of vessels at the placental site. The other choices do. (c)

139. (3) The term "stillborn" is used to describe a dead fetus of more than 24 weeks' gestation, weighing 600 or more grams. (c)

140. (2) Based on the family's decision, extraordinary care does not have to be employed. The child's basic needs are met, and nature is allowed to take its course. Euthanasia is a deliberate intervention to cause death. (c)

141. (4) Grunting is caused by the infant's attempts to keep alveoli open with back pressure and permit greater oxygen exchange. (c)

142. (3) Flaccid muscle tone is the only abnormal finding. All other choices indicate a normal newborn response and would be higher on the Apgar scale. (b)

143. (2) Intracranial bleeding may occur in the subdural, subarachnoid, or intraventricular spaces of the brain, causing pressure on vital centers. Clinical signs are related to the area and degree of cerebral involvement. (a)

144. (1) Serum bilirubin normally accumulates in the neonatal period due to the short life span of fetal erythrocytes, reaching levels of 7 mg/100 ml of the second to third day, when jaundice appears. If jaundice develops earlier, it is evidence of disease. (c)

145. (2) The tonic neck reflex (fencing position) is a spontaneous postural reflex of the newborn that may or may not be present during the first days of life. Once apparent, it persists until the third month. (a)

146. (3) Informing parents of the birth of an abnormal child as early as possible, and preferably in the delivery room when staff is present to support and assist them in mobilizing resources, prevents fantasizing about the problem. (b)

147. (4) Androgen-estrogen preparations inhibit the release of lactogenic hormone from the pituitary. (c)

148. (4) Ovulation is anticipated approximately 14 days prior to menstruation; however, it is more reliable to avoid using a specific number of days and calculate it on the basis of an individual's cycle rather than an average 28-day cycle. (c)

149. (2) As ovulation approaches, there may be a drop in the basal temperature due to an increased production of estrogen. When ovulation occurs, there will be a rise in the basal temperature due to an increased production of progesterone. (b)

150. (3) Stress or infection alters the body's metabolism, causing an elevation in temperature. A rise in temperature due to these causes may be misinterpreted as ovulation. (b)

151. (2) Ectopic pregnancy is one of the leading causes of first trimester bleeding. An embryo and placenta located outside the uterus cannot grow for more than 10 to 12 weeks without showing the classic signs of pressure and bleeding, unless they are located in the abdominal cavity. (b)

152. (1) Staining in the first trimester may indicate that the pregnancy is in jeopardy. Bed rest, sedation, and avoidance of physical and emotional stress are recommended. Abortion is usually inevitable if the bleeding is accompanied by pain and dilation and effacement of the cervix. (a)

153. (2) Following a spontaneous abortion the fundus should be checked for firmness, which would indicate effective uterine tone. If the uterus is not firm it is hypotonic, and hemorrhage may occur. It may also indicate retained placental tissue. (a)

154. (2) Hemorrhage may occur due to retained placental tissue or uterine atony. Infection may occur due to the introduction of contamination into the warm moist environment, which is favorable to microbial growth. (a)

155. (4) Allows husband and wife to comfort one another while letting them know you are available and recognize and accept their feelings of loss. (b)

156. (1) The association of toxemia with placental bleeding is frequent. This may be related to the hypertension during pregnancy. (c)

157. (1) Overdistention of the uterus due to a large baby, multiple gestation, or hydramnios predisposes a woman to uterine atony, which may cause postpartum hemorrhage. (b)

158. (2) In a breech delivery the head is not the presenting part bearing the brunt of the pressure against the pelvic floor during delivery. (b)

159. (2) Observation and record keeping are independent nursing functions and necessary for implementing safe care, since hemorrhage and shock can be life-threatening. (a)

160. (2) A fallopian tube is unable to contain and sustain a pregnancy to term. As the fertilized ovum grows, there is excessive stretching or rupture of the fallopian tube causing pain. (c)

161. (3) A position in which the mother's head is below the

level of the hips helps to decrease compression of the cord and therefore increase blood supply to the infant. (a)

162. (2) Infertility is the inability of a couple to conceive after at least 1 year of adequate exposure to the possibility of pregnancy. (b)

163. (2) At this time, due to increased estrogen levels, the cervical mucus is abundant and its equality changes in such a way as to optimize sperm survival time. (b)

164. (1) A past infection may cause tubal occlusions, most of which are due to postinfection adhesions. (c)

165. (2) Human chorionic gonadotropin (HCG), an LH-like hormone, is produced by the trophoblasts of the early embryo to promote continued metabolism of the corpus luteum (source of estrogen and progesterone); HCG can be detected as early as 6 days after fertilization (by non-routine, immunofluorescent techniques) and appears in measurable amounts in urine within about 14 days. (b)

166. (4) A bluish color results from the increased vascularity and blood vessel engorgement in the vagina. (a)

167. (4) The average weight gain during pregnancy is 20 to 25 lb (9 to 11.25 kg). Of this, the fetus accounts for 7½ lb, the blood volume 2 to 4 lb, fluid retention 5 lb, amniotic fluid 2 lb, uterus 2½ lb, and breasts 3 lb. The remainder of weight gain is fat. (c)

168. (1) Statistically CPD (cephalopelvic disproportion) is the most common indication. (a)

169. (1) The diagonal conjugate is an estimation of the true conjugate using the lower edge of the symphysis pubis as its anterior point and the sacral promontory posteriorly. The true conjugate uses the upper ridge of the symphysis pubis anteriorly but cannot be measured on a living woman. (c)

170. (2) X-ray pelvimetry is more definitive than digital pelvimetry, but because of radiation hazards it should be limited to patients in labor, where it is clearly essential to the outcome of pregnancy. (b)

171. (1) Asymmetry of the gluteal dorsal surface of the thighs and inguinal folds indicates congenital dislocation of the hip. Folds on the affected side appear higher than those on the unaffected side. (a)

172. (3) Human milk contains 42% carbohydrate and cow's milk contains 30% carbohydrate. The carbohydrate in cow's milk is further diluted when water is added to the formula, and additional sugar is required to supplement it. (b)

173. (1) Blood loss depletes the normal cellular response to infection and trauma provides an excellent medium for bacteria to grow. (c)

174. (4) The oxytocin challenge test provides data concerning the circulatory-respiratory reserve of the fetoplacental unit. A positive OCT usually indicates uteroplacental insufficiency. An OCT is contraindicated unless there is a specific indication of a problem. (b)

175. (1) Administration of oxytocin too early in pregnancy can cause induced labor and premature delivery. (c)

176. (1) Respiratory depression occurs with the use of meperidine (Demerol) and produces significant depression of the infant at birth if circulating levels are high at delivery. (a)

177. (1) Brachial palsy results from excessive stretching of the nerve fibers that run from the neck and through the shoulder and down toward the arm. The muscles of the upper arm are involved and the infant holds the arm at the side with the elbow extended and the hand rotated inward. (b)

178. (3) There is extensive activation of blood clotting factor after delivery. This, together with immobility, trauma, or sepsis, encourages thromboembolization, which can be limited through activity. (b)

179. (2) Mothering is not an inborn instinct but rather learned behavior based on past experiences. (c)

180. (3) Heart development occurs between the second and eighth week of gestation. (b)

181. (2) The increased pulmonary blood flow raises the pressure in the left atrium and functionally forces the septum to close the foramen ovale. (c)

182. (3) There is anatomic obliteration of the lumen by fibrous proliferation leading to the term "ligamentum arteriosum." (b)

183. (1) Bacteria, especially *E. coli*, produce and synthesize prothrombin. (c)

184. (3) The fundus is easily displaced upward and sideward by a distended bladder. (a)

185. (2) In the immediate postpartum period a slower than normal pulse rate can be anticipated as a result of a combination of factors—horizontal position, emotional relief and satisfaction, enforced rest after strenuous activity of labor and delivery, etc. (c)

186. (3) Rentention of urine with overflow will manifest in small, frequent voidings. The bladder should be palpated for distention. (a)

187. (4) Parenting can begin only when the baby and mother get to know each other. The nurse should carefully assess their interactions for normal development. (b)

188. (2) Cephalohematoma is a collection of blood between the skull bone and its periosteum as the result of trauma that resolves spontaneously in 3 to 6 weeks. (c)

189. (1) Nursing care is directed toward supporting the parents and reassuring them that their child is not permanently damaged. (c)

190. (3) The immunity is that which has developed from an antigen-antibody response in the mother and is passed to the fetus. (b)

191. (4) The congenital absence of a vessel in the umbilical cord is usually associated with life-threatening congenital anomalies. (b)

192. (1) Medical supervision requires treatment with an ap-

propriate antibiotic drug for 2 to 3 weeks until 2 negative cultures are obtained. Retreatment may be necessary if there is a recurrence. (c)

193. (1) The pressure exerted anywhere in a mass of fluid is transmitted equally in all directions. (c)

194. (4) Progesterone acts to reduce contractility of uterine musculature and to maintain the decidual bed. (b)

195. (3) The polypeptide, a melanocyte stimulating hormone, becomes elevated from the end of the second month of pregnancy until term. (a)

196. (2) If the woman had a hemophilic father, she must have his X chromosome, which carries the recessive gene for hemophilia (if she had his Y chromosome, she would have been male). Since her blood clots normally, her other X chromosome carries the dominant gene for normal blood clotting. She is represented by Hh. Her normal mate is represented by HY. The cross:

$$\begin{array}{c} & \overset{\Large\male}{\begin{array}{cc} H & Y \end{array}} \\ \female\begin{array}{c} H \\ h \end{array} & \begin{array}{|c|c|} \hline HH & HY \\ \hline Hh & hY \\ \hline \end{array} \end{array} \quad (c)$$

197. (1) Anemia decreases the capacity of the blood to carry oxygen and thus increases the demands on the heart. (b)

198. (2) The pregnant woman's increased hormones, metabolic rate and increased blood volume place additional demands on the pancreas, thus altering carbohydrate and lipid metabolism. (b)

199. (1) Since spillage of glucose into the urine occurs in normal women who are pregnant, dietary or insulin management in a diabetic who is pregnant must be based on blood glucose levels rather than urine glucose values. (c)

200. (4) Increased metabolic demands on the body during pregnancy require an increased ingestion of glucose. Appropriate levels of insulin must be administered to permit normal glucose utilization by the body. (c)

201. (2) The fetal pancreas, in diabetic mothers, responds to the mother's hyperglycemia by secreting more than normal amounts of insulin. This results in infant hypoglycemia after birth. (b)

202. (2) The higher than normal glucose levels in a fetus of a diabetic mother results in increased fat synthesis and deposition. Increased glucose utilization is also promoted by the combination of pituitary growth hormone and placental somatotropin. (c)

203. (1) Normal periods of marked change and adjustment are called developmental crises and predispose to situational crisis. (a)

204. (2) The ability to express one's feelings is often a first step in the recognition and resolution of crisis. (b)

205. (2) Chorionic gonadotropin is present in the urine during early pregnancy and is the basis for pregnancy tests. Since this hormone appears only during early pregnancy, its presence is taken as a clear-cut sign of pregnancy. (a)

206. (2) Nurses with positive attitudes toward abortion should counsel women who are thinking of having the procedure. They should know what services are available and the various methods that are used to induce abortion. (b)

207. (2) The uterus and the bladder occupy the pelvic cavity and lie very close together. As the uterus enlarges with the growing fetus, it impinges on the space normally occupied by the bladder and thereby diminishes its capacity. (a)

208. (2) Morning sickness seldom persists beyond the first trimester because of changes in the hormone levels. (a)

209. (2) Subsequent to IUD insertion, menstrual periods may have an excessive flow for several cycles, probably due to an increase in blood supply (inflammatory process), since the IUD is really a foreign body. (c)

210. (1) Oral contraceptives contain varying kinds and dosages of synthetic estrogen and progestogen compounds that mimic natural cyclic hormone changes and prolong the menses. (c)

211. (3) Untreated ophthalmia neonatorum becomes apparent on the third or fourth postnatal day and is evidence that the mother has gonorrhea. Conjunctivitis due to silver nitrate instillation develops on the first day. (b)

212. (4) Multiple pregnancy thins the uterine wall due to overstretching, thus reducing efficiency of contractions. (b)

213. (3) A fruity odor may indicate that the patient is becoming acidotic. (c)

214. (3) This response provides the patient with a comfort measure white giving her an opportunity to verbalize her fears about having an abnormal labor. (b)

215. (3) The oxytocic effect of Pitocin increases the intensity and duration of contractions. Prolonged contractions will jeopardize the safety of the fetus and necessitate discontinuing the Pitocin. (c)

216. (3) IV Pitocin is used to enhance postpartum uterine contractions after cesarean sections, since palpation of the fundus is difficult and painful after surgery. This drug produces effective clamping down on the vessels. (c)

217. (1) Normal infants require 2 to 3 oz of fluid per pound and 60 calories a day per pound for growth. (b)

218. (1) The cardiac sphincter in the newborn is poorly developed. If the stomach is too full, formula backs up through the sphincter and the infant regurgitates. (b)

219. (4) Clotting mechanisms are not fully effective in the infant before the eighth day of life. (a)

220. (4) The patient's rights were violated. The patient has the right to a complete and accurate explanation of treatment. (a)

221. (3) Patients must be continuously monitored for blood

loss by observing for external bleeding and counting and weighing pads to prevent further maternal and fetal complications. (b)

222. (2) A vaginal examination may precipitate severe bleeding that will be life-threatening to mother and infant, necessitating an immediate cesarean section. (b)

223. (3) An infant should receive 60 calories and 3 oz of fluid per pound daily. (b)

224. (4) Development of jaundice before 48 hours after birth may indicate a blood dyscrasia requiring immediate medical investigation. Jaundice occurring between 48 and 72 hours after birth is a consequence of the normal physiologic breakdown of fetal red cells and immaturity of the liver. (c)

225. (1) Gonorrhea transmitted from the mother is usually manifested in the infant as an eye infection. It becomes apparent on the third or fourth postnatal day unless silver nitrate has been instilled in the eyes at birth. (a)

226. (3) The spirochete *Treponema pallidum* is able to cross the placenta and cause early manifestations of syphilis after the sixteenth week of pregnancy. (c)

Pediatric nursing

1. (2) Common developmental norms of the toddler, who is struggling for independence, are inability to share easily, egotism, egocentrism, and possessiveness. (b)

2. (1) Four-year-olds boast, exaggerate, are impatient, noisy, and selfish; they are definitely not easy to get along with while they struggle to master social development. (c)

3. (4) The child 9 to 12 months of age can stand alone with support. By 15 months the child's strength and balance improve, and he can stand and walk alone. (b)

4. (2) Six-year-olds are aware of their hands as tools and can build simple structures. This is also an activity they enjoy. (b)

5. (4) In the infant, physical growth is cephalocaudal and progresses from proximal to distal and from the general to the specific. Play during infancy (solitary) allows physical development to emerge; for example, use of mobiles to strengthen eye movement, large beads to promote fine finger movement, and soft toys to encourage tactile sense. (a)

6. (3) Walking is the primary developmental task of this age group. The other choices are not developmental tasks, nor are they applicable to this age group. (b)

7. (1) Role playing encourages expression of feelings through behavior, since their ability to verbalize feelings is limited. (b)

8. (1) Although there is a time range for developmental tasks, there is no specific time for a development task; in addition, learning takes place in spurts rather than in a uniform manner. (b)

9. (2) Helps and encourages parents to put their fears and feelings into words. Once they are expressed, they can at least be examined and dealt with. (b)

10. (1) These children frequently have difficulty in handling secretions as well as breathing following surgery. Nursing measures such as using the partial side lying position or gently aspirating secretions from the mouth or nasopharynx may be necessary to prevent aspiration and respiratory complications. (a)

11. (2) Crying should be prevented, since it places tension on the suture line. Frequently an appliance called a Logan bow is taped to the cheeks to relax the operative site, which helps prevent trauma. (b)

12. (4) The 2-year-old is still attached and dependent on parents, and fear of separation is a great stress. Encouraging parents to become involved with care, providing care by the same staff members, and maintaining similar routines all help to promote security. (b)

13. (1) A priority during the immediate postoperative period is protecting the operative site. The mouth is usually rinsed with water before and after each feeding. (a)

14. (4) David is anemic. A diet of milk only is not sufficient to meet iron needs. Raisins and meat are high in iron, and finger foods meet developmental tasks. (b)

15. (1) Fetal iron reserves are depleted by the fourth to fifth month in the full-term infant and considerably earlier in the premature infant. When exogenous sources of iron are not supplied following depletion of fetal iron stores, iron-deficiency anemia results. (a)

16. (1) Milk is a very poor source of iron; if fed in large amounts to the exclusion of solid foods after 4 to 6 months of age, iron-deficiency anemia results. (b)

17. (4) Folic acid acts as a necessary coenzyme in the formation of heme, the iron-containing protein in hemoglobin. Folic acid deficiency results in megaloblastic anemia. (c)

18. (3) Egg yolk is a rich source of iron and is easily digested by infants. (a)

19. (3) The child should be taken to the dentist between 2 and 3 years of age when all the deciduous teeth (20) have erupted. (a)

20. (3) Proteins are essential for the synthesis of the blood proteins, albumin, fibrinogen, and hemoglobin. Ascorbic acid influences the removal of iron from ferritin (making more iron available for production of heme) and influences the conversion of folic acid to folinic acid. (b)

21. (2) If food is used early as praise or punishment, the older child or adult will either undereat or overeat at times of stress to decrease anxiety. (b)

22. (1) The early school-age child has become a cooperative member of the family and will mimic parents' attitudes and food habits readily. (b)

23. (4) The adult pinworm lives in the rectum or colon and

emerges onto the perirectal skin during hours of sleep, depositing her eggs during this time. (b)

24. (4) The worm attaches itself to the bowel wall in the cecum and appendix and can damage the mucosa, causing appendicitis. (c)

25. (1) Forty pounds = 18 kg. Therefore 5 mg per kilogram × 18 kg = 90 mg. (b)

26. (3) Pyrvinium pamoate, a cyanine dye, is a deep red, relatively insoluble crystalline powder that stains the stool, vomitus, and most materials. (b)

27. (2) Pyrvinium pamoate, a cyanine dye, is a deep red relatively insoluble crystalline powder which stains the stool, vomitus, and most materials. In this instance, red-stained excreta would not be significant. (b)

28. (4) School-age children lose primary, or "baby," teeth, which could be aspirated during surgery. The anesthesiologist must take special precautions to maintain patient safety. (a)

29. (4) The seeping of blood from the operative site increases secretions, which the child adapts to by swallowing frequently. (b)

30. (2) Acetaminophen relieves pain and does not cause bleeding tendencies, as does aspirin. The correct dosage for this age is 300 mg. (c)

31. (2) A myelomeningocele sac is thinly covered and can be partially open, allowing a portal of entry for organisms directly to the central nervous system. The sac should be protected. (b)

32. (3) The surgical closure of the sac eliminates the route by which the spinal fluid drains. Skull bones are soft and will expand as fluid increases, causing hydrocephalus. (b)

33. (2) Sucking meets oral needs, which are primary during infancy. (c)

34. (3) Fluids prevent dehydration. Dehydration under conditions of decreased oxygen promotes the sickling of erythrocytes. (c)

35. (1) High levels of fetal hemoglobin prevent sickling of red blood cells. The newborn has from 44% to 89% fetal hemoglobin, but this rapidly decreases during the first year. (c)

36. (2) Under conditions of decreased oxygen the relatively insoluble hemoglobin S changes its molecular structure to form long slender crystals and eventually the crescent, or sickled, shape. (b)

37. (2) Sickling is also related to the concentration of hemoglobin within the cell. Since hypertonicity of the blood plasma increases the intracellular concentration of hemoglobin, dehydration promotes sickling. (c)

38. (2) Both have poor resistance; with sickling it is due to low oxygen levels, and with celiac disease it is due to malnourishment and immunologic defects.

39. (2) The first phase of separation anxiety is protest, which is characterized by loud crying, rejection of all strangers, and inconsolable grief. (a)

40. (3) The child has progressed to the third phase, detachment, in which he resigns himself to the loss of his mother and superficially appears adjusted to his environment. One future characteristic of these children is their inability to form intimate, interpersonal attachments to significant others. (c)

41. (2) Hearing is a sense that is not greatly influenced by emotional response in the young child. (b)

42. (1) The child experiencing long-term hospitalization is forced to relate to a variety of significant adults providing mothering instead of a single figure; the lack of continuity creates anxiety. (a)

43. (1) The child learns to love others by the love he receives; when he receives love, he feels he is worthy of being loved and can share this feeling with others. (a)

44. (4) The child will be unable to develop an emotional tie to his mother until trust has been reestablished. (b)

45. (4) When the causative organism is isolated, it is tested for antimicrobial susceptibility (sensitivity) to various antimicrobial agents. When an organism is sensitive to a medication, the medication is capable of destroying the organism. (b)

46. (2) The tetracyclines are not recommended during periods of tooth development (children under 8 years of age or in pregnant women during the latter half of pregnancy) because they may permanently discolor teeth yellow, gray, or brown. (b)

47. (3) Babies with Down's syndrome have decreased muscle tone, which compromises respiratory expansion as well as an adequate drainage of mucus; these factors contribute to increased suceptibility to upper respiratory tract infections. (b)

48. (4) Simian creases are the only symptom always observable. Other physical characteristics may suggest Down's syndrome. (a)

49. (2) Parents' responses to the child may greatly influence decisions regarding future care. Learning about their child and Down's syndrome may help lessen guilt feelings. (a)

50. (2) Babies with Down's syndrome have a high incidence of congenital heart disease, especially atrial defects. Their muscle tone is usually hypotonic, and their head and trunk are of normal size. Deafness is more common in rubella syndrome. (b)

51. (3) When the parents can verbalize the need to change plans they had made for their infant, it usually signifies they are beginning to face reality. (a)

52. (2) A child who is moderately retarded is unable to follow complicated procedures or remember detailed directions; simple repetitive tasks provide all the challenge needed. (b)

53. (3) When one's efforts toward meeting a goal are blocked or thwarted, frustration results. The child with Down's syndrome may be constantly thwarted in trying to meet

his needs, especially in an environment that expects certain achievements beyond his ability. (a)

54. (1) Rubeola, or measles, is generally a viral-induced childhood disease, beginning clinically in much the same way as the common cold and diagnosed on or about the second day by the presence of Koplik's spots—small white spots surrounded by a narrow zone of inflammation; they are most numerous on the inside of the cheeks. (a)

55. (3) Invasion of the posterior (dorsal) root ganglia by the same virus that causes chickenpox can result in pain followed by a rash following the cutaneous distribution of the affected nerve root(s). This condition, known as herpes zoster or shingles, may occur due to reactivation of a previous chickenpox virus that has lain dormant in the body or by fresh contact with an individual with chickenpox. (a)

56. (4) Corticosteroids (e.g., cortisol) cause involution of lymphatic tissue and resultant depression of the immune response. Antineoplastic drugs or high-energy radiation preferentially destroys tissues with high mitotic rates, including neoplastic tissue as well as lymphatic tissue and bone marrow, the latter 2 being active sites of antibody production and other immune responses. (a)

57. (1) The injected bacteria in the vaccine have been so modified that they do not cause active infection but still elicit an immune response. (b)

58. (2) The recommended immunization schedule for infants is administration of the combined diphtheria, pertussis, and tetanus vaccine and the trivalent oral polio virus at ages 2, 4, and 6 months. (b)

59. (3) The body's immune system constructs proteins called antibodies that possess a specificity toward another protein called the antigen. The combination of antibody with antigen may neutralize or precipitate the antigen or activate the complement system, which damages the antigen (e.g., part of a bacterial wall) and renders it harmless. (c)

60. (2) Maternal antibodies to measles infection persist in the infant until approximately 15 months of age. Measles live attenuated virus given prior to this time is inactivated by the maternal antibodies. (b)

61. (2) Because of the infant's increasing mobility, high level of oral activity, and relative lack of fear or appreciation for danger, accidents are the primary cause of death in children above 1 year of age. (c)

62. (4) In passive artificial immunity an antibody made in another organism is injected into the infected or presumed infected person to provide immediate immunity to the invading organism. (b)

63. (1) In active, natural immunity the infected person's immune system responds to the invading organism by producing antibodies specific for the invader. (c)

64. (1) Rubeola, or measles, produces coldlike respiratory symptoms and, after 3 or 4 days, a dark red macular or maculopapular skin rash. Complications include convulsions in young children and secondary infection with hemolytic streptococci, pneumococci, or staphylococci. Such infection can result in otitis media and pneumonia, which are especially dangerous in children under 2 years of age. (c)

65. (1) Adequate immunizations for normal infants and children include DPT at 2 months, 4 months, 6 months, 18 months, and 4 to 6 years and TOPV at 2 months, 4 months, 6 months, 18 months, and 4 to 6 years. Measles, rubella, and mumps vaccine is given at 12 months if the mothers are not pregnant (mother can be infected by live virus from her immunized children with resultant fetal damage). (c)

66. (2) Antibodies received in utero through the placenta and in the neonate through the mother's milk provide the baby with immunity against most bacterial, viral, and fungal infections during the first several weeks after birth. Then, as the titer of maternal antibodies drops and is not replaced by the child's own antibodies, prolonged and repeated infection occurs. (a)

67. (3) Supporting and slightly flexing the knee joint with a pillow relieves tension (and pain) in the joint; elevation of the leg will promote venous return, reducing joint swelling and pain. (b)

68. (2) Rest reduces the strain on the heart and minimizes metabolic needs during the acute, febrile stage of the disease. (a)

69. (4) Nonstrenuous, diversional activities involving interpersonal relationships with another person provide better support and resting conditions than does more active play. (a)

70. (3) A bland high-protein, high-carbohydrate diet provides adequate nutrition in the face of infection and fever. (a)

71. (1) The attack by autoantibodies on the heart valves can cause immediate impairment of heart function and lifelong valvular insufficiency. (b)

72. (4) A few minutes provides the child with an opportunity to begin to feed herself. The nurse should provide both physical and emotional support, since the child's request for help indicates the need for dependence during a period of stress. (a)

73. (3) Regression is the retreat to a past level of behavior as a way of minimizing stress or controlling anxiety. Increased dependence, such as being fed by another person, is a form of regression. (a)

74. (3) Dinner is frequently a family activity. Having her parents visit during mealtime may provide her with additional emotional, social, and physical support, resulting in an improved nutritional intake. (a)

75. (3) A predominant clinical sign of croup is reactive spasm of the laryngeal muscles, which produces partial respiratory obstruction. Cough is tight, with a barking metallic sound. (b)

76. (2) Syrup of ipecac is a nonprescription emetic causing vomiting, which helps to interrupt the laryngospasm characteristic of croup. (c)

77. (3) Ipecac causes forceful vomiting; the reversal of peristalsis puts pressure on the glottis and interrupts the spasm. (b)

78. (2) The toddler is in Erikson's stage of acquiring a sense of autonomy. The negativism is the result of the child's need to express his will and test out his environment. (a)

79. (4) Children who are expressing negativism need to have a feeling of control. One way of achieving this within reasonable limits is to give the child a choice of 2 items, rather than forcing one on him. (a)

80. (2) The parents' attitude, approach, and understanding of the child's physical and psychologic readiness are essential to letting the child proceed at his own pace with appropriate interventions by the parent. (a)

81. (4) Children learn socially acceptable behavior when consistent reasonable limits that provide guidelines are established. (b)

82. (3) In PKU the absence of the hepatic enzyme phenylalanine hydroxylase prevents normal metabolism (hydroxylation to tyrosine) of the amino acid phenylalanine. The increased body fluid levels of phenylalanine and alternate metabolic byproducts (phenylketones) are associated with severe mental retardation (exact mechanism not known). (b)

83. (1) The Guthrie blood test reliably detects abnormal phenylalanine levels as early as 4 days of age, provided the infant has been fed a milk diet. (a)

84. (2) The deficient product can be supplied, but, in most cases, limiting the intake of the substance the body cannot metabolize reduces toxic buildup. (b)

85. (3) Reducing dietary phenylalanine will hopefully prevent brain damage; diets are planned to attempt to maintain the serum phenylalanine level between 5 and 10 mg/100 ml. (c)

86. (3) Maintaining low phenylalanine levels is recommended until brain growth is almost completed, usually by 6 to 8 years of age. (b)

87. (4) Shivering increases the metabolic rate, which increases the body's need for O_2 and raises the body temperature. (c)

88. (3) Febrile convulsions are not necessarily associated with major neurologic problems but often accompany high fever. Such convulsions may be partially accounted for by the overall brain immaturity in children. (b)

89. (4) First convert the grains to milligrams:

$$\frac{1 \text{ gr}}{60 \text{ mg}} \times \frac{1.25 \text{ gr}}{x \text{ mg}}$$

$$x = 75.00 \text{ mg}$$

Then perform the computation for the correct dosage:

$$\frac{150 \text{ mg}}{75 \text{ mg}} \times \frac{x \text{ tablets}}{1 \text{ tablet}}$$

$$75 \, x = 150$$
$$x = 2 \text{ tablets} \quad \text{(b)}$$

90. (1) Meningococcal meningitis is identified by its epidemic nature and purpuric skin rash. It is treated with sulfadiazine. (c)

91. (3) Peripheral circulatory collapse (the Waterhouse-Friderichsen syndrome) is a serious complication of meningococcal meningitis caused by bilateral adrenal hemorrhage. The resultant acute adrenocortical insufficiency causes profound shock, petechiae and ecchymotic lesions, vomiting, prostration, and hypotension. (b)

92. (1) Since part of a nurse's responsibility is to foresee potential harm and prevent risks, it is imperative that the nurse not only take a health history and perform a physical assessment on each patient but also ensure the safety of the patient. (c)

93. (2) A common side effect of long-term phenytoin (Dilantin) therapy is hyperplasia of the gingiva. (c)

94. (1) Chickenpox, mumps, and rubeola are all caused by a virus and may be followed by encephalitis. (c)

95. (3) Viral multiplication damages the anterior horn cells of the spinal cord with a typical irregular and asymmetric pattern. The cervical and lumbar regions contain more anterior horn cells, and therefore the extremities are more frequently affected than is the trunk. (b)

96. (3) Pain is paroxysmal due to persitaltic action; abdominal distention pushes up the diaphragm, causing respiratory distress characterized by grunting respirations. (c)

97. (1) Sucking is a primary need of infancy. It decreases anxiety and does not interfere with gastric decompression. (b)

98. (3) If the circulation is overloaded with too much fluid or the rate is too rapid, the stress on the heart becomes too great and cardiac embarrassment may occur. (b)

99. (2) By 4 months of age infants are able to turn over and can easily fall from an inadequately guarded height. (a)

100. (3) Identifying feelings and providing support during stressful times are both ways of demonstrating concern during a crisis. (a)

101. (3) Allowing the patient time to talk about her feelings and staying with her when she sees the baby for the first time provide support, acceptance, and understanding. (c)

102. (2) The usual initial response to a crisis situation such as this is denial that it could occur and that they could produce a less than normal child. Mrs. Handler's response is her way of dealing with the reality of the situation. (a)

103. (3) An infant is a totally dependent human being; the infant with a congenital anomaly usually has additional physical and emotional needs. An initial major concern is that the mother is physically and emotionally capable of caring for the infant. (b)

104. (4) The congenital defect prevents the infant from creating a tight seal with the lips to promote sucking. As a result the infant swallows large amounts of air when feeding. The mother should be taught to provide frequent rest periods and to bubble the infant often to expel the excess air in the stomach. (b)

105. (3) The decreased filtration of plasma in the glomeruli results in an excess accumulation of water and sodium, producing edema that is first evident around the eyes. Hypertension is thought to be due to the hypervolemia, although its exact cause is unclear. (b)

106. (4) During the acute stage, anorexia and the loss of protein lower the child's resistance to infection. (b)

107. (3) Piaget stresses that age 7 is the turning point in mental development. New forms of organization appear at this age that mark the beginning of logic, symbolism, and abstract thought. (a)

108. (2) Once urinary test findings are normal, such as no evidence of hematuria or proteinuria, the child is allowed to resume his pre-illness activities. (b)

109. (4) Rheumatic fever is an inflammatory disease involving the joints, heart, central nervous system, and subcutaneous tissue. It is believed to be an autoimmune process that causes connective tissue damage. (b)

110. (4) Impetigo is a bacterial infection of the skin caused by streptococci or staphylococci. *Streptococcus* is the causative organism of rheumatic fever and glomerulonephritis. (b)

111. (3) Respiratory tract obstructions usually occur in the larynx, trachea, or major bronchi (usually right). Hoarseness may indicate vocal cord injury; unintelligible speech may indicate an interference in the flow of air out of the respiratory tract and/or obstruction or injury to the larynx. (b)

112. (4) During the acute phase, body movement causes pain and should therefore be avoided; immobility in rheumatic fever does not result in joint deformity, since the acute phase is not prolonged. (c)

113. (2) The child with rheumatic fever needs to be kept happy to decrease his oxygen needs. The school-age child has an interest in hobbies or collections of various kinds as a means of gathering information and knowledge about the world in which he lives. (b)

114. (1) C-reactive protein, which indicates the presence of an inflammatory reaction, is never present in normal blood and disappears as the child's condition improves. (c)

115. (1) Cystic fibrosis is characterized by overproduction of viscid mucus by exocrine glands in the lungs. The mucus traps bacteria and foreign debris but adheres to the lining and cannot be expelled by the cilia, thus obstructing the airway and favoring growth of organisms and infection. (a)

116. (2) The first usual indication of cystic fibrosis is meconium ileus. The small intestine is blocked with a thick, tenacious mucilaginous meconium, usually near the ileocecal valve. This causes intestinal obstruction with abdominal distention, vomiting, and fluid and electrolyte imbalance. (b)

117. (2) Production of tenacious mucus in the pancreas blocks the ducts, leading to cystic dilations of the acini, which then undergo degeneration and fibrosis. As a result, pancreatic enzyme production is greatly impaired; thus fats, proteins, and, to a lesser extent, carbohydrates cannot be absorbed. (b)

118. (1) In cystic fibrosis the mucous glands secrete thick mucoid secretions that accumulate and dilate the small passages in the affected organs. In the lungs there is reduced ciliary action, a slow mucus flow, and reduced expectoration. Postural drainage promotes the removal of mucopurulent secretions by means of gravity. (b)

119. (3) Because of a lack of the pancreatic enzyme lipase, fats remain unabsorbed and are excreted in excessive amounts in the stool. (a)

120. (3) Pancreatic enzymes are given as replacement for lack of production of these substances by the pancreas. Antibiotics are prescribed to prevent and control respiratory tract infection. (a)

121. (4) Rectal prolapse is the most common GI complication and is due to wasting of perirectal supporting tissues, secondary to malnutrition. (c)

122. (2) The nurse recognizes the child's protest over his mother's absence and tries to comfort him by staying near him until he feels more comfortable in her presence. The nurse should delay the bath until he has had time to test out his environment and is less anxious. (b)

123. (4) The second stage of separation anxiety is despair, in which the child is depressed, lonely, and disinterested in his surroundings. (b)

124. (1) Detachment is the result of trying to escape the emotional pain of desiring the mother by repressing feelings for her. (c)

125. (4) Once the child has progressed to detachment as a method of coping with the separation, reunion of child and mother will necessitate a period of time before the child is again willing to experience his emotional feelings because of his memory of the pain during their separation. (a)

126. (2) The hyperextension required in swimming aids in strengthening back muscles and increases deeper respirations, which are both necessary prior to surgery and/or wearing a brace or cast. (a)

127. (1) Continuing growth causes changes in muscle and bone structure and position. Adolescent girls have a rapid growth spurt. The brace is worn for 6 months after physical maturity, which is proved by x-ray examination to show cessation of bone growth. (b)

128. (4) The hypothalamic-pituitary-gonadal-adrenal mechanism is responsible for the physiologic and structural

changes that occur at puberty. The female adrenal glands secrete androgens that are responsible for the appearance of axillary and pubic hair, usually between 11 and 14 years of age. Menarche usually occurs 2 years after initial pubescent changes. (b)

129. (2) Thrush, also called moniliasis, usually affects the mucous membranes of the oral cavity, causing painful white patches. Individuals with immunologic deficiencies or those receiving prolonged antibiotic therapy are particularly susceptible to this organism. (b)

130. (2) Grunting and rapid respirations are abnormal behaviors in the infant. Grunting is a compensatory mechanism whereby the infant attempts to keep air in the alveoli to increase arterial oxygenation; increased respirations increase the amount of oxygen and carbon dioxide exchange. (b)

131. (4) In heart failure there is a decrease in the blood flow to the kidneys, causing sodium and water reabsorption and resulting in peripheral edema. Peripheral edema indicates severe cardiac decompensation. The other responses are the body's early adaptations in an attempt to handle the initial stress of decreased cardiac output. (b)

132. (2) Crying increases the amount of air being brought into the lung. The flow of air coming into the lung creates an increase in positive pressure, which helps to expand the alveoli and improve oxygen exchange, thereby decreasing cyanosis. In atelectasis some of the alveoli do not expand, which is evidenced by a lack of chest expansion on the affected side. (c)

133. (3) Chalasia is an incompetent cardiac sphincter, which allows a reflux of gastric contents into the esophagus and eventual regurgitation. Placing the infant in an upright position keeps the gastric contents in the stomach by gravity as well as limiting the pressure against the cardiac sphincter. (b)

134. (1) Hypertrophy of the pyloric sphincter, at the distal end of the stomach, causes partial and then complete obstruction. Nonprojectile vomiting progresses to projectile vomiting, which rapidly leads to dehydration. (c)

135. (2) In excessive vomiting there is an increased loss of hydrogen ions (hydrochloric acid), which results in a lowered serum pH (metabolic alkalosis) and an excess of base bicarbonate. (b)

136. (4) The percentage of total body water is related to the amount of body fat. The newborn's proportion of total body water is 20% greater than that of the adult; it rapidly diminishes in the neonatal period and continues to decline steadily until about 2 years of age, when it almost equals that of the adult. In addition, infants have very little fluid volume reserve. (c)

137. (1) An infant's intravascular compartment is fairly limited and cannot accommodate large volumes of fluid administered in a short period of time. Equipment such as minidroppers, volume control chambers, and infusion pumps should be used, since they help to control or limit the volume of fluid to be infused. (b)

138. (4) Initial feedings of glucose in water or electrolyte solutions are given 4 to 6 hours after surgery. Once clear fluids are retained, usually within 24 hours, diluted formula feedings are begun. (c)

139. (3) Children who have been abused quickly learn that attention-seeking behavior such as crying for comforting provokes more abuse. Therefore they learn to accept the battering silently. (c)

140. (1) Typically, abusing parents have difficulty in showing concern for their child. They are unable to comfort him, such as through touch, and give little indication of realizing how he feels. (b)

141. (4) In an attempt to block the hospital staff from discovering what really happened, abusing parents frequently provide inconsistent accounts. (c)

142. (2) Assault is a threat or an attempt to do violence to another. Implementing an action that requires informed consent prior to obtaining the consent is grounds for the charge of assault. (c)

143. (3) Battery means touching in an offensive manner or the actual injuring of another person. (b)

144. (2) Tetralogy of Fallot classically consists of 4 defects. Three of them are anatomic—ventricular septal defect, pulmonic stenosis, and overriding aorta. However, a fourth defect, right ventricular hypertrophy, is secondary to increased resistance to blood flow in the right ventricle. (b)

145. (4) Oxygen is necessary for growth of cells. Decreased oxygen in the developing child causes a slow growth rate. Adults do not have this adaptation because their growth is complete. (b)

146. (2) The purpose of digoxin (Lanoxin) is to slow and strenghten the apical rate. The normal apical rate for a child of 5 years is 90 to 110 beats per minute. If the apical rate is already slow (10 to 20 beats below normal), administration of the drug could lower the apical rate to an unsafe level. (a)

147. (4) Decreased tissue oxygenation stimulates erythropoiesis, resulting in excessive production of red blood cells. (a)

148. (1) Forceful evacuation results in the child's taking a deep breath, holding it, and straining (Valsalva maneuver). This increased intrathoracic pressure puts excessive strain on the heart sutures. (b)

149. (2) Polycythemia reflected in an elevated hematocrit level is a direct attempt of the body to compensate for the decrease in oxygenation to all body cells due to the mixture of oxygenated and unoxygenated circulating blood. (c)

150. (3) In the fetus, oxygenated blood is shunted directly into the systemic circulation via the ductus arteriosus, a connection between the pulmonary artery and the aorta.

Normally after birth the increased oxygen tension causes a functional closure of the ductus arteriosus. Occasionally, particularly in premature infants, this vessel remains open and is known as patent ductus arteriosus. (c)

151. (4) In acyanotic heart disease there is a narrowing of the vessels and/or pinpoint holes in the septum of the heart that cause a murmuring sound as the blood is pumped through. These interfere primarily with the circulation of oxygenated blood. (c)

152. (2) Coarctation of the aorta is a narrowing, usually in the thoracic segment, causing decreased blood flow below the constriction and increased blood volume above it. This results in full, bounding pulses and increased blood pressure in the upper extremities and weak or absent pulses and decreased blood pressure in lower extremities. (c)

153. (3) The nurse's data collection was not adequate because no questions were asked concerning the recency of the previous tetanus inoculation. The nurse failed to support the life and well-being of a patient. (c)

154. (4) The slightest stimulation sets off a wave of very severe and very painful muscle spasms involving the whole body. Nerve impulses cross the myoneural junction and stimulate muscle contraction due to the presence of exotoxins produced by *C. tetani*. (c)

155. (4) Gluteal folds should by symmetric, as should all planes and folds of the body. Any abnormality of the hips will cause asymmetry and/or a shorter leg on the affected side. (a)

156. (1) Hypostatic pneumonia can develop from decreased activity. Also, the cast prevents full chest expansion. (a)

157. (2) Pillows under the head or shoulders of a child in a spica cast will thrust the chest forward against the cast, causing discomfort and respiratory distress. Therefore, when elevation of the head is desired, the entire mattress and spring should be elevated at the head of the bed. (b)

158. (1) Because phenylalanine is an essential amino acid, it must be provided in quantities sufficient for promoting growth while maintaining safe blood levels. (c)

159. (2) Congenital cretinism is caused by an insufficiency of the secretion of the thyroid gland due to an embryonic defect. The gland is either absent or rudimentary and unable to produce the thyroid hormone. Therefore the decreased thyroid hormone has been affecting the infant long before birth. If treatment is delayed, the infant may become more retarded in growth and mental development. (a)

160. (2) $\dfrac{0.35 \text{ mg}}{0.25 \text{ mg}} \times \dfrac{x \text{ minims}}{15 \text{ minims}} = 21 \text{ minims}$ (b)
     (15 or 16 minims = 1 ml)

161. (3) This is due to the fact that celiac patients have a gluten-induced enteropathy and are unable to absorb fats from the intestinal tract. (b)

162. (1) Rubeola signs and symptoms include a high fever, photophobia, Koplik's spots (white patches on mucous membranes of the oral cavity), and a rash. Rubella usually does not cause a high fever, runs a 3- to 6-day course, and never causes Koplik's spots. (c)

163. (1) Infants are almost 85% water in composition. An elevated temperature causes increased absorption of fluid via the bowel and may upset the balance of fluid. It could also interfere with K^+ balance, the electrolyte that can be lost via the large intestine. A tap water enema should never be repeated without a physician's order. In addition, no more than 300 ml of fluid should be instilled without a physician's order. (a)

164. (2) Steroids have an anti-inflammatory effect. It is believed that resistance to certain viral diseases, including chickenpox, is greatly decreased when the child is taking steroids regularly. (b)

165. (3) Mumps can cause orchitis (inflammation of the testes) in males and oophoritis (inflammation of ovaries) in females; both can render the postpubescent child sterile. (b)

166. (3) Secondary syphilis, occurring 1 to 3 months after healing of the primary lesion and lasting for several weeks to as long as a year, is the stage at which the individual is most infectious. This stage is characterized by influenza-like symptoms, lymphadenopathy, and a generalized skin eruption. Communicability gradually diminishes after the first year. (b)

167. (1) Syphilis is caused by a spirochete, *Treponema pallidum*. The organism is readily destroyed by mild disinfectants such as soap and water. (b)

168. (2) Based on the history of exposure and clinical manifestations, it was during the last 6 months to the present time when the patient was most communicable. (c)

169. (1) Hemophilia is carried on the X chromosome but is recessive. Therefore the female is the carrier (a normal X_O and an affected X_H). If the male receives the affected X_H ($X_H Y_O$), the disease is manifest. This mode of transmission is sex-linked recessive. (a)

170. (2) The mating of a carrier female ($X_O X_H$) and an unaffected male ($X_O Y_O$) results in the following possible offspring: a carrier female ($X_O X_H$), a normal female ($X_O X_O$), a normal male ($X_O Y_O$), or an affected male ($X_H Y_O$). (b)

171. (4) Bleeding is greatly influenced by activity. In the active school-age child, bleeding into weight-bearing joints, especially the knees, is the most common site. (b)

172. (2) Salicylates in large doses causes irritation of the gastric mucosa (gastric distress, nausea, vomiting) and also affect the CNS (tinnitus, dizziness, disturbances in hearing and vision). Gastric disturbances can be limited by administering the drug with large amounts of water or with milk or food. (a)

173. (2) Salicylates act as analgesics by protecting peripheral pain receptors from bradykinin, a component in the in-

flammatory process. Salicylates act as antipyretics by affecting the heat-regulating center in the hypothalamus and increasing the elimination of heat through peripheral blood vessel dilation and evaporation of increased perspiration. (a)

174. (2) Rheumatic fever is almost always preceded by a group A *Streptococcus* infection, which is most often associated with upper respiratory tract infections. Therefore upper respiratory tract infections should be treated early to prevent the development of rheumatic fever. (b)

175. (1) Choanal atresia is a lack of an opening between the nasal passages and the nasopharynx. (c)

176. (2) Since there is no opening between the nasal passages and the nasopharynx, the infant can only breathe through the mouth. When feeding, the infant cannot breathe without aspirating some of the fluid, which causes choking. (b)

177. (4) An Apgar score of 3 indicates neonatal distress and should signal the nurse that the infant requires close supervision and support. (b)

178. (4) Infection is a constant threat because of poor general state of nutrition, tendency toward skin breakdown in edematous areas, corticosteroid therapy, and lowered immunoglobulin levels. (c)

179. (3) Children with nephrosis have a characteristic pale, overweight appearance from the malnutrition and edema and become very sensitive about these changes as they grow older. (b)

180. (1) Bed-wetting accidents are not uncommon in this age group, especially during hospitalization when regression may occur. Therefore the best approach is to ignore the event. (b)

181. (2) Fear of mutilation and intrusive procedures is most common at this age because of fantasies and active imagination. These children also connect illness with being bad and view intrusion as punishment. (c)

182. (2) The restricted ventilation accompanying an asthmatic attack limits the body's ability to blow off CO_2. As CO_2 accumulates in the body fluids, it reacts with H_2O to produce carbonic acid (H_2CO_3); the result is respiratory acidosis. (b)

183. (2) Prednisone causes atrophy of the thymus, decreases the number of lymphocytes, plasma cells, and eosinophils in the blood, and decreases the formation of antibodies. Therefore prednisone reduces the individual's resistance to certain infectious processes and viral diseases. Also, it is an anti-inflammatory drug that masks infection. (b)

184. (2) Aminophylline relaxes smooth muscle of the vasculature, causing peripheral vasodilation that can lead to hypotension. (b)

185. (1) Cold can precipitate bronchospasm, and increased exercise depletes oxygen. (b)

186. (2) Peak crying times are early evening and night, which

exhaust the mother. She needs time away from the baby to rest and should be encouraged to hire a sitter or make some arrangements for time alone. (a)

187. (3) The traditional efforts to explain and treat colic center around control of gas in the intestinal tract that is causing the paroxysmal pain. Crying starts abruptly with loud screams, clenched fists, and legs that are drawn up to the abdomen. (a)

188. (3) Muscular coordination and perception are developed enough at 6 months so that the infant can roll over. If unaware of this ability of the infant, the nurse could leave the child unattended for a moment to reach for something and the child could roll off the crib. All safety precautions should be enforced. (b)

189. (3) Touching the palms of the hands causes flexion of the fingers, (grasp reflex); this reflex usually lessens after 3 months of age. An unexpected loud noise causes abduction of the extremities and then flexion of the elbows (startle reflex); this reflex usually disappears by 4 months of age. Persistence of primitive reflexes usually is indicative of a cerebral insult. (b)

190. (4) By law, a nurse cannot administer medications without a prescription from a physician. This is a dependent function of the nurse. (a)

191. (1) An individual is legally unable to sign a consent until age 18 years. The only exception is the emancipated minor, a minor who is self-sufficient or married. (a)

192. (4) The nurse made the assessment that the medication was ineffective in relieving Loren's pain for the duration ordered. This information should be communicated to the physician for his evaluation. Legally the nurse cannot administer another dose of the medication; however, the nurse should not ignore the patient's need for relief from pain. (a)

193. (1) Chlorpheniramine (Chlor-Trimeton) is an antihistaminic that prevents histamine from reaching its site of action by competing for the receptors. (b)

194. (3) Assault is a threat or an attempt to do violence to another, and battery means touching an individual in an offensive manner or the actual injuring of another person. (a)

195. (4) Tetracycline is potentially hepatotoxic, especially in anyone with liver dysfunction, since it is metabolized in the liver. Signs of hepatotoxicity are lethargy, anorexia, behavioral changes, jaundice, and fatty necrosis. (c)

196. (3) The principle of Bryant's traction is bilateral Buck's extension applied to legs. It is skin traction and does not require surgery. Its purpose is to decrease the fracture, maintain alignment, and immobilize both legs. (a)

197. (3) No more than 300 ml of solution should be administered to an infant or child unless specifically ordered, since fluid and electrolyte balance in an infant or child is easily disturbed. (c)

198. (3) A patient cannot legally be locked in a room (isolated)

unless there is a threat of danger involved either to the patient or to other patients. (b)

199. (2) A pounding board is a safe toy for toddlers, since it is fairly large, easy to manipulate, and sturdy. A pounding board provides a way for anger to be sublimated. (b)

200. (3) Decision making fosters and supports independence, a developmental need of the adolescent. It also increases a sense of self-worth. (b)

201. (3) A plaster cast is not flexible and can inhibit circulation. Cold toes, loss of sensation in toes, pain, and inability to move toes should be reported to the physician immediately. (b)

202. (1) Using the formula, convert grains to milligrams (grains 1/300 = 0.2 mg); then using the formula:

$$\frac{0.2 \text{ mg}}{0.4 \text{ mg}} \times \frac{x}{1 \text{ ml}}$$

$0.4x = 0.2$
$x = 0.5$ ml will contain the desired dose of 0.2 mg atropine. (c)

203. (3) Since young children have difficulty verbalizing their fears or anxiety, play is a therapeutic way for these feelings to be expressed. The school-age child also likes to role play. (b)

204. (3) Regression is normal in times of stress. It is a transient need that should be accepted, since it helps to reduce anxiety. (a)

205. (2) The drug must be given in the exact amount at the times directed to maintain the desired blood level. If the blood level of the drug falls, the organisms have an opportunity to build up resistance to the drug. (b)

206. (3) Isoniazid (INH) is the most potent tuberculostatic drug available at this time. It is given in conjunction with para-aminosalicylic acid (PAS), since PAS potentiates the action of INH as well as limits bacterial resistance to the drugs. (b)

207. (3) Tubercle bacilli multiply in caseous lesions, which have a poor vascular supply. These areas receive lower levels of the drugs, and as a result therapy must be prolonged. (b)

208. (2) Family members who have been exposed are at high risk and should receive prophylactic therapy with INH and PAS. (b)

209. (4) Mineral oil coats the mucosal lining of the stomach and retards absorption of the poison. (c)

210. (3) Lye, a basic solution, is neutralized by administration of a weak acid such as vinegar. (c)

211. (2) Ipecac exerts its effect through direct stimulation of the vomiting control center and local irritation of the gastric mucosa, which is enhanced through dilution of the drug in large quantities of fluid. (c)

212. (2) One of the most universal characteristics of minimally brain damaged children is distractability. They are highly reactive to any extraneous stimuli such as noise and movement and are unable to inhibit their responses to such stimuli. (c)

213. (2) Because of short attention span and distractability, specific limit setting consistently employed is crucial toward providing an environment that promotes concentration, prevents confusion, and minimizes conflicts for the child. (a)

214. (3) Prednisone is a synthetic glucocorticoid that has an active anti-inflammatory effect by stabilizing lysosomal membranes and thus inhibiting proteolytic enzyme release. (b)

215. (1) Vincristine is highly neurotoxic, causing paresthesias, muscle weakness, ptosis, diplopia, paralytic ileus, vocal cord paralysis, and loss of deep tendon reflexes. (c)

216. (4) Excessive crying and clinging are the usual responses of an infant that expects to be comforted, not one that has been separated from a parent because of illness. (a)

217. (2) Infants who have experienced maternal deprivation usually exhibit failure to thrive; i.e., weight below third percentile, developmental retardation, clinical signs of deprivation, and malnutrition. These physical and emotional factors predispose the infant to a variety of illness. (b)

218. (2)
$$\frac{20 \text{ mg}}{50 \text{ mg}} \times \frac{x}{15 \text{ minims}}$$
$50x = 300$
$x = 6$ minims   (a)
(15 or 16 minims = 1 ml)

219. (3) This defect interferes with the normal diaphragmatic respirations of the newborn. Respirations are further affected by stomach and intestinal distension, a mediastinal shift, atelectasis, and the presence of abdominal organs in the thoracic cavity. Oxygen should be administered to prevent, limit, or correct respiratory distress and acidosis. (a)

220. (4) Following a thoracotomy, negative intrathoracic pressure is reestablished and the alveoli reexpand within 12 to 48 hours. (b)

221. (3) $\dfrac{\text{Total milliliters to be infused} \times \text{Drop factor}}{\text{Total time to be infused in minutes}}$

$\dfrac{1000 \times 60}{1440} = \dfrac{60000}{1440} = 41.6$ gtt/minute   (a)

222. (3) When taking a health history, any areas of concern should be explored fully before making a nursing diagnosis. (a)

223. (2) Normally there may be a weight gain caused by the influence of hormones prior to the growth spurt. Also, 10- to 12-year olds eat an adult-size meal without the increased metabolic needs of adolescence. (b)

224. (1) Hepatitis virus B is in the blood during the late incu-

bation and acute stages of the disease. It may also persist in the carrier state for years. It is transmitted when the blood of an infected individual comes in contact with the blood or mucous membranes of another individual. Post-transfusion hepatitis has been reduced now that the surface antigen of hepatitis B (HB$_s$Ag) can be identified in the blood of carriers of type B virus. (a)

225. (3) Positioning on right side after feeding facilitates digestion because the pyloric sphincter is on this side and gravity aids in emptying the stomach. (c)

226. (2) The correct placement of the tube will be verified by the return of the gastric contents. If over half the previous feeding is aspirated, the next feeding must be withheld. (b)

227. (3) Isotonic saline is compatible with body fluids. It is neither hypertonic or hypotonic so it does not cause a change in osmotic pressure and upset the balance of intracellular and extracellular fluid and electrolytes. (b)

228. (4) In strabismus one eye is generally not used as much as the other, and therefore poor central vision in that eye results from disuse. (c)

COMPREHENSIVE TEST 1

1. (4) Gentle pressure is applied against the baby's head as it emerges so that it is not delivered too rapidly. The head is never held back and it should be supported as it emerges to prevent vaginal lacerations. (b)

2. (2) Position baby with head lower than chest and rub infant's back to stimulate crying so that infant can oxygenate lungs. (a)

3. (1) Precipitate delivery may be injurious to both mother and infant. Maternal morbidity is increased due to infection and/or hemorrhage resulting from the trauma of the rapid forceful delivery in a contaminated field. (b)

4. (2) The first hour following delivery is called the fourth stage of labor. During this time the uterus is at the level of the umbilicus, and each day after delivery it descends one finger breadth. (c)

5. (3) The Nurse Practice Act requires nurses to diagnose human responses. (b)

6. (4) Mucus must be removed from the respiratory tract to maintain a patent airway to promote the processes of respiration and gaseous exchange. (b)

7. (1) Respiratory distress is a frequent response indicative of possible immaturity of the infant's respiratory tract, such as smaller lumen, weakness of respiratory musculature, paucity of functional alveoli, and insufficient calcification of bony thorax. (b)

8. (1) The tonic neck reflex is normal in the newborn and disappears within 3 to 6 months. (b)

9. (2) Allowing the mother time to inspect the child permits viewing, touching, and holding, promoting bonding. (b)

10. (3) Some mothers will respond to mores and pressures by trying to nurse in spite of the fact that they would prefer to give the baby a bottle. The nurse should elicit more information before responding. (b)

11. (4) Daily washing of the breasts and nipples with water is sufficient for cleanliness; soap may be drying. (b)

12. (3) The pressure and tenderness due to the accumulated milk can be relieved by manually expressing some of the fluid. (b)

13. (1) The emotional excitement of going home frequently diminishes lactation and/or the letdown reflex for a brief period. When the mother has knowledge that this may happen and how to cope with it, the problem is apt to be a minor one that is easily overcome. (b)

14. (3) Most average size babies regulate themselves on an approximate 4-hour schedule, although a wide variation does exist. (b)

15. (3) Anovulation occurs in nursing mothers for varying periods. Lactation does effect a degree of infertility but it is generally not a reliable method of birth control. (a)

16. (1) The common bile duct enters the duodenum. The pyloric sphincter is located between the end of the stomach and the beginning of the duodenum; therefore, when it is hypertrophied, the tight sphincter prevents any mixing of formula with bile. (b)

17. (1) The hypertrophied muscle becomes elongated and is palpable as an olive-shaped mass. Because of its normal anatomic location, it is felt in the upper right quadrant of the abdomen. (b)

18. (2) Prior to inserting the tube the nurse measures the anatomic pathway the tube will follow; i.e., from the nose to the earlobe (corresponding to the nasopharynx) to the epigastric area of the abdomen (lower end of stomach). The tube is marked and then inserted to this point. (b)

19. (2) If the nasogastric tube is accidently passed into the trachea rather than the esophagus, it will occlude the airway, causing cyanosis. (b)

20. (4) During and after feeding, the position most favoring gravity is employed to promote retention of fluid and prevent vomiting. (c)

21. (3) Offering a new food after giving formula associates this activity with eating and takes advantage of the child's unsatisfied hunger. (b)

22. (1) The first solid foods added to the infant's diet should be easily digestible, such as fruits and cereals, and rich sources of iron, such as cereals and egg yolk. Egg yolks are added last because of the allergic reactions often associated with them. (b)

23. (2) Signs of mild to moderate separation include uterine discomfort and tenderness due to concealed bleeding. Visible bleeding may be scant, moderate, or heavy. (b)

24. (4) The blood cannot escape from behind the placenta; thus the abdomen becomes boardlike and painful due to the trapped retroplacental blood. (b)

25. (1) Clotting defects are common in moderate and severe abruptio placentae because of loss of fibrinogen from severe internal bleeding. (b)

26. (4) Parents must be helped to identify their feelings. (a)

27. (1) Excess thyroid hormones increase the metabolic rate, causing nervousness, weight loss, increased appetite, heat intolerance, and tachycardia. (a)

28. (1) Radioactive iodine uptake, which involves administration of trace amounts of ^{131}I and subsequent evaluation of uptake, and T_3 (triiodothyronine) levels in the blood are both increased in hyperthyroidism. (b)

29. (3) Promotion of rest to reduce metabolic demands is an essential and challenging task for the patient with hyperthyroidism. (b)

30. (1) Propylthiouracil, used in the treatment of hyperthyroidism, blocks the synthesis of thyroid hormones by preventing iodination of tyrosine. (b)

31. (4) Lugol's Solution provides iodine, which aids in decreasing the vascularity of the thyroid gland, decreasing the risk of hemorrhage. (b)

32. (1) Medication is regulated to maintain the normal blood levels of thyroxin; therefore ovulation is not affected and future pregnancy is possible. (c)

33. (4) Thyroid surgery sometimes results in accidental removal of the parathyroid glands. A resultant hypocalcemia may result in contraction of the glottis, causing airway obstruction; edema also causes obstruction. (b)

34. (3) Thyroid storm refers to a sudden and excessive release of the thyroid hormones causing pyrexia, tachycardia, and exaggerated symptoms of thyrotoxicosis. Surgery or infection will generally precipitate this life-threatening condition. (b)

35. (2) Thyroid trauma, thyroid surgery, or psychologic stress in a patient with hyperthyroidism may result in release of an abnormally high level of thyroid hormone. This intensifies all symptoms of hyperthyroidism–thyroid storm (increased pulse, elevated temperature, restlessness, vomiting, and often death). (b)

36. (1) Glaucoma refers to a disease of the eye in which there is increased intraocular pressure resulting from narrowing

of the canal of Schlemm. This can lead to blindness due to compression of nutritive blood vessels supplying rods and cones. (a)

37. (2) Retinal damage caused by increased intraocular pressure of glaucoma is permanent and is progressive if the disease is not controlled. (b)

38. (3) In chronic glaucoma there is a loss of peripheral vision long before the central vision is affected. The patient may also complain of seeing halos around lights. (b)

39. (4) Atropine causes pupils to dilate, leading to increased intraocular pressure in the patient with glaucoma. Any such order must be questioned because permanent damage may result. (b)

40. (2) The prone position stretches the flexor muscles, thus preventing hip flexion contractures. (b)

41. (2) Muscles that originate on the vertebrae or pelvic girdle and insert on the femur act to abduct, adduct, flex, extend, and rotate the femur. Normal body alignment should be maintained because it facilitates safe and efficient use of muscle groups for balance and stability. (b)

42. (3) Subcutaneous fat is reduced due to the pressure of the initial constrictive bandage and the socket of the prosthesis. (c)

43. (4) The patient is usually instructed to push forcefully yet gently over the bone to toughen the limb for weight-bearing. This process is begun by pushing the stump against increasingly harder surfaces. (a)

44. (2) Since Mrs. Kraft has severe diabetes, it is essential that the nurse test her urine before meals for sugar and ketones to evaluate the success of control of diabetes and the possible need for insulin coverage. (c)

45. (4) Exercise should not include bending and the Valsalva maneuver, which may cause an increase in intraocular pressure. (b)

46. (4) In small children prior to physical maturity the eustachian tube is shorter, wider, and straighter. Pulling the auricle down and back facilitates passage of fluid to the drum. (b)

47. (2) The middle ear contains the 3 ossicles—the malleus, incus, and stapes. Together with the tympanic membrane and oval window they form an amplifying system. The pressure of sound waves striking the relatively large tympanic membrane is amplified 22 times as it is transmitted through the lever systems of the ossicles and the relatively small oval window to the fluids in the cochlea; the amplified signal is then detected by the organ of Corti within the cochlea (inner ear). (b)

48. (4) Myringotomy is a surgical procedure to relieve pressure and prevent spontaneous rupture of the eardrum. After incision is made, pus and fluid escape from middle ear into the external auditory canal from which the exudate drains. (b)

49. (4) Toddlers are ritualistic and do not tolerate change well. Any change in diet should be done matter-of-factly.

Because of their characteristic struggle for independence, toddlers should not be forced to eat. (b)

50. (1) The toddler is still dependent on the mother, is narcissistic, and still plays alone but is aware of others playing next to him. (a)

51. (4) Appropriate limit setting and discipline are necessary for children to develop self-control while learning the boundaries of their abilities. (c)

52. (4) Introducing May Ann to the nurse who will be primarily working with her on a one-to-one basis is extremely important because the withdrawn patient can be assisted back to reality by a caring individual (nurse) who is interested in everything that happens to her. (b)

53. (2) A simple statement that the patient is not understood provides feedback to the patient and points out reality. (b)

54. (3) May Ann needs someone who has been working with her and whom she trusts to stay with her until she is calmer. She has lost control and needs the protection of another person who will observe, anticipate, and prevent her from acting out her destructive impulses. (c)

55. (1) The nurse demonstrates that she knows her own perceptions and can accept the patient's, even though they are hallucinatory. (b)

56. (2) Once May Ann realizes that the staff does not recognize her negative behavior (which is a defense against feelings of inferiority) but praises her for real accomplishments, she will no longer need the superior attitude; she will have gained recognition and self-esteem for socially acceptable behavior. (b)

57. (3) The caffeine in coffee acts as a stimulant to counteract the drowsiness she may experience during the first week of treatment. After the first week, drowsiness may be replaced by a feeling of calmness. (c)

58. (1) Tranquilizers reduce anxiety levels and make patients more amenable to looking at new approaches to handling stress. (b)

59. (2) Maladaptive behavior that may be accepted in the hospital will not be approved in the community. The nurse's observations can help to determine which patients are ready to cope with life's realities and which need further help. The nurse can report the observations to the medical team and appropriate actions can be taken. (c)

60. (2) Third-degree burns extend into the subcutaneous tissue and are not painful because of nerve destruction. (c)

61. (3) Using the rule of nines, each arm is 9%, each leg is 18%, and the head is 9%. Therefore the total percentage of burned area is 36%. (a)

62. (3) In the first 48 hours after a severe burn, fluid moves into the tissue surrounding the injured area. Fluid is also lost in drainage and from evaporation. This results in a decreased blood volume and could lead to shock. (a)

63. (1) The severe pain experienced by the patient during debridement of burns places an emotional strain on the nurse. (a)

64. (2) The mucous membranes of the respiratory tract may be charred after inhalation burns. This is evidenced by the production of sooty sputum. (c)

65. (3) The shift of plasma proteins into the burned area increases the tissue colloid osmotic pressure (TCOP). This results in fluid diffusion from the intravascular to the interstitial fluid compartment. The result is decreased blood volume and hypovolemic shock. (c)

66. (3) Cellular catabolism, as in burns, results in loss of potassium from cells; this raises the K^+ level in the extracellular fluid (normal range from 3.5 to 5.5 mEq per liter). Such hyperkalemia may lead to arrhythmias (peaked T wave at 6 mEq per liter) and, as a terminal event, cardiac arrest. (c)

67. (2) Showing understanding and identifying the patient's feelings by giving feedback helps in establishing a therapeutic relationship. (b)

68. (4) Emotional support and close surveillance can demonstrate the staff's caring and their attempt to prevent acting out of suicidal ideation. (b)

69. (3) The staff's presence provides continued emotional support and helps relieve anxiety. (b)

70. (3) The relatively massive electrical energy passing through the cerebral cortex during ECT results in a temporary state of confusion following treatment. (b)

71. (1) Succinylcholine (Anectine) causes paralysis of muscles, including the intercostals and diaphragm, so artificial support of respirations is required to sustain life. (a)

72. (2) Succinylcholine temporarily paralyzes the muscles, including those of respiration; some artificial means of respiration is necessary until the drug is metabolized and excreted. (b)

73. (2) Depressed patients have difficulty expressing anger and hostility because they have internalized these feelings and turned them on themselves. (b)

74. (1) Severely depressed patients are not motivated to take action or to plan ahead, since they are unable to direct their energy on the environment. (c)

75. (2) Breathing techniques should be demonstrated preoperatively to increase compliance with the postoperative regime. (c)

76. (2) Poor dental hygiene may predispose to oral infections but would only be remotely involved in laryngeal neoplasms. (c)

77. (2) The outer tube is not removed, since the stoma may close, and it is usually sutured in place. The inner tube may be cleaned prn. (b)

78. (2) Food should be avoided until the area is totally healed to avoid contamination and irritation and generally to promote healing. Tube feedings are usually discontinued within 2 weeks. (c)

79. (4) Slow feeding of reduced carbohydrate content food helps to prevent rapid peristalsis and subsequent diarrhea. (c)

80. (2) The patient's concerns will be reduced if he knows the stoma will stay open until another tube can be inserted. (b)

81. (3) The procedure should be explained so the patient understands that the tracheostomy can serve as an entrance for bacteria and that cleanliness is imperative. (b)

82. (3) Inactivity over an extended period of time increases stiffness and pain in joints. (a)

83. (3) Polyarthritis of rheumatic fever is transitory and does not cause deformity. Rheumatoid arthritis is chronic and causes changes in joints. (a)

84. (2) Aspirin interferes with platelet aggregation, thereby lengthening bleeding time. (b)

85. (1) Ten-year-old boys prefer the company of the same sex and age group. Also, Mark needs to avoid stressful situations that would tend to increase exacerbations. (b)

86. (2) Valium is a tranquilizer and anticonvulsant used to relax smooth muscles during seizures. (a)

87. (1) Serum albumin is administered to maintain serum levels and normal oncotic pressures by pulling fluid from the interstitial spaces into the intravascular compartment, thus decreasing the hematocrit level. (c)

88. (1) Albumin acts to elevate the blood pressure to normal levels when it is administered slowly and oral fluid intake is restricted, since fluid is pulled from interstitial spaces into the circulatory system. (b)

89. (4) Paraldehyde is excreted through the lungs and gives off a specific identifiable odor. (c)

90. (2) Neomycin aids in reducing intestinal flora that act on protein substances, causing the production of ammonia. Ammonia is detoxified in the liver. When the liver is unable to perform this function adequately, blood ammonia levels rise, causing encephalopathy. (c)

91. (2) When the bladder contains large amounts of urine, it becomes distended and may extend upward into the abdominal cavity where it may be punctured. (a)

92. (4) Elixir terpin hydrate should be avoided because it contains alcohol and will cause an Antabuse reaction. (a)

93. (3) Psychoemotional factors related to chronic illness often affect an individual's compliance with medical regimen. These feelings must be explored and worked out for acceptance of the treatment plan. (b)

94. (2) Before planning and instituting a teaching plan, the nurse must assess patient attitudes, experience, knowledge, and understanding of the health problem. (b)

95. (1) The acquiring of knowledge or understanding aids the development of concepts rather than skills or attitudes and is a basic learning task in the cognitive domain. (b)

96. (2) As a result of hormones involved in growth and development, patients with juvenile diabetes have different and changing needs regarding nutrition and exogenous insulin. (a)

97. (4) An insulin-dependent diabetic patient must carry sugar or candy as a ready source of carbohydrate in the event of signs of hypoglycemia. (a)

98. (2) The protein in milk and cheese may be slowly converted to carbohydrate (gluconeogenesis), providing the body with some glucose during sleep while the NPH is still acting. (b)

99. (3) In the later stages of adaptation an individual is better able to understand and integrate information. A patient or family member asking for information is a clue identifying readiness for learning. (b)

100. (3) A diagnosis of cancer and a colostomy alter a person's body and self-image drastically. People react differently to this stress, often finding it difficult to verbally express their concerns, although their actions may demonstrate an awareness of the situation. (b)

101. (4) Insomnia is often caused by anxiety. By stating an observation about a patient's activity, the nurse communicates her concern and recognition that the patient may have more covert problems that he wishes to verbalize. (a)

102. (1) Daily colostomy irrigations at the same time help establish normal patterns of bowel evacuation. The diet should be as close to normal as possible. (b)

103. (4) Patients who have radical changes in their body image as a result of surgery are usually best able to relate to someone who has faced the same stress and has successfully adapted. (b)

104. (4) Rapid instillation of fluid into the colon may cause abdominal cramps. By clamping off the tubing, the cramps will generally subside so the enema can be continued. (b)

105. (1) A colostomy located on the left side of the abdomen would involve the descending colon. Since the descending colon contains stool from which most fluid has been absorbed, the stool quality would be moist and formed. (c)

106. (2) A diet as close to normal as possible after a colostomy is recommended for the stated reason; individuals will discover their own food intolerances and should eat accordingly. (b)

107. (3) Ischemia causes tissue injury and release of chemicals such as bradykinin, which stimulate sensory nerves producing pain. (b)

108. (3) Administration of oxygen increases the transalveolar O_2 gradient, which improves the efficiency of the cardiopulmonary system; this increases the oxygen supply to the heart. (b)

109. (1) Until the patient's condition has reached some degree of stability after myocardial infarction, routine activities such as changing sheets are avoided to minimize patient movements and help reduce cardiac workload. (b)

110. (2) Acute care of the patient with a myocardial infarction is aimed at reducing the cardiac workload. Foods that are easily digested help reduce this workload. Sympathetic nervous system involvement causes decreased peristalsis and gastric secretion, so limiting food intake will help prevent gastric distention. (b)

111. (2) The body's general inflammatory response as a result of myocardial necrosis causes an elevation of temperature within 24 hours and leukocytosis. (b)
112. (3) Visits by family members can allay anxiety and consequently reduce emotional stress, an important risk factor in cardiovascular disease. (a)
113. (3) Presence of a P wave before each QRS complex indicates a sinus rhythm. A heart rate over 100 beats per minute is referred to as tachycardia. (a)
114. (1) Signs of digitalis toxicity include cardiac arrhythmias, anorexia, nausea, vomiting, and visual disturbance. Cardiac arrhythmias result from the inhibition, by digitalis, of myocardial Na^+, K^+, and ATP. Extracardiac effects may be due to CNS or local actions. (a)
115. (3) By 2 years of age the child should demonstrate an interest in others, communicate verbally, and possess the ability to learn from the environment; before these skills develop, autism is difficult to diagnose. (b)

116. (2) Autistic behavior turns inward; the child does not respond to the environment and attempts to maintain emotional equilibrium by rubbing and manipulating self and displaying a compulsive need for behavioral repetition. (a)
117. (3) One begins by trying to enter the world where the child's attention is currently focused; this is a way of making human contact, since the child's usual contacts are inanimate objects. (b)
118. (2) Isolated, unrelated activities predominate; child's behavior reflects withdrawal or feelings of destructive rage. (b)
119. (2) Self-isolation and disinterest in interpersonal relationships lead the autistic child to find security in nonthreatening, impersonal objects. (c)
120. (4) The rhythmic movement of the merry-go-round provides soothing, nonthreatening comfort to the autistic child who cannot reach out to his environment. (c)

COMPREHENSIVE TEST 2

1. (2) The nurse fulfilled the expectation in the Nurse Practice Act, which includes teaching. In this case she had knowledge of dietary needs and their relation to well-being during pregnancy. (b)
2. (3) The longer matter remains in the GI tract, the more water is reabsorbed, and constipation results. (b)
3. (2) Rupture of the membranes and the gush of fluid can carry the umbilical cord downward. Immediate placement in lithotomy position and inspection may lead to identification of prolapse and prevention of fetal distress. (b)
4. (3) Hypertonic contractions of the uterus, if allowed to continue, can lead to uterine rupture. Therefore the infusion should be discontinued so that the hypertonic contractions cease. (b)
5. (3) As cervical dilation nears completion, labor is intensified with an increase in pain and energy expenditure. (b)
6. (2) A relaxed uterus is the most frequent cause of bleeding in the early postpartum period. The uterus can be returned to a state of firmness by intermittent gentle fundal massage. (a)
7. (1) A distended bladder will easily displace the fundus upward and laterally. (a)
8. (4) Forcing the family to be involved at the nurse's convenience will interfere with the development of a productive relationship and affect cooperation of the family. (a)
9. (1) The role of stranger is the initial role in any relationship. (a)

10. (3) The first step in the problem-solving process would be exploration so family needs could be identified. (b)
11. (4) Inclusion in the interview will avoid a feeling of ostracism by Mr. Wyer and will foster his cooperation. (b)
12. (4) This allows Mr. Wyer to express his feelings and is nonjudgmental. All other choices place him on the defensive. (a)
13. (3) The schedule for immunization of children not immunized in early infancy is altered and adapted from the schedule followed for infants. The tuberculin test normally given at 1 year is added to the first of the DTP and TOPV series. The combined measles, rubella and mumps vaccine is then given 1 month later. It is never given before 15 months. The Td toxoid is given to children 6 years and older and contains less diphtheria antigen. (c)
14. (2) These children have difficulty reaching out to the environment and tend to be withdrawn. They get little response from parents and do not learn how to respond to others. (b)
15. (4) A consistent caregiver enhances the formation of a trusting and mutually satisfying relationship between child and nurse. Stimulation must be moderate and geared to the child's present developmental level to promote age-appropriate learning without overstimulation. (b)
16. (3) Head control and rolling over are achieved at 4 to 5 months, respectively. Transferring objects from one hand

to another and sitting unsupported are achieved at 7 and 8 months, respectively. (b)

17. (4) Fine motor coordination is inadequately developed to manipulate snap toys. (a)

18. (3) Mothers of failure-to-thrive children are usually insecure of their mothering ability and easily threatened. Teaching them by example is a nonthreatening approach that allows them to proceed at their own pace. Satisfying the parents' needs allows them emotional reserves to give to the child. (b)

19. (4) Paraplegia is the paralysis of both the lower extremities and lower trunk resulting from damage to the spinal cord from the thoracic to the lumbar segments. (b)

20. (2) The priority of care at this time is to protect the spinal area from strain to prevent additional damage to the traumatized area while it heals. (c)

21. (1) Patients with early spinal cord damage experience an atonic bladder, which is characterized by the absence of muscle tone, an enlarge capacity, no feeling of discomfort with distention, and overflow with a large residual. This leads to urinary stasis and infection. High fluid intake limits urinary stasis and infection by diluting urine and increasing urinary output. (b)

22. (3) The Circ-O-lectric bed facilitates frequent vertical turning of the patient to prevent decubiti, which can form within 24 hours due to pressure. (b)

23. (2) The patient should have a nasogastric tube to prevent aspiration and keep the stomach decompressed. (b)

24. (1) These signs could be indicative of hemorrhage due to perforation and require immediate surgical intervention. (a)

25. (3) Trauma of surgery results in some seeping or oozing into the remaining gastric area, which is being immediately suctioned out of the body via the nasogastric tube. (c)

26. (2) Too rapid administration can result in hyperkalemia, which can cause a long refractory period in the cardiac cycle and can result in cardiac arrhythmias and arrest. (c)

27. (4) The nurse should not only count the rate but also inspect the infusion site no matter who starts the IV. Failure to do so constitutes negligence. (c)

28. (2) When high osmotic fluid passes rapidly into the small intestine, it causes hypovolemia. This results in a sympathetic response resulting in tachycardia, diaphoresis, and dizziness. The symptoms are also attributed to a sudden rise and subsequent fall in blood sugar. (b)

29. (4) Small feedings reduce the amount of bulk passing into the jejunum and therefore reduce the symptom. (b)

30. (4) John's denial is a pattern of defense often demonstrated in the self-protective stage of adaptation to illness. John's thoughts and feelings are so painful and anxiety provoking that he rejects the existence of his paraplegia. (b)

31. (3) Absent or diminished gag reflex could be life threatening because the infant might aspirate mucus or formula. (b)

32. (2) Milia commonly occur, are not indicative of any illness, and eventually disappear. (a)

33. (1) The brick-red color is caused by albumin and urates that are concentrated due to dehydration, which is normal in the first 10 days. (c)

34. (1) Jaundice occurs due to the normal physiologic breakdown of fetal red blood cells and the immaturity of the infant's liver. (a)

35. (2) Eye patches are applied to prevent drying of the conjunctiva, injury to the retina, and alterations in biorhythms. (c)

36. (3) Head lag in an infant 6 months old is abnormal and is frequently a sign of cerebral damage. (c)

37. (1) Increased intracranial pressure results in pressure exerted against the cranium, which is especially evident in areas with less confinement, such as the fontanels (bulges), the orbits (pushed forward so that eyelids are pulled taut and upper lids are above the iris [sunset eyes]), and brain (vomiting center stimulated regardless of activity of eating). (b)

38. (2) Child can be positioned on back or abdomen to allow for a routine change of head position. The head is elevated to decrease the intracranial pressure through gravity. (b)

39. (4) Mental retardation is the result of brain cell death. Cellular destruction occurs as the brain is pressed against the unyielding skull, thus occluding blood vessels and depriving the cells of oxygen. (a)

40. (2) Sedatives and analgesics are avoided because they can mask signs of impending loss of consciousness. (c)

41. (2) Shunts need to be revised; as child grows, the length of tubing needs to be changed. The shunts are also prone to malfunction and may need revision. (a)

42. (3) Varicose veins are dilated veins that occur as a result of incompetent valves. Varicosities may be due to a variety of factors, including heredity, prolonged standing, which puts strain on the valves, and abdominal pressure on the large veins of the lower abdomen. (b)

43. (4) Because of the dilation in the veins and concomitant decrease in arterial flow, the patient may experience heaviness or muscle cramps in the legs. Edema, if present, can be relieved by elevating the legs. (b)

44. (1) The Trendelenburg test evaluates the backflow of blood through defective valves. If, after raising the legs to empty the veins, the patient stands and the veins fill from above the site of the suspected varicosity, the diagnosis is supported. (c)

45. (2) Since the superficial vein (saphenous) will be ligated, it is first necessary to determine if the deep veins will be capable of supporting the return circulation. (a)

46. (4) Hypersecretion of the mucous glands provides an excellent warm, moist medium for microorganisms. (b)

47. (1) The legs should be elevated to promote venous return by gravity. (a)
48. (4) Muscle contraction of the legs helps promote venous return and prevent thrombus formation. (c)
49. (1) Asthma involves spasms of the bronchi and bronchioles as well as an increased mucus production. This decreases the size of the lumen, interfering with inhalation and exhalation. (b)
50. (1) In addition to dilating the bronchi, treatment is aimed at expectoration of mucus because it interferes with gas exchange in the lungs. (a)
51. (3) Aminophylline relaxes the smooth muscles, causing bronchodilation and thereby relieving respiratory distress and promoting rest. (a)
52. (3) When an IV infusion is infiltrated, it should be removed to prevent swelling of the tissues and pain. (b)
53. (1) During sleep mucus secretions in the respiratory tract move more slowly toward the throat. On awakening, increased ciliary motion raises such secretions more vigorously; this facilitates expectoration and collection of sputum specimens. (a)
54. (2) Individuals who have difficulty asking for help may ''cry for help'' through a psychosomatic illness. (b)
55. (3) Although dust cannot be avoided completely, use of a damp cloth helps eliminate the amount of air-borne particles that might be inhaled. (a)
56. (3) The purpose of the support hose is to apply external pressure on the veins, preventing retrograde pressure or flow that may occur in standing or sitting positions. By putting on the stockings before arising, the veins do not have the chance to engorge. (a)
57. (4) Marked jaundice generally indicates liver damage or excessive hemolysis and is not a sign of leukemia, unless hepatic damage from late effects of the disease or drugs has occurred. Edema is not a manifestation of the disease, since the pathophysiology does not involve transport of fluids. (a)
58. (3) Acute leukemia is an excessive, uncontrolled production of immature white blood cells that compete for nutrients and eventually crowd the bone marrow, preventing formation of other blood cells. (b)
59. (4) A side effect of vincristine is alopecia, or hair loss. To adolescents, who are very concerned with identity, this represents a tremendous threat to their self-image. (a)
60. (1) Infection from lowered resistance is a constant threat from the disease and from the immunosuppressant drugs, both of which affect white blood cells. (b)
61. (3) Constipation from adynamic ileus can be prevented with high-fiber foods and liberal fluids, which keep the stool bulky and soft, thus promoting evacuation. (c)
62. (1) Low platelet count predisposes to bleeding, which may be evident in urine. Red blood cells are seen microscopically in the sediment. (b)

63. (1) The protective blood-brain barrier initially screens leukemic cells from the CNS. However, in advanced stages leukemic infiltration occurs. The chemotherapeutic agents, also screened out by the blood-brain barrier, are ineffective. (c)
64. (3) Children at early school age are not yet able to comprehend death's universality and inevitability but fear it, often personifying death as a bogey-man or death-angel. They need to be told of the seriousness of the illness at least to let them know that recovery may not be possible. (b)
65. (2) The individual cannot resolve the conflict consciously because of emotional pressure pulling him in both directions; as anxiety increases, the unconscious seeks a solution; the conversion selected usually resolves the initial conflict by making action impossible, thus removing the need to select one or the other choice. (c)
66. (1) The development of physical symptoms without a physical cause is an anxiety-reducing mechanism specific to the psychoneurotic pattern of behavior. (b)
67. (2) The development of the symptom is the unconscious method of reducing the anxiety; as the symptom is meeting this need, it does not create anxiety itself but is passively accepted. (b)
68. (3) The psychosomatic response (hyperfunction or hypofunction) creates actual tissue change; hypochondria is an exaggerated body concern unrelated to organic changes. (b)
69. (3) Response focuses the patient on the relationship between emotion and physical symptoms in a nonthreatening accepting manner. (b)
70. (4) Until the patient learns new ways of dealing with anxiety, he will continue to use this pattern of behavior; learning new ways to operate will break the pattern. (b)
71. (4) Helps patient to identify behavior and feelings in a nonthreatening manner. (c)
72. (2) The mismatched blood cells are attacked by antibodies, and the hemoglobin released from the ruptured erythrocytes plugs the kidney tubules; such kidney involvement results in backache. (c)
73. (2) The cessation of renal function is usually evidenced by a decrease in output to less than 400 ml/24 hours. (b)
74. (1) Perspiration is an involuntary physiologic response; it is mediated by the autonomic nervous system under a variety of circumstances, such as rising ambient temperature, high humidity, stress, and pain. (a)
75. (1) The patient is assessed and observed, and the dialysis solutions are intilled, equilibrated, and drained by the nurse. (b)
76. (3) Peritoneal dialysis uses the peritoneal membrane as a selectively permeable membrane for diffusion of toxins and wastes from the blood into the dialyzing solution. (a)
77. (4) Hyperkalemia occurs in renal failure, since the body does not excrete K^+ due to damage of the kidneys. (b)

78. (2) Potassium is always low to prevent hyperkalemia. (c)
79. (3) If fluid is not draining properly, the patient should be positioned from side to side or with the head raised, or manual pressure should be applied to the lower abdomen to facilitate drainage by means of external pressure and gravity. (c)
80. (2) When respiratory embarrassment occurs, possibly due to pressure of the dialysate on the diaphragm, fluid should be removed and the patient's vital signs and status should be observed. (c)
81. (3) All patients who are confined to bed for any considerable period risk losing calcium from bones. This is precipitated in the urine and causes calculi. (b)
82. (2) Constriction of circulation results in decreased venous return and increased pressure within the vessels. Fluid then moves into the interstitial spaces, causing edema. (a)
83. (1) Immunosuppressive agents are administered to decrease the immune system's tendency to reject the transplanted organ. (b)
84. (2) Exposure to infection, cold, or overexertion in a patient with chronic adrenocortical insufficiency (Addison's disease) can cause circulatory collapse. (b)
85. (2) Deficiency of the glucocorticoids causes hypoglycemia in the patient with Addison's disease. Signs of hypoglycemia include weakness, dizziness, cool moist skin, hunger, tremors, and nervousness. (c)
86. (4) Patients with Addison's disease must take glucocorticoids regularly to enable them to physiologically adapt to stress and prevent Addisonian crisis, a medical emergency similar to shock. (b)
87. (1) Due to diminished mineralocorticoid secretion, patients with Addison's disease are prone to developing hyponatremia; therefore addition of salt to the diet is advised. (c)
88. (2) When there is not enough circulating glucocorticoids and mineralocorticoids to sustain normal functioning of the body, hypotension, fever, pallor, tachycardia, and cyanosis result (Addisonian crisis). (b)
89. (2) Prolonged steroid therapy may produce Cushing's syndrome. Signs include slow wound healing, buffalo hump, hirsutism, weight gain, hypertension, acne, moon face, thin arms and legs, and behavioral disturbances. (c)
90. (2) Some cortisol derivatives possess 17 ketosteroid (androgenic) properties, which result in masculinization. (c)
91. (1) Development of mood swings and psychosis is possible from overdose of glucocorticoids as a result of fluid and electrolyte alterations. (b)
92. (3) An interpersonal relationship based on trust must be established before patients can be helped back to reality. (a)
93. (2) Provides support and security without rejecting the patient or placing value judgments on behavior. (b)

94. (2) This behavior reflects the early fetal position; the individual curls up for both protection and security. (c)
95. (4) When the patient who is out of control feels someone is assuming control, it promotes a feeling of security; when this continues, a feeling of trust in this individual is established. (c)
96. (3) Trust is basic to all other therapy; without trust a therapeutic relationship cannot be established. (b)
97. (2) Response reassures that the staff member is able to help and that the patient's feelings are accurate. (b)
98. (3) Yellow sclera is a sign of jaundice, indicating liver damage, which can be irreversible if drug therapy is continued. (b)
99. (2) Close follow-up and continued monitoring of medication, behavior, and emotional state are necessary to enable the patient to maintain positive behavioral change. (a)
100. (4) If the patient does not have a tracheostomy after radical neck surgery, tracheal edema may cause an obstructed airway after the endotracheal tube is removed. (a)
101. (2) Inadequate oxygenation to the brain may produce restlessness or behavioral changes. The pulse and respiratory rate will increase as a compensatory mechanism for hypoxia. (b)
102. (3) The cuff should be inflated to the minimum occlusive volume that allows desired volume to be achieved but does not press against the trachea, constricting circulation. This can be judged by using a stethoscope to listen for a slight air leak at the back of the throat. (c)
103. (4) To facilitate entry of the suction catheter into the bronchi, the patient's head should be turned from side to side. For entry into the left bronchus the head should be turned to the right; the head should be turned to the left for entry into the right bronchus. (c)
104. (2) The tracheotomy site is a portal of entry for microorganisms. Sterile technique must be used. (c)
105. (2) Drugs such as atropine and opiates are contraindicated because the effects of drying secretions and depressing the cough reflex are undesirable. (c)
106. (3) The inner cannula must be removed, cleansed with peroxide, and rinsed with saline to prevent mucus accumulation and occlusion of the tube. (b)
107. (2) Apple juice and pear nectar have low sodium content; tomato juice is high in sodium. (b)
108. (2) $\dfrac{0.2 \text{ mg}}{0.5 \text{ mg}} \times \dfrac{x}{2 \text{ ml}}$ 0.2 mg: x = 0.5 mg: 2 ml

    $0.5x = 0.4 \text{ ml}$ *or* $0.5x = 0.4$
    $x = 0.8 \text{ ml}$ $x = 0.8 \text{ ml}$ (a)
109. (2) Elevation of an extremity promotes venous and lymphatic drainage by gravity. (a)

110. (2) This combination of foods has the highest sodium content. (b)
111. (4) Fluctuation of IV fluid in the manometer with respirations is due to alterations of intrathoracic pressure during inhalation and exhalation. (c)
112. (1) Furosemide (Lasix) inhibits sodium reabsorption in the ascending loop of Henle, whereas chlorothiazide (Diuril) inhibits the reabsorption of sodium and chloride. As a result, water and potassium are not reabsorbed by the distal renal tubules and dehydration and hypokalemia may result. (b)
113. (1) Digitalis increases the strength of the contraction of the myocardium (positive inotropic effect) and alters the electrophysiologic properties of the heart, slowing the heart rate (positive chronotropic effect). (a)
114. (2) The nurse was negligent by not providing close supervision, since she knew Mr. Norman was combative. A reasonable, prudent nurse would have closely observed Mr. Norman to protect him from himself as well as to protect others. (a)

115. (4) Lithium carbonate alters sodium transport in nerve and muscle cells and causes a shift toward intraneuronal metabolism of catecholamines. Since the range between therapeutic and toxic levels is very small, the patient's serum lithium level should be monitored closely. (b)
116. (3) Sets appropriate limits for patient who cannot set them for himself; rejects behavior but accepts the patient. (b)
117. (2) Activities that release tension and use up energy can decrease anxiety. (b)
118. (2) A threat is a type of an assault that is an intentional tort. (c)
119. (1) Patients who are hyperactive are easily diverted. It is best to use this characteristic behavior rather than precipitate a confrontation. (a)
120. (1) Patient is asking for help to prevent suicide; response focuses on feelings and does not challenge or deny these feelings. (a)

COMPREHENSIVE TEST 3

1. (2) A rapid delivery does not give the fetal head adequate time for molding, so pressure against the head is increased. (b)
2. (3) Lacerated tissue does not heal as quickly as a smooth, closely approximated surgical incision. (c)
3. (3) Tears in the tentorial membrane result in bleeding into the cerebellum, pons, or medulla oblongata, in which the respiratory regulation center is located. (c)
4. (1) The newborn's immature neuromuscular development normally causes dorsal flexion of the big toe and fanning of the remaining toes. A positive Babinski sign is abnormal in the adult. (b)
5. (2) Elevation of the head helps decrease intracranial pressure by gravity. (c)
6. (3) Sitting down shows the patient you care enough to spend time and opens up channels of communication. (a)
7. (2) Braces are used to enable the spastic child to control his motions and prevent deformities from poor alignment. (a)
8. (1) The choice of gait is based on the wight-bearing capabilities of each of the 4 extremities. (b)
9. (3) The 4-point alternate crutch gait is a simple, slow, but stable gait because there are always 3 points of support of the floor with equal but partial weight-bearing on each limb. (b)
10. (4) When sensory perceptions are impaired with resultant

lack of effective specific motor responses, an individual will be more vulnerable to skin irritation and trauma. (a)
11. (2) Many behaviors require a background of knowledge, skills, and attitudes (experiential readiness). If this background is not available, then more learning must take place before the individual can function. (c)
12. (1) When the patient's thermoreceptive senses are impaired, the patient will be unable to detect changes or degrees of temperature. The patient must be taught to test the temperature in any water-related activity to prevent scalding and burning. (a)
13. (3) Cerebral palsy ranges from mild to severe. There is no common cause. The damage is fixed and does not become progressively greater. (c)
14. (4) Devices such as side rails can help patients increase mobility by facilitating movement in bed. Side rails, an immovable object, provide a hand hold for leverage when changing positions. (c)
15. (4) Explaining procedures and routines decreases the patient's anxiety about the unknown. (a)
16. (3) Patients and their families should be included in dietary teaching. (a)
17. (4) Processed foods generally have sodium (usually in the form of sodium chloride) added to enhance the taste and help preserve the food. (a)
18. (3) A lowered concentration of extracellular sodium ef-

fects a decrease in the release of ADH, resulting in an increase in urine excretion. (b)

19. (2) Fluid in the interstitial spaces impairs circulation, leading to poor absorption of drugs as well as predisposition for skin breakdown. (b)

20. (2) Range of motion exercises keep muscles in good tone and prevent venous stasis through physical compression of veins; such compression propels venous blood toward the heart, facilitated by venous one-way valves. (b)

21. (4) The wheelchair should be angled close to the bed so that the patient should only have to make a simple pivot on the stronger leg. When the wheelchair is within the patient's visual field, the patient will be aware of the distance and direction that the body has to navigate to transfer safely and avoid falling. (c)

22. (3) In crutch walking the patient uses the triceps, trapezius, and latissimus muscles. A patient who has been in bed may need to implement an exercise program to strengthen these shoulder and upper arm muscles before initiating crutch walking. (a)

23. (3) When ambulating a patient, the nurse walks on the patient's stronger or unaffected side. This provides a wide base of support and therefore increases stability during the phase of ambulation that calls for weight-bearing on the affected side as the unaffected limb moves forward. (c)

24. (4) An extended care facility would best meet the patient's convalescent needs, since a wide range of services beyond acute care are provided at a lower cost than hospital care. Its health services are more appropriate for this patient because they are greater than those provided in an adult facility but less than those provided in a nursing home. (a)

25. (3) Preoperative skin preparation includes washing the operative site with an antiseptic agent several times to reduce the number of microorganisms on the skin. (c)

26. (3) Women facing breast surgery often have many feelings relating to their sexuality, change in body image, etc. The nurse plays a vital role in helping the patient to verbalize feelings. (a)

27. (4) Postoperatively the arm on the operated side is elevated on pillows with the hand higher than the arm to prevent muscle strain and edema. (b)

28. (1) Postmastectomy exercises should be bilateral, using both arms simultaneously to prevent shortening of muscles and contracture of joints. (b)

29. (1) Chemotherapeutic agents are not specific for malignant cells; they generally interfere with protein synthesis and cell division in all rapidly dividing cells, including those regenerating traumatized tissue (as in wound healing), bone marrow, and cutaneous and alimentary tract epithelial tissue. (b)

30. (2) When there is increased pressure within the cranial cavity, the body adapts by increasing the blood pressure and decreasing the pulse. (c)

31. (4) Rotating tourniquets are used to decrease venous return to the heart and have no value in the treatment of increased intracranial pressure. (b)

32. (3) If there is no obstruction, pressure on the jugular vein causes increased intracranial pressure, and this in turn causes an increased spinal fluid pressure. (b)

33. (2) The cerebellum is involved in the synergistic control of muscle action. Below the level of consciousness it functions to produce smooth, steady, coordinated, and efficient movements. (b)

34. (3) Consent must be obtained before a patient's head may be shaved because of cosmetic concerns. (b)

35. (3) Yellow drainage may be CSF and should be reported immediately. (a)

36. (2) Near term, most mothers are tired of the pregnant state and anxious for labor to begin. It is helpful to know that this is a common reaction. (c)

37. (2) Preparation for parenthood classes should help couples have realistic expectations of the laboring process, including associated discomfort and ways of dealing with it. (b)

38. (3) Tension of the patient is related to expectation and perception of pain, which is based on cultural norms and past experience. (a)

39. (2) It is important to listen to the FHR during contraction even though it may be difficult to hear. If the FHR slows during contraction and then resumes the normal rate within 30 seconds after acme, it is not serious. (c)

40. (1) In the advanced stage of labor the presenting part is low in the birth canal and may cause strong sensations of pressure on the rectum. (c)

41. (3) Immediate action to prevent excessive bleeding is to massage the fundus until it is firm, since this stimulates muscle contraction. (b)

42. (1) The tremendous visual impact of cleft lip on parents may significantly affect the parent-child attachment process and is often considered a reason for early surgical intervention. (c)

43. (4) An almost universal reaction to birth of an imperfect child is guilt. Encouraging the parents to discuss such feelings, without actually asking if they feel guilty, allows them an opportunity to express such thoughts. (b)

44. (1) Cleft lip and palate demonstrate a familial pattern of inheritance that is significantly increased when a close relative is similarly affected. However, neither condition follows mendelian laws of inheritance. (b)

45. (1) Because infants with cleft lip and palate are unable to form the vacuum needed for sucking, they are fed with a rubber-tipped syringe or dropper, which allows formula to flow along the side and back of the mouth, minimizing the danger of aspiration. (a)

46. (3) Infants with cleft lip breathe through their mouth, bypassing the natural humidification provided by the nose. As a result, the mucus membranes become dry, cracked, and are easily infected. (b)

47. (4) Although thrombophlebitis is suspected, prior to a definitive diagnosis the patient should be confined to bed to prevent further complications. (a)

48. (2) Following cleft lip repair, children are always placed supine or slightly on their side to prevent damage to the suture line. (b)

49. (1) Due to excess secretions of glucocorticoids, patients with Cushing's syndrome will develop hyperglycemia and resultant polyuria. (c)

50. (1) Excess adrenocorticoids cause hyperglycemia, hypertension, acne, weight gain, hirsutism, buffalo hump, moon face, and emotional lability due to fluid and electrolyte changes. (c)

51. (2) Steroid therapy is usually instituted preoperatively to prepare for the acute adrenal insufficiency following surgery. (b)

52. (4) Because of the instability of the vascular system and the lability of circulating adrenal hormones following adrenalectomy, hypotension frequently occurs until the hormonal level is controlled by replacement therapy. (c)

53. (3) Administration of adrenocortical hormones causes sodium retention by the kidneys; dietary intake of salt must therefore be limited. (b)

54. (3) Patients with adrenocortical insufficiency who are receiving steroid therapy usually require increased amounts of medication during periods of stress, since they are unable to produce the excess needed by the body. (c)

55. (4) The 2-year-old child is extremely fearful of separation as well as intrusive procedures. If parents are present, they should be encouraged to stay and give comfort. (b)

56. (3) If able to handle personal anxiety and give comfort to the child, parents can be a real help to the staff as well as the child. If the parents are extremely anxious, their anxiety can be transmitted, making the child even more anxious. (b)

57. (3) Infants and small children have small buttocks with a very proximal sciatic nerve. (b)

58. (4) It is difficult to apply adequate pressure to this vascular site, so observation for early signs of bleeding is imperative. (b)

59. (1) Patients with Cushing's syndrome or those who are receiving cortical hormones must limit their intake of salt and increase their potassium intake because the kidneys are retaining sodium and excreting potassium. (b)

60. (2) Excess glucocorticoids cause hyperglycemia, and signs of diabetes mellitus may develop. (c)

61. (4) Warm water will often relax the urinary sphincter, enabling a patient to void. (b)

62. (4) A suprapubic prostatectomy involves an abdominal incision to gain access to the prostate through the bladder. Postoperatively the patient has a suprapubic cystotomy tube to drain urine, as well as a Foley catheter. (b)

63. (1) Because of the vascularity of the involved tissue, hemorrhage and shock constitute the immediate postoperative danger after a prostatectomy. (a)

64. (3) Pulling on the urethral catheter after a prostatectomy may cause bleeding, which could block the tubing and lead to urine retention. Adequate drainage of the bladder must be ensured, since a distended bladder can lead to hemorrhage and shock. (a)

65. (4) After a suprapubic prostatectomy there is generally leakage of urine around the suprapubic tube, creating an environment in which bacteria can flourish if the dressing is not changed frequently. (b)

66. (3) Pain after a suprapubic prostatectomy may denote retention of urine as a result of blocked drainage tubes or infection as well as a normal response to surgery. The possibility of any complication must first be investigated. (a)

67. (3) Straining applies pressure to the operative site. (c)

68. (3) Superego development reflects the internalized norms of the family and society; the sociopath has never achieved this internalization. (b)

69. (1) A sincere, cautious, and consistent attitude limits the sociopath's ability to manipulate both situations and staff members. (b)

70. (4) Sets realistic limits on behavior without rejecting the patient. (b)

71. (4) Helps the patient focus on feelings rather than just pointing out that current behavior is unacceptable. (b)

72. (1) Accepts the patient while rejecting and setting limits on the behavior the patient is using. (b)

73. (2) Sets limits, points out reality, and places responsibility for behavior on the patient. (b)

74. (2) Demonstrates patient's acceptance of the professional role of the nurse as well as the ability to end dependent relationships. (b)

75. (2) Intermittent positive pressure breathing is used to provide full expansion of the lungs, to loosen secretions, and to administer medication. (a)

76. (3) As a result of increased pressure in the pulmonary circulation, the right side of the heart hypertrophies. This is called cor pulmonale and may lead to congestive heart failure. (b)

77. (4) Productive coughing can cause nausea and vomiting induced by IPPB treatment. (b)

78. (2) The fluid level and time must be marked to evaluate the amount of drainage in a closed drainage system (such as with chest tubes). (a)

79. (3) Atmospheric pressure is greater than the pressure inside the pleural space. If a chest tube were not attached to underwater seal drainage, air would enter the pleural space and collapse the lung (pneumothorax). (b)

80. (1) Turning and positioning prevent pooling of secretions in lungs and maximize lung expansion. Cupping and clapping, as well as postural drainage, are dependent nursing functions. (c)

81. (2) There are several modes for the administration of oxygen. Selection is based on the disease and the patient's adaptations. (b)

82. (2) Oxygen can dry the mucous membranes of the respiratory tract and must be humidified for administration; drying of mucous membranes can predispose to infection. (a)
83. (2) Any arrhythmia should be documented by an ECG strip. Frequent PVCs indicate ventricular irritability, which may progress to ventricular fibrillation requiring emergency precordial shock. (c)
84. (4) The T wave is the period of repolarization of the ventricles; stimulation of the ventricles during this vulnerable period often causes ventricular fibrillation. (c)
85. (1) A defibrillator delivers a massive electric charge to the myocardium simultaneously depolarizing and then throwing into refractory all heart regions; rhythmic contractions due to SA node depolarization may then restore normal heart action. The defibrillating current reaches the heart from the body surface through the electric conductivity of the body fluids containing many ions. (b)
86. (1) Levarterenol bitartrate (Levophed) acts on alpha receptors, causing vasoconstriction of superficial and splanchnic arterioles and leading to the desired response of a rise in blood pressure. (c)
87. (2) Because of potential hypertension from arteriole constriction, administration of levarterenol must be monitored carefully. The flow rate must be exact, and a second clamp or infusion control device should be used as a safeguard to prevent inaccurate infusion rates. (b)
88. (2) Knowing that nausea and vomiting are possible signs of digitalis toxicity, the nurse should withhold the drug and call the physician. (c)
89. (2) After a myocardial infarction it generally takes 6 to 8 weeks for replacement of necrotic tissue by scar tissue. (c)
90. (2) Procainamide is rapidly absorbed from the GI tract and excreted in the urine. It must be taken at prescribed intervals to maintain a therapeutic blood level. (b)
91. (2) Fetal death usually occurs in diabetic mothers after 36 weeks gestation due to acidosis and placental dysfunction. The fetus may be delivered by cesarean section or induction as necessary. (c)
92. (1) Usually, as pregnancy progresses, there are alterations in glucose tolerance and insulin metabolism and utilization resulting in an increased need for exogenous insulin. (a)
93. (3) Although the effects of insulin on the fetus are known, since the fetal pancreas secretes insulin, the effects of oral hypoglycemics are not well known and such agents may be teratogenic. (b)
94. (4) Feeding difficulties are due to hypoglycemic effects on the fetal CNS. (c)
95. (4) The infant of a diabetic mother is a newborn at risk because of the interplay between the maternal disease and the developing fetus. (b)
96. (2) When the intestine cannot be returned to the body cavity, the hernia is incarcerated. (c)
97. (3) A possible complication of hernias is intestinal obstruction. If an obstruction occurs, there will be no passage of flatus or normal bowel movements. (b)
98. (4) Hernioplasty involves not only the reduction of a hernia but also an attempt to change or strengthen the structure to prevent future occurrence. (b)
99. (1) After inguinal hernia repair, the scrotum frequently becomes edematous and painful. Drainage is facilitated by elevating the scrotum on a rolled towel or using a scrotal support. (c)
100. (3) Placing the feet apart creates a wider base of support and brings the center of gravity closer to the ground. This improves stability. (b)
101. (1) Response demonstrates an understanding of the patient's feelings and encourages the patient to share feelings, which is an immediate need at this time. (b)
102. (4) You cannot argue a patient out of a delusion. Statements made by the nurse show a lack of knowledge and really constitute a threat, which is a form of assault. (c)
103. (2) Response recognizes patient's feelings and provides the patient with the assurance that the staff member will stay with him. (a)
104. (3) Delusions are protective and can only be abandoned when the individual feels secure and adequate. This response is the only one directed at building the patient's security and reducing anxiety. (b)
105. (2) Patients losing control feel frightened and threatened. They need external controls and a reduction in external stimuli. (b)
106. (4) Jaundice signifies liver cell damage, a side effect of the phenothiazine drugs, which can be irreversible and life threatening. The nurse should immediately stop the medication if this side effect is noted. (b)
107. (2) This response supports reality and self-awareness while helping the patient to look to the future rather than focusing on the past. (c)
108. (2) The phenothiazine drugs cause photosensitivity, and severe burning can occur on exposure to the sun. (b)
109. (3) Patients with internal radiation for cervical cancer are placed on low-residue diets and are often given medications to suppress peristalsis to prevent pressure from bowel movements. (c)
110. (2) A total abdominal hysterectomy in the premenopausal woman produces artificial onset of menopause. (a)
111. (3) Accidental ligation of a ureter is a serious complication of a total abdominal hysterectomy. A decrease in urine output should be reported immediately to the surgeon. (c)
112. (3) Abdominal distention, caused by retention of flatus, is a frequent postoperative problem. A rectal tube will usually accomplish expulsion of flatus in 20 to 30 minutes. Application of heat, in addition to its vasodilating effect, will relax tensed muscles. (b)
113. (4) Postoperatively a patient may wear a girdle to provide

support and/or do exercises to strengthen the abdominal muscles. (a)

114. (1) Patients use delusions as a defense and cannot be argued out of them. The nurse's response did not demonstrate acceptance of the patient and only added to her anxiety and agitation. (b)

115. (3) Electroconvulsive therapy helps relieve severe depression by interrupting established patterns of behavior, thereby limiting possible suicide attempts. (a)

116. (3) Feelings of hopelessness, helplessness, and of isolation dominate the emotional state of the depressed patient; the ability to attempt to act out suicide ideation frequently does not occur until psychomotor depression begins to lift. (a)

117. (4) Patients who are preoccupied are usually not aware of events in the environment. The patient has not refused to eat but has simply not responded to external stimuli. Taking her by the hand to the dining hall simply puts her where she needs to be. (c)

118. (1) Spending time with patients communicates to them that the staff members feel they are worthy of their attention and that someone cares. (b)

119. (2) Although MAO inhibitors are not stimulants but antidepressants, they can cause an increase in psychomotor activity and appetite as the depression lifts. (c)

120. (4) Wine and cheese, which contain the amino acid tyramine, are contraindicated when taking MAO inhibitors, since they can react with the drug to cause a severe hypertensive crisis. (c)

COMPREHENSIVE TEST 4

1. (2) A low-residue diet limits stool formation. (a)

2. (3) Sitz baths provide moist heat, which dilates blood vessels and promotes circulation. It also relieves local inflammation and itching. (b)

3. (1) Moist cotton is the most soothing to the anal mucosa. Since the rectum is a contaminated area, pads do not have to be sterile. (b)

4. (3) The carotid pulse, because of its proximity to the heart, is used to determine whether the ventricles are contracting effectively. The absence of a carotid pulse, in the absence of other vascular problems, indicates ventricular fibrillation or standstill, and immediate cardiopulmonary resuscitation is required to prevent death. (a)

5. (3) CPR carried out by one person is less efficient than that performed by 2. Approximately 80 compressions per minute are needed to provide adequate tissue perfusion. (b)

6. (2) This position provides the best leverage to depress the sternum so that the heart is adequately compressed, forcing blood into the arteries. Grasping the fingers keeps them off the chest and concentrates the energy expended into the heel of the hand while minimizing the possibility of fractured ribs. (a)

7. (1) Hair and oils in the skin may interfere with conduction of electric impulses; therefore the chest hair immediately around the site may need to be shaved and the area must be scrubbed to remove oils and debris. (c)

8. (3) The first intervention when ventricular fibrillation is verified is defibrillation, since it is the only measure that will terminate this lethal arrhythmia. (b)

9. (3) In the absence of O_2 the body will supply energy anaerobically, causing a buildup of lactic acid. Sodium bicarbonate, an alkaline drug, will help neutralize this acid, raising the pH of the body back to normal. (a)

10. (2) An oral contraceptive program requires taking 1 tablet daily from the fifth day of the cycle and continuing for 20 or 21 days. Interrupting the monthly dosage program may permit release of LH, then ovulation, and possible pregnancy. (b)

11. (3) Knowing that others share the same problems may be comforting. The second part of the nurse's statement is open ended and allows the patient to describe her physical and emotional feelings. (a)

12. (4) Before health teaching is instituted, the nurse should ascertain the patient's past experiences, since they will influence the teaching plan. (b)

13. (3) In calculating the expected date of delivery, subtract 3 months and add 7 days to the date of the last menstrual period. (b)

14. (2) Successful dietary teaching usually incorporates, as much as possible, the patient's food preferences and dietary patterns. (c)

15. (4) Maintaining the sitting position for prolonged periods may constrict the vessels of the legs, particularly in the popliteal spaces, as well as diminish venous return. Walking contracts the muscles of the legs, which apply gentle pressure to veins in the legs promoting venous return. (b)

16. (4) When the membranes rupture, the potential for infection is increased; when the contractions are 5 to 8 minutes apart they are usually of sufficient force to warrant medical supervision; therefore, for the safety of the mother and fetus, the mother should go to the hospital. (b)

17. (3) The fetal heart rate is usually between 120 and 160

beats per minute. This is a normal expectation, and the mother should be made aware of this fact. (a)

18. (2) Lets him know that the nurse understands adjustments will have to be made and is open ended enough to let him talk about feelings. (b)

19. (2) The sensitive and dependent individual who has a conflict accepting the need for dependence frequently develops ulcerative colitis; the exact neural mechanism resulting in colonic inflammation is unknown. (c)

20. (4) Since the mucosa of the intestinal tract is damaged, its ability to absorb vitamins taken orally is greatly impaired. (a)

21. (1) $\dfrac{\text{Amount to be infused} \times \text{Drop factor}}{\text{Amount of time in minutes}}$ (b)

22. (1) This grouping of foods does not contain high-residue fruits, vegetables, or whole grains, which are irritating to the intestinal mucosa, cause bulk, and increase peristalsis. (c)

23. (2) The key in treatment of this disease is to prevent spastic intestinal activity. (a)

24. (4) The affected areas of the intestines are in need of repair; protein is required in the building and repairing of tissues. (a)

25. (1) Since her diabetes appears out of control, dietary indiscretions or changes should be ruled out first. (b)

26. (2) Taking a pill may give the patient a false sense that the disease is under control, and this could lead to dietary indiscretion. (b)

27. (4) An understanding of the diet is imperative for compliance. A balance of carbohydrates, proteins, and fats usually apportioned over 3 main meals and 2 between-meal snacks needs to be tailored to the patient's specific needs, keeping in mind activity, diet, and insulin therapy. (b)

28. (4) Past experiences are the most meaningful influence on present learning. (b)

29. (2) Nonjudgmentally identifying the patient's feelings encourages further verbalization about her feelings and the diet. (a)

30. (2) Fasting prior to the test is indicated for accurate and reliable results, since food will elevate the blood glucose levels due to metabolism of the nutrients. (b)

31. (2) Cough syrup contains a sugar base, which must be taken into account by diabetic patients. (b)

32. (4) In diabetes mellitus the progressive thickening of capillary basement membranes and medial sclerosis of small arteries leading to the eyes gradually occlude the vessel lumina. This significantly reduces retinal perfusion and leads to blindness. (b)

33. (3) Damage to Broca's area, located in the posterior frontal region of the dominant hemisphere, causes problems in the motor aspect of speech. (a)

34. (4) Giving the patient adequate time to respond and employing a calm, accepting, deliberate, and interested

manner will reduce the patient's anxiety and tension as well as increase her self-esteem. (a)

35. (1) Assuming a normal position for voiding reduces tension (physical and psychologic), facilitates the movement of urine into the lower main portion of the bladder, and relaxes the external sphincter, increasing pressure and initiating the micturition reflex. (c)

36. (2) Ambulation causes a change in the position of the center of gravity, which can upset balance. Using a cane provides a wider base of support and therefore greater stability. (a)

37. (3) The body is supported partially on the affected limb and partially on the cane as the unaffected limb moves forward. (b)

38. (4) Orienting the patient to the hospital provides knowledge that might reduce the strangeness of the environment, whereas introducing staff members lets the patient know who will be caring for her as well as providing a personal touch. (b)

39. (4) Atherosclerosis begins with the accumulation of fatty deposits (plaques) within the inner lining (intima) of the arteries, leading to a narrowing of the lumen. Later on the plaques enlarge, cause greater occlusion, and harden by deposition of calcium; the narrowing and hardening increase the work of the heart. (b)

40. (1) Each person is a unique individual and the nurse should avoid making the patient feel dehumanized. (b)

41. (4) Identifying and accepting feelings helps to open lines of communication with the patient. (b)

42. (1) Nitroglycerine is sensitive to light and moisture and must be stored in a dark air-tight container. (b)

43. (1) Alzheimer's disease is insidious and causes irreversible brain changes. The individual maintains the ability to make socially correct comments, but the intellect diminishes. (c)

44. (2) Since these patients do experience a lability of mood, it is best to attempt to establish a relationship and give care when they are in a receptive mood. (c)

45. (4) Sameness provides security and safety and reduces stress for the patient. (b)

46. (4) A consistent approach and consistent communication from all members of the health team help the patient with a chronic brain syndrome remain a bit more reality oriented. (b)

47. (3) Patients with long-term psychiatric problems who have limited contact with reality can usually still become involved with a remotivation therapy group, since the demands of this type of group are limited and self-confining. (c)

48. (3) Remotivation therapy is designed to encourage patients to interact with their environment by focusing their attention on some common routine "emotionally safe" article that most patients can recognize and talk about. (b)

49. (2) Vitamin K stores are almost absent in the newborn

because the intestinal flora that produce this vitamin are not present. Vitamin K is an essential precursor of prothrombin, which supports the clotting mechanism. (b)

50. (2) Drug dependence in the neonate is physiologic. As the drug is cleared from the body, symptoms of drug withdrawal become evident. Tremors, irritability, difficulty sleeping, twitching, and convulsions may result. (b)

51. (3) Drug-dependent neonates are poor feeders because of hyperactivity, nausea, vomiting, respiratory distress, excessive mucus, and pyrexia. Small frequent feedings should be given to prevent dehydration. (c)

52. (3) The nurse should attempt to support the mother-child relationship. The mother is experiencing a developmental crisis while having to deal with drug addiction and possibly guilt. (a)

53. (4) The immediate postburn period is marked by dramatic alterations in circulation due to large fluid losses through the denuded skin, vasodilation, edema formation, and a direct response on the contractility of the heart muscle. The precipitous drop in cardiac output causes shock. (a)

54. (3) Body weight is used in the calculation of body surface area, the main criterion used in determining drug dosage and fluid requirements. (b)

55. (3) High fever and disorientation may be initial indications of infection and/or an early sign of hypoxia from respiratory complications. (c)

56. (2) The minimum urine volume is 10 to 20 ml per hour in children under 2 years and 20 to 30 ml per hour in children over 2 years of age. (b)

57. (4) Children act out their feelings via play, since their verbal ability is limited. (a)

58. (2) By having the patient lie on the affected side, the unaffected lung can expand to its fullest potential. Elevation of the head facilitates respirations by reducing the pressure of the abdominal organs on the diaphragm and allowing the diaphragm to descend with gravity. (c)

59. (1) The rate and characteristics of respirations should be assessed to determine the amount of exertion required for breathing. The nurse should also evaluate signs such as unilateral chest movements, which may indicate pneumothorax and tachypnea, which are associated with hypercapnea and acidosis. (b)

60. (4) Maintains negative intrathoracic pressure by limiting amount of air rushing in from outside, which can result in total pneumothorax and mediastinal shift, severely embarrassing respirations. (b)

61. (4) $\dfrac{\text{Total amount to be infused} \times \text{Drop factor}}{\text{Total time for infusion in minutes}}$ (b)

62. (1) Deep breathing maximizes gaseous exchange, ridding the body of excess CO_2. Retention of CO_2 in the blood lowers the pH, causing respiratory acidosis. (b)

63. (2) Leakage of air into the subcutaneous tissue is evi-

denced by a crackling sound when the area is gently palpated. This is referred to as crepitus. (c)

64. (2) Many analgesics administered for postoperative pain act by depressing the CNS; an assessment of vital signs is necessary to determine if any contraindications to analgesic administration exist, such as hypotension or a respiratory rate of 12 or less. (c)

65. (1) Talking in the third person reflects poor ego boundaries and a dissociation from the real self. (a)

66. (2) The patient needs sensory stimulation to maintain orientation and should be encouraged to do as much as possible for self, depending on ability. (c)

67. (4) When patient's perceptions are especially frightening, the nurse must let the patient know that her fears are recognized as real and frightening to her even if the nurse does not share her perceptions. Staying with the patient will convey concern as well as reduce her fears. (b)

68. (3) This response points out reality while attempting to let the patient understand that the nurse sees her as a person of worth. (c)

69. (2) Major tranquilizers tend to make the patient listless or drowsy and can interfere with the patient's ability to participate in the therapeutic regimen. (b)

70. (1) Liver damage is a well-documented toxic side effect of the major tranquilizers. By continuing to administer the drug, the nurse failed to use her professional knowledge in the performance of her responsibilities as outlined in the Nurse Practice Act. (b)

71. (4) The delusional patient can never be argued out of a delusion, since they serve as a defense against reality and are the patient's reality. It is best to simply accept the delusion without discussion. (c)

72. (1) When an individual expresses interest in physical appearance, it demonstrates a rebuilding of the self image, feelings of worth, and concerns for how others see them. (a)

73. (1) One of the characteristic differences between juvenile and adult diabetes is the disease's rapid onset in children. Diabetes is often first diagnosed during acute ketoacidosis. (a)

74. (3) Helping families understand their feelings about juvenile diabetes is essential in assisting them in developing positive attitudes for optimal control of the disease and promotion of a normal life for the child. (a)

75. (2) Equation no. 1

$$40 \text{ units} : 1 \text{ ml} = 12 \text{ units} : x$$
$$40x = 12$$
$$x = 0.3 \text{ ml}$$

Equation no. 2

$$1 \text{ ml} = 15 \text{ minims}$$
$$0.3 \text{ ml} \times 15 \text{ minims/ml} = 4.5 \text{ minims} \quad \text{(b)}$$

76. (2) A bedtime snack is needed for the evening. NPH in-

sulin peaks in 10 to 20 hours and lasts for 28 to 30 hours. Carbohydrate ingestion prior to sleep prevents hypoglycemia during the night, when the action of NPH insulin will be at its highest. (a)

77. (4) Exercise reduces the body's need for insulin because increased muscle activity accelerates the transport of glucose into the muscle cells, thus producing an insulin-like effect. (b)

78. (3) The sitting position allows the diaphragm to lower by gravity, allowing for greater lung expansion. (b)

79. (4) Emphysema involves destructive changes in the alveolar walls, leading to dilation of the air sacs with subsequent air trapping and difficulty with expiration. (a)

80. (1) Epinephrine acts on both alpha and beta receptors; however, it is the stimulation of the beta receptors that causes bronchial relaxation and increased heart rate and contractility. (c)

81. (1) Patients with COPD must be given only low concentrations of oxygen because a decreased O_2 blood level is their only stimulus for breathing. (b)

82. (3) Isoproterenol (Isuprel) is a catecholamine that acts on the beta receptors, leading to increased heart rate and contractility, as well as dilation of the arteries of the skeletal muscles. (b)

83. (2) Isoproterenol is a potent bronchodilator used in the treatment of asthmatic attacks. Indiscriminant use leads to heart palpitations, nausea, tremors, and precordial pain. (c)

84. (1) In addition to the desired effect of bronchodilation, isoproterenol inhalation can lead to tachycardia and palpitations, so use of the drug should be limited to periods of dyspnea. (b)

85. (4) Aminophylline, a theophylline derivative, causes relaxation of the smooth muscle of the bronchi, interrupting spasms and constriction. (b)

86. (3) After the needs to survive (air, food, water) the need for comfort and freedom from pain closely follow. Care should be given in order of patient needs. (b)

87. (2) The anti-inflammatory action of acetylsalicylic acid (A.S.A.) is effective in reducing the discomfort and pain associated with rheumatoid arthritis. (b)

88. (4) Maintenance fo joint extension offsets the deformity of joints often seen in rheumatoid arthritis and frequently prevents potentially deforming contractures. (b)

89. (1) Incontinence without a physiologic basis is an act of hostility that the individual uses to deal with anxiety-producing situations. (a)

90. (2) For psychologic equilibrium Mrs. Ryan's environment must be one of novel and changing stimuli, promoting physical activity and effective interaction with others. (b)

91. (1) Since air-conduction hearing aids utilize the person's own middle ear, they increase hearing sensitivity in cases of diminished sensitivity of the cochlea; the amplified signal from the hearing aid gives the cochlea greater stimulation and promotes hearing. (b)

92. (4) IV fluids are necessary, since severe dehydration and fluid and electrolyte imbalance occur rapidly and can lead to death in infancy because of the infant's large fluid content. (b)

93. (2) Loss of fluid as a result of dehydration is most objectively assessed by measuring the child's weight, since total body water accounts for approximately 60% of body weight. (c)

94. (1) Sodium, potassium, and bicarbonate are the electrolytes most often lost due to diarrhea, since they are excreted before they can be absorbed. (b)

95. (3) $\dfrac{\text{Total amount} \times \text{Drop factor}}{\text{Total time in minutes}}$ (a)

96. (2) Clear liquids with sugar added provide glucose without bulk. Fruit juices may cause fermentation, which can stimulate peristalsis, and ginger ale adds a great deal of unnecessary carbonation. (c)

97. (2) Weight is the best measurement of fluid loss if measured each day at the same time, on the same scale, and with the same amount of clothes. (b)

98. (3) By 12 months of age a child can usually drink from a cup, although fluid may spill and a bottle may be preferred at times. (c)

99. (1) An interference in the flow of bile into the intestine will result in increasing inability to tolerate fatty foods. The unemulsified fat remains in the intestine for prolonged periods, resulting in inhibition of stomach emptying and possible formation of gas. (a)

100. (2) Vitamin K is necessary to form prothrombin to prevent bleeding. Vitamin K, a fat-soluble vitamin, is not absorbed from the GI tract in the absence of bile. (a)

101. (2) A nasogastric tube attached to suction removes gastric secretions and prevents vomiting. However, if it becomes clogged, secretions may accumulate leading to distention, nausea, and vomiting. (b)

102. (3) Bleeding disorders are common when bile does not flow through the intestines; vitamin K is a fat-soluble vitamin requiring bile salts for absorption. Vitamin K is required for the liver's synthesis of prothrombin. (a)

103. (1) An incision close to the diaphragm (as in surgery of the biliary tract) causes a great deal of pain when the patient coughs and deep breathes. These patients tend to take shallow breaths, which leads to inadequate expansion of the lungs, the accumulation of secretions, and infection. (a)

104. (3) A full fluid diet ordered by the physician following a cholecystectomy should be verified by the nurse, since there are different schools of thought concerning the use of creamed fluids. Providing a correct diet is the shared responsibility of the physician and nurse. (b)

105. (4) Although the gallbladder has been removed, the liver

will continue to produce and secrete the bile necessary for the emulsification of fatty foods. Once any inflammation affecting the common bile duct subsides, the bile will flow into the duodenum, but not in concentrated form. (a)

106. (2) In an attempt to ward off anxiety, the manic patient runs headlong into it, becoming totally involved in everything that goes on in the environment. (b)

107. (2) Overactive individuals are stimulated by environmental factors. A responsibility of the nurse is to simplify their surroundings as much as possible. (c)

108. (3) Patients in the manic phase of manic-depressive psychosis are easily distracted. Rather than placing emphasis on their behavior, staff members should use their easy distractability to redirect the patient's behavior to more constructive channels. (a)

109. (2) This approach incorporates the principles of starting where the patient is and helping the patient verbalize feelings. It also provides for more data collection to carry out the nursing process. (b)

110. (4) Because of the severity of side effects and the stress it places on the renal as well as cardiovascular system, its administration is contraindicated in patients with renal or cardiovascular diseases. (b)

111. (4) Albumin in the urine is a sign of toxemia, as are an elevated blood pressure and a weight gain of more than 2 lb per week. (c)

112. (1) Weight gain due to fluid retention is the earliest objective sign of mild preeclampsia. (c)

113. (1) The latest concept concerning preeclampsia or eclampsia is that this condition is a consequence of salt loss during pregnancy and poor protein intake. The recommendations therefore call for a diet containing normal sodium, high protein, and sufficient number of calories. (c)

114. (1) The cumulative effects of magensium sulfate include depressed respirations and an absent or weak knee-jerk reflex. (b)

115. (2) Magnesium sulfate given by deep IM injection is very painful. One percent procaine may be mixed with the drug with a physician's order or established hospital protocol. (c)

116. (4) In severe preeclampsia fluid is drawn from plasma into the tissue and the blood becomes more concentrated. This is reflected in the elevated hematocrit level. (b)

117. (4) The patient's exact compliance in carrying out the compulsive ritual relieves anxiety, at least temporarily, so it does meet a need and is necessary to the patient. (a)

118. (3) The neurotic personality is characterized by anxiety and minor distortions of reality; the anxiety results in an inability to reach a decision, since all alternatives are threatening. (a)

119. (4) Rituals are an individual's means for controlling anxiety. If not permitted to carry out the ritual, the patient will probably experience unbearable anxiety. (c)

120. (2) Since the compulsive ritual is used to control anxiety, any attempt to prevent the action would greatly increase the anxiety. (c)

BIBLIOGRAPHY

MEDICAL-SURGICAL NURSING

Andreoli, K. G.: Comprehensive cardiac care: a text for nurses, physicians, and other health practitioners, ed. 4, St. Louis, 1979, The C. V. Mosby Co.

Anthony, C. P., and Thibodeau, G. A.: Textbook of anatomy and physiology, ed. 10, St. Louis, 1979, The C. V. Mosby Co.

Barber, J. M., et al.: Adult and child care: a client approach to nursing, ed. 2, St. Louis, 1977, The C. V. Mosby Co.

Barrett-Connor, E., et al.: Epidemiology for the infection control nurse, St. Louis, 1978, The C. V. Mosby Co.

Bates, B.: A guide to physical examination, ed. 2, Philadelphia, 1979, J. B. Lippincott Co.

Beland, I. L., and Passos, J. Y.: Clinical nursing, ed. 3, New York, 1975, Macmillan, Inc.

Bergersen, B. S.: Pharmacology in nursing, ed. 14, St. Louis, 1979, The C. V. Mosby Co.

Brooks, S. H.: Fundamentals of operating room nursing, ed. 2, St. Louis, 1979, The C. V. Mosby Co.

Brundage, D. J.: Nursing management of renal problems, ed. 2, St. Louis, 1980, The C. V. Mosby Co.

Brunner, L. S., et al.: Textbook of medical-surgical nursing, ed. 4, Philadelphia, 1980, J. B. Lippincott Co.

Burrell, Z. L., and Burrell, L. O.: Critical care, ed. 3, St. Louis, 1977, The C. V. Mosby Co.

Byrne, J., et al.: Laboratory tests: implications for nurses and allied health professionals, Menlo Park, Calif., 1981, Addison-Wesley Publishing Co., Inc.

Conover, M. B.: Understanding electrocardiography: physiological and interpretive concepts, ed. 3, St. Louis, 1980, The C. V. Mosby Co.

Conway, B. L.: Carini and Owens' neurological and neurosurgical nursing, ed. 7, St. Louis, 1978, The C. V. Mosby Co.

Dison, N.: Clinical nursing techniques, ed. 4, St. Louis, 1979, The C. V. Mosby Co.

Ellis, P. D., and Billings, D. M.: Cardiopulmonary resuscitation: procedures for basic and advanced life support, St. Louis, 1980, The C. V. Mosby Co.

Fardy, P. S., et al.: Cardiac rehabilitation: implications for the nurse and other allied health professionals, St. Louis, 1980, The C. V. Mosby Co.

Garfield, C. A.: Stress and survival: the emotional realities of life-threatening illness, St. Louis, 1980, The C. V. Mosby Co.

Gröer, M. E., and Shekleton, M. E.: Basic pathophysiology: a conceptual approach, St. Louis, 1979, The C. V. Mosby Co.

Gruendemann, B. J., et al.: The surgical patient: behavioral concepts for the operating room nurse, ed. 2, St. Louis, 1977, The C. V. Mosby Co.

Hilt, N. E., and Cogburn, S. B.: Manual of orthopedics, St. Louis, 1979, The C. V. Mosby Co.

Holloway, N. M.: Nursing the critically ill adult, Menlo Park, Calif., 1979, Addison-Wesley Publishing Co., Inc.

Johanson, B. C., et al.: Standards for critical care, St. Louis, 1981, The C. V. Mosby Co.

Jones, D. A.: Medical-surgical nursing: a conceptual approach, New York, 1978, McGraw-Hill Book Co., Inc.

Kozier, B. B., and Erb, G. L.: Fundamentals of nursing: concepts and procedures, Menlo Park, Calif., 1979, Addison-Wesley Publishing Co., Inc.

Luckmann, J., and Sorensen, K. C.: Medical surgical nursing: a psychophysiologic approach, ed. 2, Philadelphia, 1980, W. B. Saunders Co.

Malasanos, L., et al.: Health assessment, ed. 2, St. Louis, 1981, The C. V. Mosby Co.

Marriner, A.: The nursing process: a scientific approach to nursing care, ed. 2, St. Louis, 1979, The C. V. Mosby Co.

Phipps, W. J., et al.: Medical-surgical nursing: concepts and clinical practice, St. Louis, 1979, The C. V. Mosby Co.

Phipps, W. J., et al.: Shafer's medical-surgical nursing, ed. 7, St. Louis, 1980, The C. V. Mosby Co.

Rhodes, M. J., et al.: Alexander's care of the patient in surgery, ed. 6, St. Louis, 1978, The C. V. Mosby Co.

Saxton, D. F., Ercolano, N. H., and Walter, J. F.: Programmed instruction in arithmetic, dosages, and solutions, ed. 4, St. Louis, 1977, The C. V. Mosby Co.

Saxton, D. F., and Hyland, P. A.: Planning and implementing

nursing intervention: stress and adaptation applied to patient care, ed. 2, St. Louis, 1979, The C. V. Mosby Co.

Sundeen, S. J., et al.: Nurse-client interaction: implementing the nursing process, ed. 2, St. Louis, 1981, The C. V. Mosby Co.

Thompson, J. M., and Bowers, A. C.: Clinical manual of health assessment, St. Louis, 1980, The C. V. Mosby Co.

Tilkian, S. M., Conover, M. B., and Tilkian, A. G.: Clinical implications of laboratory tests, ed. 2, St. Louis, 1979, The C. V. Mosby Co.

Tucker, S. M.: Patient care standards, ed. 2, St. Louis, 1980, The C. V. Mosby Co.

Vinsant, M. O., et al.: Commonsense approach to coronary care, ed. 3, St. Louis, 1980, The C. V. Mosby Co.

Vitale, B. A., Latterner, N. S., and Nugent, P. M.: A problem-solving approach to nursing care plans, ed. 2, St. Louis, 1978, The C. V. Mosby Co.

Wade, J. F.: Respiratory nursing care: physiology and technique, ed. 2, St. Louis, 1977, The C. V. Mosby Co.

Warner, C. G.: Emergency care: assessment and intervention, ed. 2, St. Louis, 1978, The C. V. Mosby Co.

Williams, S. R.: Nutrition and diet therapy, ed. 3, St. Louis, 1977, The C. V. Mosby Co.

Zander, K. S.: Practical manual for patient teaching, St. Louis, 1978, The C. V. Mosby Co.

PSYCHIATRIC NURSING

Aguilera, D. C.: Review of psychiatric nursing, St. Louis, 1977, The C. V. Mosby Co.

Aguilera, D. C., and Messick, J. M.: Crisis intervention: theory and methodology, ed. 3, St. Louis, 1978, The C. V. Mosby Co.

Burgess, A. W., and Lazare, A.: Psychiatric nursing in the hospital and the community, ed. 2, Englewood Cliffs, N.J., 1976, Prentice-Hall, Inc.

Dreyer, S., Bailey, D., and Doucet, W.: Guide to nursing management of psychiatric patients, ed. 2, St. Louis, 1979, The C. V. Mosby Co.

Haber, J., et al.: Comprehensive psychiatric nursing, New York, 1978, McGraw-Hill Book Co., Inc.

Jasmin, S., and Trygstad, L. N.: Behavioral concepts and the nursing process, St. Louis, 1979, The C. V. Mosby Co.

Kyes, J., and Hofling, C. K.: Basic psychiatric concepts in nursing, ed. 4, Philadelphia, 1980, J. B. Lippincott Co.

Lancaster, J.: Community mental health nursing: an ecological perspective, St. Louis, 1980, The C. V. Mosby Co.

Loomis, M. E.: Group process for nurses, St. Louis, 1979, The C. V. Mosby Co.

Marram, G. D.: The group approach in nursing practice, ed. 2, St. Louis, 1978, The C. V. Mosby Co.

Mereness, D. A., and Taylor, C. M.: Essentials of psychiatric nursing, ed. 10, St. Louis, 1978, The C. V. Mosby Co.

Pasquali, E. A., et al.: Mental health nursing: a bio-psycho-cultural approach, St. Louis, 1981, The C. V. Mosby Co.

Pothier, P. C.: Psychiatric nursing: a basic text, Boston, 1980, Little, Brown & Co.

Saxton, D. F., and Haring, P. W.: Care of patients with emotional problems, ed. 3, St. Louis, 1979, The C. V. Mosby Co.

Sedgwick, R.: Family mental health: theory and practice, St. Louis, 1981, The C. V. Mosby Co.

Stuart, G. W., and Sundeen, S. J.: Principles and practice of psychiatric nursing, St. Louis, 1979, The C. V. Mosby Co.

Sundeen, S. J., et al.: Nurse-client interaction, St. Louis, 1976, The C. V. Mosby Co.

Topalis, M., and Aguilera, D. C.: Psychiatric nursing, ed. 7, St. Louis, 1978, The C. V. Mosby Co.

Wilson, H. S., and Kneisl, C. R.: Psychiatric nursing, Menlo Park, Calif., 1979, Addison-Wesley Publishing Co., Inc.

MATERNITY NURSING

Clark, A. L., and Affonso, D.: Childbearing: a nursing perspective, ed. 2, Philadelphia, 1979, F. A. Davis Co.

Clausen, J. P., Flook, M., and Ford, B.: Maternity nursing today, ed. 2, New York, 1977, McGraw-Hill Book Co., Inc.

Ingalls, A. J., and Salerno, M. C.: Maternal and child health nursing, ed. 4, St. Louis, 1979, The C. V. Mosby Co.

Iorio, J.: Family-centered nursing, ed. 3, St. Louis, 1975, The C. V. Mosby Co.

Jensen, M. D., Benson, R. C., and Bobak, I. M.: Maternity care: the nurse and the family, ed. 2, St. Louis, 1981, The C. V. Mosby Co.

Jensen, M. D., and Bobak, I. M.: Handbook of maternity care: a guide for nursing practice, St. Louis, 1980, The C. V. Mosby Co.

Klaus, M. H., and Kennell, J. H.: Maternal-infant bonding: the impact of separation or loss on family development, St. Louis, 1976, The C. V. Mosby Co.

Lerch, C., and Bliss, V. J.: Maternity nursing, ed. 3, St. Louis, 1978, The C. V. Mosby Co.

Lipkin, G. B.: Parent-child nursing: psychosocial aspects, ed. 2, St. Louis, 1978, The C. V. Mosby Co.

McNall, L. K.: Contemporary obstetric and gynecologic nursing, St. Louis, 1980, The C. V. Mosby Co.

Olds, S. B., et al.: Obstetric nursing, Menlo Park, Calif., 1980, Addison-Wesley Publishing Co., Inc.

Phillips, C. R.: Family-centered maternity/newborn care: a basic text, St. Louis, The C. V. Mosby Co.

Phillips, C. R., and Anzalone, J. T.: Fathering: participation in labor and birth, St. Louis, 1978, The C. V. Mosby Co.

Reeder, S. R., Mastroianni, M. L., and Fitzpatrick, E.: Maternity nursing, ed. 14, Philadelphia, 1980, J. B. Lippincott Co.

Tucker, S. M.: Fetal monitoring and fetal assessment in high-risk pregnancy, St. Louis, 1978, The C. V. Mosby Co.

Varney, H.: Nurse midwifery, Boston, 1980, Blackwell Scientific Publishers, Inc.

Wiggins, J. D.: Childbearing: physiology, experiences, needs, St. Louis, 1979, The C. V. Mosby Co.

Woods, N. F.: Human sexuality in health and illness, ed. 2, St. Louis, 1979, The C. V. Mosby Co.

Worthington, B. S., et al.: Nutrition in pregnancy and lactation, ed. 2, St. Louis, 1981, The C. V. Mosby Co.

PEDIATRIC NURSING

Alexander, M., and Brown, M.: Pediatric physical diagnosis for nurses, New York, 1974, McGraw-Hill Book Co., Inc.

Barnard, K. E., and Erickson, M. L.: Teaching children with developmental problems: a family care approach, ed. 2, St. Louis, 1976, The C. V. Mosby Co.

Chinn, P. L.: Child health maintenance: concepts in family-centered care, ed. 2, St. Louis, 1979, The C. V. Mosby Co.

Chinn, P. L., and Leitch, C. J.: Child health maintenance: a guide to clinical assessment, ed. 2, St. Louis, 1979, The C. V. Mosby Co.

Endres, J. B., and Rockwell, R. E.: Food, nutrition, and the young child, St. Louis, 1980, The C. V. Mosby Co.

Erickson, M. L.: Assessment and management of developmental changes in children, ed. 2, St. Louis, 1981, The C. V. Mosby Co.

Korones, S. B.: High-risk newborn infants: the basis for intensive nursing care, ed. 2, St. Louis, 1976, The C. V. Mosby Co.

Marlow, D. R.: Textbook of pediatric nursing, ed. 5, Philadelphia, 1977, W. B. Saunders Co.

Pierog, S. H.: Medical care of the sick newborn, ed. 2, St. Louis, 1976, The C. V. Mosby Co.

Pipes, P. L.: Nutrition in infancy and childhood, ed. 2, St. Louis, 1981, The C. V. Mosby Co.

Scipien, G. M., et al.: Comprehensive pediatric nursing, ed. 2, New York, 1979, McGraw-Hill Book Co., Inc.

Shirkey, H. C.: Pediatric therapy, ed. 6, St. Louis, 1980, The C. V. Mosby Co.

Vaughn, V. C., et al.: Nelson textbook of pediatrics, ed. 11, Philadelphia, 1979, W. B. Saunders Co.

Whaley, L. F.: Understanding inherited disorders, St. Louis, 1974, The C. V. Mosby Co.

Whaley, L. F., and Wong, D. L.: Nursing care of infants and children, St. Louis, 1979, The C. V. Mosby Co.

Wong, D. L., and Whaley, L. F.: Clinical handbook of pediatric nursing, St. Louis, 1981, The C. V. Mosby Co.

HISTORY AND LEGAL TRENDS

Abu-Saad, H.: Nursing: a world view, St. Louis, 1979, The C. V. Mosby Co.

Creighton, H.: Law every nurse should know, ed. 3, Philadelphia, 1975, W. B. Saunders Co.

Deloughery, G. L.: History and trends of professional nursing, ed. 8, St. Louis, 1977, The C. V. Mosby Co.

Flynn, B. C., and Miller, M. H.: Current perspectives in nursing: social issues and trends, vol. 2, St. Louis, 1979, The C. V. Mosby Co.

George, J. E.: The law and emergency care, St. Louis, 1980, The C. V. Mosby Co.

Gibbon, J. M., and Mathewson, M. L.: Three centuries of Canadian nursing, Toronto, 1947, The Macmillan Co.

Good, S., and Kerr, J.: Contemporary issues in Canadian law for nurses, Toronto, 1973, Holt, Rinehart & Winston.

Hemelt, M. D., and MacKert, M. E.: Dynamics of law in nursing and health care, Reston, Va., 1978, Reston Publishing Co., Inc.

Kelly, L. Y.: Dimensions of professional nursing, ed. 3, New York, 1975, Macmillan Publishing Co.

Kramer, M.: Reality shock: why nurses leave nursing, St. Louis, 1974, The C. V. Mosby Co.

Mauksch, I. G., and Miller, M. H.: Implementing change in nursing, St. Louis, 1980, The C. V. Mosby Co.

Miller, M. H., and Flynn, B. C.: Current perspectives in nursing: social issues and trends, vol. 1, St. Louis, 1977, The C. V. Mosby Co.

Murchison, I.: Legal accountability in the nursing process, St. Louis, 1978, The C. V. Mosby Co.

Murchison, I., and Nichols, T.: Legal foundations of nursing practice, New York, 1970, The Macmillan Co.

INDEX

A

Aarane; *see* Cromolyn sodium
Abdominal perineal resection, 136
Abnormalities, congenital; *see* Congenital abnormalities
ABO incompatibility, 389-390
Abortion, 384, 394
Abruptio placentae, 384-385
Abscesses
    bone, 235-236
    brain, 225
    intestinal, 133, 135
    lung, 97
    pancreatic, 129
Absolute temperature, 24
Absorption, gastrointestinal, 109
Abstract for Action, 482
Academy of Nursing, 482
Academy for Nursing Practice, 482
Acceptance, 332-333
    of illness, 334
Accident prevention, 421, 440, 461
Accreditation
    of health care facilities, 501
    of nursing programs
        in Canada, 502-503
        in United States, 489
Acedapsone, 35
Acetaminophen, 28
Acetazolamide, 219
Acetic acid, 47, 160, 442
Acetohexamide, 173
Acetophenazine maleate, 341
Acetophenetidin, 28
Acetosulfone sodium, 35
Acetylcholine, 184, 198, 214, 230
Acetylcysteine, 92
Acetylsalicylic acid; *see also* Salicylates
    in arthritis, 218, 458
    colostomy care and, 123
    excretion of, 143
    infectious mononucleosis and, 85
    mixing of, with other drugs, 17
    pain and, 28
    peptic ulcer and, 126
    toxicity of, 442, 459
Achromycin; *see* Tetracycline
Acid-base balance, 43-46; *see also* Acidosis; Alkalosis
Acid-fast stain, 20
Acidosis, 43
    diabetic coma and, 180
    metabolic, 46, 436
    respiratory, 44-45, 453

Acids, 47
Acne vulgaris, 254
Acoustic neuroma, 224
Acoustics, 57
Acromegaly, 175
ACTH; *see* Adrenocorticotropic hormone
Acticort; *see* Hydrocortisone
Actinomycetales, 19
Actinomycin D; *see* Dactinomycin
Action potential, 184
Acupuncture, 237
Acute care facilities, 6
Ad Hoc Committee on Nursing Education, Department of Public Health, Province of Saskatchewan, 494
Adams-Stokes syndrome, 72
Adapin; *see* Doxepin hydrochloride
Adaptation
    communication and, 11
    to extrauterine life, 378-381
Addiction, 336, 346-347
Addison's disease, 181-182
Adenocarcinoma of kidneys, 154; *see also* Carcinoma
Adenohypophysis, 173
Adenoidectomy, 454
Adenomas, 177, 180
Adenomyosis, 161
Adenosine diphosphate, 117
Adenosine triphosphate, 117, 198
Adenoviruses, 91
ADH; *see* Antidiuretic hormone
Adjustment reactions, 349
Adolescence, 460-461
    adjustment reaction of, 349
    behavioral disorders of, 349-351
    personality development and, 328
    problems of, 461
ADP; *see* Adenosine diphosphate
Adrenal glands, 167, 169-170
    cortex of, 169, 170
        hormones of, 111, 181, 182; *see also* Corticosteroids
    diseases of, 180-182
    medulla of, 169
    metabolism and, 111
Adrenalectomy, 164, 181, 182
Adrenaline; *see* Epinephrine
Adrenocorticotropic hormone, 171, 174
    excessive, 181
    metabolism and, 111
    myasthenia gravis and, 232
    placenta and, 372
    tests and, 182

Adrenocorticotropic hormone—cont'd
    ulcers and, 127
Adriamycin; *see* Doxorubicin
Adult facility, 7
Adult respiratory distress syndrome, 104-105
Adulthood
    adjustment reaction of, 349
    later
        adjustment reaction of, 349
        personality development and, 329
    young, 329
Advanced degree nursing programs, 486, 499
Aerobes, 20
Aerosporin; *see* Polymyxin B sulfate
Affective disorders, 338-340
Afferent neurons, 183
Agar, 120
Agar-agar, 114
Agencies
    government, 5, 395
    for parent-child health services, 395
    voluntary, 5-6, 395
Agglutination, 63
Aggressive behavior, 335, 338-340, 345
Aggressive reaction of childhood and adolescence, 350
$AgNO_3$; *see* Silver nitrate
Agranulocytosis, 83-84
Airways, suctioning of, 94
Akineton; *see* Biperiden
Albacide; *see* Benzyl benzoate lotion
Albumin, 115
    in blood, 49
    chemistry of, 59
    nephrosis and, 452
    toxemias of pregnancy and, 383
Albuminoids, 115
Alcohol
    dependence on, 336, 346-347
    drug potentiation and, 339, 344
    ethyl, 22
    injections of, 230, 231
    isopropyl, 22
    newborn and, 390
    organic brain syndromes and, 337
Aldactone; *see* Spironolactone
Aldehyde, 113
Aldomet; *see* Methyldopa
Aldosterone, 141, 143
    adrenal gland and, 169, 170
    cirrhosis and, 132
    feedback mechanism and, 42
    primary aldosteronism and, 180-181
Aldosteronism, primary, 180-181

Alkali metals, 214-215

Alkaline-ash diet, 235

Alkaloids, 39

   rauwolfia, 67, 225

Alkalosis, 43

   metabolic, 46, 436

   respiratory, 45

Alkeran; *see* Melphalan

Alkylating agents, 39, 164; *see also* specific drug

Alleles, 148

Allen, M., 493

Allergy

   blood transfusions and, 29

   in children, 452-454

   diarrhea and, 436

   diet and, 420, 438

   eczema and, 438

   rhinitis and, 452

Allopurinol, 151, 218

Almetropin; *see* Chorionic gonadotropin

Al (OH)$_3$; *see* Aluminum hydroxide

Alpha cells, 107

Alpha globulins, 49

Alpha lipoproteins, 171

Alpha particle, 61

ALS; *see* Amyotrophic lateral sclerosis

Aluminum

   and magnesium hydroxides, 119

   tetracyclines and, 33

Aluminum carbonate gel, basic, 119

Aluminum hydroxide, 47

   with magnesium trisilicate, 119

Aluminum hydroxide gel, 119

Aluminum phosphate gel, 119

Alupent; *see* Metaproterenol

Alurate; *see* Aprobarbital

Alveolar ducts, 87

Alveoli, 87

Alzheimer's disease, 337

Amantadine hydrochloride, 34, 216, 217

Ambenonium chloride, 217, 232

Ambulatory care, 491

Amebiasis, 36

Amelia, 434

American Association of Colleges of Nursing, 484

American Association of Industrial Nurses, 483

American Association of Nurse Anesthetists, 484

American hookworm, 118

American Hospital Association, 491

American Journal of Nursing, 483

American Nurses' Association, 482-483

   Position Paper on Nursing Education of, 487

American Nurses' Foundation, 483

American Society for Psychoprophylaxis in Obstetrics, 395

Amethopterin; *see* Methotrexate

Ametropia, 213-214

Amicar; *see* Aminocaproic acid

Amid-Sal; *see* Salicylamide

Amikacin sulfate, 33

Amiken; *see* Amikacin sulfate

Amines, 214

Amino acids, 113; *see also* Proteins

   nerves and, 184, 214

   renal tubules and, 141

Aminocaproic acid, 226, 456

Aminoglycosides, 33

Aminophylline, 91, 92, 453

Aminosalicylates, 36

Amitriptyline hydrochloride, 339

Ammonia, 45, 46, 166

Ammonium chloride, 247

Ammonium hydroxide, 47

Amnesia, 343

Amnestrogen; *see* Esterified estrogens

Amniocentesis, 373

Amnion, 147

Amobarbital, 27, 353

Amodiaquine hydrochloride, 37

Amoxicillin, 32

Amoxil; *see* Amoxicillin

amp; *see* Amperes

Amperes, 24

Amphetamines, 118-119

   hyperactivity and, 350, 351, 460

Amphiarthrotic joints, 203

Amphicol; *see* Chloramphenicol

Amphojel; *see* Aluminum hydroxide gel

Amphotericin B, 36

Ampicillin, 32

Amputations, 78-80, 236

Amygdala, 189

Amylase, 448

Amyotrophic lateral sclerosis, 233

Amytal; *see* Amobarbital

Anabolism, 107, 108, 110

Anacel; *see* Tetracaine hydrochloride

Anaerobes, 20

Anaphylactic shock, 82

Anatomy and physiology

   of bony pelvis, 374

   of circulatory system, 48-55

   of endocrine system, 166-173

Anatomy and physiology—cont'd

   of gastrointestinal system, 105-111

   of genitourinary system, 140-148

   of integumentary system, 248-249

   of muscular system, 197-199

   of nervous system, 183-197

   of respiratory system, 86-89

   of skeletal system, 199-206

Anbesol; *see* Benzocaine

Ancef; *see* Cefazolin sodium

Ancylostoma duodenale, 117

Androgens, 144, 166-168, 169; *see also* Testosterone

   adrenal gland and, 169

   in chemotherapy, 38, 157

     breast carcinoma and, 164

   fertility and, 392

   metabolism and, 111

Androlan; *see* Testosterone

Andronaq; *see* Testosterone

Andronate; *see* Testosterone

Anectine; *see* Succinylcholine chloride

Anemia, 82-83

   adolescence and, 461

   blood viscosity and, 57

   in children, 440, 447-448, 449-450

     hemolytic disease of newborn and, 389

   sickle cell, 449-450

Anesthesia, 25-27

   drug potentiation and, 339

Aneurysmectomy, 77

Aneurysms, 81

   cerebral, 225

   removal of, 77

Anger, illness and, 333

Angina pectoris, 74-75, 348

Angiography, 72

Angiotensin II, 143

Angstrom unit, 209

Angular gyrus, 189

Anions, 41-42

Anorexiants, 118-119

Anspor; *see* Cephradine

Antabuse; *see* Disulfiram

Antacids, 17, 119

Antagonists, 198

Antepar Citrate; *see* Piperazine citrate

Antepartal period, 371-373

Anterior pituitary hormones, 110-111; *see also* specific hormone

Anterior segment disorders of eye, 243-244

Anthelmintics, 447

Anthropology, 322-323

Antianxiety drugs, 344; *see also* specific drug

Antiarrhythmic drugs, 64-66; *see also* specific drug
Antibiotics, 32; *see also* specific drug
  antineoplastic, 39
  integumentary system and, 250
  intestinal, 121
  radioactive, 39
  sensitivity and, 22
Antibodies, 62-63
  anti-Rh, 50
  infant and, 422
  neutralizing, 63
Anticholinergics, 119, 218; *see also* specific drug
  drug potentiation and, 339
  Parkinson's disease and, 216-217
Anticoagulants, 70; *see also* specific drug
  drug interactions and, 34, 36, 353, 458, 459
Anticonvulsants, 215-216, 228-229; *see also* specific drug
Antidepressants, 339; *see also* specific drug
Antidiarrheal agents, 119-120
Antidiuretic hormone, 59, 172; *see also* Vasopressin
  diabetes insipidus and, 176
  as drug, 175
  hypothalamus and, 188
  kidneys and, 141, 143
  lithium carbonate and, 340
Antidote, universal, 442
Antiemetics, 118
Antifungals, 36, 250; *see also* specific drug
Antigens, 62, 63
  contact dermatitis and, 254
  immune serum, 131
Antihemophilic factor, 456
Antihemophilic plasma, 456
Antihistamines, 93; *see also* specific drug
  as cough suppressants, 92
  drug potentiation and, 339
Anti-infective drugs, 22, 32-38; *see also* specific drug
Anti-inflammatory agents, 251; *see also* specific drug
Antimalarials, 37
Antimetabolites, 38; *see also* specific drug
  breast carcinoma and, 164
  mechanism of, 16
Antiminth; *see* Pyrantel pamoate
Antineoplastic drugs, 38-40; *see also* specific drug
Antiparasitics, 36-38
Antiparkinsonism drugs, 216-217, 231, 342
Antiprotozoan preparations, 160-161

Antipruritics, 251
Anti-Rh antibodies, 50
Antiseptic, 21
Antisera, 64
Antisocial personality, 345
Antistreptolysin-O titer, 457
Antithyroid drugs, 173-174, 177
Antitoxins, 63, 64
  botulism and, 140
Antitussives, 92
Antivirals, 34
Antrectomy, 126
Antuitrin-S; *see* Chorionic gonadotropin
Anuria, 143
Anus, 106
  imperforate, 380, 425-426
Anxiety, 327, 335, 343
  behavior and, 330-331
  levels of, 330
  separation, 422
Anxiety reactions, 335, 343
Aorta
  coarctation of, 427
  overriding, 427-428
Aortic stenosis, 427
Apamide; *see* Acetaminophen
Apatite salts, 202
Apgar score, 379
Aphasia, 226, 227
Aphthous stomatitis, 124
A.P.L.; *see* Chorionic gonadotropin
Aplastic anemia, 83
Apocrine glands, 248
Apoenzyme, 59
Appendix, 106
Apresoline Hydrochloride; *see* Hydralazine hydrochloride
Aprobarbital, 27, 353
Aquadiol; *see* Estradiol
Aqualin; *see* Theophylline
Arachnoid membrane, 189
Aralen Phosphate; *see* Chloroquine phosphate
Aramine; *see* Metaraminol bitartrate
ARDS; *see* Adult respiratory distress syndrome
Arector pili, 248-249
Aristocort; *see* Triamcinolone
Arnold-Chiari syndrome, 430
Arrhythmias, 71, 72, 75, 426-430
Arsenic, 131
Artane; *see* Trihexyphenidyl
Arteries, 52; *see also* Blood vessels
Arterioatherosclerosis, 74
Arteriosclerosis, 74

Arthritis
  drugs in, 217-218
  gouty, 235
  osteoarthritis and, 234-235
  rheumatic fever and, 457
  rheumatoid, 234
    juvenile, 458-459
Arthrodesis, 235
Arthropan; *see* Choline salicylate
A.S.A.; *see* Acetylsalicylic acid
Ascaris lumbricoides, 117
Aschheim-Zondek test, 373
Aschoff bodies, 457
Ascites, 76, 132, 452
ASD; *see* Atrial septal defect
Asepsis, 31-32
Asphyxia neonatorum, 388
Aspiration of foreign objects, 443
Aspirin; *see* Acetylsalicylic acid
A.S.P.O.; *see* American Society for Psychoprophylaxis in Obstetrics
Assault, 507
Associate degree nursing programs, 485-486, 497, 498
Association of Collegiate Schools of Nursing, 483
Association of Operating Room Nurses, 484
Asteric; *see* Acetylsalicylic acid
Asthenic personality, 345
Asthma, 100, 452-454
  psychogenic factors and, 348
Astigmatism, 213
Astrocytes, 184
Asystole, 71
Atarax; *see* Hydroxyzine hydrochloride
Ataxia, 445
Atelectasis, 98, 388
Atherosclerosis, 74
Athetosis, 445
Athlete's foot, 459
Atonic nonreflex bladder, 243
ATP; *see* Adenosine triphosphate
Atresia
  choanal, 426
  tricuspid, 428
Atrial septal defect, 427
Atrioventricular block, 72
Atrioventricular bundle of His, 51-52
Atrioventricular node, 51-52
Atrophic vaginitis, 160
Atropine sulfate, 66, 119, 217, 218
[198]Au; *see* Gold, radioactive
Audiometry, speech, 207-208

Aureomycin; *see* Chlortetracycline hydrochloride

Autistic psychosis, 351

Autoclave, 25

Autografts, 251

Autoimmune defects, 257-258

Automatic bladder, 243

Autonomic nervous system, 193-195

Autonomous bladder, 243

AV bundle of His; *see* Atrioventricular bundle of His

AV node; *see* Atrioventricular node

Aventyl; *see* Nortriptyline hydrochloride

Avlosulfon; *see* Dapsone

Axon, 183

Azathioprine, 38

Azulfidine; *see* Sulfasalazine

B

Babinski reflex, 380

Baby; *see also* Fetus; Newborn

antepartal growth and development of, 371-372

labor and, 374-375

Baccalaureate degree nursing programs

in Canada, 496, 498-499, 504

in United States, 486, 490

Bacid; *see* Lactobacillus acidophilus

Bacillus of Calmette-Guérin, 39, 256

Bacillus anthracis, 19

Bacitracin, 250, 389

Bacteria, 18-20

circulatory system and, 457

destruction of, 21, 32

diarrhea and, 436

food poisoning and, 139

gastrointestinal system and, 117, 139, 436

genitourinary system and, 149-150, 161

impetigo and, 459

meningitis and, 437

neuromusculoskeletal systems and, 215, 235, 437

pelvic inflammatory disease and, 161

resistance and, 32

respiratory system and, 91, 437

rheumatic fever and, 457

Bacterial endocarditis, subacute, 76

Bactericide, 21, 32

Bacteriostatic effect, 32

Bactocill; *see* Oxacillin sodium

BAL; *see* Dimercaprol

Balantidium coli, 117

Bárány's caloric test, 223

Barbital, 27, 353

Barbiturates; *see also* specific drug

as anesthetics, 25-26

drug interactions and, 339, 353

lipoid tissue affinity of, 353

overdosage of, 353

as sedatives, 27, 352-353

Bargaining, 333

Barium sulfate, 48

enemas and, 112, 121-122

Baroreceptors, 195-196

Bartholin's glands, 146

Basal cell carcinoma, 256

Basal metabolic rate, 111

growth and, 415

Basaljel; *see* Aluminum carbonate gel, basic

Base bicarbonate, 43, 44

Bases, 46-47

in acid-base balance, 43-46

Basic needs, 329-330

BaSO₄; *see* Barium sulfate

Battered child syndrome, 443-444

Battery, 507

BCG; *see* Bacillus of Calmette-Guérin

Beef tapeworm, 118

Behavior

addictive, 336, 346-347

aggressive, 335, 338-340, 345

socially, 335-336, 345

anxiety and, 330-331

childhood and adolescent disorders of, 349-351

deviate patterns of, 334-336

emotions and, 331-332

illness and, 333-334

motivation and learning and, 331-332

projective, 334-335, 342-343, 345

psychoneurotic, 335, 343-344

withdrawn, 334, 340-342, 345

Behavioral disorders of childhood and adolescence, 349-351

Behavioral sciences, 322-332

anthropology in, 322-323

psychology in, 326-332

sociology in, 323-326

Bell's palsy, 229-230

Belladonna leaf, tincture, 119

Benadryl; *see* Diphenhydramine

Benedict's test, 113

Benemid; *see* Probenecid

Benign prostatic hypertrophy, 159

Benoxinate hydrochloride, 26

Bentyl; *see* Dicyclomine hydrochloride

Benylate; *see* Benzyl benzoate lotion

Benzalkonium, 22

Benzedrine; *see* Amphetamines

Benzocaine, 26, 251, 254

Benzodiazepines, 344

Benzonatate, 92

Benzphetamine hydrochloride, 118

Benztropine mesylate, 216, 217, 342

Benzyl benzoate lotion, 250

Beta cells, 107

Beta-Chlor; *see* Chloral betaine

Beta globulins, 49

Beta lipoproteins, 171

Beta particle, 61

Betamethasone, 251

Betamethasone valerate, 174, 251

Bicarbonate, 42, 43, 44

Bicarbonate sodium; *see* Sodium bicarbonate

Bile, 107, 109

Bile acids, 115

Bile ducts, common, 107

Bile salts, 131

Bilopaque, 129

Bilroth I and II surgery, 126

Binocular vision, 214

Biofeedback, 237

Biperiden, 342

Birth injuries, 388-389

Bisacodyl, 120

Bismuth subcarbonate, 119, 123

Biuret test, 116

Black light, 255

Black lung, 101

Blackheads, 254

Bladder; *see* Urinary bladder

Blalock-Hanlon procedure, 428

Blalock procedure, 428

Blalock-Taussig procedure, 428

Blastocoele, 147

Blastocyst, 147, 371

Bleeding; *see* Hemorrhage

Blenoxane; *see* Bleomycin

Bleomycin, 39, 103

Blepharitis, 243

Blindness; *see* Eye

Blockain Hydrochloride; *see* Propoxycaine hydrochloride

Blood, 48-50

buffer mechanisms and, 61

carbon dioxide transport and, 89

circulating volume of, drugs for decrease of, 68-69

coagulation of, 50

drugs for preventing; *see* Anticoagulants

studies of, 75

fluid pressures and, 40

Blood—cont'd
  kidney and, 141
  myocardium and, 51
  oxygen transport and, 89
  pH of, 43
    respiration and, 88, 89
  in stool specimen, 122
Blood dyscrasias, 83-84
Blood factor replacement, 456
Blood groups, 50, 148
  incompatibility in newborn and, 389-390
Blood pressure, 53-54
  elevated, 73-74, 132, 348
  growth and, 415
Blood serum enzymes, 74
Blood serum isoenzymes, 74
Blood sugar
  excessive; *see* Diabetes mellitus
  growth and, 415
  low, 180, 455
Blood transfusions; *see* Transfusions, blood
Blood types; *see* Blood groups
Blood vessels, 52; *see also* Veins
  adrenal glands and, 170
  drugs and, 64-70
  transposition of great, 428
Bloody show, 375
Blueprint Committee, 488
BMR; *see* Basal metabolic rate
Body defense, 327
Body fluids, pH of; *see* pH
Body image, changes in, 10-11, 334
Body weight; *see* Weight
Boiling, 25
The Bolton Act, 488
Bone marrow aspiration, 72
Bones, 199-202
  abscesses of, 235-236
  age and, 205-206
  cancellous, 202-203
  compact, 202-203
  formation of, 202-203
  growth of, 203
  list of, 204-205
  repair of, 206
Bonine; *see* Meclizine hydrochloride
Bony pelvis anatomy, 374
Bordetella pertussis, 91
Boric acid, 47
Borrelia vincentii, 124
Bottle-feeding, 382-383, 419
Botulism, 139-140
Bowel; *see also* Intestines
  resection of, 134, 135, 435

Bowel—cont'd
  retraining and, 242-243
Boyle's law, 90, 112
Braces, 222
Brachial palsy, 389
Brain, 187-190
  abscess of, 225
  and spinal cord coverings, 189
  surgery of, 224-225
  tumors of, 224-225
    pressures and, 206
Brain stem, 187
Brain syndromes, organic, 337-338
Braxton-Hicks contractions, 375
Breast-feeding, 381-382, 383, 419
Breasts, 146
  carcinoma of, 163-164
  care of, 382
Breathing; *see* Respirations
Brethine; *see* Terbutaline
Brevital Sodium; *see* Methohexital sodium
Bricanyl; *see* Terbutaline
Bridgman, M., 481
British Thermal Unit, 25
Brompheniramine maleate, 93
Bronchial asthma, 100, 348, 452-454
Bronchial tree, 87
Bronchioles, 87
Bronchitis, 100, 437
Bronchodilators, 91-92, 453
Bronchogenic carcinoma, 102-103
Bronchoscopy, 93-94
Bronkephrine; *see* Ethylnorepinephrine hydrochloride
Brown, E. L., 481, 497
The Brown Report, 481, 486, 487, 497
Brucella, 117
Bryant's traction, 239, 433, 443
BTU; *see* British Thermal Unit
Bubartal Sodium; *see* Butabarbital sodium
Buccal cavity, 105-106
  inflammation and, 124-125
Buck's extension, 239
BudOpto; *see* Tetracaine hydrochloride
Buerger's disease, 80
Buffers, 43-44, 61
  gastrointestinal system and, 113
Bu-Lax; *see* Sodium carboxymethylcellulose
Bulbourethral glands, 144
Bulla, 252
Bupivacaine hydrochloride, 26
Burgess, M. A., 481
Burns, 252-254
  in children, 441-442

Bursae, 199
Busulfan, 39, 83
Butabarbital sodium, 27, 353
Butacaine sulfate, 26
Butazolidin; *see* Phenylbutazone
Butesin Picrate; *see* Butyl aminobenzoate
Butisol Sodium; *see* Butabarbital sodium
Butyl aminobenzoate, 26
Butyn Sulfate; *see* Butacaine sulfate
Butyrophenones, 342

C

$CaCO_3$; *see* Calcium carbonate
Cafergot; *see* Ergotamine with caffeine
Calamine, 251
Calciferol, 178, 216; *see also* Vitamins, D
Calcitonin, 166
Calcium
  adolescence and, 461
  bone and, 199
  children and, 440
  drugs for increasing, 216
  fluid and electrolyte balance and, 41
  lead poisoning and, 443
  neuromusculoskeletal systems and, 198, 199, 215
  parathyroid glands and, 42-43, 166
  stones of, 151
  tetracyclines and, 33
Calcium aminosalicylate, 36
Calcium carbonate, 48, 178, 216
Calcium chloride, 178, 216
Calcium disodium edetate, 443
Calcium Disodium Versenate; *see* Calcium disodium edetate
Calcium gluconate, 216
  in hypoparathyroidism, 177, 178
  magnesium sulfate and, 384
Calcium hydroxide, 47
Calcium iodide, 92, 454
Calcium ion replacement, 216
Calcium phosphate, 47
Calcium sulfate, 48
Calculi
  in gallbladder, 128
  renal and ureteral, 151
Calories, 24, 111
Calurin; *see* Carbaspirin calcium
Cameron, S., 491
Camoquin Hydrochloride; *see* Amodiaquine hydrochloride
Camphorated opium tincture, 120
Canada, nursing in; *see* Nursing in Canada

Canadian Association of University Schools of Nursing, 496
Canadian Council on Hospital Accreditation, 501
Canadian Council of Nurse Researchers, 504
Canadian Hospital Association, 501
Canadian Hospital Directory, 503
The Canadian Nurse Journal, 499
Canadian Nurses' Association, 495-496, 503
Canadian Nurses' Association Position on Accreditation, 503
Canadian Nurses' Association Position Paper on Nursing Education, 500
Canadian Nurses' Association Testing Service, 496, 500, 509
Canadian Testing Service Examination, 500
Canadian University Nursing Student Association, 496
Cancer; *see* Carcinoma
Candida albicans, 21
    mouth and, 124
    newborn and, 389
    superinfection and, 32, 457
    vagina and, 160
Candidiasis; *see Candida albicans*
Canes, 220
Cantor tube, 136, 137
Ca(OH)₂; *see* Calcium hydroxide
Capastat Sulfate; *see* Capreomycin sulfate
Capillaries, 52
    Starling's law of, 40
Capillarity, 57
CaPO₄; *see* Calcium phosphate
Capreomycin sulfate, 36
Caprokol; *see* Hexylresorcinol
Caput succedaneum, 388
Carbachol, 218
Carbamazepine, 28, 216, 230
Carbaspirin calcium, 28, 458
Carbenicillin disodium, 32
Carbhemoglobin, 89
Carbinoxamine maleate, 93
Carbocaine Hydrochloride; *see* Mepivacaine hydrochloride
Carbohydrates, 113-114
    absorption of, 109
    liver and, 107
    metabolism of, 110
Carbon dioxide
    adrenal gland and, 169
    pH and, 44, 88, 89
    respiratory system and, 88, 89
Carbon monoxide poisoning, 105
Carbon tetrachloride, 131

Carbonic acid, 43, 44, 47, 61, 166
Carbonic anhydrase inhibitors, 219
Carcinoma; *see also* Tumors
    of breast, 163-164
    bronchogenic, 102-103
    of cervix, 159-160
    in children, 451-452
    of esophagus, 128
    immunotherapy for, 39
    of intestines, 136-137
    of kidneys, 154
    of larynx, 103-104
    lasers and, 209-210
    of liver, 133
    of mouth, 125
    Paget's, 163
    of pancreas, 130-131
    of prostate, 158-159
    of skin, 255-256
    of stomach, 127
Cardiac arrhythmias, 71, 72, 75, 426-430
Cardiac cycle, 52
Cardiac glycosides, 64; *see also* Digitalis
Cardiac monitoring, 71
Cardiac muscle, 197
Cardiac output, 53, 170
Cardiac pacemakers, 24, 58, 72
Cardiac skeleton, 51
Cardiac surgery, 77-78
Cardiaquin; *see* Quinidine polygalacturonate
Cardilate; *see* Erythrityl tetranitrate
Cardiogenic shock, 81
Cardiovascular system; *see* Circulatory system
Carditis, 76, 457-458
Cardrase; *see* Ethoxzolamide
Career ladder, 489, 504
Cariolipids, 115
Carisoprodol, 217
Carmustine, 39
Carotid endarterectomy, 227
Carriers, 23
Caryolysine; *see* Mechlorethamine
Cascara sagrada, 120
CaSO₄; *see* Calcium sulfate
Castor oil, 120
Casts
    care of, 239-240
    spica, 433-434
    wedge, 433
Catabolism, 109-110
Catapres; *see* Clonidine hydrochloride
Cataracts, 245
Catecholamines, 111, 169
Cathartics, 120-121

Catheters
    suprapubic, 156
    Swan-Ganz, 72-73
Cations, 41
C.A.U.S.N.; *see* Canadian Association of University Schools of Nursing
Cecostomy, 136, 137
Cecum, 106, 136, 137
Cedilanid; *see* Lanatoside C
Cefazolin sodium, 32
Celestoderm-V; *see* Betamethasone valerate
Celestone; *see* Betamethasone
Celiac disease, 420, 448
Cellophane tape test, 447
Cellothyl; *see* Methylcellulose
Celontin; *see* Methsuximide
Celospor; *see* Cephacetrile
Cells
    alpha, 107
    beta, 107
    of bone, 199-202
    chief, 106, 173
    goblet, 100
    islet, 107
    memory, 62
    of nervous system, 183-184
    parietal, 106
    plasma, 62
    Reed-Sternberg, 85
    Schwann, 183
Cellulose, 114
Celsius temperature, 24
Centigrade temperature, 24
Central auditory hearing disorders, 446
Central canal of spinal cord, 189
Central nervous system; *see* Nervous system
Central venous pressure, 73
Cephacetrile, 32
Cephalexin monohydrate, 32
Cephalins, 115
Cephaloglycin, 32
Cephalohematoma, 388
Cephaloridine, 32
Cephalosporins, 32-33
Cephalothin sodium, 33, 253
Cephradine, 33
Cerebellum, 187
Cerebral aneurysm, 225
Cerebral aqueduct, 189
Cerebral cortex, 189
Cerebral hemispheres, 189
Cerebral hemorrhage, 224, 225-228
Cerebral palsy, 445-446
Cerebral stimulants, 339

Cerebral tracts, 189
Cerebral vascular accident, 226-228
Cerebrospinal fluid, 190
    hydrocephalus and, 431-432
    lumbar puncture and, 222-223
    pressures and, 206
Ceruminous glands, 248
Cervical disc herniation, 238
Cervix, carcinoma of, 159-160
Cesarean section, 384, 385, 386
Cestodes, 118
Chadwick's sign, 372
Chalasia, 436
Chalazion, 244
Change
    in body image, 10-11, 334
    of state of matter, 25
Ch₃CHOHCOOH; *see* Lactic acid
Chel-Iron; *see* Ferrocholinate
Chemical poisoning, 442
Chemistry
    circulatory system and, 58-62
    fluid and electrolytes and, 46-48
    gastrointestinal system and, 112-117
    genitourinary system and, 149
    integumentary system and, 249
    metabolism and, 109-111
    neuromusculoskeletal systems and, 214-215
    respiration and, 88
Chemosurgery for skin cancer, 256
Chemotherapy, 14; *see also* specific drug
    bladder tumors and, 155
    brain tumors and, 224
    breast carcinoma and, 164
    bronchogenic carcinoma and, 103
    combination, 39-40
    cystitis and, 151
    esophageal cancer and, 128
    eye tumors and, 244
    Hodgkin's disease and, 85
    hormones in, 38, 154, 157, 158, 164
    intestinal cancer and, 137
    kidney cancer and, 154
    laryngeal cancer and, 103
    leukemias and, 84, 451, 452
    microbial control and, 22
    in multiple myeloma, 237
    osteogenic sarcoma and, 236
    pancreatic cancer and, 131
    paranoid states and, 342
    skin cancer and, 256
    stomach carcinoma and, 127
Chest injuries, 102
Chest tubes, 95-96

CHF; *see* Congestive heart failure
Chief cells, 106, 173
Childbirth, injuries in, 386-387
Children; *see also* Pediatric nursing
    adjustment reactions of, 349
    behavioral disorders of, 349-351
    death and, 451-452
    defective, parent reactions to, 422-423
    and parents, relationship disturbances and, 414
    personality development and, 328
    schizophrenia and, 351
Children's Bureau, 395
Chlophedianol hydrochloride, 92
Chloral betaine, 27, 352
Chloral hydrate, 27, 352
Chlorambucil, 39, 85, 164
Chloramphenicol, 34, 250
Chlordiazepoxide hydrochloride, 344
Chlorides, 41-42
Chlorine and chlorine-releasing compounds, 22
Chlormezanone, 217
Chloroguanide hydrochloride, 37
Chloromycetin; *see* Chloramphenicol
Chloroprocaine hydrochloride, 26
Chloroquine phosphate, 37
Chlorothen citrate, 93
Chlorothiazide, 68
Chlorotrianisene, 157, 392
Chlorphenesin carbamate, 217
Chlorpheniramine maleate, 93
Chlorphentermine hydrochloride, 119
Chlorpromazine hydrochloride, 341
Chlorpropamide, 173
Chlorprothixene, 342
Chlortetracycline hydrochloride, 33
Chlorthalidone, 68
Chlor-Trimeton; *see* Chlorpheniramine maleate
Chlorzoxazone, 217
Choanal atresia, 426
C₂H₃O₂H; *see* Acetic acid
Cholangiogram, intravenous, 128-129
Cholecystectomy, 129
Cholecystitis, 128-129
Cholecystojejunostomy, 131
Cholecystokinin, 117
Cholecystotomy, 129
Choledochotomy, 129
Choledyl; *see* Oxtriphylline
Cholelithiasis, 128
Cholesterol, 115
Choline salicylate, 28, 458
Cholinergics, ophthalmic, 218
Cholinesterase, 198

Cholinesterase inhibitors, 217
Chorea
    Huntington's, 234
    organic brain syndromes and, 338
    Sydenham's, 457
Chorex; *see* Chorionic gonadotropin
Chorigon; *see* Chorionic gonadotropin
Chorion, 147
Chorionic gonadotropin, 148, 372, 373, 393
Chorionic villi, 147
Chromoproteins, 115
Chromosomes, 147, 148
    alterations in, 148, 423-424
Chronic brain syndrome, 337
Chronic obstructive pulmonary disease, 100-101
Chvostek's sign, 178
Circ-O-lectric bed, 219-220
Circulatory system, 48-86
    anatomy and physiology of, 48-55
    arrhythmias and, 71, 72, 75, 416-430
    cardiac output and, 53, 170
    chemistry and, 58-62
    congenital defects of, 426-430
    diseases of, 73-86
        anemia in, 82-83
        aneurysms in, 81
        angina pectoris in, 74-75
        arterioatherosclerosis in, 74
        blood dyscrasias in, 83-84
        cardiac surgery for, 77-78
        congestive heart failure in, 76-77
        emboli in, 78-80
        Hodgkin's disease in, 85
        hypertension in, 73-74
        infectious mononucleosis in, 84-85
        inflammations in, 76, 457-458
        leukemias in, 84
        lymphosarcoma in, 85-86
        myocardial infarction in, 75-76
        peripheral vascular, 80-81
        pregnancy and, 387
        shock in, 81-82
        thrombophlebitis in, 78-80
        varicose veins in, 80
    efficiency and, 56
    of fetus, 52, 372
    fluid volume and, 42
    growth and, 415
    hepatic portal, 53
    microbiology and, 62-64
    newborn and, 380
    pacemakers and, 24, 58, 72
    pharmacology and, 64-70
    physics and, 55-58

Circulatory system—cont'd
  postpartal period and, 377
  pregnancy and, 373, 387
  procedures and, 71-73
  pulmonary, 52
  rheumatic fever and, 457-458
Cirrhosis, hepatic, 132-133
Citanest Hydrochloride; *see* Prilocaine hydrochloride
Citric acid, 113
Cleft lip, 424
Cleft palate, 424-425
Cleocin Hydrochloride; *see* Clindamycin hydrochloride
Clindamycin hydrochloride, 33
Clinical specialists, 487, 490, 505
Clinitest, 113
Clistin; *see* Carbinoxamine maleate
Clitoris, 146
  cleft, 432
Clofazimine, 35
Clomid; *see* Clomiphene citrate
Clomiphene citrate, 393
Clonidine hydrochloride, 67
Clonorchis sinensis, 118
Clorazepate dipotassium, 344
Clostridium botulinum, 19, 139
Clostridium perfringens, 112
Clostridium tetani, 19, 215
Clotrimazole, 250
Clotting of blood; *see* Blood, coagulation of
Clubfoot, 432-433
C.M.C.; *see* Sodium carboxymethylcellulose
CNATS; *see* Canadian Nurses' Association Testing Service
Coagulation of blood; *see* Blood, coagulation of
Coal tar ointments, 255
Coarctation of aorta, 427
Cocaine, 26, 339
Cochlea, 197
Cochlear nerve, 197
Code of Ethics, 503-504
Codeine sulfate, 28
CODFU regimen, 40
Codone; *see* Hydrocodone bitartrate
Coenzyme, 59
Cogentin; *see* Benztropine mesylate
Cognitive functioning, 326
Coherin, 172
Coitus interruptus, 393
Colace; *see* Dioctyl sodium sulfosuccinate
Colchicine, 218
Colectomy, 135, 136
Colic, 436-437

Colistimethate sodium, 34
Colistin sulfate, 34
Colitis
  psychogenic factors and, 348
  ulcerative, 135
Collagen, 202
Collagen diseases, 457, 458
Collective action or bargaining, 489, 501, 509
Collegiate education
  changes in, 490, 498-499, 504
  early developments in, 485, 496-497
Collegiate Education for Nursing, 481
Colliculi, 188
Colloid particle, 61
Colloid solutions, 61
Cologel; *see* Methylcellulose
Colon, 106; *see also* Colostomy
  irrigation of, 112, 121-122
    high, 122
  megacolon and, 435
  resection of, 135, 136
Color, 210
Color blindness, 210
Colostomy, 136, 137
  care of, 123, 426
  imperforate anus and, 426
  megacolon and, 435
Colporrhaphy, 162
Coly-Mycin M; *see* Colistimethate sodium
Coly-Mycin S; *see* Colistin sulfate
Coma
  diabetic, 180
    in child, 455
  hepatic, 132, 133
Combination chemotherapy, 39-40
Comedo extractor, 254
COMFU-P regimen, 40
Committee on the Healing Arts, 494
Common bile duct, 107
Common law, 506
Communication, 9-11, 326-327, 329
Community
  health services delivery and, 326
  society and, 325
Community College Education for Nursing, 481, 485
Community college systems, 485-486, 497, 498
Community Colleges and Nursing Education in Ontario, 494-495
Community Health Center Project, 505
Community health nurse, 504, 505
Community mental health services, 351-352
Compazine; *see* Prochlorperazine
Compensation, 331

Complaints of patient, 509
Complement-fixation, 63
Complete heart block, 71, 72
Compounds, 113-117
Compromise, 331
Concentrated solution, 60
Conception, 147, 371
  drugs for
    enhancement of, 392-393
    prevention of, 146, 147, 157-158, 393
Conchae, 86
Concussion, 224
Condom, 147, 393
Conduction of nerve impulse, 184-185
  motor pathways for, 190-193
  sensory pathways for, 190
Conduction system of heart, 51-52
Conductive hearing disorders, 446
Conductors, 57-58
Cones of retina, 210
Conestron; *see* Conjugated estrogens
Conflict resolution, 324
Congenital abnormalities, 389, 423-434
  chromosomal aberrations in, 422-423
  inborn errors of metabolism in, 420, 434
  malformations in, 424-434
    choanal atresia in, 426
    cleft lip in, 424
    cleft palate in, 424-425
    exstrophy of bladder in, 432
    facial, 424
    heart defects and, 426-430
    hydrocephalus in, 431-432
    intestinal, 425-426
    laryngeal stridor in, 426
    orthopedic, 432-434
    spina bifida in, 430-431
    tracheoesophageal, 425
    urethral opening displacement in, 432
  parent reactions and, 422-423
Congestive heart failure, 76-77
Congress of Nursing Practice, 482
Conjugated estrogens, 38, 392
Conjunctivitis, 243
Conjutab; *see* Conjugated estrogens
Conn's syndrome, 180-181
Conscious level, 327
Consensual validation, 327
Consent, informed, 508
Conservation of energy, law of, 56; *see also* Energy
Constipation, 120-121
  in children, 437
  diet and, 420

Contact dermatitis, 254
Contact lenses, 214, 245
Continued patient care, 7
Continuing education, mandatory, 489, 503
Contraception methods, 146, 147, 157-158, 393
Contractions of uterus
  Braxton-Hicks, 375
  induction of, 376, 385-386
Contractures, 249
Contusions, 224
Convergence principle, 191
Converging lens, 212
Conversion, 331
Conversion reactions, 335, 343
Convex lenses, 212
Convulsive disorders, 228-229
  drugs for, 215-216, 228-229
  febrile, 438
Cooperative play, 450-451
COP regimen, 40
COPD; *see* Chronic obstructive pulmonary disease
Cordotomy, 237
Cordran; *see* Flurandrenolone
Coronary bypass surgery, 77
Coronary occlusion, 51, 75-76
  psychogenic factors and, 348
Coronary vessels, 51
  drugs for dilation of, 66-67
Coronaviruses, 91
Corpus albicans, 371
Corpus callosum, 189
Corpus luteum, 371
Corpus striatum, 189
Corrosive chemical poisoning, 442
Cortef; *see* Hydrocortisone
Corticospinal tracts, 191
Corticosteroids, 115, 174; *see also* specific drug
  acne vulgaris and, 254
  adrenal gland and, 169, 170
  after adrenalectomy, 181, 182
  adult respiratory distress syndrome and, 104
  in arthritis, 218, 234, 459
  asthma and, 454
  blood dyscrasias and, 83
  brain tumors and, 225
  breast carcinoma and, 164
  cerebral hemorrhage and, 226
  chronic obstructive pulmonary disease and, 100
  contact dermatitis and, 254
  drug potentiation and, 339
  eye inflammations and, 244
  in Guillain-Barré syndrome, 233

Corticosteroids—cont'd
  heart inflammations and, 76
  herpes zoster and, 256
  infectious mononucleosis and, 85
  in leukemia, 451
  in multiple sclerosis, 231
  myasthenia gravis and, 232
  nephrosis and, 452
  pemphigus and, 255
  polyarteritis nodosa and, 257
  psoriasis and, 255
  sarcoidosis and, 99
  scleroderma and, 258
  systemic lupus erythematosus and, 257
  ulcerative colitis and, 135
Corticosterone, 111, 169, 170
Corticotropin; *see* Adrenocorticotropic hormone
Cortigel; *see* Andrenocorticotropic hormone
Cortisol, 111, 169, 170, 182
Cortisone, 100
Cortril; *see* Hydrocortisone
Corynebacterium diphtheriae, 19
Corynebacterium parvulum, 39
Cosmegen; *see* Dactinomycin
Cotazym; *see* Pancrelipase
Coulomb, 24
Coumadin; *see* Warfarin sodium
Courts, 509
Cow's milk, 383, 419
Cowper's glands, 144
Coxiella burnetii, 91
CPK; *see* Creatinine phosphokinase
Cranial nerves, 191
  Bell's palsy and, 229-230
  trigeminal neuralgia and, 230
Craniosacral nervous system, 193-195
Craniotomy, 225
Crawl reflex, 380
C-reactive protein, 457
Creatine phosphate, 198
Creatinine phosphokinase, 74
Credé maneuver, 243, 431
Cremothalidine; *see* Phthalylsulfathiazole
Cresols, 22
Cretinism, 176
Crib death, 436
Crimes, 507-508
Criminal conspiracy, 508
Crises intervention groups, 6
Criteria for College Education, 498
Crohn's disease, 134-135
Cromolyn sodium, 17, 453
Cross-contamination, 31-32
Croup, 437

Crutch walking, 220-222
Crutchfield tongs, 239
Cryoprecipitate, 456
Cryosurgery, 231, 246, 256
Cryotherapy in acne, 254
Cryptococcus neoformans, 215
Crystalloids, 61
Crysticillin A.S.; *see* Penicillin G procaine
Crystodigin; *see* Digitoxin
Crystoids; *see* Hexylresorcinol
CSF; *see* Cerebrospinal fluid
Culture inhibition, 22
Cultures
  microbiology and, 19, 22
    urine and, 150
  sociology and, 322-323
Curettage of uterus, 384, 394
Curling's ulcer, 252
Currant jelly stool, 435
Current electricity, 24
Curriculum change in baccalaureate programs, 490, 504
Cushing's syndrome, 181
Custom, 506
CVA; *see* Cerebral vascular accident
CVP; *see* Central venous pressure
Cyanocobalamin; *see* Vitamins, B$_{12}$
Cyanotic heart defects, 427-428
Cyantin; *see* Nitrofurantoin
Cyclaine Hydrochloride; *see* Hexylcaine hydrochloride
Cyclandelate, 68
Cyclogyl; *see* Cyclopentolate
Cyclomethycaine, 26
Cyclopentolate, 218
Cyclophosphamide, 39, 40
  breast carcinoma and, 164
  in leukemia, 451
  side effects of, 452
Cyclopropane, 25
Cycloserine, 36
Cyclospasmol; *see* Cyclandelate
Cyclothymic personality, 345
Cyproheptadine hydrochloride, 93
Cystectomy, 155
Cystic duct, 107
Cystic fibrosis, 448-449
Cystine stones, 151
Cystitis, 150-151
Cystocele, 162-163, 386
Cystoscopy, 150
Cysts, 252
Cytarabine, 38
Cytolysis, 63

Cytomel; *see* Liothyronine sodium
Cytosar; *see* Cytarabine
Cytoxan; *see* Cyclophosphamide

D

Dactinomycin, 39, 40
Dalmane; *see* Flurazepam hydrochloride
Dalton's law, 90
Dance reflex, 380
Dapsone, 35
Daranide; *see* Dichlorphenamide
Daraprim; *see* Pyrimethamine
Darbid; *see* Isopropamide
Darvon; *see* Propoxyphene hydrochloride
Daunomycin, 39
Daunorubicin, 451
Davis Social Adequacy Index, 208
Davoxin; *see* Digoxin
Day-care facilities, 7
DBI; *see* Phenformin hydrochloride
Deafness, 208, 425, 446
Deamination, 107
Death, child and, 451-452
Debridement, 253
Decadron; *see* Dexamethasone
Decapryn; *see* Doxylamine succinate
Declomycin; *see* Demeclocycline
Defecation, 108; *see also* Constipation; Diarrhea
    retraining and, 242-243
Defective child, parent reactions to, 422-423;
        see also Congenital abnormalities
Defense mechanisms, 330, 331
Defibrillator, 58
Dehydration
    diarrhea and, 436
    integumentary system and, 249
    sickle cell anemia and, 449
Delalutin; *see* Hydroxyprogesterone caproate
Delatestryl; *see* Testosterone enanthate
Delivery
    of baby; *see* Maternity nursing
    of health services, community and, 326
    of nursing care, methods of, 8
Demecarium, 218
Demeclocycline, 33
Demerol; *see* Meperidine hydrochloride
Demulen; *see* Ethinyl estradiol and ethynodiol
        diacetate
Denaturation of proteins, 116
Dendrites, 183
Denial, 331, 333
Denis Browne splint, 432
Deoxyribonucleic acid, 116-117
    testes and, 166

Deoxyribose, 113
Department of Family and Children's Services,
    395
Depo-Heparin Sodium; *see* Heparin sodium
Depo-Provera; *see* Medroxyprogesterone acetate
Depo-Testosterone; *see* Testosterone cypionate
Depression
    illness and, 334
    involutional psychosis and, 340
    manic-depressive psychosis and, 338-340
    in neurotic reactions, 344
    psychotic depressive reactions and, 340
Dermabrasion, 254
Dermatitis, contact, 254
Dermis, 248
Dermoplast; *see* Benzocaine
DES; *see* Diethylstilbestrol
Deserpidine, 67
Desiccation, 21
Desipramine hydrochloride, 339
Detached retina, 246
Development
    communication and level of, 10
    of fetus, 371-372
    growth and; *see* Growth and development
    of individual, 147-148
    of personality, 327-330
    timetables of
        for adolescent, 460
        for infant, 416-418
        for preschool-age child, 450
        for school-age child, 454
        for toddler, 438-439
Deviate patterns of behavior, 334-336
Dexamethasone, 174
Dexedrine; *see* Dextroamphetamine sulfate
Dextran, 69
Dextran 40, 69
Dextran 70, 69
Dextroamphetamine sulfate, 119
Dextromethorphan hydrobromide, 92
Dextrose, 114; *see also* Glucose
    50%, in hypoglycemia, 180
Diabetes insipidus, 176
Diabetes mellitus, 178-180
    in child, 455-456
    pregnancy and, 387-388
Diabetic coma, 180, 455
Diabinese; *see* Chlorpropamide
Dialysis, 153
Diamox; *see* Acetazolamide
Diaper rash, 459
Diaphragm for contraception, 147, 393
Diaphragmatic hernia, 426

Diapid; *see* Lypressin
Diarrhea, 436
    diet and, 420
    drugs for, 119-120
    epidemic, 389
Diarthrotic joints, 203-205
Diasone Sodium; *see* Sulfoxone sodium
Diazepam, 216, 217, 229, 344
Diazoxide, 67
Dibucaine, 26
DIC; *see* Disseminated intravascular coagulation
Dichlorphenamide, 219
Diclonine hydrochloride, 26
Dicodid; *see* Hydrocodone bitartrate
Dicumarol, 34, 70
Dicyclomine hydrochloride, 119
Didrex; *see* Benzphetamine hydrochloride
Diencephalon, 188
Dienestrol, 392
Diet; *see also* Feeding; Nutrition
    alkaline-ash, 235
    in celiac disease, 420, 448
    in cirrhosis, 132-133
    in cystic fibrosis, 449
    in diabetes mellitus, 179
        for child, 455, 456
    in diarrhea, 436
    in hepatitis, 131-132
    infant and modifications of, 420
    liquid, 31
    low-phenylalanine, 420, 434
    renal failure and, 152, 153
    in renal and ureteral calculi, 151
    soft, 31
Diethyl ether, 25
Diethylpropion hydrochloride, 119
Diethylstilbestrol, 157
    cancer and, 38, 158
Diffraction, 211-212
Diffusion
    gastrointestinal system and, 113
    respiratory system and, 88, 89
Digestion, 108-109
Digestive system; *see* Gastrointestinal system
Digitaline; *see* Digitoxin
Digitalis, 64
    adverse effects of, 428-429
    congenital heart defects and, 428-429
    congestive heart failure and, 77
    hyperthyroidism and, 177
    myocardial infarction and, 75
    pregnancy and, 387
    pulmonary edema and, 96
Digitalization, 428-429

Digitoxin, 64
Digits, developmental anomalies of, 434
Digoxin, 17, 64, 428, 429
Dihycon; *see* Phenytoin
Dihydroindolone, 342
Dihydrotachysterol, 178, 216
Dihydroxyacetone, 113
Di-Lan; *see* Phenytoin
Dilantin; *see* Phenytoin
Dilation and curettage of uterus, 384, 394
Dilaudid; *see* Hydromorphone hydrochloride
Dilor; *see* Dyphylline
Dilute solution, 60
Dimenhydrinate, 118
Dimercaprol, 443
Dimetane; *see* Brompheniramine maleate
Dimethisoquin hydrochloride, 26
Dimethone; *see* Dipyrone
Dinoprost tromethamine, 394
Dioctyl calcium sulfosuccinate, 120
Dioctyl sodium sulfosuccinate, 120
Diothane Hydrochloride; *see* Diperodon hydro-
    chloride
Diperodon hydrochloride, 26
Diphenhydramine, 92, 93, 342
Diphenidol hydrochloride, 118
Diphenoxylate hydrochloride, 120
Diphtheria, tetanus, and pertussis, 420, 421
Diphtheria and tetanus toxoids, 420
Diphtheria toxoid, 420, 421
Diphyllobothrium latum, 118
Diplococci, 18; *see also Diplococcus pneu-
    moniae*
Diplococcus pneumoniae, 18, 19, 91, 437
Diploma nursing programs, 486, 497-498
Dipyrone, 28
Disaccharide, 113
Disc, slipped, 238
Discipline, 439
Discomfort, need for relief from, 329
Diseases; *see also* Syndromes
    Addison's, 181-182
    Alzheimer's, 337
    Buerger's, 80
    celiac, 420, 448
    Crohn's, 134-135
    Graves', 176-177
    Hanson's, 35
    hemolytic, of newborn, 389-390
    Hirschsprung's, 435
    Hodgkin's, 85
    hyaline membrane, 388
    Meniere's, 247
    Parkinson's, 228, 230-231

Diseases—cont'd
    pelvic inflammatory, 161-162
    Pick's, 337
    Raynaud's, 80
    Simmonds', 175-176
Disinfection, 21
Dislocations, 380, 389, 433
Disopyramide phosphate, 65
Displacement
    as defense mechanism, 331
    of uterus, 386
Disseminated intravascular coagulation, 70, 84
Dissociative reactions, 343
Distillation, 25
Disulfiram, 346
Diuresis, 143
Diuretics, 68-69, 216; *see also* specific drug
Diuril; *see* Chlorothiazide
Diurnal-Penicillin; *see* Penicillin G procaine
DNA; *see* Deoxyribonucleic acid
DNA viruses, 91, 215
Doctoral degree programs, 486
Dog tapeworm, 118
Dominant traits, 148
Dopamine, 184, 214, 230
Dopar; *see* Levodopa
Doppler effect, 207
Doriden; *see* Glutethimide
Dormethan; *see* Dextromethorphan hydrobro-
    mide
Dorsacaine; *see* Benoxinate hydrochloride
Dorsal column stimulator, 237
Dosage-response relationships, 16
Douches, 160, 161
Down's syndrome, 148, 423
Doxepin hydrochloride, 339
Doxinate; *see* Dioctyl sodium sulfosuccinate
Doxorubicin, 39, 85, 164
Doxycycline hyclate, 33
Doxylamine succinate, 93
Dramamine; *see* Dimenhydrinate
Dramicillin; *see* Penicillin G potassium
Drenison; *see* Flurandrenolone
Drolban; *see* Androgens
Droperidol, 342
Drug dependency, 336, 347
    newborn and, 390
Drug dosage forms, 16-17
Drug interactions, 16
    acetylsalicylic acid and, 17
    alcohol and, 339, 344
    anesthetics and, 339
    anticholinergics and, 339
    anticoagulants and, 34, 36, 353, 458, 459

Drug interactions—cont'd
    antihistamines and, 339
    barbiturates and, 36, 339, 353, 429
    central nervous system depressants and, 339
    chloramphenicol and, 34
    cocaine and, 339
    corticoids and, 339
    digitalis and, 429
    indomethacin and, 459
    iron and, 448
    magnesium trisilicate and, 448
    methotrexate and, 458
    narcotics and, 339
    oral hypoglycemics and, 458
    penicillins and, 457
    phenobarbital and, 17, 36, 429
    phenylbutazone and, 429
    phenytoin and, 34, 215, 429
    probenecid and, 457, 459
    salicylates and, 17, 457, 458-459
    sedatives and, 344, 353
    sodium bicarbonate and, 33
    sulfonamides and, 457, 458, 459
    sympathomimetic drugs and, 339
    tetracycline and, 17, 448
Drugs; *see also* specific drug
    actions of, 15-16
    addiction and, 336, 346-347
    administration of, 14-18
    for anesthesia, 25-27, 339
    antianxiety, 344
    antiarrhythmic, 64-66
    antibiotic; *see* Antibiotics
    anticholinergic; *see* Anticholinergics
    anticonvulsant, 215-216, 228-229
    antidepressant, 339
    antidiarrheal, 119-120
    antiemetic, 118
    antifungal, 36, 250
    antihistaminic, 92, 93, 339
    anti-inflammatory, 251
    antimalarial, 37
    antimetabolic, 16, 38, 164
    antineoplastic, 38-40; *see also* Chemotherapy
    antiparasitic, 36-38
    antiparkinsonism, 216-217, 342
    antiprotozoan, 160-161
    antipruritic, 251
    antithyroid, 173-174, 177
    antitussive, 92
    antiviral, 34
    for bronchial relaxation, 91-92, 453
    cardiac glycosides and, 64
    circulatory system and, 64-70

Drugs—cont'd
for constipation, 120-121
effects of, 15
endocrine disorders and, 173-175
expectorants as, 92, 453-454
for eye, 218-219, 223
forms of, 16-17
gastrointestinal system and, 118-121
infection control and, 32-38
infertility and sterility and, 392-393
integumentary system and, 250-251
interactions of; see Drug interactions
legislation and, 14
for *Mycobacterium tuberculosis,* 35-36
neuromusculoskeletal systems and, 215-219
nomenclature and, 16
for pain control, 37-38
preoperative and postoperative care and, 25-28
psychiatric nursing and; see Psychiatric nursing
reproductive system and, 156-158
respiratory system and, 91-93
for sedation and sleep, 27, 344, 352-353
sources of, 16
standards for, 14-15
Dry phlebotomy, 77, 96-97
DT toxoids; see Diphtheria and tetanus toxoids
DTP; see Diphtheria, tetanus, and pertussis
Ducts
of liver, 107
of male reproductive system, 144
Ductus arteriosus, 372, 426
patent, 427
Ductus venosus, 372, 426
Dulcolax; see Bisacodyl
Dumping syndrome, 126, 127
Dunant, H., 484
Duodenum, 106
Duphaston; see Dydrogesterone
Dura mater, 189
Durabolin; see Nandrolone phenpropionate
Duracillin A.S.; see Penicillin G procaine
Durandro; see Testosterone cypionate
DV; see Dienestrol
Dwarf tapeworm, 118
Dyclone; see Dyclonine hydrochloride
Dyclonine hydrochloride, 26
Dydrogesterone, 146
Dymelor; see acetohexamide
Dyphylline, 91, 453
Dyrenium; see Triamterene
Dyspareunia, 395
Dystocia, 385-386

E

Eardrops, 437
Ears, 197
deafness and, 208, 425, 446
disorders of, 246-247
eardrops and, 437
irrigations of, 223
Eccrine glands, 248
Echinococcus granulosa, 118
Echothiophate, 218
Eclampsia, 383-384
Economic factors, nursing and, 488-489, 490-491, 501, 505-506
Ecotrin; see Acetylsalicylic acid
Ectoderm, 147
Ectopic pregnancy, 384
Eczema, 438, 452
Edecrin; see Ethacrynic acid
Edema
congestive heart failure and, 76
nephrosis and, 452
pulmonary, 96-97
Edrophonium, 217, 232
Education for nurses
in Canada, 496-501
in United States, 485-487, 489-490
The Education of Nursing Technicians, 481, 485
Efferent neurons, 183
Effervescent sodium phosphate, 121
Ego, 328
Ejaculation, 370
Ejaculatory ducts, 144
EKKO; see Phenytoin
Elasticity, concept of, 56, 149, 249
Elavil; see Amitriptyline hydrochloride
Electric force, 47
Electricity, 23-24, 57-58
Electrocardiograms, 24, 58
Electroconvulsive therapy, 338, 341, 342
Electrolytes
balance of, 40-43
maintaining concentration of, 42-43
strength of, 46
Electromagnetic radiation, 58
light and, 208-209
neuromusculoskeletal systems and, 207
wavelengths of, 58, 209
Electronic stimulation, 237
Electronic thermometers, 24
Electrons, 46, 57
Electrosurgery, 24
Elixir of terpin hydrate, 453-454
Elixophyllin; see Theophylline
Elkosin; see Sulfisomidine

Emboli, 78-80
pulmonary, 96
Embryonic period, 147
Emetine hydrochloride, 37
Emmetropia, 213
Emotions
behavior and, 331-332
color and, 210
Emphysema, 100
Employee, nurse as, 509
Empyema, 97-98
E-Mycin; see Erythromycins
Endarterectomy, carotid, 227
Endocarditis, subacute bacterial, 76
Endocardium, 51, 76
Endocrine system, 166-182; see also specific gland
anatomy and physiology of, 166-173
diseases of, 175-182
pregnancy and, 387-388
newborn and, 381
pharmacology of, 173-175
pregnancy and, 372
Endoderm, 147
Endometriosis, 161
Endoplasmic reticulum, 198
Endorphins, 185
Endoscopy, 121
Endothyrin; see Thyroglobulin
Endotoxins, 23
Endoxan; see Cyclophosphamide
Enduron; see Methyclothiazide
Enemas, 122
barium, 112, 121-122
Energy
circulatory system and, 56
conservation of, 56
gastrointestinal system and, 111-112
genitourinary system and, 149
neuromusculoskeletal systems and, 206
respiratory system and, 90
Enflurane, 25
Enkephalins, 185
Enkide; see Potassium iodide
Enovid; see Mestranol-norethynodrel
Entamoeba histolytica, 117
Enteritis, regional, 133-134
Enterobacter, 32, 149
Enterobius vermicularis, 118
Enterocrinin, 117
Enterogastrone, 117
Entry, portals of, 23
Enucleation, 244
Enuresis, 349

Environment
  teaching-learning, 11-14
  transient situational disturbances and, 349
Enzymes
  chemistry of, 59
  debridement and, 253
  gastrointestinal system and, 117
  pancreatic, cystic fibrosis and, 448, 449
  serum, 74
Ephedrine sulfate, 92
Epidemic diarrhea, 389
Epidermis, 248
Epididymis, 144, 159
Epididymitis, 159
Epidural hemorrhage, 224
Epifrin; *see* Epinephrine
Epiglottitis, 437
Epilepsy, 215-216, 228-229
Epinephrine
  adrenal gland and, 169, 170
  aqueous, 92
  in asthma, 453
  heart rate and, 66
  metabolism and, 111
  pheochromocytoma and, 182
  respiratory system and, 92
Episiotomy, 386
Epispadias, 380, 432
Episilon-aminocaproic acid, 226, 456
Epsom salt; *see* Magnesium sulfate
Epstein-Barr virus, 99
Equanil; *see* Meprobamate
Equgen; *see* Conjugated estrogens
Erb-Duchenne paralysis, 389
Ergonovine maleate, 377
Ergosterol, 115
Ergotamine with caffeine, 223
Ergotamine tartrate, 223
Ergotrate Maleate; *see* Ergonovine maleate
Erikson, E., 328, 329
ERV; *see* Expiratory reserve volume
Erythrityl tetranitrate, 66
Erythrocin; *see* Erythromycins
Erythrocin Ethylsuccinate; *see* Erythromycin
    ethylsuccinate
Erythrocyte sedimentation rate, 457
Erythrocytes, 49
  drugs affecting building of, 70
  sedimentation rate and, 457
  synthetic, 105
Erythromycin ethylsuccinate, 33
Erythromycins, 33, 457
Escherichia coli, 19, 20
  bladder and, 150

Escherichia coli—cont'd
  epidemic diarrhea and, 389
  gastrointestinal system and, 117
  osteomyelitis and, 235
  pyelonephritis in pregnancy and, 388
  urethritis and, 156
Esidrix; *see* Hydrochlorothiazide
Eskalith; *see* Lithium carbonate
Esophagectomy, 128
Esophagogastrostomy, 128
Esophagus, 106
  absence or atresia of, 425
  cancer of, 128
Essential hypertension, 73, 348
Esterified estrogens, 157, 392
Estimated date of delivery, 373
Estinyl; *see* Ethinyl estradiol
Estradiol, 371, 392
Estradiol cypionate, 157
Estradiol valerate, 157
Estrifol; *see* Esterified estrogens
Estrogen and progesterone sequential contraceptives, 158
Estrogen and progesterone tablets, 158
Estrogens, 156-157
  abortion and, 394
  breast carcinoma and, 164
  in chemotherapy, 38
  esterified, 157, 392
  lactation and, 146
  menopause and, 395
  menstrual cycle and, 146, 371
  osteoporosis and, 236
  ovaries and, 168, 169
  placenta and, 372
  pregnancy and, 148
  and progestins, combined, 158, 393
  prostatic cancer and, 158
  sterility and infertility and, 392
  vaginitis and, 161
Estrone, 157, 392
Estrusol; *see* Estrone
Ethacrynic acid, 69
Ethambutol hydrochloride, 36
Ethamide; *see* Ethoxzolamide
Ethchlorvynol, 27, 353
Ether, 25
Ethics, code of, 503-504
Ethinamate, 27, 353
Ethinyl estradiol, 38, 157, 392
    and ethynodiol diacetate, 158, 393
    and norethindrone acetate, 158, 393
    and norgestrel, 158, 393
Ethionamide, 36

Ethisterone, 146
Ethopropazine hydrochloride, 216, 217
Ethosuximide, 216, 229
Ethoxzolamide, 219
Ethrane; *see* Enflurane
Ethyl alcohol, 22
Ethyl chloride, 25
Ethylene, 25
Ethylene oxide, 22
Ethylnorepinephrine hydrochloride, 92
Eubacteriales, 18-19
Eucatropine, 218
Evaluation, learning and, 14
Evaluation of the Metropolitan School of Nursing, 491-492
Evaporation, 25, 249
Evex; *see* Esterified estrogens
Examination, preparation for, 1-3
Exchange transfusion, 390
Excretory system; *see* Genitourinary system
Exhibitionism, 346
Exit, portals of, 23
Exotoxins, 23
Expandex; *see* Dextran
Expectorants, 92, 453-454
Expert witness, 509
Expiration, 87
Expiratory reserve volume, 88
Exploratory thoracotomy, 103
Explosive personality, 345
Exstrophy of bladder, 432
Extended care facilities, 6-7, 491
External degree program, 489-490
Exteroceptors, 195
Extracellular fluid, 40, 41
  pH of, 48
Extrapyramidal symptoms, 342
Extrapyramidal tracts, 191-193
Extrauterine life, adaptation to, 378-381
Extremities, developmental anomalies of, 434
Eye, 196-197
  disorders of, 243-246, 446-447
  drugs for, 218-219
    instillation of, 223
  examination of, 214
  lasers and, 209
  light principles and, 208-214
  physiology of vision and, 196-197
  tumors of, 244-245

F

Facial malformations, 424
Facial paralysis of newborn, 389
Facilitatory tracts, 193

Factor replacement, 456
Fahrenheit temperature, 24
Failure to thrive syndrome, 435-436
Fallopian tubes, 145
　ligation of, 147, 158
　rupture of, 384
Fallot's tetralogy, 427-428
Family, 414
　individual in, 324
　in society, 324
　structure and functions of, 414
Family planning, 146, 147, 157-158, 393
Fantasy, 331
Fasciola hepatica, 118
Fasciolopsis buski, 118
Fathering, 378
Fat-soluble solutions, 249
Fats, 114; *see also* Lipids
　absorption of, 109
　liver and, 107
Fatty acids, 114, 170
Fears
　in children, 451
　illness and, 333
Febrile convulsions, 438
Febrile reaction to blood transfusion, 29
Febrolin; *see* Acetaminophen
Fecal fat test, 134
Feces; *see* Defecation; Stools
Federal legislation, 488-489
Federal Security Agency Appropriations Act, 488
Feeding; *see also* Diet; Nutrition
　blindness and, 447
　cerebral palsy and, 445
　cleft lip and, 424
　cleft palate and, 424-425
　of infant, 418-420
　　schedules for, 383
　laryngeal stridor and, 426
　pyloric stenosis and, 435
Feet, fungal infection of, 459
Fellozine; *see* Promethazine hydrochloride
Felsules; *see* Chloral hydrate
Female
　bone structure of, 205
　infertility and sterility in, 392-393
　puberty in, 370
　reproductive system of, 145-146; *see also* Reproductive system
　role patterns of, altered, 324
　sex hormones of, 168-169
　sterilization of, 393
Feminone; *see* Ethinyl estradiol

Femogen; *see* Esterified estrogens
Femoral hernias, 138
Femoropopliteal bypass grafting, 80-81
Femur, dislocation of, 433
Fendon; *see* Acetaminophen
Fenfluramine hydrochloride, 119
Fermentation, 19
Ferric chloride urine test, 434
Ferro Drops; *see* Ferrous lactate
Ferrocholinate, 70, 448
Ferrolip; *see* Ferrocholinate
Ferrous fumarate, 70, 448
Ferrous gluconate, 70, 448
Ferrous lactate, 70, 448
Ferrous sulfate, 70, 448
Fertilization, 147, 371
$FeSO_4$; *see* Iron (II) sulfate
Fetal alcohol syndrome, 390
Fetal circulation, 52, 372
Fetishism, 346
Fetus, 147
　alcohol and, 390
　androgens and, 168
　circulation of, 52, 372
　growth and development of, 147, 371-372
Fever
　convulsions and, 438
　transfusion reactions and, 29
Fibrillation, ventricular, 71
Fibrin, 50
Fibrinogen, 50, 456
Fibroplasia, 249
Fidler, N., 491
Filtration, microbes and, 21
Final common path principle, 190-191
Fish tapeworm, 118
Fistulas
　rectovaginal, 162
　tracheoesophageal, 425
　ureterovaginal, 162
　vaginal, 162
　vesicovaginal, 162
Flaccidity
　bladder and, 243
　cerebral palsy and, 445
　paralysis and, 241
Flagella, 19
Flagyl; *see* Metronidazole
Flail chest, 102
Flavoquin; *see* Amodiaquine hydrochloride
Fleet Phospho-Soda; *see* Effervescent sodium phosphate
Florinef Acetate; *see* Fludrocortisone acetate
Floropryl; *see* Isoflurophate

Floxuridine, 38
Fludrocortisone acetate, 174
Fluids; *see also* Water
　and electrolytes
　　balance of, 40-43
　　chemistry and, 46-48
　　maintaining body volume of, 42
Flukes, 118
Fluocinolone acetonide, 251
Fluocinonide, 251
Fluonid; *see* Fluocinolone acetonide
Fluorescence, 209
Fluoride, infants and, 419
Fluorine, 215
Fluoromar; *see* Fluroxene
Fluoroscopy, 112
Fluorouracil, 38, 40
　breast cancer and, 164
　laryngeal carcinoma and, 103
　stomach cancer and, 127
Fluosol; *see* Erythrocytes, synthetic
Fluothane; *see* Halothane
Fluoxymesterone, 157, 392
Fluphenazine, 234, 341
Flurandrenolone, 251
Flurazepam hydrochloride, 27, 353
Fluroxene, 25
Focal-motor seizures, 228
Focal point, 212
Focusing, 213-214
Folate sodium, 70
Folic acid, 49, 70, 374
Folic acid antagonist, 38
Follicle-stimulating hormone, 146, 171
　conception enhancers and, 392, 393
　menstrual cycle and, 371
Follutein; *see* Chorionic gonadotropin
Folvite; *see* Folic acid
Folvite Sodium; *see* Folate sodium
Food poisoning, 139-140
Foramen ovale, 372, 426
　failure to close, 427
Forebrain, 188
Foreign objects, aspiration of, 443
Formulas for infants, 382, 419
Foster frame, 219
Four-point alternate crutch gait, 221
Fractures, 239-240
　in children, 443
　head trauma and, 224
　of hip, 240-241
　of jaw, 125
　newborn and, 380, 389
　reduction of, 239, 240

Fractures—cont'd
  types of, 239
  of vertebrae, 241
Fraud, 507
Fredet-Ramstedt procedure, 435
Freezing of tissue, 231, 246, 256
Frejka pillow, 433
Freud, S., 328, 329
Friction, 56, 249
Friedländer's bacillus, 91, 98
Friedman's test, 373
Frontal lobes of brain, 189
Fructose, 114
FSH; see Follicle-stimulating hormone
5-FU; see Fluorouracil
Fulvicin-U/F; see Griseofulvin
Functional nursing, 8
Functional psychoses, 338-343
Fungi, 20-21
  drugs for, 36, 250; see also specific drug
  mouth and, 124
  neuromusculoskeletal systems and, 215
  newborn and, 389
  respiratory system and, 91, 98
  skin infections in children and, 459
  superinfection and, 32, 457
  vaginitis and, 160
Fungi Imperfecti, 21
Fungicide, 21
Fungizone; see amphotericin B
Furacin; see Nitrofurazone
Furadantin; see Nitrofurantoin
Furalan; see Nitrofurantoin
Furazolidone-nifuroxime, 161
Furosemide, 69, 77

G

GABA; see Gamma-aminobutyric acid
Gaits for crutch walking, 221-222
Galactose, 114, 420, 434
Galactosemia, 420, 434
Galeazzi's sign, 433
Gallbladder, 128, 129
Gametes, 147
Gamma-aminobutyric acid, 184, 214
Gamma benzene hexachloride, 250
Gamma globulins, 49, 62-63
Gamma ray, 61
Ganglia, 185
Ganphen; see Promethazine hydrochloride
Gantanol; see Sulfamethoxazole
Gantrisin; see Sulfisoxazole
Garamycin; see Gentamicin sulfate
GAS; see General adaptation syndrome

Gases
  circulatory system and, 57
  gastrointestinal system and, 112
  respiratory system and, 88, 89, 90
Gastrectomy, 126, 127
Gastric analysis, 122
Gastric gavage, 123-124
Gastric juice, 48, 109
Gastrin, 109, 117
Gastritis, 125-126
Gastrointestinal series, 112, 121
Gastrointestinal system, 105-140
  active transport and, 113
  anatomy and physiology in, 105-111
  chemistry and, 112-117
  diseases of, 124-140
    cholecystitis in, 128-129
    cirrhosis in, 132-133
    Crohn's disease and, 134-135
    esophageal cancer in, 128
    food poisoning in, 139-140
    gastritis in, 125-126
    hemorrhoids in, 138
    hepatitis in, 131-132
    hernias in, 138-139
    hiatus hernia in, 127-128
    intestinal cancer in, 136-137
    intestinal obstruction in, 135-136
    jaw fracture in, 125
    liver carcinoma in, 133
    mouth cancer in, 125
    pancreatic cancer in, 130-131
    pancreatitis in, 129-130
    peptic ulcer in, 126-127
    peritonitis in, 137-138
    regional enteritis in, 133-134
    stomach carcinoma in, 127
    stomatitis in, 124-125
    ulcerative colitis in, 135
  growth and, 415
  microorganisms and, 117-118
  newborn and, 380-381
  pharmacology and, 118-121
  physics and, 111-112
  postpartal period and, 377
  pregnancy and, 372
  procedures and, 121-124
Gastrostomy, 128
Gelusil; see Aluminum hydroxide with magnesium trisilicate
General adaptation syndrome, 5, 327
Generalist, 486
Genes, 148
Genitourinary system, 140-165

Genitourinary system—cont'd
  anatomy and physiology of, 140-148
  chemistry and, 149
  diseases of, 150-156
  growth and, 415
  infection of, in children, 452
  microorganisms and, 149-150
  newborn and, 380
  physics and, 148-149
  postpartal period and, 377
  pregnancy and, 372-373
  procedures and, 150
  reproductive system in; see Reproductive system
Gentamicin sulfate, 33, 253
Gentian violet, 160, 250, 389
Geopen; see Carbenicillin disodium
Germicide, 21
Gesterol; see Progesterone
Gexane; see Gamma benzene hexachloride
GH; see Growth hormone
GI series; see Gastrointestinal series
Giardia lamblia, 117
Gigantism, 175
Ginsberg, E., 481
The Ginsberg Report, 481
Giordano-Giovannetti regimen, modified, 153
Girard, A. M., 496, 499
Gitaligin; see Gitalin
Gitalin, 64
Glands
  adrenal; see Adrenal glands
  of endocrine system; see Endocrine system
  female reproductive, 145-146
    ovaries as, 167, 168-169
  of integumentary system, 248
    cystic fibrosis and, 449
  male reproductive, 144
    testes as, 167-168, 169
  mammary, 146, 248
    carcinoma of, 163-164
  salivary, 106
  of stomach, 106
Glaucoma, 245-246
Glen procedure, 428
Gliomas, 224
Globulins, 59, 115
  gamma, 49, 62-63
Globus pallidus destruction, 231
Glomerular filtration, 141, 142, 143
Glomerulonephritis, 155
Glucagon, 110, 172, 173, 180
Glucocorticoids, 115, 169, 170
  in Addison's disease, 181-182

Glucocorticoids—cont'd
  excessive, 181
  metabolism and, 111
Gluconeogenesis, 107, 110
Glucose, 114
  50%, carbon monoxide poisoning and, 105
  diabetes mellitus and, 179, 180
  drugs and assimilation of, 173
  muscles and, 198
  pancreas and, 172
  renal tubules and, 141
  transport of, 110
  in urine, tests for, 113
Glucotropin-Forte; *see* Chorionic gonadotropin
Glucuronyl transferase, 422
Glutamic acid, 184, 214
Gluteline, 115
Gluten, 420, 448
Glutethimide, 27, 353
Glycerin, 219
Glycerol, iodinated, 92
Glycerose, 113
Glyceryl guaiacolate, 92, 454
Glycine, 184, 214
Glycogen, 114, 169
Glycogenesis, 107, 108, 110
Glycogenolysis, 107, 110
Glycolysis, 110
Glycoproteins, 115
Glyestrin; *see* Esterified estrogens
Glyrol; *see* Glycerin
Goblet cells, 100
Goiter, 177
Gold
  compounds of, 131, 217, 218
  neuromusculoskeletal systems and, 215
  radioactive, 39
Goldmark, J., 481
The Goldmark Report, 481
Gonadal dysgenesis, 423
Gonadotropic hormones
  menopause and, 395
  pituitary gland and, 188
  placenta and, 372
Gonadotropins
  chorionic, 148, 372, 373, 393
  menopause and, 395
Gonads; *see also* Reproductive system
  female, 145
  fertility and, 392-393; *see also* Reproductive
    system
  male, 144
Gonococci; *see* Neisseria gonorrhoeae
Gonorrhea, 165; *see also Neisseria gonorrhoeae*

Goodell's sign, 372
Gooseflesh, 249
Gout, 218, 235
Gouty arthritis, 235
Government agencies, 5, 395
Graafian follicles, 145
The Grading Committee Report, 481
Grading Committee Study, 487
Graduate degree nursing programs, 486, 499
Grafts
  femoropopliteal bypass, 80-81
  of skin, 251-252
Gram-negative bacilli, 18, 19, 91, 150; *see also*
    specific organism
Gram-negative cocci, 19, 91
Gram-positive bacilli, 19
Gram-positive cocci, 18, 62, 91, 139
Gram stain, 20
Grand mal seizures, 228
Grasp reflex, 380
Graves' disease, 176-177
Gravindex, 373
Gravitation, law of, 55, 89, 111, 206
Gray baby syndrome, 34
Gray matter, 185, 186, 187
Great vessels, transposition of, 428
Greenstick fractures, 239, 443
Grey Nuns, 496, 498
Grifulvin V; *see* Griseofulvin
Grisactin; *see* Griseofulvin
Griseofulvin, 36, 353, 459
Groups, 325
  peer, 324-325, 460
Growth
  characteristics of, 415-416
  and development, 414-416; *see also* Devel-
    opment
    of adolescent, 460
    of infant, 416-418
    infant feeding and, 418
    of preschool-age child, 450
    of school-age child, 454
    of toddler, 438-439
  potential for, 332
  principles of, 414-415
Growth charts, 418
Growth hormone, 111, 171, 372
Guaiac, 122
Guaifenesin; *see* Glyceryl guaiacolate
Guanethidine sulfate, 67
Guillain-Barré syndrome, 233
Gummas, 165
Guthrie blood test, 434
Gynergen; *see* Ergotamine tartrate

Gynorest; *see* Dydrogesterone

H

Habituation, 347
Haemophilus aegyptius, 215
Haemophilus ducreyi, 149-150
Haemophilus influenzae, 91, 98, 437
Hair, 248-249
Hair dye, 254
Haldol; *see* Haloperidol
Halogens, 215
Haloperidol, 234, 342
Halotestin; *see* Fluoxymesterone
Halothane, 25, 131
Hansen's disease, 35
Harmonyl; *see* Deserpidine
Harris flush or drip, 122
The Hasting Report, 505
H_3BO_3; *see* Boric acid
HCG; *see* Human chorionic gonadotropin
HCl; *see* Hydrochloric acid
H_2CO_3; *see* Carbonic acid
Head injuries, 224
Headaches, migraine, 223-224
Health
  basic concepts of, 4-5
  culture and, 323
  definition of, 4
  sociology and, 325-326
Health Amendments Act, 488
Health Disciplines Act, 501-502
Health field concept, 505-506
Health-illness continuum, 4-5
Health problems
  of infants, 422-438; *see also* Infant
  preschool-age child and, 451-454
  school-age child and, 455-460
Health promotion
  for adolescent, 461
  during childhood, 440
Health resources, 5-7
Health services
  delivery of, 326
  personnel and, 7
    increase in number and type of, 491
Hearing, 197
  loss of, 208, 425, 446
  physiology of, 197
Hearing aids, 208
Heart, 50-52; *see also* Circulatory system
  congenital defects of, 426-430
  congestive failure of, 76-77
  inflammations of, 76
  Starling's law of, 53

Heart block, 71, 72

Heart failure, congestive, 76-77

Heart rate, 54
    antiarrhythmics and, 64-66; *see also* specific drug
    drugs for increasing, 66
    growth and, 415

Heart sounds, 52

Heat, 24-25, 112, 249

Hegar's sign, 372

Height
    of infant, 416, 417
    of school-age child, 454
    of toddler, 439

Heimlich maneuver, 443

Hemangioblastomas, 224

Hematinics, 70

Hematocrit, 50

Hemicolectomy, 136

Hemiplegia, 226

Hemodialysis, 153

Hemofil; *see* Antihemophilic factor

Hemoglobin, 49
    growth and, 415
    sickle cell anemia and, 449-450

Hemolytic disease of newborn, 389-390

Hemolytic reactions to blood transfusion, 29

Hemophilia, 456-457

Hemopoiesis, 199

Hemorrhage
    cerebral, 224, 225-226
    head trauma and, 224
    intracranial, of newborn, 388-389
    during maternity cycle, 384-385

Hemorrhoids, 138

Hemostasis, 50

Hemothorax, 101

Henry's law, 90

Heparin sodium, 70, 84

Hepatic cirrhosis, 132-133; *see also* Liver

Hepatic coma, 132, 133

Hepatic duct, 107

Hepatic portal circulation, 53

Hepatitis, 131-132

Heredity, 148

Hering-Breuer reflex, 88

Hernias, 138-139
    diaphragmatic, 426
    hiatus, 127-128
    of intervertebral disc, 238
    muscle weakness and, 199

Hernioplasty, 139

Herniorrhaphy, 139

Herpes genitalia, 165

Herpes simplex, 124

Herpes zoster, 256-257

Herpesviruses, 215

Hexadrol; *see* Dexamethasone

Hexastrol, 392

Hexobarbital, 27, 352

Hexylcaine hydrochloride, 26

Hexylresorcinol, 447

Hiatus hernia, 127-128

Hierarchy of needs, 10

Higher degree nursing programs, 486, 499

Hill-Burton Act, 489

Hindbrain, 187

Hip
    dislocation of, 380, 433
    fractures of, 240-241

Hiprex; *see* Methenamine hippurate

Hirschsprung's disease, 435

Histadyl; *see* Methapyrilene hydrochloride

Histamine, 63, 214

Histaspan; *see* Chlorpheniramine maleate

Histone, 115

Histoplasma capsulatum, 91

History
    family, newborn and, 377-378
    of nursing, 480-509; *see also* Nursing
    of patient, 11

Hodgkin's disease, 85

Holocaine Hydrochloride; *see* Phenacaine hydrochloride

Holoenzyme, 59

Holotestin; *see* Androgens

Homans' sign, 78

Homatropine hydrobromide, 218

Home care, 7

Homografts, 251

Homosexuality, 346

Hookworm, 117

Hopkins-Cole test, 116

Hordeolum, 244

Hormale Aqueous; *see* Testosterone

Hormale Oil; *see* Testosterone propionate

Hormone-releasing hormones, 184-185

Hormones
    adrenal; *see* Adrenal glands
    adrenocorticotropic; *see* Adrenocorticotropic hormone
    antidiuretic; *see* Antidiuretic hormone; Vasopressin
    in chemotherapy, 38, 154, 157, 164
    endometriosis and, 161
    estrogens as; *see* Estrogens
    follicle-stimulating; *see* Follicle-stimulating hormone

Hormones—cont'd
    gastric juice and, 109
    gonadotropic, 188, 372, 395; *see also* Gonadotropins
    growth, 111, 171, 372
    hormone-releasing, 184-185
    lactogenic, 372, 377
    luteinizing, 171, 371, 376, 392, 393
    luteinizing hormone-releasing, 188
    male sex; *see* Androgens; Testosterone
    melanocyte-stimulating, 172
    menstrual cycle and, 146
    metabolism and, 110-111
    oxytocin as; *see* Oxytocin
    pancreatic juice and, 109
    pituitary and
        anterior, 110-111, 171
        deficiency of, 175-176
        excessive, 175
        posterior, 172
    pregnancy and, 148
    progesterone as; *see* Progesterone
    prolactin as, 146, 171, 376, 382
    steroid, 115; *see also* specific hormone; Corticosteroids
    thyroid, 173, 176-177
    thyroid-stimulating, 171, 188
    thyrotropin-releasing, 188
    in urine, 143

Hospitals
    increase in beds of, 491
    infants and, 422
    preschool-age child and, 451
    society and, 326
    toddler and, 440-441

HPL; *see* Human placental lactogen

Human chorionic gonadotropin, 148, 372, 373, 393

Human growth and development; *see* Growth and development

Human placental lactogen, 372

Humorsol; *see* Demecarium

Huntington's chorea, 234, 338

Hyaline membrane disease, 388

Hyaluronidase, 147

Hydatidiform mole, 384

Hydralazine hydrochloride, 67

Hydriodic acid, 453

Hydrocele, 379

Hydrocephalus, 206, 431-432

Hydrochloric acid, 47
    anemia and, 448
    growth and, 415
    pancreatic juice and, 109

Hydrochloric acid—cont'd
peptic ulcer and, 126
Hydrochlorothiazide, 68
Hydrocodone bitartrate, 92
Hydrocortisone, 169, 170, 174, 251
Hydrocortisone succinate, 174
Hydrocortone; *see* Hydrocortisone
HydroDiuril; *see* Hydrochlorothiazide
Hydrogen, parathyroid glands and, 166
Hydrogen ion concentration; *see* pH
Hydrogen peroxide, 22, 94
Hydrolose; *see* Methylcellulose
Hydrolysis, 58, 114, 116
Hydromorphone hydrochloride, 28
Hydronephrosis, 151-152
Hydrostatic pressure, 40, 56
Hydrothorax, 101
Hydroxocobalamin, 70; *see also* Vitamins, B$_{12}$
Hydroxyamphetamine, 69, 219
Hydroxychloroquine sulfate, 37
Hydroxyprogesterone caproate, 38, 146, 157
17-Hydroxysteroids, 181, 182
Hydroxyurea, 38
Hydroxyzine hydrochloride, 93, 118, 344
Hydroxyzine pamoate, 93, 118, 344
Hygroton; *see* Chlorthalidone
Hymenolepsis nana, 118
Hyperactivity, 349, 350, 351, 460
Hyperalimentation, 31, 124
Hyperexcitability, reflex, 241
Hyperkeratosis of follicular orifices, 254
Hyperkinetic reactions, 349; *see also* Hyperactivity
Hyperopia, 213-214
Hyperparathyroidism, 177-178
Hyperpituitarism, 175
Hyperstat IV; *see* Diazoxide
Hypertension, 73-74
portal, 132
psychogenic factors and, 348
Hyperthyroidism, 176-177
Hypertonicity
microbes and, 21
solutions and, 60
Hypertrophy of muscle, 199
Hyperventilation syndrome, 348
Hyphae, 20
Hypnotics, 344, 352-353
Hypodermic medications, 17-18
Hypoglycemia, 180, 455
Hypoglycemics
insulin as; *see* Insulin
oral, 173
chloramphenicol and, 34

Hypoglycemics—cont'd
oral—cont'd
diabetes mellitus and, 179
drug interactions and, 458
mechanism of, 16
Hypoparathyroidism, 178
Hypophysectomy, 164, 175, 181
Hypopituitarism, 175-176
Hypoplastic anemia, 83
Hypospadias, 380, 432
Hypothalamus, 59, 188-189
Hypothyroidism, 176
Hypotonic solutions, 60
Hypovolemic shock, 81, 253
Hysterectomy, 160, 161, 163, 386
Hysterical personality, 345
Hysterosalpingo-oophorectomy, 160
Hysterotomy, 384, 394
Hytakerol; *see* Dihydrotachysterol
Hytone; *see* Hydrocortisone
Hyzyd; *see* Isoniazid

I

^{131}I; *see* Iodine, radioactive
Ibuprofen, 218
Id, 328
Identification as defense mechanism, 331
Igs; *see* Immunoglobulins
Ileal conduit, 155, 156
Ileostomy, 122, 135, 136
Ileum, 106
Ileus, paralytic, 135
Illness
behavior and, 333-334
behavioral disorders and, 350
psychogenic factors and, 347
type of, communication and, 10
Ilopan; *see* Pantothenyl alcohol
Ilotycin; *see* Erythromycins
Imferon; *see* Iron-dextran
Imipramine hydrochloride, 339
Immune serum antigen, 131
Immunity, 63-64
thymus and, 172
Immunizations, 420-421
Immunoglobulins, 62-63
Immunotherapy, cancer, 39; *see also* specific
drug
blood dyscrasias and, 83
Imperforate anus, 380, 425-426
Impetigo, 389, 459-460
Implantation after fertilization, 147, 371
Improvement of Nursing Education in the Clinical Field, 491

Impulse conduction, 184-185
Imuran; *see* Azathioprine
Inadequate personality, 345
Inapsine; *see* Droperidol
Inborn errors of metabolism, 420, 434
Incisional hernias, 138
Incus, 197
Independence, need for, 329
Independent contractor, 509
Inderal; *see* Propranolol hydrochloride
Index of refraction, 211
Indifference to illness, 333
Individual
development of, 147-148; *see also* Growth
and development
in family, 324
Indocin; *see* Indomethacin
Indomethacin, 126, 218, 235, 459
Induction of labor, 376, 385-386
Industrial Revolution, 324
Infant, 416-438; *see also* Newborn
adjustment reaction of, 349
congenital abnormalities of, 422-434; *see also*
Congenital abnormalities
defective, parent reactions to, 422-423
of diabetic mother, 387-388
feeding of, 418-420; *see also* Feeding
growth and development of, 416-418
health problems of, 422-438
health promotion and, 418-422
hospitalization of, 422
low birth weight, 390-391
noncongenital conditions of, 434-438
and parent relationships, 377, 378
personality development of, 328
play and, 418
premature, 390-391
Infarction
cerebral vascular accident and, 226
myocardial, 51, 75-76
psychogenic factors and, 348
pulmonary, 96
Infection, 22-23; *see also* Inflammations
of bladder, 150-151
brain abscess and, 225
circulatory system and, 62-64, 76
control of, 31-38
infants and, 389, 436, 437-438
of kidneys, 155
neuromusculoskeletal systems and, 233-234,
235-236, 243-244, 246-247
organic brain syndromes and, 337
preschool-age child and, 452
puerperal, 377

Infection—cont'd
  respiratory system and, 91, 97-100, 104
  in school-age child, 457-458, 459-460
  of skin, 256-257
  of urethra, 156
  urinary tract, 150-151, 155, 156, 452
  of vagina, 160-161
Infectious mononucleosis, 84-85
Infertility, 391-393
Inflammations; *see also* Infection
  agents for, 251
  of bladder, 150-151
  of buccal mucosa and tongue, 124-125
  of ear, 246
  of epididymis, 159
  of eye, 243-244
  of gallbladder, 128
  of heart, 76
  of intestines, 133-134
  of pancreas, 129-130
  of pelvic cavity, 161-162
  of peritoneal cavity, 137-138
  of pleura, 97
  poliomyelitis and, 233
  of prostate gland, 158
  psoriasis and, 255
  rheumatoid arthritis and, 234
  of skin, 254-257
  of stomach, 125-126
  in tissue repair, 249
  of urethra, 156
  of vagina, 160-161
Informed consent, 508
Inguinal hernias, 138
INH; *see* Isoniazid
Inhalation anesthetics, 25
Inhibitory tracts, 193
Injuries; *see* Trauma
Inositol hexanitrate, 66
Inspiration, 87
Inspiratory reserve volume, 88
Institutions, 323
  health agencies as social, 326
  licensure of, 490
Insulators, 57-58
Insulin, 107-108, 173
  antagonist to, 173
  diabetes mellitus and, 178-180
    in diabetic coma, 180
    juvenile, 455, 456
  hypoglycemia and, 180, 455
  mechanism of, 16
  metabolism and, 110
  pancreas and, 172

Insulin—cont'd
  types of, 174
Insulin antagonist, 173
Insulin shock, 180, 455
Insurance, malpractice, 508
Intal; *see* Cromolyn sodium
Integumentary system, 248-258
  anatomy and physiology of, 248-249
  cancer and, 255-256
  chemistry and, 249
  diseases of, 252-258
  grafts and, 251-252
  infection of, in children, 459-460
  newborn and, 380
  pharmacology and, 250-251
  physics and, 249
  postpartal period and, 377
  pregnancy and, 373
  primary lesions of, 252
  procedures and, 251-252
Intellectualization, 331
Intelligence quotient, 444
Intensive care, 6
Intercalated neurons, 183
Interferon, 62
Intermediate care, 6
Intermittent positive pressure breathing, 90
Internal reflection, total, 90-91, 211
International Childbirth Education Association,
    395
International Council of Nurses, 484
International Red Cross, 484-485
Interneurons, 183
Internuncial neurons, 183
Intestitial fluid, 40, 41
Intertrigo, 459
Intervertebral disc herniations, 238
Intestinal antibiotics, 121
Intestinal cramps, paroxysmal, 436-437
Intestinal parasites, 447
Intestines; *see also* Gastrointestinal system
  anomalies of, 425-426
  antibiotics and, 121
  bowel retraining and, 242-243
  carcinoma of, 136-137
  cystic fibrosis of pancreas and, 448
  intussusception and, 135, 435
  large, 106
    cancer of, 136-137
  malabsorption and, 448
  megacolon and, 435
  obstruction of, 135-136, 425
  parasites and, 447
  paroxysmal cramps of, 436-437

Intestines—cont'd
  resection of, 134, 135, 435
  small, 106
    cancer of, 136-137
Intracellular fluid, 40, 41
Intracranial hemorrhage, 225
  of newborn, 388-389
Intracranial pressure
  hydrocephalus and, 431
  increased, 225
Intractable pain, 237-238
Intradermal medications, 18
Intramuscular medications, 18
  nonbarbiturate anesthetics and, 26
Intraocular pressure, increased, 245
Intrapartal period, 374-376; *see also* Maternity
    cycle
  injuries in, 386-387
Intrauterine device, 147, 393
Intrauterine transfusion, 390
Intravascular clot formation, 70, 84
Intravenous cholangiogram, 128-129
Intravenous nonbarbiturate anesthetics, 26
Intravenous pyelography, 150
Intravenous therapy, 28-29
Introjection, 331
Intussusception, 135, 435
Inulin, 114
Invasion of privacy, 507
Involution, 376, 377
Involutional depressive psychosis, 340
Iodinated glycerol, 92, 454
Iodine, 22
  as antithyroid medication, 177
  and iodine-releasing compounds, 22
  radioactive, 39, 177
Ionization, 46
Ions
  chemistry and, 46
  fluid and electrolyte balance and, 41-42
  hydrogen; *see* pH
Ipecac syrup, 442
IPPB; *see* Intermittent positive pressure breath-
    ing
Ipral; *see* Probarbital calcium
IQ; *see* Intelligence quotient
Ircon; *see* Ferrous fumarate
Iridectomy, 245
Iron
  adolescent and, 461
  breast milk and, 419
  children and, 440
  deficiency of, 82; *see also* Anemia
  drugs for sources of, 70

Iron—cont'd
  supplements of, 448
    anemia and, 82
    in celiac disease, 448
    pregnancy and, 374, 383
    tetracyclines and, 33
    tissue effects of, 17
Iron deficiency anemia, 82
Iron-dextran, 18, 70, 448
Iron sorbitex, 70, 448
Iron (II) sulfate, 48
Irradiation; *see* Radiation
Irrigations
  colonic, high, 122; *see also* Enemas
    of ear, 223
  of nasogastric tube, 122-123
IRV; *see* Inspiratory reserve volume
ISG; *see* Immune serum antigen
Islands of Langerhans, 107
Islet cells, 107
Ismelin; *see* Guanethidine sulfate
Iso-Bed; *see* Isosorbide dinitrate
Isocarboxazid, 339
Isoenzymes, blood serum, 74
Isoflurophate, 218
Isometric contractions, 199
Isoniazid, 35-36, 99
Isopropamide, 119
Isopropyl alcohol, 22
Isoproterenol hydrochloride, 66, 71, 92, 453
Isordil; *see* Isosorbide dinitrate
Isosorbide dinitrate, 66, 67
Isotonic contractions, 199
Isotonic solutions, 60
Isoxsuprine hydrochloride, 68
Isuprel; *see* Isoproterenol hydrochloride
Itch mite, 459
IUD; *see* Intrauterine device
IV therapy; *see* Intravenous therapy
IBP; *see* Intravenous pyelography

J

Jacksonian seizures, 228
Jaw fracture, 125
Jectofer; *see* Iron sorbitex
Jejunum, 106
Jewett, P., 495
Joints, 203-206
Juvenile diabetes, 455-456
Juvenile rheumatoid arthritis, 458-459

K

Kafocin; *see* Cephaloglycin
Kalium; *see* Potassium aminosalicylate
Kanamycin sulfate, 33, 121

Kantrex; *see* Kanamycin sulfate
Kaolin and pectin, 119
Kaopectate; *see* Kaolin and pectin
Karaya, 123
KCl; *see* Potassium chloride
Keflex; *see* Cephalexin monohydrate
Keflin; *see* Cephalothin sodium
Kefzol; *see* Cefazolin sodium
Keloid, 249
Kelvin temperature, 24
Kenalog; *see* Triamcinolone
Keratitis, 244
Kernicterus, 390
Kerotin, 249
Ketaject; *see* Ketamine hydrochloride
Ketamine hydrochloride, 26
Ketoacidosis, 180, 455-456
Ketogenesis, 107
Ketone, 113
17-Ketosteroids, 181, 182
Khorion; *see* Chorionic gonadotropin
Kidney, 140-143
  acid-base balance and, 44, 45-46
  adenocarcinoma of, 154
  anti-infectives and, 35
  calculi and, 151
  diseases of, 151-156
  failure of, 152-154
  hypertension and, 73
  renal colic and, 151-152
  renal tubules and, 44, 45, 46, 141, 142
  transplantation of, 154
Kidney-specific anti-infectives, 35
Kilowatt, 24
Kinetic energy, 111-112
Kirschner wire, 239
Klebsiella pneumoniae, 91, 98
Klinefelter's syndrome, 148, 424
Koch's postulates, 22
Koch-Weeks bacillus, 215
KOH; *see* Potassium hydroxide
Korsakoff's syndrome, 337
Krebs' citric acid cycle, 110
Kussmaul breathing, 455
Kveim test, 99
kW; *see* Kilowatt
Kwell; *see* Gamma benzene hexachloride

L

La belle indifférence, 343
La Leche League, 395
Labia majora and minora, 145
Labor, 374-376
  abnormal, 385-386
  changes in mother during, 375

Labor—cont'd
  danger signs and symptoms during, 376
  induction of, 376, 385-386
  mechanisms of, 375
  position of baby during, 375
  precipitate, 385
  stages of, 375
Labor relations, 501
Labyrinth, 197, 247
  test for function of, 223
Labyrinthectomy, 247
Lactation, 146, 376-377, 381-382
Lactic acid, 47, 113
Lactic dehydrogenase, 75
Lactinex; *see* Lactobacillus bulgaricus
Lactobacillus acidophilus, 119
Lactobacillus bulgaricus, 119
Lactogenic hormone, 377
Lactose, 114
  intolerance to, 420, 434
Lactulose, 132
Laminectomy, 238, 241
Lamprene; *see* Clofazimine
Lanatoside C, 64
Lanoxin; *see* Digoxin
Lanugo, 380
Large intestine, 106, 136-137; *see also* Intestines
Largon; *see* Propiomazine hydrochloride
Larocin; *see* Amoxicillin
Larodopa; *see* Levodopa
Laryngeal stridor, congenital, 426
Laryngectomy, total, 103-104
Laryngomalacia, 426
Laryngotracheobronchitis, 437
Larynx, 86-87
  cancer of, 103-104
  congenital abnormalities and, 426
  inflammation of, 437
Lasers, 209-210
Lasix; *see* Furosemide
Later adulthood, 329, 349
Laws; *see also* Legislation
  Boyle's, 90, 112
  common, 506
  of conservation of energy, 56; *see also* Energy
  Dalton's, 90
  drug, 14, 508
  of gases, 90, 112; *see also* Gases
  of gravitation, 55, 89, 111, 206
  Henry's, 90
  of motion, 111, 148-149
  Newton's, 55, 148-149
  nursing and, 487-489, 501-503, 506-509
  Ohm's, 24

Laws—cont'd
    society and, 325, 480, 506
    Starling's
        of capillaries, 40
        of heart, 53
    statutory, 506
    of thermodynamics, 56, 112
    typology of, 506
LDH; *see* Lactic dehydrogenase
Lead poisoning, 442-443
Leadership, 325
Learning, 11-14, 331-332
Learning disturbances, 349
Lecithins, 115
Legal aspects of nursing, 480-509; *see also*
        Nursing
Legal status of nurse, 509
Legislation, 325, 387-389, 501-503, 506-509
    drug, 14, 508
Lenses, 212-214
    cataracts and, 245
    chromatic aberration of, 213
    contact, 214
    defects in, 212-213
    implants of, 245
    spherical aberration of, 213
Leptospira icterohaemorrhagiae, 117
Letdown reflex, 376, 381-382
Letter; *see* Levothyroxine sodium
Leukemias, 84, 451-452
Leukeran; *see* Chlorambucil
Leukocytes, 49
Leucovorin calcium, 70
Levallorphan, 93, 384
Levarterenol bitartrate, 69
Levers, 206
Levin tube irrigation, 122-123
Levodopa, 216, 217, 231, 234
Levo-Dromoran; *see* Levorphanol tartrate
Levoid; *see* Levothyroxine sodium
Levophed Bitartrate; *see* Levarterenol bitartrate
Levoprome; *see* Methotrimeprazine hydrochlo-
        ride
Levopropoxyphene napsylate, 92
Levorphanol tartrate, 28
Levothyroxine sodium, 173
Levulose, 114
LH; *see* Luteinizing hormone
LHRH; *see* Luteinizing hormone-releasing hor-
        mone
Liability, 508
Liberal Education and Nursing, 481
Libigen; *see* Chorionic gonadotropin
Librium; *see* Chlordiazepoxide hydrochloride
Lice, 459

Licensed practical nurse programs, 486-487,
        500
Licensing examination, preparation for, 1-3
Licensure
    institutional, 490
    legislation and, 487-489, 502, 508-509
    mandatory, 509
    permissive, 509
Lidex; *see* Fluocinonide
Lidocaine hydrochloride
    as anesthetic, 26
    as antipruritic, 251
    circulatory system and, 65, 71
    herpes zoster and, 256
Life-support systems, legislation and, 508
Ligation of veins, 80
Light, 58, 208-214
    emission of, 209
    gastrointestinal system and, 112
    integumentary system and, 249
    respiratory system and, 90-91
Lightening, 375
Limbs, absence of, 434
Lincocin; *see* Lincomycin hydrochloride mono-
        hydrate
Lincomycin hydrochloride monohydrate, 33
Liothyronine sodium, 173
Lipase, 448
Lipids, 114-115; *see also* Fats
    neuromusculoskeletal systems and, 214
    ovaries and, 168
Lipo-Hepin; *see* Heparin sodium
Lipo-Lutin; *see* Progesterone
Lipoproteins, 115, 171
Liquid diets, 31
Liquids, physical properties of, 56-57; *see also*
        Fluids; Water
    gastrointestinal system and, 112
    genitourinary system and, 149
    respiratory system and, 90
Liquiprin; *see* Salicylamide
Lithane; *see* Lithium carbonate
Lithium carbonate, 338, 340
Litholapaxy, 151
Lithonate; *see* Lithium carbonate
Liver, 107
    carcinoma of, 133
    circulation and, 53
    cirrhosis and, 132-133
    cystic fibrosis and, 449
    inflammation of, 131-132
Liver injection, 70
Lobectomy, 103
Local anesthetics, 26-27
Lochia, 376, 377

Lofenalac, 420, 434
Log-rolling turning, 238
Lomotil; *see* Diphenoxylate hydrochloride
Long-term services, 7
Lopress; *see* Hydralazine hydrochloride
Lord Report, 491-492
Lorfan; *see* Levallorphan
Loridine; *see* Cephaloridine
Lorinal; *see* Chloral hydrate
Loss, communication and, 11
Lotrimin; *see* Clotrimazole
Lotusate; *see* Talbutal
Loudness, 207; *see also* Sound
Low birth weight infant, 390-391
Low-phenylalanine diet, 420, 434
Lumbar puncture, 222-223
Lumbosacral disc herniation, 238
Luminal; *see* Phenobarbital
Lumpectomy, 164
Lungs, 87; *see also* Respiratory system
    capacity of, 95
    carcinoma of, 102-103
Lupus erythematosus, 257
Luteinizing hormone, 171
    conception enhancers and, 392, 393
    menstrual cycle and, 146, 371
    postpartal period and, 376
Luteinizing hormone-releasing hormone, 188
Luton; *see* Chorionic gonadotropin
Lye poisoning, 442
Lymph, 55
Lymph nodes, 54-55
Lymphatic system, 54-55
Lymphosarcoma, 85-86
Lynoral; *see* Ethinyl estradiol
Lypressin, 175
Lysozyme, 62
Lyteca; *see* Acetaminophen

M

M; *see* Molar solution
Maalox; *see* Aluminum and magnesium hydrox-
        ides
MAC regimen, 40
MacLaggan, K., 493
Macrodantin; *see* Nitrofurantoin
Macrodex; *see* Dextran 70
Macrophages, 62
Macule, 252
Mafenide acetate, 250-251, 253
Magaldrate, 119
Magnesium
    neuromusculoskeletal systems and, 202,
        215
    parathyroid glands and, 166

Magnesium—cont'd
  tetracyclines and, 33
Magnesium citrate solution, 121
Magnesium hydroxide, 47, 121
Magnesium sulfate, 48, 121, 216, 384
Magnesium trisilicate, 448
Malabsorption syndrome, 420, 448
Male
  bone structure of, 205
  infertility and sterility in, 391-392
    drugs and, 392-393
  puberty in, 370
  reproductive organs of, 144-145; see also Reproductive system
  role patterns of, altered, 324
  sex hormones of, 144, 167-168, 169; see also Androgens; Testosterone
    metabolism and, 111
  sterilization of, 147, 158, 393
Malformations, congenital; see Congenital abnormalities, malformations in
Malignant hypertension, 73
Malignant melanoma, 256
Malleus, 197
Malogen; see Testosterone
Malogen CYP; see Testosterone cypionate
Malogen LA; see Testosterone cypionate
Malpractice, 506-507
  insurance and, 508
Maltose, 114
Mammary glands, 146, 248
  carcinoma of, 163-164
Mammography, 163
Mandatory continuing education, 489, 503
Mandatory licensure, 509
Mandelamine; see Methenamine mandelate
Manic-depressive psychosis, 338-340
Mannitol, 105, 216, 219
Mannitol hexanitrate, 66
MAO inhibitors; see Monoamine oxidase inhibitors
Maolate; see Chlorphenesin carbamate
Marcaine Hydrochloride; see Bupivacaine
Marplan; see Isocarboxazid
Marrow aspiration, 72
Masochism, 346
Mastectomy, 164
Master's degree nursing programs, 486, 499
Mastoidectomy, 246-247
Mastoiditis, 246-247
Maternal deprivation syndrome, 435-436
Maternal separation, 422
Maternity cycle, 371-377
  antepartal period in, 371-372

Maternity cycle—cont'd
  bleeding during, 384-385
  deviations from
    in mother, 383-388
    in newborn, 388-391
  intrapartal period in, 374-376
  postpartal period in, 376-377
  prenatal period in, 373-374
Maternity nursing, 370-413; see also Pregnancy
  abortion and, 394
  agencies and, 395
  family planning and, 393
  grief responses in pregnancy and, 394
  infertility and sterility and, 391-393
  maternity cycle and, 371-377; see also Maternity cycle
  menopause and, 394-395
  newborn and, 377-383
  puberty and, 370-371
  review questions for, 395-413
Matter
  change of state of, 25
  physical properties of
    circulatory system and, 56-57
    gastrointestinal system and, 112
    genitourinary system and, 149
    integumentary system and, 249
    neuromusculoskeletal systems and, 206-214
    respiratory system and, 90
Matulane; see Procarbazine
Maximal expiratory flow rate, 89
MBD; see Minimal brain dysfunction
Measles vaccine, 420, 421
Mebaral; see Mephobarbital
Mechanical ventilation, 94-95
Mechanics
  circulatory system and, 55-56
  genitourinary system and, 148-149
  integumentary system and, 249
  neuromusculoskeletal systems and, 206
  respiratory system and, 89
Mechlorethamine, 39, 85
Mecholyl; see Methacholine chloride
Meclizine hydrochloride, 118
Meconium, 380
Mediastinal shift, 102
Medical asepsis, 31-32
Medical Care Act, 501
Medical practice, changes in, 491
Medical-surgical nursing, 4-321
  antineoplastic drugs and, 38-40
  circulatory system in, 48-86; see also Circulatory system

Medical-surgical nursing—cont'd
  conceptual introduction to, 4-18
    health-illness continuum in, 4-5
    health resources and, 5-7
    nurse's role and, 7-18
  endocrine system in, 166-182; see also Endocrine system
  fluid, electrolyte, and acid-base balance in, 40-48
  gastrointestinal system in, 105-140; see also Gastrointestinal system
  genitourinary system in, 140-165; see also Genitourinary system
  infection control in, 31-38; see also Infection
  integumentary system in, 248-258
  neuromusculoskeletal systems in, 183-247; see also Neuromusculoskeletal systems
  preoperative and postoperative care in, 18-31; see also Preoperative and postoperative care
  respiratory system in, 86-105; see also Respiratory system
  review questions in, 258-321
Medicare, 488
Medications; see Drugs
Medihalers, 17
Medroxyprogesterone acetate, 38, 146, 154, 157
Medulla of brain, 187
Mefenamic acid, 28
Magace; see Megestrol acetate
Megacolon, 435
Megestrol acetate, 38, 157
Melanin, 249
Melanocyte-stimulating hormone, 172
Melanoma, 244, 256
Melatonin, 173
Mellaril; see Thioridazine hydrochloride
Melozets; see Methylcellulose
Melphalan, 39, 237
Memory cells, 62
Menarche, 370
Menest; see Esterified estrogens
Menformon; see Estrone
Meniere's disease, 247
Meninges, 189
Meningioma, 224
Meningitis, 437-438
Meningocele, 430
Meningomyelocele, 430
Menopause, 394-395
Menotabs; see Conjugated estrogens
Menotropins, 392
Menstrual cycle, 146, 371

Mental disorders; *see also* Psychiatric nursing
 classification of, 336-337
 nonpsychotic, 343-347
 psychotic; *see* Psychoses
Mental retardation, 444-445
Meparin; *see* Heparin sodium
Meperidine hydrochloride, 17, 28
Mephenesin, 217
Mephentermine sulfate, 69
Mephenytoin, 216, 228
Mephobarbital, 216
Mephson; *see* Mephenesin
Mepivacaine hydrochloride, 26
Meprane Dipropionate; *see* Promethestrol dipro-
 pionate
Meprobamate, 344
Meprospan; *see* Meprobamate
Meprotabs; *see* Meprobamate
Meratran; *see* Pipradrol hydrochloride
Mercaptomerin sodium, 68
Mercaptopurine, 38, 40, 451
Mercurials, 68-69
Mersalyl with theophylline, 68
Mesantoin; *see* Mephenytoin
Mesoderm, 147
Mesophiles, 20
Mestinon; *see* Pyridostigmine bromide
Mestranol-ethynodiol diacetate, 393
Mestranol-norethynodrel, 158, 393
Metabolic acidosis, 46, 436
Metabolic alkalosis, 46, 436
Metabolism, 109-111
 of carbohydrates, 110
 hormones and, 110-111
 inborn errors of, 420, 434
 rate of, 111, 415
 of skeletal muscle, 199
 thyroid gland and, 166
Metalloproteins, 116
Metals, 214-215
Metamine; *see* Trolnitrate phosphate
Metamucil; *see* Psyllium hydrophilic mucilloid
Metandren; *see* Methyltestosterone
Metaprel; *see* Metaproterenol
Metaproterenol, 92, 453
Metaraminol bitartrate, 69
Metaxalone, 217
Methacholine chloride, 218
Methadone, 347, 390
Methallenestril, 392
Methapyrilene hydrochloride, 93
Methaqualone, 27, 353
Methazolamide, 219
Methdilazine hydrochloride, 93

Methenamine, 35
Methenamine hippurate, 35
Methenamine mandelate, 35
Methenamines, 34, 35
Methergine; *see* Methylergonovine maleate
Methiacil; *see* Methylthiouracil
Methicillin sodium, 32
Methimazole, 174, 177
Methionine, 151
Methocarbamol, 217
Methohexital sodium, 26
Methotrexate, 38, 40
 breast carcinoma and, 164
 drug interactions and, 458
 laryngeal cancer and, 103
 in leukemia, 451
 psoriasis and, 255
Methotrimeprazine hydrochloride, 27, 352
Methoxamine hydrochloride, 69
Methoxsalen, 255
Methoxyflurane, 25
Methoxyphenamine hydrochloride, 453
Methsuximide, 216
Methulose; *see* Methylcellulose
Methyclothiazide, 68
Methylcellulose, 120
Methyldopa, 67
Methylergonovine maleate, 377
Methylphenidate hydrochloride, 339
Methylprednisolone sodium succinate, 174
Methylrosaniline chloride, 447
Methyltestosterone, 392
Methylthiouracil, 174
Methyprylon, 27, 353
Methysergide maleate, 223
Metolazone, 69
Metronidazol, 36-37, 160
Metycaine Hydrochloride; *see* Piperocaine hy-
 drochloride
$Mg(OH)_2$; *see* Magnesium hydroxide
$MgSO_4$; *see* Magnesium sulfate
Microbiology, 18-23; *see also* specific organism
 circulatory system and, 62-64
 gastrointestinal system and, 117-118
 genitourinary system and, 149-150
 neuromusculoskeletal systems and, 215
 respiratory system and, 91
Microphages, 62
Midbrain, 188
Migraine headache, 223-224
Milia, 380
Milk, 383, 419
Milk of Magnesia; *see* Magnesium hydroxide
Miller-Abbott tube, 136, 137

Millimicron, 209
Millon's test, 116
Mineral oil, 120, 437, 442
Mineralocorticoids, 115, 169, 170
 in Addison's disease, 182
 kidney and, 141
 primary aldosteronism and, 180-181
Minimal air, 88
Minimal brain dysfunction, 460
Minipress; *see* Prazosin hydrochloride
Miotics, 218, 245
Mithracin; *see* Mithramycin
Mithramycin, 39
Mitomycin, 39
Mitral commissurotomy, 77
Mitral valve replacement, 77
Mitral valvotomy, 77
Moban; *see* Molidone hydrochloride
Moderil; *see* Rescinnamine
Molal solution, 60
Molar solution, 60
Molds, 20
Moldes, hydatidiform, 384
Molidone hydrochloride, 342
Momentum, 56, 89-90, 149
Mongolian spots, 380
Mongolism, 148, 423
Moniliasis, 160
Monitoring, cardiac, 71
Monoamine oxidase inhibitors, 339
Monoamines, 184, 214
Mononeuritis, 229
Mononucleosis, infectious, 84-85
Monosaccharide, 113
Mons veneris, 145
Montag, M. L., 481, 485
MOPP regimen, 39
Moro reflex, 380
Morphine sulfate, 28
 congestive heart failure and, 77
 myocardial infarction and, 75
 newborn and, 390
 pulmonary edema and, 96
Morula stage, 371
Mosaicism, 423
Mother, pregnancy and, 372-373; *see also* Ma-
 ternity nursing
Mothering, 378
Motion, law of, 55, 111, 148-149
Motivation, 13-14, 331-332
Motoneural pathways, 190-193
Motoneurons, 183
Mouth, 105-106
 carcinoma of, 125

Mouth—cont'd
   fungi and, 124, 389
MSH; *see* Melanocyte-stimulating hormone
MTX; *see* Methotrexate
Mucilose; *see* Psyllium hydrophilic mucilloid
Mucolytics, 92, 454
Mucomyst; *see* Acetylcysteine
Multifuge; *see* Piperazine citrate
Multiple choice questions, 3
Multiple myeloma, 237
Multiple personalities, 343
Multiple sclerosis, 231-232
Muracil; *see* Methylthiouracil
Muscles
   anatomy and physiology of, 197-199
   chemistry and, 214-215
   diseases of; *see* Neuromusculoskeletal sys-
      tems, diseases of
   of eye, 196
   microorganisms and, 215
   pharmacology and, 215-219
   physics and, 206-214
   procedures and, 219-223
   skeletal
      metabolism of, 199
      motoneural pathways for, 190-193
      origins, insertions, and functions of, 200-
         202
      relaxants for, 217
Mussallem, H. K., 492, 493, 497
Mustard, 442
Mustard procedure, 428
Mustargen; *see* Mechlorethamine
Mutamycin; *see* Mitomycin
Mutations, 148
Myambutol; *see* Ethambutol hydrochloride
Myasthenia gravis, 232-233
Mycelium, 20
Mychel; *see* Chloramphenicol
Mycifradin Sulfate; *see* Neomycin
Mycobacterium leprae, 19, 35
Mycobacterium tuberculosis, 19, 35-36, 91, 99,
   161
Mycoplasmatales, 19
Mycostatin; *see* Nystatin
Mydriacyl; *see* Tropicamide
Mydriatics, 218-219, 244, 245
Myelin sheaths, 183
Myeloma, multiple, 237
Myleran; *see* Busulfan
Myocardial infarction, 51, 75-76
   psychogenic factors and, 348
Myocarditis, 76

Myocardium, 51, 76
Myopia, 213
Mysoline; *see* Primidone
Mytelase; *see* Ambenonium chloride
Myxedema, 176

N

N; *see* Normal solution
^{32}Na; *see* Sodium phosphate, radioactive
NaCl; *see* Sodium chloride
NAD; *see* Nicotinamide adenine dinucleotide
NADP; *see* Nicotinamide adenine dinucleotide
   phosphate
Nafcillin sodium, 32
Nagele's rule, 373
NaHCO$_3$; *see* Sodium bicarbonate
Nalidixic acid, 35
Nalline; *see* Nalorphine hydrochloride
Nalorphine hydrochloride, 93
Naloxone hydrochloride, 93
Nandrolone phenpropionate, 157
NaOH; *see* Sodium hydroxide
Narcan; *see* Naloxone hydrochloride
Narcotic analgesics, 28
Narcotics, 28
   as antitussives, 92
   diarrhea and, 120
   drug potentiation and, 339
   drugs antagonizing effects of, 92-93
   legislation and, 508
   newborn and, 390
Nardil; *see* Phenelzine sulfate
Narone; *see* Dipyrone
Nartate; *see* Dipyrone
Nasogastric tube irrigation, 122-123
National Association for Colored Graduate
   Nurses, 483
National Association for Practical Nurse Educa-
   tion Service, Inc., 484
National Council of State Boards, Inc., 488
National Federation of Licensed Practical
   Nurses, Inc., 484
National Health Insurance, 501
National Institutes of Health, 395
National League for Nursing, 483-484
   accreditation and, 489
National League for Nursing Education, 483
National League for Nursing Test Construction
   Unit, 488
National Organization of Public Health Nursing,
   483
National Student Nurses' Association, 484
Nationality, 322

Navane; *see* Thiothixene
N-CAP; *see* Nurses Coalition for Action in Poli-
   tics
NCSBN; *see* National Council of State Boards,
   Inc.
Nebcin; *see* Tobramycin sulfate
Nebs; *see* Acetaminophen
Necator americanus, 118
Nectadon; *see* Noscapine
Needs
   basic, 329-330
   hierarchy of, 10
   of newborn, 381
NegGram; *see* Nalidixic acid
Negligence, 506-507
Neisseria gonorrhoeae, 19, 150, 165
   newborn and, 389
   pelvic inflammatory disease and, 161
Neisseria meningitidis, 19, 215, 437
Nemasol; *see* Para-aminosalicylic acid
Nematodes, 117, 215
Nembutal; *see* Pentobarbital sodium
Neobiotic; *see* Neomycin
Neo-Hombreol; *see* Testosterone propionate
Neo-Hombreol-F; *see* Testosterone
Neo-Hombreol-M; *see* Methyltestosterone
Neomycin, 33
   cirrhosis and, 132
   impetigo and, 389
   integumentary system and, 250
   as intestinal antibiotic, 121
Neonatal respiratory distress, 388; *see also*
   Newborn
Neostigmine, 217
   intestinal obstruction and, 136
   myasthenia gravis and, 232
   ophthalmic, 218
Neo-Synephrine Hydrochloride; *see* Phenyl-
   ephrine hydrochloride
Neothylline; *see* Dyphylline
Neo-Tric; *see* Metronidazol
Nephrectomy, 154
Nephrolithotomy, 151
Nephron, 141, 142
Nephrosis, 452
Nephrostomy, 155
Nephrotic syndrome, 452
Neptazane; *see* Methazolamide
Nerve blocks, 26-27, 230, 231, 256
Nerve fiber, 183
Nerve impulse conduction, 184-185
Nerves; *see also* Nervous system
   autonomic, 193-195

Nerves—cont'd
  cochlear, 197
  cranial, 191
    Bell's palsy and, 229-230
    trigeminal neuralgia and, 230
  to heart, 51
  optic, 224
  pancreatic juice and, 109
  parasympathetic, 193-195
  respiration and, 87-88
  salivary secretion and, 108
  spinal, 190
  sympathetic, 193-195, 327
  vestibular, surgical destruction of, 247
Nervous system; see also Nerves
  anatomy and physiology of, 183-197
  autonomic, 193-195
  chemistry and, 214-215
  diseases of; see Neuromusculoskeletal sys-
    tems, diseases of
  growth and, 415-416
  microorganisms and, 215
  minimal brain dysfunction and, 460
  newborn and, 380
  organs of, 185-190
  pharmacology and, 215-219
  physics and, 206-214
  procedures and, 219-223
  receptors of, 195-197
  sympathetic, 193-195, 327
Nesacaine; see Chloroprocaine hydrochloride
Neural pathways, 190-193
Neurilemma, 183
Neurogenic bladder, 243, 431
Neurogenic shock, 81-82, 253
Neuroglia, 184
Neurohypophysis, 59, 173
Neuroma, acoustic, 224
Neuromuscular junction, 198
Neuromusculoskeletal systems, 183-247
  anatomy and physiology of, 183-206
    muscular system in, 197-199
    nervous system in, 183-197
    skeletal system in, 199-206
  cerebral palsy and, 445-446
  chemistry and, 214-215
  diseases of, 223-247
    amyotrophic lateral sclerosis in, 233
    Bell's palsy in, 229-230
    brain abscess in, 225
    brain tumor in, 224-225
    cerebral aneurysm in, 225
    cerebral hemorrhage in, 225-226

Neuromusculoskeletal systems—cont'd
  diseases of—cont'd
    cerebral vascular accident in, 226-228
    epilepsy in, 228-229
    eye disorders in, 243-246
    fractures in, 239-241
    gouty arthritis in, 235
    Guillain-Barré syndrome in, 233
    head injuries in, 224
    hip fractures in, 240-241
    Huntington's chorea in, 234
    intractable pain in, 237-238
    mastoiditis in, 246-247
    migraine headache in, 223-224
    mononeuritis in, 229
    multiple myeloma in, 237
    multiple sclerosis in, 231-232
    myasthenia gravis in, 232-233
    osteoarthritis in, 234-235
    osteogenic sarcoma in, 236
    osteomyelitis in, 235-236
    osteoporosis in, 236
    otitis media in, 246
    otosclerosis in, 247
    paralysis agitans in, 230-231
    poliomyelitis in, 233-234
    polyneuritis in, 229
    rheumatoid arthritis in, 234
    ruptured nucleus pulposus in, 238
    spinal cord injury in, 241-243
    trigeminal neuralgia in, 230
  growth and, 415-416
  microorganisms and, 215
  newborn and, 381
  pharmacology and, 215-219
  physics and, 206-214
  pregnancy and, 373
  procedures and, 219-223
Neuronal cell membrane, 183
Neuronidia; see Barbital
Neurons, 183, 193
Neuropeptides, 184-185
Neuroses, 343-344
  behavioral disorders and, 350
Neurotic traits, 330
Neutralization, 63
Neutralizing antibodies, 63
Neutrapen; see Penicillinase
A New Perspective on the Health of Canadians,
  505-506
Newborn, 377-383; see also Infant
  appraisal of, 378-381
  diseases of, 388-391

Newborn—cont'd
  family history and, 377-378
  feeding schedules for, 383; see also Feeding
  needs of, 381
  nutrition and, 381-383
Newton's laws of motion, 55, 148-149
NH_3; see Ammonia
NHO_3; see Nitric acid
NH_4OH; see Ammonium hydroxide
Niconyl; see Isoniazid
Nicotinamide adenine dinucleotide, 117
Nicotinamide adenine dinucleotide phosphate,
  117
Nightingale, F., 480
Nikolsky's sign, 255
Nilevar; see Norethandrolone
Nilstat; see Nystatin
Ninhydrin test, 116
Nipride; see Sodium nitroprusside
Nitranitol; see Mannitol hexanitrate
Nitrates, 66-67
Nitric acid, 47
Nitro-Bid ointment, 67
Nitrofurantoin, 35
Nitrofurazone, 250
Nitrogen monoxide, 25
Nitrogen mustard; see Mechlorethamine
Nitroglycerin, 17, 66, 74
Nitrol ointment, 67
Nitrong ointment, 67
Nitrous oxide, 25
Noctec; see Chloral hydrate
Nodule, 252
Noise level, 207; see also Sound
Noludar; see Methyprylon
Nomenclature, drug, 16
Nonverbal communication, 327
Norepinephrine
  adrenal gland and, 169
  antidepressants and, 339
  metabolism and, 111
  neuromusculoskeletal systems and, 184, 214
  pheochromocytoma and, 182
Norepinephrine blockers, 339
Norepinephrine release stimulators, 339
Norepinephrine uptake accelerator, 339-340
Norethandrolone, 157
Norethindrone, 146
Norethindrone acetate, 146
Norlestrin; see Ethinyl estradiol and norethin-
  drone acetate
Norlutate; see Norethindrone acetate
Norlutin; see Norethindrone

Normal saline, 94, 230
Normal solution, 60
Norpace; *see* Disopyramide phosphate
Norpramin; *see* Desipramine hydrochloride
Northern Health Service nurse, 505
Northwest Territories Registered Nurses' Association, 502
Nortriptyline hydrochloride, 339
Noscapine, 92
Nose, 86
    choanal atresia and, 426
Novaflor; *see Lactobacillus bulgaricus*
Novaldin; *see* Dipyrone
Novocaine; *see* Procaine hydrochloride
Novochlorocap; *see* Chloramphenicol
Novonidazol; *see* Metronidazol
Novrad; *see* Levopropoxyphene napsylate
$N_2S_{O_4}$; *see* Sulfuric acid
Nucleoprotiens, 115, 116-117
Nucleus pulposus, ruptured, 238
Numorphan; *see* Oxymorphone hydrochloride
Nupercaine; *see* Dibucaine
Nurse practice acts, 502
Nurse practitioner, 489, 490, 504, 505
Nurse Training Acts, 488, 489
Nurses; *see also* Nursing
    collective action or bargaining and, 489, 501, 509
    in courts, 509
    as employees, 509
    as independent contractors, 509
    legal status of, 509
    legislation and, 487-489, 501-503, 506-509
    nonuniversity programs for preparation of, 499-500
    role of, 7-18
        communication and, 9-11
        delivery of nursing care and, 8
        medication administration and, 14-18
        problem-solving and, 8-9
        responsibilities in, 7-8
        teaching-learning environment and, 11-14
    shortages of, 491
Nurses' Acts, 502, 503
Nurses Coalition for Action in Politics, 489
Nursing; *see also* Nurses
    in Canada, 491-506
        accreditation and, 502-503
        Code of Ethics and, 503-504
        current developments and, 503-506
        educational advances and, 496-500, 504-505
        legislation and, 501-503
        nursing service and, 500-501, 505-506

Nursing—cont'd
    in Canada—cont'd
        organizations and, 495-496, 503
        research and, 504
        studies affecting, 491-495
        twentieth century and, 491-501
    legal definition of, 489, 503
    legislation and, 487-489, 501-503, 506-509
    research in, 504
    in United States, 480-491
        accreditation and, 489
        current developments and, 489-491
        educational advances and, 485-487, 489-490
        institutional licensure and, 490
        international organizations and, 484-485
        legislation and, 487-489
        nursing organizations and, 482-484
        nursing service and, 487, 490
        studies affecting, 480-482
        twentieth century and, 480-489
Nursing for the Future, 481, 486, 487, 497
Nursing and Nursing Education in the United States, 480
Nursing assistant programs, 500-501
Nursing education
    in Canada, 496-500, 504-505
    in United States, 485-487, 489-490
Nursing Education in Canada, 497
Nursing homes, 7, 491
Nursing organizations
    in Canada, 495-496
    international, 484-485
    in United States, 482-484
Nursing Outlook, 489
Nursing relationship, therapeutic, 332-334
Nursing Schools Today and Tomorrow, 481
Nursing service
    in Canada, 500-501, 505-506
    in United States, 487, 490
Nursing team, 487, 501
Nutramigen, 434
Nutrition; *see also* Diet; Feeding
    of adolescent, 461
    childhood, 440
    infant, 418-419
    newborn and, 381-383
    postoperative, 31
    pregnancy and, 373-374
    premature infants and, 391
N.W.T.R.N.A.; *see* Northwest Territories Registered Nurses' Association
Nydrazid; *see* Isoniazid
Nystatin, 36, 160, 250, 389

O

Oatmeal baths, 255
Obesity, 440, 461
Obsessive-compulsive personality, 345
Obsessive-compulsive reactions, 335, 343-344
Obstructive pulmonary disease, chronic, 100-101
Occipital area of brain, 189
Occult blood in stool, 122
Ohm's law, 24
Old tuberculin, 99
Olfaction, 196
Oliguria, 143, 152
Olive oil, 120
Omnipen; *see* Ampicillin
Oncovin; *see* Vincristine
Ontario Council of Health Report, 495
Oogenesis, 145
Oophorectomy, 161, 164
Oophoritis, 161
Operant conditioning, 14
Ophthaine; *see* Proparacaine hydrochloride
Ophthalmia neonatorum, 165, 389
Ophthalmic drugs, 218-219
Ophthalmoscope, 214
Ophthetic; *see* Proparacaine hydrochloride
Opiates; *see* Narcotics
Opisthotonos, 437
Opium, tincture of, 120
Opsonification, 63
Optic chiasm, 189
Optic nerve spongioblastoma polare, 224
Optic vesicles, 188
Oracen; *see* Estrogen and progesterone sequential contraceptives
Oral contraceptives, 146, 157-158, 393
Oral hypoglycemic agents; *see* Hypoglycemics, oral
Oral poliovirus vaccine, 420, 421
Ora-Testryl; *see* Fluoxymesterone
Oratrol; *see* Dichlorphenamide
Orchiectomy, 158
Oretic; *see* Hydrochlorothiazide
Oreton; *see* Testosterone
Oreton-M; *see* Methyltestosterone
Oreton Propionate; *see* Testosterone propionate
Organic acids, 113-114
Organic brain syndromes, 337-338
Organidin; *see* Iodinated glycerol
Organizations
    in Canada, 495-496
    international, 484-485
    in United States, 482-484
Orinase; *see* Tolbutamide

Ortho-Novum; *see* Estrogen and progesterone tablets
Orthopedic deformities, 432-434
Orthoxine; *see* Methoxyphenamine
Ortolani's sign, 433
Os-Cal; *see* Calcium carbonate
Oscillator, 24
Osmitrol; *see* Mannitol
Osmoglyn; *see* Glycerin
Osmoreceptor system, 42
Osmosis, 60, 113
Osmotic agents, 219
Osmotic diuretics, 216; *see also* specific drug
Osmotic pressure, 40, 60
Ossification, 203
Osteoarthritis, 234-235
Osteoblasts, 199
Osteoclasts, 202
Osteocytes, 202
Osteogenic sarcoma, 236
Osteomyelitis, 235-236
Osteoporosis, 236
Ostomy, 136, 137
    bladder tumors and, 155, 156
    care of, 123, 426
    imperforate anus and, 426
    megacolon and, 435
OT; *see* Old tuberculin
Otitis media, 246, 437
Otosclerosis, 247
Ouabain, 64
Ova, 145, 146, 371
    chromosomes and, 147
Ovaries, 145, 167, 168-169
Overanxious reaction of childhood and adolescence, 349
Oviducts, 145
    rupture of, 384
Ovral; *see* Ethinyl estradiol and norgestrel
Ovulation, 145, 146, 371
Ovulen; *see* Mestranol-ethynodiol diacetate
Oxacillin sodium, 32
Oxazepam, 344
Oxidation-reduction, 112
Oxtriphylline, 91, 453
Oxycodone, 28
Oxygen
    administration of, 93
        birth injuries and, 389
        neonatal respiratory distress and, 388
        sickle cell anemia and, 449
    adrenal gland and, 169
    bacteria and, 20
    in blood, 88, 89

Oxygen—cont'd
    respiratory system and, 88, 89
Oxyhemoglobin, 89
Oxymorphone hydrochloride, 28
Oxyphenbutazone, 235
Oxytetracycline, 33
Oxytocics, 385, 387; *see also* Oxytocin
Oxytocin, 172
    hypothalamus and, 188
    induction of labor and, 376, 385
    lactation and, 146, 381
    pregnancy and, 148

P

P_{CO_2}; *see* Partial pressure of carbon dioxide
Pacemakers, 24, 58, 72
Paget's carcinoma, 163
Pain
    drugs for, 27-28
    intractable, 237-238
Palate, 105
Palonyl; *see* Ethinyl estradiol
Palsy, Bell's, 229-230; *see also* Paralysis
Paludrine; *see* Chloroguanide hydrochloride
Pancreas, 107-108, 167, 172
    carcinoma of, 130-131
    cystic fibrosis of, 448-449
    diabetes mellitus and, 178-180
    inflammation of, 129-130
    metabolism and, 110
Pancreatic enzymes
    cancer and, 131
    cystic fibrosis and, 448, 449
Pancreatic juice, 109
Pancreatic polypeptide, 172
Pancreatin, 121
Pancreatitis, acute, 129-130
Pancrelipase, 121
Pancreozymin, 109, 117
Panheprin; *see* Heparin sodium
Panhysterectomy, 160
Panmycin; *see* Tetracycline
Pantopium, 28
Pantopon; *see* Pantopium
Pantothenyl alcohol, 136
Panwarfin; *see* Warfarin sodium
Papanicolaou cytologic findings, 160
Papule, 252
Para-aminosalicylic acid, 36, 99
Paracentesis, 123, 132
Paradione; *see* Paramethadione
Paraflex; *see* Chlorzoxazone
Parafon Forte, 217
Paragonimus westermani, 118

Paraldehyde, 352
Parallel play, 439-440
Paralysis
    Erb-Duchenne, 389
    facial, of newborn, 389
    flaccid, 241
    spastic, 241
Paralysis agitans, 216-217, 230-231, 338
Paralytic ileus, 135
Paramethadione, 216
Paranoid personality, 345
Paranoid states, 342-343
Paraphenylenediamine, 254
Parasal Sodium; *see* Sodium aminosalicylate
Parasites, 19
    drugs for, 36-38
    gastrointestinal system and, 117-118, 447
    neuromusculoskeletal systems and, 215
Parasympathetic nerves, 193-195
Parathormone, 42, 166, 168
    deficiency of, 178
    high levels of, 177-178
    injections of, 178
Parathyroid glands, 166, 167, 168
    calcium regulation and, 42-43, 166, 168
    hyperfunction of, 177-178
    removal or trauma of, 177, 178
Paredrine; *see* Hydroxyamphetamine
Paregoric; *see* Opium, tincture of
Parenogen; *see* Fibrinogen
Parent Report, 498
Parenteral nutrition, total, 31, 124
Parenteral preparations, administration of, 17-18
Parents
    of defective child, reactions of, 422-423
    nursing responsibilities and, 421-422
    relationships with child of, 377, 378
        disturbances in, 414
Parietal cells, 106
Parietal lobes of brain, 189
Parkinson's disease, 216-217, 230-231
    organic brain syndromes and, 338
Parnate; *see* Tranylcypromine sulfate
Parsidol; *see* Ethopropazine hydrochloride
Partial pressure of carbon dioxide, 88, 89
Partial thromboplastin time, 75
P.A.S.; *see* Para-aminosalicylic acid
Pascal's principle, 56-57, 112, 149, 206
Pasdium; *see* Sodium aminosalicylate
Passive-aggressive personality, 345
Passive positioning, assistive devices for, 219-220
Pasteurization, 21
Patent ductus arteriosus, 427

A Path to Quality, 493
Pathogenicity, 20, 23
Pathogens, 22-23; *see also* Microbiology
Patient Bill of Rights, 491
Patient complaints, 509
Patient history, communication and, 11
Patient positioning, assistive devices for, 219-220
Patient transfer, 219
PDA; *see* Patent ductus arteriosus
Pedacillin; *see* Penicillin G potassium
Pediamycin; *see* Erythromycin ethylsuccinate
Pediatric nursing, 414-479; *see also* Children; Infant; Newborn
  adolescent in, 460-461; *see also* Adolescence
  basic concepts in, 414
  family and, 414
  growth and development and, 414-416; *see also* Growth and development
  infant in, 416-438; *see also* Infant
  preschool-age child in, 450-454
  review questions for, 461-479
  school-age child in, 454-460
  toddler and, 438-450; *see also* Toddler
Pediculicides, 250
Pediculosis, 459
Pedophilia, 346
PEEP; *see* Positive and expiratory pressure
Peer groups, 324-325, 460
Peer review, 490, 505
Pelvic inflammatory disease, 161-162
Pelvis, anatomy of, 374
Pemphigus, 255
Penbritin; *see* Ampicillin
Penicillin G potassium, 32
Penicillin G procaine, 32
Penicillin V, 32
Penicillinase, 32, 457
Penicillins, 32
  burns and, 253
  cystitis and, 151
  excretion of, 143
  glomerulonephritis and, 155
  in rheumatic fever, 457
  for syphilis, 165
    of newborn, 389
  venereal disease and, 165
Penis, 144
  short, 432
Pentaerythritol tetranitrate, 66
Pentazocine hydrochloride, 28
Penthrane; *see* Methoxyflurane
Pentids; *see* Penicillin G potassium
Pentids-P; *see* Penicillin G procaine

Pentobarbital sodium, 27, 353
Pentothal Sodium; *see* Thiopental sodium
Pen-Vee; *see* Penicillin V
Peptic ulcer, 126-127, 252, 348
Percent solution, 60
Perception, 326
Percodan, 28
Percutaneous stimulator, 237
Pergonal; *see* Menotropins
Periactin Hydrochloride; *see* Cyproheptadine hydrochloride
Pericarditis, 76
Pericardium, 50-51
  inflammation of, 76
Periclor; *see* Petrichloral
Peri-Colace, 120
Perineum, lacerations of, 386
Peripheral vascular disorders, 80-81
  drugs for, 67, 69
Peristalsis, 108
Peristaltin; *see* Cascara sagrada
Peristim; *see* Cascara sagrada
Peritoneal cavity inflammation, 137-138
Peritoneal dialysis, 153
Peritonitis, 137-139
Peritrate; *see* Pentaerythritol tetranitrate
Permissive licensure, 509
Pernicious anemia, 82-83
Perphenazine, 341
Personality, 344-345
  defenses for, 331-332
  development of, 327-330
  disorders of, 344-347
  traits of, anxiety and, 330
Personnel, health services, 7
  increase in number and types of, 491
Pertofrane; *see* Desipramine hydrochloride
Pertussis vaccine, 420, 421
Pessary, 163, 386
Petit mal seizures, 228
Petrichloral, 27, 352
Petroleum distillates, 442
Pfizerpen; *see* Penicillin G potassium
pH, 48
  bacteria and, 20
  blood, 43, 88, 89
  of body fluids, 43, 48, 61
  carbon dioxide and, 44
  gastrointestinal system and, 113
  of urine, 149
  of vagina, 161
Phagocytosis, 62
Phantom limb, 79
Pharmacodynamics, 15

Pharmacology; *see* Drugs
Pharmacotherapeutics, 15
Pharynx, 86
Phenacaine hydrochloride, 26
Phenaglycodol, 344
Phenazopyridine, 151
Phenelzine sulfate, 339
Phenergan; *see* Promethazine hydrochloride
Phenformin hydrochloride, 173
Phenmetrazine hydrochloride, 119
Phenobarbital
  drug interactions and, 17, 36, 429
  epilepsy and, 229
  hyperthyroidism and, 177
  menopause and, 395
  as sedative, 27, 353
Phenol coefficient, 21
Phenols, 251
  substituted, 22
Phenothiazines, 27, 341, 352; *see also* specific drug
Phensuximide, 228
Phenylalanine, 420, 434
Phenylbutazone
  in arthritis, 217, 218
  drug interactions and, 429
  in gout, 235
  ulcers and, 127
Phenylephrine hydrochloride, 69, 219
Phenylketonuria, 420, 434
Phenylpropranolamine hydrochloride, 453
Phenytoin, 216, 228
  circulatory system and, 65
  drug interactions and, 34, 215, 429
Pheochromocytoma, 73, 182
pHisoHex, 389
Phlebotomy, dry, 77, 96-97
Phobic reactions, 335, 343
Phosphaljel; *see* Aluminum phosphate gel
Phosphate, 42, 44
Pholine; *see* Echothiophate
Phospholipids, 115
Phosphoproteins, 116
Phosphorescence, 209
Phosphorus
  bone and, 199
  lead poisoning and, 443
  parathyroid glands and, 166
  radioactive, 83
Photocoagulation, 246
Phthalylsulfathiazole, 34
Physical properties of matter; *see* Matter, physical properties of
Physician's associate, 505

Physics
  circulatory system and, 55-58
  gastrointestinal system and, 111-112
  genitourinary system and, 148-149
  integumentary system and, 249
  neuromusculoskeletal system and, 206-214
  preoperative and postoperative care and, 23-25
  respiratory system and, 89-91
Physiology; *see* Anatomy and physiology
Physostigmine, 218
Pia mater, 189
Pica, 442
Pick's disease, 337
Picornaviruses, 91
Piggyback medications, 18
Pilocarpine hydrochloride or nitrate, 218
Pineal body, 188
Pineal gland, 167, 172-173
Pinworms, 118, 447
Piperazine citrate, 447
Piperocaine hydrochloride, 26
Pipobroman, 39
Pipradrol hydrochloride, 339
Pitch of sound, 208
Pitocin; *see* Oxytocin
Pitressin; *see* Vasopressin
Pituitary gland, 167, 171-172, 173
  diseases and, 175-176
  hormones of, 171
    deficiency of, 175-176
    excessive, 175
    metabolism and, 110-111
  hypothalamus and, 188
  lesions of, 181
PKU; *see* Phenylketonuria
Placenta, 147, 372
Placenta previa, 384
Placidyl; *see* Ethchlorvynol
Plan for the Development of Nursing Education Programs Within the General Educational System of Canada, 493
A Plan for the Education of Nurses in the Province of New Brunswick, 493-494
Plane polarized light, 212
Plant alkaloids, 39
Plantar reflex, 380
Plaquenil Sulfate; *see* Hydroxychloroquine sulfate
Plasma, 48-49
  antihemophilic, 456
  burns and, 253
  electrolytes and, 40, 41
Plasma cells, 62

Plasma substitute, 253
Plasma volume expanders, 69-70
Plasmodium, 37
Play, 416
  during infancy, 418
  preschool-age child and, 450-451
  school-age child and, 454
  of toddler, 439-440
Pleural effusion, 97
Pleurevac, 95
Pleurisy, 97
Pleuropneumonia-like organisms, 19
Pneumoencephalogram, 207
Pneumonectomy, 103
Pneumonia, 98, 437
Pneumothorax, 90, 101-102
Poison ivy, 254
Poisoning
  carbon monoxide, 105
  in children, 442-443
  food, 139-140
Polarization, 212
Polaroid filters, 212
Poliomyelitis, 233-234
  vaccines for, 420, 421
Polyarteritis nodosa, 257
Polycillin; *see* Ampicillin
Polycythemia, 57, 83
Polydactyly, 434
Polymycins, 33-34
Polymyxin B sulfate, 34
Polyneuritis, 229
Polysaccharide, 113, 202
Polysporin, 250
Polyuria, 143
POMP regimen, 40
POMR; *see* Problem oriented medical record
Pondimin; *see* Fenfluramine hydrochloride
Pons, 187
Ponstel; *see* Mefenamic acid
Pontocaine Hydrochloride; *see* Tetracaine hydrochloride
Pork tapeworm, 118
Portal caval shunt, 132
Portal circulation, 53
Portal hypertension, 132
Portals of entry and exit, 23
Portrait of Nursing, 493-494
Positioning of patient, 219-220
Positive end expiratory pressure, 104
Posterior pituitary hormones, 172
Postoperative care; *see* Preoperative and postoperative care
Postoperative complications, 30-31

Postpartal period, 376-377
  hemorrhage in, 385
Postural drainage, 89
Potassium
  congestive heart failure and, 77
  Cushing's syndrome and, 181
  digitalis and, 429
  fluid and electrolyte balance and, 40-41
  neuromusculoskeletal systems and, 184, 214
  pancreas and, 172
  parathyroid glands and, 166
Potassium aminosalicylate, 36
Potassium chloride, 47
Potassium hydroxide, 47
Potassium iodide, 92, 454
Potassium permanganate, 250, 255
Potassium-sparing drugs, 68
Potts procedure, 428
Povan; *see* Pyrvinium pamoate
Power, 24
PPD; *see* Purified protein derivative
PPLO; *see* Pleuropneumonia-like organisms
Practical nurse programs, 486-487, 500
Practitioners, 489, 490, 504, 505
Pramoxine hydrochloride, 26
Prazosin hydrochloride, 68
Preadolescence, 328
Precedent, 506
Precipitate labor, 385
Precipitation, 63
Prednisone, 174
  Bell's palsy and, 230
  breast carcinoma and, 164
  in combination chemotherapy, 39, 40
  Hodgkin's disease and, 85
  in leukemia, 451
Preeclampsia, 383
Pregnancy; *see also* Maternity nursing
  changes in mother during, 372-373
  course, signs, and diagnosis of, 373
  development of individual and, 147-148
  ectopic, 384
  grief responses in, 394
  medical diseases during, 387-388
  medical supervision during, 373
  nutrition and, 373-374
  tests for, 373
  toxemias of, 383-384
Pregnosticon, 373
Pregnyl; *see* Chorionic gonadotropin
Preludin; *see* Phenmetrazine hydrochloride
Premarin; *see* Conjugated estrogens
Premature ventricular contractions, 71
Prematurity, 390-391

Premocel; *see* Methylcellulose
Prenatal period, 373-374
Preoperative and postoperative care, 18-31
  congenital heart defects and, 429-430
  microbiology and, 18-23
  nursing care and, 29-31
  pharmacology and, 25-28
  physics and, 23-25
  procedures and, 28-29
Presamine; *see* Imipramine hydrochloride
Pre-Sate; *see* Chlorphentermine hydrochloride
Preschool-age child, 328, 450-454
Presentation of baby, 374
Pressoreceptors, 195-196
Pressure
  blood, 40, 53-54, 415
  central venous, 73
  hydrostatic, 40, 56
  intracranial, 225
  intraocular, 245
  osmotic, 40, 60
Prilocaine hydrochloride, 27
Primaquine phosphate, 37
Primary aldosteronism, 180-181
Primary health care worker, 505
Primary nursing, 8, 487, 490
Prime movers, 198
Primidone, 216, 228
Principen; *see* Ampicillin
Privacy, invasion of, 507
Private practice, 489, 490, 504
Pro-Banthine; *see* Propantheline bromide
Probarbital calcium, 27, 353
Probenecid, 218, 235, 457, 459
Problem oriented medical record, 8-9, 490, 505
Problem-solving approach, 8-9
Procainamide hydrochloride, 65
Procaine hydrochloride, 27
Procarbazine, 39
Prochlorperazine, 118, 341
Procidentia, 163
Proctosigmoidoscopy, 134
Professional Code, 502
Progesterone, 157
  in chemotherapy, 38
  lactation and, 146
  menopause and, 395
  menstrual cycle and, 146, 371
  ovaries and, 168, 169
  placenta and, 372
  pregnancy and, 148
  in progestogen replacement, 146
Progestin; *see* Progesterone
Progestines, 157

Progestins and estrogens, combined, 393
A Program for the Nursing Profession, 481, 487
Progressive systemic sclerosis, 257-258
Progynon; *see* Estradiol
Projection, 331
Projective behavior, 334-335, 342-343, 345
Prolactin, 146, 171, 376, 382
Prolamines, 115
Prolapse of uterus, 163, 386
Prolixin; *see* Fluphenazine
Proloid; *see* Thyroglobulin
Proluton; *see* Progesterone
Promacetin; *see* Acetosulfone sodium
Promazine hydrochloride, 27, 341, 352
Promethazine hydrochloride, 118
Promethestrol dipropionate, 392
Promizole; *see* Thiazolsulfone
Pronestyl; *see* Procainamide hydrochloride
Propadrine; *see* Phenylpropanolamine hydrochloride
Propanediol compounds, 344
Propantheline bromide, 119
Proparacaine hydrochloride, 26
Properdin, 62
Propiomazine hydrochloride, 27, 352
Propionic acid gel, 160
Proposed Curriculum for Schools of Nursing, 491
Propoxycaine hydrochloride, 27
Propoxyphene hydrochloride, 28
Propranolol hydrochloride, 65-66, 177
Proprioceptors, 195
Propylthiouracil, 174, 177
Prostaglandins, 185, 385
Prostaphlin; *see* Oxacillin sodium
Prostate gland, 144, 158-159
Prostatectomy, 158
Prostatitis, 158
Prostheses, 79-80, 235
Prostigmin; *see* Neostigmine
Prostin F$_2$ Alpha; *see* Dinoprost tromethamine
Protamines, 115
Protein buffer, 43
Proteins, 115-116; *see also* Amino acids
  absorption of, 109
  bone and, 202
  chemistry of, 59, 115-116
  liver and, 107
  nephrosis and, 452
  neuromusculoskeletal systems and, 214
  ovaries and, 168
  testes and, 166
Proternol; *see* Isoproterenol hydrochloride
Proteus bacilli, 20, 98

Prothrombin, 50
Prothrombin time, 75
Protons, 57
Protozoa, 117, 150, 160, 215
Protriptyline hydrochloride, 339
Provera; *see* Medroxyprogesterone acetate
Provest; *see* Estrogen and progesterone tablets
Pseudoephedrine hydrochloride, 92, 453
Pseudomonas
  cephalosporins and, 32
  genitourinary system and, 150
  pneumonia and, 98
  superinfection and, 32, 457
  urethritis and, 156
Psoriasis, 255
Psychiatric nursing, 322-369
  affective disorders and, 338-340
  alcoholism and, 346-347
  basic principles of, 332
  behavioral disorders of childhood and adolescence and, 349-351
  behavioral sciences and, 322-332
    anthropology in, 322-323
    psychology in, 326-332
    sociology in, 323-326
  classification of mental disorders and, 336-337
  community mental health services and, 351-352
  conditions without manifest psychiatric disorders and nonspecific conditions and, 351
  deviate patterns of behavior and, 334-336
  drug dependence and, 347
  drugs for sedation and sleep and, 352-353
  neuroses and, 343-344
  organic brain syndrome and, 337-338
  paranoid states and, 342-343
  personality disorders and, 344-346
  psychophysiologic disorders and, 347-349
  psychoses in; *see* Psychoses
  review questions and, 354-369
  schizophrenia and, 340-342
  sexual deviations and, 346
  special symptoms and, 349
  therapeutic relationship in, 332-334
  transient situational disturbances and, 349
Psychology, 326-332
Psychomotor seizures, 228
Psychoneurotic behavior, 335, 343-344
Psychophysiologic disorders, 347-349
Psychoses, 337-343
  autistic, 351
  behavioral disorders and, 350

Psychoses—cont'd
depressive reactions and, 340
functional, 338-343
symbiotic, 351
Psychotic traits, 330
Psychrophiles, 20
Psyllium hydrophilic mucilloid, 120
PT; *see* Prothrombin time
Pterygium, 244
PTT; *see* Partial thromboplastin time
Puberty, 370-371
Public Health Nursing, 483
Puerperal infection, 377
Puerperium, 376-377
Pulleys, 206
Pulmonary circulation, 53; *see also* Respiratory
system
banding of arteries and, 428
embolism and infarction and, 96
stenosis and, 427
Pulmonary disease, chronic obstructive, 100-101
Pulmonary edema, 96-97
Pulmonary function tests, 95
Pulmonary tuberculosis, 99-100
Pulse; *see* Heart rate
Purified protein derivative, 99
Purine, 116, 151, 235
Purine antagonist, 38
Purinethol; *see* Mercaptopurine
Purkinje fibers, 51-52
Pustule, 252
PVCs; *see* Premature ventricular contractions
Pydirone; *see* Dipyrone
Pyelography, intravenous, 150
Pyelonephritis, 388
Pyloric stenosis, 434-435
Pyopen; *see* Carbenicillin disodium
Pyral; *see* Dipyrone
Pyramidal tracts, 191
Pyrantel pamoate, 447
Pyrazinamide, 36, 99
Pyribenzamine Citrate; *see* Tripelennamine citrate
Pyridium; *see* Phenazopyridine
Pyridostigmine bromide, 217, 232
Pyridoxine, 35, 231; *see also* Vitamins, B_6
Pyrilamine maleate, 93
Pyrilgin; *see* Dipyrone
Pyrimethamine, 37
Pyrimidine, 116
Pyrimidine antagonist, 38
Pyrvinium pamoate, 447
PZA; *see* Pyrazinamide

Q

Quaalude; *see* Methaqualone
Quebec Nurses' Act, 502
Queckenstedt's test, 222
Questions
multiple choice, 3
types of, 1-2
Quickening, 372
Quinaglute; *see* Quinidine gluconate
Quinidex; *see* Quinidine sulfate
Quinidine, 64-65
Quinidine gluconate, 65
Quinidine hydrochloride, 65
Quinidine polygalacturonate, 65
Quinidine sulfate, 65
Quinine sulfate, 37-38
Quinora; *see* Quinidine sulfate
Quotane Hydrochloride; *see* Dimethisoquin hydrochloride

R

Race, 322
Radiation
electromagnetic, 58
light and, 208-209
neuromusculoskeletal systems and, 207
wavelengths of, 58, 209
hazards of, 207
integumentary system and, 249
microbes and, 21
to pituitary, 175, 181
in therapy
bladder tumors and, 155
brain tumors and, 224
breast carcinoma and, 164
bronchogenic carcinoma and, 103
cervical cancer and, 160
esophageal cancer and, 128
eye tumors and, 244
Hodgkin's disease and, 85
intestinal cancer and, 137
kidney cancer and, 154
laryngeal cancer and, 103
mouth cancer and, 125
multiple myeloma and, 237
myasthenia gravis and, 232
osteogenic sarcoma and, 236
pancreatic cancer and, 131
prostatic cancer and, 158
psoriasis and, 255
skin cancer and, 256
stomach carcinoma and, 127
to thymus, 232
Radical neck dissection, 103-104

Radioactive antibiotics, 39
Radioactive elements, 39, 61-62, 83, 177
bone and, 202
Radioactive iodine, 39, 177
Radioactive phosphorus, 83
Radiography, pregnancy and, 373
Radiotherapy; *see* Radiation in therapy
Rashkind procedure, 428
Raspberin; *see* Salicylamide
Rastelli's operation, 428
Rationalization, 331
Raudixin; *see* Rauwolfia serpentina
Rau-Sed; *see* Reserpine
Rautina; *see* Rauwolfia serpentina
Rauwolfia alkaloids, 67, 225
Rauwolfia serpentina, 67
Raynaud's disease, 80
Reaction formation, 331, 333
Receptors, 195-197
Recessive traits, 148
Recovery room, 31
Rectocele, 162-163, 386
Rectovaginal fistula, 162
Rectum, 106
herniation of, 162-163, 386
varicosities of, 138
Red blood cells; *see* Erythrocytes
Reduction of fractures, 239, 240
Reed-Sternberg cells, 85
Reflection
of light, 210-211
total internal, 90-91, 211
Reflex arcs, 184, 185; *see also* Reflexes
Reflex bladder, 243
Reflex hyperexcitability, 241
Reflexes, 184, 185
Hering-Breuer, 88
letdown, 376, 381-382
newborn and, 380
Refraction of light, 210-211
gastrointestinal system and, 112
Refrigeration, microbes and, 21
Regional enteritis, 133-134
Registration of nurses, 508
Regression, 331
Rehabilitation, 5, 7
Reinforcement, learning and, 14
Rela; *see* Carisoprodol
Relief from discomfort, need for, 329
Religion, 323
Renal artery and vein, 141
Renal calculi, 151
Renal colic, 151-152
Renal diseases, 151-156; *see also* Kidney

Renal hypertension, 73
Renal failure, 152-154
Renal tubules, 44, 45, 46, 141, 142
Renin, 143
Reoviruses, 91
Repetition, learning and, 14
Report on the Canadian Nurses' Association School Improvement Program, 492-493
Report of the Committee on Nurse Practitioners, 504
Report on the Experiment in Nursing Education at the Atkinson School of Nursing of the Toronto Western Hospital, 492
Report of the Nursing Education Survey Committee for the Province of Alberta, 492
Report of the Ontario Health Council on Health Care Delivery Systems, 495
Report of the Pilot Project for the Evaluation of Schools of Nursing in Canada, 492
Report on the Project for the Evaluation of the Quality of Nursing Service, 494
Report of Royal Commission on Health Services, 492
Report of the Royal Commission of Inquiry on Education, 498
Repo-Test; *see* Testosterone enanthate
Repression, 331
Reproductive system, 144-146
    development of individual and, 147-148
    diseases of, 158-165
    female, 145-146; *see also* Female
    heredity and, 148
    male, 144-145; *see also* Male
    pharmacology and, 156-158
    postpartal period and, 376-377
    pregnancy and, 372
    procedures for, 158
Rescinnamine, 67
Research in nursing, 504
Reserpine, 67
Reserpoid; *see* Reserpine
Residual air, 88
Resistance to infection, 22-23, 62-63; *see also* Infection
Resolution of conflict, 324
Respirations; *see also* Respiratory system
    acid-base balance and, 44-45
    air exchanged in, 88-89
    Boyle's law and, 90
    growth and, 415
    physiology of, 87-89
Respiratory acidosis, 44-45, 453
Respiratory alkalosis, 45
Respiratory distress syndrome, adult, 104-105

Respiratory system, 86-105; *see also* Respirations
    anatomy and physiology of, 86-89
    cystic fibrosis and, 449
    diseases of, 96-105, 437
    growth and, 415
    infections and, 437
    microorganisms and, 91
    newborn and, 380
    pharmacology and, 91-93
    physics and, 89-91
    pregnancy and, 373
    procedures and, 93-96
Respondeat superior doctrine, 506, 508
Resting potential, 184
Retardation, mental, 444-445
Retina, 196-197
    cones of, 210
    detached, 246
    tumor of, 244
Retinoblastoma, 244
Retinoscope, 214
Rh blood groups, 50
    incompatibility and, 389-390
Rheomacrodex; *see* Dextran 40
Rheumatic fever, 457-458
Rheumatoid arthritis, 234
    juvenile, 458-459
Rhinitis, allergic, 452
Rhizotomy, 237
RhoGAM, 376, 390, 394
Rhythm method of contraception, 393
Ribonucleic acid, 116-117, 166, 168
Ribose, 113
Rickettsials, 91
Rifadin; *see* Rifampin
Rifampin, 36
Rigidity, 445
Rigor mortis, 199
Rimactane; *see* Rifampin
Ringer's lactate, 253
Ringworm, 459
Riogon; *see* Chorionic gonadotropin
Riopan; *see* Magaldrate
Ritalin; *see* Methylphenidate hydrochloride
RNA; *see* Ribonucleic acid
RNA viruses, 91, 215
Robaxin; *see* Methocarbamol
Robitussin; *see* Glyceryl guaiacolate
Rocking beds, 89
Roles
    altered patterns of, 324
    of nurse, 7-18; *see also* Nurses, role of
Rolsul; *see* Succinylsulfathiazole

Romeph; *see* Mephenesin
Romilar; *see* Dextromethorphan hydrobromide
Rooting reflex, 380
Roquine; *see* Chloroquine phosphate
Rotating tourniquets, 77, 96-97
Rothalid; *see* Phthalylsulfathiazole
Roundworms, 117
Rowsell, G. S., 493
Royal Commission on Health Services, 501
Royal Commission on Health Services Briefs, 492
Royal Commission on Health Services in Canada, 498, 499
Royal Commission on Health Services Nursing Education in Canada, 493
Royal Commission Inquiry into Civil Rights, 501
Rubella vaccine, 420, 421
Runaway reaction, 349
Rupture
    of bladder, 156
    of fallopian tube, 384
    of nucleus pulposus, 238
    of uterus, 386-387
Russell, K., 492
Russell traction, 239

S

SA node; *see* Sinoatrial node
Saccharomyces cerevisiae, 20-21
Sadism, 346
SAI; *see* Social Adequacy Index
St. Vitus' dance, 457
Salamide; *see* Salicylamide
Salicim; *see* Salicylamide
Salicylamide, 28, 458
Salicylates; *see also* Acetylsalicylic acid
    in arthritis, 217, 218, 458
    drug interactions and, 457, 458-459
    pain control and, 27-28
    poisoning from, 442, 459
Salicylic acid, 113
Saline injection abortion, 394
Saliva, 108
Salivary glands, 106
Salmonella, 19, 20, 40, 140, 235
Salpingectomy, 161
Salpingitis, 161
Salrin; *see* Salicylamide
Salts, 47-48
Salyrgan-Theophylline; *see* Mersalyl with theophylline
Sandril; *see* Reserpine
Sansert; *see* Methysergide maleate
Saponification, 114

Saprophytes, 19
Sarcoidosis, 99
Sarcolemma, 198
Sarcomas, osteogenic, 236
Saturated solution, 60
Scabanca; *see* Benzyl benzoate lotion
Scabicides, 250
Scabies, 459
Scalp, ringworm and, 459
Scarlett Report, 492
Scars, 249
Schizoid personality, 345
Schizophrenia, 340-342, 351
School-age child, 328, 454-460
Schwann cells, 183
Science for Health Services, 505
Scleral buckling, 246
Scleroderma, 257-258
Sclerosis
    multiple, 231-232
    progressive systemic, 257-258
Scopolamine, 218, 387
Scrotum, 144
Search warrants, 508
Seatworm, 118
Sebaceous glands, 248
Secobarbital, 27, 353
Seconal; *see* Secobarbital
Second-degree AV block, 72
Secretin, 109, 117
Security, need for, 329
Sedatives, 27, 352-353; *see also* specific drug
    drug interactions and, 344, 353
    excess ingestion of, 353
Seizures, 215-216, 228-229, 438
Self-care, 6
Self-concept, 329
Self-help groups, 6
Selye's general adaptation syndrome, 5, 327
Semicircular canal, 197
Seminal ducts, 144
Seminal vesicles, 144
Senescence, 329, 349
Sengstaken-Blakemore tube, 132, 133
Senna, 120
Senokot; *see* Senna
Sense organs, 195-197
Sensorineural hearing disorders, 446; *see also*
    Hearing
Sensory neural pathways, 190
Sensory neurons, 183
Separation anxiety, 422
Septic shock, 82
Sequestrectomy, 236

Serax; *see* Oxazepam
Seromycin; *see* Cycloserine
Serotonin, 184, 214
Serous otitis, 437
Serpasil; *see* Reserpine
Serum, 48
Serum enzymes, 74, 75
Serum glutamic oxaloacetic transaminase, 75
Serum isoenzymes, 74
Sex determination, 148
Sex hormones, 167-168, 169
    female, 168-169; *see also* specific hormone
    male, 144, 167-168, 169; *see also* Androgens;
        Testosterone
    metabolism and, 111
Sex-linked genes, 148
Sexual deviations, 346
SGOT; *see* Serum glutamic oxaloacetic trans-
    aminase
Sheaths
    of nervous system, 183
    of tendons, 199
Shigella, 19, 20, 117
Shingles, 256-257
Shivering, 199
Shock, 81-82
    anaphylactic, 82
    cardiogenic, 81
    hypovolemic, 81, 253
    insulin, 180, 455
    neurogenic, 81-82, 253
    spinal, 241
Sickle cell anemia, 449-450
SIDS; *see* Sudden infant death syndrome
Sight; *see* Vision
Sigmoid implantation of ureters, 155, 156, 432
Signs
    Chadwick's, 372
    Chvostek's, 178
    Galeazzi's, 433
    Goodell's, 372
    Hegar's, 372
    Homans', 78
    Nikolsky's, 255
    Ortolani's, 433
    of labor, 375
    of pregnancy, 373
    Trousseau's, 178
Silicosis, 101
Silvadene; *see* Silver sulfadiazine
Silver, 215
Silver nitrate, 22
    burns and, 251, 253
    chemistry of, 48

Silver nitrate—cont'd
    ophthalmia neonatorum and, 165, 376, 378-
        379
Silver sulfadiazine, 250, 251, 253
Simmonds' disease, 175-176
Sinequan; *see* Doxepin hydrochloride
Single-lens reflex, 212
Singoserp; *see* Syrosingopine
Sinoatrial node, 51-52, 72
Sinuses, 86
Skelaxin; *see* Metaxalone
Skeletal muscles; *see also* muscles
    metabolism of, 199
    motoneural pathways to, 190-193
    origins, insertions, and functions of, 200-202
    relaxants for, 217
Skeletal system
    anatomy and physiology of, 199-206
    chemistry and, 214-215
    diseases of; *see* Neuromusculoskeletal sys-
        tems, diseases of
    microorganisms and, 215
    pharmacology and, 215-219
    physics and, 206-214
    pregnancy and, 373
    procedures and, 219-223
Skeletal traction, 239
Skene's glands, 146
SK-Estrogens; *see* Esterified estrogens
Skin; *see* Integumentary system
Skin grafts, 251-252
Skin traction, 239
SK-Soxazole; *see* Sulfisoxazole
SLE; *see* Systemic lupus erythematosus
Sleep, drugs for, 27, 352-353
    drug interactions and, 344, 353
Sleepwalking, 343, 349
Slipped disc, 238
SLR; *see* Single-lens reflex
Small intestine, 106
    carcinoma of, 136-137
Smell, sense of, 196
Smooth muscle, 197; *see also* muscles
SOAP format, 9
Soapsuds enema, 122
Social Adequacy Index, 208
Social factors, nursing and, 490-491, 505-506;
    see also society
Social Security Act, 488-489
Socially aggressive behavior, 335-336, 345
Society, 323-324
    communities in, 325
    family in, 324
    health and, 325-326

Society—cont'd
  hospitals and, 326
  nursing and, 490-491, 505-506
Sociology, 323-326
Sociopathic personality, 345
Sodium
  bone and, 199, 202
  fluid and electrolyte balance and, 40-41
  neuromusculoskeletal systems and, 184, 214
  pancreas and, 172
Sodium aminosalicylate, 36
Sodium bicarbonate
  as antacid, 119
  buffer mechanisms and, 43, 44, 61
  as salt, 48
  tetracyclines and, 33
Sodium bromide, 27, 353
Sodium carboxymethylcellulose, 120
Sodium chloride, 47
Sodium hydroxide, 47
Sodium iodide, radioactive, 39; *see also* Iodine,
    radioactive
Sodium nitroprusside, 67
Sodium phosphate
  effervescent, 121
  radioactive, 39
Sodium pump, 184
Sodium salicylate, 28, 218, 458
Sodizole; *see* Sulfisoxazole
Soft diet, 31
Solacen; *see* Tybamate
Solar irradiation, 255
Solarcaine; *see* Benzocaine
Solids, physical properties of, 56, 90, 112
Solitary play, 418
Solubility, 60
Solu-Cortef; *see* Hydrocortisone succinate
Solu-Medrol; *see* Methylprednisolone sodium
    succinate
Solute, 60
Solutions, 60-61
  integumentary system and, 249
Solvent, 60
Soma; *see* Carisoprodol
Somatostatin, 172
Sombucaps; *see* Hexobarbital
Sombulex; *see* Hexobarbital
Somnambulism, 343, 349
Somnos; *see* Chloral hydrate
Sopor; *see* Methaqualone
Sorbitrate; *see* Isosorbide dinitrate
Sosol; *see* Sulfisoxazole
Sound, 207-208
  interpretation of, 207-208
  principles of, 57

Sound—cont'd
  quality of, 208
Soxomide; *see* Sulfisoxazole
Sparine; *see* Promazine hydrochloride
Sparteine sulfate, 376, 385
Spartocin; *see* Sparteine sulfate
Spastic bladder, 243
Spastic paralysis, 241
Spasticity, 445
Special Committee on Nurse Education, 491
Specialty nurse practitioner, 490, 504-505
Specific gravity of urine, 149
Specific heat, 25
Speech appliance, 425
Speech audiometry, 207-208
Speech disturbances, 349
Speech reception threshold, 208
Spermatic cords, 144-145
Spermatogenesis, 144
Spermatozoa, 144, 147
Spermicidal creams, jellies, foam tablets, and
    vaginal suppositories, 393
Sphingomyelins, 115
Spica cast, 433-434
Spina bifida, 380, 430-431
Spinal cord, 185-187
  coverings of, 189
  injury to, 241-243
  intervertebral disc herniation and, 238
  lumbar puncture and, 222-223
Spinal fluid; *see* Cerebrospinal fluid
Spinal fusion, 238, 241
Spinal nerves, 190
Spinal shock, 241
Spine
  fractures of, 241
  fusion of, 238, 241
  malformations of, 430-431
Spirochete, 19, 150, 165, 389
Spirometer, 88
Spironolactone, 68, 181
Spleen, 55
Splints, 222
Spontaneous pneumothorax, 101
Spores, 19, 20
Spotlight on Nursing Education, 492
Squamous cell carcinoma of skin, 255-256
SRT; *see* Speech reception threshold
SSE; *see* Soapsuds enema
Stages of development, 328-329
Staining, 20
Stapedectomy, 247
Stapes, 197
  removal of, 247
Staphcillin; *see* Methicillin sodium

Staphylococci, 18
  food poisoning and, 139
  impetigo and, 389, 459
  newborn and, 389
  osteomyelitis and, 235
  otitis media and, 437
  penicillins and, 32
  pneumonia and, 98
  pyelonephritis in pregnancy and, 388
  urethritis and, 156
Staphylococcus aureus, 18, 32, 98, 139, 235
Starch, 114
Starling's law
  of capillaries, 40
  of heart, 53
State of matter; *see* Matter
State Board Test Pool Examination, 488, 509
Statement of Delivery of Nursing Care, 501
Statement of the Expanded Role of the Nurse,
    504
Statement on Specialization in Nursing, 504-505
Static electricity, 23-24
Station of baby, 375
Status asthmaticus, 100, 453, 454
Status epilepticus, 228
Statutory law, 506
Steatorrhea, 448
Steinmann pin, 239
Stelazine; *see* Trifluoperazine
Stemultrolin; *see* Chorionic gonadotropin
Stenosis
  of aorta, 427
  pulmonary, 427
  pyloric, 434-435
Step reflex, 380
Stereotypes, 322
Sterility, 391-393
Sterilization
  asepsis and, 21
  family planning and, 147, 158, 393
Steroid hormones, 115; *see also* specific hor-
    mone; Corticosteroids
Sterotate; *see* Testosterone
Stimulants, cerebral, 339
Stimulators, intractable pain and, 237
Stocking and glove anesthesia, 343
Stomach, 106
  carcinoma of, 127
  inflammation of, 125-126
Stomatitis, 124-125
Stools; *see also* Defecation
  currant jelly, 435
  of newborn, 380
  specimens of, 122
Strabismus, 446-447

Streptococci, 18
  circulatory system and, 62, 76
  glomerulonephritis and, 155
  impetigo and, 389, 459
  osteomyelitis and, 235
  otitis media and, 437
  pelvic inflammatory disease and, 161
  pneumonia and, 98
  pyelonephritis in pregnancy and, 388
  rheumatic fever and, 457
  urethritis and, 156
Streptococcus pyogenes, 18, 62
Streptococcus viridans, 62, 76
Streptomycin, 33, 36, 99
Stresses, 5
  transient situational disturbances and, 349
Striae gravidarum, 248
Striated muscle, 197
Stridor, laryngeal, 426
Stroke, 226-228
Strontium, 215
Structure Study of the Canadian Nurses' Association, 495
Strycin; *see* Streptomycin
Stryker frame, 219
Student Nurses' Association, 496
Studies of nursing and nursing education, 480-482, 491-495
The Study of Credentialing in Nursing, 482
A Study of the Development of a Diploma Program in Nursing at the Ryerson Institute of Technology, Toronto, 493
Study of Nursing Education in New Brunswick, 492
Stump care, 79
Subacute bacterial endocarditis, 76
Subarachnoid hemorrhage, 225
Subarachnoid space, 189
Subconscious, 327
Subcutaneous medications, 17-18
Subcutaneous nodules, 457
Subdural hemorrhage, 224, 226
Sublimation, 331
Substitution, 331
Succinylcholine chloride, 338
Succinylsulfathiazole, 34
Sucking reflex, 380
Sucrets; *see* Dextromethorphan hydrobromide
Sucrose, 114
Suctioning of airways, 94
Sudafed; *see* Pseudoephedrine hydrochloride
Sudden infant death syndrome, 436
Sulfa drugs, 34, 35, 388; *see also* specific drug; Sulfonamides
Sulfabid; *see* Sulfaphenazole

Sulfadiazine, 34, 457-458
Sulfamethizole, 34
Sulfamethoxazole, 34, 35
Sulfamides, 34, 35, 388; *see also* specific drug; Sulfonamides
Sulfamylon; *see* Mafenide acetate
Sulfaphenazole, 34
Sulfasalazine, 34
Sulfasuxidine; *see* Succinylsulfathiazole
Sulfathalidine; *see* Phthalylsulfathiazole
Sulfinpyrazone, 151, 459
Sulfisocon; *see* Sulfisoxazole
Sulfisomidine, 34
Sulfisoxazole, 34, 35
Sulfonamides, 34-35, 388; *see also* specific drug
  cystitis and, 151
  drug interactions and, 457, 458, 459
  rheumatic fever and, 457-458
Sulfones, 35
Sulfonylureas, 16; *see also* Hypoglycemics, oral
Sulfoxone sodium, 35
Sulfuric acid, 47
Sullivan, H. S., 328, 329
Sumycin; *see* Tetracycline
Sunset eyes, 431
Superego, 328
Superinfection, 32, 457
Supersaturated solution, 60
Suppression, 331
Suprapubic catheter, 156
Surfacaine; *see* Cyclomethycaine
Surface tension, 90, 112
Surfactant, 87
Surfak; *see* Dioctyl calcium sulfosuccinate
Surgical asepsis, 32
Surgical nursing; *see* Medical-surgical nursing
Surital Sodium; *see* Thiamylal sodium
Survey of Nursing Education in Canada, 491
Sus-Phrine; *see* Epinephrine, aqueous
Swan-Ganz catheter, 72-73
Sweat glands, 449
Swine flu, 233
Swing crutch gaits, 221
Sydenham's chorea, 457
Symbiotic psychosis, 351
Symmetrel; *see* Amantadine hydrochloride
Sympathectomy, 80, 237
Sympathetic amines, 91-92
Sympathetic nervous system, 193-195, 327
Sympathomimetic drugs, 339
Synalar; *see* Fluocinolone acetonide
Synapse, 183-184
  conduction across, 184-185
Synarthrotic joints, 203
Syncelose; *see* Methylcellulose

Syncytium, 197
Syndactyly, 434
Syndromes; *see also* Diseases
  Adams-Stokes, 72
  adult respiratory distress, 104-105
  Arnold-Chiari, 430
  battered child, 443-444
  Conn's, 180-181
  Cushing's, 181
  Down's, 148, 423
  dumping, 126, 127
  failure to thrive, 435-436
  fetal alcohol, 390
  general adaptation, 5, 327
  gray baby, 34
  Guillain-Barré, 233
  hyperventilation, 348
  Klinefelter's, 148, 424
  Korsakoff's, 337
  malabsorption, 420, 448
  maternal deprivation, 435-436
  nephrotic, 452
  organic brain, 337-338
  sudden infant death, 436
  Turner's, 148, 423
  Zollinger-Ellison, 126
Synergists, 198
Synestrol; *see* Dienestrol
Synovectomy, 235
Synthroid; *see* Levothyroxine sodium
Syntocinon; *see* Oxytocin
Syphilis, 165, 389; *see also Treponema pallidum*
Syrosingopine, 67
Syrup of ipecac, 442
Systemic lupus erythematosus, 257
Systemic sclerosis, progressive, 257-258

T

T tube, 129
Tacaryl; *see* Methdilazine hydrochloride
Tace; *see* Chlorotrianisene
Tachycardia, ventricular, 71
Taenia marginata, 118
Taenia solium, 118
Tagathen; *see* Chlorothen citrate
Talbutal, 27, 353
Talipes equinovarus, 432
Talwin; *see* Pentazocine hydrochloride
Tandearil; *see* Oxyphenbutazone
Tap water enema, 122
Tapazole; *see* Methimazole
Tapeworm, 118
Taractan; *see* Chlorprothixene
Tardive dyskinesias, 342

Tars, 251

Task Force Reports on Cost of Health Service in Canada, 495

Task Force Reports on Cost of Health Services in Canada-Public Health Services, 495

Taste, 196

Taurine, 184

Ta-Verm; *see* Piperazine citrate

Td; *see* Tetanus and diphtheria toxoids, combined

Teaching, 11

Teaching-learning environment, 11-14

Team nursing, 8, 487, 501

Teebacin; *see* Potassium aminosalicylate

Teebacin Calcium; *see* Calcium aminosalicylate

Teeth, 105
  cleft palate and, 425
  of infant, 417, 418
  school-age child and, 454
  of toddler, 439

Tegretol; *see* Carbamazepine

Teldrin; *see* Chlorpheniramine maleate

Telepaque, 129

Temperature
  absolute, 24
  bacteria, 20
  conversions of, 24
  elevated
    convulsions and, 438
    transfusions and, 29

Temporal lobes of brain, 189

Tempra; *see* Acetaminophen

Tendon sheaths, 199

Tensilon; *see* Edrophonium

Tension pneumothorax, 101

Tenuate; *see* Diethylpropion hydrochloride

Tepanil; *see* Diethylpropion hydrochloride

Terbutaline, 92, 453

Terpin hydrate elixir, 92, 453-454

Terramycin; *see* Oxytetracycline

Teslac; *see* Androgens

Tessalon; *see* Benzonatate

Test questions; *see also* Tests
  multiple choice, 3
  types of, 1-2

Testate; *see* Testosterone enanthate

Testes, 144, 166-168, 169
  undescended, 432

Testonate; *see* Testosterone propionate

Testosterone, 144, 157, 167-168, 169, 392
  chemotherapy and, 38, 158
  metabolism and, 111

Testosterone cypionate, 392

Testosterone enanthate, 157, 392

Testosterone propionate, 392

Testostroval-P.A.; *see* Testosterone enanthate

Tests
  adrenocorticotropic hormone, 182
  Aschheim-Zondek, 373
  Bárány's caloric, 223
  Benedict's, 113
  biuret, 116
  Clinitest, 113
  fecal fat, 134
  ferric chloride urine, 434
  Friedman's, 373
  for glucose in urine, 113
  Guthrie blood, 434
  Hopkins-Cole, 116
  Kveim, 99
  Millon's, 116
  ninhydrin, 116
  pregnancy, 373
  pulmonary function, 95
  Queckenstedt's, 222
  in rheumatic fever, 457
  Thorn, 182
  Trendelenburg, 80
  tuberculin, 99, 420, 421
  of urine, 113, 150, 181, 182
  xanthoproteic, 116
  D-xylose tolerance, 134

Tetanus and diphtheria toxoids, combined, 420, 421

Tetanus toxoid, 253, 420, 421

Tetany, 177, 178

Tetracaine hydrochloride, 26

Tetracycline, 33
  acne vulgaris and, 254
  cystitis and, 151
  drug interactions and, 17, 448
  trachoma and, 244

Tetrahydrofolic acid, 70

Tetralogy of Fallot, 427-428

Thalamus, 188
  destruction of, 231

Theelin; *see* Estrone

Theogen; *see* Conjugated estrogens

Theophylline, 91, 453

Therapeutic index, 16

Therapeutic nursing relationship, 332-334

Thermodynamics, laws of, 56, 112

Thermography, 163

Thermometers, electronic, 24

Thermophiles, 20

Thiamine in neuritis, 229

Thiamylal sodium, 26

Thiazides, 68

Thiazolsulfone, 35

Thioguanine, 38

Thiomerin; *see* Mercaptomerin sodium

Thiopental sodium, 26

Thiophosphoramide, 39, 85, 164

Thioridazine hydrochloride, 341

Thiosulfil; *see* Sulfamethizole

Thio-TEPA, 39, 85, 164

Thiothixene, 342

Thioxanthenes, 342

Thirst mechanism, 42

Thoracentesis, 95

Thoracolumbar nervous system, 193-195

Thoracoplasty, 103

Thoracotomy, exploratory, 103

Thorazine; *see* Chlorpromazine hydrochloride

Thorn test, 182

Three-point gait, 221

Thrombi, 78

Thrombin, 456

Thromboangiitis obliterans, 80

Thrombocytes, 49-50

Thrombophlebitis, 78-80

Thrush, 124, 389

Thymus, 167, 172
  x-ray therapy of, 232

Thyrar; *see* Thyroid

Thyrocalcitonin, 168

Thyroglobulin, 173

Thyroid, 173
  deficiency of, 176
  excessive, 176-177

Thyroid gland, 166, 167, 168
  diseases of, 176-177
  drugs and, 173-174

Thyroid-stimulating hormone, 171, 188

Thyroid storm, 177

Thyroidectomy, 177

Thyrotomy, 103

Thyrotropin-releasing hormone, 188

Thyroxine, 168

T.I.; *see* Therapeutic index

TIA; *see* Transient ischemic attacks

Tic douloureux, 230

Tidal air, 88

Tidal volume, 95

Tigan; *see* Trimethobenzamide hydrochloride

Timolol maleate, 218

Timoptic; *see* Timolol maleate

Tincture
  belladonna leaf, 119
  of opium, 120

Tindal; *see* Acetophenazine maleate

Tinea capitis, 459

T-Ionate-P.A.; *see* Testosterone cypionate
Tissue repair, 249
Titroid; *see* Levothyroxine sodium
Tobramycin sulfate, 33
Tocosamine; *see* Sparteine sulfate
Toddler, 438-450
  accident prevention and, 440
  anemia and, 447-448
  aspiration of foreign objects and, 443
  battered child syndrome and, 443-444
  burns and, 441-442
  celiac disease and, 448
  cerebral palsy and, 445-446
  cystic fibrosis of pancreas and, 448-449
  fractures and, 443
  growth and development of, 438-439
  health problems of, 440-450
  health promotion and, 440
  hearing disorders and, 446
  hospitalization of, 440-441
  mental retardation and, 444-445
  nutrition of, 440
  pinworms and, 447
  play of, 439-440
  poisoning and, 442-443
  sickle cell anemia and, 449-450
  visual disorders and, 446-447
Tofranil; *see* Imipramine hydrochloride
Togaviruses, 215
Toilet training, 439
Tolanate; *see* Inositol hexanitrate
Tolax; *see* Mephenesin
Tolazamide, 173
Tolbutamide, 173
Tolerance, 347
Toleron; *see* Ferrous fumarate
Tolinase; *see* Tolazamide
Tolserol; *see* Mephenesin
Tongue, 105-106
Tonic contractions, 199
Tonsillectomy, 454
Tonsillitis, 437
Tonsils, 86, 106
  inflammation of, 437
  removal of, 454
Topical drugs, 250-251
  anesthetics as, 26
TOPV; *see* Trivalent oral poliovirus vaccine
Torts, 506-507
Total internal reflection, 90-91, 211
Total lung capacity, 95
Total parenteral nutrition, 31, 124
Tourniquets, rotating, 77, 96-97
Toxemias of pregnancy, 383-384

Toxic products of microorganisms, 23
Toxicology, 15
Toxoids, 63, 253, 420, 421
Toys, 416
T.P.N.; *see* Total parenteral nutrition
Trace; *see* Chlorotrianisene
Trachea, 87
  diseases of, 425
  opening into, 94, 104
Tracheoesophageal anomalies, 425
Tracheoesophageal fistula, 425
Tracheostomy, 94, 104
Trachoma, 244
Traction, 239
  in children, 443
  dislocated hip and, 433
  patient care and, 240
Tracts
  extrapyramidal, 191-193
  facilitatory, 193
  inhibitory, 193
  nervous system and, 185, 191-193
  pyramidal, 191
Trancopal; *see* Chlormezanone
Tranquilizers; *see also* specific drug
  drug dependence and, 347
  major
    adverse effects of, 342
    psychoses and, 341-342
  minor
    behavioral disorders and, 350, 351
    neuroses and, 344
Transfer of patients, 219
Transference, 331
Transfusions, blood, 29
  exchange, 390
  intrauterine, 390
  in leukemia, 451
Transient ischemic attacks, 226
Transient situational disturbances, 349
Transitional stools, 380
Translocation 15/21, 423
Transplantation of kidneys, 154
Transposition of great vessels, 428
Transvestism, 346
Trantoin; *see* Nitrofurantoin
Tranxene; *see* Clorazepate dipotassium
Tranylcypromine sulfate, 339
Tratracyn; *see* Tetracycline
Trauma
  bladder, 156
  chest, 102
  childbirth and, 386-387
  to head, 224

Travase ointment, 253
Trecator S.C.; *see* Ethionamide
Trematodes, 118
Tremin; *see* Trihexyphenidyl
Tremor, 230, 445
Trench mouth, 124
Trendelenburg test, 80
Treponema pallidum, 19, 150, 165, 389
Treppe, 199
TRH; *see* Thyrotropin-releasing hormone
Triamalone; *see* Triamcinolone
Triamcinolone, 251, 256
Triamterene, 68
Trichinella spiralis, 215
Trichloroacetic acid, 27, 352
Trichloroethylene, 25
Trichomonas vaginalis, 36, 150, 160
Trichuris trichiura, 118
Tricofuron; *see* Furazolidone-nifuroxime
Tricuspid atresia, 428
Tridione; *see* Trimethadione
Triethylenethiophosphoramide, 39, 85, 164
Trifluoperazine, 341
Triflupromazine hydrochloride, 341
Trigeminal neuralgia, 230
Trihexyphenidyl, 216, 217, 342
Triiodothyronine, 168
Trilafon; *see* Perphenazine
Trilene; *see* Trichloroethylene
Trimethadione, 216, 228
Trimethobenzamide hydrochloride, 118
Trimethylene, 25
Tripelennamine citrate, 93
Tripod crutch gaits, 221
Trisomy 18, 423
Trisomy 21, 148, 423
Trivalent oral poliovirus vaccine, 420, 421
Trocosone; *see* Esterified estrogens
Trolnitrate phosphate, 66
Tronothane Hydrochloride; *see* Pramoxine hydrochloride
Trophoblast, 371
Trophoderm, 147
Tropicamide, 218, 219
Trousseau's sign, 178
Truncus arteriosus, 428
Trypanosoma, 215
Trypsin, 448
TSH; *see* Thyroid-stimulating hormone
Tubal ligation, 147, 158
Tube feeding, 123-124
Tubercle bacillus, 19, 35-36, 91, 99, 161
Tuberculin tests, 99, 420, 421

Tuberculosis, pulmonary, 99-100; *see also* Tubercle bacillus
Tubules, renal, 44, 45, 46, 141, 142
Tumors, 252; *see also* Carcinoma
    bladder, 155-156
    brain, 224-225
        pressures and, 206
    of eye, 244-245
Turbinates, 86
Turner's syndrome, 148, 423
Turning patient by log-rolling, 238
TWE; *see* Tap water enema
Two-point alternate crutch gait, 221
Tybamate, 344
Tylenol; *see* Acetaminophen
Tympanoplasty, 246
Tyndall effect, 61
Tyramine, 339
Tyrosine, 420, 434

U

Ulcerative colitis, 135, 348
Ulcers
    Curling's, 252
    intestinal, 133-134
    peptic, 126-127, 252, 348
    psychogenic factors and, 348
Ulo; *see* Chlophedianol hydrochloride
Ultandren; *see* Fluoxymesterone
Ultran; *see* Phenaglycodol
Ultrasonography, 208, 231, 373
Ultraviolet light, 249, 255
Umbilical cord, 147, 372
Umbilical hernias, 138
Unconscious, 327-328
Unconscious patient, 226
Underweight, 420, 440, 448, 461
Unipen; *see* Nafcillin sodium
Unisulf; *see* Sulfisoxazole
Universal antidote, 442
University education
    changes in, 490, 498-499, 504
    early developments of, 485, 496-497
United States, nursing in; *see* Nursing, in United States
Unsaturated solution, 60
Unsocialized aggressive reaction, 350
Urea, 20, 107, 219
Ureaphil; *see* Urea
Uremia, 153
Ureteral calculi, 151
Ureterosigmoidostomy, 155, 156, 432
Ureterostomy, 155

Ureterovaginal fistula, 162
Ureters, 143
    calculi in, 151
    opening into, 155
    sigmoid implantation of, 155, 156, 432
    vaginal fistulas and, 162
Urethra, 143-144
    displacement of opening of, 432
    inflammation of, 156
Urethritis, 156
Urevert; *see* Urea
Uric acid, 151, 235
Urinalysis, 150
Urinary bladder, 143
    exstrophy of, 432
    flaccid, 243
    herniation of, 162-163
    inflammation of, 150-151
    neurogenic, 243, 431
    retraining and, 243
    spastic, 243
    trauma or rupture of, 156
    tumors of, 155-156
Urinary meatus, female, 146
Urinary system; *see* Genitourinary system
Urine
    acidification of, 44, 46
    chemistry of, 149
    composition of, 143
    normal, 149
    tests for, 150
        glucose, 113
        17-ketosteroid and 17-hydroxysteroid, 181, 182
    volume of, 143
Uritone; *see* Methenamines
Uteracon; *see* Oxytocin
Uterine tubes, 145
    ligation of, 147, 158
    rupture of, 384
Uterus, 145
    contractions of, 375
        Braxton-Hicks, 375
        induction and control of, 376, 385-386
    displacement of, 386
    endometriosis and, 161
    prolapse of, 163, 386
    rupture of, 386-387
Uveitis, 244

V

V; *see* Volts
Vaccines, 63, 420, 421

Vacuum aspiration abortion, 394
Vagina, 145
    absent, 432
    fistulas and, 162
    inflammation of, 160-161
    orifice of, 146
    outlet relaxation of, 386
    pH of, 161
    repair of, 386
Vaginal pessary, 163
Vaginitis, 160-161
Vaginoplasty, 386
Vagotomy, 126
Validation, consensual, 327
Valisone; *see* Betamethasone valerate
Valium; *see* Diazepam
Vallestril; *see* Methallenestril
Valmid; *see* Ethinamate
Valsalva maneuver, 244
Valves of heart, 51
Vaponefrin; *see* Epinephrine
Varicose veins, 80
    of rectum, 138
Vas deferens, 144
Vasectomy, 147, 158, 393
Vasodilan; *see* Isoxsuprine hydrochloride
Vasopressin, 69, 172, 175; *see also* Antidiuretic hormone
    body water regulation and, 59
    diabetes insipidus and, 176
Vasopressin tannate, 175, 176
Vasoxyl; *see* Methoxamine hydrochloride
V-Cillin; *see* Penicillin V
V.D.; *see* Venereal disease
Veins, 52; *see also* Blood vessels
    central venous pressure and, 73
    ligation of, 80
    varicose, 80, 138
Velban; *see* Vinblastine sulfate
Velosef; *see* Cephradine
Venereal disease, 165
Ventilation, mechanical, 94-95
Ventilators, 94
Ventricles
    of brain, 189-190
    of heart, 51, 71, 427, 428, 431
Ventricular fibrillation, 71
Ventricular hypertrophy, right, 428
Ventricular septal defect, 427
Ventricular tachycardia, 71
Ventriculoatrial shunt, 431
Ventriculoperitoneal shunt, 431
Vercyte; *see* Pipobroman

Vermidol; *see* Piperazine citrate
Vermiform appendix, 106
Vertebrae
   fractures of, 241
   fusion of, 238, 241
   malformations of, 430-431
Vertigo, 247
Vesicle, 252
Vesicovaginal fistula, 162
Vesprin; *see* Triflupromazine hydrochloride
Vessels; *see* Blood vessels
Vestibular labyrinthine function test, 223
Vestibular nerve, surgical destruction of, 247
Vestibule of ear, 197
Vibramycin Hyclate; *see* Doxycycline hyclate
Vibrio cholerae, 117
Vinblastine sulfate, 39
Vincent's angina, 124
Vincristine, 39, 40, 85, 164, 452
Vinegar, 47, 160, 442
Vinethene; *see* Vinyl ether
Vinyl ether, 25
Viocin; *see* Viomycin sulfate
Viokase; *see* Pancreatin
Viomycin sulfate, 36
Virtual images, 211
Virucide, 21
Viruses, 20
   diarrhea and, 436
   Epstein-Barr, 99
   herpes simplex and, 124
   herpes zoster and, 256
   neuromusculoskeletal systems and, 215, 233, 437
   respiratory system and, 92, 98, 99, 437
Visceroceptors, 195-196
Vision, 196-197; *see also* Eye
   binocular, 214
   disorders of, in children, 446-447
   physiology of, 196-197
Vistaril; *see* Hydroxyzine pamoate
Vital capacity, 88-89, 95
   growth and, 415
Vitamins
   A
      acne vulgaris and, 254
      adolescent and, 461
      childhood and, 440
      hepatitis and, 132
      integumentary system and, 249
      liver and, 107
   B_1, 229

Vitamins—cont'd
   B_3, 107
   B_6
      cerebral palsy and, 445
      isoniazid and, 35
      paralysis agitans and, 231
      tuberculosis and, 100
   B_{12}
      blood and, 49
      Crohn's disease and, 134
      with intrinsic factor concentrate, 70
      liver and, 107
      pernicious anemia and, 82
      replacement of, 70
      stomach carcinoma and, 127
   C
      adolescent and, 461
      anemia and, 448
      birth injuries and, 389
      childhood and, 440
      wound healing and, 31
      in celiac disease, 448
      cystic fibrosis and, 449
   D
      breast milk and, 419
      calcium regulation and, 42, 166
      ergosterol and, 115
      hepatitis and, 132
      in hypoparathyroidism, 178
      integumentary system and, 248, 249
      lead poisoning and, 443
      liver and, 107
      osteoporosis and, 236
      parathyroid glands and, 166
      replacement of, 216
      as steroid, 116
   E, 132, 249
   K
      birth injuries and, 389
      blood coagulation and, 50
      cholecystitis and, 129
      hepatitis and, 132
      liver and, 107
      pancreatic cancer and, 131
      polymycins and, 34
      salicylate poisoning and, 442
      renal tubules and, 141
      in urine, 143
Vivactil; *see* Protriptyline hydrochloride
Vocal cords, 86-87
Volts, 24
Voluntary agencies, 5-6, 395
Volvulus, 135

Vomiting
   induction of, 442
   infants and, 436
Vontrol; *see* Diphenidol hydrochloride
Voyeurism, 346
VSD; *see* Ventricular septal defect
Vulva, 145-146
   lacerations of, 386

W

W; *see* Watts
Walkers, 222
Wallace, W. S., 492
War crises for nursing, 485, 500
Warfarin sodium, 70
Water; *see also* Fluids
   avenues of, for entering and leaving body, 42
   body regulation of, 59
   chemistry of, 58-59
   as conductor, 58
   importance of, 58-59
   integumentary system and, 249
   ionization and, 46
   physical properties of, 58
   as standard, 59
Waterston-Cooley procedure, 428
Watts, 24
Wavelengths of electromagnetic radiation; *see* Electromagnetic radiation
Waxes, 114
Weaning, 419-420
Wedge cast, 433
Wedge section of lung, 103
Weight, 111
   excess of, 440, 461
   inadequate, 420, 440, 448, 461
   of infant, 416, 417, 418
   of toddler, 439
Weir Report, 491
Wharton's jelly, 472
Wheal, 252
Wheelchairs, 220
   transfer of patient from, 219
Whipple's procedure, 131
White blood cells, 49
White matter, 185, 186, 187
Winslow, C. E. A., 480
Withdrawal reaction of childhood and adolescence, 349
Withdrawn behavior, 334, 340-342, 345
Witnesses, 509
Wolfina; *see* Rauwolfia serpentina
Women's Bureau, 395

Work, physics of, 56
Works Progress Administration, 488
World Health Organization, 395, 485
Worms, 118, 215, 447
Wounds
 contractures and, 249
 healing of, 31, 249
Wyamine Sulfate; *see* Mephentermine sulfate
Wycillin; *see* Penicillin G procaine
Wynestron; *see* Estrone

X

Xanthoproteic test, 116

Xenografts, 251
Xeroradiography, 163
X rays, 90
 diffraction of, 212
 gastrointestinal system and, 112
 in therapy of thymus, 232; *see also* Radiation
 in therapy
Xylocaine; *see* Lidocaine hydrochloride
D-Xylose tolerance test, 134

Y

Yeasts, 20-21
Yolk sac, 147

Young adulthood, 329

Z

Zarontin; *see* Ethosuximide
Zaroxolyn; *see* Metolazone
Zephiran; *see* Benzalkonium
Zeste; *see* Esterified estrogens
Zinc, 31
Zinc chloride, 256
Zollinger-Ellison syndrome, 126
Zygote, 147
Zyloprim; *see* Allopurinol

ANSWER SHEETS

MEDICAL-SURGICAL NURSING

Review questions 1-160, pp. 258-269

NAME_____ GRADE_____ SEX_____ DATE OF BIRTH_____
LAST   FIRST   MIDDLE   M OR F   YEAR MONTH DAY

DATE_____ AGE_____ SCHOOL_____ CITY_____
YEAR MONTH DAY

INSTRUCTOR_____

NAME OF TEST_____

IDENTIFICATION NUMBER

BE SURE TO MAKE YOUR MARKS
HEAVY AND BLACK

ERASE COMPLETELY ANY ANSWERS
YOU WISH TO CHANGE

1	2	3	4
1	2	3	4
5	6	7	8	9

(Identification number columns: 0 1 2 3 4   5 6 7 8 9, repeated for ten rows)

1 2 3 4	2 2 3 4	3 2 3 4	4 2 3 4
5 2 3 4	6 2 3 4	7 2 3 4	8 2 3 4
9 2 3 4	10 2 3 4	11 2 3 4	12 2 3 4
13 2 3 4	14 2 3 4	15 2 3 4	16 2 3 4
17 2 3 4	18 2 3 4	19 2 3 4	20 2 3 4
21 2 3 4	22 2 3 4	23 2 3 4	24 2 3 4
25 2 3 4	26 2 3 4	27 2 3 4	28 2 3 4
29 2 3 4	30 2 3 4	31 2 3 4	32 2 3 4
33 2 3 4	34 2 3 4	35 2 3 4	36 2 3 4
37 2 3 4	38 2 3 4	39 2 3 4	40 2 3 4
41 2 3 4	42 2 3 4	43 2 3 4	44 2 3 4
45 2 3 4	46 2 3 4	47 2 3 4	48 2 3 4
49 2 3 4	50 2 3 4	51 2 3 4	52 2 3 4
53 2 3 4	54 2 3 4	55 2 3 4	56 2 3 4
57 2 3 4	58 2 3 4	59 2 3 4	60 2 3 4
61 2 3 4	62 2 3 4	63 2 3 4	64 2 3 4
65 2 3 4	66 2 3 4	67 2 3 4	68 2 3 4
69 2 3 4	70 2 3 4	71 2 3 4	72 2 3 4
73 2 3 4	74 2 3 4	75 2 3 4	76 2 3 4
77 2 3 4	78 2 3 4	79 2 3 4	80 2 3 4
81 2 3 4	82 2 3 4	83 2 3 4	84 2 3 4
85 2 3 4	86 2 3 4	87 2 3 4	88 2 3 4
89 2 3 4	90 2 3 4	91 2 3 4	92 2 3 4
93 2 3 4	94 2 3 4	95 2 3 4	96 2 3 4
97 2 3 4	98 2 3 4	99 2 3 4	100 2 3 4
101 2 3 4	102 2 3 4	103 2 3 4	104 2 3 4
105 2 3 4	106 2 3 4	107 2 3 4	108 2 3 4
109 2 3 4	110 2 3 4	111 2 3 4	112 2 3 4
113 2 3 4	114 2 3 4	115 2 3 4	116 2 3 4
117 2 3 4	118 2 3 4	119 2 3 4	120 2 3 4
121 2 3 4	122 2 3 4	123 2 3 4	124 2 3 4
125 2 3 4	126 2 3 4	127 2 3 4	128 2 3 4
129 2 3 4	130 2 3 4	131 2 3 4	132 2 3 4
133 2 3 4	134 2 3 4	135 2 3 4	136 2 3 4
137 2 3 4	138 2 3 4	139 2 3 4	140 2 3 4
141 2 3 4	142 2 3 4	143 2 3 4	144 2 3 4
145 2 3 4	146 2 3 4	147 2 3 4	148 2 3 4
149 2 3 4	150 2 3 4	151 2 3 4	152 2 3 4
153 2 3 4	154 2 3 4	155 2 3 4	156 2 3 4
157 2 3 4	158 2 3 4	159 2 3 4	160 2 3 4

Continued.

MEDICAL-SURGICAL NURSING—cont'd

Review questions 161-320, pp. 269-281

NAME_____ GRADE_____ SEX_____ DATE OF BIRTH_____
LAST   FIRST   MIDDLE   M OR F   YEAR MONTH DAY

DATE_____ AGE_____ SCHOOL_____ CITY_____
YEAR MONTH DAY

INSTRUCTOR_____   IDENTIFICATION NUMBER _____

NAME OF TEST_____

0 ::::: 1 ::::: 2 ::::: 3 ::::: 4 :::::   5 ::::: 6 ::::: 7 ::::: 8 ::::: 9 :::::
0 ::::: 1 ::::: 2 ::::: 3 ::::: 4 :::::   5 ::::: 6 ::::: 7 ::::: 8 ::::: 9 :::::
0 ::::: 1 ::::: 2 ::::: 3 ::::: 4 :::::   5 ::::: 6 ::::: 7 ::::: 8 ::::: 9 :::::
0 ::::: 1 ::::: 2 ::::: 3 ::::: 4 :::::   5 ::::: 6 ::::: 7 ::::: 8 ::::: 9 :::::

**BE SURE TO MAKE YOUR MARKS
HEAVY AND BLACK**

**ERASE COMPLETELY ANY ANSWERS
YOU WISH TO CHANGE**

0 ::::: 1 ::::: 2 ::::: 3 ::::: 4 :::::   5 ::::: 6 ::::: 7 ::::: 8 ::::: 9 :::::
0 ::::: 1 ::::: 2 ::::: 3 ::::: 4 :::::   5 ::::: 6 ::::: 7 ::::: 8 ::::: 9 :::::
0 ::::: 1 ::::: 2 ::::: 3 ::::: 4 :::::   5 ::::: 6 ::::: 7 ::::: 8 ::::: 9 :::::
0 ::::: 1 ::::: 2 ::::: 3 ::::: 4 :::::   5 ::::: 6 ::::: 7 ::::: 8 ::::: 9 :::::
0 ::::: 1 ::::: 2 ::::: 3 ::::: 4 :::::   5 ::::: 6 ::::: 7 ::::: 8 ::::: 9 :::::
0 ::::: 1 ::::: 2 ::::: 3 ::::: 4 :::::   5 ::::: 6 ::::: 7 ::::: 8 ::::: 9 :::::

161 1 2 3 4	162 1 2 3 4	163 1 2 3 4	164 1 2 3 4
165 1 2 3 4	166 1 2 3 4	167 1 2 3 4	168 1 2 3 4
169 1 2 3 4	170 1 2 3 4	171 1 2 3 4	172 1 2 3 4
173 1 2 3 4	174 1 2 3 4	175 1 2 3 4	176 1 2 3 4
177 1 2 3 4	178 1 2 3 4	179 1 2 3 4	180 1 2 3 4
181 1 2 3 4	182 1 2 3 4	183 1 2 3 4	184 1 2 3 4
185 1 2 3 4	186 1 2 3 4	187 1 2 3 4	188 1 2 3 4
189 1 2 3 4	190 1 2 3 4	191 1 2 3 4	192 1 2 3 4
193 1 2 3 4	194 1 2 3 4	195 1 2 3 4	196 1 2 3 4
197 1 2 3 4	198 1 2 3 4	199 1 2 3 4	200 1 2 3 4
201 1 2 3 4	202 1 2 3 4	203 1 2 3 4	204 1 2 3 4
205 1 2 3 4	206 1 2 3 4	207 1 2 3 4	208 1 2 3 4
209 1 2 3 4	210 1 2 3 4	211 1 2 3 4	212 1 2 3 4
213 1 2 3 4	214 1 2 3 4	215 1 2 3 4	216 1 2 3 4
217 1 2 3 4	218 1 2 3 4	219 1 2 3 4	220 1 2 3 4
221 1 2 3 4	222 1 2 3 4	223 1 2 3 4	224 1 2 3 4
225 1 2 3 4	226 1 2 3 4	227 1 2 3 4	228 1 2 3 4
229 1 2 3 4	230 1 2 3 4	231 1 2 3 4	232 1 2 3 4
233 1 2 3 4	234 1 2 3 4	235 1 2 3 4	236 1 2 3 4
237 1 2 3 4	238 1 2 3 4	239 1 2 3 4	240 1 2 3 4
241 1 2 3 4	242 1 2 3 4	243 1 2 3 4	244 1 2 3 4
245 1 2 3 4	246 1 2 3 4	247 1 2 3 4	248 1 2 3 4
249 1 2 3 4	250 1 2 3 4	251 1 2 3 4	252 1 2 3 4
253 1 2 3 4	254 1 2 3 4	255 1 2 3 4	256 1 2 3 4
257 1 2 3 4	258 1 2 3 4	259 1 2 3 4	260 1 2 3 4
261 1 2 3 4	262 1 2 3 4	263 1 2 3 4	264 1 2 3 4
265 1 2 3 4	266 1 2 3 4	267 1 2 3 4	268 1 2 3 4
269 1 2 3 4	270 1 2 3 4	271 1 2 3 4	272 1 2 3 4
273 1 2 3 4	274 1 2 3 4	275 1 2 3 4	276 1 2 3 4
277 1 2 3 4	278 1 2 3 4	279 1 2 3 4	280 1 2 3 4
281 1 2 3 4	282 1 2 3 4	283 1 2 3 4	284 1 2 3 4
285 1 2 3 4	286 1 2 3 4	287 1 2 3 4	288 1 2 3 4
289 1 2 3 4	290 1 2 3 4	291 1 2 3 4	292 1 2 3 4
293 1 2 3 4	294 1 2 3 4	295 1 2 3 4	296 1 2 3 4
297 1 2 3 4	298 1 2 3 4	299 1 2 3 4	300 1 2 3 4
301 1 2 3 4	302 1 2 3 4	303 1 2 3 4	304 1 2 3 4
305 1 2 3 4	306 1 2 3 4	307 1 2 3 4	308 1 2 3 4
309 1 2 3 4	310 1 2 3 4	311 1 2 3 4	312 1 2 3 4
313 1 2 3 4	314 1 2 3 4	315 1 2 3 4	316 1 2 3 4
317 1 2 3 4	318 1 2 3 4	319 1 2 3 4	320 1 2 3 4

MEDICAL-SURGICAL NURSING—cont'd

Review questions 321-480, pp. 281-292

NAME_____ LAST   FIRST   MIDDLE   GRADE_____ SEX____ M OR F   DATE OF BIRTH_____ YEAR MONTH DAY

DATE_____ YEAR MONTH DAY   AGE____ SCHOOL_____ CITY_____

INSTRUCTOR_____

NAME OF TEST_____

IDENTIFICATION NUMBER

BE SURE TO MAKE YOUR MARKS HEAVY AND BLACK

ERASE COMPLETELY ANY ANSWERS YOU WISH TO CHANGE

321 322 323 324
325 326 327 328
329 330 331 332
333 334 335 336
337 338 339 340
341 342 343 344
345 346 347 348
349 350 351 352
353 354 355 356
357 358 359 360
361 362 363 364
365 366 367 368
369 370 371 372
373 374 375 376
377 378 379 380
381 382 383 384
385 386 387 388
389 390 391 392
393 394 395 396
397 398 399 400
401 402 403 404
405 406 407 408
409 410 411 412
413 414 415 416
417 418 419 420
421 422 423 424
425 426 427 428
429 430 431 432
433 434 435 436
437 438 439 440
441 442 443 444
445 446 447 448
449 450 451 452
453 454 455 456
457 458 459 460
461 462 463 464
465 466 467 468
469 470 471 472
473 474 475 476
477 478 479 480

Continued.

NAME _____ GRADE _____ SEX _____ DATE OF BIRTH _____
LAST   FIRST   MIDDLE   M OR F   YEAR MONTH DAY

DATE _____ AGE ____ SCHOOL _____ CITY _____
YEAR MONTH DAY

INSTRUCTOR _____

NAME OF TEST _____

**BE SURE TO MAKE YOUR MARKS
HEAVY AND BLACK**

**ERASE COMPLETELY ANY ANSWERS
YOU WISH TO CHANGE**

IDENTIFICATION NUMBER

0 ::::: 1 ::::: 2 ::::: 3 ::::: 4 ::::: 5 ::::: 6 ::::: 7 ::::: 8 ::::: 9 :::::
0 ::::: 1 ::::: 2 ::::: 3 ::::: 4 ::::: 5 ::::: 6 ::::: 7 ::::: 8 ::::: 9 :::::
0 ::::: 1 ::::: 2 ::::: 3 ::::: 4 ::::: 5 ::::: 6 ::::: 7 ::::: 8 ::::: 9 :::::
0 ::::: 1 ::::: 2 ::::: 3 ::::: 4 ::::: 5 ::::: 6 ::::: 7 ::::: 8 ::::: 9 :::::
0 ::::: 1 ::::: 2 ::::: 3 ::::: 4 ::::: 5 ::::: 6 ::::: 7 ::::: 8 ::::: 9 :::::
0 ::::: 1 ::::: 2 ::::: 3 ::::: 4 ::::: 5 ::::: 6 ::::: 7 ::::: 8 ::::: 9 :::::
0 ::::: 1 ::::: 2 ::::: 3 ::::: 4 ::::: 5 ::::: 6 ::::: 7 ::::: 8 ::::: 9 :::::
0 ::::: 1 ::::: 2 ::::: 3 ::::: 4 ::::: 5 ::::: 6 ::::: 7 ::::: 8 ::::: 9 :::::
0 ::::: 1 ::::: 2 ::::: 3 ::::: 4 ::::: 5 ::::: 6 ::::: 7 ::::: 8 ::::: 9 :::::
0 ::::: 1 ::::: 2 ::::: 3 ::::: 4 ::::: 5 ::::: 6 ::::: 7 ::::: 8 ::::: 9 :::::

481 1 2 3 4	482 1 2 3 4	483 1 2 3 4	484 1 2 3 4
485 1 2 3 4	486 1 2 3 4	487 1 2 3 4	488 1 2 3 4
489 1 2 3 4	490 1 2 3 4	491 1 2 3 4	492 1 2 3 4
493 1 2 3 4	494 1 2 3 4	495 1 2 3 4	496 1 2 3 4
497 1 2 3 4	498 1 2 3 4	499 1 2 3 4	500 1 2 3 4
501 1 2 3 4	502 1 2 3 4	503 1 2 3 4	504 1 2 3 4
505 1 2 3 4	506 1 2 3 4	507 1 2 3 4	508 1 2 3 4
509 1 2 3 4	510 1 2 3 4	511 1 2 3 4	512 1 2 3 4
513 1 2 3 4	514 1 2 3 4	515 1 2 3 4	516 1 2 3 4
517 1 2 3 4	518 1 2 3 4	519 1 2 3 4	520 1 2 3 4
521 1 2 3 4	522 1 2 3 4	523 1 2 3 4	524 1 2 3 4
525 1 2 3 4	526 1 2 3 4	527 1 2 3 4	528 1 2 3 4
529 1 2 3 4	530 1 2 3 4	531 1 2 3 4	532 1 2 3 4
533 1 2 3 4	534 1 2 3 4	535 1 2 3 4	536 1 2 3 4
537 1 2 3 4	538 1 2 3 4	539 1 2 3 4	540 1 2 3 4
541 1 2 3 4	542 1 2 3 4	543 1 2 3 4	544 1 2 3 4
545 1 2 3 4	546 1 2 3 4	547 1 2 3 4	548 1 2 3 4
549 1 2 3 4	550 1 2 3 4	551 1 2 3 4	552 1 2 3 4
553 1 2 3 4	554 1 2 3 4	555 1 2 3 4	556 1 2 3 4
557 1 2 3 4	558 1 2 3 4	559 1 2 3 4	560 1 2 3 4
561 1 2 3 4	562 1 2 3 4	563 1 2 3 4	564 1 2 3 4
565 1 2 3 4	566 1 2 3 4	567 1 2 3 4	568 1 2 3 4
569 1 2 3 4	570 1 2 3 4	571 1 2 3 4	572 1 2 3 4
573 1 2 3 4	574 1 2 3 4	575 1 2 3 4	576 1 2 3 4
577 1 2 3 4	578 1 2 3 4	579 1 2 3 4	580 1 2 3 4
581 1 2 3 4	582 1 2 3 4	583 1 2 3 4	584 1 2 3 4
585 1 2 3 4	586 1 2 3 4	587 1 2 3 4	588 1 2 3 4
589 1 2 3 4	590 1 2 3 4	591 1 2 3 4	592 1 2 3 4
593 1 2 3 4	594 1 2 3 4	595 1 2 3 4	596 1 2 3 4
597 1 2 3 4	598 1 2 3 4	599 1 2 3 4	600 1 2 3 4
601 1 2 3 4	602 1 2 3 4	603 1 2 3 4	604 1 2 3 4
605 1 2 3 4	606 1 2 3 4	607 1 2 3 4	608 1 2 3 4
609 1 2 3 4	610 1 2 3 4	611 1 2 3 4	612 1 2 3 4
613 1 2 3 4	614 1 2 3 4	615 1 2 3 4	616 1 2 3 4
617 1 2 3 4	618 1 2 3 4	619 1 2 3 4	620 1 2 3 4
621 1 2 3 4	622 1 2 3 4	623 1 2 3 4	624 1 2 3 4
625 1 2 3 4	626 1 2 3 4	627 1 2 3 4	628 1 2 3 4
629 1 2 3 4	630 1 2 3 4	631 1 2 3 4	632 1 2 3 4
633 1 2 3 4	634 1 2 3 4	635 1 2 3 4	636 1 2 3 4
637 1 2 3 4	638 1 2 3 4	639 1 2 3 4	640 1 2 3 4

NAME_____ LAST FIRST MIDDLE ___ GRADE_____ SEX __ M OR F __ DATE OF BIRTH_____ YEAR MONTH DAY

DATE_____ YEAR MONTH DAY ___ AGE_____ SCHOOL_____ CITY_____

INSTRUCTOR_____

NAME OF TEST_____

IDENTIFICATION NUMBER

0	1	2	3	4	5	6	7	8	9
0	1	2	3	4	5	6	7	8	9
0	1	2	3	4	5	6	7	8	9
0	1	2	3	4	5	6	7	8	9
0	1	2	3	4	5	6	7	8	9
0	1	2	3	4	5	6	7	8	9
0	1	2	3	4	5	6	7	8	9
0	1	2	3	4	5	6	7	8	9
0	1	2	3	4	5	6	7	8	9
0	1	2	3	4	5	6	7	8	9

**BE SURE TO MAKE YOUR MARKS
HEAVY AND BLACK**

**ERASE COMPLETELY ANY ANSWERS
YOU WISH TO CHANGE**

641 1 2 3 4	642 1 2 3 4	643 1 2 3 4	644 1 2 3 4
645 1 2 3 4	646 1 2 3 4	647 1 2 3 4	648 1 2 3 4
649 1 2 3 4	650 1 2 3 4	651 1 2 3 4	652 1 2 3 4
653 1 2 3 4	654 1 2 3 4	655 1 2 3 4	656 1 2 3 4
657 1 2 3 4	658 1 2 3 4	659 1 2 3 4	660 1 2 3 4
661 1 2 3 4	662 1 2 3 4	663 1 2 3 4	664 1 2 3 4
665 1 2 3 4	666 1 2 3 4	667 1 2 3 4	668 1 2 3 4
669 1 2 3 4	670 1 2 3 4	671 1 2 3 4	672 1 2 3 4
673 1 2 3 4	674 1 2 3 4	675 1 2 3 4	676 1 2 3 4
677 1 2 3 4	678 1 2 3 4	679 1 2 3 4	680 1 2 3 4
681 1 2 3 4	682 1 2 3 4	683 1 2 3 4	684 1 2 3 4
685 1 2 3 4	686 1 2 3 4	687 1 2 3 4	688 1 2 3 4
689 1 2 3 4	690 1 2 3 4	691 1 2 3 4	692 1 2 3 4
693 1 2 3 4	694 1 2 3 4	695 1 2 3 4	696 1 2 3 4
697 1 2 3 4	698 1 2 3 4	699 1 2 3 4	700 1 2 3 4
701 1 2 3 4	702 1 2 3 4	703 1 2 3 4	704 1 2 3 4
705 1 2 3 4	706 1 2 3 4	707 1 2 3 4	708 1 2 3 4
709 1 2 3 4	710 1 2 3 4	711 1 2 3 4	712 1 2 3 4
713 1 2 3 4	714 1 2 3 4	715 1 2 3 4	716 1 2 3 4
717 1 2 3 4	718 1 2 3 4	719 1 2 3 4	720 1 2 3 4
721 1 2 3 4	722 1 2 3 4	723 1 2 3 4	724 1 2 3 4
725 1 2 3 4	726 1 2 3 4	727 1 2 3 4	728 1 2 3 4
729 1 2 3 4	730 1 2 3 4	731 1 2 3 4	732 1 2 3 4
733 1 2 3 4	734 1 2 3 4	735 1 2 3 4	736 1 2 3 4
737 1 2 3 4	738 1 2 3 4	739 1 2 3 4	740 1 2 3 4
741 1 2 3 4	742 1 2 3 4	743 1 2 3 4	744 1 2 3 4
745 1 2 3 4	746 1 2 3 4	747 1 2 3 4	748 1 2 3 4
749 1 2 3 4	750 1 2 3 4	751 1 2 3 4	752 1 2 3 4
753 1 2 3 4	754 1 2 3 4	755 1 2 3 4	756 1 2 3 4
757 1 2 3 4	758 1 2 3 4	759 1 2 3 4	760 1 2 3 4
761 1 2 3 4	762 1 2 3 4	763 1 2 3 4	764 1 2 3 4
765 1 2 3 4	766 1 2 3 4	767 1 2 3 4	768 1 2 3 4
769 1 2 3 4	770 1 2 3 4	771 1 2 3 4	772 1 2 3 4
773 1 2 3 4	774 1 2 3 4	775 1 2 3 4	776 1 2 3 4
777 1 2 3 4	778 1 2 3 4	779 1 2 3 4	780 1 2 3 4
781 1 2 3 4	782 1 2 3 4	783 1 2 3 4	784 1 2 3 4
785 1 2 3 4	786 1 2 3 4	787 1 2 3 4	788 1 2 3 4
789 1 2 3 4	790 1 2 3 4	791 1 2 3 4	792 1 2 3 4
793 1 2 3 4	794 1 2 3 4	795 1 2 3 4	796 1 2 3 4
797 1 2 3 4	798 1 2 3 4	799 1 2 3 4	800 1 2 3 4

Continued.

MEDICAL-SURGICAL NURSING—cont'd

Review questions 801-871, pp. 316-321

NAME ______ LAST FIRST MIDDLE ______ GRADE ______ SEX ______ M OR F ______ DATE OF BIRTH ______ YEAR MONTH DAY

DATE ______ YEAR MONTH DAY ______ AGE ______ SCHOOL ______ CITY ______

INSTRUCTOR ______

NAME OF TEST ______

BE SURE TO MAKE YOUR MARKS HEAVY AND BLACK

ERASE COMPLETELY ANY ANSWERS YOU WISH TO CHANGE

IDENTIFICATION NUMBER

0 1 2 3 4 5 6 7 8 9
0 1 2 3 4 5 6 7 8 9
0 1 2 3 4 5 6 7 8 9
0 1 2 3 4 5 6 7 8 9
0 1 2 3 4 5 6 7 8 9
0 1 2 3 4 5 6 7 8 9
0 1 2 3 4 5 6 7 8 9
0 1 2 3 4 5 6 7 8 9
0 1 2 3 4 5 6 7 8 9
0 1 2 3 4 5 6 7 8 9

801 1 2 3 4	802 1 2 3 4	803 1 2 3 4	804 1 2 3 4
805 1 2 3 4	806 1 2 3 4	807 1 2 3 4	808 1 2 3 4
809 1 2 3 4	810 1 2 3 4	811 1 2 3 4	812 1 2 3 4
813 1 2 3 4	814 1 2 3 4	815 1 2 3 4	816 1 2 3 4
817 1 2 3 4	818 1 2 3 4	819 1 2 3 4	820 1 2 3 4
821 1 2 3 4	822 1 2 3 4	823 1 2 3 4	824 1 2 3 4
825 1 2 3 4	826 1 2 3 4	827 1 2 3 4	828 1 2 3 4
829 1 2 3 4	830 1 2 3 4	831 1 2 3 4	832 1 2 3 4
833 1 2 3 4	834 1 2 3 4	835 1 2 3 4	836 1 2 3 4
837 1 2 3 4	838 1 2 3 4	839 1 2 3 4	840 1 2 3 4
841 1 2 3 4	842 1 2 3 4	843 1 2 3 4	844 1 2 3 4
845 1 2 3 4	846 1 2 3 4	847 1 2 3 4	848 1 2 3 4
849 1 2 3 4	850 1 2 3 4	851 1 2 3 4	852 1 2 3 4
853 1 2 3 4	854 1 2 3 4	855 1 2 3 4	856 1 2 3 4
857 1 2 3 4	858 1 2 3 4	859 1 2 3 4	860 1 2 3 4
861 1 2 3 4	862 1 2 3 4	863 1 2 3 4	864 1 2 3 4
865 1 2 3 4	866 1 2 3 4	867 1 2 3 4	868 1 2 3 4
869 1 2 3 4	870 1 2 3 4	871 1 2 3 4	872 1 2 3 4
873 1 2 3 4	874 1 2 3 4	875 1 2 3 4	876 1 2 3 4
877 1 2 3 4	878 1 2 3 4	879 1 2 3 4	880 1 2 3 4
881 1 2 3 4	882 1 2 3 4	883 1 2 3 4	884 1 2 3 4
885 1 2 3 4	886 1 2 3 4	887 1 2 3 4	888 1 2 3 4
889 1 2 3 4	890 1 2 3 4	891 1 2 3 4	892 1 2 3 4
893 1 2 3 4	894 1 2 3 4	895 1 2 3 4	896 1 2 3 4
897 1 2 3 4	898 1 2 3 4	899 1 2 3 4	900 1 2 3 4
901 1 2 3 4	902 1 2 3 4	903 1 2 3 4	904 1 2 3 4
905 1 2 3 4	906 1 2 3 4	907 1 2 3 4	908 1 2 3 4
909 1 2 3 4	910 1 2 3 4	911 1 2 3 4	912 1 2 3 4
913 1 2 3 4	914 1 2 3 4	915 1 2 3 4	916 1 2 3 4
917 1 2 3 4	918 1 2 3 4	919 1 2 3 4	920 1 2 3 4
921 1 2 3 4	922 1 2 3 4	923 1 2 3 4	924 1 2 3 4
925 1 2 3 4	926 1 2 3 4	927 1 2 3 4	928 1 2 3 4
929 1 2 3 4	930 1 2 3 4	931 1 2 3 4	932 1 2 3 4
933 1 2 3 4	934 1 2 3 4	935 1 2 3 4	936 1 2 3 4
937 1 2 3 4	938 1 2 3 4	939 1 2 3 4	940 1 2 3 4
941 1 2 3 4	942 1 2 3 4	943 1 2 3 4	944 1 2 3 4
945 1 2 3 4	946 1 2 3 4	947 1 2 3 4	948 1 2 3 4
949 1 2 3 4	950 1 2 3 4	951 1 2 3 4	952 1 2 3 4
953 1 2 3 4	954 1 2 3 4	955 1 2 3 4	956 1 2 3 4
957 1 2 3 4	958 1 2 3 4	959 1 2 3 4	960 1 2 3 4

PSYCHIATRIC NURSING

Review questions 1-160, pp. 354-366

NAME_____ LAST   FIRST   MIDDLE   GRADE_____ SEX___ M OR F ___ DATE OF BIRTH_____ YEAR MONTH DAY

DATE_____ YEAR MONTH DAY   AGE_____ SCHOOL_____ CITY_____

INSTRUCTOR_____

NAME OF TEST_____

**BE SURE TO MAKE YOUR MARKS
HEAVY AND BLACK**

**ERASE COMPLETELY ANY ANSWERS
YOU WISH TO CHANGE**

IDENTIFICATION NUMBER

0 1 2 3 4   5 6 7 8 9
0 1 2 3 4   5 6 7 8 9
0 1 2 3 4   5 6 7 8 9
0 1 2 3 4   5 6 7 8 9
0 1 2 3 4   5 6 7 8 9
0 1 2 3 4   5 6 7 8 9
0 1 2 3 4   5 6 7 8 9
0 1 2 3 4   5 6 7 8 9
0 1 2 3 4   5 6 7 8 9
0 1 2 3 4   5 6 7 8 9

1 1 2 3 4	2 1 2 3 4	3 1 2 3 4	4 1 2 3 4
5 1 2 3 4	6 1 2 3 4	7 1 2 3 4	8 1 2 3 4
9 1 2 3 4	10 1 2 3 4	11 1 2 3 4	12 1 2 3 4
13 1 2 3 4	14 1 2 3 4	15 1 2 3 4	16 1 2 3 4
17 1 2 3 4	18 1 2 3 4	19 1 2 3 4	20 1 2 3 4
21 1 2 3 4	22 1 2 3 4	23 1 2 3 4	24 1 2 3 4
25 1 2 3 4	26 1 2 3 4	27 1 2 3 4	28 1 2 3 4
29 1 2 3 4	30 1 2 3 4	31 1 2 3 4	32 1 2 3 4
33 1 2 3 4	34 1 2 3 4	35 1 2 3 4	36 1 2 3 4
37 1 2 3 4	38 1 2 3 4	39 1 2 3 4	40 1 2 3 4
41 1 2 3 4	42 1 2 3 4	43 1 2 3 4	44 1 2 3 4
45 1 2 3 4	46 1 2 3 4	47 1 2 3 4	48 1 2 3 4
49 1 2 3 4	50 1 2 3 4	51 1 2 3 4	52 1 2 3 4
53 1 2 3 4	54 1 2 3 4	55 1 2 3 4	56 1 2 3 4
57 1 2 3 4	58 1 2 3 4	59 1 2 3 4	60 1 2 3 4
61 1 2 3 4	62 1 2 3 4	63 1 2 3 4	64 1 2 3 4
65 1 2 3 4	66 1 2 3 4	67 1 2 3 4	68 1 2 3 4
69 1 2 3 4	70 1 2 3 4	71 1 2 3 4	72 1 2 3 4
73 1 2 3 4	74 1 2 3 4	75 1 2 3 4	76 1 2 3 4
77 1 2 3 4	78 1 2 3 4	79 1 2 3 4	80 1 2 3 4
81 1 2 3 4	82 1 2 3 4	83 1 2 3 4	84 1 2 3 4
85 1 2 3 4	86 1 2 3 4	87 1 2 3 4	88 1 2 3 4
89 1 2 3 4	90 1 2 3 4	91 1 2 3 4	92 1 2 3 4
93 1 2 3 4	94 1 2 3 4	95 1 2 3 4	96 1 2 3 4
97 1 2 3 4	98 1 2 3 4	99 1 2 3 4	100 1 2 3 4
101 1 2 3 4	102 1 2 3 4	103 1 2 3 4	104 1 2 3 4
105 1 2 3 4	106 1 2 3 4	107 1 2 3 4	108 1 2 3 4
109 1 2 3 4	110 1 2 3 4	111 1 2 3 4	112 1 2 3 4
113 1 2 3 4	114 1 2 3 4	115 1 2 3 4	116 1 2 3 4
117 1 2 3 4	118 1 2 3 4	119 1 2 3 4	120 1 2 3 4
121 1 2 3 4	122 1 2 3 4	123 1 2 3 4	124 1 2 3 4
125 1 2 3 4	126 1 2 3 4	127 1 2 3 4	128 1 2 3 4
129 1 2 3 4	130 1 2 3 4	131 1 2 3 4	132 1 2 3 4
133 1 2 3 4	134 1 2 3 4	135 1 2 3 4	136 1 2 3 4
137 1 2 3 4	138 1 2 3 4	139 1 2 3 4	140 1 2 3 4
141 1 2 3 4	142 1 2 3 4	143 1 2 3 4	144 1 2 3 4
145 1 2 3 4	146 1 2 3 4	147 1 2 3 4	148 1 2 3 4
149 1 2 3 4	150 1 2 3 4	151 1 2 3 4	152 1 2 3 4
153 1 2 3 4	154 1 2 3 4	155 1 2 3 4	156 1 2 3 4
157 1 2 3 4	158 1 2 3 4	159 1 2 3 4	160 1 2 3 4

Continued.

NAME_____ GRADE_____ SEX_____ DATE OF BIRTH_____
　　　　　LAST　　FIRST　　MIDDLE　　　　　　　　M OR F　　　　　YEAR MONTH DAY

DATE_____ AGE____ SCHOOL_____ CITY_____
　　　YEAR MONTH DAY

INSTRUCTOR_____

NAME OF TEST_____

IDENTIFICATION NUMBER

0 ::::: 1 ::::: 2 ::::: 3 ::::: 4 :::::　5 ::::: 6 ::::: 7 ::::: 8 ::::: 9 :::::
0 ::::: 1 ::::: 2 ::::: 3 ::::: 4 :::::　5 ::::: 6 ::::: 7 ::::: 8 ::::: 9 :::::
0 ::::: 1 ::::: 2 ::::: 3 ::::: 4 :::::　5 ::::: 6 ::::: 7 ::::: 8 ::::: 9 :::::
0 ::::: 1 ::::: 2 ::::: 3 ::::: 4 :::::　5 ::::: 6 ::::: 7 ::::: 8 ::::: 9 :::::
0 ::::: 1 ::::: 2 ::::: 3 ::::: 4 :::::　5 ::::: 6 ::::: 7 ::::: 8 ::::: 9 :::::
0 ::::: 1 ::::: 2 ::::: 3 ::::: 4 :::::　5 ::::: 6 ::::: 7 ::::: 8 ::::: 9 :::::
0 ::::: 1 ::::: 2 ::::: 3 ::::: 4 :::::　5 ::::: 6 ::::: 7 ::::: 8 ::::: 9 :::::
0 ::::: 1 ::::: 2 ::::: 3 ::::: 4 :::::　5 ::::: 6 ::::: 7 ::::: 8 ::::: 9 :::::
0 ::::: 1 ::::: 2 ::::: 3 ::::: 4 :::::　5 ::::: 6 ::::: 7 ::::: 8 ::::: 9 :::::
0 ::::: 1 ::::: 2 ::::: 3 ::::: 4 :::::　5 ::::: 6 ::::: 7 ::::: 8 ::::: 9 :::::

**BE SURE TO MAKE YOUR MARKS
HEAVY AND BLACK**

**ERASE COMPLETELY ANY ANSWERS
YOU WISH TO CHANGE**

161 1 ::::: 2 ::::: 3 ::::: 4 :::::　162 1 ::::: 2 ::::: 3 ::::: 4 :::::　163 1 ::::: 2 ::::: 3 ::::: 4 :::::　164 1 ::::: 2 ::::: 3 ::::: 4 :::::
165 1 ::::: 2 ::::: 3 ::::: 4 :::::　166 1 ::::: 2 ::::: 3 ::::: 4 :::::　167 1 ::::: 2 ::::: 3 ::::: 4 :::::　168 1 ::::: 2 ::::: 3 ::::: 4 :::::
169 1 ::::: 2 ::::: 3 ::::: 4 :::::　170 1 ::::: 2 ::::: 3 ::::: 4 :::::　171 1 ::::: 2 ::::: 3 ::::: 4 :::::　172 1 ::::: 2 ::::: 3 ::::: 4 :::::
173 1 ::::: 2 ::::: 3 ::::: 4 :::::　174 1 ::::: 2 ::::: 3 ::::: 4 :::::　175 1 ::::: 2 ::::: 3 ::::: 4 :::::　176 1 ::::: 2 ::::: 3 ::::: 4 :::::
177 1 ::::: 2 ::::: 3 ::::: 4 :::::　178 1 ::::: 2 ::::: 3 ::::: 4 :::::　179 1 ::::: 2 ::::: 3 ::::: 4 :::::　180 1 ::::: 2 ::::: 3 ::::: 4 :::::
181 1 ::::: 2 ::::: 3 ::::: 4 :::::　182 1 ::::: 2 ::::: 3 ::::: 4 :::::　183 1 ::::: 2 ::::: 3 ::::: 4 :::::　184 1 ::::: 2 ::::: 3 ::::: 4 :::::
185 1 ::::: 2 ::::: 3 ::::: 4 :::::　186 1 ::::: 2 ::::: 3 ::::: 4 :::::　187 1 ::::: 2 ::::: 3 ::::: 4 :::::　188 1 ::::: 2 ::::: 3 ::::: 4 :::::
189 1 ::::: 2 ::::: 3 ::::: 4 :::::　190 1 ::::: 2 ::::: 3 ::::: 4 :::::　191 1 ::::: 2 ::::: 3 ::::: 4 :::::　192 1 ::::: 2 ::::: 3 ::::: 4 :::::
193 1 ::::: 2 ::::: 3 ::::: 4 :::::　194 1 ::::: 2 ::::: 3 ::::: 4 :::::　195 1 ::::: 2 ::::: 3 ::::: 4 :::::　196 1 ::::: 2 ::::: 3 ::::: 4 :::::
197 1 ::::: 2 ::::: 3 ::::: 4 :::::　198 1 ::::: 2 ::::: 3 ::::: 4 :::::　199 1 ::::: 2 ::::: 3 ::::: 4 :::::　200 1 ::::: 2 ::::: 3 ::::: 4 :::::
201 1 ::::: 2 ::::: 3 ::::: 4 :::::　202 1 ::::: 2 ::::: 3 ::::: 4 :::::　203 1 ::::: 2 ::::: 3 ::::: 4 :::::　204 1 ::::: 2 ::::: 3 ::::: 4 :::::
205 1 ::::: 2 ::::: 3 ::::: 4 :::::　206 1 ::::: 2 ::::: 3 ::::: 4 :::::　207 1 ::::: 2 ::::: 3 ::::: 4 :::::　208 1 ::::: 2 ::::: 3 ::::: 4 :::::
209 1 ::::: 2 ::::: 3 ::::: 4 :::::　210 1 ::::: 2 ::::: 3 ::::: 4 :::::　211 1 ::::: 2 ::::: 3 ::::: 4 :::::　212 1 ::::: 2 ::::: 3 ::::: 4 :::::
213 1 ::::: 2 ::::: 3 ::::: 4 :::::　214 1 ::::: 2 ::::: 3 ::::: 4 :::::　215 1 ::::: 2 ::::: 3 ::::: 4 :::::　216 1 ::::: 2 ::::: 3 ::::: 4 :::::
217 1 ::::: 2 ::::: 3 ::::: 4 :::::　218 1 ::::: 2 ::::: 3 ::::: 4 :::::　219 1 ::::: 2 ::::: 3 ::::: 4 :::::　220 1 ::::: 2 ::::: 3 ::::: 4 :::::
221 1 ::::: 2 ::::: 3 ::::: 4 :::::　222 1 ::::: 2 ::::: 3 ::::: 4 :::::　223 1 ::::: 2 ::::: 3 ::::: 4 :::::　224 1 ::::: 2 ::::: 3 ::::: 4 :::::
225 1 ::::: 2 ::::: 3 ::::: 4 :::::　226 1 ::::: 2 ::::: 3 ::::: 4 :::::　227 1 ::::: 2 ::::: 3 ::::: 4 :::::　228 1 ::::: 2 ::::: 3 ::::: 4 :::::
229 1 ::::: 2 ::::: 3 ::::: 4 :::::　230 1 ::::: 2 ::::: 3 ::::: 4 :::::　231 1 ::::: 2 ::::: 3 ::::: 4 :::::　232 1 ::::: 2 ::::: 3 ::::: 4 :::::
233 1 ::::: 2 ::::: 3 ::::: 4 :::::　234 1 ::::: 2 ::::: 3 ::::: 4 :::::　235 1 ::::: 2 ::::: 3 ::::: 4 :::::　236 1 ::::: 2 ::::: 3 ::::: 4 :::::
237 1 ::::: 2 ::::: 3 ::::: 4 :::::　238 1 ::::: 2 ::::: 3 ::::: 4 :::::　239 1 ::::: 2 ::::: 3 ::::: 4 :::::　240 1 ::::: 2 ::::: 3 ::::: 4 :::::
241 1 ::::: 2 ::::: 3 ::::: 4 :::::　242 1 ::::: 2 ::::: 3 ::::: 4 :::::　243 1 ::::: 2 ::::: 3 ::::: 4 :::::　244 1 ::::: 2 ::::: 3 ::::: 4 :::::
245 1 ::::: 2 ::::: 3 ::::: 4 :::::　246 1 ::::: 2 ::::: 3 ::::: 4 :::::　247 1 ::::: 2 ::::: 3 ::::: 4 :::::　248 1 ::::: 2 ::::: 3 ::::: 4 :::::
249 1 ::::: 2 ::::: 3 ::::: 4 :::::　250 1 ::::: 2 ::::: 3 ::::: 4 :::::　251 1 ::::: 2 ::::: 3 ::::: 4 :::::　252 1 ::::: 2 ::::: 3 ::::: 4 :::::
253 1 ::::: 2 ::::: 3 ::::: 4 :::::　254 1 ::::: 2 ::::: 3 ::::: 4 :::::　255 1 ::::: 2 ::::: 3 ::::: 4 :::::　256 1 ::::: 2 ::::: 3 ::::: 4 :::::
257 1 ::::: 2 ::::: 3 ::::: 4 :::::　258 1 ::::: 2 ::::: 3 ::::: 4 :::::　259 1 ::::: 2 ::::: 3 ::::: 4 :::::　260 1 ::::: 2 ::::: 3 ::::: 4 :::::
261 1 ::::: 2 ::::: 3 ::::: 4 :::::　262 1 ::::: 2 ::::: 3 ::::: 4 :::::　263 1 ::::: 2 ::::: 3 ::::: 4 :::::　264 1 ::::: 2 ::::: 3 ::::: 4 :::::
265 1 ::::: 2 ::::: 3 ::::: 4 :::::　266 1 ::::: 2 ::::: 3 ::::: 4 :::::　267 1 ::::: 2 ::::: 3 ::::: 4 :::::　268 1 ::::: 2 ::::: 3 ::::: 4 :::::
269 1 ::::: 2 ::::: 3 ::::: 4 :::::　270 1 ::::: 2 ::::: 3 ::::: 4 :::::　271 1 ::::: 2 ::::: 3 ::::: 4 :::::　272 1 ::::: 2 ::::: 3 ::::: 4 :::::
273 1 ::::: 2 ::::: 3 ::::: 4 :::::　274 1 ::::: 2 ::::: 3 ::::: 4 :::::　275 1 ::::: 2 ::::: 3 ::::: 4 :::::　276 1 ::::: 2 ::::: 3 ::::: 4 :::::
277 1 ::::: 2 ::::: 3 ::::: 4 :::::　278 1 ::::: 2 ::::: 3 ::::: 4 :::::　279 1 ::::: 2 ::::: 3 ::::: 4 :::::　280 1 ::::: 2 ::::: 3 ::::: 4 :::::
281 1 ::::: 2 ::::: 3 ::::: 4 :::::　282 1 ::::: 2 ::::: 3 ::::: 4 :::::　283 1 ::::: 2 ::::: 3 ::::: 4 :::::　284 1 ::::: 2 ::::: 3 ::::: 4 :::::
285 1 ::::: 2 ::::: 3 ::::: 4 :::::　286 1 ::::: 2 ::::: 3 ::::: 4 :::::　287 1 ::::: 2 ::::: 3 ::::: 4 :::::　288 1 ::::: 2 ::::: 3 ::::: 4 :::::
289 1 ::::: 2 ::::: 3 ::::: 4 :::::　290 1 ::::: 2 ::::: 3 ::::: 4 :::::　291 1 ::::: 2 ::::: 3 ::::: 4 :::::　292 1 ::::: 2 ::::: 3 ::::: 4 :::::
293 1 ::::: 2 ::::: 3 ::::: 4 :::::　294 1 ::::: 2 ::::: 3 ::::: 4 :::::　295 1 ::::: 2 ::::: 3 ::::: 4 :::::　296 1 ::::: 2 ::::: 3 ::::: 4 :::::
297 1 ::::: 2 ::::: 3 ::::: 4 :::::　298 1 ::::: 2 ::::: 3 ::::: 4 :::::　299 1 ::::: 2 ::::: 3 ::::: 4 :::::　300 1 ::::: 2 ::::: 3 ::::: 4 :::::
301 1 ::::: 2 ::::: 3 ::::: 4 :::::　302 1 ::::: 2 ::::: 3 ::::: 4 :::::　303 1 ::::: 2 ::::: 3 ::::: 4 :::::　304 1 ::::: 2 ::::: 3 ::::: 4 :::::
305 1 ::::: 2 ::::: 3 ::::: 4 :::::　306 1 ::::: 2 ::::: 3 ::::: 4 :::::　307 1 ::::: 2 ::::: 3 ::::: 4 :::::　308 1 ::::: 2 ::::: 3 ::::: 4 :::::
309 1 ::::: 2 ::::: 3 ::::: 4 :::::　310 1 ::::: 2 ::::: 3 ::::: 4 :::::　311 1 ::::: 2 ::::: 3 ::::: 4 :::::　312 1 ::::: 2 ::::: 3 ::::: 4 :::::
313 1 ::::: 2 ::::: 3 ::::: 4 :::::　314 1 ::::: 2 ::::: 3 ::::: 4 :::::　315 1 ::::: 2 ::::: 3 ::::: 4 :::::　316 1 ::::: 2 ::::: 3 ::::: 4 :::::
317 1 ::::: 2 ::::: 3 ::::: 4 :::::　318 1 ::::: 2 ::::: 3 ::::: 4 :::::　319 1 ::::: 2 ::::: 3 ::::: 4 :::::　320 1 ::::: 2 ::::: 3 ::::: 4 :::::

MATERNITY NURSING

Review questions 1-160, pp. 395-408

NAME _____
LAST   FIRST   MIDDLE   GRADE _____ SEX _____ DATE OF BIRTH _____
     M OR F   YEAR MONTH DAY

DATE _____ AGE _____ SCHOOL _____ CITY _____

     YEAR MONTH DAY

INSTRUCTOR _____

NAME OF TEST _____

IDENTIFICATION NUMBER

0 1 2 3 4   5 6 7 8 9 (× 10 rows)

BE SURE TO MAKE YOUR MARKS HEAVY AND BLACK

ERASE COMPLETELY ANY ANSWERS YOU WISH TO CHANGE

1 1 2 3 4	2 1 2 3 4	3 1 2 3 4	4 1 2 3 4
5 1 2 3 4	6 1 2 3 4	7 1 2 3 4	8 1 2 3 4
9 1 2 3 4	10 1 2 3 4	11 1 2 3 4	12 1 2 3 4
13 1 2 3 4	14 1 2 3 4	15 1 2 3 4	16 1 2 3 4
17 1 2 3 4	18 1 2 3 4	19 1 2 3 4	20 1 2 3 4
21 1 2 3 4	22 1 2 3 4	23 1 2 3 4	24 1 2 3 4
25 1 2 3 4	26 1 2 3 4	27 1 2 3 4	28 1 2 3 4
29 1 2 3 4	30 1 2 3 4	31 1 2 3 4	32 1 2 3 4
33 1 2 3 4	34 1 2 3 4	35 1 2 3 4	36 1 2 3 4
37 1 2 3 4	38 1 2 3 4	39 1 2 3 4	40 1 2 3 4
41 1 2 3 4	42 1 2 3 4	43 1 2 3 4	44 1 2 3 4
45 1 2 3 4	46 1 2 3 4	47 1 2 3 4	48 1 2 3 4
49 1 2 3 4	50 1 2 3 4	51 1 2 3 4	52 1 2 3 4
53 1 2 3 4	54 1 2 3 4	55 1 2 3 4	56 1 2 3 4
57 1 2 3 4	58 1 2 3 4	59 1 2 3 4	60 1 2 3 4
61 1 2 3 4	62 1 2 3 4	63 1 2 3 4	64 1 2 3 4
65 1 2 3 4	66 1 2 3 4	67 1 2 3 4	68 1 2 3 4
69 1 2 3 4	70 1 2 3 4	71 1 2 3 4	72 1 2 3 4
73 1 2 3 4	74 1 2 3 4	75 1 2 3 4	76 1 2 3 4
77 1 2 3 4	78 1 2 3 4	79 1 2 3 4	80 1 2 3 4
81 1 2 3 4	82 1 2 3 4	83 1 2 3 4	84 1 2 3 4
85 1 2 3 4	86 1 2 3 4	87 1 2 3 4	88 1 2 3 4
89 1 2 3 4	90 1 2 3 4	91 1 2 3 4	92 1 2 3 4
93 1 2 3 4	94 1 2 3 4	95 1 2 3 4	96 1 2 3 4
97 1 2 3 4	98 1 2 3 4	99 1 2 3 4	100 1 2 3 4
101 1 2 3 4	102 1 2 3 4	103 1 2 3 4	104 1 2 3 4
105 1 2 3 4	106 1 2 3 4	107 1 2 3 4	108 1 2 3 4
109 1 2 3 4	110 1 2 3 4	111 1 2 3 4	112 1 2 3 4
113 1 2 3 4	114 1 2 3 4	115 1 2 3 4	116 1 2 3 4
117 1 2 3 4	118 1 2 3 4	119 1 2 3 4	120 1 2 3 4
121 1 2 3 4	122 1 2 3 4	123 1 2 3 4	124 1 2 3 4
125 1 2 3 4	126 1 2 3 4	127 1 2 3 4	128 1 2 3 4
129 1 2 3 4	130 1 2 3 4	131 1 2 3 4	132 1 2 3 4
133 1 2 3 4	134 1 2 3 4	135 1 2 3 4	136 1 2 3 4
137 1 2 3 4	138 1 2 3 4	139 1 2 3 4	140 1 2 3 4
141 1 2 3 4	142 1 2 3 4	143 1 2 3 4	144 1 2 3 4
145 1 2 3 4	146 1 2 3 4	147 1 2 3 4	148 1 2 3 4
149 1 2 3 4	150 1 2 3 4	151 1 2 3 4	152 1 2 3 4
153 1 2 3 4	154 1 2 3 4	155 1 2 3 4	156 1 2 3 4
157 1 2 3 4	158 1 2 3 4	159 1 2 3 4	160 1 2 3 4

Continued.

MATERNITY NURSING—cont'd

Review questions 161-226, pp. 408-413

NAME_____ LAST FIRST MIDDLE GRADE_____ SEX____ M or F DATE OF BIRTH_____ YEAR MONTH DAY

DATE_____ YEAR MONTH DAY AGE____ SCHOOL_____ CITY_____

INSTRUCTOR_____

NAME OF TEST_____

BE SURE TO MAKE YOUR MARKS HEAVY AND BLACK

ERASE COMPLETELY ANY ANSWERS YOU WISH TO CHANGE

IDENTIFICATION NUMBER

0 1 2 3 4 5 6 7 8 9
0 1 2 3 4 5 6 7 8 9
0 1 2 3 4 5 6 7 8 9
0 1 2 3 4 5 6 7 8 9
0 1 2 3 4 5 6 7 8 9
0 1 2 3 4 5 6 7 8 9
0 1 2 3 4 5 6 7 8 9
0 1 2 3 4 5 6 7 8 9
0 1 2 3 4 5 6 7 8 9

161 1 2 3 4	162 1 2 3 4	163 1 2 3 4	164 1 2 3 4
165 1 2 3 4	166 1 2 3 4	167 1 2 3 4	168 1 2 3 4
169 1 2 3 4	170 1 2 3 4	171 1 2 3 4	172 1 2 3 4
173 1 2 3 4	174 1 2 3 4	175 1 2 3 4	176 1 2 3 4
177 1 2 3 4	178 1 2 3 4	179 1 2 3 4	180 1 2 3 4
181 1 2 3 4	182 1 2 3 4	183 1 2 3 4	184 1 2 3 4
185 1 2 3 4	186 1 2 3 4	187 1 2 3 4	188 1 2 3 4
189 1 2 3 4	190 1 2 3 4	191 1 2 3 4	192 1 2 3 4
193 1 2 3 4	194 1 2 3 4	195 1 2 3 4	196 1 2 3 4
197 1 2 3 4	198 1 2 3 4	199 1 2 3 4	200 1 2 3 4
201 1 2 3 4	202 1 2 3 4	203 1 2 3 4	204 1 2 3 4
205 1 2 3 4	206 1 2 3 4	207 1 2 3 4	208 1 2 3 4
209 1 2 3 4	210 1 2 3 4	211 1 2 3 4	212 1 2 3 4
213 1 2 3 4	214 1 2 3 4	215 1 2 3 4	216 1 2 3 4
217 1 2 3 4	218 1 2 3 4	219 1 2 3 4	220 1 2 3 4
221 1 2 3 4	222 1 2 3 4	223 1 2 3 4	224 1 2 3 4
225 1 2 3 4	226 1 2 3 4	227 1 2 3 4	228 1 2 3 4
229 1 2 3 4	230 1 2 3 4	231 1 2 3 4	232 1 2 3 4
233 1 2 3 4	234 1 2 3 4	235 1 2 3 4	236 1 2 3 4
237 1 2 3 4	238 1 2 3 4	239 1 2 3 4	240 1 2 3 4
241 1 2 3 4	242 1 2 3 4	243 1 2 3 4	244 1 2 3 4
245 1 2 3 4	246 1 2 3 4	247 1 2 3 4	248 1 2 3 4
249 1 2 3 4	250 1 2 3 4	251 1 2 3 4	252 1 2 3 4
253 1 2 3 4	254 1 2 3 4	255 1 2 3 4	256 1 2 3 4
257 1 2 3 4	258 1 2 3 4	259 1 2 3 4	260 1 2 3 4
261 1 2 3 4	262 1 2 3 4	263 1 2 3 4	264 1 2 3 4
265 1 2 3 4	266 1 2 3 4	267 1 2 3 4	268 1 2 3 4
269 1 2 3 4	270 1 2 3 4	271 1 2 3 4	272 1 2 3 4
273 1 2 3 4	274 1 2 3 4	275 1 2 3 4	276 1 2 3 4
277 1 2 3 4	278 1 2 3 4	279 1 2 3 4	280 1 2 3 4
281 1 2 3 4	282 1 2 3 4	283 1 2 3 4	284 1 2 3 4
285 1 2 3 4	286 1 2 3 4	287 1 2 3 4	288 1 2 3 4
289 1 2 3 4	290 1 2 3 4	291 1 2 3 4	292 1 2 3 4
293 1 2 3 4	294 1 2 3 4	295 1 2 3 4	296 1 2 3 4
297 1 2 3 4	298 1 2 3 4	299 1 2 3 4	300 1 2 3 4
301 1 2 3 4	302 1 2 3 4	303 1 2 3 4	304 1 2 3 4
305 1 2 3 4	306 1 2 3 4	307 1 2 3 4	308 1 2 3 4
309 1 2 3 4	310 1 2 3 4	311 1 2 3 4	312 1 2 3 4
313 1 2 3 4	314 1 2 3 4	315 1 2 3 4	316 1 2 3 4
317 1 2 3 4	318 1 2 3 4	319 1 2 3 4	320 1 2 3 4

PEDIATRIC NURSING

Review questions 1-160, pp. 461-473

NAME _____ GRADE _____ SEX _____ DATE OF BIRTH _____
　　　　　LAST　　FIRST　　MIDDLE　　　　　　　　　　M OR F　　　　　　　YEAR MONTH DAY

DATE _____ AGE _____ SCHOOL _____ CITY _____
　　　　YEAR MONTH DAY

INSTRUCTOR _____

NAME OF TEST _____

IDENTIFICATION NUMBER

0	1	2	3	4	5	6	7	8	9
0	1	2	3	4	5	6	7	8	9
0	1	2	3	4	5	6	7	8	9
0	1	2	3	4	5	6	7	8	9
0	1	2	3	4	5	6	7	8	9
0	1	2	3	4	5	6	7	8	9
0	1	2	3	4	5	6	7	8	9
0	1	2	3	4	5	6	7	8	9
0	1	2	3	4	5	6	7	8	9
0	1	2	3	4	5	6	7	8	9

**BE SURE TO MAKE YOUR MARKS
HEAVY AND BLACK**

**ERASE COMPLETELY ANY ANSWERS
YOU WISH TO CHANGE**

1　1 2 3 4	2　1 2 3 4	3　1 2 3 4	4　1 2 3 4
5　1 2 3 4	6　1 2 3 4	7　1 2 3 4	8　1 2 3 4
9　1 2 3 4	10　1 2 3 4	11　1 2 3 4	12　1 2 3 4
13　1 2 3 4	14　1 2 3 4	15　1 2 3 4	16　1 2 3 4
17　1 2 3 4	18　1 2 3 4	19　1 2 3 4	20　1 2 3 4
21　1 2 3 4	22　1 2 3 4	23　1 2 3 4	24　1 2 3 4
25　1 2 3 4	26　1 2 3 4	27　1 2 3 4	28　1 2 3 4
29　1 2 3 4	30　1 2 3 4	31　1 2 3 4	32　1 2 3 4
33　1 2 3 4	34　1 2 3 4	35　1 2 3 4	36　1 2 3 4
37　1 2 3 4	38　1 2 3 4	39　1 2 3 4	40　1 2 3 4
41　1 2 3 4	42　1 2 3 4	43　1 2 3 4	44　1 2 3 4
45　1 2 3 4	46　1 2 3 4	47　1 2 3 4	48　1 2 3 4
49　1 2 3 4	50　1 2 3 4	51　1 2 3 4	52　1 2 3 4
53　1 2 3 4	54　1 2 3 4	55　1 2 3 4	56　1 2 3 4
57　1 2 3 4	58　1 2 3 4	59　1 2 3 4	60　1 2 3 4
61　1 2 3 4	62　1 2 3 4	63　1 2 3 4	64　1 2 3 4
65　1 2 3 4	66　1 2 3 4	67　1 2 3 4	68　1 2 3 4
69　1 2 3 4	70　1 2 3 4	71　1 2 3 4	72　1 2 3 4
73　1 2 3 4	74　1 2 3 4	75　1 2 3 4	76　1 2 3 4
77　1 2 3 4	78　1 2 3 4	79　1 2 3 4	80　1 2 3 4
81　1 2 3 4	82　1 2 3 4	83　1 2 3 4	84　1 2 3 4
85　1 2 3 4	86　1 2 3 4	87　1 2 3 4	88　1 2 3 4
89　1 2 3 4	90　1 2 3 4	91　1 2 3 4	92　1 2 3 4
93　1 2 3 4	94　1 2 3 4	95　1 2 3 4	96　1 2 3 4
97　1 2 3 4	98　1 2 3 4	99　1 2 3 4	100　1 2 3 4
101　1 2 3 4	102　1 2 3 4	103　1 2 3 4	104　1 2 3 4
105　1 2 3 4	106　1 2 3 4	107　1 2 3 4	108　1 2 3 4
109　1 2 3 4	110　1 2 3 4	111　1 2 3 4	112　1 2 3 4
113　1 2 3 4	114　1 2 3 4	115　1 2 3 4	116　1 2 3 4
117　1 2 3 4	118　1 2 3 4	119　1 2 3 4	120　1 2 3 4
121　1 2 3 4	122　1 2 3 4	123　1 2 3 4	124　1 2 3 4
125　1 2 3 4	126　1 2 3 4	127　1 2 3 4	128　1 2 3 4
129　1 2 3 4	130　1 2 3 4	131　1 2 3 4	132　1 2 3 4
133　1 2 3 4	134　1 2 3 4	135　1 2 3 4	136　1 2 3 4
137　1 2 3 4	138　1 2 3 4	139　1 2 3 4	140　1 2 3 4
141　1 2 3 4	142　1 2 3 4	143　1 2 3 4	144　1 2 3 4
145　1 2 3 4	146　1 2 3 4	147　1 2 3 4	148　1 2 3 4
149　1 2 3 4	150　1 2 3 4	151　1 2 3 4	152　1 2 3 4
153　1 2 3 4	154　1 2 3 4	155　1 2 3 4	156　1 2 3 4
157　1 2 3 4	158　1 2 3 4	159　1 2 3 4	160　1 2 3 4

Continued.

NAME_____ LAST FIRST MIDDLE GRADE_____ SEX_____ M OR F DATE OF BIRTH_____ YEAR MONTH DAY

DATE_____ YEAR MONTH DAY AGE_____ SCHOOL_____ CITY_____

INSTRUCTOR_____

IDENTIFICATION NUMBER

NAME OF TEST_____

**BE SURE TO MAKE YOUR MARKS
HEAVY AND BLACK**

**ERASE COMPLETELY ANY ANSWERS
YOU WISH TO CHANGE**

161	162	163	164
165	166	167	168
169	170	171	172
173	174	175	176
177	178	179	180
181	182	183	184
185	186	187	188
189	190	191	192
193	194	195	196
197	198	199	200
201	202	203	204
205	206	207	208
209	210	211	212
213	214	215	216
217	218	219	220
221	222	223	224
225	226	227	228
229	230	231	232
233	234	235	236
237	238	239	240
241	242	243	244
245	246	247	248
249	250	251	252
253	254	255	256
257	258	259	260
261	262	263	264
265	266	267	268
269	270	271	272
273	274	275	276
277	278	279	280
281	282	283	284
285	286	287	288
289	290	291	292
293	294	295	296
297	298	299	300
301	302	303	304
305	306	307	308
309	310	311	312
313	314	315	316
317	318	319	320

COMPREHENSIVE TEST 1

Questions 1-120, pp. 510-521

NAME_____ GRADE_____ SEX_____ DATE OF BIRTH_____
　　　LAST　　FIRST　　MIDDLE　　　　　　　　M OR F　　　　　YEAR MONTH DAY

DATE_____ AGE_____ SCHOOL_____ CITY_____
　　YEAR MONTH DAY

INSTRUCTOR_____

NAME OF TEST_____

**BE SURE TO MAKE YOUR MARKS
HEAVY AND BLACK**

**ERASE COMPLETELY ANY ANSWERS
YOU WISH TO CHANGE**

IDENTIFICATION NUMBER

0 ····· 1 ····· 2 ····· 3 ····· 4 ····· 5 ····· 6 ····· 7 ····· 8 ····· 9 ·····
0 ····· 1 ····· 2 ····· 3 ····· 4 ····· 5 ····· 6 ····· 7 ····· 8 ····· 9 ·····
0 ····· 1 ····· 2 ····· 3 ····· 4 ····· 5 ····· 6 ····· 7 ····· 8 ····· 9 ·····
0 ····· 1 ····· 2 ····· 3 ····· 4 ····· 5 ····· 6 ····· 7 ····· 8 ····· 9 ·····
0 ····· 1 ····· 2 ····· 3 ····· 4 ····· 5 ····· 6 ····· 7 ····· 8 ····· 9 ·····
0 ····· 1 ····· 2 ····· 3 ····· 4 ····· 5 ····· 6 ····· 7 ····· 8 ····· 9 ·····
0 ····· 1 ····· 2 ····· 3 ····· 4 ····· 5 ····· 6 ····· 7 ····· 8 ····· 9 ·····
0 ····· 1 ····· 2 ····· 3 ····· 4 ····· 5 ····· 6 ····· 7 ····· 8 ····· 9 ·····
0 ····· 1 ····· 2 ····· 3 ····· 4 ····· 5 ····· 6 ····· 7 ····· 8 ····· 9 ·····
0 ····· 1 ····· 2 ····· 3 ····· 4 ····· 5 ····· 6 ····· 7 ····· 8 ····· 9 ·····

1 1 2 3 4	2 1 2 3 4	3 1 2 3 4	4 1 2 3 4
5 1 2 3 4	6 1 2 3 4	7 1 2 3 4	8 1 2 3 4
9 1 2 3 4	10 1 2 3 4	11 1 2 3 4	12 1 2 3 4
13 1 2 3 4	14 1 2 3 4	15 1 2 3 4	16 1 2 3 4
17 1 2 3 4	18 1 2 3 4	19 1 2 3 4	20 1 2 3 4
21 1 2 3 4	22 1 2 3 4	23 1 2 3 4	24 1 2 3 4
25 1 2 3 4	26 1 2 3 4	27 1 2 3 4	28 1 2 3 4
29 1 2 3 4	30 1 2 3 4	31 1 2 3 4	32 1 2 3 4
33 1 2 3 4	34 1 2 3 4	35 1 2 3 4	36 1 2 3 4
37 1 2 3 4	38 1 2 3 4	39 1 2 3 4	40 1 2 3 4
41 1 2 3 4	42 1 2 3 4	43 1 2 3 4	44 1 2 3 4
45 1 2 3 4	46 1 2 3 4	47 1 2 3 4	48 1 2 3 4
49 1 2 3 4	50 1 2 3 4	51 1 2 3 4	52 1 2 3 4
53 1 2 3 4	54 1 2 3 4	55 1 2 3 4	56 1 2 3 4
57 1 2 3 4	58 1 2 3 4	59 1 2 3 4	60 1 2 3 4
61 1 2 3 4	62 1 2 3 4	63 1 2 3 4	64 1 2 3 4
65 1 2 3 4	66 1 2 3 4	67 1 2 3 4	68 1 2 3 4
69 1 2 3 4	70 1 2 3 4	71 1 2 3 4	72 1 2 3 4
73 1 2 3 4	74 1 2 3 4	75 1 2 3 4	76 1 2 3 4
77 1 2 3 4	78 1 2 3 4	79 1 2 3 4	80 1 2 3 4
81 1 2 3 4	82 1 2 3 4	83 1 2 3 4	84 1 2 3 4
85 1 2 3 4	86 1 2 3 4	87 1 2 3 4	88 1 2 3 4
89 1 2 3 4	90 1 2 3 4	91 1 2 3 4	92 1 2 3 4
93 1 2 3 4	94 1 2 3 4	95 1 2 3 4	96 1 2 3 4
97 1 2 3 4	98 1 2 3 4	99 1 2 3 4	100 1 2 3 4
101 1 2 3 4	102 1 2 3 4	103 1 2 3 4	104 1 2 3 4
105 1 2 3 4	106 1 2 3 4	107 1 2 3 4	108 1 2 3 4
109 1 2 3 4	110 1 2 3 4	111 1 2 3 4	112 1 2 3 4
113 1 2 3 4	114 1 2 3 4	115 1 2 3 4	116 1 2 3 4
117 1 2 3 4	118 1 2 3 4	119 1 2 3 4	120 1 2 3 4
121 1 2 3 4	122 1 2 3 4	123 1 2 3 4	124 1 2 3 4
125 1 2 3 4	126 1 2 3 4	127 1 2 3 4	128 1 2 3 4
129 1 2 3 4	130 1 2 3 4	131 1 2 3 4	132 1 2 3 4
133 1 2 3 4	134 1 2 3 4	135 1 2 3 4	136 1 2 3 4
137 1 2 3 4	138 1 2 3 4	139 1 2 3 4	140 1 2 3 4
141 1 2 3 4	142 1 2 3 4	143 1 2 3 4	144 1 2 3 4
145 1 2 3 4	146 1 2 3 4	147 1 2 3 4	148 1 2 3 4
149 1 2 3 4	150 1 2 3 4	151 1 2 3 4	152 1 2 3 4
153 1 2 3 4	154 1 2 3 4	155 1 2 3 4	156 1 2 3 4
157 1 2 3 4	158 1 2 3 4	159 1 2 3 4	160 1 2 3 4

COMPREHENSIVE TEST 2

Questions 1-120, pp. 522-533

NAME_____ GRADE_____ SEX_____ DATE OF BIRTH_____
    LAST   FIRST   MIDDLE   M OR F   YEAR MONTH DAY

DATE_____ AGE_____ SCHOOL_____ CITY_____
    YEAR MONTH DAY

INSTRUCTOR_____

NAME OF TEST_____

BE SURE TO MAKE YOUR MARKS HEAVY AND BLACK

ERASE COMPLETELY ANY ANSWERS YOU WISH TO CHANGE

IDENTIFICATION NUMBER

0 1 2 3 4 5 6 7 8 9
0 1 2 3 4 5 6 7 8 9
0 1 2 3 4 5 6 7 8 9
0 1 2 3 4 5 6 7 8 9
0 1 2 3 4 5 6 7 8 9
0 1 2 3 4 5 6 7 8 9
0 1 2 3 4 5 6 7 8 9
0 1 2 3 4 5 6 7 8 9
0 1 2 3 4 5 6 7 8 9
0 1 2 3 4 5 6 7 8 9

1 1 2 3 4	2 1 2 3 4	3 1 2 3 4	4 1 2 3 4
5 1 2 3 4	6 1 2 3 4	7 1 2 3 4	8 1 2 3 4
9 1 2 3 4	10 1 2 3 4	11 1 2 3 4	12 1 2 3 4
13 1 2 3 4	14 1 2 3 4	15 1 2 3 4	16 1 2 3 4
17 1 2 3 4	18 1 2 3 4	19 1 2 3 4	20 1 2 3 4
21 1 2 3 4	22 1 2 3 4	23 1 2 3 4	24 1 2 3 4
25 1 2 3 4	26 1 2 3 4	27 1 2 3 4	28 1 2 3 4
29 1 2 3 4	30 1 2 3 4	31 1 2 3 4	32 1 2 3 4
33 1 2 3 4	34 1 2 3 4	35 1 2 3 4	36 1 2 3 4
37 1 2 3 4	38 1 2 3 4	39 1 2 3 4	40 1 2 3 4
41 1 2 3 4	42 1 2 3 4	43 1 2 3 4	44 1 2 3 4
45 1 2 3 4	46 1 2 3 4	47 1 2 3 4	48 1 2 3 4
49 1 2 3 4	50 1 2 3 4	51 1 2 3 4	52 1 2 3 4
53 1 2 3 4	54 1 2 3 4	55 1 2 3 4	56 1 2 3 4
57 1 2 3 4	58 1 2 3 4	59 1 2 3 4	60 1 2 3 4
61 1 2 3 4	62 1 2 3 4	63 1 2 3 4	64 1 2 3 4
65 1 2 3 4	66 1 2 3 4	67 1 2 3 4	68 1 2 3 4
69 1 2 3 4	70 1 2 3 4	71 1 2 3 4	72 1 2 3 4
73 1 2 3 4	74 1 2 3 4	75 1 2 3 4	76 1 2 3 4
77 1 2 3 4	78 1 2 3 4	79 1 2 3 4	80 1 2 3 4
81 1 2 3 4	82 1 2 3 4	83 1 2 3 4	84 1 2 3 4
85 1 2 3 4	86 1 2 3 4	87 1 2 3 4	88 1 2 3 4
89 1 2 3 4	90 1 2 3 4	91 1 2 3 4	92 1 2 3 4
93 1 2 3 4	94 1 2 3 4	95 1 2 3 4	96 1 2 3 4
97 1 2 3 4	98 1 2 3 4	99 1 2 3 4	100 1 2 3 4
101 1 2 3 4	102 1 2 3 4	103 1 2 3 4	104 1 2 3 4
105 1 2 3 4	106 1 2 3 4	107 1 2 3 4	108 1 2 3 4
109 1 2 3 4	110 1 2 3 4	111 1 2 3 4	112 1 2 3 4
113 1 2 3 4	114 1 2 3 4	115 1 2 3 4	116 1 2 3 4
117 1 2 3 4	118 1 2 3 4	119 1 2 3 4	120 1 2 3 4
121 1 2 3 4	122 1 2 3 4	123 1 2 3 4	124 1 2 3 4
125 1 2 3 4	126 1 2 3 4	127 1 2 3 4	128 1 2 3 4
129 1 2 3 4	130 1 2 3 4	131 1 2 3 4	132 1 2 3 4
133 1 2 3 4	134 1 2 3 4	135 1 2 3 4	136 1 2 3 4
137 1 2 3 4	138 1 2 3 4	139 1 2 3 4	140 1 2 3 4
141 1 2 3 4	142 1 2 3 4	143 1 2 3 4	144 1 2 3 4
145 1 2 3 4	146 1 2 3 4	147 1 2 3 4	148 1 2 3 4
149 1 2 3 4	150 1 2 3 4	151 1 2 3 4	152 1 2 3 4
153 1 2 3 4	154 1 2 3 4	155 1 2 3 4	156 1 2 3 4
157 1 2 3 4	158 1 2 3 4	159 1 2 3 4	160 1 2 3 4

COMPREHENSIVE TEST 3

Questions 1-120, pp. 534-546

NAME_____ GRADE_____ SEX_____ DATE OF BIRTH_____
LAST   FIRST   MIDDLE   M OR F   YEAR MONTH DAY

DATE_____ AGE_____ SCHOOL_____ CITY_____
YEAR MONTH DAY

INSTRUCTOR_____

NAME OF TEST_____

IDENTIFICATION NUMBER

0 :::: 1 :::: 2 :::: 3 :::: 4 ::::   5 :::: 6 :::: 7 :::: 8 :::: 9 ::::
0 :::: 1 :::: 2 :::: 3 :::: 4 ::::   5 :::: 6 :::: 7 :::: 8 :::: 9 ::::
0 :::: 1 :::: 2 :::: 3 :::: 4 ::::   5 :::: 6 :::: 7 :::: 8 :::: 9 ::::
0 :::: 1 :::: 2 :::: 3 :::: 4 ::::   5 :::: 6 :::: 7 :::: 8 :::: 9 ::::
0 :::: 1 :::: 2 :::: 3 :::: 4 ::::   5 :::: 6 :::: 7 :::: 8 :::: 9 ::::
0 :::: 1 :::: 2 :::: 3 :::: 4 ::::   5 :::: 6 :::: 7 :::: 8 :::: 9 ::::
0 :::: 1 :::: 2 :::: 3 :::: 4 ::::   5 :::: 6 :::: 7 :::: 8 :::: 9 ::::
0 :::: 1 :::: 2 :::: 3 :::: 4 ::::   5 :::: 6 :::: 7 :::: 8 :::: 9 ::::
0 :::: 1 :::: 2 :::: 3 :::: 4 ::::   5 :::: 6 :::: 7 :::: 8 :::: 9 ::::
0 :::: 1 :::: 2 :::: 3 :::: 4 ::::   5 :::: 6 :::: 7 :::: 8 :::: 9 ::::

**BE SURE TO MAKE YOUR MARKS
HEAVY AND BLACK**

**ERASE COMPLETELY ANY ANSWERS
YOU WISH TO CHANGE**

1 1 2 3 4   2 1 2 3 4   3 1 2 3 4   4 1 2 3 4
5 1 2 3 4   6 1 2 3 4   7 1 2 3 4   8 1 2 3 4
9 1 2 3 4   10 1 2 3 4   11 1 2 3 4   12 1 2 3 4
13 1 2 3 4   14 1 2 3 4   15 1 2 3 4   16 1 2 3 4
17 1 2 3 4   18 1 2 3 4   19 1 2 3 4   20 1 2 3 4
21 1 2 3 4   22 1 2 3 4   23 1 2 3 4   24 1 2 3 4
25 1 2 3 4   26 1 2 3 4   27 1 2 3 4   28 1 2 3 4
29 1 2 3 4   30 1 2 3 4   31 1 2 3 4   32 1 2 3 4
33 1 2 3 4   34 1 2 3 4   35 1 2 3 4   36 1 2 3 4
37 1 2 3 4   38 1 2 3 4   39 1 2 3 4   40 1 2 3 4
41 1 2 3 4   42 1 2 3 4   43 1 2 3 4   44 1 2 3 4
45 1 2 3 4   46 1 2 3 4   47 1 2 3 4   48 1 2 3 4
49 1 2 3 4   50 1 2 3 4   51 1 2 3 4   52 1 2 3 4
53 1 2 3 4   54 1 2 3 4   55 1 2 3 4   56 1 2 3 4
57 1 2 3 4   58 1 2 3 4   59 1 2 3 4   60 1 2 3 4
61 1 2 3 4   62 1 2 3 4   63 1 2 3 4   64 1 2 3 4
65 1 2 3 4   66 1 2 3 4   67 1 2 3 4   68 1 2 3 4
69 1 2 3 4   70 1 2 3 4   71 1 2 3 4   72 1 2 3 4
73 1 2 3 4   74 1 2 3 4   75 1 2 3 4   76 1 2 3 4
77 1 2 3 4   78 1 2 3 4   79 1 2 3 4   80 1 2 3 4
81 1 2 3 4   82 1 2 3 4   83 1 2 3 4   84 1 2 3 4
85 1 2 3 4   86 1 2 3 4   87 1 2 3 4   88 1 2 3 4
89 1 2 3 4   90 1 2 3 4   91 1 2 3 4   92 1 2 3 4
93 1 2 3 4   94 1 2 3 4   95 1 2 3 4   96 1 2 3 4
97 1 2 3 4   98 1 2 3 4   99 1 2 3 4   100 1 2 3 4
101 1 2 3 4   102 1 2 3 4   103 1 2 3 4   104 1 2 3 4
105 1 2 3 4   106 1 2 3 4   107 1 2 3 4   108 1 2 3 4
109 1 2 3 4   110 1 2 3 4   111 1 2 3 4   112 1 2 3 4
113 1 2 3 4   114 1 2 3 4   115 1 2 3 4   116 1 2 3 4
117 1 2 3 4   118 1 2 3 4   119 1 2 3 4   120 1 2 3 4
121 1 2 3 4   122 1 2 3 4   123 1 2 3 4   124 1 2 3 4
125 1 2 3 4   126 1 2 3 4   127 1 2 3 4   128 1 2 3 4
129 1 2 3 4   130 1 2 3 4   131 1 2 3 4   132 1 2 3 4
133 1 2 3 4   134 1 2 3 4   135 1 2 3 4   136 1 2 3 4
137 1 2 3 4   138 1 2 3 4   139 1 2 3 4   140 1 2 3 4
141 1 2 3 4   142 1 2 3 4   143 1 2 3 4   144 1 2 3 4
145 1 2 3 4   146 1 2 3 4   147 1 2 3 4   148 1 2 3 4
149 1 2 3 4   150 1 2 3 4   151 1 2 3 4   152 1 2 3 4
153 1 2 3 4   154 1 2 3 4   155 1 2 3 4   156 1 2 3 4
157 1 2 3 4   158 1 2 3 4   159 1 2 3 4   160 1 2 3 4

COMPREHENSIVE TEST 4

Questions 1-120, pp. 547-558

NAME_____ LAST   FIRST   MIDDLE ___ GRADE_____ SEX ___ M or F ___ DATE OF BIRTH_____ YEAR MONTH DAY

DATE_____ YEAR MONTH DAY ___ AGE____ SCHOOL_____ CITY_____

INSTRUCTOR _____

NAME OF TEST _____

**BE SURE TO MAKE YOUR MARKS
HEAVY AND BLACK**

**ERASE COMPLETELY ANY ANSWERS
YOU WISH TO CHANGE**

IDENTIFICATION NUMBER

0 1 2 3 4   5 6 7 8 9
0 1 2 3 4   5 6 7 8 9
0 1 2 3 4   5 6 7 8 9
0 1 2 3 4   5 6 7 8 9
0 1 2 3 4   5 6 7 8 9
0 1 2 3 4   5 6 7 8 9
0 1 2 3 4   5 6 7 8 9
0 1 2 3 4   5 6 7 8 9
0 1 2 3 4   5 6 7 8 9
0 1 2 3 4   5 6 7 8 9

1 2 3 4	2 2 3 4	3 2 3 4	4 2 3 4
5 2 3 4	6 2 3 4	7 2 3 4	8 2 3 4
9 2 3 4	10 2 3 4	11 2 3 4	12 2 3 4
13 2 3 4	14 2 3 4	15 2 3 4	16 2 3 4
17 2 3 4	18 2 3 4	19 2 3 4	20 2 3 4
21 2 3 4	22 2 3 4	23 2 3 4	24 2 3 4
25 2 3 4	26 2 3 4	27 2 3 4	28 2 3 4
29 2 3 4	30 2 3 4	31 2 3 4	32 2 3 4
33 2 3 4	34 2 3 4	35 2 3 4	36 2 3 4
37 2 3 4	38 2 3 4	39 2 3 4	40 2 3 4
41 2 3 4	42 2 3 4	43 2 3 4	44 2 3 4
45 2 3 4	46 2 3 4	47 2 3 4	48 2 3 4
49 2 3 4	50 2 3 4	51 2 3 4	52 2 3 4
53 2 3 4	54 2 3 4	55 2 3 4	56 2 3 4
57 2 3 4	58 2 3 4	59 2 3 4	60 2 3 4
61 2 3 4	62 2 3 4	63 2 3 4	64 2 3 4
65 2 3 4	66 2 3 4	67 2 3 4	68 2 3 4
69 2 3 4	70 2 3 4	71 2 3 4	72 2 3 4
73 2 3 4	74 2 3 4	75 2 3 4	76 2 3 4
77 2 3 4	78 2 3 4	79 2 3 4	80 2 3 4
81 2 3 4	82 2 3 4	83 2 3 4	84 2 3 4
85 2 3 4	86 2 3 4	87 2 3 4	88 2 3 4
89 2 3 4	90 2 3 4	91 2 3 4	92 2 3 4
93 2 3 4	94 2 3 4	95 2 3 4	96 2 3 4
97 2 3 4	98 2 3 4	99 2 3 4	100 2 3 4
101 2 3 4	102 2 3 4	103 2 3 4	104 2 3 4
105 2 3 4	106 2 3 4	107 2 3 4	108 2 3 4
109 2 3 4	110 2 3 4	111 2 3 4	112 2 3 4
113 2 3 4	114 2 3 4	115 2 3 4	116 2 3 4
117 2 3 4	118 2 3 4	119 2 3 4	120 2 3 4
121 2 3 4	122 2 3 4	123 2 3 4	124 2 3 4
125 2 3 4	126 2 3 4	127 2 3 4	128 2 3 4
129 2 3 4	130 2 3 4	131 2 3 4	132 2 3 4
133 2 3 4	134 2 3 4	135 2 3 4	136 2 3 4
137 2 3 4	138 2 3 4	139 2 3 4	140 2 3 4
141 2 3 4	142 2 3 4	143 2 3 4	144 2 3 4
145 2 3 4	146 2 3 4	147 2 3 4	148 2 3 4
149 2 3 4	150 2 3 4	151 2 3 4	152 2 3 4
153 2 3 4	154 2 3 4	155 2 3 4	156 2 3 4
157 2 3 4	158 2 3 4	159 2 3 4	160 2 3 4